W9-CCN-046

THE HEALTH BUILDER

THE
Health Builder

Formerly Called Volume Two of the Health Finder

An Encyclopedia of Health Information from the Preventive Point-of-View

Self-contained from A to Z

Subject Index, pages 999-1024

Edited by **J. I. RODALE**

With the Collaboration of RUTH ADAMS *and* CHARLES GERRAS

RODALE BOOKS, Inc.

Emmaus, Pennsylvania

PRINTED IN UNITED STATES

LIBRARY OF CONGRESS CATALOG CARD NO.: 54-12539

EIGHTH PRINTING—NOVEMBER, 1971

H-67

INTRODUCTION

The material in these pages continues the search we started with the first issue of our health magazine *Prevention*—a search for a way of life that will prevent disease.

As the magazine grew, month after month and year after year, we realized that we must provide for the material we had uncovered some more permanent form than bound copies of the back issues of the magazine. We collected the most significant articles from the first two years of *Prevention* and put them in encyclopedic form, alphabetically arranged and cross-referenced. After the first printing, we realized that we must provide a complete index, so this was added to all printings thereafter.

The first volume, called the Health Finder, had a phenomenal sale. Because of the kind of book it is, it was not listed on newspaper and magazine best seller lists, but we believe that it probably outsold many of these best sellers.

We knew we would have to publish a second volume—and a third. This is the second volume.

Prevention is a magazine devoted to the conservation of human health. New discoveries in nutrition and medicine are being made faster than any magazine can keep up with them. The Health Builder contains articles under many headings that did not appear anywhere in the Health Finder. And much additional material on subjects covered only partially in the first volume.

We have made a deliberate effort to include material not covered before, so that by owning both the Health Finder and the Health Builder you can have thorough coverage of many important health matters.

We do not take up in this book every disease or every condition of ill-health known to man. No one volume could do this with any degree of thoroughness. Besides we have not had time to do research on all diseases, nor have we been able to find significant material on all subjects.

We don't write articles in *Prevention* the way "health" articles are written in most other magazines which go like this: an outline of the symptoms of the disease and how widespread it is, with a note on the various drugs that may be used to quell some of the symptoms and a final caution to see your doctor early and let him do what he can to give you some help. We don't think that this kind of article is very helpful, especially to someone interested as we are in *preventing* disease. All our research is slanted in this direction.

If we turn up enough evidence in medical and scientific journals to indicate that certain vitamins, minerals, enzymes, kinds of food, or other factors in living have been used successfully to treat a disease, we believe we are justified in writing an article saying that perhaps enough of these certain vitamins, minerals, enzymes, kinds of food or way of life will prevent the disease. We also make comparisons of diets as related to disease. If a certain disease is unknown in a certain locale, why not study the diet there and compare it with the diet in another place where the disease is rampant? It is amazing the facts one uncovers in research of this kind.

In general, you will find that articles in the Health Builder fall into several categories—first, information on preventing different conditions of ill-health—varicose veins, prostate gland troubles, menopause difficulties, asthma, heart trouble, hardening of the arteries, colds, gall bladder diseases, and so forth. Then you will find many articles on various foods, giving you the vitamin and mineral content of the food and an estimate of just what place it should have in your diet. You will find many articles on various parts of the body—the nerves, the heart, the skin, the hair, the stomach, the lungs and so forth. Then you will find articles dealing with more abstract aspects of health—exercise, chiefly, and the effect of the emotions on health, habits with vitamins and minerals, some suggestions on sleep and posture, how and when to eat, what to do about harmful chemicals in food, air and water.

Finally you will find articles on the elements of diet themselves—proteins, starches, fats, minerals, vitamins, enzymes, hormones. Here again, we have not been able to present a complete picture of all the information known at present about nutrition. This would fill many volumes. But, adding the articles in the Health Builder to those in the Health Finder, you will have, we believe, everything that you need to steer a successful path through the maze of contradiction, confusion and half-truth that constitutes the information most of us have on nutrition.

With this knowledge too, you will be able to attain better health. If you are well, we believe you will be able to stay well. If you are ill, we believe you can greatly improve your health and perhaps achieve perfect well-being once again, by following the information in the Health Builder.

Good luck and good health to you!

J. I. Rodale, *Editor*
Ruth C. Adams, *Assistant Editor*
Charles Gerras, *Assistant Editor*

Acerola

According to reports, this fruit, new to us, will be used to enrich the vitamin C content of various fruit juices.

The group of Puerto Rican laboratory technicians nibbled on the fruit one of them had brought as a treat. They were chatting about the tree the fruit grows on—called "the health tree" by the Puerto Ricans who declare that you will never have a cold if you have such a tree growing in your back yard. The laboratory people, working under the direction of Dr. Conrado F. Asenjo, had been testing various fruits for their vitamin C content. Someone suggested testing the fruit they were eating which grows wild on the island. The vitamin C content was too high to be measured with their usual equipment. Eagerly they diluted the juice and tried again. Still it registered too high. Again and again they tried. Finally they discovered that the fruit of the acerola tree is the world's richest known source of vitamin C.

This was a number of years ago. Dr. Asenjo wrote articles about his discovery which were duly printed in scientific magazines and read soberly by other scientists. Nutritionists, school teachers and doctors became interested. They confirmed in their own laboratories the fantastically high vitamin C content of the acerola cherry. Civic and health-minded people in Puerto Rico saw to it that acerola trees were planted in school yards so that the children would eat plenty of the fruit. More years went by. Yet, apparently it occurred to no one that such a discovery as this could revolutionize a large section of the food industry. Everyone who knew of the fruit and its precious vitamin content expressed interest, but that was all.

Eventually word came to Harvey Greenspan, a citrus grower in Florida. He went to Puerto Rico and put the machinery into motion for planting orchards. Five years later there were thousands of acerola trees producing the fabulous little red cherries that may mean so much in the way of good health to many of us. The acerola juice is bottled close to the orchards so that none of the precious vitamin is lost.

The fruits, which look like cherries produce a reddish-orange juice with a pleasant tart flavor. Just before the cherries ripen is the time when their vitamin C content is highest. So they are picked just as the green fruit begins to turn red. The juice is canned within an hour from the time it leaves the tree. Stainless steel is used for the processing, for the high ascorbic acid content would corrode any softer and more permeable metal.

The government of Puerto Rico is encouraging their people to plant acerola trees and use the fruit. Teachers now give each school child two acerolas daily, and enough trees have been planted that the juice is now available commercially. Supposedly the first use to be made of it is to reinforce infant foods. That is, it will be added to apple, orange or pear juice to increase the vitamin C content. There is also a suggestion that it may be used in soft drinks—perish the thought! To throw away this fine, natural vitamin-rich substance on soft drinks seems to us almost criminal. To be sure, the soft drinks have at present no nutritional value at all, and, if children are going to continue to drink them, the added vitamin C will be welcome, nutritionally speaking. But we shudder to think of the advertising campaign that will ensue once the soft drink industry can prove that there is a vitamin—a real, live vitamin—in their product. Even the most reluctant mother will then probably stock up on soft drinks. Of course the sugar content, the artificial flavorings and colors, the acids and the caffeine will still work their inestimable harm on the drinkers of soft drinks, no matter how reinforced they may be with vitamin C.

Comparing Acerola and Rose Hips

However, we are delighted to know that a brand new, and, we suppose, inexpensive source of vitamin C has been discovered and developed. Exactly how good a source of vitamin C is it?

Just to refresh our memories, here is a list of foods high in vitamin C, along with their vitamin C content in milligrams per 100 grams. We indicate in each case approximately what 100 grams means in the way of an individual serving. We are told that the juice of acerola or "C-rola" as it is sometimes called, contains as much as 80 times more vitamin C than orange juice. According to the figures we have on rose hips, some species of rose hips contain far, far more vitamin C than that.

Broccoli	90	milligrams in ¾ cup or 100 grams.
Cantaloupe	50	milligrams in ½ small cantaloupe or 100 grams.
Collards	70	milligrams in ½ cup or 100 grams.
Grapefruit	45	milligrams in ½ grapefruit or 100 grams.
Guavas	125	milligrams in 1 guava or 100 grams.
Honeydew	90	milligrams in ¼ honeydew or 100 grams.
Kale	96	milligrams in ¾ cup.
Mustard Greens	125	milligrams in ½ cup.
Orange	50	milligrams in 1 medium orange.
Orange Juice	59	milligrams per 100 grams.
Peppers, green	125	milligrams in 1 medium pepper.
Peppers, pimento	200	milligrams in 2 medium peppers.
Rose hips	500	to 6000 milligrams in 100 grams.
Turnip tops	130	milligrams in ½ cup.

Rose hips are the fruit of the rose bush which appear after the flower is gone. Their vitamin C content varies according to the kind of rose and the climate where it is grown. Roses native to northern countries contain far more vitamin C. We have been singing the praises of rose hips for several years as the finest possible source of vitamin C. Our advertisers sell rose hip products—tablets or powder. These are made by drying the hips at very low heat to conserve all the precious vitamin C.

According to the way we figure, rose hips are still a far better source of vitamin C than acerola juice. Orange juice contains approximately 60 milligrams of vitamin C per 100 grams. Rose hips contain anywhere from 500 to 6000 milligrams of vitamin C per 100 grams. We are told that acerola juice is 80 times richer in vitamin C than orange juice. But rose hips are 10 to 100 times richer!

Rose hips do not, of course, fill exactly the same need as the acerola juice. You can't—or most people wouldn't want to—serve rose hip purée in a glass for breakfast. You can add the purée to other fruit drinks, a teaspoon or a tablespoon at a time. You wouldn't want to use even fresh rose hips as your only fruit, for they somehow are not that appealing in taste. To gather rose hips you must first find them where they are growing wild, or grow them in your garden. They must be picked at exactly the right time and then made into a syrup or purée.

Acerola juice you will be able to buy already processed in a can, we are told. This is convenient, but canning at the high temperature necessary destroys enzymes and much else that is valuable in a fruit juice. Perhaps some day when all the growing and marketing problems have been solved, readers who live in the south can grow their own acerola trees or buy fresh acerola fruit in their own home town. Until then we suggest that you watch for the acerola juice when it appears on the market. Use it as you would other fruit juice. But continue to take your rose hips as the best and surest source of vitamin C.

Just so you will be sure to recognize it, the acerola cherry goes by several other names, too: the Puerto Rican cherry, West Indian cherry, Barbados cherry or (its botanical name) *Malpighia punicifolia.*

Acne

Acne disappeared in from two and a half to six months under treatment with large doses of vitamin A, according to an article in the *Journal of the Indian Medical Association,* March 1954. In all, seventy-five patients were treated. All other kinds of treatment had failed, even those continued over long periods of time. During the time the doctors gave vitamin A, they gave no other treatment. The dosage was 100,000 units per day. All patients could be "regarded as cured."

It is the belief of the two authors of this article, K. D. Lahiri and F. J. Scandrett, that the vitamin A is effective not only because of its direct action on the skin, but also, they feel, because it probably has some effect on the lack of balance of the sex hormones, which appears to be characteristic of acne, coming as it generally does, at the time of puberty. Perhaps, say these researchers, large doses of vitamin A may eventually restore the proper ratio of androgen and estrogen—that is, the male and female sex hormones.

The author of a paper in the *Archives of Dermatology and Syphilology,* volume 70, page 363, 1954, gave massive doses of vitamin C to 53 acne patients, 43 of whom improved. Fifteen of these had been treated for months or years by all the usual methods, without success. Ten patients failed to improve and seven did not return for a check-up.

The vitamin C consisted of an eight-ounce glass of citrus juice twice daily as well as three grams (3000 milligrams) of ascorbic acid per day.

We assume that this was synthetic ascorbic acid, since nothing in the article indicates that it could have been from natural sources.

In addition, the patients were put on a diet free of chocolate, nuts and peanut butter, were told to clean their skin three times a day and were given *lotio alba* to apply at night. As we know, vitamin C has a lot to do with skin health. It has also been found that persons deprived of vitamin C entirely are likely to suffer from a worsening of their acne, if they are subject to it. It seems as if plenty of vitamin C in the diet might play a big part in preventing acne. And it is well-known that the diet of teen-agers (most susceptible to acne) is likely to be short on this vitamin.

Alcoholism

Is Alcoholism a Disease of Starvation?

Within the past thirty years perhaps no change in thinking in this country has been so great as the change in our thinking about alcoholism. In the last century the "drunk" was a figure of fun, abuse or contempt. Popular songs spoke righteously of the disgrace he brought on his family, the poverty, broken homes, deaths, illness and misery. Ministers railed in their pulpits against the evils of the demon rum. Temperance workers steadied the steps of confirmed alcoholics as they tottered forward to take the pledge. Wives nagged, children wept, doctors scolded, saloon keepers got rich, and through it all the agonized and helpless alcoholic suffered more shame, pain and bewilderment than anyone involved.

In those days apparently no one suspected that an alcoholic was ill, just as ill as respectable people who contracted tuberculosis, scarlet fever or diabetes. In those days it was believed that the alcoholic was the result of pure cussedness and that he could give up drinking if he would just pull himself together. Somewhat the same theories had prevailed earlier about mental disease. Mental patients were beaten, chained and exposed to all kinds of outrages in the belief that this would cast out the devils that possessed them.

Today we know that mental disease and alcoholism are illnesses. There no longer remains a shred of doubt on which an uncharitable lecture can be hung. The true alcoholic is just as helpless in the grip of his illness as is the diabetic or the sufferer from heart disease. It is only within the last twenty-five or thirty years that science has gotten busy on the problem of alcoholism and has come up with some astounding discoveries. And high time it is, too, for if things go on at their present rate we can soon expect that today's alarming statistics will go completely out of bounds. As it is, there are an estimated 600,000 chronic alcoholic addicts in this country today. There are about two million "heavy" drinkers and 40 million "social" drinkers. As another statistician puts it, about four million Americans today drink to excess. About 750,000 have severely damaged their health through alcohol. In 1949 this nation spent eight billion, eight hundred million dollars for alcoholic beverages. By 1948 the per capita consumption of alcohol had risen to 1.98 gallons per year. The potential wage losses incurred as a result of drinking came to an estimated one billion dollars. Between 1941 and 1947 drinking by high school students rose 30.2 per cent, 58 per cent of which took place in the homes of the students, not in bars.

Who Is the Alcoholic?

What kind of people are alcoholics? Do personality and physical make-up give us any clue as to which people can "take it or leave it alone" and which people have a compulsive need to drink to excess? Many studies have been done on this aspect of the problem. Dr. James T. Smith of Bellevue Hospital in New York in a General Electric Science Forum radio program on January 9, 1952, said that an alcoholic is a person who becomes socially or financially irresponsible because of drinking, the person who gets an excessive effect from alcohol. . . . If he takes alcohol, he has lit a fuse which will inevitably lead on to the explosion of acute intoxication. In a detailed study of over 2,000 male alcoholics it was found that they show physical characteristics differing from the average healthy male. Baldness is rare among alcoholics; they usually have a full head of hair, often prematurely gray. Acne, so common in adolescent boys, occurs seldom in history of alcoholics. Such physical characteristics are dependent on the chemical functioning of the body.

Another investigator, Jackson T. Smith, M.D., of Houston, Texas, has this to say in an article in the *American Practitioner and Digest of Treatment* for July, 1953: "More often than not the alcoholic is from a 'broken home,' either there has been a separation or divorce by the time he reached his teens or else one or both parents will have died. The alcoholic may be very labile emotionally, tending to express his moods without average restraint. There may be a continuously vacillating attitude toward whatever authority he is faced with; at one time he is openly defiant (particularly when drinking) and at another totally dependent. It would appear that the individual's confidence in himself varies from time to time, but is always increased by his taking a drink. . . . Intellectually he may be above average, but may have repeatedly failed to utilize his innate abilities to achieve any particular goal . . . he is apt to be more self-conscious than average. . . ."

Harold W. Lovell, M.D. and John W. Tintera, M.D., of New York, writing in *Modern Medicine,* for May 15, 1951, say "Two distinct groups of alcoholics are recognized. One group comprises the constitutionally hypoadrenocortic (suffering from diminished activity of the adrenal glands). Such individuals are tall, asthenic (inclined to be weak physically) men who usually report low tolerance for alcohol from the outset. These men are predisposed to alcoholism from an early age.

"In the second group are those with acquired adrenocortical insufficiency. Initially, these individuals have good tolerance for alcohol, but prolonged overindulgence damages the adrenal cortex and reduces cortical function. Consequently alcohol tolerance is lowered and addiction results."

In an earlier issue of *Modern Medicine,* Dr. Tintera had this to say: "For many years we have maintained that an adrenocortical deficiency is as much of a genetic factor as the well-established diabetic hereditary factor. Individuals manifesting this genetic influence . . . usually show a decreased metabolism, marked hypotension (low blood pressure) and orthostatic (caused by standing upright) changes in blood pressure, a characteristic hair distribution and a fondness or even a real craving for salt and carbohydrates. . . . It is so often found that the offspring of alcoholic parents either become alcoholics themselves or teetotalers because they realize their inability to handle or tolerate alcohol. These same individuals are the ones who retain their leanness and asthenia throughout life since they are not able to metabolize carbohydrates properly. Like their teetotaler forbears they may expect to have longevity much beyond the average with the assurance that senility due to arteriosclerotic changes will not usually ensue."

What do all these statements and big words boil down to? Well, the typical alcoholic seems to be a thin, not-very-energetic person, who is insecure and self-conscious. He may be above average in intelligence; he probably thinks of himself as a failure whether or not he is. His body seems to have a chronic inability to handle carbohydrates properly and this is the reason why alcohol spells his downfall. This is what is involved in hypoadrenocortical function. And we will explain later on just how this mechanism for regulating the digestion of carbohydrates seems to work.

What Alcohol Does in the Body

First let us investigate how alcohol behaves in the body—what it does and what it does not do. Alcohol is a carbohydrate—that is, it is made of carbon, hydrogen and oxygen with a certain proportion and arrangement of molecules that differentiate it from other carbohydrates. Says John J. O'Neill in the *New York Herald-Tribune* for June 10, 1951, "alcohol acts in the body the way gasoline acts in an automobile engine. The gasoline is burned to provide heat and power but it contributes nothing to the maintenance and growth of the engine. Alcohol acts as a fuel, not as a food." Dr. Lovell in his book *Hope and Help for the Alcoholic* (Doubleday and Co., 1951), says that alcohol is a depressant. The impression of a stimulating effect after a few drinks is the result of the temporary lift in blood sugar. But this is followed by a sharp decline if drinking is continued. A drink dilates the tiny blood vessels at the surface of the skin, bringing with the increased amount of blood a sensation of warmth. But if the skin is exposed to cold while these vessels are dilated, body heat is lost and the whole body temperature goes down. "Alcohol is not directly responsible for any disease except alcoholism," says Dr. Lovell, "alcoholics and other excessive drinkers may impair their resistance to many diseases by allowing themselves to become undernourished, but it is the bad nutrition and not the alcohol which is the direct cause."

Alcoholism is a Glandular Disorder

Perhaps one reason why we keep coming back to the comparison of alcoholism with diabetes is this—diabetes is also a disease of those who cannot properly metabolize carbohydrates. In the case of diabetics, not enough insulin is produced by the pancreatic gland which has this function, so the patient suffers from high blood sugar. This is why he must be given insulin to reduce his blood sugar. In the case of alcoholics, there is *too much insulin* rather than too little, with the result that the alcoholic has low blood sugar. Now the answer would be simple if it were possible just to drain off this extra insulin, but we find it is much more complicated than that. What causes the extra insulin that causes the low blood sugar? Apparently the function of at least two glands is involved—the *adrenals* (and it is the *cortex* or covering of these glands that is involved) and the *pituitary* (which regulates the adrenals).

Says E. M. Abrahamson, M.D., in his book *Body, Mind and Sugar* (Henry Holt and Co., 1951), "Alcoholism is caused by a deficiency in the adrenal cortical hormones—those hormones whose action is antithetical to insulin. The trouble may not be in the adrenal cortical itself, however, but in the master gland, the pituitary, which for some reason fails to stimulate the adrenal cortical glands as it does in normal operation of the endocrine system. It is believed, moreover, that this disability of the pituitary is not caused by the alcoholism itself but antedates its development." Dr. Abrahamson goes on to tell us that physicians have achieved almost miraculous results by giving injections of ACTH and cortisone to alcoholics in their very worst condition of delirium tremens or hangovers. ACTH and cortisone are the gland extracts of the adrenal glands, in which the alcoholic is deficient. "These spectacular 'cures' are a great step forward," says Dr. Abrahamson, "and they provide evidence in reverse for the theory which the medical and the lay members of this collaboration arrived at independently; that hyperinsulinism, with its chronic partial blood sugar starvation, is an essential underlying condition of alcholism."

It all sounds almost impossibly complicated, doesn't it? And yet the answer, as Dr. Abrahamson gives it, is so remarkably simple that we feel it should be blasted from loud speakers in every metropolis in the country and headlined in newspapers and magazines. The answer is a diet which regulates the blood sugar so that it does not fall below safe levels. This is a diet high in fat and protein and low in carbohydrates which will result—and *has* resulted in many cases treated by Dr. Abrahamson—in a complete lack of desire for alcohol. The alcohol was needed to raise the low blood sugar level which is responsible for the "jitters," the uneasiness, the lack of confidence, the restlessness of the alcoholic, which caused him to crave alcohol.

We then arrive at the question—did the alcoholic become an alcoholic because of his low blood sugar, or did the use of alcohol bring about the low blood sugar to begin with? The answer seems, at present, to be that both these suppositions are correct. That is, the individual who has a tendency, (perhaps inherited) toward an improper functioning of the glands that regulate blood sugar may take to alcohol because it raises his blood sugar and thus relieves his jitters and nervousness. On the other hand, an individual who begins to drink early in life simply because of the exhilarating effect of liquor, may so damage the functioning of these glands (by drinking to excess) that he eventually gets a bad case of low blood sugar in which case of course he feels an overpowering compulsion to go on drinking to keep his blood sugar high.

Vitamins and Alcoholism

Another important aspect of the question, it seems to us, is the part that vitamins, especially the B vitamins, may play in the whole story. Dr. Roger J. Williams of the University of Texas is our authority for most of the work that has been done along these lines. Dr. Williams believes, according to *Time* for June 11, 1951, that "While all men need the same vitamins and minerals, they do not need them in the same amounts or the same proportions. Many human disorders, he thinks, arise because some people (partly because of heredity) need some life-essential substances in far greater quantities than normal diets supply." The craving for alcohol is one such disorder, he believes. In his experiments with rats, he found that those animals whose diet was deficient in vitamins developed a craving for alcohol, while rats fed on a diet which supplied the necessary vitamins developed a dislike for alcohol.

Dr. Williams treated one human alcoholic patient with massive doses of vitamins A, C, D and E and all of the B vitamins. The patient went without alcohol without any difficulty and even, finally, demonstrated that he could take one or two beers and then quit. "This individual," says Williams, "probably constitutes the first case on record in which an alcoholic has become a moderate drinker." Up to this time there has been unanimous agreement that the true alcoholic could never become a moderate drinker, no matter what the "cure"—he would always have to be a teetotaler. But Dr. Williams has apparently proved otherwise. "Since then," says *Time,* "doctors at Boston's Peter Bent Brigham Hospital have tested the method with 85 alcoholics, giving some of them dummy capsules to rule out the psychological factor, and report at least one-third better results in the vitamin treated cases."

It seems to us that this discovery ties in well with Dr. Abrahamson's plea for a diet containing little or no carbohydrate. White sugar and white flour that constitute more than 50 per cent of the average American diet, are carbohydrates, but they are also carbohydrates from which all the vitamins have been removed by processing. Carbohydrates must be accompanied by B vitamins or the body cannot handle them, so to digest white sugar and white flour foods, the body is robbed of B vitamins until a deficiency is produced. Most drinkers also smoke, which practically guarantees them a shortage of vitamin C. Vitamin A deficiencies are extremely common, as military doctors discovered among men in service.

Now, let us imagine an individual—man or woman—whose body naturally requires far more vitamins than the average. Perhaps this might be because of unusual gland activity of some kind—who knows? Right from the start this individual is getting less vitamins than he needs. As he grows up, on a diet 50 per cent of which is de-vitaminized white flour and sugar, his vitamin deficiency grows worse. In addition, if he is predisposed to the adrenal disorders Dr. Abrahamson mentioned, his blood sugar level is bound to fall to dangerous depths. Not knowing any better, he continues to eat a diet high in carbohydrates, because they raise his blood sugar level giving him some comfort for an hour or so. If alcohol is at hand—and where in this country is it not at hand?—he soon finds that alcohol gives him release from jitters and self-consciousness. From then on, he is a gone gosling, for his body cannot handle alcohol any better than it can handle other carbohydrates. As he drinks more, he eats less and less. What food he does eat certainly does not supply the necessary protein and vitamins, so he must drink more—not because he is depraved or lacks will power, but because his body is starving for food which he does not give it.

Stress and the Alcoholic

One other factor enters in to which many researchers have devoted a lot of time. Says George N. Thompson, M.D., of the University of Southern California, writing in *Industrial Medicine and Surgery* for June, 1951, "The alcoholic is a person who, because he cannot stand the strain and tension of life without developing strong anxieties, escapes from responsibilities into oblivion . . . we are quick to state that the human organism can tolerate just so much stress. *But in spite of this knowledge, and in spite of the realization that our mental hospitals are filled with those who have fallen under the stress of their environments, under working situations intolerable to them . . . we continue to place workers in jobs for which they are unsuited, to enforce factors of stress to which we would not subject a mechanical contrivance and to expect performance beyond the capacity of the emotionally handicapped person.*"

Such a statement arouses another question in our minds—is the alcoholic a person who cannot stand stress because of his glandular make-up, or does his constant anxiety and nervousness disorder his glands? And if so, what causes the original anxiety? Could it not be lack of those vitamins whose chief function is to safeguard the health of the nervous system? One of the chief treatments for alcoholism is, and for some time has been, psychotherapy and drugs which will make alcohol repugnant to him. The question in our minds is: is it possible to rehabilitate an alcoholic by removing the frustrations and stresses in his life, without at the same time repairing the functions of his glands that affect and are affected by these emotions? Quite apart from this, of course, is the question of how many of us can afford psychotherapy, even if it is available in our home town. And how many of us can afford hospitalization which the taking of Antabuse and other drugs necessitates?

It is noteworthy that practically all writers on alcoholism mention Alcoholics Anonymous. It appears to be one organization to which unanimous approval and support is given. But it has been pointed out that the word *Alcoholic* is always used by a member when he introduces himself. He does not qualify himself as a "cured alcoholic." For he knows that, unless and until he corrects the body disorder that creates his craving for alcohol, he must remain a teetotaler—at whatever cost to his peace of mind—and can never again touch alcohol. We are in agreement that, for the confirmed alcoholic, this organization offers much in the way of psychotherapy. Socializing with people who are in the same boat and who are dedicated with fanatic fervor to helping other alcoholics appears to us to be a healthful and sound step to take.

We are convinced, moreover, that an alcoholic can be returned to health by diet, and vitamin and mineral supplements, administered at home without expense and without upsetting the family's way of life. The diet we outline at the end of this article is the one Dr. Abrahamson publishes in his book which, incidentally you can buy at your local bookstore or direct from the publishers–*Body, Mind and Sugar,* published by Henry Holt and Co., 383 Madison Ave., New York City. Two other books on alcoholism we want to recommend are *Hope and Help for the Alcoholic* by Harold W. Lovell, published by Doubleday and Company, Garden City, New York and *Nutrition and Alcohol* by Roger J. Williams, published by the University of Oklahoma Press, Norman, Oklahoma.

For those of you may have had alcoholics in the family or who, for some other reason, fear that some member of the family may have inclinations this way, we would say don't try to prevent alcoholism by scolding, lecturing and forbidding alcohol in the house. Liquor is easily available at almost any corner of the street these days. Instead, try putting the whole family on a high protein diet with as few sweet and starchy foods as possible. This means meat, fish, eggs, nuts, cheese, fresh vegetables and fruits, supplemented by brewer's yeast or desiccated liver for vitamin B, rose hips or some other natural food supplement for vitamin C, fish liver oil for vitamins A and D, bone meal for calcium and other minerals and wheat germ for vitamin E.

This is the diet for curing or preventing low blood sugar, as outlined by Dr. Abrahamson:

On arising–Medium orange, half grapefruit or four ounces of fruit juice.

Breakfast–Fruit or 4 ounces of juice, 1 egg with or without 2 slices of ham or bacon; only one slice of bread or toast with plenty of butter, beverage.

2 hours after breakfast–4 ounces of juice.

Lunch–Meat, fish, cheese or eggs; salad (large serving of lettuce, tomato or Waldorf salad with mayonnaise or French dressing) ; vegetables if desired; only one slice of bread or toast with plenty of butter; dessert; beverage.

3 hours after lunch–8 ounces of milk.

1 hour before dinner–4 ounces of juice.

Dinner–Soup if desired (not thickened with flour) ; vegetables; liberal portion of meat, fish or poultry; only one slice of bread if desired; dessert; beverage.

2-3 hours after dinner–8 ounces of milk.

Every two hours until bedtime–4 ounces of milk or a small handful of nuts.

Allowable vegetables: Asparagus, avocado, beets, broccoli, Brussels sprouts, cabbage, cauliflower, carrots, celery, cucumbers, corn, eggplant, lima beans, onions, peas, radishes, sauerkraut, squash, string beans, tomatoes, turnips.

Allowable fruits: Apples, apricots, berries, grapefruit, pears, melons, oranges, peaches, pineapple, tangerines. May be cooked or raw with or without cream but without sugar. Canned fruits should be packed in water, not syrup.

Lettuce, mushrooms and nuts may be taken as freely as desired.

Juice: Any unsweetened fruit or vegetable juice except grape juice or prune juice.

Beverages: Weak tea (tea ball not brewed); decaffeinated coffee, coffee substitutes.

Desserts: Fruit, unsweetened gelatin, junket (made from tablets, not mix).

Alcoholic and soft drinks: Club soda, dry ginger ale, whiskey and other distilled liquors.

Avoid Absolutely

Sugar, candy and other sweets, such as cake, pie, pastries, sweet custards, puddings, and ice cream.

Caffeine: Ordinary coffee, strong brewed tea, beverages containing caffeine. (Your doctor will tell you what these are.)

Potatoes, rice, grapes, raisins, plums, figs, dates and bananas.

Spaghetti, macaroni and noodles. (We add crackers, pretzels, biscuits, etc.)

Wines, cordials, cocktails and beer.

(We have included bacon, ham, soft drinks and distilled liquors in this list, as Dr. Abrahamson does, but we assume that you will automatically have crossed these off as you read the list. Of course alcoholic beverages do not belong on a diet list for an alcoholic, *but we contend that he will soon not want them.* Also note that we do not recommend using citrus fruits as freely as Dr. Abrahamson suggests and we do not approve of drinking citrus fruit juice or milk. Any lack of Vitamin C can be made up by taking rose hips.)

Alfalfa

Alfalfa has long been thought of as food for herbivorous farm animals, but more recently it has assumed considerable importance as food for human beings. It is a legume, as beans and peas are. But we eat the leaves, stems and seeds, rather than just the seeds. Alfalfa is one of the oldest of the legume family, its history going back for thousands of years. It seems likely that one of the main reasons for its richness in food value is the fact that its roots burrow deep into the earth, seeking out minerals that are buried in the soil. The average alfalfa seed has roots 10 to 20 feet long and reports have been found of phenomenally long roots—even as long as 128 feet.

It is a perennial plant, by which we mean that it need not be resowed every year, as corn must be, for example. It grows readily in almost any land and climate and is produced most abundantly in the southern and western parts of our country. For cattle it is used as hay, pasture, silage and alfalfa meal.

We have long believed that foods that are valuable for stock feed are likely to be good for human beings, too. And such is indeed the case with alfalfa. Frank W. Bower of Sierra Madre, California, has done a great deal to popularize alfalfa for human consumption, according to an article in *Physical Culture* magazine for February, 1948. Mr. Bower who has devoted most of his life to research on alfalfa, makes bread, muffins, flapjacks, and tea from alfalfa, to name but a few of the ways he advocates eating it. It is available, too, from many other health food producers in tablet form, as a food supplement, and as seeds or leaves from which to make tea.

Alfalfa is perhaps most valuable for its vitamin A content. Vitamin A is a fat soluble vitamin, so it is not lost to any great extent when the alfalfa is dried. Alfalfa contains about 8000 International Units of Vitamin A for every hundred grams. This compares favorably with apricots (7500 units per hundred grams) and with beef liver (9000 units per hundred grams). In addition, alfalfa is a good source of pyridoxine, one of the B vitamins, and vitamin E, whose great importance for the health of muscles and heart is well known. Alfalfa is regarded as the most reliable source of vitamin E for herbivorous animals. In addition it is extremely rich in vitamin K, ranking along with spinach, kale and carrot tops as a good source of this vitamin which protects against hemorrhaging and helps the blood to clot properly. In animals vitamin K prevents and cures high blood pressure, so it may be far more important for the health of human beings than we know. Alfalfa contains from 20,000 to 40,000 units of vitamin K for every hundred grams.

Here are some further interesting nutritional facts: We are accustomed to thinking of foods from animal sources as being richest in protein, so it is surprising to find that the protein content of alfalfa is extremely high—18.9 per cent as compared to 3.3 per cent in milk, 13.8 per cent in whole wheat, 13.1 per cent in eggs and 16.5 per cent in beef.

In mineral content, too, alfalfa shows up well, with the following analysis, in comparison with other products:

	Calcium	*Phosphorus*	*Iron*
Alfalfa	34.9	7.35	1.30
Soy flour	3.45	17.50	.28
Kelp	1.20	.27	.16
Whole wheat flour	.75	10.90	.30
Corn meal	.36	8.44	.15
Rolled oats	1.10	8.10	.05

It is, of course, perfectly possible to go out into an alfalfa field, pick yourself some stalks and leaves and chew them for dinner. But since we do not, generally speaking, have the same gastronomical preferences as cows, it is possible that the taste may not appeal. So we would suggest getting your alfalfa in meal which you can use in the kitchen, in tablets which you can take as food supplements or as seeds or leaves, which you can make into tea. It was our search for healthful beverages that led us to our research on alfalfa. One further bit of advice—be certain that the seeds you buy have been prepared for human consumption. Seeds prepared for planting may have been treated with chemicals which would not be the best thing for one's digestive tract.

Almonds

Nuts in general seem to be one of our best foods. They come to us enclosed in a thick shell through which neither dirt nor insecticides can penetrate. They contain wonderfully fine food elements—carbohydrates, proteins and fats and a wealth of vitamins and minerals. Not only can they be eaten raw, but they taste better raw than cooked. This means we get valuable enzymes from nuts.

The almond is one of the oldest nuts historically. It came to us originally from western Asia and Morocco. The word "Luz" in Genesis has been translated as "Hazelnut" but is generally thought to mean almond. Almond trees are referred to often in the Bible. The sweet almond tree has pink flowers. The bitter almond has white. Sweet almonds are the ones we eat and they have been developed into a soft-shelled nut which is easy to crack.

Almonds are high in calories—good news for those of us who are trying to put on weight. One-half ounce of almond nutmeats contains about 100 calories—not starch incidentally, for the calories come in the fats of the nutmeat. As you know, we speak of the quality of different proteins. Vegetable proteins are in general not so good as meat proteins. That is, they are not so likely to contain the amino acids that are necessary for proper nourishment. But the protein of the almond compares very favorably with that of meat. So if you are contemplating a high protein diet, put almonds on the list!

There is an idea that nuts are hard to digest. This misconception may arise from the fact that we do not chew them well enough, or from the fact that we eat them generally at the end of a big meal. Since they contain a lot of fat, they remain in the stomach longer than carbohydrates or proteins. And if they are not thoroughly chewed the digestive juices cannot penetrate their rather dense structure and they may be excreted without being digested. This is the main reason why so many recipes call for chopping or grinding nuts. When we eat them they should be combined with foods that are not high in fats, so that the total amount of fat eaten at one time will not be too high to be digested. An excellent reason for having raw fruits and nuts for a special dessert.

Almonds contain an extremely small amount of a substance that changes to hydrocyanic acid so they should not be eaten to excess, or to the exclusion of other foods. Almond extract is made from oil of bitter almonds from which the hydrocyanic acid has been removed. Because of its soothing effect almond oil is sometimes used in cough medicines.

When the holidays approach and when the youngsters clamor loudly for sweets, and festive refreshments must be provided for holiday guests, it's well to keep a bowl of nuts handy, especially almonds which, for most people, are a real delicacy. Serve them just as they are, with a nutcracker. Blanching (removing the dark outer skin) can be accomplished by soaking them for a minute or so in hot water. But skip all the roasting, frying and salting processes which do nothing but detract from the nuts' nutritional value. Blanched almonds mixed with raisins or dates are a real holiday treat. Or you can make marzipan. Marzipan is a favorite European delicacy which is made up for the holidays in entrancing shapes of tiny fruits, vegetables and animals. It is simply almond paste, made by grinding up blanched almonds and shaping the paste into desired shapes.

Here are the words of a famous nutrition expert, Dr. J. H. Kellogg, on the subject of nuts: "They supply for a given weight nearly twice the amount of nutriment of any other food."

These are the vitamins and minerals contained in 10 almonds:

Vitamin A	7 international units
B Vitamins	
Thiamin	15 micrograms
Riboflavin	10 micrograms
Niacin	.5 milligrams
Vitamin C	1 milligram
Calcium	25 milligrams
Phosphorus	45 milligrams
Iron	.4 milligrams
Copper	.1 milligram
Magnesium	.2 milligrams
Chlorine	.3 milligrams
Potassium	7 milligrams

Aluminum

ALUMINUM COOKING UTENSILS

The evidence is so conclusive against aluminum utensils that there is not the slightest question in my mind about it, one should ban them from the kitchen. I am fully aware that the American Medical Association, the U. S. Government, the Better Business Bureau and Frederick Carleton believe that the use of aluminum utensils is not harmful to human health, but we have so much material that shows them to be wrong that it would be a grievous sin for us to remain quiet about it.

Canadian Rose Hip Experiment

In the *Canadian Journal of Research,* Volume 21, Section C, is described an experiment in the cooking of rose hips in vessels of various materials. Quoting from this article we find that, "Dried, powdered flesh (of rose hips), 0.5 gram, was placed in the vessel being used in the experiment. This was covered with 20 ml. water and the mixture boiled for 15 minutes, then cooled, centrifuged, and acidified aliquots (equal parts) were titrated. . . . Tests with vessels of glass and enamel showed practically no loss of ascorbic acid (Vitamin C). The loss in the copper vessel is very marked, and in the aluminum less, but appreciable."

This would indicate that cooking in copper and aluminum would cause losses in vitamins, and that glass and enamelware are safest. The fact that glass and enamel are better than aluminum was shown in cases described by Arthur F. Coca, M.D., in his book, *Familial Nonreaginic Food Allergy,* published in 1945 by Charles C. Thomas, Springfield, Illinois. Coca quotes from the book *Practice of Allergy,* P. 831, by Vaughan, stating that the author mentions "the cure of cases of long-standing refractory colitis following change from aluminum cooking utensils to enamel or glass vessels."

An experiment was performed at the University of Colorado which adds some additional light to this question of the effect on aluminum of contact with certain liquids. It was written up in the journal, *Food Technology* of December, 1951. It showed that orange juice dissolved on the average 37 parts per million of the aluminum of the pot in which it was contained. In the case of grapefruit juice the average was about 23 parts. When we consider that in fluoridation of water great care is taken not to use more than 1 part per million we can see how dangerous it is to use a substance as toxic as aluminum in as high as 37 parts. And bear in mind this is cold orange juice. There was no cooking involved.

Another worker against aluminum is Dr. Leo Spira who in 1933 published a monograph on the subject called *The Clinical Aspect of Chronic Poisoning by Aluminum and its Alloys,* which gives his experience with the subject over a period of ten years.

Dr. Spira not only cured himself by discontinuing the use of aluminum cooking utensils but also dozens of others. As symptoms of aluminum poisoning in various patients which were cleared up by not using aluminum utensils were constipation, flatulence, colicky pain, impairment of appetite, nausea, many forms of skin ailments, neuralgia, twitching of legs, giddiness, excessive perspiration, loss of energy, etc. Dr. Spira not only has his patients discontinue the use of aluminum utensils, but also has them stop using tap water, for in many cities alum (which is a form of aluminum) is placed in city water supplies to purify it. Dr. Spira has found also that many brands of aluminum ware contain poisonous impurities such as copper, antimony, fluorine, zinc, lead, tin, etc.

When in 1935 Dr. Spira discussed the aluminum question in the columns of *The London Times,* many persons wrote in confirming Dr. Spira's experiences by describing their own cases of cure.

Dr. F. Von Halla, in "Aluminum und Darm," *Deutsche Aertze Zeitung,* pp. 195 and 201, describes twenty-five cases of patients with severe constipation who could not be cured by regular medical procedures but whose condition dramatically yielded when they gave up cooking in aluminum.

Dr. O. Putensen, in the *Deutsche Aertze Zeitung,* pp. 223, 231, 242, describes the case of a dog with rash sores and intense itching who was cured only when the aluminum pans from which he was fed were thrown out. Dr. Putensen describes experiences with many patients showing cures of gastric and skin disturbances caused by cooking food in aluminum.

Dr. Coram James writing in the *British Medical Journal* of April 9, 1932, in describing some cases of gastric disturbances which he was able to cure by substituting enamel or iron pots for aluminum, said, "It seems like riding coincidence too hard to suppose that a sequence of a score or more relieved could all have been hypersensitive to aluminum."

What the doctor means is that the aluminum people and their medical friends believe that only *some* people are allergic to aluminum.

Dr. Alexander Francis, writing in the April 16, 1932, issue of the *British Medical Journal,* describes how he cured his own case of severe abdominal pain by discontinuing the use of aluminum. The pain had been so bad that at times it completely incapacitated him. Several times later, the pain returned but in every case he found that he had eaten something cooked in aluminum. The abdominal pain caused by aluminum, says the doctor, is of such nature that it cannot be relieved by the usual sedatives. Dr. Francis, in this article, also reports six cases in which he cured abdominal pain by ordering the disuse of aluminum cooking utensils.

Dr. E. H. Rink, writing in the August 6, 1932, issue of the *British Medical Journal* describes how he treated two patients who were suffering respectively from abdominal pain which was thought to be appendicitis, and a case of colitis. Following the method of Dr. Spira he had them stop using aluminum ware, and he gave them charcoal tablets to absorb some of the accumulated aluminum with striking cures in each case.

Dr. Eric Pritchard in the *British Medical Journal* of Oct. 29, 1932, says, "I have had plenty of evidence of chronic aluminum poisoning among members of my own family and among my personal friends, and also in the case of a dog, and several large groups of infants in institutions under my charge. Except in the case of infants, who appear to be very susceptible to the acute effects of aluminum poisoning, symptoms do not usually arise in the case of adults until after prolonged exposure to its effects."

The Mellon Institute of Industrial Research issued Bulletin No. 3, to show that aluminum was safe for household use.

The following table shows various food products cooked in aluminum and glassware:

Aluminum content in parts per million.

Foodstuffs	*Cooking Time in Minutes*	*Glass*	*Aluminum*	*Average Increase in Aluminum in Parts per Million*
Boiled ham	120	.78	2.1	1.32
Creamed chicken	120	.95	2.43	1.48
Oatmeal	150	1.51	9.13	7.62
Stewed tomatoes (bright pan)	20	.12	4.36	4.24
Stewed tomatoes (dark pan)	20	.14	15.6	15.46
Creamed cabbage	45	.34	90.8	90.5
Cranberry sauce	10	.52	28.0	27.48
Rhubarb	5	.94	41.8	40.9
Apricots	40	24.6	73.3	48.7
Lemon pie filling	2	.31	118.0	117.69

Please note the tremendous increase in aluminum.

What To Use

My suggestion as first choice for the cooking and storage of food is Pyrex glassware. It has the added advantage of cooking food evenly all through. It may be expensive because it is so expendable, but what is a little money compared to health, and you may stave off the undertaker's bill for many years. Think of the interest that can be earned on such a sum.

Next comes enamelware, but get only the best. Third in line is stainless steel. Porcelainware is perfect for food storage. Keep lemons and other citrus and acid fruit juices only in glass, enamel, or porcelain.

I have written much more on aluminum and its dangers in cooking utensils in my booklet *Poison in Your Pots and Pans* (available from Rodale Press for one dollar).

J. I. RODALE

Antibiotics

Our file on antibiotics contains many articles. According to an editorial in *The Lancet* for July 11, 1953, there are supposedly three general types of reaction to penicillin—"the least toxic of the antibiotics." Most serious of these is the anaphylactic shock which may result in death within a matter of minutes. Six per cent of everyone who receives penicillin develops a "serum-sickness-like" disease.

Speaking before the Southern California State Dental Association on April 21, 1953, Dr. Donald A. Kerr of the University of Michigan told of a woman who lost all of her skin, from head to foot—even the lining of her mouth, as a result of sensitivity to penicillin which she took by mouth. He said further that the incidence of gum disease is increasing sharply all over the country because of the habit of taking antibiotics, especially penicillin, by mouth. There has been a notable increase in *thrush,* he said—an ulcerative infection of the mouth which causes white patches there.

"The same type of sensitivity can result from taking large doses of penicillin to curb pneumonia and other serious diseases," said Dr. Kerr. "It's quite definite now that the indiscriminate use of antibiotics is a bad and dangerous thing. The gum trouble it may produce is difficult for dentists to heal. Metabolism difficulties such as those caused by diabetes and a shortage of vitamin C also damage the gums."

Dentistry in relation to antibiotics comes up again in a note in *Today's Health* for February 1954. Antibiotics are now added to the dental cements and resins used in filling teeth, because they apparently help to prevent decay from recurring under the fillings. What will be the effect of this additional use of antibiotics on those who are sensitive to them already?

In an article in the Journal of the *American Medical Association* for September 12, 1953, Charles W. Fairlie and Ralph E. Kendall, M.D., write as follows: "Fatal staphylococcus enteritis (inflammation of the intestines), following antibiotic therapy is now a familiar entity." The article goes on to describe in detail five patients, three of whom died. The patients were all in hospital for operations, some of them minor. They were given antibiotics as a routine thing. When they developed alarming symptoms the antibiotics were increased, apparently with the notion that antibiotics will cure anything. The two patients whose dosages of antibiotics were stopped as soon as the symptoms began, lived.

A survey done in England in 1953 revealed the fact that, of the hospitals queried, between one and five per cent of the nurses using antibiotics became sensitized to them! Streptomycin and penicillin were the two drugs responsible for most of the sensitizing. In most cases skin sensitivity was involved—on the hands, arms, face and neck. This seems to point to local contact with the antibiotics—in handling sponges or bandages and swabs or in expelling the air from syringes before giving injections. An article in *The Lancet* for July 11, 1953 indicates that such sensitization may be permanent, especially if it is not caught in the early stages. In this case, of course, the nurse cannot continue in her profession.

The editorial in *The Lancet* goes on to say "Too often it seems not to be recognized that uncomplicated recovery is the rule after minor surgical operations done with proper regard for asepsis; even before antibiotics were used it was exceptional for clean operation wounds to show signs of infection. . . . In process of evolution microorganisms generally have proved their power to adapt themselves to many changes in their environment; and it is improbable that we shall fundamentally improve our position by affording them uncalled-for opportunities to grow accustomed to our antibiotics. Uncritical use of antibiotic 'umbrellas' is likely to lead to an increase in both resistant bacteria and sensitized patients."

This was written in 1953. Have you heard of any decrease in the use of antibiotics during the years since 1953? We do not have the figures for these years, but we do know (*Chemical Week,* October 9, 1954) that production of penicillin increased from 318,622 billion units in 1951 to 371,589 billion units in 1953.

Sudden Fatalities from Penicillin

Perhaps most disturbing of all are the stories of penicillin (given for colds) causing sudden death. Penicillin has no beneficial effect whatsoever on colds. Says Dr. Sheppard Siegal writing in *The New York State Journal of Medicine* for April 15, 1955, "In viral respiratory illness there exists no indication for penicillin apart from patient pressure for the 'magic shot'." In other words the doctor, giving his patient penicillin for a cold or "flu," knows perfectly well that it will do no good. Why does he not give plain water, if the patient insists on a shot? Dr. Siegal tells us that reaction to penicillin has been reported after a penicillin lozenge, after an instillation of the drug in the antrums (for sinus trouble, we suppose) and even after the use of an eye ointment containing the antibiotic.

Listen to the account of a couple of cases of individuals who became suddenly sensitive to penicillin without knowing it. A 67-year-old woman with chronic asthma, sinus disease and aspiring allergy had received penicillin many times for "colds." On her last visit to the doctor's office, she was given the antibiotic and within thirty seconds had collapsed and died. A twenty-seven year old physician had had penicillin frequently without any ill effects. One day he reacted with a rash. Some months later he had trouble breathing after an injection. Two months later he was given penicillin again, went into collapse within thirty seconds, fell unconscious and would undoubtedly have died had a powerful drug and oxygen not been administered immediately. This was a physician, mind you, who had a family history of allergy.

A woman of thirty-five had had penicillin often for respiratory illnesses. On the last occasion she complained of itching in the palms of her hands fifteen minutes after the injection had been given. This patient's physician was a sensible man. He sought advice from an allergist who gave the patient skin tests for allergy to penicillin. Up to a dose of 6000 units she was fine. But at that dosage she had an immediate reaction. If her physician had paid no attention to her first mild reaction but had gone on giving her penicillin at the usual dosage she would undoubtedly have died of shock.

One thing to keep in mind about reaction to penicillin—the fact that you have never been sensitive to it is no indication that you will not be—*the next time*. Says Dr. Siegal, "The majority of patients with penicillin shock have given a negative history as to previous penicillin allergy." A reaction need scarcely be feared in patients never before exposed to the drug, says he. The most hazardous injection is the first given after an interval since previous administration of the drug. You should watch for immediate reactions such as itching or rash, faintness, generalized tingling, chokiness or difficulty in breathing, asthma or pain or constriction across the chest.

"Allergic reactions to the antibiotics . . . constitute a major problem in current medical practice," says Dr. Siegal.

Avoid Antibiotics if You Can

Our conclusion in regard to taking the antibiotics—any of them, but penicillin in particular—is, don't. Don't let your doctor give you any of the antibiotics if there is any possible way to avoid it. It has been known for a long time that using the antibiotics off and on for minor illnesses and infections will make them completely ineffective for major illnesses. But we have not had, until fairly recently, the rash of sudden fatalities from the antibiotics. If, for an extreme emergency, you must take one of the antibiotics, by all means give your doctor a full history of how much of it you have had in the past and also what your past history as to allergy has been. If you have or ever have had asthma, it would be especially important to tell him that.

But suppose you know you are sensitive to antibiotics and must avoid them at all costs—how are you going to do it? That's a harder question to answer, for antibiotics are becoming almost as common as DDT in almost everything we eat. Says the *Drug Trade News* for August 3, 1953: "The Food and Drug Administration is faced with a serious problem as a result of use of drugs to treat animals subsequently slaughtered for human consumption." Antibiotics are of course given to treat diseased animals. And in addition they are now being added to the feed of healthy animals because it appears that the animals grow faster if a little antibiotic is added to their food. How much of the antibiotic is left in the meat? Your guess is as good as ours. We do know that antibiotics in milk (coming, of course, from those that have been fed to the cow) have caused trouble in the cheese industry, for so much remains in the milk that the bacteria responsible for making the cheese are killed and cannot perform their function.

Even vegetarians have cause to worry. An undated article from a Madison, Wisconsin, paper tells us that the "wonder drugs" are now being used to fight fruit diseases. Streptomycin and terramycin are used to treat apple and pear orchards.

At last notice (*Journal of the American Medical Association for March* 14, 1953) the Food and Drug Administration was forbidding the use of antibiotics as preservatives in food, explaining that "consumption of food so treated may cause sensitization of the consumer to such antibiotics and may result in the emergence of strains of . . . (bacteria) resistant to these drugs." We do not know whether the FDA still holds this viewpoint, but does it matter very much, especially when meats, vegetables and fruits have all been treated with antibiotics by their producers before they even reach the processing or canning establishments?

In an article in the British journal called *Nutrition* J. S. Willcox, Senior Lecturer in Agricultural Chemistry at the University of Leeds, says that the value of the sale of antibiotics for animal feeds exceeds the value of all the antibiotics used for medical purposes in the United States!

On the basis of such a report as this, how much chance do you think there is of getting the antibiotic-makers to stop selling their products for use on food? What can you do about antibiotics in food? Raise your own food if it's humanly possible. Or get a farmer friend to raise it for you, organically. If you must eat food bought at the local market check as closely as you can with the people who produce it. Buy food that has not been treated in any way with antibiotics if you can get it. And protest! Protest to your grocer, your doctor, your congressman, your board of health!

Antibiotics and Cancer

A new theory about the possible relationship between the taking of the new medicines and cancer incidence.

In the United States, recorded deaths from lung cancer for the period 1935 to 1948 increased over 140 per cent. The mortality rate for all other forms of cancer increased by only 31 per cent. In England somewhat the same thing has happened and according to projections made by statisticians the rate will continue to increase at about the same speed. On the other hand, the primitive races in Asia and Africa show no increase in the incidence of cancer. Why should such a situation exist?

Many authorities have placed the blame for the terrible increase in lung cancer on air pollution and smoking. Indeed the evidence against these two villains is overwhelming. And it appears that the more we study the matter, the more information we discover leading us to the inescapable conclusion that these two factors have at least a large share of responsibility for the present frightening status of lung cancer incidence.

However, say B. A. Meyer and J. D. Benjafield of London, writing in *The Medical Press* for August 31, 1955, there has been no comparable increase in cancer of the larynx. If you are inhaling the smoke of a cancer-causing cigarette or a cancer-causing layer of smog, the concentrated strength of the deadly agent would seem to be brought to bear on the larynx or voice box. By the time this puff of whatever-it-is reaches the lungs, it has been somewhat diluted and furthermore it is then spread out over thousands of little cells in the lungs. How does it happen, then, that cancer of the larynx has not increased at the same rate as lung cancer?

In 1928 penicillin was discovered, say Doctors Meyer and Benjafield. In 1935 sulfanilamide therapy was born. Since then we have had all manner of antibiotics and the list grows almost daily. Sir Arthur Fleming, discoverer of penicillin, showed that it is a powerful killer of bacteria in concentrations that were harmless to the tissues of the body. "Antibiotics are by far the greatest life-saving discovery in the history of medicine, and most of the antibiotics are relatively innocuous when compared with antiseptics, but it seems that a minority of patients are sensitive or allergic to some of them. The impairment of their therapeutic value through reckless and indiscriminate use is a very serious matter, for they are too frequently given for mild infections, such as coughs, colds, coryza (sniffles) sinusitis and many respiratory infections, no matter how trivial they may be. Patients often demand penicillin injections from their doctors and many a doctor is forced to give them lest he should offend the patient and be thought not to be keeping abreast of modern methods," say Drs. Meyer and Benjafield.

Now antibiotics have no killing effect at all on viruses, so any disease caused by a virus will not be cured by a dose of antibiotic. But is it not possible, ask these thoughtful and probing writers, that, if cancer is due to a virus, the antibiotics may damage tissue in such a way that the body does not feel the need to bring into play the normal mechanism that protects against viruses—a mechanism that has been acquired over the many thousands of years that man has lived on the earth! Perhaps in addition the antibiotic may upset the virus-bacteria balance and so predispose the tissues to invasion by cancer cells.

Doesn't it seem to you that this theory may explain *in part* at least the seeming immunity of some individuals to cancer? Here is a man, let's say, who boasts that he has always smoked many cigarettes, yet he has no disposition toward cancer. Might not his apparent immunity stem from the fact that he has never been ill with the kind of disorder for which antibiotics are used? On the other hand, you can find additional evidence that seems to back up the theory in the fact that smokers in general *do* suffer from frequent colds and often chronic coughs—the very kind of thing for which the antibiotics are given. People who live in areas where there is air pollution may get more frequent colds. Might the antibiotics they take for the colds be partly responsible for their incidence of lung cancer?

To get back to the article in the *Medical Press,* our theorists remind us that town dwellers have more cancer of the lung than country-dwellers. And the primitive countries show no increase in lung cancer such as the so-called "civilized" countries show. Town dwellers have more and closer doctors than rural folks. Since antibiotics are fashionable, they are freely given in cities where doctors are up-to-date and patients are demanding. In the country, with its few and far-between doctors and its complete lack of medical clinics, how many people insist on having antibiotics for slight colds? And in the primitive countries, of course, doctors and antibiotics are both so rare that there would be no such problem there.

We feel that this theory should be thoroughly investigated by research organizations. Perhaps it may reveal something very significant. And meanwhile, it certainly behooves all of us to keep our bodies so healthy that we will never have to take antibiotics for some serious illness. Certainly none of us should *ever* take them for a minor illness.

Antihistamines

For quite a long time Americans took up the fad of antihistamines for colds. Medical journals were full of pros and cons. Experiments were conducted in hospitals and universities and among private patients. Reports came in of high percentage of "cures" for a while, then further investigation revealed that these were not cures at all. Symptoms had disappeared for a while, but nothing more. Then the reports of serious side effects began to come in. A death was finally scored up to the credit, or discredit of the antihistamines.

In the July 23, 1950, issue of *The Journal of the American Medical Association,* Hugh G. Rives, M.D., and associates report on the death of a 16-month old girl in Dubuque, Iowa, who was poisoned "accidentally" one day in March, 1949, was rushed to the hospital and died the following morning. The poison which the unguarded child took *within the limits of the average adult dose* was one of the antihistamines, so-called because they reduce the efficiency of the action of "histamines" a vaguely understood substance formed in and released from body tissues during allergic reactions such as those incidental to hay fever, colds and so forth.
The dictionary defines histamine as an amine (that is, a compound

prepared from ammonia) containing 5 atoms of carbon to 9 of hydrogen and 3 of nitrogen. When produced in the body, it is a powerful stimulant to the female uterus and also lowers the blood pressure. Other reactions include those of the allergy group, for the treatment of which these "antihistamine" drugs were originally created.

Dr. Rives' article states that the incidence of unfavorable reactions following use of the antihistamines is estimated at ranging from 24 per cent to 46 per cent, even the average of which is surely sufficiently high to question the validity of calling them remedial, if not to justify their being banned. Other complaints against them are given in an article in *The Annals of Allergy* for May-June, 1950, by S. W. Jennes, M.D. He announces that two men patients were made sexually impotent as a result of treatment with two different types of antihistamine drugs. Though the impotence disappeared with discontinuance of the medicine, they might have been rendered permanently sterile if the dosage had been continued.

In addition Dr. Jennes gives up an imposing list of other disastrous results including dizziness, heart palpitations, nervousness, nausea, diarrhea, dryness in the mouth, headaches and general weakness. A somewhat smaller number of patients were afflicted with rectal bleeding, abdominal pains and premature menstruation in women. More recently added to this list in other articles are: fainting spells, severe prostration and mental conditions varying in gravity from simple confusion to serious mental illness. Concludes Dr. Rives: "That present indiscriminate use of these antihistaminic agents needs a critical review is evidenced in the medical literature. Although we have found no (other) report of a fatality, there have been serious reactions."

It appears clear to us that the discomfort of a common cold, while it may bother you for several days, is certainly not painful enough to warrant taking chances on any of the above-mentioned side effects. Perhaps you will not have any bad after effects at all. But considering the serious nature of some that have been reported, do you want to make it a practice to take any substance which, in other people, has such drastic results?

Finally we have the report of Drs. Howard S. Triasman and L. Martin Hardy of the Children's Memorial Hospital in Chicago who, according to an Associated Press dispatch tested 159 cold patients in their hospital with two treatments. One group was given Grandma's remedy—bed rest, fluids in abundance and (we must report it truthfully!) aspirin if needed The other group received the same treatment plus sulfa drugs and antibiotics All patients had the same symptoms. Of the group receiving Grandma's remedy, 56 per cent recovered in one week, 34 per cent in two weeks and the remaining 10 per cent took longer. Of the drug-treated group only 39 per cent recovered in one week, 48 per cent in two weeks and 13 per cent took more than two weeks.

So why spend money for a drug that will not cure you any faster than no drug at all and may in addition start all kinds of unwholesome processes to work inside you?

Apples

Winesap, Delicious, Rome Beauty, Russet—they are names to conjure with! Since the earliest days of history, apples have been one of man's favorite foods and deservedly so. Here is a fruit we can recommend without reservations. Whether you are young or old, sick or well, reducing or trying to gain weight, apples are good for you. The natural sugars in apples are easily digested. And apples do not have such a high sugar content as some fruits such as grapes, figs, dates, and prunes, etc. In green apples there is no sugar, but starch, which is converted to sugar as the fruit ripens. A fully ripe apple contains little or no starch.

Apples have been used as medicine by physicians for many years. In cases of infant diarrhea apple pulp alone given with no other food resulted in remarkable cures. On the other hand, the laxative qualities of the apple are well known and stubborn cases of constipation often yield to this same prescription of apple pulp, or scraped apple. Scientists do not know which ingredient of the apple is responsible—is it the acid that detoxifies the system in cases of diarrhea or is it the pectin of the apple that solidifies watery stools? Any one of the ingredients of the apple tried separately does not have the same good effect, so we must believe that there is something else in these crisp, juicy beauties that is so very beneficial for the digestive tract as a whole.

Someone on a reducing diet may find that raw apples will solve most of his problems. One small apple contains only 64 calories, in spite of its sweet taste. (An avocado contains well over 500.) The bulk of an apple is hunger-satisfying. Reducers should eat apples between meals instead of pining for chocolate bars they may not have. An apple, or perhaps, two, eaten before dinner does such an excellent job of satisfying hunger that you can easily pass up all those tasty dishes the rest of the family is eating, which are not on your diet. But beware of the treacherous apple pie, or even applesauce or baked apple. You obtain all the splendid vitamins and minerals there are in a raw apple, when you eat it raw. But when you cook it you lose these food elements. Then, too, you must add sugar and up goes your calorie count! So, taken altogether, apple pie, no matter how good it smells coming out of the oven, is a worthless kind of food compared to a raw apple!

For some reason, possibly their acid content, apples aid the body in absorbing iron from food, which is an important factor, considering our widespread national anemia. In addition, tests have shown that the decalcifying effect of apples is less than that of any other food except carrots. In other words, all foods are apparently hard on one's teeth to a certain extent, but apples and carrots to a much less degree than any other foods. So eating an apple after a meal not only cleans one's teeth, but actually helps preserve the body's store of calcium.

The sunny side of an apple (that is, the side next to the sun while the apple is growing) contains more sugar and more vitamin C than the other side. The skin contains more vitamin C than the pulp. Apples lose a certain amount of food value in storage—especially vitamin C. Storage at 40 degrees Fahrenheit results in greater loss than storage at

32 degrees. Regardless of temperature, an apple may lose as much as 17 per cent of its vitamin C after three months' storage, or 25 per cent after six months' storage.

The only unpleasant thing about our delicious apples in present-day America is the very considerable residue of insecticides they may carry. For this reason we must sadly caution you to peel apples before you eat them. Even if you are cooking them, be sure to peel them, for cooking does not destroy the spray residue. Of course, if you possibly can, eat only organically grown apples. If you live in the country raise your own, of course. If you live in the city, try to find some farmer not too far away who is not using sprays and will sell you apples. Yes, even if you find a worm from time to time, a worm is a lot less of a menace than a couple of grains of lead and arsenic.

And remember, too, that vitamins and minerals protect you against the poisons in these sprays. So if you must buy commercially raised fruit, make doubly sure you take natural food supplements for vitamins and minerals.

Here is the vitamin and mineral content of apples, in terms of 100 grams. One small apple weighs 100 grams.

Calcium	6 Milligrams
Phosphorus	10 Milligrams
Iron	.3 Milligrams
Copper	.10 Milligrams
Vitamin A	90 Int. Units
Thiamin	.04 Milligrams
Riboflavin	.02 Milligrams
Niacin	.2 Milligrams
Vitamin C	5 Milligrams

Arteries

The arteries are the elastic tubes through which fresh blood, reinforced with oxygen, is carried from the heart to the various parts of the body. They are elastic so that they can contract or expand as the heart beat forces more or less blood into them. Blood in the arteries is always under pressure, like air in a balloon. After death the pressure goes down, of course, which is why ancient anatomists thought that the arteries were for the purpose of transporting oxygen. This is the reason why they named them "arteries" from a Latin word meaning "windpipe."

The main heart artery is the aorta which is about one-half inch to one inch wide at the place where it leaves the left section of the heart and begins to branch out into smaller arteries, which carry blood to the head, the abdomen, the arms, legs and so forth. We have heard that women's arteries are wider than men's, possibly because of the greater strains women are called on to endure in childbirth and so on. We do not know whether this is so. Nor do we know what determines the width of one's arteries—is it hereditary?

Hardening of the arteries or arteriosclerosis is a disorder generally associated with growing old, though it occurs quite frequently in people below middle age. It is difficult to diagnose or to study hardening of the arteries, for naturally the process is going on inside the walls of the arteries where it cannot be observed first hand in a living person. However, it is generally accepted that what happens first is a fatty deposit on the inside of the walls which gradually becomes thicker and attracts mineral deposits as well. Now as anyone can see, a hollow tube whose inside walls are heavily crusted with fat and minerals will not continue to supply enough room for the blood to move along at the normal rate. As the space inside the arteries grows smaller, more pressure is exerted on the blood and we have "high blood pressure."

Danger Signals

Symptoms may be tingling or cramps, aches or sharp pains when you are using your arms or legs. As the deposits gather on the arteries leading to the brain there may be partial loss of mental ability, disorders of memory and so forth. Of course the arteries leading to the heart itself, the kidneys, the liver and brain are extremely important for good health and the final stages of hardening of the arteries may be complicated with diseases of these organs, since they are simply not receiving enough blood to stay healthy.

As lumps of fatty material collect on artery walls they may project so far into the blood stream as to form a barrier to the blood flow. Or they may break off in chunks and float around in the blood. When they reach a smaller blood vessel, they become jammed between the walls and a serious condition develops.

What causes hardening of the arteries? Medical authors admit they do not know. Some say it is too much cholesterol in the diet. Cholesterol is a fatty substance that occurs in animal fats, such as milk, butter, fat meat and so forth. Others say that the amount of cholesterol in the diet is not important. The important thing is how the body uses the cholesterol. Why does it deposit on the artery walls in some people and not in others? Is it not something about the whole metabolism of the person, *or something else in the food he may eat* that protects him from hardening of the arteries?

Good Diet is Important

We believe that an all-round good diet is by far the most important thing to be considered, if you would avoid disorders of the arteries. And we believe that completely natural unprocessed foods will not produce cholesterol or calcium deposits on the artery walls. It is difficult to plan such a diet in today's world. But it can be done. Such a diet would exclude all processed fats, animal or vegetable. No hydrogenated shortenings—the thick, white shortenings that are regularly used in such quantities for baking and frying.

Research indicates that several of the B vitamins are vitally concerned with the fate of cholesterol in the body—particularly choline and inositol, which occur abundantly in foods that are rich in other B vitamins and are especially plentiful in brewer's yeast and liver. The unsaturated fatty acids (sometimes called vitamin F) are important, too. These occur in natural fats and oils, but they are destroyed by processing. Lecithin, a fatty substance now being extracted from soy beans, is another important protection against cholesterol deposits. Choline and unsaturated fatty acids both appear in lecithin. Vitamin E, so important for heart and blood vessel health, is necessary too. If you eat baker's bread the vitamin E has been removed from it and you must supplement your diet with wheat germ oil or vitamin E or both, if you would be healthy. A healthful diet—the kind of diet *Prevention* is always recommending—will protect you against disorders of the arteries.

Arteriosclerosis

New and startling research seems to indicate that processed foods—especially processed fats—may be responsible for this baffling disorder of civilized man.

One of the most exciting and hopeful suggestions on the subject of diet and hardening of the arteries is made in the pages of an important British medical magazine by an M.D. who, after announcing the theme of his article, says "Your readers with stereotyped minds should stop reading at this point." So we are given ample warning that his theory is daring and provocative. It is also one of the most sensible ideas we've run across in a long time.

As it appears in *The Lancet* for April 7, 1956, the idea of Dr. H. M. Sinclair goes like this: cholesterol deposits on the walls of the arteries may be caused by two circumstances relating to diet in modern civilized countries:

First, our diets are deficient in the *unsaturated* fatty acids which are necessary to keep cholesterol on the move.

Second, our diets are rich in *saturated* fatty acids, whose sources are the large amounts of animal fat we eat and the processed fats—the hydrogenated vegetable oils and the fat heated to a high temperature as in deep-fat drying.

A third angle to his theory is that one of the B vitamins, pyridoxine, is closely related to the chemical activities of all these fatty substances. It is vitally important for us to have plenty of pyridoxine in our meals. But modern refining removes most of it.

Sounds complicated, doesn't it? But actually it is not. Basically all that Dr. Sinclair is saying is that modern food processing may be almost entirely responsible for the disease that is today's number one killer in "civilized" countries.

An experiment with laboratory rats led Dr. Sinclair and his associate, Dr. V. Basnayake, to their theory. They fed the rats a diet that contained no fats at all, but which was a good diet in other respects. What did they find? Large cholesterol deposits in the arteries of the animals. The longer the diet went on the more cholesterol accumulated. Now we are told that cholesterol deposits come from too much fat in the diet. How then could these rats, who were getting no fat at all, develop cholesterol deposits? Dr. Sinclair tells us that their bodies were manufacturing it—and we know that cholesterol is indeed manufactured in our bodies as well as coming from our food. And the reason that it accumulated had to be simply that a fat-free diet prevented the rats from getting any of the unsaturated fatty acids, which must be present in order to keep the cholesterol from depositing where it is not wanted.

It is impossible for us to imagine a daily diet for human beings entirely free from fat, so there is little danger that we may have the same experience the rats had. But, as Dr. Sinclair goes on to say, the more cholesterol and the more *saturated* fat you have in your diet the more *unsaturated* fat you need, if you want to avoid cholesterol deposits. Then, too, if you have enough pyridoxine in your diet, you are likely to avoid trouble, for this vitamin can help out when the important fatty acids are not there.

What Kind of Diets Produce Cholesterol?

So, says Dr. Sinclair, we might expect cholesterol deposits (which we speak of generally as atherosclerosis or arteriosclerosis, or hardening of the arteries) when the diet is high in cholesterol or unnatural fats, low in the unsaturated fatty acids, and/or deficient in B vitamins. "Are such diets encountered?" he asks.

We believe that such diets are the usual ones in this country, rather than the exception. Dr. Sinclair says, "For many years, and particularly in recent years, animal fats and more especially vegetable fats have become increasingly oxidized and deprived of E. F. A. (Essential Unsaturated Fatty Acids) before being eaten. Vegetable oils, in many cases rich in E. F. A., are hardened by hydrogenation; margarine and shortenings are produced by hydrogenation of cottonseed and soybean oil, some peanut-oil and certain other oils; during this hydrogenation much of the E. F. A. are destroyed and unnatural *trans* fatty acids are formed. Unnatural fatty acids are formed not only during hydrogenation but also during the practice of deep-frying."

How else do we lose these important food elements? Well, they occur in the germ of cereals which our food processors carefully remove and discard when they make white flour and packaged cereals. In addition, the flour "improvers," the bleaches, and many other chemicals that go into baked goods these days undoubtedly have some destructive action on the fatty acids. We have no idea how extensive this may be. In addition, when foods are refined, pyridoxine, the B vitamin, that might get in a few good licks to help the situation, is also removed and discarded.

The next time somebody tries to tell you that "enriched" cereals are just as good as completely whole grain ones, remember what we have said above. Remember how complex the whole thing is and how little of it we understand as yet. The only thing we know for certain is that the essential unsaturated fatty acids and the B vitamins are intimately and certainly involved in what happens to cholesterol in your body. Once you have deprived your body of these two precious food elements, you can expect the worst.

In the next article we are going to go on with Dr. Sinclair's theory relating to lung cancer, skin diseases, leukemia, ulcers and mental disorders in relation to a possible deficiency of the unsaturated fatty acids.

Now, however, we want to talk just about heart and blood vessel disorders in their relation to processed fats. Dr. Sinclair tells us that he worked with Dr. Ancel Keys (one of the world's greatest authorities on the subject of fat in nutrition) and Dr. Keys came to the conclusion that the total amount of fat in the diet was responsible for hardening of the arteries and also coronary thrombosis, or heart attack. Dr. Keys said, in essence, "it doesn't matter what kind of fat it is—we must stop eating so much fat. If we cut down on the fat in our diets, we will cut down on the cholesterol deposits in our arteries."

The Kind of Fat You Do or Do Not Eat Is the Important Thing

Dr. Sinclair tells us that he now believes this theory is wrong. "What matters," he says, "is, I believe, the amount and structure of the dietary fatty acids." That is, the important thing is *not how much* fat you get but *what kind*. In the final paragraphs of his article Dr. Sinclair pleads for more research. Heart and vascular diseases are wiping out hundreds of thousands who might still continue to live healthy lives if research showed the truth of Sinclair's theory. At any rate, he pleads, let us not make matters possibly worse by taking even more of the B vitamins and fatty acids from our flour and our processed fats.

Dr. Sinclair, handicapped as he says he is, by lack of time and a laboratory to continue his researches, can only urge British medical men to listen to his theory and, if possible, do more research along these lines. And he has already met with opposition. Dr. Ancel Keys, whose theory he disagreed with, replied to him in the April 28, 1956 issue of *The Lancet*. Dr. Keys says that a number of other researchers have had Dr. Sinclair's theory, but he still does not agree with it and he devotes a page and a half of very small type to disagreeing. He does admit that the more sophisticated, richer nations consume more fats of all kinds and he says, "The problem has been complicated by the enterprise and ingenuity of food producers and technologists who provide a superabundance of all kinds of fats and then persuade us to eat them." But what are we going to do, he asks. Are we going to persuade them to add unsaturated fatty acids to their processed products? Or are we going to try to persuade people to eat lots of vegetable, cereal and fish oil, "fresh and in the virgin liquid state?"

We don't know what Dr. Keys or Dr. Sinclair plan to do. We do know what *Prevention* plans to do about a theory like Dr. Sinclair's. We think that the theory makes very good sense. It adds still another weapon in the war we are conducting against processed foods. It provides still another possible explanation for why civilized diet produces diseases unknown among more primitive people.

And this is what we are going to do about it. We urge those who are worried about hardening of the arteries and heart disease, to adjust the fatty part of their diets *to eliminate all processed fats* and to make sure they are getting enough of the unsaturated fatty acids and the B vitamins.

How can you best do this? First of all, cross off your grocery list permanently anything that has been "hydrogenated." The label will tell you. Solid shortenings are hydrogenated. Commercial peanut butter is. Margarine is. Furthermore, factory-made foods contain hydrogenated fats. Don't eat them. This means crackers, prepared "mixes," noodles, roasted and salted nuts, popcorn and so forth. It means any foods fried in deep fat—potato chips, french fries, doughnuts and so forth. Before you buy anything in a grocery, stop and consider whether or not it may contain hydrogenated or highly-heated fats. And don't buy it if it does.

What can you do if you eat in restaurants? Don't order anything fried. Don't eat anything which might contain the wrong kind of fat. What do we mean by that? The crackers that come with your tomato juice or soup, for instance. Muffins, roasted nuts, piecrust, cake—these are not for you.

On the positive side—how can you be certain you are getting enough of the essential unsaturated fatty acids? Regardless of how much or how little fat you eat, get unhydrogenated vegetable fat somehow in your diet—eat sunflower seeds or other raw seeds, like wheat seeds. Take wheat germ oil and fish liver oil—both rich sources of unsaturated fatty acids, or take a food supplement made up chiefly of unsaturated fatty acids. Lecithin contains the unsaturated fatty acids. Take a food supplement containing lecithin.

About salad oils—rich sources of the unsaturated fatty acids. Cold pressed oils—available so far as we know, only from health food stores—are best. If you can't get these, buy and eat the regular salad oils your grocery carries—corn oil, peanut oil and so forth. We are assured by the people who make these that they contain the essential unsaturated fatty acids.

One last thing—the B vitamins. Even though you pay the strictest attention to your diet from a health standpoint, we don't believe it's possible for you to get enough of the B vitamins unless you take a natural supplement that contains them—brewers yeast, wheat germ or desiccated liver. Although there is no official standard, it has been estimated that we need from ½ to 5 milligrams of pyridoxine alone, every day. A natural food supplement is your best source.

We received a clipping from the Oakland (California) *Tribune* for May 20, 1956, revealing that a California scientist has completely tamed cholesterol and prevented unwanted deposits of it in his patients by giving them a "cocktail," chief ingredients of which are unsaturated fat from vegetable and fish liver oils, pyridoxine and an essential amino acid or form of protein.

Arthritis, (or Rheumatism)

Rheumatism is a disease older than man. Prehistoric man suffered from rheumatism and the animals who lived on the earth for millions of years before man suffered from rheumatism. Evidence of rheumatism has been found in the skeletons of dinosaurs. Animals, either in captivity or in their natural wild state, may develop rheumatism; it is common to both meat-eating and vegetarian animals. In America it is estimated that approximately 7,500,000 individuals have one form or another of rheumatism. Of these 147,000 are considered permanently invalided!

Rheumatism is not a dramatic quick killer like heart disease. It has not the slow but certain malignancy of cancer. Patients with rheumatism may live to a great age and in fact seldom die of this disease. It is a "chronic" disease. But considering that it afflicts more people than any of the other chronic diseases and that its one common symptom is excruciating pain, it seems strange that medical science has not come any nearer to finding a cure. Most of us think of rheumatism as a disease of later life. While it is quite true that most elderly people suffer to a certain degree from rheumatic symptoms, it is also true that fifty per cent of the disability incidental to rheumatism is found among persons under forty-five.

Since symptoms may come and go without any apparent cause, some physicians believe that rheumatism may have a psychosomatic origin. This means that the disease itself is real enough, but that the reasons for it lie in some unresolved conflict in the patient's life. According to *Time* Magazine for June 13, 1949, Dr. Edward Weiss of Philadelphia theorizes that the patient may be troubled with "chronic resentment"—an unhappy marriage, some bitter disappointment in his career, some frustration against which he subconsciously battles every day.

Physicians are certain by now that there is a definite relationship between hormones (gland secretions) and rheumatism. The emotions affect the glands that manufacture hormones; in turn the hormones affect the emotions. While we do not minimize the importance to health of a happy adjustment to one's life environment, we are inclined to take hold of it the other way around. We believe that healthy people don't meet with as many conflicts and frustrations, or, if they do, they find ways to overcome them. We have a notion that most frustrations and conflicts exist in sick minds, and sick minds are at least partly caused by sick bodies in which, for instance, hormones may not be functioning properly for some very sound physical reason. Animals as well as men suffer from psychosomatic illness, true, but honestly now, isn't it just a bit far-fetched to imagine a dinosaur wasting away with rheumatism just because of some unbearable frustration in his life with the other dinosaurs?

It seems to us that rheumatism must have certain definite physical reasons for being. About a year ago we set out to collect all the material we could find on this subject. Medical and scientific journals are crammed with information. Back over the years probably no one subject has received the attention devoted to rheumatism. In clinics, rest homes, hospitals, spas and laboratories, here and abroad, noted scientists have devoted themselves to the study of rheumatism. Why is it that, over all these centuries, no answer has been found? We believe it may be because each investigator is looking for some one answer—which he *has* to do in order to be scientifically accurate. But perhaps one answer will not solve the problem—more things may be involved.

The Different Kinds of Rheumatism

There are many kinds of rheumatism, all of them related. In *The Medical Clinics of North America* for November, 1940, rheumatic diseases are classified as follows: atrophic (rheumatoid or proliferative) arthritis, and hypertrophic (osteo or degenerative) arthritis. Those patients who show symptoms of both are said to have "mixed arthritis." Then there are types of arthritis caused by definite, known poisoning, such as tuberculous, pneumococcal and so forth. Rheumatic fever, muscular rheumatism (fibrositis) and menopausal neuralgia are other related diseases in which actual joint involvement is not so great.

In atrophic or rheumatoid arthritis there is evidence of "atrophic" or "wasting" manifestations in the bone and muscle system of the body as well as disorder in other body tissues. Victims of rheumatoid arthritis are usually individuals from 30 to 50, more women than men. Exhaustion, anemia, nervous disturbances, digestive disorders and sometimes liver trouble are accompanying symptoms, aside from the swelling and pain in the joints. Osteoarthritis is generally considered a degenerative disease—that is, a disease of old age, resulting from wear and tear on the body generally and strain or injury in some particular part of the body. For instance, the hands of farmers, craftsmen and housewives are particularly susceptible to osteoarthritis because they have worked so hard and gotten so many knocks and bumps.

Experiments With Cures For Rheumatism

In 1950 Dr. Granirer of Queens General Hospital, Jamaica, Long Island, reported on a new therapy involving the injection of blood drawn from women 48 hours after childbirth. It is known that rheumatism often disappears completely during pregnancy. It also disappears when the patient contracts jaundice. So physicians reasoned that some substance present in the blood of pregnant women, or in jaundice patients, might be antagonistic to rheumatism. According to the one report we read, all arthritis patients treated with the new substance showed great improvement in symptoms, half of them maintaining their gains after treatment had been discontinued for a year. One patient had no symptoms of arthritis 22 months after the injections were stopped.

A year or so later a new remedy for osteoarthritis was announced by Dr. W. S. Collins and his associate of Maimonides Hospital, Brooklyn. This consisted of an extract derived from the livers of pregnant cows. In many cases this substance brought relief from pain and joint stiffness.

Among the various cures experimented with through the years most have been aimed at alleviating the symptoms of the disease—that is, stopping or lessening the pain, improving the stiffness and preventing deformities. Shock treatment, ozone therapy, massage, percussion therapy, sulfur baths, thermal therapy, injections of sulfur have been used. Counter-irritants have been tested, injections of proteins, bee and cobra venom have been tried. Gold salts have been given orally and injected.

In preventing deformities from the twisting and crippling of the disease, physicians have used surgery, splints, plaster casts, exercise, massage, heat treatments, underwater exercise, various kinds of baths—the list is almost endless.

How Much Have We Learned About Preventing Rheumatism?

Under the heading of possible preventives of rheumatism there seem to be two aspects of living that might be involved—diet and posture. What do we know up to now of the relation of diet to rheumatism? Arthritis does not seem to be a disease in which there is a gross deficiency of vitamin A, yet certainly some deficiency is suggested by the following symptoms: the frequency of respiratory tract infections in conjunction with rheumatism—colds, bronchitis, laryngitis, etc. Could these not result from a lack of vitamin A to strengthen these delicate tissues against bacterial invaders? The frequency of liver disorder in arthritics suggests that the liver might be unable to do its work of transforming carotene into vitamin A, so that a greater quantity of vitamin A would be necessary in the patient's diet.

Most arthritics have difficulty assimilating carbohydrates—that is, starches and sugars. This suggests a deficiency of vitamin B which is the vitamin necessary to accompany these substances on their way through the digestive tract. There also may be lack of appetite, another symptom of vitamin B deficiency. There may be neuritis or edema (swelling) both of which may indicate need for vitamin B. Digestive disorders point to deficiency of niacin, one of the B vitamins; anemia and nervousness both indicate need for niacin. The B vitamins will also relieve the frequent constipation of arthritics. In the early part of 1952 the *American Practitioner* reported remarkable results in the treatment of osteoarthritis and osteoporosis with vitamin B12—the fabulous new vitamin occurring most abundantly in liver. Of 33 cases of arthritis, 20 patients benefited from the treatment within the first week, seven of whom obtained complete relief. By the end of the third week, all but three of the patients showed some benefit. Three cases of rheumatoid arthritis did not react at all to the vitamin.

Vitamin C is found to be abnormally low in the blood of arthritics. Charles W. Buckley, M.D., F.R.C.P., writing in *The Practitioner* for September, 1938, has this to say about the importance of vitamin C in the diet of arthritics: "From available evidence this deficiency (of vitamin C) is the result rather than the cause of the infection and it has been found that the amount of vitamin C required to raise the level in a normal individual to saturation point is much below what is required to produce the same effect in one suffering from acute rheumatism or rheumatoid arthritis. It seems probable that there is an increased destruction of this vitamin owing to a greater metabolic demand. There is however no definite evidence as yet that vitamin C has any curative effect on the disease." Dr. C. Wesler Scull, writing in the *Medical Clinics of North America,* tells us that placing animals on a diet low in vitamin C results in conditions similar to human arthritis. So, although vitamin C will not apparently cure these symptoms after they have appeared, does it not seem possible that they may be brought on by lack of vitamin C?

In osteoarthritis a de-mineralization of the bones takes place which is similar to that occurring in rickets, a disease due entirely to vitamin D deficiency. So it is considered good clinical practice generally, to give ample vitamin D to all arthritic patients.

Vitamin E Is Important In Preventing Rheumatic Diseases

Considerable investigation has been carried out on the subject of vitamin E and rheumatism. C. L. Steinberg, physician in charge of the Arthritis Clinic, Rochester General Hospital, tells us in the *Annals of the New York Academy of Science* for October 3, 1949, of his success in giving vitamin E to rheumatic patients. Treating fibrositis (muscular rheumatism) in 300 patients with vitamin E, he found that relief was obtained in the vast majority of cases. He cautions that the patient should keep on taking a "maintenance" dose, after the symptoms have disappeared.

He also treated rheumatic fever with vitamin E. He relates five case histories of young people whose rheumatic fever symptoms were relieved by vitamin E. It is interesting to note that he gave natural (not synthetic) vitamin E throughout the experiment.

Dr. Morris Ant of Kings County Hospital, Brooklyn, treats muscle diseases and industrial injuries with wheat germ oil directly applied to the painful spot. Reporting on his experiences in *Industrial Medicine* for June, 1946, he tells us he used a 55 per cent ointment of wheat germ oil and food supplementation by wheat germ oil, as well as a diet rich in vitamin E foods. Out of 20 cases treated successfully, he reports in detail on four—one a housewife whose hands were swollen and stiff. Local application of wheat germ oil soon returned the hands to their normal condition. A physician with swelling of his knees and back so painful that he could not walk was given wheat germ oil locally and internally and was soon able to resume his practice once more. An elevator operator who had had a serious fall developed pain and stiff muscles in his chest and legs along with bronchial asthma. After several months of wheat germ oil therapy both locally and internally he went back to work free from all symptoms except for a slight occasional limp. Incidentally the asthma disappeared, too. A clerk who had fallen against the sharp corner of a desk suffered from a long-standing pain over her ribs, so violent that she was unable to sleep. Wheat germ oil locally and internally left her symptom-free within several months.

In a later article in *The Annals of the New York Academy of Science* Dr. Ant, along with Erwin DiCyan describes the use of vitamin E in rheumatic diseases—this time given orally, intramuscularly and locally. In a series of 100 patients, there was relief from pain, improvement or disappearance of physical symptoms and increased mobility of joints. In addition to the therapy which these patients received at the doctor's office they were placed on diets high in vitamin E—for instance, a tablespoon of wheat germ was taken at breakfast, one-fourth head of lettuce with peanut oil dressing and one banana were added to the lunch menu. At dinner lean beef, spinach and lettuce with peanut oil dressing contributed to the vitamin E content of the day's meals.

The Raw Food Diet For Rheumatism

Dorothy C. Hare, C.B.E., M.D., writing in the British journal, *Proceedings of the Royal Society of Medicine,* volume 30, 1936, contributes what seems to us the most convincing piece of evidence on diet influencing the course of chronic rheumatism. Dr. Hare describes an experiment at the Royal Free Hospital in which rheumatic patients received a diet of raw fruits and vegetables with results that were, it seems to us, spectacular. Dr. Hare is apparently a conservative physician who indicates that she does not advise this diet to replace other forms of medical therapy nor does she advise it in all cases. She simply reports on it and suggests that further research would be valuable.

Twelve patients were selected for the experiment—all were sent to the hospital for this purpose. They represented the main types of rheumatic disorders—muscular, osteoarthritis and rheumatoid arthritis. No other treatment was given them aside from the diet; they were encouraged to be up and around, whenever the severity of their ailment allowed. Some of them were bed-ridden.

After they became accustomed to the hospital life, eating the diet usually served in the wards for one week, they were placed for two weeks on a diet consisting of nothing but fresh raw fruits and vegetables, nuts, cream, salad oil, milk and raw oatmeal.

A day's menu went like this:

BREAKFAST—apple porridge made of grated apple, soaked raw oatmeal, grated nuts, cream, fresh orange, tea with milk and cream
MID-MORNING—tomato puree with lemon
DINNER—salad of lettuce, cabbage, tomato, root vegetables
salad dressing with oil
mixed fruit salad and cream
TEA—dried fruits, nuts and tea with milk and cream
SUPPER—fruit porridge, prune, apricot or apple
salad dish with dressing
BEDTIME—lemon and orange juice with hot water

After two weeks, the following cooked foods were added to this diet:

vegetable soup
one egg
2 ounces of meat
2 ounces of bacon
2 ounces of bread
butter, cheese and milk

At no time during the weeks of the diet was any salt added to either the raw or cooked foods. The dried fruits and raw oatmeal were soaked in water, the vegetables were shredded, nuts crushed or whole. All food was prepared fresh for every meal and was served attractively.

Eight of the patients began to feel better in one to four weeks on this diet. Two improved up to five or six weeks, then relapsed. Two showed no improvement at all. In the follow-up, after the patients who improved had gone home, it was found that seven of them continued to improve to a marked degree. For example, one patient aged 46 had suffered for four years with occasional pain and swelling of the knees, but for the three months before she was admitted to the hospital, she had general pain and stiffness in shoulders, arms, hands, knees and legs. She had been in bed for ten weeks. There was fluid in both knee joints, swelling and pain in other joints. She was discharged from the hospital after being on the diet for three weeks. Seven weeks later, after continuing with the diet for seven more weeks, she was free from all pain and able to do her housework.

All of the patients lost considerable weight during the first week on the diet, but those who continued to lose in the following weeks lost much less and in every case except very obese patients weight was properly maintained on the diet. For the obese patients, of course, losing weight was extremely helpful, as overweight adds greatly to the problems of an arthritic.

In commenting on her diet and its success, Dr. Hare remarks on the fact that the rawness of the food seemed to be the one outstanding factor that brought about results. The fact that the food was raw made a great impression on the patients themselves and on observers. She tells us that a Zurich physician who used raw diets similar to this in treating rheumatism claimed that the diet was successful "because of the absorption of the unaltered solar energy of plant life." Says Dr. Hare "science has so far revealed nothing . . . of this occult solar energy, as something apart from vitamin and chemical constituents (of food)."

Prevention has made no study of "occult solar energy" but it seems that science will soon have to be convinced of the healthfulness of raw foods, for every day we are finding out more and more about the vitamins and enzymes destroyed by heating foods. May there not be many other elements in food, unknown as yet to science, that we destroy when the food is heated above body temperature?

Then, says Dr. Hare, such a diet contains a lot of vitamin C and B (as well as A, we can add). Protein and fat is lacking in the vegetables and fruits. This deficiency is partly made up for by the cream, nuts, and salad oil, later by the meat, eggs and cheese. Finally, Dr. Hare remarks, we must consider how much of the effectiveness of the diet depends on the fact that it was low in sodium. Vegetables contain little sodium and considerable potassium. No salt (sodium chloride) was added at any time during the diet, so that, even though bacon and other foods were added later on, the diet was still extremely low in sodium compared to the usual diet.

An Abundance of Raw Foods and Vitamins and Very Little Salt Seem To Be the Answer

As we found in reviewing symptoms of vitamin deficiency in rheumatic patients, many vitamins appear to be in short supply. Vitamin C (found in fresh fruits and vegetables) is most abundant in its natural form in rose hips which also contain vitamins A and E and several of the B vitamins. Vitamin A is in the yellow foods—butter, carrots, sweet potatoes, and most abundant in fish liver oil. Vitamin B12 has produced almost miraculous results in cases of osteoarthritis. B12 is found most abundantly in liver along with the other members of the B complex of vitamins. Desiccated liver tablets or capsules are the one sure way of getting enough B12 every day. We hardly need to add that all of us—adults and children alike—must have ample vitamin D, the sunshine vitamin, which is also plentiful in fish liver oil.

We have shown many times in these pages the nutritive value of raw foods. Dr. Hare's success in treating rheumatic patients with raw foods does not surprise us at all and we are firmly convinced that the results would have been even better had these been organically raised foods, brought fresh from the garden to the trays of these patients. We do not advise going on such a diet on your own, as an experiment. Undoubtedly your need for animal protein (meat, eggs, butter, cheese and especially organ meats like liver) is great, and some of these foods are not palatable eaten raw. But we have before and do again urge you to include raw foods as part of the menu at every meal. Eat fruits raw, always. Don't cook any vegetable that you can eat raw. At breakfast be certain you have raw fruit. Make sure that lunch includes salad, raw carrot, celery, cauliflower or tomato, etc. For dinner serve as many vegetables raw as you can and develop your skill in combining them and seasoning them with herbs, butter and dressing, so that your family will ask for more.

Remember, too, that the low sodium diet appears to be helpful in treating rheumatism. As you know, we believe that most of us use far, far too much salt and advise cutting it down to a minimum. Try leaving the salt shaker off the table for a week. Then the next week begin to omit salt from some dishes as you prepare them in the kitchen. You'll soon find how easy it is to do without salt altogether. You'll discover, too, how much better the food tastes when you're tasting it, instead of the salt.

Our sincere gratitude for translations from foreign medical journals to: Rolla Myer, Olympia, Washington; Dr. Jacob Kasen, McKeesport, Pa.; P. Heidt, Masonville, N. J.; Vasilie Sofronescu.

Arthritis and Foot Disability

This is from the sixth chapter in Dr. Simon J. Wikler's book *Your Feet Are Killing You,* available from Dr. Wikler, 210 S. E. First Avenue, Miami (32) Fla.

Arthritis is the term applied to many different diseases affecting the joints of the body. It is irritation and inflammation of the bony joints. The most common types are called degenerative arthritis and rheumatoid arthritis. Of these two, rheumatoid arthritis is the more dangerous and deforming, but it is less common. Degenerative arthritis is less severely crippling, but it is a leading cause of chronic illness.

It is the purpose of this chapter to demonstrate that modern foot disability may be the commonest cause of rheumatoid and degenerative arthritis. Foot trouble of course is not an exclusive cause. Stressful occupations, injuries, and aging processes are important predisposing factors. Arthritis has been found in the bones of Egyptian mummies and the joints of wild animals where, naturally, influence of the modern shoe is no factor.

Rheumatoid Arthritis

The cause of rheumatoid arthritis is still unknown. It is uncommon where people go barefoot or wear non-deforming footgear. In most cases a postural factor can be demonstrated before the onset of this disease. In its later stages it causes permanent damage and contraction of the various joints, making any movement difficult and free use of the hands and feet often impossible.

Women outnumber men in the ratio of three to one in contracting the disease. It may be pointed out that, in considering foot disability as a cause, we find that also more common among women. The typical person contracting rheumatoid is between the ages of twenty and forty, inclined to be asthenic, chronically fatigue-ridden, with poor posture and imbalance, strained feet. The usual history then reveals that such an individual is subjected to a physically stressful period when joint coverings become actively inflamed and the disease first manifests. If the strain continues, the disease progresses at a rapid rate. However, in the cases which this author has reviewed, if the patient recognized the postural source of the illness and avoided undue stress or use of the feet, the progress of rheumatoid arthritis became subdued. Sufferers of this disease are less prone to cancer, as though their difficulty in movement protects their tissues from further injury.

Undoubtedly previous illnesses, nutritional factors, and emotional crises all play a role in the contraction of rheumatoid arthritis. The recent success of cortisone in ameliorating the symptoms strongly indicates that the disease is essentially one of unusual physical stress, and, as previous arguments have shown, extensive use of disabled feet is the most important and malignant source of stress today.

In an asthenic (weak) individual, the most important preventive measure as considered here is avoidance of strain and the rehabilitation of disabled feet. In the case histories here presented, it will also be seen that once the process of rheumatoid arthritis has begun, care of the feet is an important aspect of treatment.

Degenerative Arthritis

Degenerative arthritis is very common in modern shoe-wearing societies, and it is estimated to affect over 75 per cent of the population over forty years of age. It is characterized by a chronic destruction of the joint cartilages, and by excessive growth of bone around the joint. These changes are not necessarily painful, but they limit movement.

The constant pulling of joint ligaments in an imbalanced foot acts as a perpetuating agent of inflammation to the edges of the joint surface, which eventually take on a lipped and irregular appearance. The pulling of tendons and larger ligaments can be so intense with imbalanced feet that bone can be pulled away from the normal outline in the form of an osteophyte (bony outgrowth). Joints in the center of the foot (which are tighter and have a smaller range of movement) are the first to show evidence of these injuries. When the metatarsal and toe joints are affected, however, complete dislocations of the toes commonly take place, thus destroying irretrievably the balance of the foot.

Degenerative arthritis of the foot may have a serious secondary influence on degenerative arthritis changes in other parts of the body. If we should assume that the injuries from foot disabilities are a direct cause of arthritis in the feet and lower limbs, it is still difficult to account for the concurrent appearance of arthritis processes in the joints of the fingers, elbows and shoulders which obviously are not influenced by any direct postural factors originating in the feet. It can be speculated that the syndrome of chronic stress and fatigue that disabled feet originate can cause humoral (fluid) imbalance and tissue irregularities throughout the body; that in such individuals minor injuries of the joints of the upper limbs will develop into arthritic degeneration. This author has found on a number of occasions that an individual, upon being relieved of arthritic severity in the feet after rehabilitation, likewise experienced relief of arthritis in the fingers upon which no local therapeutic measures had been taken.

In the usual case of osteoarthritis in the lower limbs, not enough attention has been paid to the contributing factors of foot disability. The following case is offered in illustration.

When this patient consulted me she complained of painful feet. Previously there was X-rayed and diagnosed arthritis in the feet, that made walking only barely possible. Activity caused muscular pain throughout the body. Chronic fatigue after the slightest activity became more intense. The feet were grossly deformed with the toes extended 30 degrees beyond a horizontal line, with movement impossible. The joints throughout the foot had little mobility and pained on palpation. The feet were somewhat swollen and painful to the touch; deep calluses were present on the ball; a sparse musculature on the plantar (sole of the foot) surface permitted the cuneiform bones (three wedge shaped bones in inner center of the foot) to be readily palpable. Steel arch supports were being worn, with a heavy corrective shoe having a heel an inch and a half high. Marked stooped shoulders were also observed.

Past history of the patient revealed that she had suffered with unusual foot discomfort since early adolescence. At the age of thirteen she found walking difficult, especially because of pain in the ball of the foot. The toes had been deformed at an early age; probably due to the fact that the family income did not permit frequent replacement of shoes for growing children; together with the radical styles and disinterest in foot prophylaxis. At eighteen she began work as a salesgirl. Her feet commenced to ache continuously and became worse than ever. Arch supports were secured and they gave some relief.

Marriage at nineteen released the patient from the necessity of being continuously on her feet, and, while she still suffered from moderate foot pains and chronic fatigue, gross symptoms were largely quiescent for a period of ten years. At the age of thirty the patient resumed her occupation as a salesperson, and her feet shortly became sore once more. For a period of twenty years subsequently all sorts of arch supports and corrective shoes were tried, with only moderate relief. One Christmas season the patient had a particularly strenuous time on her feet, pursuing her vocation. The pains became intolerable and finally she was unable to walk at all. Joints and muscles throughout the body were stiff and acutely painful, with the result that complete bed-rest became obligatory. She remained in bed for fourteen weeks, including four in a hospital, during which time thorough examinations left the attending physicians with the opinion that the patient suffered from some form of acute degenerative arthritis. However, no definite diagnosis was reached. On becoming ambulatory she began taking physical therapy and corrective exercises, but they seemed to exaggerate the symptoms.

Treatment consisted of first making it plain to her that her feet were woefully inadequate to meet her daily physical need, and that she must immediately cut down all activity that required her to stand or walk up steps. She was permitted walks of short duration. The arch supports were discarded and the feet were bandaged with adhesive tape with a view toward limiting lateral motion, by firmly holding the foot in an approximation of a normal attitude. The calluses were pared on each visit and felt pads were inserted behind them. Moderate manipulative therapy was used in an attempt to produce a progressively greater range of movement in the feet. In preparation for the future use of flat-heeled shoes she was given stretching exercises which would lengthen the shortened calf muscles. At first she wore flat shoes for only a few minutes each day, and within two months flat shoes could be worn the entire day with perfect comfort.

Her feet slowly achieved greater mobility until within six months her toes had almost a complete range of movement. The toes were still extended considerably but had become flexible. The calluses had decreased, so that a metatarsal pad was no longer necessary. The patient began taking on some weight, and symptoms progressively reduced until, another two months later, all symptoms of chronic fatigue, nervousness, and pain in the feet had disappeared entirely. The subject now spoke of being able to walk free of pain and fatigue for the first time in her adult life, and of experiencing a well-being she had never known before. She was cautioned against subjecting herself to any activity that her feet could not endure comfortably, since it is felt that the results of extensive damage to foot tissues over a period of forty years will leave a limitation to capacity. However she resumed her saleswoman's position with ease.

Degenerative Arthritis in the Knee

This, when caused by imbalanced feet, is usually seen in middle-aged and elderly women who have habitually worn heeled and pointed shoes. In the typical foot posture, with weight thrust on the inner side of the foot, the leg is compensatingly turned out in a degree of genel-valgum (knock-knee). This causes unusual pressure to be exerted against the soft tissues. The fact that this condition becomes relieved by balancing of the foot indicates that its precipitating cause may be foot imbalance.

An older woman patient, who came regularly to have her corns treated, complained of a chronic aching in the knees which within the past year had become so acute that she was hardly able to climb steps or rise from a chair. She was no longer able to stoop in order to take care of her garden, which had been her greatest source of pleasure.

This woman had been in the custom of wearing three-inch heel pumps. Various arthritic changes had taken place in her feet, which became stiffer with the combination of constant effects of injury from such footgear and advancing age. Finally her feet had become so limited in movement that, in order to sustain her weight, they had to turn outward more than ever. This created strain and irritation to the inner part of the knee. She had consulted various specialists and had even tried whirlpool-bath treatment, diathermy, massage and some cortisone, only to find no relief. I advised her that the pain in her knees could be relieved but not completely removed, since it was part of the wear and tear of growing old with disabled feet and a protective mechanism to keep her from activity on those feet which could overstrain her body. Her daughter was present and promised to see that with relief to the knee her mother did not become too active.

I applied an adhesive bandage to the foot and leg, to hold the inner side of the foot and ankle firm, thus permitting the weight on the foot to be placed in such a manner that no straining leverage action had to take place on the inner side of the knee. The patient walked around my office and exclaimed "Eureka! It no longer hurts!" Because of the age and degree of arthritic changes that were present in her feet, no hope was held out that the condition could be permanently relieved. However, as in other similar cases when the strain to the knee is temporarily relieved, elements of inflammation disappeared and the knee was somewhat improved even after the bandages were removed.

One day when the patient called at my office she reported that the past week had been her best in over a year. She had even been able to start her spring garden. I did not like the flushed look to her face, and I feared her blood pressure might mount.

I communicated with her daughter to ask if her mother was being moderate. The daughter admitted that the patient had attacked the garden work too vigorously and we agreed that no further correction to the knee would be attempted. Such a pronouncement was a keen disappointment to the patient, because of the relief she experienced when bandaged, but she could see the wisdom of our decision. Six months later her knees were still better than they had formerly been—evidently because they had not been over-used—and her general physical condition was good—evidently because she had not overtaxed her strength.

Aspirin

Not only does the aspirin not help your cold, but it may produce unpleasant results.

Cold remedies have been with us since the time of the first cold. And lucky indeed is the man who can meet a friend, tell him he has a cold and not be greeted with this most cheerless and ubiquitous counsel, "I'll tell you exactly what to do for it. Clear it up in a matter of hours!" He then proceeds to describe one or another of the hoary remedies that have long since proved utterly useless—it's either baking soda in water, or hot lemon juice and whiskey or hot milk with pepper in it. Or he may be from the modern school in which case he will drag you off to the nearest drugstore and exhort you to buy one or several of the new remedies attractively displayed with a great deal of advertising meant to prove that such and such a tablet will rid you of your cold within a matter of hours.

Remember, please, it's all just advertising. Ten thousand cold remedies have been patented in this country, and the only result has been an axiom famous in medical circles—*with a remedy* you can get rid of a cold in seven days. *Without any remedy at all* it will take one week. We read in *Chemical Week* for September 26, 1953, that the people who make Four-Way Cold Tablets are suing the people who make Seven-Way Cold Tablets for deceiving the public (into thinking that seven ways to cure a cold are better than four ways, we guess). Most horrifying angle to the story is the fact that the four-way cold tablet people have sold twenty million dollars worth of their product during the past five years! Their advertising expenses have been about $700,000 per year. Are any of your dollars among that 20 million? We hope not.

Foremost among so-called cold "cures" these days are aspirin, the antibiotics and the antihistamines. We have extensive files on all these preparations. It is now commonly accepted in medical journals that not one of the three "cures" a cold. Any of them may relieve symptoms temporarily. Aspirin may lessen the pain of that throbbing headache, antihistamines may make you so groggy that you won't realize how your bones aches. But as "cold cures" they are all completely discredited.

Why then should we warn against them? Because you may be tempted to nip into a drugstore and pick up one of these inexpensive boxes of pills just to relieve symptoms. And your cold may go on and on and even develop into pneumonia while you are apparently feeling better because your symptoms have lessened. Then, too, all of these drugs have side-effects that—let's face it—may be fatal.

We review for you here what has been said in *Prevention* about aspirin, antibiotics and antihistamines, along with new information we have gathered. Let's discuss aspirin first.

Aspirin Is Not a Harmless Home Remedy

Introduced into this country from Germany some forty-odd years ago, the original Bayer patent expired in 1917 but continues even today to harvest rich financial rewards from a product that now is being manufactured by many other laboratories over fundamentally the same prescription. Nowadays advertising of the chemical ingredients of most of these aspirin-containing derivatives is given second place to their more easily pronounced trade names. Doctors often prescribe aspirin (or acetylsalicylic acid) in a variety of forms without a patient's knowledge, acting on the assumption that in moderate and regulated dosage it can do no harm in its two-fold general action of fever-reducer and pain-soother.

Bruce's *Materia Medica,* an authoritative teaching manual recognized by leading American medical schools, has this to say about aspirin:

"Salicylic acid is rapidly absorbed and circulates as sodium salicylate . . . a moderate dose causes a more rapid heart beat, a rise in blood pressure, flushing and warmth of the surface, perspiration, fullness in the head, tinnitus (ringing in the ears) deafness, impairment of vision and possibly a slight fall in temperature. Larger doses may cause delirium, especially with visual hallucinations; respiration is disturbed; the heart is slowed and weakened; the vessels are relaxed and the blood pressure falls; and perspiration is increased. . . . Occasionally it induces an . . . eruption . . . sometimes (albumin or blood in the urine)."

As long ago as October 5, 1940, an editorial in the *Journal of the American Medical Association* reasoned that the main safeguard against overdose lay in a ringing sensation in the ears of aspirin users, "so that the drug may be discontinued before these persons become seriously poisoned." The editorial admitted that "No doubt much harm indirectly has probably followed its indiscriminate use, in that conditions for which it was used were not remedied. . . . Many reports have appeared on the adverse effects which may follow its unwise use. These have included depression of the heart, habit formation, miscarriage in pregnancy, and idiosyncrasy (allergic reaction) causing such alarming symptoms as urticaria (hives), pruritis (itching), erythema (redness of skin) and generalized angioneurotic edema (swelling of the skin due to a blood vessel disorder) . . . even ulceration and gangrene have been attributed to its use."

The editorial goes on to quote figures from *The Lancet* on a wave of fatalities that occurred in England from the use of aspirin. "According to this source, in England and Wales in 1938 the number of deaths due to poison was reported to be 735 of which 591 were suicides, 92 accidental and the remaining doubtful. The agent responsible for 43 of the suicides, for eight of the accidental deaths and for 14 of the doubtful group of deaths was said to be aspirin; thus aspirin was reported as the cause of death in 65 of the 735 fatal poisonings."

The list of undesirable after-effects of aspirin also includes asthmatic attacks, as related in an article entitled *Allergy to Aspirin* by C. H. A. Walton, M.D., and H. W. Bottomley, M.D., of Winnipeg in the *Canadian Medical Association Journal* for March, 1951. Stating that "in relation to its very wide use the number of cases of aspirin sensitivity is small, but the effects are so striking and often dangerous that physicians should be familiar with its character," the authors include hives and skin puffiness from disordered blood vessels among those already known manifestations of allergy following small intake of the drug. But its relation to asthma is their special interest and among such patients they cite estimates of from two to ten per cent as demonstrating this type of sensitivity.

In the September 8, 1951, issue of the *Journal of the American Medical Association,* two physicians from Cornell University Medical College report on the case of a 74-year old man who experienced eight years of continuous intestinal bleeding as the result of the prolonged use of aspirin. We know now that aspirin or other drugs containing salicylic acid block the action of vitamin K in our bodies. And vitamin K is chiefly concerned with the ability of our blood to clot properly. Now probably one aspirin will not cause an instantaneous and fatal hemorrhage.

But we know people who take aspirin every day of their lives and especially when they have colds!

The United States Armed Forces Medical Journal for January, 1952, publishes an article describing six cases of salicylate poisoning of children, for two of whom the aspirin had been prescribed by physicians. In one case a five month old child who was already taking (for a cold) several different kinds of medicine including penicillin was given aspirin every four hours in addition by her parents who did not even mention to the doctor that they were giving her aspirin! This child died of salicylate poisoning four days after she became violently ill.

We would say very positively that aspirin is not for you, if you would be healthy. And we especially deplore the giving of aspirin to children. Within the past year aspirin especially for children has been getting a big play in the family magazines. It is temptingly flavored so that the child can chew it like candy. Here is another alarming hazard. Mother persuades Junior to take the aspirin "candy" to make him well. And what is to prevent Junior from seeking out the aspirin box and swallowing a lethal dose of the "candy" when mother isn't around? Why not go through your medicine chest today and just quietly throw away all the half empty bottles of aspirin?

Appendicitis

Sometime ago we ran an article on the relationship of appendicitis to diet. Our authority believed that lack of cellulose in food is the main cause of the modern high incidence of appendicitis. Corroboration of this opinion comes from the pages of the *British Medical Journal* for September 6, 1952, in a letter from a New Zealand physician, H. M. Karn. Dr. Karn tells us that he served in West Africa, the Sudan and Egypt during the war and was impressed with the complete lack of acute appendicitis among the native troops. However, when they were transferred to other countries and had to eat European diet, their susceptibility to appendicitis went up.

"I am convinced," says Dr. Karn, "that the disease is not a racial one, but rather has its origin in a disturbance of the habitual intestinal bacterial flora occasioned by a high carbohydrate, high protein, but low cellulose diet as adopted by the so-called civilized races of the world since about 1850 when flour was bleached and roller-ground and meat subjected to mass refrigeration and exportation on a large scale." This would suggest that *Prevention's* raw vegetable and whole grain cereal recommendations have even another element in their favor. Raw vegetables and whole grains are high in cellulose. That is, they contain the tough fibrous cell-walls which refining and cooking break down. And apparently we need this cellulose for a healthy appendix.

Asthma

Presenting two conservative views and one new and revolutionary outlook on preventing asthma.

Asthma is a disease which has been known from very ancient times. Hippocrates, who lived in the fifth century B. C., described it and warned that asthmatics should guard against anger, because it was well known that such a violent emotion increased the severity of asthmatic attacks.

Because of its close relation to emotional states of mind, asthma has been blamed on psychological reasons down through the years. Even medical dictionaries that are not very up-to-date define asthma as "a paroxysmal affection of the bronchial tubes characterized by difficulty in breathing, cough and a feeling of constriction and suffocation. *The disease is probably a neurosis.*" It is equally common in children and adults, but so are many neuroses these days. It is not fatal in itself. That is, people do not die from it as they might die from cancer or heart trouble. But they may die from other complications as a result of having asthma. For instance, someone with a desperately bad heart condition might die in the throes of an asthma attack, because of the extra strain imposed on his heart by the violent gasping and wheezing that go with an attack. Someone suffering from one disease or another might be seriously weakened by asthmatic attacks which would not permit him to sleep at night.

What does the conservative medical press say about asthma? A leading article in the *Journal of the American Medical Association* for October, 1952, by Leon Unger, M. D., and Albert Howard Unger, M. D., of Northwestern University Medical School deals first with preventive treatment for bronchial asthma. They tell us that children of allergic parents are quite likely to have allergic diseases. If therefore mother and father are hay fever or asthma sufferers, or demonstrate symptoms of distress at the sight, touch, taste or feel of some allergenic substances, it is best to provide the children with a home as protected as possible against any substance that might produce allergies.

Pets should be removed from the house, they tell us, for cat and dog hairs are allergy-producing to some people. The house should be kept free from dust. By this they do not mean that it should be dusted frequently—quite the opposite, for dusting with a dry dust cloth usually only creates more dust and spreads around whatever dust is there. Mattresses, pillows and furniture upholstery should be made of rubber or covered with plastic material tightly zippered so that dust cannot enter. Clean curtains, drapes and rugs collect dust very rapidly. They should be thoroughly cleaned with vacuum attachments or should be eliminated entirely. Linoleum makes an eminently satisfactory floor covering—non-allergenic. The usual stuffed toy may be filled with kapok to which some individuals are sensitive.

Since molds cause allergies, the house should be dry, and moisture should not be permitted to collect in the basement. Cosmetics made from orris root (your druggist can tell you which these are) should be forbidden in the house. Certain foods may produce symptoms of coughs, wheezing, "runny nose." Eggs, milk, wheat products, seafoods, nuts are some of the common allergenic foods. Your doctor can easily give you a diet in which each of these foods in turn has been omitted. Then by including each food once again you can easily find out which one it was that caused the symptoms.

Asthma and Pollen

Pollen is the villain we all think of first in terms of hay fever, asthma and related allergies. The best ways of avoiding pollen are unfortunately all very expensive, unless you happen to live in a pollen-free locality. There is not as much pollen in the city as in the country, although plots of ragweed and other allergenic growths are becoming more and more common even in cities. One hundred miles from the shore on an ocean liner one can breathe air practically free from pollen. High mountain slopes and certain parts of our country, such as Arizona, California and so forth, are almost free from pollen. You can have your home air-conditioned which will bring relief from wheezing at night. But it is certainly neither possible nor wise for anyone, adult or child, to stay all day in an air-conditioned house during the summer months when pollen is most abundant. Skin tests given by your doctor can reveal much about your sensitivity to allergenic substances and once you have decided what you are allergic to, you must see to it that as little contact as possible takes place between that substance and you, from then on.

Allergy specialists have also discovered ways of immunizing sensitive persons to the things that bring on their symptoms. You can now be injected with, at first, small and then ever-increasing amounts of prepared serums which will supposedly render you insensitive to your allergens eventually. Let's say you have an allergy to goldenrod pollen. You can take injections long before the goldenrod season. Your doctor will give you first a very little bit of goldenrod serum, then a little more and a little more. As the serum builds up in your body, your own immunity to it also builds up and by the time the goldenrod is golden you can walk through a field of it without the slightest discomfort.

The two doctors Unger, whose article is of course addressed to the other doctors who read the *Journal of the American Medical Association,* go on to relate the various kinds of medicine that can be given to asthmatics (and there are a lot of them) mostly concerned with expectorants, sleeping pills and sedatives. They also mention the fact that the psychological factor is extremely important in asthma. Oversympathy on the part of the family may make symptoms much worse. Nervous tension due to fear, coughing and so forth can sometimes be relieved by a sympathetic doctor who encourages his patient to talk about the things that are bothering him.

The Psychological Side of Asthma

An article in the *Canadian Medical Journal* for August, 1952, deals with the psychological aspects of asthma in more detail. Peter G. Edgell, M. D., of the Department of Psychiatry of the Montreal General Hospital, tells us there are two kinds of asthma—extrinsic and intrinsic. Extrinsic asthma is quite clearly related to one or another of the various allergens. Intrinsic asthma may be the result of a number of different complicating causes; and both kinds may occur in the same person at the same time.

In a survey of 1129 asthmatic persons, 50 per cent showed definite and typical allergic reactions in skin tests with various substances. For 23 per cent of the 1129, no cause at all could be found for the asthma. In a further investigation 21 per cent appeared to have personality maladjustments which seemed to precipitate the asthma. At a round table conference in 1947, psychiatrists and allergenists agreed that a badly adjusted personality might not be the direct cause of asthma, but emotions might very well bring on attacks and aggravate the symptoms of susceptible persons.

Everyone agrees, says Dr. Edgell, that asthmatics have in common a "deep-seated emotional insecurity and an intense need for parental love and protection." One can see such traits more easily in children who have not as yet learned to disguise their emotions. They cling to their mothers, they are self-centered, usually of high intelligence, but often unable to perform well in school because of their continual anxiety that they may fail. The real or imagined rejection by parents is the cause of such behavior, says Dr. Edgell.

We have all heard stories of the psychological importance of asthma, such as the classic story of the man who suffered from an allergy to roses. The sight of a rose would set him to coughing, sneezing and weeping, *even if the rose happened to be made of paper.* And medical science contains some astounding stories of the relation of emotion to asthmatic attacks. A girl who fell two stories while she was cleaning a window had her first asthma attack immediately after she hit the ground. A man who identified himself strongly with his father became asthmatic after his father's death, apparently from being a witness to the gasping and choking of his father's losing battle with pneumonia. Repressed sex impulses can be a cause of asthma apparently. Repressed fears or anger that cannot be spoken out may turn into an asthmatic attack.

In addition, says Dr. Edgell, a feeling of depression may bring on an attack in some susceptible individuals. In others the asthma may alternate with the depression. A patient of a famous psychiatrist was cured of his asthma by a series of Coué treatments. (This, you will remember, was the system in which you cured yourself by auto-suggestion —"Every day in every way, I'm getting better and better.") But the attacks of anxiety that came in their place distressed him so much that he asked the psychiatrist if he might not have the asthma back again! He preferred it to the anxiety!

But Is Asthma Psychological?

In an astonishing book called *Body, Mind and Sugar* by E. M. Abrahamson, M.D., and A. W. Pezet (published by Henry Holt and Company, 1951) we found an entirely different approach to the subject of asthma. We want to recommend to you Dr. Abrahamson's approach and his conclusions, for they sound remarkably sane and reasonable. The course of action he suggests for preventing or curing asthma involves no drugs, no travel, no psychiatry, no air conditioning, no expense.

Dr. Abrahamson tells us that there are about three million hay fever sufferers in this country. Including other allergenic conditions, he estimates that the total number of allergics must approach five million. Out of a vast number of possibly allergenic substances, he lists fungus spores, the dander of animals, feathers, karaya gum (used in some wave set preparations), wheat and other flours, dusts (industrial and house), orris root, flax seed, kapok, insect scales, "practically any food," poison ivy, primrose, sumac, many drugs, chemicals and dyes, many flavoring and preservative materials, tooth pastes, mouth washes. In fact, according to Dr. Abrahamson, "it is probable that the length and list of allergens is limited only by what so far has been observed and recorded."

The fact that allergies appear to run in families and that they appear only in animals of "higher intelligence" has suggested that they have a psychological origin. One test of allergic children showed that 98.4 per cent of them were "rejected" by their mothers—that is, the children felt, whether consciously or unconsciously, whether justly or unjustly, that their mothers did not want or love them. In general however the allergy specialists refuse to recognize the opinions of the psychologists that asthma has psychological origins. "The medical profession, like other segments of humanity, is composed of a minority who believe in anything that is new and a majority who refuse to believe in anything that is new. Between them, the open-minded man of science, willing to pick up crumbs from the right and the left but unwilling to put them in his mouth until he has thoroughly tested them, has a difficult time of it," says Dr. Abrahamson.

Blood Sugar Tests Show Surprising Things About Asthmatics

The "anything that is new" referred to is a fairly recent investigation of the relationship of blood sugar to asthma, in which Dr. Abrahamson played a leading part. In general, this investigation went as follows: 1. Tests showed that asthmatics have a consistently low blood sugar. Reasoning from this point it seemed to follow that diabetics (whose blood sugar is abnormally high) should not suffer from asthma. "Joslin the great authority on diabetes, had a few patients who had suffered from asthma but lost it when they acquired diabetes." 2. Asthmatics have an excessive amount of potassium in their blood. Diabetics have a low level of potassium. 3. Asthmatics become worse when they eat excessive amounts of table salt. Diabetics can get along with less insulin when they take large amounts of salt.

4. Asthmatic attacks are specially dreaded because they occur most frequently at night after the patient has been asleep for several hours. In these early hours of the morning, the blood sugar level is at its

lowest. 5. Injections of glucose are sometimes given to asthmatic patients to relieve their attacks. This of course raises their blood sugar, relieving the attack. But it does not permanently help the asthma for taking more and more glucose (or any other form of sugar) eventually results in a still further lowering of the blood sugar. 6. The drugs used for asthma, such as morphine, amytal, ephedrine and adrenalin all raise blood sugar levels. Can this be merely coincidental or is this the reason for their temporary effectiveness?

Testing the theory that low blood sugar may make one susceptible to asthma, Dr. Abrahamson put 12 asthma patients on a diet designed to prevent low blood sugar. All of them improved considerably. How then could he explain a patient who was being treated for asthma at the allergy clinic and was also taking insulin for her diabetes? This patient's asthma grew so much worse that she carried a hypodermic needle of adrenalin always with her and could not get through a day without several injections. A six-hour test of her blood sugar revealed that for the first two hours after she took the prescribed dose of glucose, her blood sugar level soared to the diabetic range. Had the test been stopped then, it would have revealed just diabetes, resulting from a high blood sugar. But during the next four hours it fell far below the normal range and at once her asthmatic wheezing began once again. In this unusual case the patient suffered from both high and low blood sugar at different times of day, depending on when and what she had last eaten. The medicine she took for her diabetes made her asthma worse. The adrenalin she took for her asthma made her diabetes worse. She was given a diet which would bring her blood sugar to normal levels and both the diabetes and the asthma finally disappeared.

How to Eliminate Low Blood Sugar

As we pointed out in a former article on blood sugar, the answer to achieving a normal blood sugar level is to eliminate those foods which bring about a sudden, but short, rise in the blood sugar. In general, these are sugars and starches and, as Dr. Abrahamson discovered with all his patients, caffeine, which gives you a "lift" by stimulating the islands of Langerhans (a part of your pancreas) to produce insulin. As a result the blood sugar level drops too far and all kinds of symptoms can result. This persistently low blood sugar which, according to Dr. Abrahamson, is responsible for asthma and other allergies, is called "hyperinsulinism" meaning, simply, too much insulin.

Dr. Abrahamson's remarkable book contains a great deal more information on hyperinsulinism and its relation to such diseases as peptic ulcer, rheumatic fever and even epilepsy, alcoholism and neuroses. We strongly advise you to read this book whether or not you are suffering from any of these disorders. Perhaps the information in it will help some friend, neighbor or member of your family. The book is *Body, Mind and Sugar,* by E. M. Abrahamson and A. W. Pezet. It is published by Henry Holt and Company, 383 Madison Ave., New York City. If you plan to buy a copy, ask your local library to get a copy, too, so that the book will be available to others.

Now for the diet—the famous diet that worked wonders for the sufferers from hyperinsulinism. It's a very simple diet, really, and involves just about the same foods that *Prevention* has recommended for years. It's an easy diet to follow, and the forbidden items will bother you very little, if you must eat at restaurants or at the homes of friends. Dr. Abrahamson suggests following the diet for three months. We suggest that, after three months are over, the only items any sensible person will put back on the menu are the vegetables and fruits that are forbidden on the diet.

On arising—Medium orange, half grapefruit or four ounces of fruit juice.

Breakfast—Fruit or 4 ounces of juice, 1 egg with or without 2 slices of ham or bacon; *only one* slice of bread or toast with plenty of butter, beverage.

2 Hours After Breakfast—4 ounces of juice.

Lunch—Meat, fish, cheese or eggs; salad (large serving of lettuce, tomato or Waldorf salad with mayonnaise or French dressing); vegetables if desired; *only one slice of bread or toast* with plenty of butter; dessert; beverage.

3 Hours After Lunch—8 ounces of milk.

1 Hour Before Dinner—4 ounces of juice.

Dinner—Soup if desired (not thickened with flour); vegetables; liberal portion of meat, fish or poultry; *only one* slice of bread if desired; dessert; beverage.

2-3 Hours After Dinner—8 ounces of milk.

Every Two Hours Until Bedtime—4 ounces of milk or a small handful of nuts.

Allowable vegetables: Asparagus, avocado, beets, broccoli, Brussels sprouts, cabbage, cauliflower, carrots, celery, cucumbers, corn, eggplant, lima beans, onions, peas, radishes, sauerkraut, squash, string beans, tomatoes, turnips.

Allowable fruits: Apples, apricots, berries, grapefruit, pears, melons, oranges, peaches, pineapple, tangerines. May be cooked or raw with or without cream but without sugar. Canned fruits should be packed in water, not syrup.

Lettuce, mushrooms and nuts may be taken as freely as desired.

Juice: Any unsweetened fruit or vegetable juice except grape juice or prune juice.

Beverages: Weak tea (tea ball, not brewed); decaffeinated coffee, coffee substitutes.

Desserts: Fruit, unsweetened gelatin, junket (made from tablets, not mix).

Alcoholic and Soft Drinks: Club soda, dry gingerale, whiskey and other *distilled* liquors.

Avoid Absolutely

Sugar, candy and other sweets, such as cake, pie, pastries, sweet custards, puddings and ice cream.

Caffeine: Ordinary coffee, strong brewed tea, beverages containing caffeine. (Your doctor will tell you what these are.)

Potatoes, rice, grapes, raisins, plums, figs, dates and bananas.

Spaghetti, macaroni and noodles.

Wines, cordials, cocktails and beer.

(We have included bacon, ham, soft drinks and distilled liquors in this list, as Dr. Abrahamson does, but we assume you will have crossed these off automatically as you read the list. Then, too, we do not recommend using citrus fruits as freely as Dr. Abrahamson suggests and we do not approve of drinking citrus juice or milk.)

Backache

Backache is not a disease, it seems. Like so many other disorders from which so many of us suffer, it is a symptom of disease. It used to be called lumbago—a term which meant little or nothing pertaining to the possible causes or cure of the complaint. Then, later, it became more fashionable to speak of backache as "sacroiliac." This is the series of vertebrae at the very bottom end of the spine, and it was generally assumed by the term "sacroiliac" that this joint had gone out of whack. As a matter of fact the sacroiliac is one of the strongest joints in the body —it has to be—and it seldom goes awry. Sciatica, another term for backache, implied that the sciatic nerve was being pressed on as a result of the sacroiliac slipping. No one knows whether or not this is so. So gradually the word sciatica has been discarded too. Backache still continues to be a symptom of, as the doctors say, "unknown etiology" which means unknown cause.

Today we speak of it as "low back pain" for generally the severe backaches occur at the bottom end of the spine. And today a wide variety of possible causes is listed in any medical article on backache. Backache may be the result of arthritis. It may arise from some unusual muscle strain, plus emotional strain. It may result from some recent or long-forgotten bump, jar or wrench occurring especially during periods of fatigue. It may indicate a slipped vertebral disc. An infection of the genital or urinary tract, an acute illness, general ill health, a local infection somewhere in the body or overweight may bring about backache. We are surprised at how often we find physicians indicating that backache may be psychosomatic—a physical symptom of some profound emotional strain or frustration. Finally—and this is the kind of backache that is most common and most easily prevented—it may be simply the result of poor posture, improper furniture or surroundings, or the wrong kind of movements in daily life.

Says W. B. Parsons, M. D., writing in the *Canadian Medical Association Journal* for July, 1951, "every joint has an optimum position of function, . . . moderate departures from that position will increase the likelihood of strain and extreme departures will almost inevitably result in pain." The lower part of the back bears almost half the weight of the body, centered chiefly in the lumbo-sacral joint. This joint connects a movable piece of anatomy—the spine—with a part that is, generally speaking, not so mobile—the pelvic structure. Anatomists seem to feel that the construction of the lower part of the back displays abundant evidence that man is not especially well equipped to walk in an upright position. The animals who walk on all fours do not, we suspect, ever have backaches.

How the Backache Comes About

Dr. Parsons continues: "In people with poor posture, the joints are at or near the limit of normal motion, but are prevented from going beyond this point by muscle power and there is no strain—the fault is compensated. As with the heart, if something breaks that compensation, the joints will be moved beyond the limits of normal, and strain or decompensation results. Clinically this is backache."

Think of it this way, he says: the normal position of the wrist is straight out in a line with the arm. When you bend the wrist as far down as you can, at right angles, there is no pain. You can even push it down with your other hand, and so long as the muscles in the arm can withstand the push, there is no pain. But if the weight becomes too great, or if the arm muscles are caught off-guard by a sudden unaccustomed movement and the wrist is bent a little further, there is strain on the supporting muscles, and pain for you. Putting this in terms of the back, you can exert pressure on the low back joint by putting up with poor posture, for perhaps many years. But a sudden unexpected twist, lifting a too-heavy object, an unaccustomed amount of work crowded into one busy day, and there will be strain on the supporting muscles of the back—and backache.

If you drag about day after day with a pretty constant backache, we suggest that you have an examination to find out whether you may be suffering from one or another of the things outlined above. If not, your backache is what doctors call "idiopathic"—a disorder for which they can find no cause. In that case, the cause is probably poor posture, the wrong kind of furniture or the wrong kind of movements.

It might be advisable to consult a chiropractor or an osteopath, as these doctors specialize in disorders of this kind. For you, as for everyone else, we suggest bone meal, too, as the perfect answer for deficiency in minerals that may be the result of our modern diet. Bone meal contains calcium, phosphorous and all the other minerals you need for good health, all in the proper proportion, as nature planned them.

Your Backache and Your Bed

If you wake up with a backache, chances are very good that your back has not been getting proper rest during the night, due to a bed that is too soft. Look at someone lying in a hammock and you will get an exaggerated idea of what a soft bed does to one's body. If you lie on your back, your chest is constricted and your back curved unnaturally. On your side, the lower half of you is extended too far and the upper half constricted. If you lie on your stomach, the spine and hips are extended into a completely unnatural curve.

Dr. Parsons tells us of a woman who went on a camping trip where she had to sleep flat on the hard ground night after night. She experienced a remarkable recovery from a backache "that had plagued her for years." Your bed should be firm and flat. In most cases, modern springs and mattresses tend to "give" too much which is why many people find it far better to sleep with a fairly thick board between the mattress and springs, so that the bed does not curve beneath your weight, no matter how you sleep. This kind of bed board can be bought or you can make one yourself from a piece of plywood.

We all must know by now that modern living room chairs in which we are expected to "lounge" have an absolutely devastating effect on one's body and one's posture. You were not meant to sit curled in a forward curve, with your knees close to your chin, your chest constricted, your abdomen cramped, your lungs crushed into a tiny space that barely permits them to breathe. Your chairs should be reasonably straight, with a length from the seat to the floor that is comfortable for you, so that your knees don't jut up into the air if you are tall, so that your feet don't hang dangling if you are short. The back of the chair should conform pretty much to the curve of your own back.

If you sit at work all day, the chair you sit in is even more important. Progressive employers today know that workers will work faster and better and there will be less absenteeism if the chairs are fitted to the workers' height and the kind of work they are doing. If you bend over your work, it will help to raise one foot to a stool or a platform from time to time.

Poor Posture the Most Common Cause of Backache

Tall, thin people are inclined to be more susceptible to backache from poor posture than are short stocky ones. Obviously the muscles that support the back have a bigger job to do—more actual back structure to support and a longer distance over which the support must be given. By and large we moderns have extremely bad posture, which makes us highly susceptible to the backache for which there seems to be no other cause. In the pregnant woman, or the woman who has had children the muscles that support the abdomen are weakened, the abdomen sags, pulling on the back to deepen the curve there and produce a full fledged case of "sway back." This can easily be corrected if you catch it soon enough. If not, backache is a likely result.

We have often wondered how many men have "pot-bellies" because they don't wear suspenders. Hence they unconsciously stick out their abdomens to hold up their belted trousers. Teenagers who grow too fast tend to slouch so that their height will not be noticed, rounded shoulders are the result.

All of us should know by now the excessive harm to posture that can be done by wearing high heels. There is no excuse for anyone to wear high heels in these days when low-heeled shoes are so attractive and popular. If you feel you simply cannot get along without high heels, wear them only when you go out in the evenings, for a very few hours at a time, and when you are not going to be on your feet a great deal.

Good posture every day, all day long can do away with backache—the ordinary kind of backache. Good posture is a matter of exercise, very simple exercise. But it is much more a matter of remembering all day to keep your posture good. The exercise will strengthen your muscles. But if you let them sag back to their original sloppy state during the day, you will have all the work to do over again next time you take your exercises.

Correcting Your Posture

Stand in front of a full-length mirror after your next bath and look at your posture. You know what good posture is—all of us do. You should be able to hang a straight plumb-line from your ear to the ball of your feet, and half of you, perfectly balanced, should be on each side of the line. You can improve the tone of your stomach muscles by lying flat on a bed or the floor and raising up to a sitting position without using your hands or arms. Or you can lie flat and lift one leg after the other into the air, slowly. It's as simple as that.

Or, if you want someting even more simple, try exercising your abdominal muscles while you go about your business. Pull up and in on them, tucking your buttocks beneath you. Hold your head high, your chin in, your shoulders up. When you lift something heavy, bend your knees, get close to the object, and when you lift, let your legs do the work rather than your back. When you bend, don't bend over at the waist, with your knees straight. (And incidentally, this kind of bending, trying to touch your toes, with legs straight, is the very worst exercise you can do, if you suffer from backache.) Bend your legs, keep your trunk straight, let your legs do the work rather than your back.

Dr. Parsons says "For those who say they get enough exercise all day long in their work, the only answer I know is that practice makes perfect, but not if you practice the wrong way."

Bananas

Yes, we have bananas, today. We have them in all kinds of diets, for infants, adults—stout and thin—and old people who have trouble with their digestion. Not so many years ago it was fondly believed that bananas were hard to digest. This was probably because the bananas were eaten before they were fully ripe, and their raw starch caused considerable digestive trouble, just as that of green apples does. Faintly green bananas look attractive and feel firm to the touch. When dark specks begin to appear on their yellow surfaces, we are inclined to turn them down as rotten. But a banana is not fully ripe until its skin shows brown specks. By then its starch has changed into completely digestible fruit sugar.

They knew about bananas way back in history, for Alexander the Great found the people of India eating bananas in 327 B. C. Within the past few years bananas have been found to be a specific remedy for several infant diseases, such as celiac disease of which the outstanding symptom is diarrhea. It has also been discovered that bananas in the diet of infants result in better growth than is achieved with either apples or cereals. We have learned that people who are allergic to bananas can eat dehydrated bananas with no distress. Banana flour is sold as a substitute for wheat flour, tapioca, oatmeal, arrowroot and so forth. You can make bread from banana flour mixed with five per cent wheat flour.

Recently, an investigation was made of the suitability of bananas in the diet of elderly people. Even those who had never eaten bananas found that they felt well with a banana or two every day, had no trouble digesting them, enjoyed their flavor and were especially pleased with how easy they are to chew in comparison with other fruits.

The average-sized banana weighs about 100 grams, contains less than 100 calories, has an alkaline reaction in the body, as do most fruits, and in addition, contains the following quantities of vitamins and minerals:

Calcium	8.	milligrams
Phosphorus	28.	milligrams
Iron	.6	milligrams
Copper	.21	milligrams
Manganese	640.	micrograms
Sodium	.5	milligrams
Vitamin A	430.	Internat. Units
Vitamin B		
Thiamin	.09	milligrams
Riboflavin	.06	milligrams
Niacin	.6	milligrams
Pyridoxine	300.	micrograms
Inositol	34.	milligrams
Biotin	4.	micrograms
Folic acid	95.	micrograms
Vitamin C	10.	milligrams
Vitamin E	.40	milligrams
Protein	1.2	grams
Fat	.2	grams
Carbohydrates	23.0	grams

You will find recipes in your cook book for baking or frying bananas. It seems to us that there is actually less excuse for cooking a banana than for cooking any other fruit. So we would advise eating them raw. We have read a good many stories about gases used in ripening bananas commercially. So we would suggest that you buy them fairly green and ripen them yourself. The best way to do this is to keep them with little or no ventilation until they begin to color rapidly. Then keep them always at room temperature until they show the brown mottling which means they are ready to eat. Like other tropical fruits, bananas should not be kept in the refrigerator.

Blackstrap Molasses

Is blackstrap molasses a wonder food, to be included in the diet every day, capable of curing or preventing almost any ailment? Or is it a filthy product, full of dirt and germs, completely lacking in nourishment and fit only as food for animals? We don't think blackstrap molasses is any of these things. But it has come to be such a controversial subject—

should you or should you not eat blackstrap molasses?—that we have done some research to try to find the answers to these questions.

Blackstrap molasses is an end product in the manufacturing of refined white sugar. According to Jacobs in his *Food and Food Products* (Interscience Publishers), it is the "lowest grade of molasses from which all possible crystallizable sugar has been removed." Those who object to blackstrap will probably declare that this sentence is enough to condemn it. All sugar has been removed from it, therefore we should not eat it. But for those of us who are health-conscious, the fact that sugar has been removed is the finest kind of recommendation. Whole, raw sugar cane appears to be an excellent food, rich in vitamins and minerals. White refined sugar, which is made from it, is completely worthless as a food, containing nothing but calories—no vitamins, no minerals. These valuable food elements of the sugar cane are left in the molasses after the sugar has been removed.

A second point in favor of blackstrap is that it is widely used as food for animals. Anyone who reads nutrition books at all cannot but be impressed with the fact that in general our animals—especially valuable stock animals—are better fed than we are. The wheat germ removed in the milling of flour is fed to animals. It is the most valuable part of the wheat. Feeds for farm and domestic animals are well fortified with grains, alfalfa, kelp, brewer's yeast, fish liver oil, vitamin E and so forth.

Folks who raise animals for profit demand that their feed be high in nutrition. There is no question of how it looks, smells or tastes; whether the color is good or whether it can be speedily and conveniently served by a busy housewife. The one purpose of animal food is to *nourish*. So when we find that some 300 million gallons of blackstrap are imported into this country annually, of which about a third is used for cattle food, we suspect that there is some very good nutritional reason for this.

Blackstrap is rich in minerals, being especially high in calcium, iron and potassium. Here is a chart showing the mineral content of molasses compared in each case, with a food also high in this particular mineral:

Milligrams per hundred grams
(5 tablespoons)

Calcium—Molasses, 258, Milk, 120; Phosphorus—Molasses, 30, Whole wheat, 374; Iron—Molasses, 7.97, Beef liver, 8.30; Copper—Molasses, 1.93, Beef liver, 2.15; Potassium—Molasses, 1500, Dry apricots, 1700.

Blackstrap is also rich in B vitamins, especially inositol. The B vitamins in 100 grams of blackstrap are:

Inositol—150 milligrams.
Thiamin—245 micrograms.
Riboflavin—240 micrograms.
Niacin—4 milligrams.
Pyridoxine—270 micrograms.
Pantothenic acid—260 micrograms.
Biotin—16 micrograms.

The Journal of the American Medical Association for July 14, 1951, answers a query as to the nutritional value of blackstrap, lists the vitamin and mineral content, then says "Note that in no instance, with the exception of inositol, does the vitamin content reach a value that makes an appreciable contribution to the human diet when compared with other recognized protective foods." We are at a loss to understand this statement, considering that blackstrap contains almost twice as much calcium as milk, weight for weight, almost as much iron as liver, almost as much potassium as dry apricots and is also so very rich in B vitamins, compared to the foods most of us get along on, day after day.

Of course one does not eat as much molasses as milk, cheese or liver by weight. So one would not get as much nourishment from a tablespoon of blackstrap as from a glass of milk or a serving of liver. But we think blackstrap molasses should be thought of as food in an entirely different way. As you know, we believe that anyone eating a good diet gets enough sugar in fresh fruits and vegetables so that he does not need to use any form of sweetening at mealtime. We do not advise using raw sugar, brown sugar or any of the other forms of sugar that are supposedly "better for you" than white refined sugar. Just let sugar alone, we say. In a very short time you will find that you have no craving at all for a sweet taste. Your fruits and vegetables provide it in abundance.

But if you are "tapering off" on sugar, if you simply feel that you cannot finish a meal without something sweet, then by all means use a little blackstrap molasses or honey instead of sugar. In either one, you will be getting nourishment aplenty as well as a sweet taste and calories. But remember to cut down gradually on the use of even these. And incidentally, put no stock at all in the statement that blackstrap is dirty or unfit for human food. Check with the Food and Drug Administration if you have any doubts. They will assure you that blackstrap molasses, prepared for human consumption, must pass all federal regulations for cleanliness and lack of adulteration, just as all other human foods must.

Blood Pressure

Many of us use the term without understanding what it means or what its relation to health may be.

The human heart beats about 104,000 times in every 24 hours. In one day it pumps about 60 barrels of blood through the blood vessels. For comparison, picture a water pump, busily engaged in pumping 60 barrels of water per day through miles and miles of rubber hose. Imagine all the things that might go wrong—with the pump, with the hose, with the water. Then imagine this pump working steadily without a moment's rest for sixty or seventy years. Any engineer can tell you of the host of technical difficulties that might arise.

First of all, in order to pump fluids, a certain pressure must be maintained. That is the purpose of the pump—to provide the pressure. When you turn on the pump, you are immediately aware of the pressure.

The hose which has been flat and empty fills with water. As the water presses against the sides of the hose, pressure is created there. In a new hose, the walls are elastic and "give" as the pressure rises and falls. Now imagine that you have put a rope around the hose at one given point. Pull the rope tighter and tighter until no water can pass through. So long as the pump goes on pumping, pressure builds up until the hose bursts. Imagine what happens when a stone lodges within the hose, shutting off a certain amount of water. In proportion to the amount of water shut off, the pressure in the hose will rise.

Now imagine that you are using an *old* hose—sixty years old, let's say. It's been left out in the weather and used so often and so hard that its walls are crumbly on the inside and hard rather than elastic. As the force of the water varies, the walls of the hose cannot swell or contract as they should. The have lost their elasticity. So the pressure of the water is further disturbed. Now imagine that your pump is pumping a thick oil, rather than water. Naturally the pump will have to pump harder or faster or both to maintain the same pressure. And the walls of the hose will be subjected to even more strain because the fluid inside is thicker and harder to pump.

The Heart is the Human Pump

Blood pressure is the pressure exerted by the human pump—the heart—against the walls of the hose (the blood vessels). We speak of blood pressure in numerals. These indicate the height of a column of mercury that can be supported by the blood pressure. The instrument used for measuring blood pressure is called a sphygmomanometer. If your doctor takes your blood pressure he may give you two figures rather than one. He may say your blood pressure is 120/75. What does this mean? When the heart is actually pumping, we call this the systole period in the heart beat—that is the 120 recorded by the doctor. When the heart is resting between beats, we call that the diastole. That is the 75 recorded. Naturally the diastole is a lower figure than the systole because when the heart is pumping it produces a larger pressure than when it is resting. But because the pause between beats is so slight, the pressure does not have time to go down very much.

By normal blood pressure we mean that the heart is pumping at the right rate, the blood vessels are contracting and relaxing with great elasticity and there is no impediment present that causes pressure to build up. What could such an impediment be? Obviously not a rope tied around the blood vessels, or a stone that is shutting off some of the blood as was the case with your water hose. But, suppose there is some difficulty in one organ or other—let's say the kidney—so that the blood is not moving along as rapidly as it should at that point. As the blood behind is pumped strongly forward pressure goes up.

Or what if your heart is trying to pump the same amount of blood through vessels much narrower than they should be? Again the pressure goes up because there is just not enough room for the blood to move at its usual pressure. And if the vessels lack elasticity, as they do frequently when they become old, then they do not have the proper amount of "give," so they cannot contract and expand to relieve pressure at any given point. Then, too, if the blood is thicker than it should be, the heart or pump encounters still another difficulty, for it must pump harder and pressure goes up accordingly.

The Heart Adjusts To Daily Circumstances

The human heart is not just a piece of machinery such as a water pump is. It is carefully adjusted to various conditions under which you are living. If you are taking violent exercise, you need more blood in various parts of your body. To meet this demand, the heart speeds up and blood pressure is raised—just so long as you continue to exercise. When you feel some emotion—fear or exaltation, for instance—your heart pumps faster, causing blood pressure to rise again.

So you see that what we speak of as "high blood pressure" is not a disease. It is only an indication that something is wrong somewhere in the body that makes the pressure rise. Correct the disorder and the pressure will go down again. But suppose you use a drug that makes your blood pressure go down without relieving any accompanying disorder? Then the heart does not have to work so hard trying to pump blood. But if the disorder is still present that made the heart work faster to begin with, then you can see what condition you have left your heart in. The drug is making the heart go more slowly, while the disease or disorder is still trying to make it go faster. So you have solved nothing.

We hear a lot of talk these days about high blood pressure or hypertension. Mostly because half a million people die in this country every year from some kind of circulatory or heart disorder and perhaps as many as 15 million Americans may be suffering from high blood pressure at this moment. There are some 63 diseases in which high blood pressure commonly appears. It usually occurs in diseases of the kidneys, the nervous system or the glands. This is apparently because kidney disease may slow up the passage of the blood as we pointed out above. The nervous system and the glands regulate the contractions of the blood vessels and also the rapidity of the heart beat. So you can see that disorders in this field would be reflected in blood pressure.

If your doctor knows what is causing your high blood pressure, he may very well be able to remove the cause and the pressure will go down. In kidney disease, for instance, one kidney may be removed, although this does not seem to be a satisfactory solution for a health-conscious person. Our aim should be to prevent any kidney trouble in the first place. If your doctor does not know what is causing your high blood pressure, he calls it "essential high blood pressure" or "essential hypertension" which is just another name for high blood pressure—cause unknown. Most patients, we are sorry to say, have this kind of high blood pressure. Hardening of the arteries, which is generally symptomatic of old age, goes along with high blood pressure usually. But sometimes apparently the arteries are wide enough so that hypertension does not occur, even though the arteries have lost their elasticity. It is also apparent how closely related are blood pressure, blood vessels and the heart. They are all involved in the business of transporting blood to all parts of the body and when one part of the system breaks down, all the other parts will suffer. Also it follows that those things which are good for the heart are good for the blood vessels and are likely to lead to a "normal blood pressure."

How Do You Know If Your Blood Pressure Is Normal?

What do we mean by "normal blood pressure?" There is no such thing. That is, no figure can be set as the absolutely correct blood pressure for all individuals. Some folks may feel their best and enjoy the most abundant health when their blood pressure is as low as 110. Others may be at their best with a blood pressure of 130. Years ago we used to hear that "normal" blood pressure could be figured as 100 plus your age. In other words, if you were twenty-five years old, 125 was your "normal" blood pressure. If you were 66, your "normal" blood pressure was 166. However these calculations were made on the basis of *prevalent blood pressure readings.* That indicates perhaps that they are the "average" pressure readings, but it does not indicate that they are "normal," if by "normal" we mean healthful as they should be. Today's research appears to indicate that a rise in blood pressure is not a natural and necessary accompaniment to middle or old age. It is instead an indication that something is wrong somewhere. The perfectly healthy person, supposedly, should have the same blood pressure at 66 that he had at 25. We are told by M. M. Rosenberg, M.D., in *Encyclopedia of Medical Self-Help* (Scholastic Book Press, 1950), that the ideal blood pressure seems to be between 105 to 125 for the systole, and between 60 to 80 for the diastole. Yet, he says, from 130 to 140 systole pressure is considered "normal" by doctors in general. Blood pressure above 140 brings a furrow to the doctor's brow and a word of caution from him to the patient.

On the other hand, we find that an article in *Time* magazine for September 11, 1950, reported a survey of 15,706 healthy men and women from 16 to 65 which resulted in findings indicating that "normal" blood pressure *may* increase with age. According to this survey, at the age of twenty, normal blood pressure should be between 105-140 for men and between 100 to 130 for women. At the age of thirty it might be 110-145 for men and 102 to 135 for women. At the age of forty it might be 110-150 for men and 105-150 for women. At the age of fifty, 115-160 for men appears to be normal, and 110-165 for women. At the age of sixty it may range from 115-170 for men and 115-175 for women.

Causes of High Blood Pressure

What seem to be some causes of high blood pressure or hypertension? As we have stated, essential hypertension does not have any one known cause. Here are some of the theories advanced: It is caused by too much salt in the diet which overloads the kidneys. It may be the result of prolonged stress or prolonged exercise, overwork or fatigue. It may be the result of overeating or constipation, both of which cause pressure to be exerted on the blood vessels of the digestive tract. It may be caused by overweight which necessitates the heart working harder to provide blood to a greatly expanded body volume. It may come from an excess of tobacco, alcohol, coffee, or from local infections, infectious diseases or heart diseases.

An article in *Time* magazine for March 24, 1947, reviews the findings of the American Foundation for High Blood Pressure which were, in general, that hypertension is caused by city living and rich food, emotional strain, and possibly the deposit of cholesterol (a fatty substance) in the walls of the blood vessels which narrows them and makes the pumping job harder. Arthur F. Coca, M.D., in an article in *The Medical Record,* December, 1950, says he believes that high blood pressure comes from allergy to different foods and that the famous rice and fruit diet for high blood pressure succeeds because it consists of foods to which most people are not allergic.

Dr. Maurice Sokolow of the University of California School of Medicine is reported in *Newsweek,* August 14, 1950, as saying that high blood pressure is apparently caused by emotional tension and is the result of personality difficulties. He believes that it can be helped by psychiatric counsel.

James Isbister, MRAP, MRACP, writing in the *Medical Journal of Australia,* January 24, 1953, quotes a survey which found "compulsive" personality traits in 50 per cent of a group of high blood pressure patients. Eighty per cent of these also had a history of high blood pressure in their families. C. M. Wilhelm, M. McDonough and H. McCarthy writing in *The American Journal of Digestive Diseases,* Vol. 20, pages 117-122, 1953, tell us that a high protein diet caused a decrease in the blood pressure of dogs. In rats a high salt diet raised the blood pressure among the normal animals, and the hypertensive ones.

What About Low Blood Pressure?

Low blood pressure is, of course, the opposite of high blood pressure. We cannot find, in all our medical research, much concern for the victim of low blood pressure. Generally, he is thought of as a lucky fellow for he will probably never have to worry about all the disorders that may plague the hypertensive patient. It seems that low blood pressure does not result in unpleasant symptoms. People in this category generally move more slowly and work under less tension. They have a longer life expectancy partly because of this slowness and lack of tension. They may tire easily and feel weak sometimes. Dr. Rosenberg tells us that taking coal tar remedies (such as aspirin, for instance) may weaken the heart sufficiently to produce low blood pressure. Exhaustion of the adrenal glands may also produce this result.

If you have read Editor Rodale's book on heart trouble, *This Pace is Not Killing Us,* you will know in advance that we believe today's "pace" is not responsible for today's high incidence of heart trouble and high blood pressure. We believe it may well be related instead to the modern American diet in which so many of the essential vitamins and minerals are deficient or completely lacking. Editor Rodale took up obesity and too much fat in the diet as possible causes of heart trouble. He discussed calcium, vitamin C, the B complex of vitamins and vitamin E as those deficient diet elements that are most closely related to the heart and blood vessel function. We have shown that garlic capsules have been responsible for lowering blood pressure in many experiments reported in medical journals. We must have an abundance of these elements in our food if we want to prevent heart and blood vessel disorders—and high blood pressure. Any good nutrition book in your local library will give you a list of foods high in these vitamins and minerals. And, in addition, you should supplement your diet with a natural food supplement for vitamin C (such as rose hips), brewer's yeast or desiccated liver for vitamin B, bone meal for calcium and other minerals and vitamin E and/or wheat germ oil. By living healthfully in other ways too, we feel you can avoid high blood pressure and keep this important function at "normal" *for you* for many years to come.

Blood Pressure, High

A review of some of the successful ways of preventing high blood pressure by diet and a healthful way of life.

High blood pressure—hypertension—is for many of us a menacing demon skulking in the background, ready to leap upon us when we pass middle-age. Or, for others of us, it is a devastating reality—an ever-present shadow that dogs our days with headaches, heart palpitations, nervousness, fatigue and the constant threat of a stroke or a heart attack.

Garlic in the Treatment of Hypertension

One of our earliest discoveries was the wealth of material in medical literature of the past fifty years on the subject of garlic and high blood pressure. So much research has been done on the subject of garlic and hypertension that writers are not concerned these days with whether or not garlic improves high blood pressure. Instead they are now disputing exactly how garlic achieves the improvement. In an article in a European publication *Praxis* for July 1, 1948, F. G. Piotrowski, visiting lecturer and member of the faculty of medicine of the University of Geneva, writes of his experience using garlic on about a hundred patients.

Dr. Piotrowski believes that garlic improves the blood pressure picture by dilating the blood vessels. He says, too, that it is difficult to conduct experiments with high blood pressure patients and hard to interpret results for high blood pressure may be the result of a wide variety of causes.

He eliminated from his experiment any patients whose conditions might further confuse the results—that is, those whose pressure dropped when other medicines were given, those who had kidney trouble and so forth. He tells us that Schlesinger, another investigator, secured a drop in pressure after 15 days of treatment with garlic. Pouillard claimed a drop within an hour after the first dose of garlic. Dr. Piotrowski claims no such sensational results and he tells us that he believes intermittent dosage with garlic just for the purpose of obtaining a drop in pressure is not wise. He prefers to administer garlic oil for three weeks. He has obtained a drop of at least 2 cm. in blood pressure in 40 per cent of the cases. These were all patients in which the drop could not possibly be attributed to any other cause. All were going to work regularly, so not even special rest could have been responsible.

He says that good results do not occur simply if the patient is young or if his pressure is not especially high. The expected drop takes place after about a week of treatment, regardless. Dr. Piotrowski gave his patients fairly large doses of garlic at first, then gradually decreased the dose over the period of three weeks. Then he gave smaller doses throughout the rest of the treatment.

The "subjective" symptoms of high blood pressure began to disappear within three to five days after the garlic treatment was begun. This means such things as headaches, dizziness, angina-like pains and pains between the shoulder blades. Most of these symptoms were relieved in many cases. Patients said, too, that they could think much more clearly and concentrate better. Piotrowski's conclusions are that garlic certainly has useful properties in the treatment of high blood pressure. It usually causes a drop in the pressure and even when it does not, its use is justified by the relief it brings for the uncomfortable symptoms the hypertensive patient has had.

Vitamins B and C are Useful, Too

It seems that vitamin C too, may have a great deal to do with lowering blood pressure that is too high. We know that the body needs more vitamin C under conditions of stress. In *Metabolism,* a medical journal, volume 1, page 197, 1952, Dr. C. L. Pirani discusses the relationship between vitamin C and stress. He says that under conditions of acute or chronic stress the vitamin should be taken in the relatively high dosage of one to two grams daily during the acute stage and as much as 300 milligrams per day thereafter.

In the *Canadian Journal of the Medical Sciences* for August, 1951, Doctors Heroux, Dugal and Paul describe investigations which show that vitamin C given in large doses reduces high blood pressure. They also give an account of their own experiments showing the same thing. In *Clinical Medicine,* volume 50, 1943, page 152, Doctors Davis and Poser describe the results they got in reducing hypertension by giving their patients vitamin C.

In this same magazine for July, 1952, W. J. McCormick, M. D., shows that a diet containing plenty of vitamin C and the B vitamins brings about dramatic decrease in the blood cholesterol. This substance has been blamed for clogging up arteries and playing no small part in the tragedy of strokes, heart attacks and other heart and blood vessel "accidents," as they are called. So vitamin C contributes to the health of the blood vessels in two ways—first by its ability to build up the actual blood vessel tissues themselves so that they are strong and flexible and its ability to decrease collections of cholesterol.

At least one of the B vitamins has been shown to be involved in the proper adjustment of blood pressure. The *American Journal of Physiology* for December, 1950, reports the production of high blood pressure in rats following only one week of deficiency in choline, one of the

B vitamins. As soon as the choline was restored to the diet, the pressure fell and could be kept at normal *unless large amounts of salt were fed which caused the pressure to rise again.* More of that later. Interestingly enough, another researcher at the Alabama Polytechnic Institute experimented with choline deficiency and cancer. His laboratory rats died in from six to twelve days when all the choline was removed from their diets. If he added just enough choline to keep them alive, 50 to 60 out of every hundred developed cancer—about fifty times more cancer than might otherwise have appeared. Brothers and sisters of these same rats eating a normal diet developed no cancer at all. Now of course none of our diets is absolutely lacking in choline. All of us get some of it every day. But no one knows how much we need for good health. These are the foods richest in choline. How much of these do you get every day? Snap beans, soy beans, beef brain, egg yolk, kidney, heart, liver, peanuts, peas, wheat germ, brewer's yeast. How often a week do you eat many of these foods?

Vitamin E and High Blood Pressure

We have said little about vitamin E in relation to blood pressure. Say Drs. Evan and Wilfrid Shute of Canada, world authorities on the use of vitamin E in heart disease, "When reading medical reports discussing the various diets and medications that have been suggested for the treatment of hypertensive patients we have been impressed with the relatively small degree of benefit usually achieved. Admittedly many patients whose pressures are lowered only a little feel much better than the actual figures would suggest. It may be true that alphatocopheral (vitamin E) therapy has as much to recommend it in these cases as many another hypotensive (pressure-lowering) agent more widely touted. At the same time we have always felt that it has fallen so far short of what is desirable that we have adopted a rather negative attitude toward its use for high blood pressure per se."

They go on to tell us (in their book *Alphatocopherol in Cardiovascular Disease*) of some of the benefits their heart patients (who were also high blood pressure patients) derived from taking vitamin E.

Of 158 moderately hypertensive or severely hypertensive patients some 56 or 35 per cent showed some improvement. Six of these returned to normal pressure. And in a period of a year's time only two patients died. In a group of 39 mildly hypertensive patients, 49 per cent showed some benefit. About 14 of these returned to normal pressure. There were no deaths. Most of these patients had heart difficulties as well. And, say the Drs. Shute, their heart symptoms improved so much more than their blood pressure symptoms that they are inclined to overlook the lesser benefits of vitamin E so far as blood pressure is concerned.

Incidentally, folks with high blood pressure should be wary of taking vitamin E in large doses when they begin to take it. Its effect on muscle tone seems to be so striking that it may increase the force of the heart beat and produce a temporary rise in blood pressure. So the Drs. Shute never start a hypertensive heart patient with more than one hundred international units (milligrams). Then they keep close watch on his blood pressure and increase the dosage of vitamin E ever so gradually until he may be able to take 150 to 400 units a day.

They believe that the hypertensive patient should take alphatocopherol or vitamin E. He fears a stroke or a heart attack, they say. Vitamin E, being the world's safest anticoagulant, can prevent this. "Here is the best insurance against cerebral or coronary accidents that he can take himself with minimal medical supervision," they say, "the mortality figure in our series speaks for itself. Alphatocopherol therapy is indicated for hypertensive patients, largely, perhaps, on account of this protective factor—but definitely demanded by that."

Rutin is Effective

There is another factor, more recently investigated, which is also important for the health of the blood vessels—rutin, a food substance which is part of a complex "something" we call vitamin P. H. K. Hollerstein, M. D., and his colleagues at several hospitals in Illinois and Ohio experimented by producing in laboratory animals blood pressure high enough that it ruptured the small blood vessels which hemorrhaged. To one group of animals they gave rutin ten days before they induced the high blood pressure. According to the *American Heart Journal* for August, 1951, those animals which received the rutin showed no evidence of hemorrhaging.

An eye doctor, Dr. L. B. Somerville-Large, gave rutin to his patients to forestall hemorrhaging of the blood vessels in the eye. He says that high blood pressure actually has no relation to the fact that blood vessels may be fragile. But he says that a considerable percentage of hypertensives who do have delicate blood vessels eventually have hemorrhages in the eye or the brain.

Vitamin P and rutin are present in fresh raw fruits and vegetables, along with vitamin C. It is interesting to note that those of us who take natural food supplements like rose hips get all the parts of vitamin P such as rutin in our supplement right along with the vitamin C. Folks who take synthetic vitamin C are getting just that—synthetic vitamin C and nothing more. Now no one knows when, some day, scientists will discover even more valuable food elements in this complicated vitamin C-vitamin P combination. Once again, those of us who take natural supplements will have been getting this substance all along. While those who take only synthetic vitamin C plus rutin will have what? Only vitamin C and rutin.

When we were talking about choline we mentioned that lowered blood pressure in laboratory rats almost immediately shot up again when they were given large amounts of salt. Throughout all of recent medical literature you will find saltless or salt-poor diets recommended in the treatment of high blood pressure. Probably the most famous diet of all is the Kempner Rice-Fruit Diet which, incidentally, should be undertaken only under the supervision of a doctor. This diet consists of literally nothing but rice and fruit, with some sugar and vitamin supplements. It is believed that the extremely low sodium content of the diet is responsible for the lowered blood pressure that does result from following the diet. Sodium is, of course, the dangerous part of sodium chloride or table salt. The chloride part of it does you no harm.

But it seems that we civilized people, with all the salt available that we might want, have taken to using too much of the stuff. It is not a food, you know. It is the only thing we eat which comes from neither animal nor plant. And the food we eat every day (especially if we eat lots of animal protein) contains plenty of sodium. We need no more for good health.

Food Allergies and Hypertension

Dr. Arthur C. Coca has a different idea as to why the rice-fruit diet is successful in lowering blood pressure. Dr. Coca believes that the foods allowed in the rice-fruit diet are foods to which most people are not allergic. That is why the diet is so successful, he says. In an article in *The Medical Record* for December, 1950, Dr. Coca tells us he believes that hypertension is caused by allergies to food. By taking one's pulse after eating a certain food one can see if the food increases the pulse. If so, this food should be omitted. By carefully testing each and every food and not eating those that raise your pulse, you can keep your blood pressure low, he says. He describes 42 hypertensive patients who were "treated" by avoiding the foods that raised their pulses. In almost every case the blood pressure was permanently reduced to a low average not attainable with any other kind of treatment.

If you would like to try out Dr. Coca's method, it goes like this: choose a time about an hour and a half after you have eaten and eat a small portion of one food that you wish to test, taking your pulse immediately before the test. Then take your pulse a half hour later and again a half hour after that. Take your pulse at your wrist, using two fingers from the other hand. You may locate two or even many more foods that cause your pulse to race. Eliminate these from your diet and watch the effect on your blood pressure.

Two other reminders for those who want to avoid high blood pressure. Overweight goes along with it, ever so often. Overweight is unhealthy. We all know that. But its particular effects are shown up mercilessly in the statistics which show that overweight individuals are far more likely to suffer from hypertension, heart trouble and all the other heart and vascular disorders. If you are overweight, you *should* worry about the possibilities of high blood pressure. The first and best preventive is to get back to your normal weight. Without any if's, and's and but's. Skip the desserts and the white flour products. Eat meals high in protein. Take your food supplements.

These same rules hold true for those who fear hypertension whether they are overweight or not. High blood pressure is a modern disease and we can't help but feel that the largest part of the responsibility for this killer must lie in our modern devitalized, refined diets. Shun processed foods—white flour, white sugar, packaged, canned, prepared foods. Eat fresh foods—out of your own garden if it is at all possible. Cook foods simply, with as little heat as possible. Eat everything raw that can be eaten raw. Take your food supplements: fish liver oil for vitamins A and D, brewer's yeast and/or desiccated liver for all the B vitamins, rose hip preparations for natural vitamins C and P, wheat germ oil, natural vitamin E and bone meal for minerals.

Blood Pressure, High and Overweight

There seems to be no doubt that they are related and furthermore that reducing one will probably also reduce the other.

Everyone knows, in general, that overweight is unhealthful. It has been called by many physicians America's number one health problem. Statistics are constantly being quoted by insurance companies to show that overweight individuals are more susceptible to the degenerative diseases of middle and old age. Or should we say that the tendency to overweight seems to accompany a predisposition to the various degenerative diseases? Or do we mean simply that people who overeat are digging their graves with their teeth?

We know that overweight individuals are much more likely to die of cancer or heart trouble. What about high blood pressure? Is it, too, a condition which overweight makes worse?

Risk Appraisal, a book published by the National Underwriter Company, is a study of "the factors that determine length of life and the fulness thereof," according to its author, Harry Dingman. In the pages of *Risk Appraisal,* we find that blood pressure is in general higher when weight is higher. In an analysis which was done of 9,926 unselected life insurance policy holders it was found that all of them showed an increase in blood pressure with increasing age and weight.

Generally, increasing weight goes along with increasing age. It doesn't have to, of course. In the table accompanying this information we find that from the age of 10 to 60 higher blood pressure went along with overweight:

Age	10	20	30	40	50	60
			Blood Pressure			
Underweight	116	120	120	122	128	135
Normal weight	117	122	123	125	133	145
Overweight	120	125	125	128	137	152

Mr. Dingman asks "if 1000 heavyweight persons average higher blood pressure than 1000 lesser weight persons, will 1000 persons show step-up of blood pressure when they become heavier? And, conversely, will there be decrease of blood pressure with decrease in weight? Answer is yes."

He goes on to tell us that decreases in blood pressure reading with loss of weight are less than increases with gain of weight. In other words, if you are overweight and should decide to lose weight partly to reduce your blood pressure, it won't be nearly so easy as it would have been to keep your weight normal or below normal—and your blood pressure, too.

He tells us that Emerson and Irving, writing in the *Journal of the American Medical Association,* volume 11, page 1174, 1938, describe an experimental study of 100 persons whose blood pressure was above 142. Fifty of these folks were overweight—an average of about 44 pounds. They reduced an average of eight pounds each and their blood pressure dropped an average of 19 points!

In an article on obesity and hardening of the arteries in the *Canadian Medical Journal* for March, 1954, we read of a study of post mortems that was done at Bellevue Hospital. S. L. Wilens studied 1,250 cases to determine whether the weight had anything to do with the progress of this disease. He found that between the age of 45 to 54, twenty per cent of obese individuals had advanced changes in the walls of their arteries. Only 6.7 per cent of those who were lean showed such changes. Between the ages of 65 to 74, the proportions were 45.4 per cent for the overweight patients and 20.2 per cent for the underweight ones.

How Fat Causes Ill Health

Another article mentioned in *Nutrition Reviews* for October, 1953, describes results of a survey among more than 3,000 employees of the Metropolitan Life Insurance Company, extending over 12 years. Between the ages of 35 to 44 high blood pressure was almost three times as common among the "fatties." Over the age of 45, it was twice as common. The article lists these three diseases as the leading causes of high mortality among the obese: diabetes, hypertension (high blood pressure) and atherosclerosis (hardening of the arteries).

How do you suppose added fat can be responsible for the much greater incidence and severity of these diseases of the blood vessels? For one thing, we must assume that obesity is an illness—the fat body is an unhealthy one. So perhaps the same things that produce fat also produce disorders of the circulation. Eating too much of the wrong kind of food is responsible for overweight. Could this also be the cause of high blood pressure? Perhaps those thin individuals who suffer from high blood pressure simply eat the wrong kind of food without eating enough of it to get fat.

Dr. D. D. Feller of the University of Washington School of Medicine is doing some research to determine, if he can, why and how fatty tissue shortens the lives of the overweight. According to *Newsweek* for April 12, 1954, Dr. Feller explains that the heart pumps blood through the vital organs about ten times as fast as it does through the muscles and fatty tissues. As the ratio of fat in the body increases, there is an even greater decrease in the rate at which the blood moves through the body.

By means of an elaborate machine, Dr. Feller is able to measure the actual volume of blood in his volunteer subjects. He has found that the amount of blood per unit of body weight is related to the sex of the individual and also to his degree of obesity. Women have less red-blood-cell volume in proportion to their weight than men. And the fatter you get, the less blood you have circulating around, in proportion to your body weight. Lean people contain about one and a half times as much blood per pound as obese people. Dr. Feller believes that the lesser amount of blood circulating in the stout people creates extra demands on the heart and probably is at least partly responsible for the tendency for heart and blood vessel disorders associated with excess weight. It's easy to see that the less blood it has to work with, in proportion to body weight, the harder time the heart would have getting it to circulate properly to all parts of the body.

We found an account of another experiment which seems to indicate, better than anything else could, just how much reduction in weight may have to do with decreased blood pressure. A. P. Fletcher, writing in *The Quarterly Journal of Medicine,* for July, 1954, describes an ambitious undertaking at the outpatient department of the London hospital in England. Overweight women were the subjects, because at this particular clinic they far outnumbered the men. Women were classified as "obese" when their weight was 20 per cent over the maximum ideal weight for their age and height. They were called "hypertensive" if their blood pressure was above 150/100.

A diet providing 600 calories a day was given to all the women, and the doctors "tried to persuade the patients to keep to it." Toward the end of the dieting period, the calory count was raised to 1000. The doctors suspected that, even in the case of the women who managed to reduce their weight considerably, the diet probably was closer to 1000 calories throughout rather than 600. But, no matter whether they ate 600 or 1000 calories a day, the women did lose weight. And as they lost weight, their blood pressure went down. The blood pressure of those who did not diet and did not lose weight did not go down. So there seems to be no doubt, according to Dr. Fletcher, that the overweight was at least partly responsible for the high blood pressure and that reducing the weight also reduced the pressure.

Reducing Weight and Blood Pressure

It seems to us that this fact is of paramount importance for all of us who are overweight and hypertensive. Regardless of what the doctor may be giving us to lower blood pressure, regardless of what we are doing in the way of rest, relaxation, special diets, and so forth, there is one ever-so-valuable thing we can do, on our own—reduce. We all know the general principles of how to lose weight. A diet high in protein, low in carbohydrates and fats will take off the pounds. There are many physicians who allow you to eat all you want on a reducing diet, provided only that you stick to certain foods and eliminate others completely.

A very simple reducing diet from the *British Medical Journal* for July 2, 1949, is by Dr. H. L. Marriott, who believes that a simplified diet where there is little or nothing to remember and no calories to count will be more successful than a complicated one. He also believes you should never go hungry on a diet. On Dr. Marriott's diet you may eat as much as you like of any of the following: lean meat, poultry, game, liver, kidney, heart, sweetbreads (cooked in any way but without the addition of bread crumbs, sauces or gravy) ; Fish (not canned. Boiled, steamed, broiled or baked only. No fats or sauces) ; Eggs (boiled or poached only) ; Potatoes (boiled, steamed, baked in skins but not fried, roasted, sauteed or chips) ; vegetables, any you wish except that no fat or butter shall be used in their preparation; salads, any and all, without mayonnaise or oil. Fruits (any kind, fresh or frozen, including bananas. Not dried fruits or fruits canned or frozen with sugar) ; clear soup, broth or bouillon, tea or coffee, up to half a pint of milk daily. No cream. No salt. Three very small slices of bread a day. *You may have absolutely nothing else whatsoever.*

Now surely such a variety of foods, of which you may eat all you wish could not impose any hardship on a dieter. In fact, we would suggest omitting the bread entirely. And of course, taking all your food supplements as usual—fish liver oils for vitamins A and D, brewer's yeast or desiccated liver for the B vitamins, rose hips for natural vitamin C, wheat germ oil and vitamin E, and bone meal. With such a diet you cannot possibly become deficient in any vitamin or mineral. Everything you eat will nourish you and you will not be cluttering up your digestive tract with refined, processed foods.

It seems to us that, if you are overweight and have high blood pressure, a diet such as this is bound to take off pounds and reduce blood pressure. If you have high blood pressure and are not overweight, try the diet anyway. We'll even go so far as to recommend the diet for folks suffering from low blood pressure as well. If disordered blood pressure is actually caused by bad eating habits, then it seems only reasonable that any disorder of blood pressure might be prevented by eating properly and healthfully.

Blood Pressure, Low

The individual who worries about his low blood pressure gets scant attention from medical researchers. Leafing through medical lists which contain just about all the medical articles published in the world, we page through whole sections devoted to high blood pressure—every aspect of it. Turning to "Low Blood Pressure" we find no articles at all listed. Apparently, down through the years, no one has considered low blood pressure of sufficient concern to do any investigating at all on the subject.

The viewpoint of the medical profession is that low blood pressure is a blessing, for if you have it you will probably never be afflicted with all the unpleasant symptoms of high blood pressure. Some physicians believe that a blood pressure of 90 is so low that something should be done about it. Others feel that a pressure of 100 to 110 is an indication that something is wrong. The insurance companies believe that a pressure as low as 100 or even 80 is perfectly compatible with good health, if that has always been your blood pressure. But if your average pressure is 120 and suddenly it goes down to 90 or 80, then probably there is something wrong.

Edward P. Jordan, M. D., expresses the feeling of the medical fraternity in his book *You and Your Health* (G. P. Putnam's Sons, 1954) when he says . . . "most of those with low blood pressure are well off and can expect a long life. There are few exceptions: there is a condition known as Addison's disease which, among other symptoms, is characterized by low blood pressure, but this is rare and there are only a few other things which have any serious significance . . . In most cases of below-normal blood pressure the cause seems to be exceptionally elastic arteries and this is a good thing. This generally means that hardening of the arteries will be slow to develop and this in turn has much to do with the expectation for a longer life."

Other medical books tell us that low blood pressure may be simply an indication of poor nutrition and it is often accompanied by low blood sugar, low basal metabolism, sub-normal temperature, anemia, or hypothyroidism (that is, a thyroid gland which does not send out enough of the gland secretion). In general, low blood pressure seems to go with people who do less of everything than other people do. That is, they may not eat enough or exercise enough which causes their glands to slow down and decrease their secretions. In cases of outright starvation, of course, the blood pressure is always low.

Postural Low Blood Pressure

One kind of low blood pressure has been dignified with a medical name—postural hypotension. Hypotension is, of course, low blood pressure, the opposite of hypertension or high blood pressure. Many of us are inclined to feel dizzy or light-headed when we stand up or sit up from a lying-down position. But the individual with postural hypotension is quite likely to have these symptoms to a serious degree. Any sudden change in posture necessitates a change in blood pressure all over the body. In some people the mechanism which adjusts this change is disordered. So, when they rise suddenly from a prostrate position the blood does not reach the brain rapidly enough, and they may faint or black out.

We must conclude, then, that hypotension is not a disease, but is rather a symptom that something may be wrong. Blood pressure may be low after a serious illness, such as an infectious disease, an acute fever or heart failure. In these cases, it disappears when the disease has been cured.

But suppose you are one of those people who feel weak and tired all the time, and suppose your blood pressure is low. The doctor may tell you that there is nothing to worry about. But do you want to go on feeling "all dragged out?" If there is indeed no disorder that is causing your low blood pressure it seems quite possible that good nutrition can easily raise it to the point where you will no longer feel tired.

In an experiment made about 12 years ago it was shown that lack of a B vitamin (thiamin) can cause low blood pressure. In this experiment, reported in the *Archives of Internal Medicine,* volume LXIX, 1942, a number of volunteers agreed to live on a diet in which there was no thiamin. They ate a diet which many people live on in America today—white bread, canned fruits and vegetables, meat, potatoes, sugar, coffee and so forth. The doctors who conducted the experiment even gave them brewer's yeast so that they would not be deficient in the other B vitamins. But they destroyed the thiamin in the brewer's yeast. In addition, the volunteers got supplements containing vitamins A and D, iron, calcium and phosphorus.

The results were astounding. Without exception the volunteers suffered from personality changes as well as physical symptoms. They became tired, grouchy, inefficient, forgetful. Physically, they became constipated and sleepless; they developed neuritis. Their hearts beat abnormally and became enlarged. Their digestive tracts developed all kinds of disorders. Most important of all, from the point of view of our discussion, *they all developed low blood pressure.* The experiment had to be stopped in less than six months for it would perhaps have been fatal had it been carried on longer. As soon as they took some thiamin the symptoms began to disappear and before long they all felt fine once again.

High Protein Diet Important

The second wrong diet that can produce low blood pressure is one in which there is not enough first-class protein. The blood vessels are made of protein, remember, as are the other parts of the body and if enough protein is not available in the diet to keep them from being flabby they will gradually waste away, just as muscles do. By protein, we mean chiefly protein from animal foods—meat, fish, and eggs, because these are the proteins that contain all of the essential amino acids or building blocks which our bodies need. Protein from vegetables, fruits and nuts is good, too, but these foods are not so rich in protein as the foods from animal sources and, too, they do not all contain all of the essential amino acids.

If you eat a diet which is lacking in protein you may possibly invite a shortage of thiamin—so there would be two good reasons for low blood pressure. For, on a low protein diet, you are bound to eat more starchy and sweet food, if you are eating anything at all. Starches and sweets must be accompanied by thiamin so that your body can use them. Hence the more starches and sweets you eat, the more thiamin you need. If you eat refined carbohydrates (white flour, white sugar and processed cereals) then you are bound to be short on thiamin, for the thiamin has been removed from all these foods along with other vitamins and minerals.

What We Recommend

If you are worried for fear your blood pressure is too low, we would suggest first of all that you make certain you have no underlying disorder that is responsible. If there seems to be no good reason for your hypotension, then concentrate on your diet and make it a good one. From the Superintendent of Documents in Washington, D. C., you can secure Agriculture Handbook Number 8 (Composition of Foods) which lists all the common foods according to protein content, giving as well their content of starch, fat, vitamins and minerals. With this book at hand you can easily figure out just how much protein you get a day and incidentally how much thiamin.

The official recommendation from the National Research Council is 70 to 100 grams of protein a day. But it is pretty generally agreed that this is a low estimate and that most of us would be a lot healthier if we got more, especially if we have had a deficiency in it. Sit down with your Handbook and a pencil and figure out everything you eat in one day in terms of its protein content. You will probably be surprised to find that you are getting far less than you should.

As you increase the protein in your diet, you will automatically increase the B vitamins, too, for they occur in foods that are high in protein—liver, eggs, milk, whole wheat and so forth. And, too, if you eat a lot of protein you will simply not have room for all the sweet and starchy foods that are bad for you. Take to serving nuts and fruit for dessert. Eat only bread made from real whole wheat flour. Eat two eggs for breakfast instead of one. These are suggestions for improving the protein content of your meals which is bound to improve your general health and hence your blood pressure.

Bone Meal After Middle Age

Calcium and other minerals seem to be even more important for the elderly than for the children.

When we were babies our mothers carefully measured every spoonful of food and followed the pediatrician's orders in respect to cod liver oil, orange juice, milk, cereal and so forth. One of the most important food elements is calcium—our mothers knew that. So most of us grew up with straight bones and fairly good teeth, regardless of what happened to those teeth later in life. But as we grow older, how many of us pay any attention at all to this extremely important matter of getting enough calcium? And, if there are older people living in the house with us, how much attention do we pay to the amount of calcium they are getting?

Of course older people don't need calcium for growing bones and teeth, as children do. But calcium has many, many uses in the body aside from healthy growth. And for all of these it must be supplied in food which, in the case of older people, is usually woefully lacking in this important mineral. We take for granted these days that a fall means a certain broken bone for an older person. Why? Their bones are brittle, we say. But must they be brittle? If proper attention is paid to diet, why is it not possible to keep the calcium level high in older people as well as in children, so that they need not suffer from broken bones that will not knit, as well as all the other distressing symptoms, such as nervousness, that lack of calcium brings about.

A recent study reported in *Nutrition Reviews,* June, 1953, showed the actual calcium intake of a group of 33 women and 5 men between the ages of 68 and 96 who were living in an institution. Most of them were suffering from heart disease, senility, central nervous system disorders or blood vessel diseases. Their daily calcium intake was between .2 and 1.1 grams, and their phosphorus intake between .45 to 1.7 grams. Of those subjects who took .5 grams or less, 74 per cent revealed X-ray evidence of loss of bone calcium, which of course would lead to "brittle bones." Among those who took every day over .5 grams of calcium the incidence of soft, brittle bones was only 14 per cent. About the same results were found when the phosphorus content of bone was investigated.

Dr. Clive McCay of the Laboratory of Animal Nutrition at Cornell University tells us in *Vitamins and Hormones,* Vol. VII, published by Academic Press, that it appears that women from the ages of 52 to 74 years need a gram of calcium per day if they are to maintain their body stores of the mineral—that is, if they want to keep their bones hard, their nerves healthy. He says that another investigation reported in the *Journal of the American Dietetic Association,* vol. 24, page 292, indicates that a group of elderly women living in an institution were getting only .4 to .7 grams of calcium daily—or only four tenths to seven tenths of the amount required. Another woman who lived alone and ate a diet which was rich in starch and sugar was losing regularly more than 100 milligrams of calcium a day. Another who was often emotionally upset lost calcium during her periods of depression and regained it again when she began to feel more cheerful.

The Older We Are the Less Likely We Are To Assimilate All the Calcium in Our Foods

In Dr. McCay's experiments with animals, the oldsters were compared with the youngsters in their ability to absorb dietary calcium. Young animals could store about 78 to 88 per cent of the calcium they ate, he found. But animals old enough to compare with human beings of fifty could not generally even maintain what calcium they had in their bodies, let alone store any more. In other words, they were constantly losing calcium.

A lot of fat in the diet of the older animals appeared to make them lose more calcium and at a faster rate. Then, too, the older animals did not seem to be able to select the proper diet when they were left to their own choice. Young rats will be very careful about their diet and will be certain they have had enough food containing the necessary vitamins and minerals, before they will touch such worthless foods as sugar. But older rats appear to lose their power of discrimination and will turn greedily to a sugar solution, neglecting the healthful food put before them. They will continue to do this even while they die of malnutrition, says Dr. McCay.

From these observations it would appear there are two absolute necessities in the care of older people—and these are just as essential, if not more so, than in the care of infants. They need large amounts of calcium in their diets, for they have just as much need of it as children have and they lose it at a faster rate. Then, too, if they have lost the ability to choose foods that are good for them, their diets must be supervised as closely as infants' diets, to make certain they are not trying to stay alive on starch and sugar.

Many researchers have found that older people tend to have less hydrochloric acid in their stomachs than younger people. This digestive juice is necessary for the assimilation of calcium, and perhaps a lack of it explains why older animals lose calcium so rapidly. A diet rich in all the vitamins, especially the B vitamins, appears to be the best guarantee of ample hydrochloric acid in the stomach. It has been found, for instance, that lack of thiamin or of niacin in the diet results in lessening the hydrochloric acid or gastric juice available for the digestion of food.

Dr. McCay then takes up the question of whether or not hardening of the arteries and calcium deposits in the kidneys can be caused by too much calcium in the diet. We are glad to repeat here exactly what Dr. McCay has to say on this subject (and remember, please, that Dr. McCay is one of the country's outstanding authorities on nutrition, with many books and articles to his credit): "In the course of two decades of research with rats we have seen groups at the time of death with heavily calcified arteries and kidneys while parallel groups were relatively free. This calcification of soft tissues was due to unknown variables in the diet and could never be related to dietary calcium."

Lack of vitamin C may be largely responsible for kidney stones and other misuses of calcium by the body. But we have never been able to find a shred of evidence to show that too much calcium could be the cause. On the contrary, all the experiments and the surveys show beyond the possibility of a doubt that our diets today are grossly deficient in calcium and that it would take many times what we receive in food or food supplements to approximate even an optimum amount!

Two Ways of Getting Plenty of Good Calcium, Very Inexpensively

Dr. McCay tells us that one of the most serious aspects of the diet of older people in institutions is the great quantity of bread they consume. This is partly because we have been led to believe that bread is the staff of life, partly because bread is cheap, and partly because older people who lack teeth or dentures can eat soft white bread more easily than most other solid foods. White bread is a mockery of good food. What then can older people eat that will be rich in calcium, easy to chew and not expensive?

We nominate marrow bone soup as the answer to the problem. Any butcher will give you a marrow bone absolutely free, especially if you tell him you want it for the dog. Beyond this you need nothing but free water (or juices in which vegetables have been cooked) and a stove to manufacture one of the most nutritious foods imaginable. Have the bone sawed or split if you can, for the more cut areas available, the more calcium will be poured out of your soup bone into the soup. Add just a dash of vinegar when you put the bone on to boil. This acid will cause more calcium to be deposited from the bone into the liquid. You can let the bone boil as long or as short a time as you wish. The calcium and other minerals from the bone will stay right there in the soup until you are ready to eat it. If you add vegetables, cut them up rapidly and let them cook just long enough to become tender. Wouldn't you say this is a remarkably cheap way of obtaining calcium?

To make certain of an ample supply of calcium every single day, whether there is marrow bone soup for dinner or not, older people should take bone meal. We wish it were possible to convince every reader thoroughly on one point—bone meal is not a medicine. It is a food. Our ancestors regarded bone as an important food. In many parts of the world today bones are eaten as regularly as any other food. Bone meal is simply whole bone ground up so that we do not have to chew it. It contains nothing more.

Now surely no one would be afraid to eat marrow bone soup every day because it might turn him into a stiff calcium deposit. So why should anyone hesitate to take bone meal for fear he might get too much calcium? In three bone meal tablets a day he gets, we suppose, just about the same amount of calcium and other minerals he would get from a two-day supply of marrow bone soup.

In the case of old people, especially, we think bone meal is the ideal answer to sufficient calcium. For they *are* fussy about what they eat. Their eating habits have been established for many years and it may take a great deal of skill and persuasion to change them. An infant can eat only what we give them, but grandma has access to the refrigerator and the candy store. So if she complains about eating foods rich in calcium, or if she really cannot properly digest milk, cheese or raw vegetables, let the marrow bone soup and bone meal tablets every day keep her calcium store up to the level where you will not have to worry about broken bones.

Bone Meal and Minerals

This inexpensive food supplement supplies all the minerals necessary for good nutrition.

Bones were used in the diet of man earlier in history than milk was used. Primitive man hunted and fished long before he domesticated any animals from which he might obtain milk. Undoubtedly he ate the fish bones and as much of the animal bones as he could chew. Then he pounded the larger bones into powder so that they could be eaten easily. In many countries today bones are eaten right along with meat or fish and bone meal is a valued food, especially for pregnant or nursing mothers who, of course, have a great demand for lots of minerals.

We have published many articles on bone meal, as well as a booklet *Bone Meal for Human Consumption* (Rodale Press, Emmaus, Pa., price 65 cents). And every time we look back through our files we find even more information on the subject of just how much good bone meal can do in human diets. We think it is in order, right here, to point out that bone meal, taken instead of milk, will supply all the minerals in a form that is just as easily assimilated by the body.

Here is an analysis of minerals in a typical sample of bone meal as furnished by the U. S. Department of Agriculture:

	Per Cent		*Per Cent*
Sodium oxide	.46	Lead oxide	.005
Potassium oxide	.20	Zinc oxide	.018
Calcium oxide	30.52	Chlorine	.22
Magnesium oxide	.73	Phosphoric oxide	22.52
Barium oxide	.001	Boron oxide	trace
Copper oxide	.0005	Fluorine	.043
Iron oxide	.004	Iodine	.00002
Manganese oxide	.0014	Sulfur	.25

It is almost impossible to compare the mineral content of milk with that of bone meal since the bone is more than half mineral while only .7 per cent of milk is mineral, due to the large amount of water, fat, carbohydrate, protein and so forth in milk.

In the *Journal of Nutrition* for February 10, 1953, two researchers from the Department of Animal Husbandry at Cornell University report on their experiments with fresh bone. They say, "Drake and others made studies on foods containing fresh bone prepared for us in Europe and, using balance trials on human subjects, compared the availability of bone calcium with that of milk and found them nearly equal under the conditions of their experiment." This research was reported in *The Journal of Nutrition,* volume 37, page 397.

Dr. McCay and Udall from Cornell go on to report that the animals fed with fresh bone in their experiments absorbed about 56 per cent of the calcium of the ground bone, and about 49 per cent of the phosphorus. These are the two basic minerals, most important from the nutritional standpoint. Of course all the trace minerals (boron, zinc, copper, etc.) were also present in the bone and, we presume, were absorbed.

The four researchers mentioned by Dr. McCay and Dr. Udall have this to say about bones in the diet: "Present human dietaries are largely dependent on milk and milk products to supply the bulk of this calcium. This, however, was obviously not the case centuries ago, as man in the past, in common with other carnivora, was dependent on animal and fish bones for a large portion of his calcium intake. Today many aboriginal people still depend on bone as their chief source of calcium. Bone also supplies many other minerals essential for normal nutrition.

"In many areas of the world the supply of milk and milk products is not sufficient to provide the recommended dietary allowances for calcium. During and immediately after the last war a large proportion of the canned meat products prepared in Canada for U. N. R. R. A. contained 15 per cent of cooked ground bone; this resulted in the final canned meat containing approximately .8 grams of calcium per 100 grams. Today all flour sold in Newfoundland, where the consumption of milk is small, contains ½ of 1 per cent bone meal. For many years bone meal has been an ingredient of certain infant cereal products."

Fluorine in Bone Meal

In the light of the present hullabaloo over water fluoridation, it is interesting to go back and read an article that appeared in the *Journal of the American Dental Association* for February 1, 1947. This article discusses the opinion of the Council on Dental Therapeutics of the A. D. A. so far as bone meal is concerned. These gentlemen say that the "basis for their use (bone meal preparations) is the assumption that active tooth decay is, to a significant extent, a manifestation of individual or combined deficiencies of calcium, phosphorus, fluorine and vitamin D. Although it may be conceded that these dietary factors, with the possible exception of fluorine, are essential during the development of the teeth, available evidence does not indicate whether they are important after tooth formation is completed. Despite the array of reports attributing to fluorine a caries-inhibiting role, analysis of the literature on this subject discloses a lack of conclusive information. This lack renders largely presumptive any course of treatment in which fluorides, natural or synthetic, are ingested to influence the incidence and severity of the disease."

Yet only a few years later, the American Dental Association was officially on record in favor of water fluoridation as the greatest find of the century for preventing tooth decay! Anyone who says a word against fluoridated water is a crackpot, according to them. Yet they themselves announced, in 1947, that fluorine probably didn't have anything to do with preventing tooth decay. They were talking of the fluorine in bone meal of course. Now if the fluorine in fluoridated water can do such a remarkable job of preventing tooth decay as the officials of the Dental Association now feel it does, why not admit officially that the fluorine in bone meal may possibly perform the same function?

It has been shown experimentally that calcium, taken along with fluorine, protects against the poisonous action of the fluorine. Drinking fluoridated water does not guarantee any calcium supply at all. But in bone meal the calcium comes right along with the fluorine. Fluorine in bone meal is in the form of calcium fluoride. The fluorine compound used for fluoridating water is sodium fluoride, which does not appear anywhere in nature. Sodium fluoride is used because it is more soluble in water. This means that your body undoubtedly assimilates more of the fluorine in this form than it could if the fluorine were in the form of calcium fluoride, which is less soluble.

Most of the foods you eat contain fluorine. Two and a half quarts of milk contain about the same amount of fluorine you would get from a day's recommended ration of bone meal. Which, incidentally, is far, far less than you will get by drinking the average amount of fluoridated water per day and which is also in the form of calcium fluoride, not nearly so soluble—meaning that your body takes up far less of it.

Bone meal is recommended for canker sores in the standard reference book, *Dietetics for the Clinician* edited by Harry J. Johnson, M. D. (published by Lea and Febiger). The editor tells us that you can generally get rid of a canker sore within forty-eight hours with a fifteen-grain dose of bone phosphate twice a day. Do you suppose that the national incidence of canker sores is nothing more or less than a symptom of our national deficiency in minerals which bone meal supplies in such abundance?

We have published in this book and in our booklet on Bone Meal, much evidence of the healthfulness of taking bone meal. Physicians have used it—not to prevent but to cure long-standing and critical cases of bone diseases; one physician used it at her hospital for new mothers and their children, to prevent cramps, growing pains, pregnancy complications and tooth decay. A dentist gave it to patients at a mental hospital with the result that tooth decay stopped overnight in these patients, without any other treatment at all. We believe that far more research of this kind should be done with bone meal. But meanwhile those of us who know about bone meal should certainly be taking it, for we cannot get in any other food the concentration of minerals—natural, well-balanced minerals—that we get in bone meal. All the minerals that are in milk are in bone meal, just as easily assimilated and just as well used by the body.

What Some People Say About Bone Meal

Here are some comments from users of bone meal:

Dr. E. H. Eden, a dentist of St. Louis, writes us:

"I have been interested in preventive dentistry for many years, and I realize you are doing a great deal to enlighten and educate readers to the cause of disease and decay of the teeth. You are to be congratulated for your good work.

"I have been interested in the use of bone meal since reading the article by Dr. Elizabeth Martin of Canada in 1944. Since 1944 a relative's boy has been taking bone meal tablets. He will be eight years old in June and the permanent teeth are so strong. The temporary teeth have had only four cavities. I have been eating bone meal since I was about seven years old. I'm now past 65 and have most of my teeth."

Lane White of Louisiana tells us:

"One suggestion contained in the magazine has proved very beneficial—the taking of bone meal as a preventive of poison ivy—plus, of course, a reduction in the amount of cereals eaten. I have not entirely refrained from eating bread and other cereals. But I have been taking bone meal and have not had poison ivy since early spring when I started taking it. Living in the middle of a field of it, I customarily have a constant case of it all summer long."

Another letter about bone meal came to us from Pearl Hunt of Napa, California:

"About eight months ago I wrote you asking if bone meal would help a broken bone. You couldn't say as to that, but you did indicate that it couldn't do any harm, or something to that effect. Three years ago I had a compound fracture. It was very slow in healing. I wish I had known about bone meal then. After a year I could walk, but had to be very careful. Last May I began taking bone meal. Two months went by and then one day I suddenly felt new strength in my leg. I could feel it getting stronger every day for three days. Today, six and a half months from the time I started on bone meal, my leg feels almost as good as ever, thanks to you. It certainly does help a broken bone. And too, for the last month my nails have not been breaking."

Bones

A modern physician finds among old commentaries on scurvy a possible clue to our many bone and joint disorders.

For people as supposedly healthy as the present-day Americans, there seems to be little reason why any of us should suffer from bone disorders. Yet how many people do you know who complain of a sacroiliac "condition," a slipping kneecap or "trouble" with the vertebral discs? These are the discs made of fibers and cartilage that are between the vertebral bones which make up our spines.

We customarily think of minerals in connection with bones and hence, mineral deficiency in connection with bone disorders. True, the bones are made up largely of minerals, but if the mechanical system whereby our bones move and work is going to function perfectly there are other elements necessary. Not the least of these is vitamin C which is intimately concerned with the health of our connective tissues. Vitamin C assists in the formation of a substance called "collagen" which maintains the stability and elasticity of all the connective tissues—bones, cartilage, muscles and the tissues of the blood vessels. Collagen is that jelly-like substance in bone from which gelatin is made.

W. J. McCormick, M.D., of Toronto, Canada, has recently published an article in *The Archives of Pediatrics,* January, 1954, which we believe might very well revolutionize our present ideas about bone and joint disorders. Not once in the article does he mention minerals. He deals entirely with the subject of the connecting tissues that hold the bone together and connect it to other bones and to muscles. He is discussing the subject of "Intervertebral Disc Lesions"—that is, disorders of the small cartilage discs that separate the vertebral bones in the spine. He tells us that we have recently become aware of how widespread are these disorders. Even though they may have been very common years ago, they were probably unsuspected because X-ray was not known then. He also tells us that the whole spinal column is so bound up with tissues and ligaments that usually post-mortem examinations or laboratory dissections are not thorough enough to sort out this mass and disclose much that is revealing about the discs themselves.

Most commonly, he tells us, vertebral discs give trouble when they "slip" (out of place) or when the outer part of the disc is ruptured and the pulpy part in the center oozes out. Either of these may disable the spinal nerves that are so close to them. Up to now we have thought that such conditions resulted from accidents or falls. Some physicians thought the condition was congenital—that is, a defect present at birth.

Then, too, some researchers say that slipping of the discs is just the result of old age—a degenerative condition that must be expected. But, says Dr. McCormick, disc disorders are most common today in the forties, are known in the twenties and have been reported even in children and adolescents. From a carefully correlated study of the nutritional background of people who have these disorders and from studying the condition of these pieces of cartilage in cases of scurvy, Dr. McCormick has come to the conclusion that deficiency of vitamin C plays an important part in these disorders.

Ancient Researches on Scurvy

He quotes Dr. James Lind of Edinborough who wrote a description of scurvy some two hundred years ago. As you know, scurvy is a disease caused by lack of vitamin C in the diet. Dr. Lind said that the muscles of a scurvy patient are so lax and tender that they readily fall apart, the muscles of the intestines are also lax and limp and, he goes on to say, "why the scurvy should so frequently and in so singular a manner affect the cartilages of the ribs, so as sometimes to separate them altogether from their connection with the breast bone, and why it seats itself so commonly in the joint of the knee, I own I am at a loss to account for."

A Dr. Willis who wrote of scurvy in 1667 in England related that many times in observing scurvy patients, he had heard a crackling of the bones even when the patient moved in bed. The great French surgeon, Poupart, writing in 1699, stated that in some scurvy patients he could hear a small grating of the bones. In others he could hear a "small low noise" when they breathed. In these latter patients he found at post mortem examination that they had "their ribs thus separated from the cartilages, and the bony part of the ribs next to the sternum was carious (dead tissue) . . . the ligaments of the joints throughout the body were corroded and loose. Instead of finding in the cavities of the joints the usual sweet oily mucilage there was only a greenish liquor."

Says Dr. McCormick, if such dreadful bone, joint and cartilage conditions were prevalent among scurvy patients in times past, why should our present-day slight deficiency of vitamin C not result in similar symptoms, only not quite so serious? Our modern difficulties with dislocated or ruptured discs are exactly like those reported in scurvy cases many years ago—only not serious enough to cause death. In every modern case, he says, there is evidence of loss of stability of the connective tissues which is apparently the plain and simple result of lack of vitamin C.

What! in our day and age when everybody is aware of how important it is to eat fresh fruits and vegetables? In our modern enlightened times when all infants get their orange juice so that they can't possibly be deficient in vitamin C? Yes, says Dr. McCormick, and this is the reason why. True, the infants are regularly fed their vitamin C. But what about the children at grade school level, at high school level? What about the young adults who substitute cokes, chocolate bars and hot dogs for the vitamin-C-rich juices their mothers made them take when they were infants? What about the adults whose diets include alcohol, tea and coffee and who finish off their meals with pastries or cake rather than fresh fruit or vegetables from which they would get at least some vitamin C?

Are We Vitamin C Deficient?

Then Dr. McCormick tells us that in fifteen years of his own practice he tested more than 5,000 patients for vitamin C status and found that less than 10 per cent of the adults had the optimum amount of vitamin C in their blood at any given time. Very few of these 5,000 folks are being treated for scurvy. They are not in bed, suffering from the complete and possibly fatal collapse that scurvy might bring on. But how many of them are going about their daily business suffering from countless bone, joint and cartilage disorders that may be the result of *just a little less vitamin C than they need?*

One reason for this widespread deficiency may very well be smoking, says Dr. McCormick. Vitamin C is rapidly used up in the presence of infections and also poisons from without the body. In his own laboratory he has found that smoking one cigarette neutralizes 25 milligrams of vitamin C in the body. An orange contains about this amount of vitamin C. He has also found, he says, that all his patients suffering from intervertebral disc disorders are heavy smokers, and, according to chemical tests, are sadly lacking in vitamin C. He suggests (for of course his article was written for doctors to read) that ample doses of vitamin C should be made part of the treatment for disorders of the vertebral discs and other cartilagenous disorders. It is conceivable, he says, that such means might result in fixing the discs, so that they would no longer "slip" or rupture.

This theory of Dr. McCormick's and the facts he presents from old medical texts, written when scurvy was a very common disease, lead us to speculate on vitamin C as a possible preventive for all kinds of joint disorders even including rheumatism and bursitis. If, as these old-time physicians found, scurvy affected the cartilages of the ribs, the knee-joint and the spine in such a way that even the fluid in the joints seemed diseased, why might not many of our modern bone, cartilage and joint disorders spring from somewhat lesser deficiency of vitamin C—just not getting enough vitamin C to keep these tissues in good repair?

Vitamin C is abundant in fresh fruits and vegetables, but it is lost rapidly after they have been picked for marketing. To assure yourself of enough vitamin C you should have as much fresh raw or frozen fruit every day as you can comfortably eat. Certainly it should be dessert at every meal. In addition, you should have at least one large salad bowl of green, leafy vegetables every day. Any good nutrition book at your local library will give you the approximate amounts of vitamin C in common foods. Check your daily diet just to make sure. Then, because most of us are exposed to tobacco smoke whether or not we smoke ourselves and because we are also exposed to many other modern poisonous substances that use up our body's vitamin C rapidly, we should all take a natural food supplement rich in vitamin C—made from rose hips or green peppers.

Boric Acid

NOTICE — DANGER

Recent evidence shows that boric acid can be very toxic and actually cause death, even when applied externally. It may be absorbed through the broken skin or mucous membranes.
Despite the fact that in the past we have advised its use, in light of this information discard boric acid solutions, ointments and powders.

This notice appears in the reception room of a pediatric clinic in Rochester, New York. It reflects the recent thinking of the medical profession in regard to one of the oldest and most familiar medicine chest remedies to be found in American homes. How many of us have not used boric acid as an eyewash or a baby powder?

We have always believed that it was a mild, harmless, soothing powder which killed germs and somehow alleviated many irritated conditions of skin and other tissue. According to the latest information in medical journals it is not soothing, harmless or mild, it has very little germ-killing ability and it makes irritations worse even to the point of causing fatal complications.

Boric acid is made of boron (a non-metallic chemical element) hydrogen and oxygen. It occurs naturally in some parts of the world, in white transparent crystals, soluble in water and alcohol. Farther along in the medical dictionary appears the word "borism," which is boric acid or borax poisoning.

We do not eat boric acid, of course. But there have been cases of boric acid taken by mistake. One day in a northeastern hospital a jar of boric acid was mistakenly labeled "dextrose" and sent to the room where baby formulas were made. Twenty babies got boric acid in their formulas that day rather than dextrose. Thirty-six hours later all of them were dead. According to an editorial in *The International Medical Digest* for September, 1953, "The most striking symptom brought out . . . was a marked irritation of the central nervous system. The appearance was that of a severe meningitis." In the babies most severely poisoned, there was also intense redness of the skin very much like a burn. The editorial pleads for a poison label on boric acid, like the labels now used in carbolic acid and mercuric chloride. Instead of which, of course, boric acid can be bought at any drugstore, with a plain label. And, since it has always been considered a necessity in infant care, boric acid can very easily be at hand in home nurseries where the same mistake may be made by unsuspecting mothers. So a poison label is the best we can ask for.

It is a common practice to "sterilize" the nipples of nursing bottles with boric acid. Fatalities have been reported from this practice, too, even though only a tiny amount of the acid remained on the nipple. In one case a baby who was being breast-fed was poisoned because the mother's breast had been washed with a boric acid solution.

Boric Acid Applied Externally

More common, however, are the cases where boric acid is used on the skin, and, especially in the case of infants, results can be fatal. In our file we have many clippings relating to the deaths of infants from boric acid used on their skin. *The American Journal of Diseases of Children* for October, 1951, tells the story of a nine-months old girl suffering from a diaper rash. Her father used nine ounces of boric acid on the diapers and skin of the child. She died 26 hours after she was admitted to the hospital. Her symptoms were terrifying. Vomiting, bloody stools, coma and convulsions were general symptoms. In addition her skin erupted into a bright red rash—not just on the area where the boric acid had been powdered, but all over her body. After the death it was found that the severest kind of damage had been done to her entire digestive tract. "Boric acid and sodium borate are sufficiently poisonous to cause severe symptoms and death when used in amounts commonly considered to be harmless. . . . Boric acid is readily absorbed by different routes and is particularly insidious in that symptoms may be minimal until a lethal or near lethal dose has been absorbed . . . there is no known specific treatment for boric acid poisoning . . ." say C. Brooke and T. Boggs, authors of the article.

In *Pediatrics,* December, 1949, Harold Abramson, M.D., of New York City writes of the poisoning of a newborn infant. When the child's buttocks became reddened from a slight case of diarrhea, her mother applied boric acid ointment and dusted boric acid powder in the child's diaper. She died twelve hours after admission to the hospital. Lungs, kidneys, bladder, brain, liver and intestines were found to be badly damaged. Says Dr. Abramson, "Boric acid is not a mild and harmless drug. It is quickly absorbed into the body and, in proper amounts, may readily cause toxicity and death. In addition, boric acid exhibits a selective affinity for certain organs, such as the brain and spinal cord. When consideration is given to the extensive use of boric acid in various forms, it is surprising that more instances of poisoning have not been reported. It is possible that many cases have occurred unsuspected. . . . The doubtful benefits that are derived therapeutically from boric acid hardly justify its continued use, particularly when many more effective drugs are available."

What Can You Do About Boric Acid?

Other writers on boric acid agree with Dr. Abramson that probably far more cases of boric acid poisoning have not been diagnosed as such, partly because its use is so taken for granted that mothers would not think to mention it as a possible contributing cause of illness.

Medical literature contains many, many more articles on boric acid poisoning, in adults as well as children. Boric acid may be used for several days or several weeks before symptoms of poisoning appear. In some cases death has occurred after the patient had stopped using the drug and also had stopped excreting it in the urine. So it appears that the action is cumulative. It seems, too, that the harm done by the poisoning cannot be reversed, even though all the boric acid is eventually excreted. Dr. Brooke and Dr. Boggs, in the article in the *American Journal of Diseases of Children,* say "It would appear that lethal quantities are found only when (boric acid) is ingested accidentally, administered parenterally (that is, by other methods than by mouth) or applied to a previously injured or diseased skin surface. The therapeutic value of boric acid is doubtful and its antiseptic quality minimal. There are better and safer substances available for uses as antiseptics, irrigations, wet dressings and ointments. For this reason, boric acid or boric acid solutions have not been stocked on any of the floors, nurseries or treatment rooms of Strong Memorial Hospital or Rochester Municipal Hospital."

Undoubtedly readers have decided by this time to throw away any boric acid in the medicine chest and not replace it. However there is more to it than that. Boron compounds are used in other products you may buy at the drug store—baby powders, for instance. Look at the label carefully. If it says that boric acid is included in the substance, or if it says that the substance is "borated," this is not for you.

Boric acid is the time-honored eye-wash to use as a home remedy for anything that goes wrong with an eye, from an embedded cinder to conjunctivitis Let's say you've just removed some pesky piece of dirt from your eye, leaving it inflamed and sore. You want to wash it soothingly in your eye cup. What should you use in place of boric acid? Doctors say use just plain water that has been boiled and cooled, nothing else. Of course if there is something more seriously wrong with the eye, you will be seeing a doctor.

Botulism

The following article, reprinted from *California's Health,* March 15, 1954, published by the California State Department of Public Health, shows us clearly that the danger of botulism poisoning is not a thing of the past and should be kept in mind, especially during the home-canning season.

Home-canned Peaches Blamed for Botulism Death

California's first recorded cases of botulism from home-canned peaches resulted in three deaths in San Diego recently. The first two fatalities were those of a man and wife whose illness had been diagnosed as due to other conditions. The tragedy was compounded when two sisters of the dead woman came to attend the funeral and presumably ate from the same jar of toxic peaches which they had found opened in the refrigerator Both became ill, and one died. A son of the dead couple, his wife and one of their two children also ate at the later meal when the peaches were served, but did not develop symptoms. The two sisters were treated with botulinus antitoxin after their symptoms appeared. The son and his family were treated prophylactically with the antitoxin.

Laboratory tests of sampled foods taken from the household yielded Clostridium botulinus toxin, Type A, from the opened jar of peaches.

According to records of botulism cases compiled for the United States and Canada by Dr. Karl F. Myer and Dr. Bernice Eddie of the George Williams Hooper Foundation, University of California, there are only two other instances reported in which canned peaches have been found to be the cause of botulism cases. Both of these instances were in New Mexico; one in 1944 when there were two fatal cases "due to home-canned peaches and pickles," and the other in 1947 when four fatal cases were traced to "home-canned peaches."

Acid fruits and vegetables are seldom the source of botulism toxin. However, if contaminating organisms which attack sugar are present the pH value may change sufficiently to produce conditions favorable for the production of botulinus toxin. When the peaches that caused these California deaths were tested the pH was found to be 5.0. At pH 4.9 and above there is practically no inhibition of toxin formation.

In the investigation of the San Diego cases, relatives and neighbors stated that the woman who died had not followed recommended procedures for canning fruits and vegetables under steam pressure.

Events as reconstructed in the investigation by the San Diego County Health Department were as follows:

The husband was the first to become ill, on the evening of January 8th. His symptoms included vomiting and paralysis of the tongue. He was admitted to the hospital at 5:30 a. m. January 9th, and died at 10:15 a. m. On the evening of January 9th, his wife developed respiratory difficulties and loss of voice. During the night she developed pronounced respiratory distress and exhibited symptoms of ocular and pharyngeal paralysis. She was dead on arrival at the hospital about noon on January 10th.

The two sisters of the dead woman arrived at the household on January 12th to attend the funeral. The son of the dead couple and his family also came for the funeral. On the afternoon of January 13th, following the funeral services, all of these people ate at the home and included in the food served was the jar of peaches which was already open when the sisters arrived.

Within 18 hours both sisters became ill with symptoms including vomiting, double vision, difficulty in swallowing, difficulty in talking and some respiratory difficulties They were admitted to a local hospital and the clinical diagnosis of botulism was made. Botulinus antitoxin was administered immediately. One sister recovered, but the other died on January 29th.

In California during the period from 1940-1953 there were 69 outbreaks involving 140 cases of botulism, with 76 deaths. Seven of these outbreaks were traced to home-canned fruit, involving 13 cases and six deaths. The fruits included apricots, pears, figs, cactus and huckleberries. Forty-one outbreaks were traced to home-canned vegetables—beets, beet greens, asparagus, chili peppers and string beans.

In 1953 there were only two cases of botulism reported in the State. Neither died. One case resulted from eating home-canned string beans and the other from home-canned huckleberry juice.

Brain

What makes you blush? That is, what exact physiological process takes place after you are embarrassed, resulting in a sudden scarlet on your face and neck? Blushing is caused by the vasoconstrictor center of your brain whose activity is temporarily shut off by your feeling of embarrassment, so that the tiny blood vessels in your face dilate with blood. This is called a "reflex" action, meaning that it happens without your conscious knowledge or consent and there is nothing you can do to stop it. So, in case you are trying to learn how not to blush—give it up. You can't.

This sample illustrates the incredible complexity of the brain. Scientists understand fairly well and are learning more every day about the physiological part of the brain—that is, they know that this vasoconstrictor device is located there, they can draw pictures of it, and they have studied it. But the psychic part of your brain is much more mysterious. In other words, what causes you to feel embarrassment? Why should you feel embarrassed over something that does not embarrass someone else? Why should the sound of certain words or music, or the sight of certain colors or forms have one effect on you and a completely different effect on someone else?

We know a number of physiologically important things about the brain. It is the most important section of the nervous system and in many, though not in all animals, it is concentrated in the head It is composed of about 16 billion cells. It consists of three main parts—the frontal part or cerebrum, the hind part or cerebellum and the medulla oblongata by which it is joined to the spinal cord and hence to all the nerves of the body. The brain of the average man weighs about 48 ounces. A woman's brain weighs a little less, but relative to body weight, there is no difference. It is true that extremely intelligent people sometimes have brains weighing a great deal more. But it is also true that brains weighing as much as 60 ounces have been found in idiots. It is believed that normal intelligence will not exist if the brain weighs less than 32 ounces.

When something happens to some part of your body, a nerve impulse travels to your brain. That is, an electrical current moves along a well-defined path to a certain part of your brain. This impulse may be permitted to die out along the way, your brain may suppress it, or may translate it into action. In your brain are centers for everything you do or feel. Perhaps the most important of these is the respiratory center which controls your breathing. There are olfactory, auditory, visual and taste centers which register your reactions to smells, sounds, sights and tastes. There are centers for speech, music, writing and other skills. There is a motor center which decides what movements you are going to make.

No single movement of any muscle of your body takes place without involving this particular center of your brain. The vasoconstrictor center keeps the walls of the blood vessels contracting. There are centers which control chewing, swallowing, coughing, sucking, sneezing, winking and so forth. The secretion of gastric juice in your stomach, the movements of the intestines during digestion are controlled from a center of the brain. Many of the activities your brain causes you to engage in are automatic or, as scientists call it, autonomic. Breathing and winking your eyelids, for example, go on all the time although you are seldom conscious of them. No one knows exactly the extent to which these centers of the brain are automatic and to what extent you can control them. After all, you can hold your breath, you can stop winking your eyelids if you concentrate on doing it. But at what point in the mechanism of your brain does your consciousness give over your feeling of embarrassment to the brain center that causes you to blush? No one knows.

We talk a lot in these pages about healthy nerves, their importance to your welfare and the things you can do to keep them healthy. Remember that whatever we say about nerves is true to an even greater extent of your brain. So what is good for your nerves is good for your brain. It has been discovered, for instance, that nerves tire more easily than muscles, for after a certain amount of effort the nerves will stop to rest. But an electrical stimulus will cause the muscles to go on working. So, like all nerve tissue, the brain gets tired. But, like all other tissues of the body, it must be exercised to stay in good trim. It's perfectly scientific for Dad to claim his brain is "rusty" when he tries to solve Junior's arithmetic problems. For perhaps Dad hasn't used those particular parts of his brain for years, while Junior probably exercises them every day at school.

Just like other cells of the body, brain cells need oxygen and food. The blood carries these to the brain, through four arteries. When there is not sufficient oxygen the brain cannot function and unconsciousness results. This may be because there is too little blood or because the blood does not contain enough oxygen. Temporary unconsciousness is called concussion. The food of the brain is chiefly blood sugar and this is why alarming symptoms of unconsciousness result when the level of sugar in the blood becomes unbalanced. Insulin shock produces unconsciousness by lowering the blood sugar.

Vitamins and minerals are important for brain nutrition, just as they are important for other parts of the body. The B vitamins are probably the most essential, for we know that they nourish nerve tissue especially. We also know that B vitamins can favorably affect some of the psychic functions of the brain. Depression, panic, anxiety are often symptoms of B vitamin deficiency. Then, too, tests have shown that at least one of the B vitamins (thiamin) influences the ability of children to learn. How? We don't know. Perhaps by supplying just the right nourishment to that part of the brain concerned with learning. A healthy brain means intelligence, a well-adjusted personality, efficiency, cheerfulness, success. If you desire these things for yourself and your family, better take another look at that dinner you're planning for tonight. Is there enough good, wholesale nourishment, are there enough B vitamins to guarantee healthy nerves and brain?

Bread

About fifty per cent of the American diet today consists of products made of white sugar and refined chemicalized white flour. We believe this may be an important reason for the enormous increase in degenerative diseases—cancer, heart disease, stomach ulcers, diabetes, arthritis, etc.

In nature every substance used for food contains vitamins and minerals. Our bodies must have these elements if we are going to use properly the starch, protein and fat of which various food products are made. Over many thousands of years the human body has been adapting itself to eating this kind of food—charged with vitamins, enzymes and minerals. This is the kind of food that builds and replaces healthy cells. What happens when three or four or five generations of people eat food from which these completely essential substances have been removed? We do not know, for at no earlier time in history has such devitalization of food gone on at such a rapid rate. Doesn't it seem possible that this changed, degerminated food that we eat nowadays may be doing us far more harm than we know?

The newly threshed grain of wheat contains practically all of its nutritious essence in the wheat germ—a little nubbin at the end of the grain. The wheat germ is fatty and highly perishable. Besides it complicates the modern milling process by which we make our fine white flour today. So it is removed during the milling process. This makes the white flour that remains almost as completely worthless a food as starch—yes, plain laundry starch, for starch is mostly what you have left in white flour. Then the flour is treated with one chemical after another, each rendering it more unfit for human consumption.

For example, the bleach used to bleach the flour pure white and to make it easy for the bakers to knead contains chlorine which destroys vitamin E whenever it comes in contact with it. A deficiency in vitamin E can apparently cause heart trouble. Can you see why the widespread consumption of bread made from white flour might be responsible for many of those heart disease death figures?

The bleach formerly used in flour (after we had used it for many years) was discovered to be a nerve poison causing fits in dogs who were fed on white flour. We no longer use this bleach. How many years and how many fatalities will it take before we discover that the bleach used today is not good for us either? Bleach is only one of many, many chemicals used in commercial flour. This means that all these chemicals are present in every product you use which contains white flour—anything made in a bakery. Or, for that matter, white flour you may use at home in gravies or sauces.

After all the vitamins (chiefly the B vitamins and vitamin E) and all the minerals and all the many probably very important nutritional elements that we have not discovered as yet have been removed from the flour (in the wheat germ) we "enrich" it by adding several of the B vitamins (synthetically made) and iron to the lifeless white flour. We have removed who knows how many natural elements and we have replaced only four or five, and those synthetic. Who can tell us that "enriched" white flour is the same, nutritionally speaking, as flour made from whole grain, complete, rich and nourishing, just as it grows in the field?

Real whole grain flour is highly perishable. It must be kept refrigerated or it will mold, become rancid or bug-infested. How could a grocer keep such flour on his shelves until a customer bought it? It must be treated with a preservative and that is exactly what the miller does to it. In most cases the commercially sold whole-wheat bread is made from this flour. And in addition, to keep the loaf from molding, especially during the summertime, the bakers add still another preservative to the bread. This may be called calcium or sodium propionate.

The commercially-sold whole-wheat flour that you buy in the store, then, has been drenched in chemicals so that it is hardly any better for you than white bread. In fact, in one experiment, laboratory animals died sooner on a diet of commercial whole wheat bread than on commercial white bread.

So what are you going to do about bread, with all these dismal facts confronting you? We recommend, first of all, that you cut down on all cereal products. Most of us eat far, far too much of them anyway. Cutting down on bread will give you the opportunity to eat more vegetables and fruits. Now, for the bread you feel you must have, buy organically-grown, stone-ground, real whole meal flour and make your own bread. It's easy and inexpensive and you will never know what a truly delicious loaf of bread is like until you bake your own.

If you must buy bread, look for bread made from stone-ground whole grain flour, with honey, butter and yeast as the other ingredients—no preservatives and no anti-mold chemicals should be present.

Breast Feeding, Lactation

In spite of hundreds of years of research, we still do not know for certain what exact mechanisms in the body are responsible for lactation. It is believed that the hormone *prolactin* which is produced by the pituitary gland actually starts the flow of milk in the mammary glands. It is thought that some part in lactation is also played by the placenta—the sac of tissue in which the unborn baby is held. This sac also makes hormones and apparently one of these hormones prepares the breasts for lactation which must begin as soon as birth takes place.

For the first few days after the baby's birth, the substance secreted is not milk, but colostrum, a yellowish fluid that contains fat, sugar and minerals. The colostrum of any other animal is extremely rich in all the food elements needed by the baby so a human mother who is determined not to nurse her baby is urged to nurse it for at least the first few days after birth so that the baby gets the great benefit of all these elements, known and unknown, that may play such an important part in his future health.

The flow of milk from the breast is initiated by the sucking of the child. In fact there are many stories in medical history of women who have never had children but who have acted as nurses to other women's children. As the child is gradually weaned, the mother's breast little by little returns to normal and lactation stops.

Those who raise animals and especially dairymen are well aware of the fact that the milk of an animal mother depends solely on the diet she has been fed. And whether or not she has enough milk for her offspring depends on her diet. Among primitive women it is unknown for a mother to be without milk for her new-born baby. In earlier days in this country it was an accepted fact that all women would and could nurse their children, except for those who were definitely ill. Nowadays many mothers find they cannot nurse their babies. It seems perfectly apparent that the reason is our modern diet from which so many valuable things have been refined.

For instance, protein is extremely important to assure an adequate flow of milk. It is recommended that a lactating woman take 100 grams of protein a day, of which at least 2/3 should be from animal sources—meat, eggs and so forth. If her diet has been deficient before pregnancy, she must get even more protein than this. (Don't forget, when we speak of protein, that many food supplements, such as brewer's yeast and desiccated liver are high in protein. Only one rounded teaspoon of yeast equals almost five grams of protein.)

The B vitamins are the other food elements most important for assuring the flow of milk. Again here is an excellent reason for the inability of American mothers to nurse their children. The B vitamins in the average modern American diet are almost non-existent. During the period when a mother is nursing her child, she may need as much as five times more of the B vitamins than she needs at other times. Inositol, included in brewer's yeast and blackstrap molasses, is especially important among the B vitamins.

The other vitamins in the mother's diet do not seem to affect the flow of milk, but of course they have all the influence in the world on the quality of the milk the baby gets. The vitamin A and vitamin C content of the milk will reflect directly the amount of these two vitamins in the mother's diet. And calcium, of course, is necessary in the mother's diet in large amounts if the baby is to be healthy.

There is great advantage to both mother and baby when the baby is breast-fed. Medical literature is full of evidence that breast-fed babies are less liable to infections; they are stronger and do not accumulate the pudgy fat of bottle-fed babies. They are better-adjusted in later life. Recent information indicates that the incidence of retrolental fibroplasia (a new disease which causes blindness in infants) is far less frequent among babies that are breast-fed.

Brewer's Yeast

Over the centuries since the days of the early Egyptians, yeast has been used by men for baking and brewing. As more and more information has been accumulated about the nature of yeast plants, the cultivation of them has developed into a major industry.

Yeast is the smallest of all plants—about 1/4000th of an inch in diameter or about the size of a human blood corpuscle. Today the cultivation and harvesting of the plant is carried on under conditions where the seed bed and the temperature are controlled. The production of present-day brewer's yeast can be guided, very much as plant specialists can guide the production of fruits and vegetables so that only the best breeds will be used to produce plants rich in vitamins, proteins and minerals.

So carefully grown are the yeast plants that we eat in brewer's yeast that the manufacturer can foretell very accurately what the content of the final product will be in terms of protein and vitamins. The yeast plants are grown in large vats until they have produced the maximum number of yeast cells possible. They are then separated from the waste products of this growing process and dried at such a temperature that none of the nutritional value is lost. Then the yeast is pulverized and made into powder or is tableted.

Baker's yeast—the kind you use to raise bread—contains yeast plants that are still alive. As the tiny plants multiply, your bread increases in size. Housewives are well aware that they must treat live yeast plants with care. They require a temperature of about 80 degrees in order to flourish. When your bread is risen and you put it into the oven the yeast plants are killed by the heat. In the same way the yeast plants in brewer's yeast are destroyed when the yeast is dried. It is not advisable to eat live yeast—baker's yeast, that is. The yeast plant needs a large amount of B vitamins to grow. Once inside your digestive tract and still alive, the yeast plant steals B vitamins from you. But, in the case of brewer's yeast, the yeast plant is no longer alive and you are able to eat all the B vitamins the plant stored up for itself.

Brewer's yeast contains all the elements of the vitamin B complex. It is also a rich source of complex proteins—that is, protein containing all the essential amino acids or building blocks of protein. Other foods containing complete proteins are meat, fish, eggs. Altogether sixteen of the twenty or so amino acids are contained in brewer's yeast.

In comparison with several other foods high in B vitamins, here is how brewer's yeast stands:

Food	*Parts of Vitamin B_1 Per 100 Grams*
Brewer's yeast	5,000 to 8,000
Lean pork	300 to 750
Dried lima beans	450 to 600
Liver	300 to 420

Food	*Parts of Vitamin B_2 Per 100 Grams*
Brewer's yeast	2,500 to 4,700
Lean pork	200
Kidney	1,700 to 2,200
Dried lima beans	790
Liver	1,800 to 2,200

Of course, one does not eat as much brewer's yeast as one might eat of liver or beans. But it is a highly concentrated food and three tablespoons of brewer's yeast a day will weigh about as much as a serving of liver and will give you almost ten times as much thiamin and about the same amount of riboflavin as liver. So you can use brewer's yeast as a bonus food—a supplement to be taken with meals or between meals to add enormously to your store of B vitamins.

In present-day America there is a widespread deficiency in the B vitamins due partly to our over-refined food, also to the fact that refined sugar and alcohol steal B vitamins very rapidly from the body. As our national consumption of both of these has increased enormously in the last fifty years, our national vitamin B deficiency has probably increased in proportion.

A lack of thiamin (B_1) results in personality changes—irritability, depression, "nerves," skin disease, muscular weakness, hives. A lack of riboflavin (another B vitamin) produces an extreme sensitivity to light, eye fatigue, sores around the mouth, nostrils, ears. An extreme deficiency in niacin produces the disease called pellagra—with sore tongue, skin trouble, painful mouth, dementia or possibly insanity, and diarrhea. When the deficiency is a little less, these symptoms may exist to a lesser extent. Choline and inositol are two B vitamins that combat hardening of the arteries and diseases associated with it. Four other members of the B complex of vitamins are also very important for good health, although not so much is at present known of exactly what functions they perform in the body.

All these vitamins exist abundantly in brewer's yeast in the natural proportions which are most important for good results. A diet poor in one vitamin is usually poor in others, too. And a dose of just one or just a few of the B vitamins without the others may bring you grief. This is the main reason why brewer's yeast is so much better as a food supplement than synthetic vitamin B preparations. Another reason is the goodly supply of protein and minerals in yeast.

Brewer's yeast is available in tablet or powder form. They are equally good, although one must take a large number of tablets to equal the amount of powdered brewer's yeast one gets in a tablespoon. So if you want to be sure you are getting enough B vitamins, take two or three heaping tablespoons of brewer's yeast daily. Sprinkle it over food or beat it into drinks. Incidentally you may have a little trouble with gas for the first week or so. Brewer's yeast affects some people this way. But within a few days this should cause no more trouble.

Bruises

Did you know that coaches and athletic trainers are using vitamin C to help prevent the black and blue marks that follow on a rough game of football, soccer, lacrosse and so forth? Dr. A. Lee Lichtman of Manhattan's Polyclinic Hospital reported according to *Science News Letter* for June 25, 1955, that runners and others who need to get more oxygen to their muscles should take the anti-anemia vitamin B12. But large doses of vitamin C before the game will strengthen the walls of the capillaries so that bruises will be minimized. If the capillaries do not burst, there will be no bruise.

Brussels Sprouts

Brussels sprouts interest us because they are such a highly satisfactory fall and winter vegetable and because they are higher in vitamin C content per serving than almost any other vegetable. Sprouts belong in the cabbage family which is, as one nutritionist puts it, an "enormous tribe"—developed mostly by Dutch gardeners from the wild *brassica maritime*. Mustard, radishes and watercress belong to the same family.

Leaves of the cabbage family spread wide to absorb energy from the sun by means of chlorophyll in their green parts. Where there is chlorophyll there is almost always vitamin A. You can expect to find iron, too, in abundance. The vitamin C is present to catalyze (or bring about) the changes in the leaf that permit the formation of carbohydrates or sugars from carbon dioxide and water. This is the purpose of that marvelous chemical factory that hums along busily in every individual piece of plant life. The greener the leaf, the more vitamin A, iron and vitamin C you can expect to find. Brussels sprouts grow very prettily upon the tall stem of their plant, decorating it almost as gladioli blossoms bedeck their stems.

Foods of the cabbage family have the reputation of being "gassy" and "strong." Entering a kitchen where cabbage has been cooking all afternoon one can easily understand why. And trying to eat this grossly over-done cabbage one will understand why many people think food of the cabbage family is indigestible.

Properly cooked cabbage has a pleasant odor, taste and effect on the stomach. Cooking cabbagy foods for a long time or over slow heat breaks down the sulfur compounds in them, releasing the objectionably strong smell. Instead, these foods should be washed and dried quickly as soon as they are brought home. They should be stored in the refrigerator if you must store them before eating. When you cook them, drop them, thoroughly chilled, into rapidly boiling water. Keep the heat high until the water comes to a boil once again, then turn it low and cook only until the sprouts are tender. This should be no longer than eight or ten minutes. The sprouts will then have a delicate and most enjoyable flavor. Remember, use as little water as possible.

Here are the food elements in brussels sprouts. They are low in calories and starch, making them an ideal food for dieters.

One cup or about 100 grams of brussels sprouts contains:

Protein	4.4 grams
Carbohydrate	8.9 grams
Calcium	34 milligrams
Phosphorus	78 milligrams
Iron	1.3 milligrams
Sodium	11 milligrams
Potassium	450 milligrams
Vitamin A	400 Int'l Units
Vitamin B	
Thiamin	08 milligrams
Riboflavin	16 milligrams
Niacin	7 milligrams
Vitamin C	94 milligrams

Buerger's Disease

It is seldom that medical men have as clear-cut and final a cause and effect set-up in dealing with any disease as they have in the case of smoking and *Buerger's Disease.* Not absolutely everyone who gets Buerger's Disease smokes, but by far the largest majority of them do. Not absolutely every patient who stops smoking in time will be cured of Buerger's Disease. But medical men everywhere are generally agreed that patients with Buerger's Disease dare not smoke. If they stop smoking symptoms generally improve, only to become worse again if the patient goes back to smoking.

Aside from the fact that smoking appears to have a great deal to do with it, no one knows what causes Buerger's Disease. Its other name is thrombo-angiitis obliterans. Dr. Leo Buerger made an intensive study of the disease about 30 years ago, so it is called after him. It is a disease of the blood vessels, in which the inner linings of both arteries and veins become inflamed. There is also clogging of the blood vessels due to blood clots. In general, the disease affects the legs and feet. It may start with pain in the legs on exertion. As the blood vessels become more and more inflamed, the pain becomes more severe and continuous. In the acute stage, there is great pain after walking a short distance. As the disease progresses and becomes chronic, the pain becomes so severe that the patient is unable to sleep. Eventually a spot develops on a toe or under a toenail and gangrene is on the way. It may take a year or ten years, but the epilogue to a case of Buerger's Disease is generally amputation of a foot or leg to save the patient's life.

Just in case there should be any doubt in the minds of smokers as to the relationship of tobacco to the disease, here are some quotes on the subject: An editor's answer to a reader's question in the *British Medical Journal* for December 22, 1951: "As a general rule, withholding cigarettes has a beneficial effect on Buerger's Disease." *In the Journal of the American Medical Association* for May 18, 1946, appeared a warning about diabetics smoking: blood vessel disease of a kind that incapacitates the patient with pain and weakness in his feet and legs so that he cannot walk or that leads to ulcers and gangrene afflicted significantly more smokers than non-smokers in a group of 301 diabetic men. Smoking constricts the blood vessels. A patient whose vessels are constricted already may have them further constricted by using tobacco.

Another article in the *Journal of the American Medical Association* for June 12, 1954, indicates that filtered cigarettes will be just as bad for the Buerger's Disease patient as the ordinary cigarette. Dr. Irving Wright of New York told of a patient with Buerger's Disease who had not smoked since 1940. So long as he did not smoke and followed treatment, he was free from symptoms. In 1954, impressed with the ads for the new filter-tip cigarettes, he began to smoke them and almost immediately his disease appeared again and soon he was faced with the prospect of gangrene in his toes. Says Dr. Wright, no one has ever found a tobacco that does not have an effect on the blood vessels. And it is believed that the dangerous element in tobacco may not be the nicotine at all, but may be something else, at least for persons who are sensitive to tobacco, as Buerger's Disease patients appear to be.

In *Risk Appraisal,* published by the National Underwriter Company, we find some appalling statistics on smoking and health. The smoking of one cigarette by a person who inhales produces a 5 to 20 increase in pulse, a rise of 10 to 25 in blood pressure, a drop of from 3 to 6 degrees Fahrenheit in the temperatures of the fingers and toes. Twenty per cent of Buerger's Disease patients have diabetes, too. Thirty-five per cent of them have hypertension or high blood pressure. There are many more males than females among the victims of this disease. And many more smokers than non-smokers.

In one series of 1000 patients studied by one physician, every patient was a smoker. In another series of 948 cases in which the average age was 42, there were only 68 who did not smoke. In 401 of these incidentally, the disease became so bad that amputation eventually was necessary.

Vitamin E for Buerger's Disease

Until recently practically nothing could be done for the Buerger's Disease patient. If he could not stop smoking, and sometimes even if he did, he was a candidate for amputation. Since the disease is a disorder of the blood vessels, it seemed logical to try vitamin E in its treatment. In the large file of material from the medical journals on the subject of vitamin E, we find that, sure enough, it has been used with success in treating Buerger's Disease. An article in the *Medical Record,* volume 161, page 83-89, 1948, by A. B. Vogelsang, and the Shute brothers, tells us that symptoms of Buerger's Disease have been relieved, as well as those of other vascular conditions where better circulation of oxygen can improve disease conditions. These researchers found that the dose of vitamin E was extremely important and might be different for each individual. Small doses were not effective. In general doses of about 500 milligrams were used to begin with, then they were reduced to about 200 milligrams as a "maintenance dose" thereafter.

Dr. E. V. Shute in *Seminar,* volume 1, 1949, describes a series of 23 consecutive cases of Buerger's Disease treated with vitamin E. Of these only 4 got no relief and two were doubtful. Seven patients were under treatment for a year or longer and all remained improved. In more recent medical literature we find an article by W. R. Cameron in *The Summary,* volume 3, 1951, describing 35 cases of Buerger's Disease who had had it for an average of six years. They were treated with vitamin E and for four years the researchers kept in touch with them. Fourteen of these patients did not follow the directions. Of the others, 15 got good results, 5 got only fair results and 5 got poor results. Two received no benefit. Says Dr. Cameron, "thus a-tocopherol therapy is the best, safest and simplest treatment for Buerger's Disease and deserves an intensive trial before other medications are used or before surgical measures are attempted."

The International Record of Medicine for July, 1951, reports on the use of vitamin E for Buerger's Disease. Of 18 patients treated with vitamin E, 17 were cured, only one was not. It was found that the medication had to be continued indefinitely.

In the *Journal of Bone and Joint Surgery,* volume 31B, 1949, there is an article by A. M. Boyd, A. H. Ratcliffe, R. P. Jepson and G. W. H. James on three different kinds of arterial disease of which Buerger's Disease is one. The authors conclude that alphatocopherol (vitamin E), 400 milligrams daily, is the only substance that has given consistently good results in treatment of these disorders. Of 72 patients, 27 were completely relieved and 32 were markedly improved. The consistency with which there is a lag period of 4 to 6 weeks before improvement was most striking. After a few months of treatment there was obvious improvement in the appearance of the feet of the patients.

Advantages to the Use of Vitamin E

These are but a few of the many references given in medical literature on the treatment of Buerger's Disease with vitamin E. Do these samples indicate that any and all cases of the disorder will respond to vitamin treatment? Not at all. They do show that in many cases it works. This is all that is expected of the treatment. The miracle drugs and all the various hormone, antibiotic and pain-killing treatments which are used by the medical profession today have no better record than this. Sometimes they work. Sometimes they don't. And most of them have serious aftereffects which means that the patient must be watched very closely to make sure that the cure is not worse than the disease. But there are no harmful aftereffects in the use of vitamin E, because it is a food substance. So its use is surely to be preferred to that of drugs. In addition, there are apparently no drugs that are the least bit effective in Buerger's Disease!

Two further notes on Buerger's Disease that came to our attention. Dr. Julius Kaunitz of New York, addressing the American Medical Association convention on June 24, 1954, presented the theory that eating too much rye bread might possibly lead to Buerger's Disease. Ergot, a poisonous fungus that grows on rye, might be responsible, he said, for the symptoms of Buerger's Disease. Even though grain in this country is closely watched for evidence of ergot, it is conceivable that just enough of the fungus escapes detection so that there is a small but fairly constant amount of it in rye bread. This wouldn't affect you, of course, if you eat rye bread only occasionally. But if you are a confirmed eater of rye bread, eat a lot of it every day and eat no other kind of bread, perhaps you would do well to cut down. Dr. Kaunitz mentioned that Buerger's Disease has a high incidence among the Jewish people of New York who are known to be heavy consumers of rye bread.

One final clipping on Buerger's Disease. From *Newsweek* for December 17, 1951, comes the suggestion that Buerger's Disease may be related in some way to lung cancer. Drs. Martin M. Fisher of New York and Lew A. Hochberg and Nathan D. Wilensky of Brooklyn report that they have a new method of detecting lung cancer. They watch for thrombophlebitis and check closely for lung cancer in anyone who has a recurring case of the blood vessel disorder. Apparently the idea occurred to them when the late King of England died, presumably from lung cancer, after he had suffered from a blood vessel disorder in his legs.

The investigators reported four cases of lung cancer in men, three of whom were suspected of having Buerger's Disease and all of whom had had more than one attack of thrombophlebitis. The attacks of the blood vessel disorders preceded the diagnosis of lung cancer by one to six months. The physicians believe that early detection of a second attack of phlebitis or Buerger's Disease should lead to a thorough examination for lung cancer. They offered no explanation as to the possible connection between the two.

As you know, we do not deal in cures for diseases. We are interested in preventing disease. It seems to us that Buerger's Disease is surely an outgrowth of our modern way of life. It seems completely possible that lack of vitamin E in the diet may be responsible for predisposing individuals to the disease. Smoking increases this susceptibility.

How then to prevent the disease? First, decide to stop smoking if you are dedicated to that habit. Then take vitamin E as part of your daily food supplements. In former days, before food was refined, we used to get enough vitamin E in our meals. Nowadays we have to watch our diets closely to make certain we are getting any at all and in addition we should, all of us, take a protective, preventive amount of vitamin E each day—about fifty or a hundred milligrams.

We know well that vitamin E in the diet confers other benefits as well. It is closely tied up with the health of all muscles and it seems to have a part in increasing their oxygen supply. It was first investigated because of its efficient way of dealing with disorders of the reproductive tract. Infertility, abortions and stillbirths are prevented in stock animals by including vitamin E in their chow. It is effective in preventing and curing menopause symptoms in women. It is being used internationally in treatment of heart and other circulatory disorders.

Can you get vitamin E in wheat germ oil? Yes, wheat germ oil is rich in vitamin E. But it contains other substances as well—all of these very good for you, too. If you take the vitamin E that has been abstracted from wheat germ oil, you are getting much more of the vitamin in a more highly concentrated state. It was alphatocopherol, the most active form of pure vitamin E, that was used in the experiments we have outlined in this article.

Burns

A number of physicians have used vitamin C in the treatment of burns with startling results. Writing in the *New York Journal of Medicine* for October 15, 1951, D. H. Klasson tells us that vitamin C alleviates pain and in minor burns hastens the healing period. It reduces the time interval necessary for skin grafting. This in turn reduces the chances of infection and long convalescence. Sixty-two cases of burns formed the basis for Dr. Klasson's conclusions.

A remedy for burns comes from Mrs. Hester Robinson of 18 Cambridge Way, Piedmont 11, California.

> "A friend told me that when she was a little girl she stepped on some hot coals. Her mother applied a poultice made of grated raw potato and her foot healed quickly without blistering.
>
> "She said that lemon juice is also good for burns. I have tried this remedy myself and find it is excellent. When I burn myself in the kitchen I rub the spot with a cut lemon and it seems to be well immediately."

Editor's Note: We wonder if it is the vitamin C in the raw potato and the lemon that do the trick?

Bursitis

From a Canadian reader we got an astounding testimonal about rose hips. This is what makes our work here so satisfying and heart-warming. We do research in many different kinds of impressive and profound medical books and magazines. There is a lot of wisdom there. But we are continually amazed by the letters readers send us concerning their own experiences which are so much more startling than anything that appears in medical journals. Mrs. W. C. Godfrey, of Duchess, Alberta, Canada, writes us:

> "You may be interested in the fact that after my husband took rose hips powder for three or four months, his bursitis left him and has not returned."

Could it be that bursitis, a complaint so widespread after middle-age, is another disorder caused largely by vitamin C deficiency?

Cabbage

Cabbage is a vegetable known from ancient times when the Greeks and Romans used a lot of it because of its health-giving qualities. They ate it at banquets where wine flowed freely, because they believed it would keep them from becoming intoxicated. Whether or not it has any potency against tipsiness we don't know; we do know that it contains large amounts of healthful vitamins and minerals.

One-half a cup of raw cabbage contains:

46 milligrams of calcium compared to 118 in a cup of fresh milk.
31 milligrams of phosphorus. There are 93 in a cup of milk.
½ milligram of iron compared to 1½ milligrams in ½ cup of spinach.
7 to 24 micrograms of cobalt compared to 40 for beet tops.
5 milligrams of sodium. An egg contains 81.
80 units of vitamin A compared to 20 units for a baked white potato.
.07 milligrams of thiamin. Whole wheat contains .56 milligrams.
.06 milligrams of riboflavin. Whole wheat contains .12.
.3 milligrams of niacin compared to 5.6 in whole wheat.
95 milligrams of inositol compared to 51 in beef liver.
250 milligrams of choline. Soy beans contain 300.
290 micrograms of pyridoxine compared to 800 in beef liver.
52 milligrams of vitamin C. A medium orange contains 49.
3.2 milligrams of vitamin K compared to 4.6 for spinach.

Since we have compared cabbage, above, with other foods that are notably high in their particular vitamins, we'd say this adds up to a mighty fine food.

The only negative aspect we have ever uncovered about cabbage is that eating much too much of it, to the great reduction of other foods, is likely to cause goiter in susceptible persons. It would not be wise to decide to live exclusively on cabbage, but we doubt that you will.

In 1950 a Stanford University doctor reported encouraging results in the healing of gastric and duodenal ulcers by the use of cabbage juice. A recent experiment reported in *Food Research* for September-October, 1952, indicates that a water extract of cabbage contains an antibiotic capable of killing certain germs. The researchers noted that it was not the vitamin C in the cabbage that produced these results.

We'd suggest using cabbage freely in your everyday menus. Cooking it destroys much of its vitamin content. Throwing away the water in which it is cooked causes further loss of minerals and vitamins. It's best served straight from the garden, crisp and raw. And when you're shredding it for slaw or salad, postpone the shredding until just before time to serve, for vitamin C oozes out of every cut surface. Store cabbage, whole, in the refrigerator, covered tightly against the air. If you must cook it, drop it, still chilled, into a little boiling water. Reduce the heat, cover the kettle and cook it no longer than 8-10 minutes.

Eat lots of cabbage, especially if you are trying to cut down on citrus fruits and still want an abundance of vitamin C.

Calcium

Any discussion of the mineral calcium must be incomplete and abridged for volumes have been written on the subject of this most important of all elements in the body—this element which one writer calls "the prime instigator of vital activity."

Calcium is in every cell of the body. About 98 per cent of body calcium is contained in bones and teeth which also contain phosphorus, fluorine, carbon and other elements.

It seems that the importance of bones is obvious, yet perhaps we do not realize just how important good bone structure is. From the moment of conception until the moment of death, healthy bones are an absolute essential. Aside from the fact that bones support the entire body structure, they also contain the marrow in which blood corpuscles are made. Nerves, muscles and various organs of the body all depend for their health on healthy bones. So when something goes wrong with the bones, the health of the entire body suffers.

Teeth are important for appearance and for chewing, and in addition, unhealthy teeth may lead to infections and other serious complications. Calcium is essential for healthy teeth. Formerly we believed that teeth were inorganic substances—not alive. We thought that after teeth were formed, no special changes were made in them except when disease caused them to decay. But we now know that bones and teeth alike are very much alive. When the body suffers from a shortage of calcium, it may be withdrawn from teeth and bones. In pregnancy, of course, the calcium for the embryo is withdrawn from the mother's store. It seems that soft or brittle bones are not just a natural accompaniment of old age. It seems now that they are the result of not enough calcium in the diet. In someone who has eaten sensibly during his life, and continues to get enough calcium as the years advance, there seems to be no reason why his bones should not continue to grow stronger year by year.

Your blood contains calcium too—not the corpuscles, but the serum, or liquid part of the blood. This calcium helps to maintain the acid-alkaline balance of the body, and, too, assists the blood to clot. If it were not for calcium, we would bleed to death at the slightest scratch. Calcium is also important to the nerves—it transports impulses along the nerves from one part of the body to another. It is urgently needed by muscles. Lack of calcium will cause cramps or convulsions. Many people who have suffered all their lives with cramps in their feet or legs have been relieved almost immediately as soon as they began to get and use enough calcium. The heart is a muscle and calcium is the body substance that regulates the rhythm of the heart beat—your heart could not beat without it. And the laboratory solution in which hearts are kept alive outside the body is largely composed of calcium. Remove the calcium from this solution and the heart stops beating.

Calcium is also important for cell division. As you know, your body is made up of billions of microscopic cells. Cancer researchers know that the secret of cancer is involved somewhere in cell life, for cancer is just a group of cells that do not grow normally, but instead reproduce themselves wildly and erratically. Any substance that releases calcium from cells causes the cells to divide. Is it possible then that calcium deficiency may be partly responsible for cancer? Perhaps circumstances of daily life rob the cells of calcium, which causes them to divide far more rapidly than they normally do, resulting in cancer. Calcium preparations are used in treatment of many diseases. In lead poisoning, for instance, calcium brings about increased excretion of lead, resulting in improvement.

How Your Body Uses Calcium

Calcium is distributed throughout your organs in a pattern something like this: Your brain contains 4 to 5 milligrams per 100 grams. Your heart 7 to 8 milligrams, kidney 19, liver 7, muscles 7-8 and skin and spleen 9-10. This means, of course, that calcium is necessary for the efficient functioning of these various organs. Now just what will become of your good health if one of these organs begins to act up for lack of calcium? Heart, brain, liver, kidney—which of these can you afford to mistreat?

Rickets is a childhood bone disease, produced by improper nutrition. Deficiencies of calcium, phosphorus and vitamins may all be involved in producing rickets. Osteomalacia, a bone disease of adults, is thought to be due also to diet deficiency. No one knows exactly what is the physiological or chemical action of vitamin D in relation to calcium. We know that vitamin D is absolutely necessary for the proper use of calcium by the body. Vitamin D is obtained from sunshine and certain animal foods (is most abundant in fish liver oils). It is supposed that vitamin D functions somehow in the intestinal tract to make the calcium available to the body.

Along with vitamin D, ample amounts of vitamins C and A are necessary in the diet to assure proper use of calcium in food. So even though your children play all day in the sunshine and soak up vitamin D, they may be deficient in calcium unless they have enough foods rich in vitamins A and C. As we grow older, we tend to eat less and less of calcium-containing foods. Green, leafy vegetables are hard to chew, milk and cheese may not appeal to us, we get far less vitamin D from the sunshine, so our supply of calcium declines steadily with the years. This is why we feel it is so essential for older folks particularly to take a natural food supplement that contains calcium.

Phosphorus, another mineral element, is also important for the proper use of calcium by the body. For some reason, calcium and phosphorus must exist in a certain proportion in the body if both of them are to be used with utmost efficiency. This ratio is about 2 to 1—that is, there must be twice as much calcium as phosphorus. Among herbivorous animals this balance is sometimes upset because most of their food, green leaves, is rich in calcium, but they sometimes have difficulty getting enough phosphorus. Man, on the other hand, tends to eat more phosphorus—high food (meat and cereals) and less food that is rich in calcium such as green leafy vegetables.

All human children are born calcium poor. That is, they do not have a reserve store of calcium and they must have a continuous and ample supply of calcium and vitamin D for the sake of their growing bones. In general, children need much more calcium than adults, for their growing bodies use so much of it that there is little left for functional use. Just stop and think for a moment of the changes that take place in bone structure—and of course nerve and muscle structure as well—during the first 20 years of life. Calcium is necessary to all these changes. So do not think that your children can stop drinking milk and taking fish liver oil as soon as they are no longer infants. They need this extra calcium and vitamin D until they have attained their full growth. And we believe they go right on needing extra calcium all their lives, for they cannot possibly get enough of it in foods.

Remember, calcium is essential for healthy bones and teeth, and healthy blood. It is intimately concerned with the way your heart beats. On calcium depends the health of your muscles and nerves. Calcium may be an essential factor in cancer prevention. Do you think you can afford to take a chance on a possible deficiency?

Absorption of Calcium

We do not yet know all the details of calcium absorption. We do know that two members of the same family may be eating exactly the same amount of calcium in their food and one may have a deficiency while the other does not. This may be due to faulty absorption. Too much phosphorus in the diet will result in less efficient use of calcium by your body. So a diet high in meat and cereals may bring about calcium deficiency.

In order to be properly absorbed, calcium must be in an acid medium. This means that there must be enough hydrochloric acid in your stomach when that calcium-rich food appears there, or the calcium may remain insoluble and be excreted without doing your body any good. Also, too much fat in the diet tends to combine with the calcium and form a substance that cannot be absorbed. In a person suffering from any form of diarrhea, calcium is being excreted rather than being absorbed.

There are two other serious hazards involved in the absorption of calcium. Foods that contain calcium are not useful to the body as a source of this mineral if at the same time they contain large amounts of oxalic acid. The oxalic acid renders the calcium unavailable and in addition affects other calcium in the digestive tract, so that oxalic-acid-rich foods are most destructive of calcium. Spinach and other greens of the same family (swiss chard and beet greens) have a large oxalic acid content, as does rhubarb. Now while these foods are not harmful if you eat them occasionally, they should not be eaten regularly day after day, and you should not depend on them as a source of calcium.

Chocolate is another food rich in oxalic acid. We are told that 90 per cent of the milk bought at school lunch cafeterias is chocolate milk. Milk is, of course, very rich in calcium. But chocolate milk contains also large quantities of oxalic acid, which render the milk calcium unavailable and furthermore destroy some of the body calcium as well. If you have carefully trained your children to drink milk, you'd better check to make certain they don't have chocolate milk away from home. As you know, carob flour is a good substitute for chocolate—it's nutritious and contains nothing harmful.

Sir Edward Mellanby has contributed richly to our present-day knowledge of nutrition. One of his most important experiments concerned calcium and phytin. Working with animals on various diets containing various amounts of the different cereals, Sir Edward discovered that there is a substance in cereals (particularly whole grain cereals) that is destructive to calcium. This substance is phytin or phytic acid. Our custom of eating large amounts of milk with cereal seems to have a very good reason—the milk supplies calcium to replace that which the cereal is destroying. There has been a great deal of controversy over Mellanby's experiments. And no nutritionist concludes from them that whole grain cereals should not be eaten. However, we do advise that, if you eat a lot of cereals, especially whole grain cereals, you should be even more careful to make certain you are getting more than enough calcium in your diet.

How Much Calcium Do You Need?

How much is "enough" calcium? Here are some quotes from Dr. H. C. Sherman, one of the world's authorities on calcium, in his book *Calcium and Phosphorus,* published by Columbia University in 1947: "There is much evidence that in the Western World also, calcium deficiencies, while seldom so drastic as to declare themselves unmistakably in the clinic, are frequently present in borderline degree. Leitch (1937), from an investigation of British patients, reported much of the 'arthritis' of middle-aged and elderly people to be a result of long-continued shortage of food calcium; while Ramsay, Thierens, and Magee found that 37 out of 101 women lacked sufficient calcium reserves to maintain normal blood calcium during pregnancy.

"The British authorities on food and nutrition, after long and careful study, speak definitely of the 'known fact' that a large proportion of family food supplies in England and Scotland have calcium contents too low to be satisfactory. This has also been found in the United States, through the food consumption studies of Stiebeling and co-workers (1939, 1941); in China, by the survey of Maynard; in tropical America, by Cowgill; in large districts of Australia, of Africa, and of India by other investigators."

There is much evidence that lack of calcium in diets of older folks is responsible for bone disease, heart disease and brittle and fragile bones that fracture so easily.

The National Research Council gives the following as the minimum requirements of calcium:

.8 grams a day for adults regardless of their activity.
1.5 grams a day for women in the last half of pregnancy.
2 grams a day for women breast-feeding their babies.
1 gram a day for children up to nine years old.
1.2 grams a day for children 10-12 years old.
1.3 grams a day for girls from 13-15.
1 gram a day for girls from 16-20.
1.4 grams a day for boys from 13-20.

Most nutritionists agree that adults need at least one gram a day and possibly much more, for good health.

What do we mean by a gram? Well, you can get about a gram of calcium by eating 3 cups of kale, or 42 oranges or 77 potatoes, or 33 eggs or 2½ cubes of cheese, or drinking 1 quart of milk. Even here there are some further cautions about calcium content of foods. The outer green leaves of head lettuce, cabbage and so forth contain more calcium than the inner leaves. Loose leaf cabbage and lettuce is still better. The white fibrous part of the orange contains most calcium. So when you juice an orange much of the calcium is lost. If you strain the juice, even more is lost. The clearer the juice when it is served to you, the less calcium it contains. Cheddar-type cheeses contain about four-fifths of the calcium of the milk of which they are made. Cottage cheeses only about one-fifth. Dried milk solids—that is, powdered skim milk contains more calcium than any other form of milk, for the fluid and fat has been removed, and the calcium is highly concentrated in the powder.

Bones As a Source of Calcium

As you know, we advise taking bone meal for calcium, phosphorus and other minerals. We have many reasons for this. As you have seen, it is almost impossible to get enough calcium in a present-day diet without relying heavily on milk, and milk products. We feel that there is a great deal to be said against including too much milk in the diet of the adult. It is a food designed by nature for infants and it is undoubtedly equipped with many substances good for babies which may not be good for adults. Then too, many people have an allergy to milk and others just plain don't like it. Unless you can buy raw, certified milk, the product you buy has been pasteurized, homogenized and goodness knows what else, so that it is far removed from a natural product. So far as we know, no extensive experimenting has been done to determine just how all these various processes affect the person who finally drinks the milk.

Bone meal contains not only calcium, but also phosphorus in, of course, the correct proportions, since bone meal is made from the bones of healthy young animals. It contains, too, all the other minerals that go to make up bone, in the right proportions. Dr. Sherman has this to say about the advisability of eating bones:

"In Mary Rowlandson's account of the food habits of the New England Indians by whom she was held for ransom in 1676, it is said that they would cut bones in pieces at the joints, boil them and drink the liquor, and then pulverize the ends of the bones in a mortar and eat the bone meal thus obtained. More recently, LaFarge, in an account of a feast made by Indians of the Southwest, speaks of long cooking of corn with beef bone in water. As we now know, this would carry a significant amount of calcium from the bone to the cooking water and the softened absorbent corn.

"The United States Bureau of Fisheries reports that the calcium in salmon is nutritionally available when the bone, which has been cooked along with the flesh and thus softened in the can, is consumed with the flesh as human food. From the Orient it has also been reported that the bones of small fish, eaten by man, may be counted as digestible and their calcium as available, regardless of the method of cooking."

Can You Get Too Much Calcium?

What about the possibilities of getting too much calcium? We hear a lot these days about calcification, about calcium deposits in arteries, about calcification in kidneys, about kidney stones. Isn't it possible that eating too much calcium will result in one of these misfortunes? Apparently not. The body is excreting calcium all the time, whether or not there happens to be a calcium deficiency. Any excess calcium will be excreted, unless there is some disorder in the body that results in deposits of unassimilable calcium. And such a disorder will come about regardless of how much calcium is in the diet. The parathyroid glands located in the neck have a great deal to do with adjustment of the body's calcium. If these glands are out of order, then difficulties with calcium are likely to occur. Probably, too, there are many other disorders that may play havoc with the body's calcium supply, but the way to remedy these disorders is certainly not to eat less calcium!

Dr. Sherman has done many experiments in his laboratory showing that amounts of calcium far above the generally accepted minimum not only do no harm, but actually make for longer and healthier life. He says: "Extended pathological investigation has shown that doubling a normal food calcium intake did not increase the incidence of abnormal calcification in the body, as of arterial walls or other soft tissues; whereas surplus intake, for example, of cholesterol, may not be so harmless."

Many of the Scandinavian people get as much as four grams of calcium daily, in their food. They are, of course, noted for their stature and excellent physiques. Oriental peoples live largely on cereal diets with little calcium. They are much shorter in stature than westerners. There is, too, the famous story of the Shetland ponies (valuable because of their tiny size) who were moved from the calcium-poor soil of the Shetland Isles to calcium-rich soil in America and soon stopped being ponies at all!

Consider the list of foods at the end of this article in terms of getting at least one or possibly two grams of calcium per day. Then take into account all the various elements in your diet or physical condition that may prevent the absorption of some of this calcium. Do you honestly believe that, without taking bone meal, you will get enough calcium day by day, every single day, to keep you in good health, ward off heart trouble, tooth and bone trouble and the ravages of old age?

Foods Rich in Calcium

(A milligram is 1/1000 of a gram. To know how much of a gram is contained in each of the following, divide by 1000. For instance, a food containing 100 milligrams would contain 1/10 of a gram.)

Foods	
Dairy Foods	*Milligrams of Calcium*
Butter	16 in 7 tablespoons
Cheese, cheddar	873 in 5 one-inch cubes
Cheese, cottage	82 in 5 tablespoons

Cheese, Swiss	1100 in 4 slices
Cream	97 in 6 tablespoons
Eggs, whole	54 in 2 eggs
Milk, dry skim	130 in 1 tablespoon
Milk, fresh whole	236 in 1 cup
Fruits	
Dried apricot	86 in ½ cup cooked apricots
Dried date	72 in 20 dates
Dried fig	223 in 6 medium figs
Dried peach	60 in ½ cup
Dried prune	54 in 12 medium prunes
Orange	33 in one small orange
Raisin, seeded	78 in 1¼ cups
Red raspberry	49 in one cup
Nuts	
Almonds	25 in 10 almonds
Brazil nuts	124 in 14 Brazil nuts
Peanut butter	74 in 6 tablespoons
Walnuts, English	8 in 10 walnuts
Cereals	
Oatmeal	54 in ¼ cup uncooked oatmeal
Rice, brown	39 in ¾ cup steamed rice
Wheat bran	77 in 5 cups
Wheat germ	84 in 12 tablespoons
Soy flour, medium fat	244 in 100 grams

Meats

Almost no calcium except in gelatin, a meat product made from bones.

Gelatin	453 in 12 tablespoons
Vegetables	
Beet greens (calcium unavailable because of oxalic acid)	118 in ½ cup steamed
Broccoli	130 in 1 cup steamed
Celery	50 in 1 cup diced celery
Chard (Calcium unavailable)	105 in ½ cup steamed
Chick peas	92 in 1½ cups
Collards	249 in ½ cup steamed
Dandelion greens	187 in 1 cup steamed
Endive	104 in 1 head of endive
Kale	225 in 1 cup steamed
Kidney beans, dried	148 in ½ cup
Lima beans	63 in ½ cup steamed
Mustard greens	220 in 1 cup steamed
Okra	82 in 10 okra pods
Parsley	290 in 100 sprigs
Parsnips	57 in 4 pieces steamed
Soy beans, dried	227 in 1 cup
Turnip greens	259 in ½ cup steamed
Watercress	168 in 1 bunch cress

Calcification

A head of cabbage, a piece of cheese and some kale leaves don't look very much like bones and teeth, do they? Yet the calcium from these foods combined with phosphorus makes up about 90 per cent of the substance of teeth and bones. How? Calcification is the process by which the minerals in our foods are "deposited" or "laid down" in the bones and teeth. The way we talk about it, you might think that calcification is a simple process, much like the scaling that takes place on the inside of your teakettle, if you have hard water. That is calcification, too, of a sort.

But your teeth and your bones are very special objects, not to be confused with the scale on the inside of a teakettle. They must be put together in a certain way so that they can function well. They must contain other minerals as well as calcium and phosphorus. And, most important of all, even though they are made chiefly of the relatively inert minerals, they are very much alive, so that an exchange of minerals goes on all the time between them and other parts of the body.

After this kind of an introduction it seems rather like an anti-climax to tell you that we do not know exactly how calcification takes place. The calcium must be present, of course, in just the right amounts. Phosphorus must be present. They must be assembled at the place where your bones and teeth are later going to be. Then something has to happen to "precipitate" the calcium and phosphorus—that is, to make them go out of solution, so that they become the relatively insoluble substances we know as teeth and bones. An enzyme known as phosphatase must be present, we know. And somehow, somewhere in the process, vitamins A, C and D are absolutely necessary too, for proper calcification.

Vitamin D, which you get from summer sunlight or from fish liver oils, controls the parathyroid glands and these glands in turn control the fate of calcium in the body. If there is too much or too little phosphorus in relation to calcium, if there is no vitamin D or too much vitamin D, calcification will not proceed according to schedule. In the unborn baby, the amount of all these vitamins and minerals depends on the mother's diet, of course. And, if it is deficient in minerals, her own body will be robbed to do the calcifying job on the infant's body.

According to *Diseases of Metabolism,* edited by Garfield G. Duncan, M. D. (W. B. Saunders Company, 1952), "In view of the repeated observations by students of nutrition, it seems superfluous to mention that deficiency diseases are still of rather common occurrence in the United States, but the importance of keeping the American physicians 'vitamin conscious' becomes evident when one realizes that probably about 75 per cent of rickets escape diagnosis and that deficiency of vitamin D is certainly the most common disorder of this type among infants of the temperate zone." Dr. Duncan goes on to say that the reason for this state of affairs is that doctors believe this disease has been eradicated so they have arrived at a "static" state of mind concerning it.

So rickets—the disease of calcium, phosphorus and/or vitamin D deficiency—is still prevalent in America where fish liver oil has supposedly been part of every infant's diet for years. The American diet is rich in phosphorus, due to the many cereals we eat. Perhaps the deficiency of calcium is responsible for these rickets.

Then, too, many things are involved in how well the calcium in your diet is used by your body. For instance, does the pasteurization of milk so change the nature of its calcium that you cannot absorb it? There are many conflicting reports in nutrition literature. One group of researchers has discovered that only a small part of the calcium in milk is absorbed. Another has found that practically all of the calcium of milk is utilized and the calcium of vegetables is not very well used by the body. If the food that contains the calcium also contains considerable amounts of oxalic acid (spinach, rhubarb, beet greens and chocolate fall in this category), the calcium will form oxalates in the intestines and will be excreted unused. If there is too much fat in the diet, there is danger of the calcium mixing with the fat to form "soap" which cannot be absorbed. Yet there must be *some* fat, for calcium is better absorbed in the presence of a certain amount of fat.

You must have ample hydrochloric acid in the stomach for proper digestion and use of calcium, for it is absorbed only in acid surroundings. Your glands must be working properly, for a disorder of the parathyroid or the adrenal glands can disrupt calcium metabolism. And you must have just the right amount of vitamin D and phosphorus.

Will Too Much Calcium Cause Stones?

What about calcification of the soft tissues of the body? We read constantly about calcium deposits on the walls of the arteries, in the heart, in the kidneys, in the joints. Do such deposits result from too much calcium in the diet? There seems to be absolutely no evidence that they do. First of all, to prove that they do, we would have to find someone who is getting too much calcium in his every day diet. This might be pretty hard in 20th century America. The official estimate as to how much calcium a grown man should have is one gram; ¾ cup of broccoli would give him about ¼ gram and ½ cup of raw green cabbage would give him about 1/5 of a gram. One quart of milk would provide a gram of calcium, if this calcium is absorbed by the body. So it seems pretty obvious that the average American, far from getting too much calcium, gets just barely enough to keep him alive.

Suppose then that he takes bone meal or some other food supplement rich in calcium. Isn't that likely to result in calcium deposits where he doesn't want them? There is general agreement among nutritionists that such is not the case. In those geographic spots where kidney stones occur in almost all the inhabitants, there are things wrong with the diet, yes. But too much calcium is not one of them. In fact, the diets are very low in calcium. They also lack vitamin A and vitamin C. This is one good reason why deficiency in these two vitamins has been linked closely with kidney stones.

Dr. Clive McCay, of Cornell University who has worked for many years on nutritional experiments says, "In the course of two decades of research with minerals and with rats we have seen groups at the time of death with heavily calcified arteries and kidneys while parallel groups were relatively free. This calcification of soft tissues was due to unknown variables in the diet *and could never be related to dietary calcium.*" The italics are ours.

If you are worried about kidney stones or calcium deposits on the arteries, we'd suggest that you concentrate on getting ample calcium and other minerals in your diet by way of bone meal, which contains all the important ones, and then make certain you are getting enough vitamin D (from fish liver oil unless you have plenty of sunshine the year round), vitamin A (from fish liver oil) and vitamin C (from fresh raw fruits and vegetables) and also rose hips or some other natural food supplement.

Camphor

Camphor nose drops are the villain in a gruesome story reported in the *Journal of the American Medical Association* for July 17, 1954. A nurse's aide with a bad cold used an inhaler about every thirty minutes during the day and in addition used about half a bottle of camphor nose drops, which she dropped into each nostril, letting the fluid trickle down her throat and then swallowing it. By five o'clock that evening she was desperately ill, fell from her chair to the floor and suffered what appeared to be an epileptic fit. She was put to bed, grew cold, clammy and restless. She was irrational, moaned and groaned and rolled from side to side. Several hours later she vomited and a strong smell of camphor was noticeable in the vomitus. Within several days she was able to go back to work. This incident illustrates well the danger of home remedies for colds—or anything else.

Such a thing happening to a young child might well prove fatal. Get rid of the bottles in your medicine chest, won't you? There is very little possibility that any of them contain anything that could make you feel better. Doctors have shown over and over again that the cold sufferer who takes nothing at all gets well just as fast as the one who doses himself with any or every cold remedy. And if you consistently follow the best possible diet, chances are you won't be subject to colds.

Cancer and Connection With Vitamin C Deficiency

We are always glad to present new theories about the possible cause and prevention of cancer. We are doubly glad when these theories have to do with nutrition and its relation to cancer. In the present instance we have a third reason for pride. The author of this theory is an old friend of *Prevention,* W. J. McCormick, M. D., of Toronto, Canada.

Dr. McCormick's treatise on this subject appears in the *Archives of Pediatrics* for October, 1954, and has some convincing material about the possible cause of cancer. It is known that cancer results when body cells "begin to grow and multiply in an abnormal way in some part of the body, relentlessly invade the surrounding tissues and extend to other parts of the body," says Dr. McCormick. The question has always been, what causes cells to behave in this way? Dr. McCormick believes he may have the answer to this abnormal behavior of certain cells.

After describing the structure of the cells that make up the skin and what lies beneath it, he tells us that the lowest layer of cells, the germinal layer, rests upon a formation of connective tissue known as "the basement membrane." These cells might be compared to the footing of the foundation of a house.

"Any breach or disarrangement of this structure could lead to a disturbance in the orderly growth pattern of the epithelial cells (those on the surface of the skin and mucous membranes) resulting potentially in an inward extension of cell growth through the breach, which is the initial stage of malignancy," says Dr. McCormick. As we understand it, greatly simplified, this means that a disorder or break in the connective tissue underlying this layer of cells can result in the cells growing in through the break.

If the individual is suffering from faulty nutrition, the repair mechanism cannot accomplish its job and the cells begin to grow wildly, finally resulting in cancer. "The most definitely established physiological function of any food substance is that of the role of vitamin C in the maintenance of stability and elasticity of connective tissue generally and the growth of new scar tissue in wound healing," says Dr. McCormick. We know that in an individual who lacks vitamin C the material between the cells—the cement that glues the cells together sometimes called the "cement of life"—will break down easily and will be very difficult to heal, unless vitamin C is given in large doses. According to an editorial in the *Journal of the American Medical Association,* volume 117, page 937, 1941, the frailty of tissues associated with the breakdown of this cement substance is brought about through the failure of a certain substance that builds protein with which to repair the tissues. This substance, according to the *Journal,* is "normally furnished by vitamin C."

In the case of certain non-malignant tumors, says Dr. McCormick, they may be well-covered with a protective barrier of tissues which prevents them from spreading if the patient is getting enough vitamin C. But if, later on, his supply of vitamin C is reduced, this tissue barrier may break down and the tumor may then begin to spread, becoming what we call malignant. Also chronic ulcers which may have healed by scar tissue can easily break open later on if the supply of vitamin C is short. He also points out that most cancers are ulcerative and have a tendency to hemorrhage—both of these symptoms are present in individuals who are deficient in vitamin C.

How Lack of Vitamin C Affects Cells and Tissues

Dr. McCormick goes on to quote from famous physicians of many years ago who wrote descriptions of scurvy—the vitamin C deficiency disease. It was extremely common in those days, no one knew what caused it, and physicians were very much concerned with investigating every possible clue as to its cause and cure. Lind in the year 1753 wrote that the muscles of scurvy victims were so lax and tender that they readily fell apart. Their digestive tract tissue was in the same disintegrating state. Old bone fractures and old wounds also fell apart. Dr. McCormick believes these might have become cancerous later on, had the patient not died of scurvy first. Martini, writing in 1609, stated that scurvy was like the plague, for it caused carbuncles, buboes (swelling of the glands) and cancer.

A more recent investigator, Hunt, writing in the *British Medical Journal* in 1941, observed that previously formed scar tissue, over old wounds, breaks down and liquefies when vitamin C is lacking. Bonney, writing in 1908, before the discovery of vitamin C, described what happens to a pre-cancerous wound. He found a constant loss of connective tissue, changes in the appearance of the tissue and fraying of the edges of the cells lining the tissue.

There is also a general opinion that certain persons are predisposed to cancer. Might this predisposition be a slight but prolonged deficiency of vitamin C? Dr. McCormick believes that it may. He illustrates, using the now well-known figures of lung cancer in relation to smokers. In the report submitted by the American Cancer Society to the American Medical Association the death rates of 187,000 men between the ages of 50 and 70 were checked for a period of 2½ years against their tobacco-smoking habits. The death rate from all causes was 60 to 102 per cent higher in cigarette smokers than in non-smokers. The death rate from lung cancer was 200 to 1500 per cent higher, depending on the degree of addiction. The rate for cancer in general was 150 per cent higher in cigarette smokers than in non-smokers.

Treating Cancer With Vitamin C

It is a well-known medical fact that various kinds of irritation—chemical and physical—wounds, burns, ultraviolet rays, radium, chronic infections and so forth increase the body's requirements for vitamin C. If the vitamin C is not present in the patient's body in ample quantities, any of these conditions may become much more serious. Furthermore, the vitamin C level of the blood in cancer patients is considerably lower than that of healthy subjects.

We think that Dr. McCormick may have something extremely important—perhaps not for advanced cancer patients, but surely for those of us who fear cancer and want to take every precautionary measure against it. How can you tell if you are deficient in vitamin C? Do you bruise easily? Do you bleed more than you should if you get a tiny cut? Do wounds heal slowly? Do your gums bleed easily? Do you have gingivitis (inflammation of the gums)? Do you have a chronic infection that you cannot get rid of? How much of your daily diet consists of fresh raw fruits and vegetables—the year 'round? How much are you exposed to tobacco smoke—whether you smoke or those around you smoke?

No one has ever heard of an individual getting too much vitamin C, even the synthetic vitamin C which doctors give as medicine, which is unaccompanied by all the various and valuable substances that go along with natural vitamin C in food. Many of us are short on vitamin C—not short enough to get scurvy, of course, but perhaps just short enough to bring about that very weakening of the cell cement that Dr. McCormick describes. Fresh raw fruits and vegetables are the best source of vitamin C—don't soak them, don't leave them unrefrigerated, don't cook them. And, because you never can know how much vitamin C is left in any food you buy at the store, make doubly certain of your supply by taking a natural vitamin C food supplement every day.

Cancer and Drosnes-Lazenby Treatment

"The battle against death is too important to condemn a single weapon without exploring its possibilities," so said Frank Edwards, news commentator for the Mutual Broadcasting System, in a broadcast on April 18, 1950. He was speaking about a clinic in Pittsburgh, Pa., where a substance developed from a mold was being used successfully to treat cancer. Edwards made a study of the clinic and its file of case histories. He gave it nation-wide publicity. Various newspapers and magazines around Pittsburgh have taken up the story.

Two lay people founded the clinic—two people who had worked for years conducting experiments with a mold substance they grew. Excited about the possibilities of using the mold for cancer treatment, they went to the Director of the National Cancer Institute who listened to them carefully and encouraged them to go ahead. Six years of hard work went by—years in which Philip Drosnes and Lillian Lazenby spent their own time and money buying laboratory equipment and working almost around the clock on experiments to prove that cancer tissue could be broken down and destroyed by the substrate of their mold. (A substrate is the liquid that drips from the mold—the extract of the mold.)

They had gotten something started that they couldn't stop. What if this were the long-sought key to the problem of cancer? Or what if it might throw some light—even if ever so little—on that problem?

This was the thought that kept them going through one discouragement after another. Finally they were convinced that they had found an organism under their microscope which existed in cancerous tissue and also existed in the mold they had grown. By injecting the substrate from their mold they could stop cancerous growth in their laboratory animals. And the organism no longer appeared in the formerly cancerous tissues.

Analysis of the mold product made by the National Institute of Health showed that it contained two substances called Rhizopus and Mucor as well as various strains of penicillium. The name of the substance—Mucorhicin—is derived from the names of these various elements. Sending in a report of this to Mrs. Lazenby, the National Institute suggested that she interest some local physician in giving the antibiotic (as it could now be called) to cancer patients and make careful studies of results over a long period of time. Paul A. Murray, M.D., of Pittsburgh, who was already using the antibiotic, proceeded enthusiastically to give it to cancer patients and to work closely with the discoverers to keep records of his patients.

Working Against Opposition

For two people who are not medical practitioners or researchers, the path to recognition is fraught with perils. One of the easiest ways to discredit any cancer "cure" is to claim that the patients treated did not have cancer at all. At the Drosnes-Lazenby Clinic a rule was made to take only "terminal" cases of cancer, that is, patients whose cases had been declared hopeless by their physicians and who had been sent home to die. They must present at the clinic a statement from their physician or hospital giving the diagnosis of cancer.

This sounds watertight. But there are always angles and loopholes. For instance, in the files of the clinic are photostats of a hospital record of Jimmy M. which was changed (in a different handwriting) *after the patient was cured at the clinic.* His diagnosis had been sarcoma—cancer of the jaw. His parents had been told that he had only a short time to live. What possible objection could there be to his coming to the clinic to see if Mucorhicin might ease the pain of his dying days? When, a month or so later, he was discharged as cured, the draining hole in his cheek grown over with new skin, the story got around. A friend of the clinic looked up Jimmy's record in the hospital file. The diagnosis of "sarcoma" had been crossed out and a diagnosis of Fibro Hemangloma, a "non-malignant tumor" had been written in.

We have in our files a series of case histories of clinic patients written by Dr. Murray and his associate Dr. Joseph W. Wilson, another Pittsburgh M.D., both of whom treat cancer patients with Mucorhicin at the clinic. Jimmy's case is not isolated. As soon as word began to get around that there might be a cancer cure over at the Drosnes-Lazenby Clinic, it became increasingly difficult to get records from hospitals and family physicians. The clinic does not diagnose.

Perhaps it is understandable that diagnosticians do not want to become involved in any action around a highly controversial cancer treatment. Certainly it would be unpleasant for a physician to diagnose a case of cancer, tell the patient he could do nothing for him and then have the patient cured by a mold preparation developed by two people who are not even physicians.

But are physicians today interested in curing cancer or are they not? If they are, then should they not seize upon any treatment that holds out even the faintest hope of a cure? Especially when, as in the case of Mucorhicin, there has never been a single toxic or harmful reaction of any kind on the part of anyone taking the substance! If the National Cancer Institute is interested in curing cancer, should they not send an immediate investigating committee if there is the slightest chance that Mucorhicin may be effective?

But the Drosnes-Lazenby Clinic did not claim to have a cancer cure. They believed whole-heartedly that they had discovered something of great value to humanity and they wanted the chance to try it out on people already given up for dead. Sounds as though it would be simple enough, doesn't it? Especially with an ever-growing file of case histories (at present well over two thousand) of patients who were treated without fees up to 1950. But it is not so simple as it sounds, and what happened to these two folks is a nightmare of run-arounds, evasions, misrepresentations and arrest. Yes, Mr. Drosnes and Mrs. Lazenby were arrested on the grounds of practicing medicine without a license.

A Case History

We spoke to the father of one patient—Karen G. who was given up as a hopeless brain tumor case, when she was eight. *Intramedullary Glioma of the brain stem and cerebellum*—that was the diagnosis her physicians made. After a series of operations, she was taken home to die. She was in a coma, unconscious, paralyzed, and toes and hands twisted backward, when her parents came to the clinic. Karen was given Mucorhicin first through a tube in her nose. Her second dose was given orally. She began to improve at once and slowly, gradually she came back to life until about eight months later, she could sit in a wheel chair and the paralysis affected only one arm which continues to improve.

Today Karen is fifteen. She is blind, for the cancer had destroyed her sight before Mucorhicin therapy. But she is happy and well. Dr. Murray, in his written case history of Karen says "Progress of this patient can only be described as amazing."

The same can be said for other patients who have been treated with Mucorhicin. While we were talking to Karen's father, he mentioned two friends of his whose cancers had also disappeared when they got the Drosnes-Lazenby treatment. Can we prove that they had cancer? This becomes increasingly difficult. For instance, Karen's hospital records have disappeared from the files at the hospital. We were told that the clinic doctors could not get them; her lawyer could not get them.

The blistering, searing campaign of ridicule, persecution and scorn that has met Mr. Drosnes and Mrs. Lazenby at every turn is more comprehensible if you think of it in terms of what might happen to you or any other lay person under similar circumstances. They had worked for many years developing their mold substrate and treating cancerous animals successfully with it before they used it on human cancers. They took only patients who had been told by their doctors that they could not be cured. There were only two of them at the clinic. There was no money except for their own personal contributions, for they treated everyone free of charge in the early years.

Growing and processing the mold substance, getting the medicine to a widely scattered group of patients, contacting hospitals and doctors to get case histories on their patients so that they would know that the diagnosis had been cancer, following up on patients over the years to check on how long death was postponed or finally outwitted—the amount of work involved in all this staggers the imagination, when you think of two people undertaking it alone for no purpose other than to use their discovery to benefit desperately sick people. Obviously these are the kinds of jobs that should be done by a full hospital staff.

What Can You Do About It?

If you inquire, you will probably be told that the Drosnes-Lazenby treatment for cancer has been thoroughly investigated and found to be worthless. This is not the case. No bona fide investigation has ever been done. No official representative of the Cancer Society, the Public Health Service, the Medical Association, or any other professional group, has ever gone over the case histories, interviewed patients or studied the formula and processing of Mucorhicin, the mold substance which is used at the Drosnes-Lazenby Clinic. There is no secret about the mold. It is grown on a mixture of various food substances. Mr. Drosnes and Mrs. Lazenby are not only willing, but eager, to turn over the formula, the processing and the treating of patients to any reputable school or organization which will carry on their work. However, they will not turn anything over to individuals who want to make a profit from it, or to those who may want to buy it and hide it away.

If you are as indignant as we feel you should be after reading this story, what can you do to see that this kind of injustice and blind disregard for human life does not continue? Your congressman should be interested in the Drosnes-Lazenby story. We suggest that you write to him, urging him to ask for a congressional investigation of this and all the other cancer treatments which are at present unrecognized by organized medicine.

There is one thing more that you can do. During the days when it appeared that the clinic would have to close for lack of funds, a group of friendly neighbors paid the rent. This was the beginning of the organization of a Woman's Auxiliary which holds meetings, collects dues and does some fund-raising for the clinic. Everyone on the board of directors knows someone who has taken the Drosnes-Lazenby treatment. They want more members. They want a membership that will extend all over the country, partly for the sake of fund-raising, but also so that word about the clinic can be circulated and more and more pressure brought to bear for an investigation.

Cancer and FitzGerald Report On Cures

In the extensive and expensive search for drugs that heal there must be, we suppose, delays, debates, disagreements and often hard feelings before a new medical procedure or a new drug is widely accepted and used. This is the way things have always gone in the scientific world and it speaks well for the caution and integrity of scientists when they do not jump on the bandwagon to hail every new discovery as a cure-all.

But, on the other hand, it seems there are gaps—unexplained and frightening—in the investigation of some procedures and "cures" which seem certainly to warrant a most thorough examination. We are speaking of certain substances that have been developed for the cure of cancer.

Our field is prevention rather than cure. And we sincerely believe that a return to natural, unprocessed foods, rich in vitamins and minerals and free from artificiality and chemicals will promote such good health that today's plagues—the degenerative diseases—can be wiped out. Meanwhile, the incidence of these diseases increases every year. Daily we receive desperate and tragic letters from people whose friends or relatives are dying of cancer. In the cases of these people there is no question of taking up a healthful way of life in order to prevent cancer. They are faced with the hourly pain and horror of a disease they already have. It seems to us that a health magazine should devote some space to some of the much maligned "treatments" for this dreadful disease.

When the late Senator Tobey headed the Senate Interstate and Foreign Commerce Committee, he engaged an investigator, Benedict FitzGerald, to gather information about a number of hospitals, clinics and other organizations to see if there was indeed a "conspiracy" to keep the products of these organizations from being sold in interstate commerce. Mr. FitzGerald began to collect material from the leading groups which are widely known, such as the American Cancer Society, the Skin and Cancer Hospital of New York, etc., and also from organizations not so well known, such as the Drosnes-Lazenby Clinic of Pittsburgh, the Hoxsey Cancer Clinic of Dallas, Texas, and the Lincoln Foundation of Medford, Massachusetts, the Dr. Gregory Clinic of Pasadena, California, to name but a few. He also went to Illinois to study the situation in regard to Krebiozen which recently caused a tempest at the University of Illinois.

The Story on Krebiozen

Here are some quotes from his reports on Krebiozen: ". . . It is my profound conviction that this substance Krebiozen is one of the most promising materials yet isolated for the management of cancer. It is biologically active. I have gone over the records of 530 cases, most of them conducted at a distance from Chicago, by unbiased cancer experts and clinics.

". . . I have concluded that in the value of present cancer research, this substance and the theory behind it deserve the most full and complete and scientific study. Its value in the management of the cancer patient has been demonstrated in a sufficient number and percentage of cases to demand further work.

"Behind and over all this is the weirdest conglomeration of corrupt motives, intrigue, selfishness, jealousy, obstruction and conspiracy that I have ever seen.

"Dr. Andrew C. Ivy, who has been conducting research upon this drug, is absolutely honest intellectually, scientifically, and in every other way. Moreover, he appears to be one of the most competent and unbiased cancer experts that I have ever come in contact with, having served on the board of the American Cancer Society and the American Medical Association and in that capacity having been called upon to evaluate various types of cancer therapy. Dr. George G. Stoddard, President of the University of Illinois, in assisting in the cessation of Dr. Ivy's research on cancer (involving Krebiozen) at the University of Illinois, and in recommending the abolishment of the latter's post as vice-president of that institution, has in my opinion shown attributes of intolerance for scientific research in general."

We do not know what further developments there have been in the struggle around Krebiozen, but we have this report from *Chemical Week* for March 27, 1954: "An Illinois state legislative committee met this week to consider proposals for winding up its inquiry into Krebiozen, a mystery-surrounded drug that turned the state university into a battleground. The plan is to have (1) a new test carried out by an impartial laboratory satisfactory to both proponents and critics of the material and (2) a limited number of further hearings."

Some Facts about the Hoxsey Cancer Clinic

Of the Hoxsey Cancer Clinic, Mr. FitzGerald says: "I have very carefully studied the court records of three cases tried in the Federal and State Courts of Dallas, Texas. . . . Dr. (Morris) Fishbein (of the American Medical Association) contended that the medicines employed by the Hoxsey Cancer Clinic had no therapeutic value; that it was run by a quack and a charlatan. (This clinic is manned by a staff of over 30 employes, including nurses and physicians.) Reprints and circulars of several million copies of articles so prepared resulted in litigation. The government thereafter intervened and sought an injunction to prevent the transmission in interstate commerce of certain medicines. It is interesting to note that in the Trial Court, before Judge Atwell, who had an opportunity to hear the witness in two different trials, it was held that the so-called Hoxsey method of treating cancer was in some respects superior to that of X-ray, radium and surgery and did have therapeutic value. The Circuit Court of Appeals of the 5th Circuit decided otherwise. This decision was handed down during the trial of a libel suit in the District Court of Dallas, Texas, by Hoxsey against Morris Fishbein, who admitted that he had never practiced medicine one day in his life and had never had a private patient, which resulted in a verdict for Hoxsey and against Morris Fishbein. The defense admitted that Hoxsey could cure external cancer but contended that his medicines for internal cancer had no therapeutic value. The jury, after listening to leading Pathologists, Radiologists, Physicians, Surgeons and scores of witnesses, a great number of whom had never been treated by any physician or surgeon except the treatment received at the Hoxsey Cancer Clinic, concluded that Dr. Fishbein was wrong; that his published statements were false, and that the Hoxsey method of treating cancer did have therapeutic value."

The Lincoln Foundation

Of the Lincoln clinic in Massachusetts, Mr. FitzGerald writes: "I have not had an opportunity to sufficiently explore the particular type of therapy employed by this institution. However, I understand it involves a unique theory of inhalant therapy and the transmission of bacteria-phage. In passing, it is important to note that this technique was the subject of particular interest to the late chairman who was a trustee of the Lincoln Foundation, following a successful treatment of his son, Charles W. Tobey, Jr. This remedy has been tried by hundreds of patients and it is alleged that these treatments have been proven beneficial."

The report goes on into other matters that Mr. FitzGerald investigated. What happened to his report is significant. Senator Tobey died before it was completed and it was turned in to Senator John Bricker, who succeeded Senator Tobey as chairman of the committee. According to *Life Today* for June-July, 1954, Senator Bricker declared that the report does not fall within the jurisdiction of his committee and that it should go to the Judiciary Committee of which Senator Langer is chairman. Senator Langer has not responded to Mr. FitzGerald's pleas for action on the report.

Nowhere does Mr. FitzGerald state that any of the treatments he investigated cures cancer. He asks instead for an impartial investigation by qualified scientists to determine whether or not they are effective against cancer. This does not seem to us to be too much to ask. From the information we have, it appears that each of these organizations has clamored incessantly for an impartial investigation from the day they opened their doors. To deny this investigation, to persecute and smear the organizations involved without making an investigation, seems to us the height of unfairness and stupidity. But, much more important than that, we are dealing with today's greatest killer. If there is *any* substance anywhere in the world that will even mitigate the pain of, let alone cure, the agonized sufferers from cancer, should not all considerations be swept aside—be they financial, professional, ethical, or what-not, so that such a substance can be made generally available?

Instead of which, a thorough investigation is denied year after year, apparently by the very people who talk loudest about their concern for cancer victims. If anyone who today claims to cure cancer with a drug is a quack and a charlatan, let us by all means expose him as such, which can of course be done only by a proper investigation. If, instead, the investigation shows that cancer *is* being cured by one, or another, or all of the organizations mentioned by Mr. FitzGerald, then for the sake of suffering humanity, let us make this treatment immediately available in all parts of the world! Probably the most helpful action to take to further such a proposal is to write to your own two senators urging that action be taken on the FitzGerald Report.

Cancer and Gardening

In the early part of 1955, while reading the January 22nd issue of *The Medical Journal of Australia,* I was jounced out of a state of tranquility by a letter which appeared in the correspondence column of that journal. As I read it, I could not believe my eyes, for it had astounding implications. Here it is:

"Sir: It is my clinical impression that patients who are active gardeners have a much greater host resistance to internal carcinoma (cancer) than do non-gardeners. Their survival period appears to be far greater in my experience. Whether this assumption is coincidental and false could be ascertained by practitioners working in city, suburban and country districts. May I, with respect, suggest this observation be made, and if established, submitted to the biochemists.

Yours, etc.
ERIC GOULSTON, M.D.,
Sydney, December 20, 1954."

You can well imagine my excitement at the discovery of this item and I lost no time in getting off a letter to Dr. Goulston, as follows:

"Dear Dr. Goulston:

"I read your letter in the January 22, 1955, issue of *The Medical Journal of Australia* and I am wondering if you could give me more information about cancer and gardeners. We publish the magazine *Organic Gardening and Farming,* which represents Sir Albert Howard's idea of farming or gardening with non-chemical fertilizers.

"Sincerely yours,
"J. I. RODALE, EDITOR."

Under date of April 4, 1955, I received the following reply from Dr. Goulston:

"Dear Mr. Rodale.

"Thank you for your letter concerning cancer and gardeners. All I can say is that I have noticed over the years that there seems to be a greater host resistance against cancer in patients who are suffering from this disease and who delve in the garden, than is the case with complete non-gardeners. This may be due to some anti-carcinogenic agent ingested from soils or from plants. We are trying to investigate this problem biochemically but haven't got very far, so that at present, it is only a clinical impression.

"I would be very interested to learn if any similar work is being done in the States. Your idea of not farming with chemical fertilizers, would make an interesting study for a surgeon in your district to investigate and compare the incidence of cancer there as with other centres.

"I would like to hear from you again. I hope to visit the States next year, and if in Pennsylvania, I should like to make your acquaintance."

Here is a doctor after my own heart, and it would be a pleasure to meet him.

Logic would seem to tell us that the good doctor is on the right track, for gardeners grow their own vegetables, thus eating fresh foods. Gardeners live more of an outdoor life, breathing the fresh air, exercising more, bending over as they weed, which improves the tone of the stomach muscles. I recall seeing some cancer figures which showed that rural folk get less cancer than city people, which could be because they garden more. But yet, I was not satisfied. I felt vaguely that these factors somehow were only a part of the whole picture and I therefore kept probing and seeking over the next few days. Then an idea struck me!

It is a known fact that the earth contains electricity and magnetism, and gives them off in a steady stream. In fact it has been said that the world is one big magnet. We know also that the body is an electrical power station, every cell being charged with electricity. Could it not be possible, therefore, that in placing the hands in the soil, an electric circuit between the body and earth is completed, and that some of the ground electricity gently begins to course through the body, invigorating the latter? In other words, if a person gardens every day, is he or she receiving a healthful daily electrical treatment?

Let us go a little further into this realm of thinking and see if we can find examples of the way the body functions electrically. That there is electricity in the body was proven by Nobel prize winner, Dr. Pauling, of the California University of Technology, who found enough electricity in the blood to light a 25 watt bulb for five minutes. This may sound like a small amount of electricity, but in terms of the body's electrical economy it could be more than enough. Dr. Frederick Golla, former professor of Pathology of Mental Diseases at the University of London, showed that the brain, like a condenser, stores up electricty in its nerve cells which is being constantly accumulated and discharged. In fact, all living matter, from the lowest bacteria to the body of man, gives off a steady current of electricity. All matter, in fact, *is* electricity. It is by an electrical process that viruses attach themselves to the walls of bacteria before they invade them. The atoms which make up the molecule consist of a positively electrified nucleus called the *proton,* surrounded by fast moving *electrons* which are charged with negative electricity. Every cell in the human body has an electrical basis of operation. Each cell is a little electrical world, a miniature factory, where it would be very cold and inactive without electricity.

Dr. Crile, the famous medical scientist, has said that "the primary function of the cell is to fabricate electrical charges." This is no doubt true, but a strong factor in this fabrication process could be a stimulation from outside electricity that comes into the cell by sundry means, one of which could be earth electricity that could enter the body by means of the hand or foot in gardening.

Being somewhat acquainted with the operation of machinery I know that there is an ideal set of conditions which is conducive to its ideal performance. And so it must be with the body and the cells of which it is composed. Too little or too much electricity might play havoc with it. I can conceive of an electrical threshhold below which the cell could go berserk and multiply wildly. That would be cancer! There might be trouble also if the life of the cell is speeded up by too much electricity.

While we are on this subject we cannot overlook atomic fall-out and its effect on the cell's electricity integrity. The intrusion of such powerful radiations cannot do it any good. It may push it in a direction harmful to the life processes of the body. In the same way, there are certain chemicals called *carcinogens,* usually coal tar products such as benzol, certain coloring chemicals, coke, illuminating gas, etc., which are known to cause cancer. Is it possible that the end-products of body chemical combinations in which they are a part invade the cell, and affect its electrical system? Does it in some way depress or increase too much the store of cell electricity, which touches off the forces that could lead to cancer?

In the days before the advent of the wonder drugs many orthodox physicians used electric machines in their practice. These are devices which send a gentle electric current into the body, and in many cases with good results. Today the practice is still resorted to, but only in emergency situations and with the use of more powerful charges of electricity. In the *New England Journal of Medicine* (Nov. 1952) there is described a situation where a person was kept alive by electricity. His heart began to fail but by means of electricity his life was saved. Dr. Paul M. Zoll, Associate in Medicine at the Harvard Medical School, who wrote the article said, "Whenever the electric stimulator was stopped, the heart failed. During a period of 52 hours not a single natural heart beat of the ventricle muscles was observed when the electrical stimulator was turned off. After 52 hours, the heart started slowly by itself . . . Eight days after the treatment began, the patient's heart was pumping adequately on its own."

In the May, 1955, issue of *Today's Health* (an American Medical Association publication) there is described a case where, after continued attacks of unconsciousness and convulsions, a man's heart began to miss some beats. He went into a coma. But when electric currents were sent into his chest, the man awoke, but became unconscious again when the electricity was shut off. After 7 days of electrical treatment his heart returned to normal, and at present, at the age of 72, he is fully recovered, having no heart symptoms whatever.

Howard W. Blakeslee, science editor of the Associated Press, in commenting on this work in a newspaper article said, "Every cell of your body is an electrical battery. The same electrical organization is true of trees and plants. In work done at Yale it has been discovered that this electrical field changes when a woman ovulates, when she has genito-urinary cancer, that it governs growth of animal embryos, that it reveals hybrid vigor in plants."

A news event which brings home the fact of how important electricity is in the cell, is a piece of research described in the *Science News Letter* for June 26, 1954. It is a new method for testing whether women have cancer of the uterus and is done by measuring the electrical difference between the inside and outside of cells cast off from the birth canal. If the electrical reading is slightly negative there is no cancer. If it is positive by a moderate amount there is some kind of cancer in the uterus.

Drs. Burr and Langman of Yale University found in examining 428 female patients that in those that had cancer of the genital tract over 98 per cent had an electro-*negative* charge on the abdominal wall, whereas in non-cancer cases over 99 per cent had a *positive* electrical charge at that point. Many years ago Dr. E. N. Goodman of the College of Physicians and Surgeons at Columbia University, in investigating the electrical properties of the stomach, found that when digestive disease was present the electrical resistance of the stomach changed. At death, he found, all measurable electricity ceased.

Many years ago a process was developed by Dr. James Homer Burgan, of Hollywood, for reducing high blood pressure by passing a weak direct electric current directly through the human blood stream for half an hour. In the case of several hundred patients, the blood pressure was reduced by a single treatment. It was thought at the time that the current in some manner dislodged certain chemical deposits that interfered with the free passage of blood, but it could be that the reduction occurred for more basic reasons. High blood pressure could be caused by some interference with the body's electric-distribution system, which in turn could have a chemical or dietary basis, such as too much salt or sugar in the diet.

In some instances, Dr. Burgan reports the electrical treatment has resulted in a rather surprising increased growth of the patient's blood cells. "The fact must be recorded," he says, "that the treatment results frequently in the building up of the body's defense mechanism. We have observed changes in the blood vessel walls in the eye which indicate some reduction of calcium deposits that play at least some part in the cause of high blood pressure tension."

The day-to-day contact with the earth by an active gardener which means the absorption of a good deal of earth electricity, could be the equivalent of electrical treatments which would set the electricity of each one of the body's cells into perfect order, thus being the means of helping all functions of the body attain normalcy. Add to this the beneficial effect of actively working in the outdoors, and you could have a double insurance against many conditions of disease.

Does any kind of physical exercise improve conditions for the better electrical functioning of the body? When my heart used to undergo symptoms, some time ago, when I would go for a walk, it would show them usually only the first fifteen minutes. After that, the exercise seemed to have the effect of opening up the big arteries leading to the heart, the coronaries, usually eliminating all further symptoms, even in climbing hills during the latter part of the walk. But how are the arteries dilated? It could be that the exercise generates electric current, as the wheels of a moving auto cause its generator to make electrical current. It could be that this manufactured electricity, produced by the steady movement of the body's parts, could open up plugged arteries. Of course there is the oxygenating effect of the blood produced by the forced breathing occurring in exercise, but can oxygen move in the blood without electricity? The active gardener, who keeps moving about, could also be making electricity by such action. A little research on this aspect of electricity in the human body could reveal interesting things.

In *Human Physiology* (Lea and Febiger) appears the statement: "Every beat of the heart, every twitch of a muscle, every state of secretion of a gland is associated . . . with electrical changes." Again he says, ". . . every functional change in a tissue has been shown to be associated with the production of differences of electrical potential. Thus, all parts of an uninjured muscle are iso-potential," which means that, "any two points may be led off to a galvanometer without any current being observed. If, however, one part of the muscle be strongly excited, as for instance by injury, so that it is brought into a state of lasting excitation, it will be found that, on leading off from this point, and a point on the uninjured surface to a galvanometer, a current flows through the latter from the uninjured to the injured surface." This would seem to indicate that a repair process has begun, and that electricity takes a part in that process.

In this regard, Dr. Roy M. Keller, writing in the September, 1953, issue of *The Journal of Medical-Physical Research,* said, "Repair of wounds is no doubt brought about by the change in the electrical potential of the traumatized (damaged) cells. Injury breaks the cell covering and allows the electrons to escape more freely, as in cutting or mashing a comb of honey, the contents escape."

Dr. Robert Voas, at the University of California, is doing research (*Science News Letter,* Dec. 5, 1952) to show how tensions in seven muscles of the body involved in frowning, gritting of teeth, clenching of fists, and in general feelings of tenseness, are reflected in the electrical activity of the muscles.

Whichever way you look at the performance of the various parts of the body you come smack up against electricity, and yet 99.999 per cent of medical researches confine themselves exclusively to a purely chemical basis of bodily operation. Should we not begin to think of checking on a sick person's body electricity? Should this not become routine practice, along with the determination of metabolism, blood counts, heart check-up, etc.? Would not accumulated, averaged data relating to the body electricity of sick and well persons tend to teach interesting facts that might lead to methods of correcting distortions or weaknesses in body electricity, thus also in its health?

In cancer we cannot rule out the effects of the foods that a body ingests and in handling that food, electricity takes a big part. To put it in popular language, electricity sparks the food elements to combine properly in various chemical combinations. Electricity is part of the combination process just as electricity is necessary in an oil furnace to break down the oil to a combustible form. Vitamins, I am sure, could not do their work without electricity entering into the picture. Vitamins have been referred to as sparks in relation to the other food elements which they activate.

All the elements of which foods are composed give off electrical radiations. Carbon, hydrogen, nitrogen, phosphorus, potassium and all the other minerals, together form the integral parts of an electric battery in the body. Some of these food elements in the digestive process absorb electrons—others release electrons. It would be a very profitable field of research to study the electrical effects of each type of food and its elements on the body, in relation to states of health and disease, and to particular kinds of disease, including cancer.

In this respect the effect of table salt should be closely researched insofar as its effect on the body's operation is concerned. In my 96 page booklet, *Cancer, Can it be Prevented?,* there is much medical evidence incriminating table salt as one of the causes of cancer. In Starling's *Principles of Human Physiology,* previously mentioned, appears the following statement, ". . . the smallest trace of salt, acid or alkali added to distilled water enormously improves its conducting power." The question is, whether such enormous increase in electrical conductivity is desirable. In the case of the earth, there is given off a gentle electrical stream. Actually salt is not a food but an inorganic chemical. It is the only item of our diet that does not come either from an animal or a plant. It is a strong stimulant to cell metabolism—too strong and no doubt interferes with its electrical operation.

L. Duncan Bulkley, M.D., writing in the July, 1927, issue of *Cancer,* has a great deal to say on the effect of salt in cancer. He quotes Frederick Marwood as follows, "What would happen to electrical storage batteries if we added sulphuric acid greatly in excess of the necessary formulas, seems to me, will happen in another degree to our internal storage batteries, if we ingest a powerful corrosive chemical, sodium chloride (table salt), to the extent of 10, 20, 30 times, or even more, than nature has prescribed."

Nature has worked out the formula for the body's storage battery, in the blood which feeds every cell in the body. Nature wants the blood components in certain amounts Calcium should be two and one-half times the phosphorus. There should be a definite relationship between the blood's sodium and potassium, but if much salt it taken, its sodium content (salt being sodium chloride) adds greatly to the blood's sodium, thus distorting the sodium-potassium relationship.

So, the next time you grab hold of the salt shaker, pause for a moment and think of what you have just read, and do not throw unnecessary clinkers into the furnace. Think of the fact that by taking in salt, you are dangerously altering the formula of the medium through which the body's electricity flows—the blood.

A few weeks ago something interesting occurred which forcefully brought home to me the fact that our body is a storehouse of electricity. A representative of the telephone company called to describe a new service, the use of a device which a person places in his pocket to keep him in touch with his office. If his secretary desires to contact him when he is away from the office, she calls the telephone company where a record is kept of the wave-length for each subscriber. By the mere push of the button they reach the man. The device in his pocket begins to buzz which is a signal for him to call his office. I asked the telephone man whether I could keep this device on the seat of my auto, but he replied in the negative. "Your body is an aerial for it. You must keep it on your person." So our body is an electrical aerial! That is interesting—isn't it? Actually Dr. Otto Rahn of Cornell has shown that there are continuous electrical radiations from people's finger tips, noses and eyes strong enough to kill certain microorganisms.

In September 1953 I visited the Delawarr Laboratory in the city of Oxford, England, where a new electronic method for diagnosing disease is being developed. There I saw photographs of radiations from various elements such as chlorine, potassium, etc. It seems that each element has its own lines of radiation, and no two are alike. Mr. George Delawarr told me that their work has shown that, similarly, each person has a certain wave force emanating from his body, the design of which never changes basically, although there may be slight variations with change in character.

I would like to pause here and quote a recent news release issued by the *American Institute of Electrical Engineers* of New York, which said, "The possibility of electricity playing an even greater role as an aid in the diagnosis of disease was forecast today.

"The possibility, contingent on new contributions by electrical engineers, was raised by Clyde A. Dubbs, of the Veterans Administration Center, Los Angeles, in a paper entitled *'Electrophoretic Techniques; Some Applications and Problems,* presented during a medical radiation instruments session at the Summer and Pacific General Meeting of the American Institute of Electrical Engineers at the Hotel Biltmore.

"Electrophoresis, the study of movements of proteins in an electrically charged fluid field, is valuable in medical practice for evaluating responses to therapy and for providing diagnostic information, the author said, pointing out that normal blood plasmas give typical normal electrophoretic patterns, and abnormal plasmas give abnormal patterns, although rarely specified for a given disease.

"These patterns," he said, "can provide more helpful information to the physician than any empirical clinical test often performed today. In certain diseases of the liver, kidney and bone marrow, and in general infectious states, patterns are quite characteristic; and for diseases distinguished by a deficiency or lack of a major protein fraction (as gamma-globulin or fibrinogen), the patterns are decisive. Moreover, proof that certain diseases can be diagnosed by the presence of specific protein components (Itano's recent work on hemoglobin proteins in some hereditary anemia), possibly forecasts a greater role for electrophoresis as a *specific* diagnostic tool.

"Citing the difficulty of using only a small amount of electrical energy for electrophoresis, which produces unwanted heat, necessitating more electrical energy for refrigeration to dissipate the heat to prevent the proteins from denaturing, the author said, 'If new contributions from electrical engineers can solve such problems more efficiently and economically the advantages of electrophoresis can be given many more laboratories.' "

This news release was issued in 1955, but in 1953, the Delawarrs were already telling me all about this method in their Oxford city laboratory. Already they had many years of experience in this field of research. With their specially developed camera which costs in the thousands of dollars, they are able to diagnose a person's disease from a tiny specimen of blood taken by pricking the finger.

When I came across the item in the Australian medical journal regarding the average gardener's host resistance to internal cancer, I immediately thought of the Delawarrs and wrote to George. Here is part of his answer, from his letter dated March 21, 1955:

"It was originally supposed that by walking barefoot on dewy ground one's body was 'earthed' in some way, but it is now known that more than this goes on—there is a contact with that basic life force that is being evoked in the living soil. Just take a brass pot, suspend on three brass wires, and fill it with moist soil and hang it on to a spot galvanometer and see the 'current' it produces. It is wired by suspending the three wires from one terminal of the galvanometer and then connecting the other terminal to a central electrode in the soil in the pot. In this way, all the electrical energy passes through the galvanometer. Precaution must be taken to keep the moisture content constant so that any variation in potential must be from causes other than those due to moisture variation.

"The shattering thing is that potentials of 192 micro.V. can be recorded during the summer, and 2½ hours later they will have fallen to 60 M.V.I. although the rainfall and sun have not varied at all. The meter used had an internal resistance of 500 Ohms. Pundits will try and say 'Electrolysis, old boy.' If that is so, it cannot be due to the difference of the material forming the pot and the electrode because each are brass. 'Internal chemical action' is probably nearer the mark, but what sort of chemical action and what makes it vary so?

"This experiment shows us the presence of 'vital force' even in a pot of soil with no plants or seeds in it. The so-called 'current' is really the aggregation of a series of electrostatic charges that are the end result of 'life' in progress. Here is the factor in health that has been overlooked by the scientist because it does not record on a geiger counter. Here is a flow of energy charges, each one having its own complex *energy pattern.* It is these energy patterns that we detect photographically. Radionics deal only with this basic energy.

"Yes, put your hands in the soil as much as you can; handle living plants and drain their health-giving electrical charges into your body."

The medical profession would do well to hot-foot it out to the Delawarr's laboratory in the city of Oxford. There they would see things that would astonish them.

Mr. Delawarr in his letter, mentioned that in the handling of living plants one could drain their health-giving electrical charges into one's body, which should remind us that the gardener in weeding does exactly that. In pulling out an undesired plant, he touches it while it is alive, and thus he drains its health-giving electrical charges into his own body. He, therefore, gets electricity both from placing his hands in the soil and also upon the plant. Mr. Delawarr in his letter, touches upon another aspect of how one can absorb earth electricity and that is by walking barefoot on dewy ground. This prompted me to think of Father Kneipp, who in 1886 wrote his book, *My Water Cure,* which gave him great fame and attracted patients from all over Europe. The basis of Father Kneipp's treatments was to walk barefooted in the dewy grass in the early morning. Let me quote from his book:

"I knew a priest who went every year to stay for a few days with a friend who owned a large garden, and there his morning walk was always taken barefooted in the wet grass. He has many times spoken in glowing terms of the excellent effects of this kind of promenade; and I could name a number of persons of the highest ranks of society, who did not despise his well-meant advice, but tried to harden themselves in the better season, by going barefooted during their morning walks in the solitary woods, or on a remote meadow.

"One of this comparatively still small number has owned to me that in former times he seldom spent a week without a catarrh, if it were only a slight one, but this simple practice had entirely cured him of this susceptibility."

Further on he says: "I can highly recommend it to young and old, healthy and sick. . . . The wetter the grass the longer one perseveres in the exercise, and the oftener it is repeated, the more perfect will be the success. This exercise is generally taken for 15 to 45 minutes. After the promenade all the improper adherents, such as leaves, or sand, must be quickly wiped off the feet; yet the feet are not to be dried, but must be left as wet as they are. Dry stockings and shoes have to be put on, however, without delay. The walking in the grass has to be followed by walking with covered feet on a dry path, at first briskly, by and by in the ordinary measure. The time of the walking depends on how long it takes the feet to get dry and warm, but should not be less than 15 minutes. I urgently call attention to the words 'dry stockings and shoes,' for wet or damp stockings must never be worn after an application. The consequences would soon be felt in head and neck. . . . This exercise, likewise the walking barefooted generally, may be taken even when the feet are cold."

Father Kneipp's work should be re-evaluated based on the possibility that in walking on the dewy grass one absorbs liberal charges of earth electricity.

On May 2, 1955, Mr. and Mrs. Emory L. Harrison and their thirteen boys posed barefoot for the New York *Herald-Tribune* photographer. They had come up from Tennessee because Mrs. Harrison had been named *Honor Mother* of 1955. Mr. Harrison did not care for New York. "New York is all right," he said, "but I like the country best. In the country we can put a big barrel of milk on the table for the boys, and it won't cost us a thing!"

I'll wager that the milk is not pasteurized.

"In the country," he went on, "we can put up 1,000 cans of fruit and put six hogs in the smokehouse and cure them—and it won't cost us a cent." I'll wager they don't use the speed-up chemicals for smoking as is the practice in modern smoke-house methods.

"I don't spend more than $13 to $14 a week for food for all of us. Our 72 acre farm gives us everything the family needs except sugar, coffee, and cereals." I'll wager that the Harrisons use very little chemical fertilizer on their farm.

"And what's more," continued Mr. Harrison, "I'd like to show these city folks how to bring up their boys. Ours can go barefoot, summer and winter, and they've never been sick."

The Harrisons, in their barefootedness, were following unconsciously the teachings of Father Kneipp. And their "primitive" diet did not hurt any either.

Today the farmer has been mechanized. He sits on a tractor so that even his shoes do not touch the ground. He has lost that health-giving contact with the good earth. Over the hundreds of centuries man went barefoot. Shoes are only a recent innovation. Man does not thrive in paved cities. He should live where he can take his shoes off occasionally and walk barefoot.

It is a known fact that cancer is far less prevalent in the south than in the north. Here are some of the figures of cancer's deaths per 100,000 population for 1947:

State	Deaths	State	Deaths
Alabama	83.6	Mississippi	86.5
Arizona	80.9	New Mexico	77.9
Arkansas	85.5	North Carolina	74.8
Georgia	86.3	South Carolina	72.2
Tennessee	95.4		

And here are some for a few of the northern states for the same year:

State	Deaths	State	Deaths
Colorado	141.1	Illinois	161.2
Connecticut	157.3	Maine	160.5
Massachusetts	173.3	Pennsylvania	141.6
New York	174.9	Washington	127.4
Wisconsin	149.6		

In my booklet *Cancer: Can it be Prevented?* (Rodale Press, 50c) it was shown that this disease increases in frequency with remoteness from the equator. I stated that it could be due to less coal smoke in the air and I still think that that is an important factor, but isn't it possible also that there is more working in gardens in the south? The people there are not stopped by winter weather. And there is more going barefoot, especially when one gets closer to the equator, where the cancer figures are the lowest of them all.

In my book *The Healthy Hunzas* (Rodale Press, $3.00) I have shown that this northern Indian race does not get cancer. Sir Robert McCarrison, the famous English research physician who was with them for more than ten years and did not come across a single case of cancer, attributed it to the unusual care these people exercise in the raising of their food. But could it not also be the fact that they go about barefooted? And the fact that they spend so much time in gardening and farming?

There is very little cancer in primitive people. Take the case of our own Navajos. A medical team that recently investigated them was startled by the reduced amount of cancer cases among them. The Navajos are another example of a people who do not eat too much refined food and who have daily contact with the soil.

That there is electricity issuing from the soil there can be no doubt, but is there a difference in this electricity as between a soil farmed or gardened by the organic method as against one operated with chemical fertilizers? We saw how salt could be a factor in doing something to the body's electricity. Chemical fertilizers are strong, soluble chemicals, some of which are salts, that enter in the soil's water solution, and may in some way affect the pattern, or quality, or amount of electricity coming from it. In the breakdown of organic matter, electricity must take a part. But it is a gentle, natural process and, therefore, it may cause a gentle stream of beneficial electricity to issue from it.

The organic gardener, working his hands in his composted soil, treading barefoot over the earth of his organically-treated garden, should have a feeling that he is receiving natural waves of electricity from the earth and not stepped-up or in some way artificialized gusts of electric waves which could throw the metabolism of his body off balance. Of course, what I am suggesting here is rank speculation, but here is a simple subject for research, one that is purely mechanical with all the equipment available. Who will do it?

The situation with regard to cancer is becoming worse each year. Here is a charted forecast of cancer deaths recently issued by the American Cancer Society:

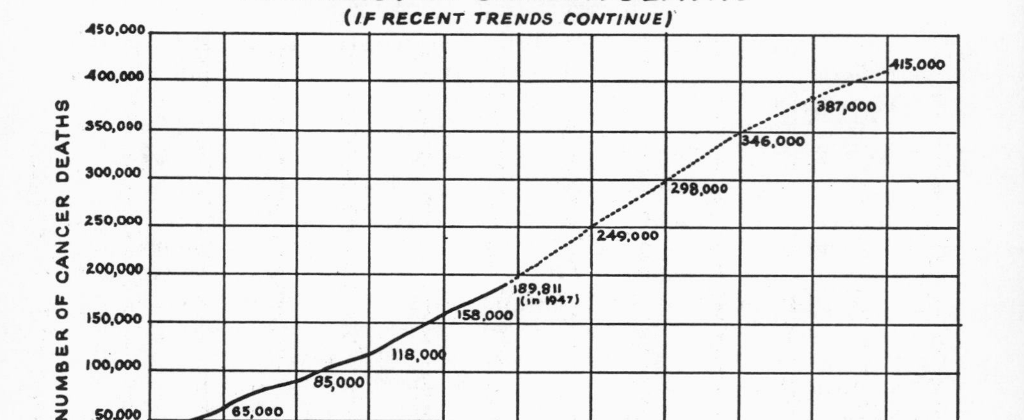

Evidentally the American Cancer Society is throwing up its hands, for up to the year 2010 its chart shows no place where cancer is checked. They expect it to go on and on and on, and it *will,* unless there comes a different mentality, one which does not fear to grasp at straws, one which does not fear to research in the primitive, one which does not fear to walk barefooted so to speak, midst the test-tubes.

What is the lesson? We must go back to nature if we wish to live long. We must garden and go barefooted. If we live in New York we must go searching for four-leaf clovers in Central Park, and no policeman will arrest you if you do it barefooted. We do not have to stop the trend of industrialization. We do not have to stop the advances of technology, but we have to learn to live with these forces. We must not permit them to overwhelm us. We must not industrialize or technologize our own bodies.

The medical profession in its researches must become aware of, and not ignore, this electrical phenomenon. They must not in observing sick people, keep on saying, we see results but we do not know causes, for some of these causes assuredly are in the realm of the electrical.

The idea that it might be earth electricity which aids the body to combat cancer might be used to help cancer cases in the hospital and in the home. An electrical connection could be made between the patient's body and the earth which would establish a circuit of earth electricity into the body. Of course this must be preceded by a thorough series of researches to establish a scientific basis for the general principle of applying earth electricity to aid the body. But, after principles are established, electrical treatment centers might be opened in every town and city in the country. Perhaps every home could own an electrical device, which would cost less than a television set and which could give the body a daily electrical charge, to counteract the effects of our citified, sedentary, artificialized way of living.

More power to Dr. Eric Goulston of Sydney, Australia, who touched off this discussion. May it be the beginning of scientific studies that will lead not only to the conquering of cancer, but diseases of all kinds.

Cancer and Gerson Treatment for

Max Gerson, M.D. of New York City, believes that cancer can be prevented and cured. His life is living testimony to that belief, for Dr. Gerson cures cancer by diet. This is a dangerous, heretical thing to say in present-day America, but from the evidence that we have studied there seems to be no doubt that Dr. Gerson cures cancer. Advanced cases. So-called "terminal" cases. What about early cases—patients who have malignant growths but who have not had surgery, X-ray or radium treatments? We are told that these cancers disappear under Doctor Gerson's treatment just about as easily and as speedily as a bad case of sniffles might.

At the pleasant convalescent home in Nanuet, New York, where Dr. Gerson's patients stay, we talked to a slim, lovely young woman, Charlotte Luchterhand of 5918 Schubert Street, Chicago, Ill. She told us her story. Breast cancer in 1945 and an operation to remove the breast at that time. In 1950 there was a recurrence. In 1952 she developed cancer of the spine. No doctor of all the specialists she visited could give her any hope. As she dragged her painful way from state to state she was met with no comment but a look of horror and the words "We can do nothing for you." She came to Dr. Gerson in 1952. In five weeks she went home, to carry out the rest of the cure at home. She was back at the clinic for a check-up when we talked to her. She was well. Her spine, which had been de-calcified, was now "strong enough to move a piano" in Dr. Gerson's words.

Harry Bess, a Gerson patient of Philadelphia, Pa., spoke to us next. With a diagnosis of enlarged heart, strangulated hernia and anemia, he had the first of a series of eight operations performed. The discovery of cancer in his stomach necessitated another operation in which most of his stomach was removed. The remaining part was still cancerous. Five years later cancer of the urine bladder was treated with X-ray. He was operated on again and again for prostate trouble. Stones appeared in his kidney. A consultation was called among several specialists in Philadelphia to decide whether or not the kidney should be removed.

The doctors and Mr. Bess' family finally agreed that doing anything about the kidney would mean just needless suffering for him. He was going to die anyway in six weeks or so—why make his last days on earth miserable? A member of Harry Bess' family told him in secret what the doctors had said. He decided he wanted to live. He wrote to every place he could think of. They answered one and all that they could do nothing for him. Finally he came to see Dr. Gerson. Dr. Gerson told him that if his liver had any life left in it, there was a chance—just the merest chance. His liver was enormously large and hard as a board. But Dr. Gerson agreed to try. In three weeks Harry Bess showed considerable improvement. Dr. Gerson has been treating him for seven months. His cancer is gone. His kidney stones have disappeared. Harry Bess—a man whose body had been riddled and honeycombed with malignant cells—asked us especially to use his name in this article. He wants the chance to tell people what has happened to him. When we told him that he might be avalanched with mail from readers, he said he wanted to be. Somehow he would manage to answer it all.

Talking to people like this makes you feel humble, awed and thankful. Talking to Dr. Gerson and his staff about his treatment is a revelation. For the treatment is living proof of our belief that the most important single factor in good health is the right food grown in the right soil. And disease occurs in bodies that have not had this kind of food. Not in a matter of days or weeks, but after years of nutritional abuse.

What the Treatment Involves

The Gerson treatment for cancer is mainly dietary. No X-ray, no surgery, no radium, are used. The diet is low in animal protein, high in vegetables and fruits. In Dr. Gerson's own words, "the liver is the center of the restoration process in those patients who improve strikingly. If the liver is too destroyed, then the treatment cannot be effective. . . . It is generally known that in cancer, especially in advanced cases, all the various metabolic systems are impaired." Vitamins, minerals, enzymes, proteins, fats, carbohydrates—the body can handle none of these properly when cancer is present.

"Diet and medication serve the purpose of restoring potassium and the minerals of the potassium group to the tissues until they are completely saturated and, conversely, of reconveying sodium and its group out of the cells and into the circulatory fluids, the connective tissues and other tissues where they belong. The retentive surplus of sodium must be eliminated. It is only on this basis that further recovery of the organs can take place," says Dr. Gerson in one of his articles.

The diet regulations forbid any stimulants such as alcohol, coffee, tobacco, refined foods such as white flour and white sugar and anything made from them, canned or frozen foods or foods processed in any other way. No fats or oils, no salt substitute—finally, no hair dyeing—relapses have occurred after hair-dyeing. Pressure cookers must not be used or any aluminum cooking utensils. Later in the treatment proteins are gradually added. Very high potassium content of the diet is obtained by taking potassium salts in the juices of fruits and vegetables which are naturally high in potassium. The cancer patient must drink many glasses of these juices every day. Thyroid tablets and iodine, vitamin B and liver are given.

The patient who is well on the road to recovery can go home and follow the diet at home. True, it is a difficult diet to follow, from the practical point of view. The vegetables and fruits must be raw, as fresh as possible and freshly juiced. No departure from the prescribed diet is permitted. Is it too much trouble for a cancer patient to follow the diet at home?

Some patients have found that it is. But think a moment. We are talking of a diet that cures cancer. Could anything be too much trouble for that? We are living in a land and a time where housewives spend uncounted hours of time rolling and cutting out cookies, baking pies, decorating cakes with colored icing, making fancy sandwiches, cutting curls into radishes, stuffing celery and so forth. *Is it possible that following a diet to cure cancer could be too much trouble?*

Meeting Dr. Gerson helps you to understand how the long patient years of research, disappointment and courage in the face of disappointment temper a man and make him strong. Dr. Gerson's presence is electric. He speaks rapidly, warmly, brilliantly. His many European years as an honored member of the medical profession there qualify him to speak in words so technical that no layman could understand them. Instead, he waves his arm around the room and says, "Here are my patients. Ask them. Get their stories. Talk to them."

We did. And we came away convinced that Dr. Gerson is curing cancer in a way little short of miraculous. We were reassured as well that those of us who want to prevent cancer are on the right track. It is interesting to note that other degeneraive diseases succumb to the diet treatment, just as cancer does. Mr. Bess found his inoperable kidney stones disappeared on the Gerson diet. Long-standing cases of arthritis, heart disease and so forth are cured along with the cancer.

Preventing Cancer with a Sensible Diet

We asked about prevention of cancer, since prevention is our field. Dr. Gerson believes that a sensible, healthful diet will prevent cancer. Children should be breast-fed if possible. Everyone should eat all food in as near the natural state as possible. Eat raw foods and shun processed and refined foods. Use no salt, no white flour or white sugar, no aluminum cookware. Avoid highly spiced foods and, of course, narcotics and stimulants. Is this such a hard diet to follow? Many thousands of readers are eating like this every day and have for years. Is it worth the extra trouble to be able to reassure yourself that you will not be one of the "one in three"?

If some member of your family or circle of friends has cancer, and you are impressed with our story of the Gerson treatment, what should you do? Your first impulse, of course, will be to go to Dr. Gerson at once. So far as we know, he has never rejected a cancer patient. But at present he has more patients than he can handle, even working "28 hours a day" as a member of his staff told us he does. He earnestly wants other doctors to learn the Gerson treatment and use it.

If a cancer patient's local doctor can be persuaded to write to Dr. Gerson and learn about the treatment, the patient can, of course, be treated at home and need not go to New York. And the more doctors who learn of the Gerson method and use it, the more lives can be saved.

Whether or not someone near you has cancer, the finest thing one can do to help along this good cause is to write to the American Medical Association, to the American Cancer Society, to your local congressman, to the magazines you read, to your newspaper telling them all about the Gerson treatment and asking *why, why* is this treatment not being used widely across the land! *Why* is it not taught in medical schools and *why* is it not investigated by the American Cancer Society and the American Medical Association?

Cancer and Hoxsey Treatment for

"This is the second jury of twelve men that has found in my court that the Hoxsey treatment cures cancer. I have sat here and listened to over fifty witnesses from all walks of life who say that they have been cured. . . . I am of the firm opinion and belief that Hoxsey has cured these people of cancer . . ." The words are those of Texas Judge W. L. Thornton in the libel suit won by Dr. Hoxsey against the (then) president of the American Medical Association, who had claimed that Dr. Hoxsey was a mountebank who did not cure cancer.

Why then should not the Hoxsey treatment be available all over the world? Why should the man who developed it and fought for recognition of it be treated like a criminal, hounded, jailed and slandered? Why should the Hoxsey cancer treatment be spoken of in popular magazines of nationwide circulation as a hoax and Hoxsey characterized as a charlatan and a quack? *Statistics released this year show that one out of every three Americans is destined to have cancer.* Why then does not the Federal Government make a full, fair and honest investigation of the Hoxsey Cancer Treatment?

The answers to all these questions are in a new and terribly exciting book *You Don't Have to Die,* written by Harry M. Hoxsey, N. D. and available from Devin-Adair, 25 East 26th St., New York City (price $3.95). Dr. Hoxsey is a fighter. Thirty-five years ago when the persecution began he could have given up the struggle, forgotten about the herb medicine developed by his father and gone into some other business or profession. But he did not. For thirty-five years he slugged it out with the American Medical Association. At the moment we write this he is engaged in still more litigation, this time suing the American Medical Association for ten million dollars for libeling him.

How Dr. Hoxsey Treats Patients

Hoxsey's treatment consists largely of herbs in a medicine whose composition he has revealed and which has been printed in the *Journal of the American Medical Association.* The A.M.A. says that nothing in the formula could possibly have any beneficial effect on the course of cancer. Questioned at various trials, individual physicians have said the same thing. Asked if they ever tried the medicine, they have all said no. They just know without any further investigation that Hoxsey's medicine could not cure cancer!

Why, Hoxsey isn't even an M.D.! That's true. He is not. But throughout his long, stormy years of treating cancer, he has worked with M.D.'s so that the charge of practicing medicine without a license has been unfounded. But it is still brought against him again and again. And of course when the licensed M.D.'s who cooperate with him have their licenses revoked just because they are working with him, he is naturally hard put to continue to treat patients with a bona fide license hanging on the wall, but he has managed to do so.

And when laboratories which make cancer biopsies tell him one after another that they cannot do any more work for him, it is difficult for him to produce biopsies, proving cancer, which have been done outside his own clinic. No one will do the biopsies for him because of the risk to themselves! So, no matter what proof he presents, the A.M.A. spokesman can always say what he always *does* say, "If Hoxsey cured the patient, he didn't have cancer; if he had cancer, Hoxsey didn't cure him."

If he cured just one person, if he cured five or ten or fifteen, would it not be the obligation of our government agencies to investigate his treatment fairly and completely? According to records at the Hoxsey Cancer Clinic, he has cured thousands! *And one out of every three Americans is destined to have cancer!*

It is difficult to believe the lengths to which persecution of Hoxsey has gone. It is hard to credit your eyes when you read of every weapon of persecution known (short of physical violence) being hurled again and again at the same man over a period of thirty-five years. It is hard to imagine a man so stubborn, so convinced of the rightness of his cause, so dedicated to the eternal hope that truth will prevail that he would not, at some time during those thirty-five years, sigh, "Oh, let's give up. It's not worth all these battle scars." But Hoxsey never gave up. And the American Medical Association never gave up.

When you stop to think of all the phoney advertising for patent medicines that goes on all the time in our newspapers and magazines and over radio and television, and when you stop to think that nobody in organized medicine seems to be the least concerned about the possible ill effects of all these harmful drugs on the American people, then you realize that the stakes in the Hoxsey vs. the A.M.A. battle must be very, very high indeed. Otherwise why would they bother?

It seems to us that the stakes are the lives of the American people. *Statistics show that one out of every three is destined to have cancer.*

Read the Book and Then Get Mad Enough to Do Something About It

It is tempting to give you some excerpts from this explosive book. But we think you should read it for yourselves and make up your own minds as to where you stand in the Hoxsey Cancer Treatment controversy.

This book is completely documented. The case histories given at the end include transcripts of tape recordings made by former patients, photographs of laboratory reports, letters from examining doctors, and so forth. Accounts of court trials include the actual wording of the testimony and the judgments made.

This amazing tale will take you behind the political scenes and will show you to what lengths we have gone in this country to make certain that no cancer cure is found. Why say "we"? Are you responsible for this situation? Am I? Yes, we are, so long as we permit it to go on without doing everything in our power to stop it.

What can you do to right this monstrous wrong and to see that a fair and impartial investigation is made of Hoxsey's claims? First, get a copy of the book. Second, get another copy and give it as a donation to your local public library. Lend your copy to everyone you know and ask them to lend it to others. Write to your congressman and your senators asking them to demand an impartial and fair investigation of the Hoxsey Cancer Clinic. Write to the National Cancer Institute, 9000 Wisconsin Ave., Bethesda, Maryland and the American Cancer Society, 47 Beaver St., New York 4, N. Y. Write to your local paper. Tell your minister, your doctor.

Don't be discouraged and don't be upset by the answers you get. You know in advance what the answers will be. Hoxsey's book tells you exactly what the orthodox answer is for people who inquire about the Hoxsey cancer treatment. With one voice, the A.M.A., the National Cancer Institute and any other official body queried will reply like this: "Mr. Hoxsey was asked to submit evidence to prove his claim of a cancer cure. So far the records submitted by Mr. Hoxsey do not show that his claims are justified. The A.M.A. has published several articles which label Mr. Hoxsey as a hoax and a charlatan." That is the kind of answer you will get. We believe that you should not settle for this kind of answer. You should write again pointing out that no fair and impartial investigation of the Hoxsey Cancer Clinic has ever been made.

You are not asking whether or not Hoxsey is a charlatan. You are asking for a complete investigation. You are asking for an answer to the charges Hoxsey makes in his book. You cannot demand these things of the A.M.A., if you are a layman, for they are not under any obligation to explain their political maneuvers to you. But the government of this country is your government. It does not belong to the A.M.A. Your money pays for organizations like the National Cancer Institute and you should resent bitterly any cent of money they spend which is not in your interest. If you believe honestly that a complete and fair and open investigation of Hoxsey is in your interest, write to them and tell them so.

Your local newspaper can tell you the names and addresses of your congressmen and senators. The address of the National Cancer Institute and that of the American Cancer Society, are given in preceding pages. The American Cancer Society is a private organization, not connected with the government, but supported by donations.

Statistics this year show that one out of three Americans will have cancer!

Cancer and Krebiozen Treatment for

"According to the Commodore, there was indeed a plot on the part of AMA treasurer J. J. Moore and businessmen Ed Moore and Kenneth Brainard to acquire distribution rights to Krebiozen and, failing that, to obtain a settlement of $2,500,000 and if not, then to wreck Krebiozen and all connected with it, finally forcing the Durovics to beg for terms. It was essentially the same story that Senor Loretani had impressed on the Durovics, as related by the Durovics—except this time there was some tangible proof. This proof was admitted as evidence in the subsequent Krebiozen Hearings and the Commodore's story was never denied—either under oath or in any specific detail *at any time, any place.*"

We are quoting from the new book *K-Krebiozen—Key to Cancer?* by Herbert Bailey. Does it sound like the plot of a grade-B movie? Villains—the treasurer of a vast and wealthy professional organization and his business buddies. Object—to buy up a new drug. If it can't be bought, destroy it. Villains brought to justice by an upright legislative investigation, and a new drug released for the public benefit. That's the way the movie plot would go. But in real life it's not that simple.

And in real life the villains have not been brought to justice (even though the legislative investigation dragged on for years) and the remedy over which the battle was being fought—Krebiozen—is still unavailable to the American people. Which might not be nearly so important except for the fact that Krebiozen, the drug in question, is a remedy for cancer.

There is little reason to relate the full story told in this astonishing book as it is spun out, excitingly as any mystery, by Herbert Bailey. You will not believe the story until you read it yourself and satisfy yourself as to its veracity. It involves men in high places in medicine—some of them incorruptible as steel; others weak, willing to go along with whoever is in the driver's seat at the moment, rather than make sacrifices for the sake of integrity; others rotted through and through by power, jealousy and greed.

The story involves Dr. Andrew Ivy, one of the foremost medical researchers of our time or any time, who was given the assignment of investigating further at his School of Medicine at the University of Illinois, a substance brought to this country from Brazil by Dr. Stevan Durovic who thought it might be effective against cancer. In Mr. Bailey's words "Krebiozen therapy was followed by favorable changes in many forms of human cancer. And most patients had been in the last stages of the disease. Further, it was non-toxic, which was not true of other chemical treatments."

What Results with Krebiozen?

As Dr. Ivy proceeded through the regular channels to make the standard reports on the effectiveness of Krebiozen, it soon became apparent that there was to be nothing "standard" about Krebiozen. Through the unbelievable confusion and turmoil of the drama that followed, two things stand out: first—the incorruptible determination of Dr. Ivy and Dr. Durovic to gain recognition for Krebiozen just to the extent that they might experiment further and have their experiments accepted objectively. The second thing that stands out is the determination of the medical hierarchy that Krebiozen shall be stigmatized as useless and its investigators disgraced and ruined. Says Mr. Bailey: "What would the AMA lose by a controlled study of Krebiozen? Nothing—except its hierarchy's jobs and the confidence of doctors and public alike. And this is why the hierarchy of the AMA cannot accept the challenge of a supervised controlled study of Krebiozen: it fears the results."

Here are some of the early comments of physicians after they had used Krebiozen on cancer patients who were either "terminal" or "far advanced."

"Clinically his condition is excellent;" "Patient alive and progressing nicely." "The results are gratifying. In fact, almost beyond belief." "Patient feeling pretty good, working daily." "Biopsy was made and no cancer cells were found." "Eleven months after first injection of Krebiozen, no cancer cells could be found. Patient feels healthy and is working every day." And so on.

But after the AMA had decided that Krebiozen was to be named a failure, after the *Journal* of the AMA had published its report declaring "these findings fail to confirm the beneficial effects reported by Ivy and associates," after the National Research Council (a government agency) had reported that they found "no evidence of any curative effect," how the reports from Krebiozen-using physicians began to change! They too began to report almost at once that Krebiozen had failed in their tests.

Dr. Ivy was suspended from the Chicago Medical Society and his position as vice-president of the University of Illinois was taken from him. He began to receive letters from his friends, begging him for his own good to denounce his early faith in Krebiozen and join the AMA in saying it was worthless. As the noose tightened around his neck, a friend tried to arrange a protest dinner. "It was then he learned that an American medical scientist or doctor keeps few friends practicing in the profession when the full fury of organized medicine is launched against him, no matter how great a scientist he is. Ivy's friend did not have the heart to tell Dr. Ivy of his dismal failure to organize a protest meeting against his suspension," says Mr. Bailey.

This is only the beginning of the Krebiozen story. Does it sound credible? Much of the substance of Mr. Bailey's book was taken from direct testimony given in the legislative committee that investigated the Krebiozen affair. Much of it is from Dr. Ivy's papers and letters. Much of it is from recorded conversations.

We urge you to read this book. You will have, as you never had before, a clear answer to the question that has probably plagued you as it has many *Prevention* readers—if there really are one or more cures for cancer (even if they are only partially effective) why do we not hear about them? Why do doctors not use them regularly? Why does not the medical profession rise up and put an end to this horror which is attacking one American in every three?

Dr. Ivy of the University of Illinois is no "quack." There is no question here of "practicing medicine without a license" or "faith healing" or giving "horse medicine" or any of the charges brought against others who have succeeded in curing cancer. Dr. Ivy's integrity cannot be doubted. The best the mud-slingers could do to besmirch his name was to throw out hints that perhaps he was senile and so didn't know what he was talking out.

We Should Support This Book

Herbert Bailey who wrote this book is a free-lance writer on medical subjects who used to do his research for magazine articles and then check with the office of the AMA to make certain he had all the facts right. Mr. Bailey is obviously, as is Dr. Ivy, a man of such forthrightness and probity that he must tell the truth no matter if he loses his livelihood, no matter if he is villified and disgraced. The book is written from a fierce burning conviction that it *had* to be written, that every fact relating to Krebiozen *had* to be brought to light.

Needless to say, it is not being promoted in the bookshops. "Too controversial" would be the excuse, we suppose. Meanwhile, Dr. Stoddard, former President of the University of Illinois, who lost his job, too, over the Krebiozen controversy, has written a book on the same subject, but not telling exactly the same story. We have not read this book, but we understand from reviews that he declares the tests made of Krebiozen show that it is unsuccessful. No doubt the book by Dr. Stoddard will get wide promotion in bookshops. So when the subject of Krebiozen is brought up, people who have seen Dr. Stoddard's book will speak as final authorities.

Cancer and Nutrition

Would you say that how much you eat has anything to do with whether or not you will get cancer? Would you say that someone who eats processed foods might be more, or less, susceptible to cancer than someone who eats foods in their natural state? Would you say that there are any vitamins which might protect you against some forms of cancer?

The answers to questions like these and many more that are intriguing to readers are to be found in a little book *Cancer, New Approaches, New Hope* by Boris Sokoloff, M.D., Ph.D., of Florida Southern College, published by Devin Adair, New York. Dr. Sokoloff is a cancer researcher and in this book, published four years ago, he tries to present and help the layman to understand more about cancer research and also help him to live so that he can possibly avoid cancer.

It is, of course, in this last matter that we are interested. And Dr. Sokoloff has done such a good job, as far as he goes, that we wish he had gone further. For instance, in his chapter on nutrition and cancer, Sokoloff relates how brewer's yeast and desiccated liver prevented liver tumors in laboratory animals who were given a cancer-causing substance.

All of the animals were kept on a diet low in protein and containing a substance called "butter yellow" which is a coal tar dye known to produce liver tumors or cancer. Adding dried liver in a proportion of about 10 per cent to the cancer-causing diet brought about a distinct decrease in the number of cancers among the animals. Adding brewer's yeast (three to five per cent of the original diet) to the animals' food also brought down the incidence of liver cancer. The investigators then began to search for what particular element in yeast and liver might be responsible. It turned out to be riboflavin, one of the B vitamins. Adding riboflavin alone, together with a protein, casein, reduced the incidence of cancer three per cent. According to Dr. Sokoloff this fact is well known by physicians who now regularly give riboflavin for cases of cirrhosis of the liver (which might of course precede cancer).

But what kind of an approach is this? Would it not be a little more helpful to discover whether or not riboflavin added to the diet of human beings helps prevent cancer? Do you know any human being who would not willingly be a subject for such an experiment—taking a B vitamin which could not possibly do him any harm and would almost certainly benefit him in many ways aside from the probability that it would protect him from cancer of the liver? It is well known among nutritionists incidentally and has been shown in many surveys that the American people are woefully short on riboflavin. Could this be one of the main reasons why cancer incidence is increasing by leaps and bounds in our country?

Sokoloff tells us that "when rats and mice are kept on natural (stock) diet, they are less predisposed to develop cancer than are animals kept on purified feed." What does he mean by that? He means that animals which get natural food in as nearly its natural state as possible are less likely to get cancer than are animals which get food that has been processed until the natural food elements are gone from it. In other words, the kind of diet many Americans live on exclusively. A diet consisting of sucrose (purified sugar), casein (a protein), degerminated corn (the kind you get in cornmeal) gave 90 per cent of rats in one experiment breast cancer and they died from six to seven months sooner than rats given "natural" foodstuffs—that is, we suppose, whole corn, meat and eggs rather than casein, fruits and vegetables rather than refined sugar.

Sokoloff says, "Why the animals kept on a purified diet are more susceptible to cancer-producing substances is not known." The fat, vitamin and mineral content was the same in both diets. Is it possible, he asks, that something happens to the food during processing which causes it to become cancer-causing? It remains an open question which deserves the full attention of investigators, says Sokoloff.

Indeed it does, sir, and, with the exception of a handful of "food faddists," there is apparently no one in this country who is willing to admit, even, that such an experiment has already been carried out.

Did you ever hear of any such experiment from the National Cancer Society which is supposedly dedicated to the prevention and cure of cancer? Did your national magazines ever carry stories about these experiments indicating that it might be wise to avoid processed food, *just in case,* even though the full laboratory proof of their effect on human beings is not available?

Why do you suppose material like this is not widely publicized? The experiments were reported in the professional magazine *Cancer Research* in 1952.

Overeating and Overweight are Dangerous

Has your Cancer Society ever warned you that overeating may be a cause of cancer? In an experiment on overeating reported as long ago as 1940 two groups of mice were used, both from a strain of mice developed purposely to be very susceptible to breast cancer. Both groups were kept on the same diet. But one group was allowed to eat all they wanted, which turned out to be about three grams a day. The other group was restricted as to diet, being allowed only two grams a day. The mice of the group whose diet was restricted *had no cancerous growths at all,* even though they came from a strain of mice highly susceptible to breast cancer. Of the mice which ate an unrestricted diet, more than half developed cancer after 90 weeks. In later experiments the same general idea was proven again and again with liver cancer, lung cancer, skin cancer. All types of tumors investigated were prevented by a restricted diet and *"as yet no tumor has been found that does not respond in this way."*

Even a slight restriction in diet affects the incidence of cancer in mice. One group given 3.2 grams of food daily developed 54 per cent cancer growth, while another group given 2.3 grams of the same food developed 22 per cent and the third group given only 2 grams developed no tumors at all.

Does this mean that you should starve yourself to a shadow? Not at all. The mice who ate less appeared to be much healthier than those who overate. Did they have to eat the restricted diet all their lives in order to be protected from cancer? No. It seems that the important time is when the mouse is approaching middle age—the time when the cancer is most likely to appear. Restricting the diet for a time just before this period will prevent the cancer and allow the mice to live to a healthy old age. But in every experiment, the more the diet is restricted in calories, the less is the incidence of cancerous growth.

In further experiments it was found that the *kind* of diet was also important. Increasing the protein and decreasing the carbohydrates *in every case* brought less cancer. What kind of lesson is this for us in modern America where more than fifty per cent of our diet is made up of refined sugar and white flour and products made from them? Why is it that our government agencies, the nutrition departments of our great universities, and the private agencies that exist for preventing cancer have not broadcast this news the length and breadth of the land—a land in which overweight from overeating is the most widespread disease of all?

In *Look* magazine for June 12, 1956, there is a big hullabaloo about a new diet for reducing—a diet on which you can eat all the goodies you supposedly long for—a diet low in protein and high in carbohydrate. Such a diet is likely to become very popular. Refined white sugar is unrestricted in this diet—you can eat as much as you want of it! What will be the toll in cancer incidence over the next decade among weak-willed followers of this so-called scientific diet, which breaks every law of nutrition we have painfully learned over the years? Do you hear the American Cancer Society protest against the publication of this diet, considering the facts they know about the experiments described above?

Chemical Poisons and Vitamin C

We know, of course, that there are many chemical substances in daily use all about us which are known to cause cancer. Arsenic is one of these. It is used on tobacco leaves which are later smoked. And of course all of the arsenic cannot possibly be removed. It is used as an insecticide on fruits and vegetables which we eat. Listen to what happens to a normal healthy mouse when its skin is painted with a substance known to cause cancer. Dr. Sokoloff is speaking, "long before this growth is detected, noticeable changes in the tissue of the mouse might be observed. The intercellular substance, which binds together the cells, undergoes peculiar changes. It loses some of its binding properties. The binding factor which holds the cells together and makes from thousands of cells an organized unit is less effective. The cells are less effective each to the other, more free to move and to live independently."

Researchers on vitamin C have told us that this is the vitamin which is responsible for the substance that holds cells together. Unless you have enough vitamin C, this intercellular cement will disintegrate gradually and the cells will fall apart.

We know, too, that vitamin C fights against poisons introduced into our bodies. And that it is used up in the battle. Could it not be that the vitamin C of a tissue painted with a cancer-causing substance is used up in a vain effort to counteract the poison, and from that point on the cells begin their disintegration which eventually leads to cancer? If so, what of us, surrounded as we are with poisons—breathing them, drinking them, eating them, every day? And, incidentally, getting less and less vitamin C every day as our food preserving, transporting and processing facilities get ever more efficient! Who would eat a piece of fresh fruit, when orange juice is available at the store in a carton, or grape juice in a can? Of course there isn't a chance that there's much vitamin C in the juice by the time it reaches you, but never mind! The important thing is to save time, and show how up-to-date you are by buying what the ads tell you to buy.

Incidentally, along with riboflavin, which we mentioned earlier, vitamin C is the element most likely to be lacking in American diet, according to nutrition surveys. Is it coincidence that pre-cancerous cells show breakdown in the substance vitamin C helps to manufacture?

We have another note on cancer prevention which is not mentioned in Sokoloff's book but which we consider vitally important—a piece of research done by Ehrenfried E. Pfeiffer at his laboratory at Threefold Farms, Spring Valley, N. Y. in 1948-49, which was financed by the Soil and Health Foundation. Two groups of mice were fed—one with food raised with chemical fertilizer and the other with organic fertilizer. The experiment proved that the group of mice fed with the organically raised food was much healthier than the other. In the strain of mice chosen for their susceptibility to cancer, the survival rate was 64 per cent in the organically-fed mice and only 35 per cent in those fed commercially-raised food.

We had meant to review other parts of the Sokoloff book as well as the chapter on nutrition, but we think the rest of it is far less significant, considering the importance of what we have outlined above. Sokoloff talks about various cures for cancer, including Dr. Gerson's, which we discussed in a previous article and which Sokoloff treats with respect if not a great deal of enthusiasm. He also mentions Hoxsey, Krebiozen, the Koch treatment and so forth, dismissing them all with the completely unscientific statement that "the secrecy about their treatment and the absence of proper clinical records so antagonize the medical profession at large that no ethical physican wants even to try their medication, and properly so."

According to this point of view, curing cancer is not the most important thing! The only important thing is observing proper scientific etiquette, writing the proper number of scientific papers with the required number of case histories presented in exactly the light the medical hierarchy prefers, and going through the "proper channels"—is that it? Otherwise the medical profession may become "antagonized!" And this point of view seems to say, let's keep from "the people" any news of laboratory experiments (or cures) which might help them to stay free from cancer—or possibly cure it if they should get it.

The time is growing short, gentlemen. By the time all these scientific proprieties are observed there may not be anybody left to experiment on.

Meanwhile, is there any conceivable reason why we do not hear, in ringing, confident, challenging words, in every publication put out by government and the cancer agencies, the astonishing facts about the relation of nutrition and cancer, presented so casually but nevertheless with scrupulous scientific accuracy by the respectable cancer researcher, Dr. Boris Sokoloff?

We do not go along with the theory that telling these facts about nutrition and cancer will "raise false hopes" in the minds of readers. We do not, of course, have positive proof that these same facts hold good for human beings. But we believe that every scrap of information about nutrition that might possibly be helpful in the fight against disease should be broadcast. How can readers use the facts we have presented here?

1. Overeating is deadly. One reason we overeat is that our food does not nourish us. Getting plenty of vitamins and minerals in our meals and in food supplements will help us to establish normal eating habits again.

2. Diets high in carbohydrates may be conducive to cancer. From the other information in the book we would say this indicates eliminating from your diet the refined carbohydrates, not good natural foods like potatoes and beans, because . . .

3. Refined and processed diets create more cancer than completely natural ones.

4. The B vitamins (of which riboflavin is a most important member) are instrumental in preventing some kinds of cancer. Most of us are deficient in B vitamins and it is almost impossible to get enough of them in modern diets without supplementing your meals with brewer's yeast, wheat germ or desiccated liver.

5. Vitamin C, so essential to help the body fight against poisons, may be a preventive of cancer. Eat fresh raw fruits and vegetables and take natural rose-hip vitamin C supplements to make sure you are getting enough.

Cantaloupe

Queen of the midsummer fruits, cantaloupe comes to us with much to recommend it from a nutritional standpoint—quite apart from its wonderful taste.

Fresh from the garden, it is an excellent source of vitamin C and vitamin A, comparing very favorably with the citrus fruits and currants without any of the citric or other acids which cause trouble for some people who find they cannot take these fruits in quantity.

The only trouble with cantaloupe is the difficulty most of us have getting vine-ripened ones. And if you have never tasted a cantaloupe ripened on the vine, then you have never tasted cantaloupe. As the melon ripens, its sugar content increases and, of course, it becomes soft and juicy. Immature melons, taken from the vine and ripened artificially, may be soft and juicy but they lack the flavor of the vine-ripened ones because they lack the sugar.

This is why it almost seems a waste of money to buy cantaloupe in winter because, no matter how carefully you choose and ripen them, they are bound to be pretty tasteless. However, their vitamin content is still there. Cantaloupe should be eaten when it is quite soft. You can generally tell by smelling the stem end of the melon when it is ripe enough to eat. You should be able to detect a good, rich, musky melon smell when it is ready to eat.

A peculiar thing about growing cantaloupes which we are sure will surprise our gardening readers. Cantaloupes raised in the light shade of a tree are a little higher in vitamin C content than those raised in full sun. The vitamin C content, of course, increases rapidly as the melon ripens. In a green melon it may be 30 milligrams per hundred grams, but will rise to forty or so in the fully ripened fruits and will decrease rapidly to twenty in the over-ripened or decomposed melon.

Editor Rodale has the following to say about cantaloupe:

"I am glad to be able to write about cantaloupe which I think is a wonderful food. Not only does it contain large amounts of vitamin C to supplement a diet in which citrus fruits have been cut down somewhat, but it also contains the natural sugars as a substitute for the artificial, and the heavy rind protects the inner portion from the insecticides used.

"I have recently come across an interesting fact, however, about cantaloupe which is worthy of being passed along. It is high in inositol which is one of the vitamin B complex. Inositol is a factor in preventing hardening of the arteries, according to some researchers that we have come across. For older persons who are worried about hardening of the arteries, we would therefore recommend cantaloupe. We would not say that this would be a definite preventive, but certainly along with a diet that contains fruit, vegetables and meat, with a reduction of such things as candies, soft drinks, pies, processed factory foods, etc., there certainly should be a smaller chance of getting hardening of the arteries."

Incidentally, inositol is also plentiful in peanuts, peas, beef brain and beef heart, and raisins. Wheat germ and brewer's yeast are its richest sources.

Here are the vitamins and minerals in one hundred grams of cantaloupe which equals about one-half cup of cantaloupe balls or about a third of a small cantaloupe:

Vitamin A	3420	Internat'l Units
Vitamin B		
Thiamin	.06	milligrams
Riboflavin	.04	milligrams
Niacin	.8	milligrams
Pyridoxine	36	micrograms
Inositol	120	milligrams
Folic acid	130	micrograms
Vitamin C	30 to 50	milligrams
Calcium	17	milligrams
Phosphorus	15	milligrams
Iron	.51	milligrams
Copper	.06	milligrams
Calories	23	

Carob Flour

"... there arose a mighty famine in that country; and he began to be in want. And he went and joined himself to one of the citizens of that country and he sent him into the fields to feed swine. And he would fain have filled his belly with the husks the swine did eat." The prodigal son in this parable from the New Testament was longing to eat the pods of the carob tree which he was feeding to the swine. What kind of tree is this and what has become of it in our modern world? Who ever heard of pods from a tree making good food for human beings? And yet, why not, when most fruits and nuts are not only edible but very nourishing?

The "husk" from the carob tree is, we are told, the bread that John the Baptist ate in the wilderness. This is the reason why it is also called "St. Johnsbread." Mohammed's armies on the march sometimes lived on "Kharub." The ancient Romans, the Spaniards, the British all knew the carob tree and lived on its pods when other food was scarce.

We became interested in the carob tree when we ran across references to it in medical and health books and when we began to see advertisements for carob flour in medical magazines. The ads indicated that carob flour is a most effective medicine for use in "non-specific" diarrheas—that is, diarrheas that are not caused by some definite bacteria or disease. Further research told us that carob flour has a pleasant taste not unlike chocolate. A sweet taste.

Then one day we received a letter from a desperate mother who was helping with the school lunch program in her community. She was very health-conscious and greatly disturbed when she contemplated the kind of food most of the children brought in their lunches and the wide variety of sweets and pastries that were served in the school lunch program. We suppose she went to work right away convincing people around her that soft drinks should be immediately eliminated. The children should drink milk, she pleaded. Milk was ordered and many of the children refused to drink it unless it was chocolate milk. Our friend was convinced that cholocate is bad for anyone, most of all, children, and in desperation she wrote us, asking what we could suggest, so that the milk could be made more appealing to the youngsters.

Believing that carob pods might be the answer, we redoubled our efforts to find out more about this elusive fruit and to find if possible, whether anyone in this country had any to sell, so that we might try it out. Letters to the Department of Agriculture brought us meager information. They knew of the carob tree (which they called the honey locust) and they kindly compiled for us all the data they could find. Then we discovered that one of our advertisers sells carob flour and could provide us with some information about the product. But we wanted to know more about carob flour than just the fact that it tastes sweet and that it can be used as a substitute for cocoa and chocolate. *What is its nutritive value?*

Nutritive Value of Carob

As readers know, we have certain criteria that we apply to all the food we eat. We don't just eat it or recommend it for the pleasant taste. Chocolate eclairs taste good, but we certainly don't advise eating them. We don't recommend eating any special foods just so that you can vary your menus or revel in some new taste sensation, or yet so that you can become known among your gourmet friends for your exotic dishes. No, indeed! We believe that every food you eat should contribute something valuable to the nourishment of your body! If it does not, you shouldn't eat it. If it contributes calories alone, or carbohydrates alone, or protein or fat alone, you shouldn't eat it. Your body must make its own good health out the food you give it. Unless every bite of food contains vitamins and minerals it is harmful to burden your body with it. So what we wanted to know about carob was the nutritive content of these brown pods. Perhaps you could make a fine-tasting hot drink from the carob flour mixed with hot water, but if the carob flour contributed nothing, why not just drink the water?

No one, it seemed, in any of the nutrition laboratories had done a thorough piece of research on carob. One advertiser offered to have the pods analyzed. The other day he sent up this analysis and, we are glad to say, carob flour meets all our requirements for an excellent food.

Here is the analysis, insofar as vitamins, minerals and other food elements are concerned:

Moisture	6.3%	Iron	.05%
Crude Protein	7.75%	Aluminum	.05%
Crude Fat	1.90%	Strontium	.05%
Nitrogen free Extract (Carbohydrates)	72.85%	Manganese	.01%
Ash (mineral matter)	2.45%	Barium	.01%
pH value of ash	10.6	Boron	.005%
Total sugars (Invert)	46.25%	Chromium	.005%
Reducing sugars	9.15%	Copper	.001%
Sucrose	37.90%	Nickel	.001%
Starch	6.30%	Carotene (Mg. per 100G)	.03
Calcium	.22%	Equivalent to Vitamin A (I. U. per pound)	227
Magnesium	.95%	Thiamin, mg. per pound	.16
Potassium	.28%	Riboflavin, mg. per pound	.25
Phosphates	.1%	Niacin, mg. per pound	12.0
Sodium	.1%	Calories, per pound	1595
Silicon	.05%		

Thiamin is that important B vitamin so necessary for proper digestion of carbohydrates—so essential for the good health of our nerves and morale. Carob flour has about ¼ as much thiamin as whole wheat, which is one of our richest sources. It has about as much thiamin as asparagus, strawberries, potatoes, dandelion greens or watercress. Niacin, another B vitamin is responsible for the health of our digestive tracts, as well as a good morale. Niacin also is involved in the assimilation of sugars and starches. Carob flour has about as much niacin as dates, bacon, sausage, lima beans, lentils, peas and so forth. Riboflavin, which guards the health of our skin and eyes, is present in carob flour in about the same proportion in which it exists in brown rice. Milk is one of our richest sources of riboflavin. Carob flour contains about ⅓ as much riboflavin as milk.

Vitamin A, the fat-soluble vitamin that protects us from night-blindness and infections, is most abundant in liver, carrots, greens and so forth. Carob flour does not compare with these foods in vitamin A content, but it does contain more vitamin A than eggplant, asparagus, beets, white potatoes, raisins, radishes, onions or rhubarb. The minerals, of course appear in "trace" amounts, as they do in all foods—that is, extremely small amounts. But we notice that there is calcium and phosphorus (for healthy teeth and bones), iron and copper (for good red blood) and magnesium—all minerals extremely necessary for good nutrition.

So we have a picture of a very good, well-balanced food that will contribute considerably to good nutrition. Carob is not as valuable a staple food as liver, or fresh greens or a number of the vegetables. It is not a food that we would insist you include on your menu every day or every week. But it very definitely seems to be a food worth eating.

Harmfulness of Using White Sugar

Now, satisfied that carob passes our test as a nutritive food, what are the special reasons why we want you to get to know it better? We are at war with sugar. And just for the record, let's look a little more closely at white granulated sugar and see where it stacks up in this nutrition game. Sugar is 99.5 per cent carbohydrate. One hundred grams of it contain one-tenth of a milligram of iron and two-hundredths of a milligram of copper. No calcium, no phosphorus, no vitamins at all. All the vitamins have been removed from white sugar in the process of refining.

This means that sugar does not nourish you, true. But it means a great deal more than that. In order to burn the sugar in your body's metabolism, certain of the B vitamins must be present. If you do not eat them with the sugar, your digestive processes must steal them from the rest of your body. So anyone who eats considerable amounts of sugar, especially if he is not concerned with getting lots of B vitamins in his food, is bound to suffer from vitamin B deficiency. Yet in this country we are consuming incredibly large amounts of white sugar every day—many, many times more than we did fifty years ago. Our sweet-tooth has been so developed that we cannot contemplate a meal without a dessert; and in addition we gorge on candy, cakes, soft drinks, chewing gum, jelly bread and so forth between meals, as well as doping our coffee, fruit and cereal with heaping tablespoonfuls of the treacherous white crystals. We believe this is one of the most obvious reasons for our national nervousness, our digestive ailments, our epidemics of colds, our alcoholism, our sleeping pill addiction.

Meal Planning Without Sugar

We are at war with sugar. Yet every day we receive letters like the one we described at the beginning of this article. Mothers trying desperately to preserve their children's health, plead with us for something they can give the children to satisfy the omniverous sweet-tooth. Housewives, trying to plan menus that don't include pastries, cakes, cookies, puddings, write asking if they can possibly get by using raw sugar, or brown sugar. What can they pack for dessert in the children's lunch? Holiday candies are an important part of the average American child's life. How can we make them without sugar? It seems to us that carob flour may be the answer to these questions. For our children particularly, carob flour can be that extra special delicacy the other children don't have. It can replace sugar in many recipes. It can replace chocolate or cocoa in all recipes.

And, while we're about it, let's just glance at chocolate and cocoa—those two prime favorites of American children. Are you in the habit of making cocoa for the youngsters at breakfast or lunch when the adults drink tea or coffee? Do you know that cocoa and chocolate contain considerable amounts of caffeine? Do you know that they contain in addition a substance called theobromine—another stimulant probably as harmful as caffeine? Chocolate and cocoa are rich in calcium—a fine mineral children need. But they contain oxalic acid, too, which not only renders this calcium unavailable to the body, but also robs the body of stored calcium. Whether the fat content or some other element in chocolate is responsible, it has been established as one of the positive causes of acne—the skin disease of adolescence. Practically all doctors today forbid chocolate to their acne patients.

Carob Flour and A Healthy Digestive Tract

The carob's chief contribution to your bodily welfare seems to be in relation to the health of the digestive tract. A letter to the Editor of *The Lancet,* British medical magazine, calls attention to the usefulness of carob flour in treating vomiting in infants. Some children seem to vomit naturally, says Dr. Theodore James of the Duchess of York Hospital for Babies in Manchester. But in many cases infants seem not to be able to keep any food on their stomachs. Naturally they become dehydrated and soon may become badly undernourished as they continue to lose the food that is so essential. Dr. James first heard of carob flour being used by a physician in Paris who treated vomiting in infants with milk thickened with carob flour. It thickens the milk without lessening its digestibility or changing its nutritive value, says Dr. James. (We suggest that it adds greatly to the nutritive value.) Dr. James used carob flour in treating nine infants all of whom were cured or remarkably improved within a very short time. If there is no relief from the vomiting after carob flour has been given, he says, it is time to suspect that there is some very serious organic disorder. This cannot be a simple case of "habitual vomiting."

The Nestlé Company which distributes carob flour in Europe announces in the *International Record of Medicine* that the potency of carob flour in treating diarrheas results from its high content of pectin and lignin. Pectin is the substance found in many fruits which offers protection against diarrhea—the same substance that causes jelly to "jell." We would suggest that the B vitamins in carob may have a lot to do with it, too, for they are well-known protectors of the health of the digestive tract.

Finally we want to call your attention to the sugar content of carob. These sugars listed in the analysis are natural sugars, such as occur in honey, fruits and vegetables. They satisfy your sweet-tooth and give you energy, for they contain calories. As you can see, the total calorie content of carob is 1595 per pound. But—and this is the important thing to remember always about naturally occurring sugars as compared to white refined sugar or synthetic sugars such as are used in candies, canned fruits, bakery products and so forth—the natural, unrefined sugars, such as the carob has, carry their own B vitamins with them for digestive purposes, so that eating this kind of sweet does not rob your body of B vitamins. As is the case with most fruits and vegetables, carob has an alkaline reaction within the body. In fact, as you can see in the analysis (page 154), its pH value is 10.6, which means that it is extremely alkaline.

Carob flour is the fruit of the carob tree, finely ground, to take the place of cocoa, chocolate and, to some extent, sugar. It contains ample vitamins and minerals to qualify as a worth-while food. It will satisfy your sweet-tooth and that of your family without doing you any of the harm done by refined and synthetic sugars. It will have an alkaline reaction in your body, as other fruits and vegetables do. You can use as much or as little of it as you like without any hesitation as to possible harmful effects.

Don't you think it would be wise to use carob flour in place of chocolate and cocoa from now on? You can make delicious drinks by beating carob flour with milk, fruit juice or water. You can use carob flour in your baking in place of both chocolate and sugar. Since it is a food fairly new to Americans (although Europeans have been using it for years) any firm from which you buy carob flour will supply you with recipes showing you the proper proportions in which to use it and suggesting all kinds of new and exotic delicacies you can make with this most unusual food.

If you suffer from diarrhea, stomach upsets, constipation or nausea, we suggest first, that you eliminate from your diet all refined sugar and synthetic sugars. This means no bakery products at all, either home-made or "boughten." No canned fruits or canned fruit juices, no candy or soft drinks. Second, if you still have a craving for something sweet, eat fruits and vegetables, preferably raw. And use carob flour for meal-time or between-meal beverages, to flavor hot breads and for any other recipes where you might use chocolate.

How to Make a Chocolate Cake

A reader, Mrs. M. Brown of Redondo Beach, Florida, has sent us a recipe for a chocolate cake that sounds delicious—a cake that contains no flour, no sugar, no baking powder. Listen!

Simply whip whole eggs and carob flour, nothing else, until double in bulk and bake carefully at about 300 degrees (no high heat, please!) for twenty to thirty minutes. You will need about eight to twelve eggs for one cup of carob flour. It depends on the size of the eggs.

Mrs. Brown uses one dozen egg whites to make chocolate angel food, then uses one dozen yolks plus one dozen eggs for the carob whole egg cake. You can frost the cake with tupelo honey, milk, rice polish, flavoring and gelatin. Sounds delicious, Mrs. Brown, and even more nutritious than delicious! And it's a natural for readers who have their own eggs.

Carob For Diarrhea

Discovery of the curative powers of the carob bean is credited to Professor Ramos, a Spanish physician. During the Spanish Civil War (1936-39) he observed that children of the poorer classes who ate large quantities of carob beans were less subject to disturbances of the digestive tract than were children of the wealthy, even though the rich children were better cared for generally. Later researchers found that the carob had indeed a marked effect on the health of the digestive organs.

Alan E. Smith, M.D. and Carl C. Fischer, writing in the *Journal of Pediatrics* for October, 1949, tell us of experiments in which thirty infants varying in age from 2 days to 15 months with acute diarrhea were given carob flour as part of their therapy. In eleven infants the stools became formed after only one day of carob flour; in twelve infants after two days; in six infants after three days. In only one infant was there no beneficial effect.

The Texas State Journal of Medicine for September 1950 relates trials with ninety-six patients with diarrhea. These children ranged in age from 2 weeks to 5 years. In the 69 patients whose diarrhea was due to intestinal organisms and/or virus infections, 47 showed "good" results in that there was an appreciable decrease in the number of and a thickening of stools within forty-eight hours. In 9 cases the results were "fair." In cases of diarrhea from other causes, the results were in general the same. Carob flour was given in a five per cent solution in water or boiled skimmed milk.

Three Canadian physicians used a 5 per cent gruel of carob flour in rice water for treating 253 children during the first 12 to 36 hours of treatment. In only three cases did they consider that the carob was ineffective. The length of time required to obtain normal stools averaged 1.8 days. Buttermilk was substituted for the carob as the infants responded to treatment. According to the *Canadian Medical Association Journal* for June 1953, these physicians say, "It is our opinion that carob flour is unexcelled by any other pectin base medication that we have heretofore employed."

Thomas R. Plowright, M.D. of Fresno, California, treated 20 infants with carob flour, reporting his results to *Pediatrics* for July, 1951. The type of diarrhea being treated was not bacterial in origin, he tells us. A "control" group of patients were not given the carob preparation, in order to compare their experience with that of the children receiving the carob. The severity of diarrhea was equally distributed in both groups.

The average number of hours for the first formed stools to be obtained in the infants who did not get carob was 174.3, compared to 47.95 in those who got carob. The average number of hospital days required for treatment of the control group was 14.15 compared to 7.85 for the carob-fed group. During a two-week follow-up period after the children went home, there was no recurrence of diarrhea in either group.

Our files contain many more instances of carob flour being used to treat diarrheas in children. For mild cases it seems to us an excellent home remedy. Apparently the pectin in the carob is what gets the results. For infants it is suggested that the dose is 2 to 4 level teaspoonsful to 4 fluid ounces of water. For children and adults, 1 to 2 level tablespoonsful in one-half glass of water every three or four hours should do the trick.

We have two cautions about using carob, particularly in the case of infants. It is, of course, a food and a good one, but a rather concentrated one for children so small. In the experience of one other physician (*Journal of the Kentucky State Medical Association,* July 1951) it was found that giving carob too long caused constipation, so he suggested watching the dosage carefully and guarding against this. Of course in the case of older children and adults where less concentrated doses are given this difficulty would probably not arise.

One further caution—a serious diarrheal condition in an infant can be fatal. Minerals and vitamins lost in diarrhea must be replaced. Do not depend on carob alone if your child has diarrhea. Consult your doctor.

Carrots

They were cultivated in very early times, but were not held in such great esteem as food until more recently—these crisp, golden roots from the garden. Then in later times they were thought of as antidotes for poisons of one kind or another. During the latter part of the 18th century carrots were made into paste and applied as poultices to open sores and wounds and apparently demonstrated great healing powers.

Today we know that these powers were probably the result of the vitamins and minerals in carrots, for they are especially rich in the alkaline minerals and carotene, which is a substance that becomes vitamin A in the body. It is the carotene that gives carrots their yellow color. Experiments have shown that only about two to five per cent of this carotene is absorbed by the body when raw or cooked carrots are eaten, no matter how well they are chewed. But from four to 36 per cent of the carotene is absorbed when the carrots are well-shredded before eating. This suggests that it is a very sound practice to drink fresh carrot juice, for in juicing the carrot the cell walls are broken down so that large amounts of carotene may be absorbed.

Carrots have considerable quantity of protein, including four of the essential amino acids, which are forms of protein. It is richest in vitamin A, containing 10,000 to 12,000 units of vitamin A in every half-cup of carrots.

Other vitamins in a half-cup of carrots are:

B Vitamins	
Thiamin	60-70 micrograms
Riboflavin	60 micrograms
Niacin	5 milligrams
Inositol	48 milligrams
Biotin	2 micrograms
Folic acid	97 micrograms
Choline	95 milligrams
Vitamin E	1.5 milligrams
Vitamin K	.1 milligrams
(Carrot tops are rich in this vitamin)	
Vitamin C	5 milligrams

The minerals in carrots are:

Calcium	46 milligrams
Phosphorus	38 milligrams
Iron	.6 milligrams
Copper	.08 milligrams
Magnesium	.06 milligrams
Chlorine	36 milligrams
Sodium	31 milligrams
Zinc	.5 to 3.6 milligrams
Cobalt	2 micrograms

In preparing carrots, as in preparing other vegetables, you should do the shredding, slicing or dicing immediately before the carrots are to be eaten, for vitamin C losses are high when foods are cut and exposed to air. Shredding carrots results in 20 per cent loss of vitamin C immediately and an additional loss of 20 per cent takes place if they are allowed to stand for an hour. However since carrots are not as rich in vitamin C as other foods, you should consider first perhaps the vitamin A value when you are preparing carrots. And since shredding or juicing makes this vitamin available for the body to use, it is apparently best to shred or juice carrots—but do it just before serving them.

You may have the wrong idea about when to pull and eat carrots. Young carrots are more tender, but actually they have less sugar and less carotene than fully mature ones, for they both increase during growth and are at their height in mid-August, if the carrots were planted in the spring. Winter-grown carrots are lower in carotene. Carrots can be stored without serious loss of food elements for six months at a temperature of 32 to 40 degrees.

We have discussed many times in these pages the value of vitamin A in protecting against infection. A diet rich in vitamin A assures the health of body tissues, such as the skin and the lining of the nose and throat. It is also essential for good eye health and protects against "night blindness" which is the inability to see well in a dim light or after dark. So if you find that you have trouble with glare when you are driving your car, if you discover that you begin to bump into things when dusk falls, vitamin A is for you! The old tradition about carrots being good for your eyes is not superstition. They really are!

Cell

Every living thing is composed of cells. By this we mean you, and all parts of your body. We mean all the animals, fish, birds, trees, flowers, grass—everything that lives. Some living things are composed of only one cell. The amoeba, for instance, is a one-celled animal that has no shape. That is, it is a microscopic blob of protoplasm that moves along in water by projecting sections of itself, so that its shape is constantly changing. The leucocytes or white blood corpuscles move through the blood with an amoeba-like movement.

At the very beginning of life, the sperm cell of the male encounters the ovum of the female and from this cell which you can see only under a strong microscope come all the cells that make up a human being. Cells are created by the division of other cells. And this cell division is a mighty complicated affair. Just think—as a cell divides itself into two cells, each of these new cells must contain all of the things which will determine what kind of cell it will be. For, of course, cells perform different functions. There are cells whose chief job is taking in oxygen, cells whose function is to receive and send stimuli, cells like muscle cells which work only by contracting or expanding, cells which secrete fluids, cells which carry substances from one part of the body to another, as red blood cells carry iron in hemoglobin. Every cell has its own special job to do. It is possible, by outside pressures or temperatures, to change the shape of a cell, but no process known to man can cause the cell to develop into anything except what it was supposed to be. In other words, a cell meant to carry hemoglobin in the blood cannot, by any wizardry of science, be made to perform any other function.

On the other hand, every cell in the body carries on all the time those most important functions which the whole body performs. That is, cells ingest oxygen and food and excrete waste matter. Cells reproduce. So you might say that the physiological activities of the body are nothing more or less than the coordinated expression of the corresponding activities of all the cells that make up the body.

The main parts of every cell are the nucleus and the cytoplasm—that is, the living substance of the cell that is not included in the nucleus. The nucleus is the controlling force of the cell. It is made of protein and nucleic acid and contains a high percentage of phosphorus. All of the body cells are constantly in the process of dying and being replaced. So, quite apart from all their essential functions for the welfare of the body as a whole, they must also be constantly repairing and replacing their own structure. This suggests the reason why protein is such a vital part of our diet.

Day and night the cells of all the different layers of our skin are busily and everlastingly working to perform their functions. They are breathing in oxygen, burning it, giving off wastes, growing old and replacing themselves with other cells. The osteoblasts are cells that form bone. The fibroblasts or fiber cells are busy keeping in repair all the fibrous or tissue parts of the body. And incidentally it has been found that the activity of these fibroblasts cannot proceed unless there is plenty of vitamin C in the diet! The blood cells are busy circulating to all parts of the body, carrying oxygen and food to other cells and meanwhile repairing and replacing their own substance.

Cytology is the science which studies cells and all the functions of cells. And you can readily see why it has become such an important science in recent years when we have just begun to realize the significance of cell life in relation to human life as a whole. You often read in the paper of some new discovery that has been made about cells and generally the headline will relate this discovery to the study of cancer. "Cell Study Gives New Cancer Hope" is the headline in the *New York Times* for May 7, 1952, and the article describes a study showing that a substance given off by cells protects animals against doses of radiation which would otherwise be fatal. The discoverers hope eventually to make possible the saving of cancer patients who could not otherwise endure the enormous doses of X-ray necessary for killing cancer tissues.

Actually, it seems quite possible that by studying the way a single cell works we may arrive at important conclusions about the way the body works. If, for instance, a certain substance is shown to be poisonous to a single cell, can we not assume that this substance, in large enough amounts, would also be poisonous to the whole body? For the body is, after all, just an orderly collection of cells. And, too, when we find that some other substance is absolutely necessary for healthy cell life, can we not assume that the body needs this substance in large quantities—enough for all its cells? This is the reason why we say so often in these pages that such and such a substance is a protoplasmic poison—do not take it into your body. It poisons cells, that's what we mean. And when we say that a certain vitamin is necessary for the proper functioning of a muscle cell, we mean that this vitamin absolutely must be eaten in large enough amounts by everyone who wants to have healthy muscles.

Then, too, if we can find from our study of cells what circumstances cause cells to reproduce abnormally, we will have found the secret of cancer, for cancerous cells are cells growing in a wild and disorderly fashion. We know what happens to human beings who live under conditions of poor nutrition, lack of fresh air, bad water, and who are subject to all kinds of poisons in food, air and water. These human beings become stunted, deformed and sluggish. Illness, immorality, crime and insanity are commonplace among them. But human beings are nothing more or less than large accumulations of cells. So doesn't it seem possible that conditions of poor nutrition, bad air and water and poisons of different kinds may react on individual cells the same way they react on communities of people? Perhaps cancer is just reaction to poor environment. Perhaps the rapid formation and spread of cancer can be compared to the spread of crime and illness in a destitute community. Perhaps cancer represents the insanity of the cell.

The research we do constantly deals often with cells. Whenever you run across some references to cells—what is good and bad for them—remember, *this means you.* What is good for your cells—every individual cell of your body—is good for you. And what is bad for your cells can't help but be bad for you.

Celery

A delectable and crisp accompaniment for fall meals is celery—so easy to prepare and healthful. The taste of celery seems to be almost universally well liked. Indeed there are few vegetables whose flavor is so outstanding that we make salt, oil, essence, and so forth, of them just for the sake of the flavor, as we do with celery.

Celery is grown on rich, moist, mucky soil and is not an easy vegetable to grow, we are told, because it needs cool temperatures, lots of moisture and, when produced commercially, a certain amount of labor involved in the blanching process.

There seems to be no reason the least bit sensible for blanching or bleaching celery. Yet large amounts of commercially grown celery are bleached. This may be done by the way it is grown—planting it in a trench and heaping earth around it as it grows, or shielding it from the light by boards while it is growing. We discovered that it is also blanched by ethylene gas, one of the constituents of illuminating gas. We are told that a concentration of one part of gas to 1000 parts of air is used to treat the celery for from six to twelve days, after which there is no chance of its turning green again before it is sold.

No one knows exactly how the ethylene gas works to achieve this modern miracle of stupidity and waste, but it is assumed that it stimulates enzymes which are concerned with breaking down various compounds in plants. The chlorophyll is completely destroyed by the use of gas or any other method of blanching celery. In our part of the country it is fashionable to eat deep green celery, so the markets have that kind for sale.

Blanching celery is almost as silly as it would be to blanch parsley. Chlorophyll is, of course, one of the most valuable elements we obtain from food. Why then should we deliberately destroy it before we eat the food? We destroy as well all the vitamin A of the celery, much of the vitamin C and a considerable portion of the B vitamins. A stalk of celery that contains 1000 units of vitamin A, green, contains from 0 to 10 units after blanching. One hundred micrograms of riboflavin in a stalk of green celery are reduced to 35 micrograms after blanching. If you can possibly get green celery in your locality, buy it, rather than blanched.

Much of the celery we buy has been on its way to us for some time. Celery can be stored for from 60 to 100 days before it begins to deteriorate. But the first time you taste your own celery right from the garden you will realize that you've never really tasted celery before. We have a lot of notes in our files about preparations used on celery in commercial growing. It is of course sprayed and otherwise treated. In fact, one letter from a grocer told us that he gets a rash on his hands from handling the celery in his store, so he must assume that the preservatives or the insecticides used are very strong indeed. You should, of course, wash celery thoroughly. But, we point out that it's next to impossible to get all of the stuff off. Your own celery from the garden or organically grown celery is the answer.

Celeriac is a celery plant of which the root is eaten. It is used widely in Europe. Its texture, after it is cooked, is much like potatoes. Celery seeds, used in salads, are chiefly imported from France. A letter from a reader tells us that she makes tea from celery seed which is a helpful natural laxative. Celery salt is dehydrated celery which is then pulverized.

Celery is popular among vegetable juice drinkers, mostly we suspect, because it makes such a fine-tasting juice. It is famous as a cure for "nerves," gout, diabetes, "sour stomach" and other disorders. There is no doubt that raw vegetables and their juices are our most healthful foods, chiefly because of the vitamins and minerals they contain, but also because they are raw and fresh and completely edible that way. A glass of (unblanched) celery juice brims over with chlorophyll and provides as well vitamins and minerals in abundance.

Here are the vitamins and minerals in about a cup of diced (unblanched) celery:

Vitamin A	1000 International Units
Vitamin B	
Thiamin	30 micrograms
Riboflavin	100 micrograms
Niacin	.4 milligrams
Vitamin C	5-7 milligrams
Calcium	50-70 milligrams
Phosphorus	40-50 milligrams
Iron	.5-.6 milligrams
Sodium	110 milligrams
Potassium	300 milligrams

Celiac Disease

Constipation has been spoken of as the national disease of America. It is indeed widespread and is caused, we believe, chiefly by our American diet of refined foods from which not only most roughage but also most vitamins and minerals have been removed. Another disorder which appears to be relatively common is diarrhea, one form of which has been the subject of much research. This is the so-called "fatty diarrhea." The medical term for it is "steatorrhea." Two closely related disorders are sprue and celiac disease. Sprue is generally found in tropical countries. Celiac disease is chiefly a disease of infants. According to most medical authorities, we have no inkling as to the cause of any of these disorders.

However, it certainly seems reasonable to relate them to what we eat. In the case of fatty diarrhea, there seems to be an inability to digest either fats or starches. Apparently the undigested starch ferments in the intestines, causing bloating, gas and distention of the abdomen. These undigested carbohydrates are then excreted along with whatever fat has been in the stools. Stools of a patient with celiac disease are frothy, bulky, fatty and ill-smelling. In addition to the ever-present diarrhea the patient is usually irritable and feverish. He suffers from lack of appetite and loss of weight. His abdomen is distended.

Why should diarrhea, especially this kind of diarrhea, be so serious an illness? Consider for a moment what happens to the whole mechanism of the body as a result of the diarrhea. Carbohydrates and fats are lost to it, so all the functions these food elements perform in the body are not performed. Calcium combines with the undigested fat in the abdomen and is carried away. So all the functions which calcium performs in the body go undone. This involves the nerves, the bone and tooth structure, the heart, the blood—all are affected by this loss of calcium. In infants prolonged diarrhea of this kind can lead to rickets and in older persons to osteomalacia or bone softening. Loss of calcium is one of the reasons for the irritability, lack of appetite and loss of weight as well. In addition to calcium other minerals are lost rapidly when the diarrhea continues for very long. No food, including minerals, stays in the digestive tract long enough to be absorbed. So potassium, iron, phosphorus and all the other important minerals are rapidly lost.

Equally important is the loss of the fat soluble vitamins. These are vitamins A, D, K and E. As the undigested fat is excreted, these vitamins go along with it and so they too are lost to the body. In the case of growing children this loss can mean the difference between straight strong bones and bones deformed with rickets. In adults and children, too, vitamin A is of the utmost importance in preventing infections and keeping the tissues healthy. Sure enough, in patients with celiac disease there is a high incidence of respiratory disorders—colds and so forth. And why not, considering that they are getting no benefit at all from all the many elements in their diets that prevent this kind of infection! We are told that one way of testing for celiac disease is to test for vitamin A in the blood. If it is far below normal then celiac disease is diagnosed.

Anemia will follow if iron continues to be lost. Anemia is another almost certain symptom of celiac disease, for it is bound to occur when iron is lost. It is interesting to note that the blood sugar level is low in these diarrheal diseases. Sugar in the blood must be kept at a certain level or all kinds of symptoms will appear—fatigue, weakness, black-outs, allergies, to name but a few. Apparently no one knows what the connection is between fatty diarrhea and blood sugar. But there seems to be no doubt that they are connected.

Treatments for Celiac Disease

There is obviously no "bug" involved in this kind of diarrhea. So the usual battery of antibiotics and sulfa drugs are not given. In general, physicians seem to agree that the disease is wholly one of nutrition and try to treat it on that basis. Some doctors report that they have had excellent results giving folic acid (one of the B vitamins) for celiac disease. Others found that they could not cure patients completely with folic acid, but that they got a good response when they gave the folic acid *along with brewer's yeast.* This strengthens our point of view that any and all of the vitamins should be taken in combination with the other vitamins and minerals that occur with it in foods.

Other physicians give diets low in carbohydrate and fat, high in protein, along with vitamins A and B and liver extract. In the case of patients who are infants taking nothing much but milk, the protein-high diet presents no problems. But in the case of older patients and adults there is a problem. What can these folks take for the carbohydrate part of their meals? It has been found that bananas (in spite of their high carbohydrate content) seem to be acceptable as food to most of these patients. Now this does not mean that the mere eating of the bananas works a cure. But they are a safe carbohydrate food, it seems, at a time when almost every other carbohydrate food causes digestive difficulty. So they are one of the first foods usually recommended when the celiac patient is gradually trying to get back to a normal diet. And they seldom cause trouble.

Recently a new aspect of celiac disease has been uncovered. Some Dutch investigators discovered that the glutinous part of wheat might be responsible for celiac disease in those who were susceptible. Other physicians began to put their patients on wheat-free diets with good results. In *The Lancet* for March 19, 1955, J. W. Gerrard and two co-workers wrote that the wheat-free diet is effective not only in the early and active phase of celiac disease which takes place usually in infancy, but also in the later stages extending on into later childhood. In some cases, it seemed to them, the diet should be continued right on into adulthood.

In a Norse medical journal *Tideskrift for Den Norse Laegeforening* for September 15, 1953, investigators disclosed the harmful effect of wheat, rye and oats in celiac disease. They reported on good results in 12 cases of the disorder, when these three cereals were omitted from the diet. In a later issue of *The Lancet* (May 28, 1955) we are told of experiments in which 30 sick children were kept on diets free from wheat gluten. Twenty-eight of them recovered completely. The other two did not respond to the diet. One of these had a deficiency in bile salts and the other was apparently allergic to fat. But in the case of 28, it appeared that the gluten of the wheat was the sole thing causing the trouble. So now it appears that, for the kind of diarrhea caused by celiac disease, one of the first things the doctor will suggest is to leave cereal products out of the diet.

The peculiar thing about the story is that the *gluten* of the wheat seems to be responsible for the damage. Gluten is a protein substance that occurs mostly in the germ part of the wheat, so it is not present in white flour in such large quantities. Gluten bread is eaten by diabetics—bread from which all the starch has been removed. In white bread, on the contrary, the germ part of the grain (containing much of the gluten) has been removed entirely. So what we are actually saying is that celiac patients get that way because their bodies cannot handle the protein whole grain cereals! And, strangely enough, *eating just the starch from the cereals* does not bring on their symptoms. It's the gluten part of the grain that does it.

What does this prove—that all of us should stop eating whole grain cereals and eat nothing but starchy refined cereals? Of course not! We know that many food elements have been removed from whole grains when they are refined to make "white" flour. By "enriching" the flour, our millers put back two or three of the B vitamins and a little iron, without any regard for what this slicing up and re-combining is going to do to the wholeness of the food. So of course our story on celiac disease does not signify that you should immediately begin to eat breads made from refined flours rather than whole grains.

Testing Foods for Yourself

What it does mean is simply that there are foods which certain people simply cannot eat happily and healthfully—no matter what good foods they happen to be nutritionally. Wheat gluten is one of these—for people who are susceptible to celiac disease.

The other lesson we learn from this story is, we think, to experiment with your food, if you happen to be suffering from some disorder that does not respond to treatment. Whether or not you have celiac disease, perhaps you were not meant to eat bread at all. Perhaps something about bread just doesn't agree with you. How will you discover this unless you stop eating bread for a while (leaving everything else in your diet just as it was). Perhaps milk is the cause of your trouble. Perhaps you just can't take citrus fruits. It won't do you a bit of harm to experiment. So long as you are eating a good diet and taking your food supplements you can leave almost any food out of your menus for three or four weeks without missing it. If your symptoms disappear, perhaps you should forget about this food permanently, so far as you personally are concerned. Just because everybody has always eaten bread is no reason why you should go on eating bread if it disagrees with you. (Editor Rodale does not eat bread.)

One caution though. You must be sure to replace, somehow, in your diet whatever food elements are plentiful in the food you decide to do without. Whole grain is rich in the B vitamins, vitamin E and iron. If you are going to stop eating it, you must make sure that you get enough of these precious substances from some other source in your food. Dried beans, lean meat, fish, liver—these are good sources of the B vitamins. Brewer's yeast is the richest source. Iron is plentiful in eggs. And so forth.

We find ourselves wondering about the kind of bread the children in these experiments were fed. It seems almost impossible that it could have been real, whole grain bread, made from freshly ground grain. This is generally not available except in the home of some "food faddist." Certainly it is not served in hospitals. Commercially processed whole grain flours must be treated with preservatives so they will keep on grocer's shelves. Do you suppose it might be the preservative in the flour that is responsible for cases of celiac disease?

Cereal

The label on the side of a commercial dry breakfast cereal caught our attention the other day. The little box was hardly big enough to contain all the long names of all the chemicals included in this breakfast dish. On the front was a strong right arm flexed to show enormous muscles suggesting we suppose, to spindly young fry that this cereal would make them certain candidates for a football team. Then the label listed all the synthetic vitamins and minerals added to the dead, refined food inside—the chemical niacin, riboflavin, calcium, iron and so forth, that had been added to take the place of the natural food elements removed in the processing. Then finally we come to a listing of the preservatives and, so help us, this is exactly what appears on that label: "not more than 1/100 of 1 per cent of propyl gallate and 2/100 of 1 per cent of butylated hydroxyanisble and 5/1000 of 1 per cent citric acid in propylene glycol." Practically all of the food value of the cereal has been removed, remember, so that there is nothing left to "spoil" or become moldy. But even so, the manufacturers must add a preservative, call it by a tricky trade name, and imply that it makes the cereal even more delicious and healthful! These are coal tar preservatives, and, as you know, we believe that they are harmful, taken over a long period of time, even in such small quantities. A box of commercial dry breakfast cereal may look inexpensive on the market shelf. Actually, it is one of the most expensive foods you can buy in terms of the false sense of security you may have in serving your children this appalling combination of starch, synthetic vitamins and coal tar preservatives!

Change of Life—Male

Is there a male "change of life?" Do middle-aged men pass through a serious physiological and psychological readjustment as women do at the time of the menopause? Are nervousness, irritability and other symptoms to be expected around fifty or sixty years of age, or are they a sign that something is wrong somewhere?

The medical experts seem to be completely divided on the subject of the "male menopause." One writer may start his article with the words "Now that it is generally accepted that the male also has a change of life around middle age . . ." Another expert will begin his article by saying "Of course, as everybody knows, there is nothing at all to this business of a male climacteric. A middle-aged man simply has a great many personal, financial and family problems. If he permits them to, they make him nervous. That's all there is to it."

A third takes the viewpoint that the term is a misnomer, for, says he, it implies that there is a definite age in males when the testes stop functioning, as the ovaries stop functioning in the female. No such thing occurs in the case of the male, therefore what is all this talk about a male climacteric?

So the one and only thing we are sure of about the male climacteric is that medical men are in complete disagreement as to whether or not it exists. Then there is the question of why some men—many men, in fact—have certain symptoms which are generally quite similar any time from fifty years on. Are these symptoms the result of a change in the reproductive system, do they come about just as a prelude to old age or are they entirely psychological? There are those who defend each of these theories.

What are the symptoms we are talking about? Nervousness is the most outstanding and characteristic. All of the articles we read mentioned the extreme nervousness of the patients. Irritability goes hand-in-hand with nervousness. Inability to concentrate, forgetfulness, loss of sleep and appetite, dizziness, numbness in fingers and toes, breathlessness, depression or melancholia, headaches, and disorders of the digestive tract and heart are common symptoms. Two writers, M. Prados and B. Ruddick writing in the *Psychiatric Quarterly* for July, 1947, say that their patients were ambitious, active, aggressive, hard workers, good family-providers; most of them were devoted husbands and fathers. They were men who held important, responsible positions. This sounds to us like a description of the kind of men who are supposedly more susceptible to ulcers—the "ulcer personality" as the medical books call it. We have always had serious doubts, however, as to whether there really is an ulcer personality—or whether the foods a man eats and the way he lives make him into a certain kind of person and are also responsible for his ulcer.

Loss of Sexual Power Most Troublesome Symptom

Almost invariably the symptom for which the "change of life" patient has come to his doctor is a decrease in sex potency. The sex urge is present, perhaps even stronger than usual, but the patient is unable to complete the sex act. There are also complaints about prostate gland function.

Dr. Richard L. Landau writing in *Medical Clinics of North America,* volume 35, page 279, says "the period of life during which 'climacteric' symptoms are presumed to occur is also that time at which the emotional and intellectual adjustment of the shift from maturity to old age must begin to be made. Usually this can be accomplished smoothly, but some men may develop neurotic reactions while accommodating to the life situation . . . Impotence and the loss of libido (sex urge) may be caused by reactive depressions and anxiety states of even the milder sort."

Could all these complaints be psychological? Is it possible that a man finding himself growing older, fearing he may be losing his grip on his business, his job, his wife's love or his place in the sun may work himself into a state of psychological panic in which physical symptoms develop? We think this is possible, but we think this kind of thing will happen only to a person whose state of health is none too good, in spite of the fact that he may be active and aggressive.

Dr. Benjamin Sieve of Boston, whose ideas we discuss at length in our article on prostate gland, was present where an article on male change of life was read. In the *Journal of the American Medical Association,* March 24, 1945, he is quoted as reminding the other professional men present that the B complex of vitamins is extremely important for the use of the body when it manufactures hormones. The role of the

B vitamins in relation to sex hormones is not fully understood, he said, but it seems that they are especially necessary for this function.

Vitamins Are Important for Sex Function

It is our belief that the degenerative diseases which attack most virulently at the time of middle age and beyond could be prevented to a large extent by a proper diet that would include natural foods and food supplements. For example the complaint of sterility and loss of potency cannot be tolerated in a stock animal used for breeding. So farmers raising such animals use the utmost care in feeding them and experiments are constantly in progress at our great agricultural universities to develop even more nourishing feeds for these animals. Vitamin E and the food elements contained in wheat germ have turned out to be extremely important for the sexual health of farm animals. Is it surprising, then, that human beings whose diet has contained little vitamin E and practically no wheat germ for more than fifty years should complain of loss of sexual power? What would a farmer say to a veterinarian who told him his prize bull could no longer fertilize cows because he was disturbed psychologically? Safe to say, the vet knows that sexual power, as well as all other aspects of bodily health depends on diet. Why are human beings so long in learning this lesson about their own health?

One last comment—we found an article in an Italian medical magazine, *Rivista di Ostetricia e ginecologia* for May, 1954, in which Dr. A. Narpozzi described the influence of the various vitamins on seminal fluid. This is the fluid which carries the sperm cells—the cells that unite with the female egg to begin the life of a new human being. Patients who suffered from a deficiency in seminal fluid were tested after being given the various vitamins. It was found that vitamin A and vitamin E, especially given together, restored to normal the number of sperm cells present. Vitamin B also improved the deficiency, due largely, it is thought, to the excellent effects of vitamin B on the liver. Vitamin C did not have any effect on the number of sperm cells but it did increase their motility and caused abnormal forms of cells to disappear. Vitamin D in average doses was beneficial—in large doses was not. Vitamin A and vitamin E were, we repeat, the two most important vitamins studied from the point of view of sperm number and health.

Is there a male "change of life"? We believe there is—for those men who have lived without regard for good diet and other important health rules. At the time of middle age or later their vitality and nervous energy are going to run down and be depleted. The symptoms will then appear—the nervousness, irritability, uncertainty and forgetfulness, the digestive disturbances, the heart pains, the loss of sexual power. Is there a male "change of life"? We believe there is not—for those men who have lived as healthfully as possible, keeping their diet and their way of life close to nature, shunning modern chemicalized and processed foods and supplementing their diets with natural food supplements to make up for the food elements that simply aren't present in modern food. We think that "change of life" is just another degenerative disorder that need not occur at all if early steps are taken to prevent it.

Chemicals

How Much Chemical Does a Man Need?

by J. I. RODALE
Editor of Prevention

This heading is a take-off of a short story from the gifted pen of Tolstoi, called, "How Much Land Does a Man Need?" which was written to epitomize man's greed for material possessions. In the story, a man is promised that he will be given all the land he can cover in a day's journeying and that the end of the day will be marked by the going down of the sun. The greedy man walks too far and as night approaches and he fears that he will not return to the marked line by sundown, he begins to run frantically and just falls over the line in time, but dies of exhaustion.

The theme of this article is, how much chemical does the human body need? How much chemical can the human body stand before it too falls over the line, dead at the sundown of a shortened life?

How much chemical does the chemical industry wish to sell in order to justify its reason for existence, satisfy its urge for continuous expansion? This of course is distantly related to how far the chemical industry can go in forcing chemicals down the American gullet before man turns into a chemical and begins to drop dead in the street from the effects of such chemicalization.

Are Poisons Needed For Full Employment?

The selling of food chemicals poses some difficult complications. There seems to be a vague fear that unless the chemical people are permitted to sell their chemicals, regardless of their effect on the human organism, short of downright killing it, that their gargantuan industry will collapse, and bread lines will form in every city. I have noted such an attitude between the lines of the thinking even of medical organizations, while in Governmental agencies it has become axiomatic. In other words we have come to the concept that man must increasingly get cancer in order to uphold the economy of this glorious America. What are a few more cases of polio if it prevents the bankruptcy of a segment of our corporate citizenry. But there is a peculiar tendency that I have taken cognizance of in Congress and in its appointed agencies. It makes a difference if you are an old, powerful company or if you are a new upstart. The intrenched, vested interests or vested concepts can get away with murder, based on the theory that we must not make too radical changes which will affect the employment of people. In the same way Congressmen and Government men generally simply worship the vested professors of science. When a man like *me* comes along, even though I have done more research and scientific reading in my field than the average agricultural professor, congressmen will heckle me unmercifully and not pay a particle of attention to my testimony and exhibits. We not only worship the golden calf but we bow down to the images in our halls of higher learning.

Which reminds me of a story! There were two wholesale diamond dealers, Jones and Brown, who sometimes bought stones from each other. One day, Jones saw a diamond that his friend possessed which caught his fancy and he bought it for $300. After he had left, Brown began to think that Jones had purchased that stone faster than he had ever made a purchase before. There must be something unusual about it that he had not noticed. The next day he visited Jones and bought back the stone for $350. But after he left, Jones began to think. Brown had never done a thing like this before so when he was at the home of Brown some time later he casually offered him $400 for the diamond. It went this way for a few weeks, the stone being sold back and forth until Jones one day paid Brown $800 for it. A few days later Brown wished to buy the diamond back again but Jones told him that he had sold it to a retail customer.

"That is too bad," said Brown mournfully, "we were making such a nice living off that stone."

Aren't we doing the same thing in our Government and in our industry? Aren't we setting up false values and fooling ourselves? The Government permits benzoate of soda to be used in various foods so that certain industries can keep their products on the store shelves longer without spoiling and thus make larger profits. As a result certain delicate stomachs are offended and the United States has to build more hospitals, like the huge one at Bethesda, Maryland, in order to study the proper ways to take care of all those outraged stomachs. To build and operate such hospitals requires money, so the Government places higher income tax on the food company which might mean that it may have to put a little more benzoate of soda into its product so that the spoilage will be reduced even further, and so that a little extra money would be forthcoming to pay the new tax. The larger amount of benzoate causes greater trouble in the customers' health which means more hospitals and higher taxes and then, of course, more benzoate of soda.

Trading Poisons Is No Picnic!

Let me give you another illustration of how artificial our relations with one another have become in the system of competitive cash culture under which we live. Mr. Brown works in a bakery where they make frankfurter rolls in which many harmful chemicals such as polyoxyethylene-monosterate are used. Even a small amount of plaster of Paris is applied to the flour in order to bleach it. His neighbor Mr. Jones works in a frankfurter factory where sodium nitrate and saltpetre are used as part of the ingredients. Jones and Brown go to a picnic where they both eat the frankfurters on a roll. You see? They are feeding each other harmful chemicals which they themselves made in order to make a living.

Mr. Smith is employed in a pickle factory where the dangerous alum is used as a firming agent and Mr. Doe works in an ice cream making plant where synthetically made, coal-tar vanilla is used as a flavoring agent. Doe sells Smith the ice cream and Smith sells Doe some pickles. Again you see the system at work. We are making such a nice living poisoning each other. Most of us are doing the same thing. We are selling things to each other which are not to our best interest, or which have a questionable value. We are involved in an economic, industrial system, a competitive cash culture, which is based on selling harmful things to each other. For every dollar we earn, directly or indirectly, we must take a certain quota of poison; otherwise the powers that control our daily destinies believe that our whole prosperity will collapse.

What a mockery! And in this crazy system is involved the use of chemical fertilizers and poisonous insecticides. I sat in on a hearing in Washington (in which I was a witness) which had for its purpose the setting of maximum tolerances of spray residues which the Government should permit on fruits and vegetables and saw this corrupting principle demonstrated. The room was filled with the chemists and attorneys of the large insecticide companies who were ready to answer any argument put forth, mechanically, so long as they continued to keep spouting words and putting the fear of economic collapse into the livers of the Government hearing officials. On the return trip by train, I sat next to one of these insecticide men and what a charming man he was. He had a large sparkling diamond which made me think of the story of the two diamond dealers. I purposely questioned him about his family without letting him know my purpose. I could see that he was dearly devoted to his wife and children, and yet he was part of a system that openly encouraged the use of dangerous chemicals in food which his own flesh and blood ate. Do the big executives think about this when they sit in church on Sunday? Is the making of any amount of money a justification of poisoning one's own family?

Is This Why Executives Died Young?

In recent years some of our very largest companies like DuPont and General Motors are finding that their executives are dying off extremely young. The medical department of DuPont believes that some of this is due to too much eating and has developed the DuPont diet which received much publicity a few years ago. I believe that too much eating is bad but am not quite in agreement with the DuPont medical men. I think the trouble is merely with eating, period. Let the DuPont people look into the amount of dangerous chemicals that their executives are eating, some of which they manufacture in their own factories. There they might find the secret of what is killing their men. Some people blame the hectic tempo and stresses of our modern business system for these deaths, but if we gave this idea some thought we would see how ridiculous it really is. The stress is much less today than it used to be. Fifty years ago a man did not take his car to go a few blocks to the grocery to buy a chemicalized loaf of bread. He walked. But come to think of it his wife baked her own bread with no chemicals in it. If a man went to a grocery store it was for something else. He did not breathe gasoline fumes. The man might be working twelve or fifteen hours a day in an unhealthful sweat-shop environment. Poverty was greater. In those days he froze in cold rooms as he slept. Today the stress is much less. Man is actually coddled more. He rarely walks. He is richer and has more comforts. Where is this modern stress that people talk about? It is only man's glib propensity for inventing excuses.

Heart Diseases Kill Many Physicians, Why?

But here is the important thing. The man we are talking about of fifty years ago ate better food than we do today. It was not raised with chemical fertilizers nor was it drenched with poison sprays. When it got into the factories it was not subjected as much to the dangerous chemicalization that our foods are subjected to today. As the Beech-Nut Company's man said at a Government hearing recently, his company is spending more than a hundred thousand dollars a year trying to eliminate some of the effects of the spray poisons from the vegetables it buys. He admitted that they cannot remove all of it. A properly nourished body can take almost any stress in its stride.

One of the most unfortunate victims of our chemical ideology is the physician, whose death rate from angina pectoris is twelve times higher than that of the farm worker. This is not because the farm worker is more active, but because in my opinion, he does not have to breathe in the chemical vapors, the ethers and other drug essences that fill the air of our hospitals. It has been shown that in the chemical industries many of the workers contract various diseases from their contacts with the products upon which they are working. For example, I have spoken about polyoxy-ethylene-monosterate used in making bread. In a medical journal that I was reading recently, I saw where workers coming in contact with ethylene amines became afflicted with asthma and skin diseases. There are thousands of volumes of medical studies showing the effect of chemicals in the factories where workers are associated with them and what it does to them, but I know of no study on the effect of physicians who have to spend a portion of each day in chemically vaporized hospitals. It is my studied opinion that this is one of the most important reasons why physicians live shorter lives than the average of their fellow-men. It is not only the walking up steps and being called in the middle of the night that does this, but it is also the effect on their bodies of the sharp hospital chemicals to which they are exposed every day.

The Case of the Bald-Headed Pharmacists

It is the effect of these same chemicals which actually make so many pharmacists bald-headed. The way I came to this peculiar conclusion was by being present at a pharmacists' convention at Atlantic City a few years ago. I was amazed at the number of bald-heads that could be seen. It was literally a sea of bald pates. But there were a few well-thatched heads there also which set me to thinking. Why do some pharmacists get bald while others do not? And here is the way I worked it out. A pharmacist works with strong chemicals. As he pulverizes, pounds and mixes some of the stuff gets onto his hands. As he works he perspires and occasionally he mops his brow with his hands, or scratches his head. In some way his chemicalized hands touch his hair. This does the damage. The chemicals seep down and attack the roots of the hair.

But why are some pharmacists not bald? In my theory these are the more phlegmatic ones, those who do not nervously bring their hands up to their head too often. Their hands are more disciplined. If this is not a scientific theory the next time you hear of a convention of pharmacists, go and see for yourself.

What was my surprise a few months ago while reading a scientific journal to learn that in a study of baldness by Peter Flesch, M.D., of the University of Pennsylvania, he mentioned the fact that workers in a synthetic rubber factory were losing their hair due to the effect of six chemical substances with which they were working. So perhaps I am not so far off base as you may have thought as you were digesting my fantastic theory.

More Chemicals, Less Religion . . . Is That Prosperity?

Coming back to our subject, "How much chemical does a man need?" the industry has reared a chemical Frankenstein which seems to be made up of a great deal of sulphuric acid. This compound is used copiously in many food and other products. It hides behind the trade-names and the skirts of chemical formulas. The consumption of sulphuric acid is so terrific in amount, over four million tons of it going into all industry in this country every year, that the financial experts use it as a gauge of prosperity. They watch the monthly figures of sulphuric acid consumption as if it were gold in the vaults of Fort Knox. On the other hand Roger Babson has used church attendance statistics to predict the future of business. When things begin to get bad people run to church. In prosperous times many forget God. It seems therefore that when the sulphuric acid consumption goes up and church attendance goes down, the financial wizards become happy. This is no reflection on Roger Babson himself, however, for I know him to be a God-fearing man. I also know him to be conservation-minded. He once sent some students from one of his business classes to hear me when I spoke to a botany class at Wellesley.

One of the places where sulphuric acid is used is in chemical fertilizers and poison sprays and I am happy that we have found a method of farming that does not need it for it seriously harms the structure and well-being of the soil. This method which we introduced into the United States more than ten years ago and which has hundreds of thousands of followers, has brought much increased health benefits to many of them. This method of producing food is the basis of the other magazine called *Organic Gardening and Farming* which is published by our organization. We advertise in this magazine many sources that sell food organically raised. I am risking sounding commercial but I advise health conscious persons to read *Organic Gardening and Farming*. Even if they do not farm nor garden, there is much of specialized interest there for them.

Chemicals In Foods and Risks That Lie in Dyes

Some years ago it was discovered that a coal tar dye (butter yellow) then being used to color butter, margarine and other yellow foods caused cancer in laboratory animals in every case in which it was given. The dye was forbidden for use in food in interstate commerce. Quite recently three dyes were declared unsafe for use in foods by the Food and Drug Administration. These three yellow and orange dyes had been used for years to color citrus fruit, candy, puddings, hot dogs, cakes, cookies, soft drinks. They had been tested many years ago by the methods then employed. They were on the "certified" list. But the Food and Drug chemists took it into their heads to test them again with methods now available, and promptly recommended that they be withdrawn from use in food.

According to the New York *Times,* reporting on a meeting of cancer specialists that took place in Brazil, in July, 1954, Dr. William E. Smith of New York University Bellevue Medical Center, announced that in the United States alone during 1953, 100,000 pounds of dyestuffs known to cause cancer in animals were approved by the F. D. A. for use in foods to be consumed by human beings. At the same meeting, Dr. Hermann Druckery of Germany observed that there was no recovery factor where substances causing cancer were concerned. "A person absorbing even infinitesimal amounts will still have the cumulative effect and when a certain level is reached and a period of latency has passed, the effect will become evident in the form of a tumor."

In 1949, the Science Editor of *The Times* reviewed the speech of a German scientist, Professor K. H. Bauer of Heidelberg, speaking before a congress of surgeons, who said that there are at present some 600,000 compounds made from carbon which were unknown a hundred years ago. Of these, we know that several hundred can cause cancer in animals and in human beings. The many cases of bladder cancer among workers in aniline dye plants finally resulted in the establishment of precautions which cut the incidence down to almost zero. But at present, said Dr. Bauer, what of the general public?

The spot most favorable for cancer growth is the digestive tract. In all of the so-called civilized countries, cancers of the mouth, throat, stomach and intestines are the commonest. The connection with food and drink is obvious. In the "backward" countries such as China where food is not doctored up with coal tar products the incidence of digestive tract cancer is much lower. Dr. Bauer demanded (and this was six years ago) that any and all substances which are known cancer-producers should not be sold in foods, over the counter or in restaurants. As we can see, nothing has been done along these lines in this country and we suppose that European countries also have made little or no progress.

The government's own top-ranking cancer expert, Dr. W. C. Hueper of the National Cancer Institute, U. S. Public Health Service, testified before the Delaney Committee in 1950 that several dyes are being used in food constantly which are known to produce cancer in animals. He mentioned a green dye used in canned peas and green maraschino cherries. A second, called yellow A. B., is used in popcorn, butter, margarine, cheese, candy and cake icings. It has been repeatedly linked to cancer of the bladder. As late as 1932 the Du Pont Company discovered 23 dye workers with cancer of the bladder. They were working with the dye which we are now using to dye popcorn, butter and other foods.

Are you as horrified by this revelation as we are?

The American Cancer Society tells us that every day of the year 620 Americans die of cancer, the most dreaded of modern diseases. Cancer, we are told, is mysterious. No one knows how it selects its victims. Formerly thought of as a disease of old age, it is at present one of the leading causes of death among children below the age of twelve.

Yet our Food and Drug Administration, charged with protecting the health of the American people, releases for human consumption 100,000 pounds of dyestuffs known to cause cancer in animals. Animal experimentation is the method used for determining whether or not a substance is dangerous to human beings. It is true that different species of animals react in different ways to various poisons and it is possible that some substances that cause cancer in some animals may not cause cancer in human beings. But it is well known that other substances *do* cause cancer in animals and in human beings, as well. Of what use is it to experiment with animals, if we are then going to release for human consumption chemicals that we know perfectly well will cause cancer in animals?

Perhaps the most shocking aspect of this whole revelation is that the substances under discussion are dyes. In respect to other chemicals, the food processors may claim that they serve some supposedly useful purpose in foods. Fats would become rancid without preservatives. Bread would become stale without softeners they tell us. But what possible excuse can there be for dyeing food? It serves no purpose whatsoever except to give the food a supposedly attractive color. Undoubtedly, it is thus possible to pass off old, tired-out vegetables, fruits and meats as fresh, wholesome foods. (Just see what a beautiful color they have!) And of course the dye in gum drops and all the other cheap candy is there to trap the eyes of the youngsters—the colors are so bright!

We wonder how long the American people are going to stand for this sort of thing. And we wonder how long they are going to contribute to cancer funds with this sort of thing going on under their noses. We are glad to see that physicians are becoming more alert and more vocal about the dangers of chemicals in foods.

For instance, an address before the Australian and New Zealand Association for the Advancement of Science appears in the May 29, 1954, issue of the *Medical Journal of Australia*. In it, R. W. W. Cunningham, Ph.C. of the Department of Health of Canberra, Australia, pleads for a better understanding of the risks we are taking and the development of other food dyes that are not dangerous to health. Cunningham is outspoken in relating chemicals in foods to cancer. He begins his address with reminding his listeners that the increase in incidence of certain diseases has gone right along with the increase in the use of processed food in which certain chemicals are used.

Can Cells Deal With These Poisons?

Living cells, he says, can deal with many, many different kinds of poisonous substances, but they may be vulnerable to new substances which differ only very slightly from things that are not poisonous at all. Aniline, from which dyes are made, and many of the chemicals made from it have been shown to cause kidney disease, to destroy red and white blood cells. Many of the substances made from aniline have been shown to cause cancer. Naphthol dyes, thought to be harmless, were recently shown to produce cancer in animal experiments. He speaks of two dyes —trypan blue and trypan red, the first of which causes cancer, the second of which does not. The only difference in the two dyes is just one chemical step that takes place in the body after ingesting the trypan blue.

All of these colors, he tells us, are authorized for use in the United States. Researchers have no way of knowing, he says, from the chemical structure of any substance whether or not it may cause cancer. Furthermore, what is cancer-causing for one kind of animal may not cause cancer in another kind. And we use these same derivatives of aniline in medicines! To be sure, says Cunningham, and physicians know perfectly well how dangerous they are and use them only for very short periods of time. But dyes in food are used possibly every day over the entire lifespan of an individual!

In Australia the death rate from leukemia has risen from 1.8 per 100,000 in 1930 to 4.4 per 100,000 in 1950. More than twice as high in a matter of twenty years! And this is what the *British Encyclopedia of Medical Practice* has to say about the relation of leukemia to chemicals: "It is well known that individuals who have been exposed to chronic benzene intoxications and many other chemical substances frequently develop leukemia. Further it has been noted that there is definite evidence that the sulphonamide group of drugs in some patients has been responsible for the onset of acute leukemia." He goes on to tell of ten cases of leukemia he has seen who had been treated with sulfa drugs, for colds or infections, just previously. He also points out that sulfanilamide, the parent substance, is widely used in the dye industry.

Cunningham gives the death rate for cancer in the United Kingdom —29.01 per 100,000 in 1851 and 188.09 per 100,000 in 1950. He believes that more people are becoming victims of cancer because of the increased period of exposure to the cancer-causing agents, whatever they may be. We know, he says, that among workers dealing with one cancer-causing chemical, the length of time it may take for the cancer to develop ranges from seven to twenty-two years. Do not forget, he says, that long-continued exposure to even small quantities of toxic substances ultimately produces recognizable cancer.

Chemicals and Dyes in Some Food Supplements

What about vitamin preparations that contain artificial coloring? We know that many readers buy vitamins. Some of them take synthetic vitamins, although we have produced ample evidence that natural vitamin products are infinitely preferable. But, natural or synthetic, vitamin preparations can and often are artificially colored.

But surely, you might say, nothing sold for health purposes will be harmful! Surely anyone who makes vitamin and mineral preparations can be relied upon to check carefully the healthfulness of everything that goes into his product! Again we quote the hearings of the Delaney Committee to Investigate Chemicals in Foods. An expert, Dr. Franklin Bing of the Public Health Association testified that, so far as could be discovered, a wetting agent or dispersing agent in a vitamin preparation was considered responsible for a relatively new disease in premature infants—retrolental fibroplasia which causes blindness and other symptoms. When the presiding physicians changed to another vitamin preparation that did not contain this particular wetting agent the incidence of this tragic disease went down from 30 to 40 per cent blindness to less than 1 per cent.

So you see that the so-called health foods can be a source of trouble. What we are especially concerned with is coloring matter in vitamin and mineral products. We check as closely as is humanly possible on all products mentioned to make certain they contain nothing that might be harmful in the way of synthetics, fillers and so forth. But some of the preparations are colored and we want to explain this color to our readers.

It is possible, of course, to color food (or food supplements) attractively without using coal tar colors. You have probably seen in your grocery the little kits of vegetable coloring used by many housewives to color icing, candy and so forth. Vegetable dyes consist of such things as a red dye made from beets, an orange dye made from carotene, which is the coloring matter of carrots, green dye made from parsley or chlorophyll and so forth. Why do not commercial food processing companies use these vegetable dyes in their foods? We are told that they are impractical for quantity production, for there are too few colors, they do not have enough intensity for commercial use and they tend to fade.

In general, makers of the natural products do not color their products at all. If they do, they use vegetable coloring.

Chemicals In the Process of Growing Foods

By Jonathan Forman, M. D.

This article is reprinted by permission from *The Columbus Dispatch* for February 12, 1956. Dr. Forman is one of the nation's leading allergists, editor of the Ohio State Medical Journal, a long-time crusader for conservation and president of Friends of the Land.

Leonard Wickenden, a retired chemist who combines the critical precision of a scientist with a rare felicity of expression, describes in a new book the disastrous effects of man's arrogant assumption that he can solve the complex biological problems of agriculture and public health by dissemination of deadly poisons.

He discusses DDT and the newer sprays, the soils they poison, the case against the addition of fluorine to the public water supply, vaporizers and fumigators, dangers of being beautified with certain cosmetics, perils of hormones and the doctoring of our daily bread.

To understand these poisons, one must gain a new and more accurate concept of life's processes and maximum health.

Each of us has a body composed of billions of tiny units called cells. Each is a living separate unit joined with other cells to make a human being. Through the process of evolution these cells have given up their independence in order to enter a cooperative state and become specialists in communication, transportation, food supply, locomotion and defense.

To carry on the life processes, each of these cells must digest food, excrete its wastes, repair itself and be ready in one-millionth part of a second to perform its specialized task.

Every reaction depends upon a chemical response triggered and controlled by a specific enzyme system. All life is merely a great number of these enzymes working together in coordination. In other words, life is the function of the protein of the cell joining with a particular vitamin and one of the mineral nutrients originally from the soil, to form an enzyme with a highly specialized function.

Every cell in the body must contain from 50,000 to 100,000 of these enzyme systems ready always to go to work in a millionth of a second. Some have been assigned the task of remembering when you had mumps or measles or diphtheria and being prepared to defend against specific germs for the rest of your life.

What most of us fail to appreciate is that each of the enzyme systems is affected by the merest trace of certain chemicals—often as little as one part in a million, or less.

The specific mineral and vitamin as well as the building stones for the proteins must be in the cell at the same time and in proper proportions if the enzyme system is to be in perfect working order. Then each cell is doing its assigned task with a minimum of wear and tear, and the body which these cells compose will live out its expectancy and fall apart of senility at about the same time.

Biologists say that under such ideal circumstances all mammals, including man, would live about five times as long as they take to mature. With man, life expectancy would be from 90 to 125 years, compared with the 68 years the average new-born baby can expect today.

According to the U. S. Department of Agriculture we of this country were using five years ago enough pesticides to kill 15,200,000 persons annually. Since that time their usage has been increased and several more deadly ones have been developed.

Before 1945 our country regularly produced crop surpluses without the use of these poisons. But now the experts in bug poisoning have convinced us that without these chemicals we cannot raise enough to eat, that millions will get sick and die from insect-borne diseases, that our flower gardens will become unsightly, our mattresses will become alive with bed-bugs and our clothes full of holes.

Such is the plight, they would have us believe, of the country which eradicated insect-borne disease from the Panama Canal Zone (without these poisons), the country which produces so much new fiber every year that it produces one crisis after another for the textile industry, the country which first produced synthetic fibers which no insect will eat!

Here we are concerned with the widespread, careless and indiscriminate use of chemicals which are introduced into our foods to preserve them and improve their texture or appearance.

Today there are nearly 800 of these chemicals found in our food. In the case of nearly 500 of them no one knows whether or not they are harmful in an accumulated way.

Man has persisted on into the age of insects, where, but for his intelligence, he would have disappeared long ago, with other prehistoric animals. We know our agricultural practices have destroyed the fertility of our soil, and it may be that without these poisons we could not produce enough to fill our stomachs. So it may be better to die a slow death by poisoning than to starve to death this year. But do we have to?

Insects demand carbonaceous food (woody fibers), while man demands proteinaceous food. So in general it holds that insects like poor, woody crops, while man thrives on rich, succulent ones. Hence it would be possible to outwit the whole insect world by good farming practices and soil conservation.

In the case of many chemicals added to our foods, we know nothing about their long-time effects. However, since they are so universally used, it is impossible to single out any one and decide whether it affects the death rate or the age at which the people die.

We are just finding out that for every vitamin there is an anti-vitamin. For every amino acid, for every purine base, and for most hormones there is an anti-metabolite—a substance almost identical chemically, but producing opposite effects.

In addition to these anti-metabolites there are hundreds of chemicals now being used by our people which have an inhibiting effect on the work of other chemicals which are essential to the functioning of enzyme systems in our bodies.

To illustrate this problem, let us consider some of the biologic antagonists to the vitamins. Three chemicals, which we take into our bodies every day, can produce a vitamin deficiency even though we may be eating a balanced diet.

Other than the anti-metabolites, these substances include all chemicals which destroy vitamins directly; inhibit activity of enzyme systems by interfering with other component proteins and minerals; enhance development of opposing enzymes, or cause excessive elimination of vitamins.

Damaging effects of these antagonists may not be complete, yet they can substantially interfere with the normal physiologic processes to the point where they produce a recognizable deficiency disease.

More often, however, the deficient person drags about half-sick, and no one, not even his physician, has any idea of the cause of his half-sickness. Occasionally excessively large doses of vitamins will turn the tide. Hence the introduction of the so-called therapeutic capsule in clinical medicine.

In some instances, where the offender may be fluorine in the drinking water, the use of distilled water for beverage and cooking purposes will bring the patient back to health. Too often these unfortunates are looked upon as pitiful neurotics and the cause of their ill health is sought in childhood experiences.

Now for a listing of the general biologic antagonists to essential vitamins:

1. Improper cooking, sterilization or pasteurization will destroy vitamins.

2. Many mineral drugs such as arsenic, mercury and bismuth have a double action, by displacing the mineral in the enzyme system and greatly increasing excretion of the vitamins.

3. Astringents, laxatives and solvents may deplete the tissues of their vitamin content.

4. Narcotics and analgesics such as nicotine, morphine, alcohol, barbiturates and aspirin are inhibitors to vitamin functioning.

5. Antibiotics kill vitamin-producing germs of the large bowel.

6. Infections with fevers burn up immense quantities of vitamins.

7. Bleaching agents, such as those used on white flour, destroy most vitamins.

8. Sulphuring of foods for preservation and the use of sulphides to "freshen" the appearance of meat are destructive to vitamins.

9. Insecticides and disinfectants often are absorbed and retained in the food, so washing and peeling are not enough to rid the food of the poison.

10. Alkaline phosphatases essential to the use of sugars and starches by our bodies are inhibited or destroyed by fluorine in the drinking

water, as are the enzymes concerned with the conduction of nerve impulses. This is a fact which those who propose to add fluorine to the drinking water to protect some children's teeth overlook.

The modern American is living under conditions conducive to the prevalence of many antagonisms to health and longevity.

These are hazards which each of us must do something about if we are to improve our health significantly now that infections are well on the way to being conquered.

Childbirth

Education for Natural Childbirth

Only three persons are inescapably involved in the launching of a new family. They are father—mother—child, an inter-dependent unit. The benefits of contemporary science, very real and very numerous though they are, have nevertheless caused us to divide this unit. Once conception has taken place, the mother and her developing child become the well-nigh exclusive concern of professional science, while the father is reduced to the dubious status of a spectator who foots the bill for a performance from which he is barred. Feeling useless, anxious, and out of place, he is shut off for the most part from the experience of birth and the first days of his child's life. Then he is abruptly expected to achieve emotional paternity. The mother at a time of greatest need for her husband's support, is sent among strangers. She is even separated from her new born baby, who has as much physiological and emotional need of her as she has of him. Unfortunately such mother-child deprivation cannot be offset by the physical care each receives, no matter what its technical excellence.

"So artificial a division of the family seems neither wise nor workable. The basic aim of the Association for Childbirth Education consequently is to restore and maintain the father-mother-child unit to the maximum degree consistent with the best obstetrical practice, and the soundest human psychology. Its program encourages the idea that a father has a continuing role to play, a supportive and participating role by no means limited to dollars and cents. The mother's role ought not to be isolated and passive. Under normal circumstances, a woman comes most fully into her own through nurturing her unborn child, actively delivering him with a minimum of intervention, and caring for him with warm responsiveness. As for the infant, his role is to seek with great persistence the satisfaction of his basic needs, and only when this satisfaction is reasonably well achieved can he progress toward maturity. The child whose infantile needs have been supplied most successfully becomes the adult best equipped to meet his mature responsibilities."

So does the Association for Childbirth Education introduce itself. We first heard of the organization through a reader who wrote us about it and about the great satisfaction she and her husband had experienced through it, in the birth of their baby. "I am confident you would find the innumerable advantages to both mother and baby (indeed the whole family) that we have found. To us it is a natural outgrowth of the philosophy of prevention," wrote Mrs. Strauss of Derby, Kansas. We have now made a study of the association and fully agree with Mrs. Strauss.

During the first quarter of this century babies were generally delivered at home and mortality among both mothers and babies was high. When it began to be practical, fashionable and handy to have babies in the hospital, a whole new era was inaugurated. According to Vance Packard writing in *The American Magazine* for June, 1952, on Education for Childbirth, hospitals began to "bring babies on a neat assembly line basis." Mother was shunted off into a dreary labor room by herself, father was left to pace the hospital waiting room and chew his nails. When delivery time came mother was probably anesthetized and knew little more until long after the baby had appeared. Baby was hustled immediately to the nursery as if any contact with his mother might harm him. Breast feeding was discouraged because it was too much trouble for hospital personnel. And altogether what should be one of the happiest and most satisfying experiences of a married couple turned into a nightmare of loneliness, anxiety and dread. Mother never even got acquainted with her child until she got home and father was still treated like someone in the way for quite a long while afterward. Perhaps all these unnecessary and painful expedients have a lot to do with modern emotional disorders in children. Perhaps the relationship between mother, father and child is the most important single thing to be considered, right from the moment of conception, no matter how much such a concept may transgress on modern medical and hospital routine.

How the Association Began

So a number of very intelligent people have been reasoning during the past few years. A woman physician in Seattle, Washington, Dr. Virginia Lawrence Larsen, decided to begin classes in education for childbirth in January, 1950. Her classes covered the entire story of conception and pregnancy, every detail of the baby's life until the moment of delivery, as well as care after delivery. Dr. Larsen believed that many of the fears of childbirth that are common to women are the result of ignorance of what is actually taking place. Education of the mother's mind on the physiology of childbirth, and education of her muscles to make birth easier might well produce a happier situation.

It seems that fears and anxieties tense the muscles that must be relaxed during childbirth. So a large part of the job was to remove the fears. Prospective fathers were invited to the classes as well as mothers, for it seemed, quite logically, that a full understanding on the part of both parents during pregnancy and childbirth would result in greater confidence and less fear. Then too, it seemed as if as great a participation as possible on the part of the father would also help everyone concerned.

A group of those women who had attended Dr. Larsen's classes met several years later to compare experiences. They had found some lack of cooperation on the part of those who did not fully understand their project. Discussing what might be done, they found that organization seemed to be the answer. So they formed the Association for Childbirth Education, inviting a group of doctors, psychiatrists and obstetricians to their first meeting. They decided on dues, set a fee for childbirth education classes, and began to work toward establishing classes for anyone who wanted to attend. Teachers had to be trained, a meeting place arranged and finances discussed.

At present the Association is a going concern located at the Y.W.C.A., Fifth and Seneca Sts., Seattle, Wash. They meet regularly, hold classes for hundreds of prospective mothers, raise money with sales of baby clothes, Christmas wrappings, home-made food and so forth. They have established a Board of Consultants of professional people—pediatricians, obstetricians, and so forth. And by now three Seattle hospitals permit husbands to be with their wives in the labor room; one permits the father to be present during delivery. From the testimony of everyone concerned, this appears to be the happiest possible arrangement. Father and mother feel in a very real sense that the baby's birth is actually their accomplishment—not a feat of professional skill on the part of the obstetrician.

What Is the Attitude of Physicians?

We suspect that one of the biggest jobs of the Association is to convince physicians of the soundness of their principles. And we are glad to find an article written with this in mind in the *New York State Journal of Medicine* for November 1, 1953. Harold B. Davidson, M.D., of the Lenox Hill Hospital, New York, calls his article "The Psychosomatic Aspects of Educated Childbirth." He points out the fallacy of using the term "natural childbirth," for he tells us that modern childbirth is not actually "natural." However, he believes that much can be accomplished to lessen the pain of childbirth by taking into account the emotional make-up of the woman, and by training her mind to a mature acceptance of what is involved, as well as training her muscles for the job of childbirth. Dr. Davidson believes that the whole process of labor and delivery should be conducted exactly as the mother wishes it to be. If she prefers no anesthesia, this wish should be fully respected. If at any time later on she feels the need of anesthesia, she should have it. At no time should she feel that she is in competition with other women or with any ideal that she has set for herself. By allaying her fears and solving her emotional problems, the co-operative physician can assure his patient of a helpful emotional attitude toward childbirth which is bound to make the experience easier for her.

He reminds us of the sad experiences of the past when deep anesthesia has resulted in an asphyxiated child or a child whose later life was unhealthful due to lack of oxygen at birth, brought about by anesthesia of the mother. Aside from the actual physical hazards involved in anesthesia there is also the psychological factor of the relief that comes often from "doing something" in a difficult situation. If the mother is conscious throughout all or nearly all of the labor and delivery of her child, she can feel very justly that she is "doing something" rather than being a "vessel" from which the attending doctor removes the baby. This "doing something" relieves her anxiety and pain and may actually make childbirth a happy and well-nigh painless experience. But since the "doing something" consists of certain movements of certain muscles, these must be trained for the occasion, as a golf player must train his muscles for a proper "follow through."

Growth of the Idea of Education For Childbirth

Exercises for training prospective mothers are available for two dollars and fifty cents from The Maternity Center Association, 48 East 92nd St., New York, N. Y. These exercises, concerned as they are with strengthening and improving the tone of abdominal muscles, seem to us so excellent that they should be studied and practiced by everyone, not just prospective mothers. There are breathing exercises, exercises for relaxing, for posture, for doing daily chores, for resting, for lifting, and most of all, for keeping abdominal, pelvic and lower back muscles in good trim—something all of us need to know. Other material is also available from the Center in New York—charts, posters, slides and books to help teach about maternity. The center also gives classes for parents, a clinic for expectant mothers and a consultation service for anyone who needs it.

The Seattle Association has widened out into a nation-wide organization, with classes being held in more than twenty cities: Albany, N. Y.; Boston; Chicago; Dayton, Ohio; Flint, Michigan; Madison and Milwaukee, Wisconsin; New Haven; New Orleans; New York; Oklahoma City; Philadelphia; Portland, Oregon; San Francisco and three other cities in the Bay Area; Seattle, Tacoma, Wash.; Cedar Rapids, Iowa; Toronto, and Vancouver, Canada. At present the Association in Seattle is teaching the facts of birth using a "foetus doll" made exactly the size and shape of a human infant at birth. Dolls are available for class work elsewhere. Association members are also in the process of making a movie on childbirth, reprints of which we hope will be available for other classes to use.

If you are planning to have a baby, or if someone in your family or neighborhood is planning to, why not get in touch with the Seattle group and ask them for suggestions and literature. They have excellent material on breast feeding and exercise as well as helpful books and pamphlets on childbirth and child raising. Perhaps there is a class on Childbirth Education functioning near you. Ask your hospital, visiting nurse association, health department, doctor, nurse or Red Cross. If there is not, consider starting such classes locally with other parents or prospective parents. You can get plenty of helpful suggestions from the Seattle Association of Childbirth Education or the Maternity Center Association in New York. The whole idea of childbirth as a cooperative and rewarding experience for both parents, the idea of little or no anesthesia, as a result of months of preparation on the mother's part, the idea of breast feeding as a natural and necessary part of the baby's start in life—all these are right in line with our program for healthful living and we cannot endorse them too highly.

Children, Muscular Development of

"When Grampa was a kid, he used to tote the firewood clear from the shed to the house—*after* he'd chopped it up to size, *after* he'd walked three miles home from school, *after* he'd licked the daylights out of the class bully. And he didn't take vitamins, either. So grampa says. He just laughs when I say I'm too tired to walk to the store for milk—and besides I want to watch television. He says I'm too soft—that boys aren't boys anymore."

Is grampa right? Are our boys "soft" or are our children physically up to the mark they should be? Are we pampering them so—making too few physical demands on them, in this day of conveniences—that we are doing them untold harm rather than the good we want for them? There is damaging evidence that all this is true.

A disheartening picture of the muscular fitness of our children is painted in a paper, "Health and Muscular Fitness," in the *Journal of the American Association for Health, Physical Education, Recreation,* Dec., 1953, by Hans Kraus, M. D., and Ruth Hirschland, of the Institute of Physical Medicine and Rehabilitation, New York University, Bellevue Medical Center: "In our studies of the muscular fitness of American children in northeastern urban and suburban communities, we reported that 56.6 per cent between the ages of six and nineteen failed to meet even a minimum standard required for health."

Of the 4,458 "normal, healthy school children" in the age group mentioned, 56.6 per cent failed one of the given tests for muscular power and flexibility, and 16.4 per cent failed two or more of the tests—giving a total figure of 78.3 per cent of tests failed.

For comparison, it was decided to make similar tests on European children. The results give us an even gloomier picture—and certainly should tear down our pride and confidence in the health of our own seemingly well-cared for, well-nourished, "well-vitaminized" children. The institute chose 1,987 school children in Italy and Austria—and they got the comparison they were looking for. Results showed that only 8.3 per cent failed one of the tests and 0.3 per cent failed twice!

Every effort was made to keep the test conditions identical. The picture grows worse, however, when we realize the circumstances under which the European tests had to be given. As the schools were closed for vacation, it was necessary to get the children from the public rest centers where welfare societies provided a month's period of good food, care, rest, and mountain air for several hundred of the neediest cases. These children were victims of war or the aftermath of war, undernourished, and in some cases minus a leg or an arm, or both. Yet the tests found them in much better muscular condition than our own much more fortunate children. Even in some of the most seemingly helpless cases the children were able to pass the tests easily.

What does all this mean? Obviously, it means that our children are *suffering* (and the word is not too strong), in many respects, from a highly mechanized society. In urban communities, Johnnie doesn't have to lead the life that "grampa" led. He doesn't need to "tote" the wood—much less chop it—he has a thermostat and furnace. He doesn't need to walk miles to school, there is a school bus or he is taken in the family car. He doesn't run wild outdoors playing, he has a television set to play for him, while he *sits* comfortably by, *watching*. We may be thankful—in a strange sense—that he still enjoys "licking" the class bully—if he has the strength. In Europe, where children still do not have such mechanized conveniences, they must walk, and their recreation is largely based on the active use of their bodies.

Half the fun of growing up is a child's discovery and use of his body. Gaining an increasing confidence in his own powers, as well as the fun he gets out of taxing himself and succeeding, are important processes in themselves to the healthy development of a child. To take the earliest examples of growth: Have you ever watched a very young child's utter delight and pride in his first steps, and then in finding the use he can make of his legs—climbing, skipping, jumping? You may say that these examples are too basic, but you can carry them straight through: watch a young boy's thrill at beating another in a race or at climbing to the highest branch of a tree, or a man of 50's pride in playing two sets of tennis without "fagging out."

Exercise and Nervous Tension

Another factor in the importance of exercise is its relation to nervous tension. A child, as well as an adult, needs an outlet for the strains of daily life, and the use of his body provides that. A game of tag or a good whack with a baseball bat in the field are the best ways for a child to get rid of bottled-up emotions. Or, better still, to keep them from bottling up. Getting physically tired and at the same time building strength accomplishes miracles in helping a child to live more happily and peacefully with himself—and hence be healthier. In the tests in both Europe and America, those who proved to be muscularly deficient were the tense, anxious, jittery ones. So it works both ways.

On this subject, in another paper, "Muscular Fitness and Orthopedic Disability," in the *New York State Journal of Medicine,* Vol. 54, No. 2, 1954, Dr. Kraus and Ruth Hirschland state that "When the individual is prevented from ridding himself of surplus energies, tension remains and often results in physical discomfort," and "Physical activity—actual physical work, walking, stair-climbing, carrying, dancing, and active sports—forms an outlet for emotional stimuli."

Though, as we have seen from the tests made on school children, the effects of too little exercise can be seen at a very early age, the damage does not stop there. It was found by a University of Virginia doctor (Dr. Charles J. Frankel) that there has been a 30 per cent increase in injuries to the players on the University's football squad. Dr. Frankel, who has kept records of all football injuries since 1935, also says that not only are the injuries running 30 per cent ahead of the average for the last 20 years, but they are more severe. In an article in the Wilmington, Delaware, *Journal* (Nov. 18, 1953), Dr. Frankel, who is also examiner for the American Board of Orthopedic Surgery, reports that "Military service examinations have shown that this generation of young men is less rugged than the last. Most boys today don't walk as much as they used to. They usually ride in an auto and consequently their legs and their bodies weaken."

Moving up a few rungs on the age ladder, we find even more severe problems arising from this early neglect. Complaints of backache in adults have been found through research to have a very positive relation to muscular fitness. Again, in their article, "Muscular Fitness and Orthopedic Disability," Dr. Kraus and Ruth Hirschland find that physical discomfort in many of these cases results from emotional tension, which in turn arises from a general condition of muscular weakness. This condition does not always limit itself to purely local discomfort, but a "minor back strain, either acute or chronic, merely designates the location for a much deeper and more complex disease." In over 3,000 cases complaining of low back pain, examined by an orthopedic surgeon, a neurosurgeon, an internist, a radiologist, and a specialist in physical medicine at the Columbia Medical Center, at the Institute of Physical Medicine and Rehabilitation of the New York University Bellevue Medical Center, and in private practice, the majority showed a combination of muscular deficiencies and nervous tension. "While the complaints were definitely 'backache,' they were not healthy people suffering from a local difficulty, nor were they neurotics somatizing (applying to their bodies) their emotional complaints. They offered a combination of both physical and emotional difficulties."

Muscular Exercise is Necessary

A good many of these patients are reported to have improved through systematic muscle training. "The pain had to be alleviated by local general treatment, but the final outcome and the permanency of relief mainly ran parallel with the muscle status."

To get back to the root of the evil, the lack of enough strenuous exercise in childhood, we should think seriously about this part of our child's health. Perhaps if we ask ourselves the following questions, and then consider the listed suggestions made by Dr. Kraus and Ruth Hirschland, we will start on the way to raising healthier, happier children, who will become healthier, happier adults.

Are we being too "careful" of our children? Are we making their lives too "soft"? Are we providing physical outlets for our children's emotions and pent-up energies? Are they getting *enough strenuous exercise?*

Suggestions:

(1) Pre-school children should have an increase of active play, to be in the best physical condition on entering school.

(2) Habits of exercise should be provided for those who don't have the necessity of walking, doing physical work, or actively entertaining themselves.

(3) We should instill a philosophy of physical effort and exercise so that we will be able to meet extreme demands on our bodies.

(4) Tests for muscular deficiency should be made in physical education departments of schools, so that individual attention may be given where needed.

(5) The time allotted for physical education in the schools should be increased.

(6) Games with formal exercise should be provided for those who for one reason or another are not fit for physical competition, and who hence lose the benefits of competitive sports.

The findings of these two scientists highlight the same theme that Editor Rodale has dealt with in his book *This Pace is Not Killing Me.* As he shows so clearly in this book, our lives today are not the hectic, mad, hurried rush we like to imagine them. We actually get far too little physical activity of a helpful kind.

But in addition to our need for exercise, Editor Rodale pointed out that the main cause of our generally substandard health is the refined, processed food we eat. He says that Dr. Pauline B. Mack, dean of the College of Household Arts and Sciences of Texas State College for Women recently said, after making a survey, that American teenagers are gravely undernourished, and that this applies even to those who come from our wealthiest families. Of 2,536 boys and girls studied, most of them showed calcium and phosphorus deficiencies as well as that of vitamins A, B and C. In other words, we are starving in the midst of plenty.

The high record of football injuries mentioned by Dr. Frankel would undoubtedly be reduced with a diet high in calcium and phosphorus. Even if it were impossible to change the actual meals eaten, a supplement of bone meal with each meal would provide the necessary minerals.

Dr. Mack also found that 49 per cent of the boys studied in her survey and 48 per cent of the girls had "nutritional nerves"—that is, nail biting, face twitchings and general nervousness. Undoubtedly, a large part of the reason is the bread they eat—bread made of flour from which all of the B vitamins have been removed and a few synthetic vitamins added. Vitamin B is the food element charged with the health of the nerves. Vitamin E, which is also removed from our grains before they are made into bread, is the vitamin that protects the health of muscles. Can this be the main reason for our children's inferiority in muscular aptitude, compared with children of those countries where the standard of living is so low (!) that they are still eating real whole grain cereals and bread, rich in the B vitamins and vitamin E?

Four things are wrong with our nutrition and we believe that these four things have far more to do with the health of American children than the amount of exercise they get or do not get: 1. Our food crops are not grown properly, 2. the important parts of our food are removed in processing, 3. various processing operations change the structure of the food so that our bodies cannot use it properly and 4. toxic chemicals are added for purposes of preservation, anti-staling, coloring and so forth. So long as American children are eating food devoid of most of the precious minerals and vitamins their bodies need, just so long will they show up poorly in competition with children whose food comes straight from the fields, orchards and gardens, untampered with and unchemicalized.

Children and Problem Eaters

"You must eat your vegetables or you can't have any dessert." "You must drink your milk and eat everything on your plate before you can leave the table." "Doctor, why is it my children won't eat?" Does any of this sound like your family or the family next door? Are you one of those fathers or mothers whose every meal is a nightmare of persuading reluctant children to eat?

When adults refuse to eat as they should, we call their condition "anorexia" (absence of appetite) and we decide that it may be due to psychological reasons, such as fatigue or anxiety or a lack of some of the vitamins that are so important for good appetite—the B complex of vitamins mostly. But when children refuse to eat, the reasons may be far more complex and may deserve a great deal of patient study to determine the cause, and wise strategy to correct the situation.

Hilda M. Davis, M.D., Ch.B., D.P.H., writing in the July, 1952, journal called *Nutrition,* which is published in England, tells us that "this problem of refusal to eat presents itself to every parent at some time and to some degree . . . The grim-faced or pleading adult hovers around the obstinate child who, glorying in the limelight, is the center of attention.

"It may be due to an over-anxious mother who, naturally wanting her baby to be perfect, is over-zealous in carrying out instructions given to her regarding the feeding routine of the baby," says Dr. Davis. When her doctor advises that the baby should eat at certain times, should eat certain foods and should obtain certain food supplements, this over-anxious mother may fret if one of the feeding times is missed or one of the food supplements forgotten. Any anxiety on her part is immediately reflected in the baby who always senses when his mother is upset. Then too the mother may have exaggerated ideas of the amount of milk the baby should have. In this case, she may force him to take more milk than he can, his stomach will rebel and he will vomit the milk. Then his mother will insist that he take more, he will refuse and the stage will be set for "scenes" at the dining table which may very well go on until the child is half-grown.

One very critical time in the baby's life when patterns for eventual bad food habits may be laid down is when the baby is beginning to eat cereal and strained vegetables. Some children want this kind of food by the age of four months; others will have none of it until they are six months old or more. Some children refuse all food but milk until they are much older than this.

Again, says Dr. Davis, "it is usually the inexperienced and anxious mother who forces food upon an unwilling baby in the belief that it is necessary. She does not appreciate a varying appetite, resistance to a flavor and feel of food met for the first time when milk was expected, or the devastating effect of a hard spoon hitting tender gums." If the mother routinely tries out the new kind of food, encouraging the child to eat it, all may go well. But if she is anxious and upset, her emotions will be transmitted to the child, who will view the whole matter with apprehension.

Let Him Feed Himself

During the baby's second year another stage in his development influences his food habits. This is the year when the baby becomes independent and wants to do things for himself—even things he is unable to do with any degree of success as yet. He decides that he wants to feed himself and the wise mother will not only permit, but will encourage this desire. True, the food will land on the baby's face, on his fingers, in his hair, on the floor and almost anywhere except in his mouth, but the mess and the breakage are all part of raising a baby. The alternative is for mother to hold the dish firmly out of reach of baby's hands and spoon-feed him, which is certain to result, says Dr. Davis, "in the turned head, refusal to eat and screams of frustration."

Once the child has discovered that a "scene" around his refusal to eat makes him the center of attraction, he will continue to refuse for this adds to his self-importance and assures him of being the center of attention at every meal. Later when he is able to feed himself, he may still from time to time overturn a cup, drop a piece of buttered bread or upset his plate of food. This is a bid for attention. "Aggravating as it is," says Dr. Davis, "the most effective way to deal with it is to let the child leave the table and return to play, assuming that no more food is wanted; then the mess can be cleaned up and no further remark made." If he finds out several times that no "scene" results and that no attention is focused on him, the child will be less inclined to create such a disturbance again.

Encouraging the child to eat new kinds of food depends also to a great extent on the point of view of the adults about him. You may be certain that if adults in the house do not like any given food, the children will not like that food either. It may also be true that some emotional upset associated with the food has turned the child against it. Remember that children are not articulate about the reasons why they like or dislike things. Perhaps your child will not eat salad greens because he once found a worm (or something he thought was a worm) in them. If the child continues to refuse a certain food, it is best to make no comment and engage in no persuasion. The next time it is served to the rest of the family, do not give any to the child. This may result in an immediate demand for it. Child psychologists agree that it is completely useless to fume and scold, as this will produce only more and more scenes, for as long as attention can be secured this way, the child will try to secure it. If a child genuinely dislikes any food, it is best not to press him to eat it, for he may be allergic or otherwise unsuited to it.

Last but not least, keep in mind that emotional upsets in the child may be his reason for refusal to eat. Many different incidents almost unnoticed by adults, can produce upsetting emotional crises in children—a disappointment, a forgotten promise, an injustice real or imagined may assume such importance to the child that he may refuse to eat.

We sometimes have letters from readers telling us of their difficulties trying to get their children to eat the kind of food that is healthful for them. How, for instance, do you persuade a child that salad, fruit and vegetables are good for him and cake, soft drinks and candy are not? We would suggest that the very best method is for the adults to omit harmful foods from all menus and smack their lips over the salads, meat, fish, fruits and vegetables. A tongue in cheek attitude gets you nowhere, for Junior recognizes it instantly. If father says "Um, this salad is good" and then leaves most of it on his plate, Junior will do the same. If mother promises a soft drink or a piece of candy as a reward, Junior will begin to think of these foods as treasures and will refuse the wholesome food until he is "bribed" with another reward.

Adult table manners are important where there are children in the family; Junior imitates everything he sees. It is just as important that adults choose their food wisely, for Junior will learn his food habits from them.

Chiropractic

This article is reprinted in its entirety by permission from *The Journal of the National Chiropractic Association*, for September 1955. We believe interested readers will be encouraged, as we were, to find that, in other countries at least, methods of healing other than orthodox medicine are finding their rightful place.

***By C. W. Weiant, D.C., Ph.D.*, Peekskill, New York**
Dean, Chiropractic Institute of New York

For a number of years now, the medical journals of Germany have been referring to the existence of a crisis in German medicine. There has been a definite mood of self-examination and self-criticism expressed in pleas for a more fundamental understanding of the disease process and its cause. Speransky's researchers on the over-all importance of the nervous system in every type of pathology have been the subject of frequent discussion. New books have appeared dealing with such unorthodox matters as zone therapy, acupuncture, and iridiagnosis. A special technical journal, devoted to empirical healing methods and wide open to nonconformist thinking in every department of therapy, has been started and is evidently a publishing success.

Nothing, however, has so completely captured the imagination of German physicians as chiropractic. It all began, it seems, when Werner Peper, D. C., a graduate of the Palmer School of Chiropractic, and L. Zukschwerdt, M. D., a German surgeon, were thrown together by the vicissitudes of the last war. Zukschwerdt, now professor of surgery at the University of Hamburg, learned about chiropractic from Peper, who at the present time practices chiropractic in Hamburg.

About 1950, Zukschwerdt delivered a lecture on chiropractic before a German medical group. In 1951 he wrote an article entitled "Chiropraktik" which appeared in the journal *Hippokrates.* His opening sentences, as I translate them, read as follows: "A new interchange between school medicine and chiropractic has become necessary. New researches in the pathological anatomy and roentgenology of the vertebral column (Schmorl, Junghanns, Toendury, Duus, Vosschulte), and above all clinical experiences with osteochondrosis of the different vertebral segments today cause much of chiropractic teaching to appear in a different light than formerly." These two sentences set the tone for the entire article, the first favorable mention of chiropractic ever to appear in a German medical publication.

In 1953, he returns to the subject in the same journal with a second article, "The Problems of Chiropractic." Here he discusses the history of chiropractic, the training of the chiropractor, the subluxation theory, factors contributing to the narrowing of intervertebral foramina, therapeutic measures which have brought relief by virtue of enlarging the foramina, the chiropractic explanation of pain, the relevancy of chiropractic to visceral disease, and the possibility of doing damage by vertebral adjustment.

On the last point, after citing three or four British and American medical writers who claimed to have observed damage, he asserts that he has practiced several thousand adjustments (or "repositions," to use his own term) without ever observing harm done in a single case. He also gives the chiropractors credit for having been the first to demonstrate that it is possible, by a thrust, to "reposition" a subluxated vertebra. He concludes with a plea to his medical colleagues not to neglect to use chiropractic, and having discovered its value, not to jump to the conclusion that it can take care of every situation which arises.

It is a little difficult to realize at once the sensational character of these two articles and their impact on German medicine. Actually, nothing remotely comparable has ever occurred in the United States. It is as though the chief of surgery at the Mayo Clinic, or an outstanding professor of surgery at one of our leading medical schools, were to write a lead article for the *Journal* of the AMA extolling chiropractic and calling upon all physicians to apply it in their respective practices.

The appeal has not been in vain. One of the first to respond was Dr. Freimut Biedermann, a young surgeon who learned chiropractic from Zukschwerdt. Abandoning a hospital post which netted him, I was told in Switzerland, a hundred to a hundred fifty dollars a month, he now practices chiropractic exclusively, in Stuttgart, and needless to say, earns a fine living. He has produced a small book of thirty-eight pages entitled Grundsatzliches zur Chiropraktik vom artzlichen Standpunkt aus (*The Foundations of Chiropractic from the Standpoint of a Physician*). This scholarly little book, listing a bibliography of more than 200 medical and chiropractic authorities, presents an extremely thorough version of the anatomical, physiological, and pathological data upon which chiropractic rests. Thanks to an excellent translation by Dr. Nathan Muchnick, of the faculty of the Chiropractic Institute of New York, it will soon be available to all English-speaking chiropractors.

Meanwhile a new periodical, *Neuralmedizin,* devoted to the neurological aspects of medical practice, has come into existence. It began publication in 1953. The June, 1954, issue contains an article by H. W. Passler, chief physician of the state hospital in Leverkusen and a specialist in rehabilitation, dealing with a typical case of postoperative pain following lumbar sympathectomy and its treatment by vertebral adjustment. The same issue contains an article by Dr. K. R. von Roques on "the necessity and form of the incorporation of chiropractic in medicine!"

Only this year the trend has been accentuated by the appearance of an illustrated book on chiropractic technic by Werner Peper, D. C., and a book called *Lehrbuch der Chiropraktik der Wirbelsaule,* a textbook of chiropractic written by a physician, Albert Cramer, for his medical colleagues. In this foreword, Dr. Cramer, the director of a large clinic in Hamburg where chiropractic has been the subject of four years of experimentation, has this to say:

"The working of the chiropractic thrust upon the patient is so deep-reaching, so widespread, goes so directly to the innermost vital circuit of the creature, that, in its ultimate consequences, it simply cannot be followed by the therapist."

In his thinking, Cramer appears to have been about equally influenced by the newer Palmer ideas and the work of Illi, of Geneva, Switzerland. This fact is reflected in two of his recent articles in *Hipprokrates:* "Statik, Dynamik, und Chiropraktik" and "Atlas, Statik, und Chiropraktik."

Prominent in the picture, also, is Dr. Sell, a German orthopedist connected with a "sports-sanitarium," who poses as an authority on chiropractic, is actively working to have chiropractic incorporated into the work of all German orthopedists, and travels about Germany offering short courses in chiropractic for physicians. His use of chiropractic has been widely publicized in German newspapers and magazines.

Much of this I already knew when I left last March for Europe to investigate the work of the famous Swiss chiropractor Fred Illi. What I did not know, until I had talked with people in Switzerland, Austria, and Germany itself, was that this new ferment in German medicine has its roots in matters purely economic. There are, it is said, 60,000 too many doctors in West Germany. Two factors have contributed to this situation. First of all, during the war years, the medical schools were the only departments of German universities which remained open. Thus, many students who would normally have entered other professions chose medicine. Incidentally, they thereby escaped immediate military service. The second factor has been the constant migration of doctors from the East to West Germany. By devious methods they have managed to escape the rule of the Soviets. The resulting surplus of doctors has greatly sharpened competition among them. The greatest hope of avoiding starvation is the acquisition of some new therapeutic technic which will differentiate a man from his nearest competitor and enable him to stand out as capable of rendering some sensational service which the next man cannot do. One of the unfortunate ones I met in Geneva. Unable to make a living in Germany, he had migrated to Switzerland, where he works as a journalist attached to a leading weekly newspaper! And this man has been trained as a specialist in neurology!

It must not be forgotten, either, that there have never been in Germany enough chiropractors to constitute an economic threat to medicine. Chiropractic being relatively unknown until recent years, there has been little occasion to deride it. Hence, there is no need to resort to the face-saving device of concealing chiropractic under the name of physical medicine. Chiropractic is openly discussed by its own name. Nor is there in Germany any such monolithic organization as the AMA. Each doctor is free to express his own opinions without fear of reprisals. True, there is an old-guard conservative faction, and this group has, in a few instances, succeeded in depriving over-enthusiastic champions of chiropractic from their university connections, but by and large it is the newer liberal groups who dominate the field.

It is no exaggeration to state that literally thousands of German physicians have demonstrated an active interest in embracing chiropractic. New study groups are constantly forming—one physician teaching ten others. A special medical society exists for the express purpose of engaging in research on chiropractic. Chiropractic tables are manufactured in Germany and advertised in German medical journals. A student who recently arrived in New York to study chiropractic reports that there are very few physicians in the entire city of Frankfort who do not attempt to practice chiropractic.

One may well be concerned about the qualifications of these men to engage in such practice. In the past year, sixteen cases of paralysis and two deaths following manipulation under anesthesia by physicians have been reported in German medical journals. The inadequacy of their training is well exemplified in the courses offered by Dr. Sell. I should like to relate how Dr. Sell learned the art of chiropractic. In the difficult days following the war, Dr. Bielefeldt, Frankfort chiropractor, staved off starvation by an arrangement under which he adjusted about thirty of Dr. Sell's patients daily for a period of exactly fifty-two days. During this time Dr. Sell used to pass through the room where the adjustments were given. He was never told what was being done or why. He saw only what any patient would see in a chiropractic clinic in this country. To this day, he cannot read and interpret a chiropractic X-ray. Repeated requests for assistance in this connection have been rejected by Dr. Bielefeldt. Nevertheless, he teaches, or pretends to teach, chiropractic to physicians.

Before I got to Germany, I was told by Swiss chiropractors that Sell's courses are of two weeks' duration. When I arrived in Frankfort, I learned that this is an exaggeration. The course lasts four days! From

Dr. Bielefeldt's stepdaughter, a physiotherapist at a local hospital, I learned some details of the last course given at the hospital. At the end of the first day's session, the members of the class expressed dissatisfaction. When would Dr. Sell tell them something they didn't already know? When would he give them something they could really use? This, they were assured, would come later. On the second day, the class heard a repetition of the first day's lectures. It was necessary, so the teacher said, to repeat and repeat, in order to have a good foundation. The third day, once more, was like the first. The fourth day would surely bring the great revelation. And what did Dr. Sell give them on the fourth day? A very fine lecture on vitamin therapy! Now the class was ready to go out and adjust vertebrae!

In fairness to the medical doctors, it must be said that they have made repeated overtures to the chiropractic profession for instruction of the proper kind. Their negotiations with the European Chiropractic Union have been well publicized in our journals. The ECU said, in effect, first create a law in Germany creating a distinct and legalized chiropractic profession. Then meet the same standards as those set up for the chiropractor.

Last year at the St. Louis convention I was the bearer of a letter from one of the top medical men of Hamburg asking the NCA to set up a school, or sponsor a school, in Germany for the express purpose of training M.D.'s in chiropractic. Otherwise, said this man, more and more of them will go to Switzerland posing as chiropractic patients in order to find out what the chiropractor does. Those who can't conveniently do that will snap up any itinerant naturopath or pseudo-chiropractor who professes to teach the new art of adjusting.

In either case, the failures experienced by inadequate preparation will give chiropractic a bad name in Germany. The National Council on Education discussed the proposal with considerable sympathy for the sincere men in German medicine who want to learn and practice chiropractic, but was unable to reach any decision other than that of the European chiropractors. Since there have been no further developments in the negotiations, it is obvious that, for the most part, the German medical profession is not ready to abandon altogether the old for the new, nor to create a rival professional group. Their position is understandable, but so also is that of the chiropractors. The latter are not disposed to sell out to the traditional enemy.

Meanwhile, the problem persists, and let no American chiropractor imagine complacently that this is purely a European problem. The prestige of German medicine is still great. Up to this point, the situation has enormous and, as yet, almost unused propaganda value for us in the United States, but once chiropractic has been fully integrated into German medicine (an intention frankly admitted by Dr. Sell in a letter now in my possession, written to one of my former students who had asked his advice about coming to Germany to practice), the repercussions in other parts of the world may become extremely serious. Already the German chiropractic epidemic is spreading to France, where it is said that no fewer than 10,000 persons—masseurs, physiotherapists, kinesiotherapists, physicians, and pure laymen—are holding forth as practitioners of chiropractic.

I can see but one solution, although, as yet, there is not the slightest indication that it will be put into effect. A responsible group of chiropractors should band together to assist two or three of their European colleagues to establish, as soon as possible, a creditable school of chiropractic on German soil, where German citizens can be trained to become bonafide chiropractors. They most certainly would not lack students. The demand for admission would be tremendous, and the financial returns all that could be desired. The naturopaths already have a school, demonstrating that such an enterprise can exist in Germany without legal interference. They are willing (even to the extent of supplying some of the needed capital) to pool their efforts with those of chiropractors.

This possibility deserves to be explored. The one thing most necessary and urgent at the present time is to flood Germany with good chiropractors. If there must be a battle, there must be soldiers. A determined minority can achieve its goal as well in Germany as in America. But the minority must not be too minor. The German chiropractors, scarcely half a dozen in number, find themselves today in somewhat the same situation as the first class to be graduated by D. D. Palmer. If their numbers can be increased, they will become increasingly strong.

Chlorine

By J. I. RODALE
Editor of Prevention

In the excitement and unholy zeal to railroad through fluoridation of our drinking waters, people seem to have forgotten all about the fact that our water is being chlorinated. They take chlorine for granted. It is a *fait accompli,* and they believe that nothing can be done about it. Chlorination has been in use for so long that time has given it a sort of complacent acceptance. The sad part of it is, however, that in the eyes of some people it has a halo. The best people are for it, aren't they? The schools and doctors and congressmen recommend it, do they not? After all, we've been drinking chlorinated water all our lives and we aren't all dead yet, so it couldn't possibly be harmful.

I have heard dentists, in public recommendations of the use of fluorine, practically predicate their entire case on the fact that since a city has the right to place chlorine in the water, it may also therefore, put in fluorine. But fluorine is used to reduce cavities in the teeth of children—while chlorination is resorted to, to kill harmful bacteria that can cause diseases like typhoid. The latter has the barest semblance of justification, but the use of fluorine would set off a new dangerous trend. Where would municipalities stop? Would they eventually put aspirin in the water to prevent headaches?

Chlorine is a powerful disinfectant—a potent poison, highly irritative to the skin and the mucous membranes. In Clorox it is used for bleaching, and it has a great many industrial uses because of its active nature as a chemical element. If house-plants are watered with chlorinated water they will not thrive, nor will guppies live in such water. Many years ago, I was told by a man who conducted a market where fish were kept alive till sold, that the day the waterworks placed a charge of chlorine into the water, all his fish died. This is a point that has been completely overlooked. In the case of fluorine, the machinery has been devised so that there is a constant change of fluorine into the water. An attempt is made to maintain a constancy of amount. But with chlorine there is an unscientific, sledge-hammer treatment. Large amounts are dumped in at one time. How about sensitive people who drink water on such a day?

Here is a happening to illustrate what I mean. I will quote from the St. Petersburg (Florida) *Times* of September 25, 1954:

"A 25-year-old mother was almost totally blinded yesterday morning when she washed her eyes out with water and found too late the water supply at the trailer park where she resides had been treated with strong chemicals during the night, police reported.

"Les Grant, manager of the trailer park, said he and Chester Hamilton, the owner, had treated the court's water supply with chlorine at midnight. He said a health inspector told him the bacteriological count was off and the pipes needed flushing.

"Grant told the *Times* he posted a big sign warning about the water over the mail boxes at the court but it was too late to notify residents personally. He said no other residents made any complaints about the water."

A sad case, but it is only one of hundreds of deadly experiences with chlorine.

Clippings from a number of New England newspapers tell us of a recent happening in a Cambridge (Massachusetts) swimming pool where a score or so of children became violently ill from chlorine poisoning. While the gasping, choking youngsters were given artifical respiration and taken to the hospital for oxygen administration, authorities were investigating the possible cause of the accident. It seems that a filter had back-fired, causing an extra amount of the purifying powder to be released into the pool. It was surmised that some of the children had swallowed some of the water; others had simply been overcome by the fumes. At any rate, they turned blue and dizzy. They choked. True, it was a big overdose of chlorine that poisoned the children. But how much is an overdose for each individual cell of our bodies, when you and I drink chlorinated water daily, year after year?

In the 1955 Pennsylvania floods many cases of diarrhea occurred in the city of Tamaqua, population 11,508, because of larger than usual amounts of chlorine used for fear of a typhoid epidemic. According to the Allentown *Morning Call* of August 30, 1955, "A state health department official has assured worried residents that an estimated 3,000 cases of diarrhea in the community are only 'seasonal' and the result of sensitivity to the increased amounts of chlorine added to the Tamaqua water supply since the flood." This sort of thing is only seasonal or incidental to a public health official, who overlooks the fact that such happenings occur many times a year when the chlorine charge is put into the water. How many are getting diarrhea under such conditions?

Physicians do not seem to be aware, nor do they care much about the effect of chlorine on the human body. One rarely sees references to it in medical literature. In his book *How to Help Your Doctor Help You* (Dell), Walter C. Alvarez, M. D., says: "It is hard to explain why many a highly sensitive person reacts strongly and in an allergic way to such simple chemical substances as aspirin or sugar or chlorine in the city water. These small molecules are very different from the huge and extremely complicated molecules of protein which were originally supposed to produce all allergic reactions."

The physicians are always ready to attribute something that they do not understand to an allergy. Chlorine is about as much an allergy causer as the left front foot of my bed. I was going to say, "as my left shoe," but shoes are sometimes allergy causers. The doctors should learn more about chlorine, and they should seek for a substitute water purifier that is safer.

In the *Journal of Allergy* for November, 1944, appears an article in which M. J. Gutmann, M. D., of Jerusalem writes of a case of giant hives in an English officer. Skin tests showed no evidence of sensitivity; testing with over 40 different food substances showed no allergy nor were there any indications of bacterial allergy.

Yet this officer's hives disappeared when he was transferred from Jerusalem to other stations. He could recollect no difference in his diet and way of life at these other stations except that he drank mineral waters. As soon as he returned to Jerusalem and once again drank the city water, he developed hives immediately. The water in Jerusalem is chlorinated. When chlorinated water is heated, for coffee, tea and so forth, the chlorine is given off into the air and can produce no symptoms. But, for those who drink the water cold, out of the faucet, a number of symptoms may arise.

Dr. Gutmann reviews an article in the *Journal of Allergy* for 1934 in which chlorine in water was found to be the cause of asthma and functional colitis. When the patient was put on distilled water exclusively for three days, he experienced no return of either disorder. Then when one drop of sodium hypochloride was placed in his drinking water, his asthma and colitis promptly returned. Dr. Gutmann tells us that he has had other patients who got hives from the addition of even the smallest amounts of chlorine to their drinking water. One was a woman of 28 who had hives from childhood. All her life she had tried the most extreme kinds of diet in an effort to locate the food which was causing the allergy. Eventually someone thought of changing her drinking water. The hives disappeared within a few days. As soon as she returned to chlorinated drinking water, the eruptions appeared within a short time.

One day I was reading the *Journal of the American Medical Association* (July 28, 1951 issue) and I saw something that astounded me. In the section where the doctors ask questions, there appeared a question to the editor which asked whether studies had ever been made to determine the harmful effects of chlorinated water used for drinking purposes. The editor's answer said that a careful check of all the literature and all available information revealed the fact that no organized investigation had ever been made of the effect of chlorine on the human body. He admitted that there had been cases of allergic skin inflammation and many outbreaks of asthma that were traced to chlorine, but the editor refers to them as allergies.

Imagine, permitting hundreds of millions of persons to drink chlorinated water without ever having made a thorough investigation of its effects on the human system! At least there should have been a comprehensive study of the subject based on the fragments of existing facts which show up here and there in the medical literature. For example in *Bridges' Dietetics for the Clinician* by Harry J. Johnson, M. D. (1949, Lea and Febiger) on page 91 appears the statement that chlorine destroys vitamin E. This is one of the most difficult vitamins to maintain a sufficiency of in the body, and it is one of the most important ones, for a lack of vitamin E will produce heart disease. Yet from the very first day of life one is given chlorinated water which slowly keeps undermining the body's dwindling store of this precious vitamin, a vitamin that is rarely included in the regular all-in-one vitamin capsules purchasable in drug stores.

Another medical bit of evidence incriminating chlorine in the causation of heart disease is contained in a book called *Poisoning* by W. F. von Oettingen, M. D., page 72 (Paul Hoeber, Inc.). The author says, "It has been claimed that injury of the mitral valve (of the heart) and cardiac (heart) insufficiency may result from severe exposure to chlorine, or carbon monoxide. Coronary thrombosis, characterized by palpitation, irregularities of the heart beat, and anxiety, has been reported in poisonings with chlorine, carbon monoxide and ferric chloride." The latter is a chlorine compound.

While this refers to severe exposures, we must not overlook the fact that taking in chlorine every day of one's life, beginning from the day of birth, will eventually accumulate into the equivalent of a severe exposure. In fact, the unborn child may already be suffering from the effects of chlorinated water its mother may be drinking during pregnancy, for why is it that 25,000 babies are born each year in the United States with heart trouble?

In connection with the relation between a lack of vitamin E and heart trouble, let us look into some sad mathematics. As we have seen, the main reason for chlorinating drinking water is to prevent typhoid. As we have also seen, the introduction into the human body of chlorine compounds results in a reduction of its vitamin E resources. So what do we have? The effect of chlorine is to reduce typhoid, but to increase heart disease.

In 1900 before chlorination was in very general use, there were 35,379 deaths from typhoid in the United States, or about 31 per 100,000 of population. In that same year, namely 1900, there were 68,439 deaths from heart disease, or 137 per 100,000 of population. Now, in 1950, as a result of the use of chlorine, plus a general improvement in the sanitation of the water supply, reduction of pollution, etc., there were only 90 deaths from typhoid in the United States, which means that it is down to practically zero. But what has happened with heart disease?

By 1950 it had skyrocketed up to 535,920 deaths or at the rate of 355 per 100,000 of population.

So what have we done with our chlorine? We have traded 35,379 typhoid deaths for 535,920 heart disease deaths. Shown in table form here is how it looks.

1900	Typhoid	35,379	31.3 per 100,000
	Heart	68,439	137.4 per 100,000
1950	Typhoid	90	(zero)
	Heart	535,920	355.5 per 100,000

This does not look like a case of good management. Of course, the medical profession will say that the increase in heart disease deaths is due to the fast pace at which we are living, but if you will read my little book *This Pace Is Not Killing Us* (Rodale Press, $1.00) you will think differently.

The case against chlorine is much worse than I have painted it. According to an article from a German magazine on this subject which we read, chlorine reduces vitamins A, B, C, E and H as well as destroying one of the amino acids of protein, namely tryptophane.

Water is not the only place where man comes in contact with chlorine in these modern times. He is breathing it in DDT, he is getting it in the chlorine dioxide that is applied to flour to bleach it. It is being used in processing potatoes to improve their dehydration qualities and to prevent them from turning brown in storage. It is contained in tobacco as a residue from insecticides. It is used in dozens of other applications throughout the present day system of industry, food processing, etc.

I am not considering table salt, which is a chloride namely, sodium chloride. In the body we know that its two elements break apart, the sodium wreaking fearful havoc in many susceptible persons, causing high blood pressure, heart and kidney involvements, etc. But what happens to the chlorine portion of table salt? No one seems to worry about it. As I say I am not considering table salt, but am merely mentioning it. However, its effects on the human body, with regard to its chloride content should be thoroughly investigated. Until this is done, no health-conscious person should use a grain of table salt.

In the meantime the problem of supplying drinking water is becoming more complicated, or is it the greed of the chemical companies who wish to sell their chemicals, for now there are available 50 different chemical compounds for processing drinking water. If you want to see what chemistry has done to our water, look at the list of chemicals reproduced herewith, 50 of them, that are used in public water treatment all over the country. We have in our possession the printed chart containing them, given to us by one of the engineers of a water-works of a large city. Here is the list of 48 chemicals:

Activated Carbon
Activated Silica
Alum. Ammonium Sulfate
Aluminum Chloride Soln.
Alum. Potassium Sulfate
Aluminum Sulfate
Alum, Liquid
Ammonia, Anhydrous
Ammonia, Aqua
Ammonium Silicofluoride
Ammonium Sulfate
Bentonite

Bromine
Calcium Carbonate
Calcium Hydroxide
Calcium Hypochlorite
Calcium Oxide
Carbon Dioxide
Chlorinated Copperas
Chlorinated Lime
Chlorine
Chlorine Dioxide
Copper Sulfate
Disodium Phosphate
Dolomitic Hydrated Lime
Dolomitic Lime
Ferric Chloride
Ferric Sulfate
Fluosilicic Acid
Hydrofluoric Acid
Ozone
Sodium Aluminate
Sodium Bicarbonate
Sodium Bisulfite
Sodium Carbonate
Sodium Chloride
Sodium Chlorite (13)
Sodium Fluoride
Sod. Hexametaphosphate
Sodium Hydroxide
Sodium Hypochlorite
Sodium Silicate
Sodium Sulfite
Sodium Thiosulfate
Sulfur Dioxide
Sulfuric Acid
Tetra-Sod. Pyrophosphate
Tri-Sodium Phosphate

The same chart gives a list of purposes for which these chemicals are used. They are:

Algae Control
Boiler Water Treatment
Coagulation
Color Removal
Corrosion and Scale Control
Dechlorination
Disinfection
Fluoridation
Iron & Manganese Removal
pH Control
Softening
Taste and Odor Control
Miscellaneous
B. O. D. Removal
Condition-Dewater Sludge
Odor Control
Chlorination
Flotation
Neutralization—Acid
Neutralization—Alkali
Oxidation
Reduction

Think of the power put into the hands of the public water works engineer. He is given 50 chemicals and instructed to use them as he sees fit. If he has problems of flotation, or neutralization, or coagulation, he can use this or that chemical, but does he worry about its effect on the coagulation of the human blood of the people who drink this water? What does he know about its effect on human health? I see no doctor standing at his elbow to advise him in this regard. The U. S. Public Health Service is too busy trying to get more public water works managers to use fluorine to worry about chlorine. It should enlist the best engineering and medical brains of the land to develop methods to give us pure drinking water without benefit of dangerous chemicals.

Recently I was in the small town of Appeldoorn in Holland and was amazed to discover that the people there drank the water without a single chemical being put into it for any purpose whatever. Upon investigation I found that the drinking water of this town of about

30,000 people is obtained from deep wells sunk for the purpose. This would seem to be an ideal solution for many American cities. The existing water lines could be maintained for non-drinking and industrial purposes, and a separate line could be used merely for drinking water.

A cheaper way would be for the city to deliver free non-chemicalized drinking water in bottles to every citizen of the city. The municipality already does certain things for the citizens such as to have a truck call at his home to take away the garbage, to clean the streets, to conduct a water works, etc. The city could acquire springs and make sure that its people drink only the purest water obtainable, because it is so basic to their health. It will save the city money in the end. I am not suggesting this for a large city like New York. Huge metropolises pose special problems. People should not live in them in the first place. There is far more cancer in such large aggregations of population.

As far as chlorination is concerned, have we re-evaluated the need for it based on the fact that the general conception of sanitation has improved so much today compared to the primitive conditions of 1900? We are treating our water based on a 1900 diagnosis. Is it not time for the medical profession to take another look?

An example of the proper attitude towards drinking water is found in the Hunza people of Northern India, a group of about 20,000 persons, one of the healthiest in the world. Let me quote from my own book *The Healthy Hunzas* (Rodale Press, $3.00): "The Hunza drinking water is kept scrupulously clean in roofed tanks or closed cisterns placed down steep steps so that animals cannot come near them. The people do not wash their clothes in the running streams from which they obtain their drinking water, but draw off water which is used especially for this purpose. They are consummate in all matters pertaining to sanitation. They are singularly careful with regard to their privies which are operated by a system that makes it impossible to contaminate any nearby water supply."

The Hunzas are absolutely free of goitre but their neighbors, the Nagyri, who are careless with their water are wretchedly afflicted with it and its companion disease, cretinism. Sir Robert McCarrison, in his medical researches, in that region, definitely connected polluted water supply with goitre. He was able to prove his point beyond any question of doubt in giving the disease to himself and fifteen others by drinking fouled water, and then calmly proceeding to cure it in every case, merely by drinking pure water.

We, on our side of the world, must keep our drinking water sources unpolluted. If we study methods to keep water as clean as possible, then chlorination, or any other chemicalization would not be required. There must be safer means. The Romans used silver to purify their water—infinitesimal amounts of it, and I have heard that some city in this country is experimenting with it. Water can also be purified by ultraviolet light. Perhaps the cities could pasteurize the water as it goes into the mains, that is, to boil it in order to kill offensive organisms. Incidentally, this may be an excellent idea for the home. Boil all chlorinated water to be used for drinking, because boiling will eliminate all traces of chlorine from it. It will not, however, get rid of the fluorine. Distillation will do that. But cities might rig up automatic pasteurizing equipment that could work economically. Where are our vaunted engineering brains? You don't see them putting chlorine in milk to kill organisms. No! Milk is a commercial product that brings dollars. But water? What care the politicians if it reeks of chlorine!

Our trouble is that we put engineers to work mainly on commercial problems that mean immediate money. For example, a certain enterprising toilet tank-ball manufacturer has placed on the market a tank-ball, the tag on which reads, "The *Water Master* tank ball is made of a special water resistant rubber which withstands chlorinated water," but who is taking pains to protect the sensitive cells and tissues of human beings who drink chlorinated water? They do not seem to be so important as a 50 cent tank-ball.

But sometimes it works in reverse from a commercial viewpoint. There's an ironic twist to the story about the calf that was to win the prize at the annual Houston (Texas) fair in 1954. Shell Oil Company, busy the year 'round making chemicals, sponsors a winning calf each year. This year they had a Hereford which, from all appearances, could win without half trying. But, according to *Chemical Week* for April 3, 1954, the Hereford had been drinking pure ranch water all his life and absolutely refused to drink the chlorinated city water when he was brought in for the fair. Result? The Hereford lost 40 precious pounds and the Shell Company lost the prize. You'd think somebody somewhere would learn the lesson which nature is trying so hard to teach us with an incident like this. But no, we go right ahead drinking chemicalized water that "dumb" animals know is not fit to drink.

What we need is pure water societies to spring up all over the United States, which could eventually grow into general health groups that could wield great power in moulding public and official opinion on health matters.

In the meantime, either boil your drinking water or buy bottled spring water, and watch carefully to observe the effects on the health of the family.

Chocolate

Four centuries ago the Aztecs of Mexico made a delicious chocolate drink by crushing the cocoa bean, beating the fluid to a froth of honey thickness, flavoring it with vanilla and serving it cold. It is said that the emperor Montezuma was so fond of this drink that he had no less that fifty jars of it prepared for his own daily consumption. Two thousand more jars were prepared for his household. There was a soda fountain on an illustrious scale!

After the Spaniards conquered Mexico, they took chocolate back to Spain. Although they supposedly guarded the secret of making the chocolate drink, knowledge of it gradually spread to other parts of Europe. By the middle of the 17th century chocolate was known in

England and Germany. It was not widely used in this country until well along in the nineteenth century, partly because it was very expensive.

An elegant little booklet, *Golden Harvest,* is available from the British Information Services, New York 20, N. Y., dealing with the cocoa trade of the African Gold Coast. From this booklet we learn much about how cocoa is grown, processed and sold. It is one of the chief products of this part of Africa which produced 248,000 tons of cocoa beans in the year 1950. In the best season yet recorded the total amount paid to the cocoa farmers in the Gold Coast for the full crop was more than thirty-four million pounds, or about $95,200,000.00 in American money. So the cocoa business is a flourishing one and, as you might expect, the United States buys about twice as much cocoa as the next country on the list. Cocoa and chocolate have become accepted, almost traditional elements of our daily menus. Chocolate cake, chocolate candy, chocolate sodas, chocolate bars, chocolate milk—would America be America without these items on the menu? Yet the story of cocoa and chocolate leads us finally to the conclusion that we would be far better off had the tasty brown substance never reached our shores.

How Cocoa Is Processed

What is cocoa and how is it related to chocolate? In the Gold Coast which produces many times more chocolate than any other region of the world, cocoa is grown by farmers on small family farms. The cocoa tree needs good, deep soil, a warm moist climate and the shelter of forests 'round about. Seed pods develop on the tree when it is about five years old. The pods are about six to eight inches long. When they are fully ripe they are harvested and piled. Then the pods are split open with a cutlass and the beans extracted. The beans are then fermented, which means simply spreading them in heaps to lie for six days. Then they are dried in the sun. After the cocoa beans are graded and packed, they are shipped, and further processing takes place in the country which is importing them.

The beans are first roasted, which brings out the characteristic chocolate flavor. Then they are cracked between rollers and ground in mills from which they emerge as a thick brown mass, for the heat of the grinding has melted the fat in the cocoa. Powerful hydraulic presses (up to 6,000 pounds per square inch) are then used to extract much of the fat, which is sold as cocoa butter. The cakes that are left contain about 20 to 30 per cent of cocoa fat or butter. This is bitter chocolate, as we know it, which may then be ground to fine powder, producing cocoa. For sweet chocolate sugar is added. For milk chocolate, milk and sugar are added. From then on, candy, chocolate bars and chocolate syrup are just a few of the hundreds of products our ingenious food processors turn out.

What Cocoa Contains

Cocoa and chocolate are among the foods highest in calories. In one pound of the original chocolate, after its first processing, there are 2,182 calories in fats, 482 calories in carbohydrates and 221 in proteins. This adds up to about 3,000 calories. In one pound of good plain processed chocolate there are about 2,500 calories. Milk chocolate has over 2,600. What else is there besides calories? Well, cocoa, as we drink it for breakfast, is one to two per cent theobromine. This is, like caffeine, an alkaloid. It is closely related to caffeine and acts like caffeine in the body. In other words, it is a drug, very active chemically and frequently used in medicine. Cocoa (and of course chocolate) also contains caffeine. One ten cent bar of chocolate, as you would buy it at the candy store, contains 78 milligrams of caffeine—about half as much as the average cup of coffee.

It is believed that the cocoa bean may develop some vitamin D while it is being dried in the sun. Cocoa, if we make it with milk, may contain vitamin A, vitamin D and two of the B vitamins, thiamin and riboflavin. But, we assume that this vitamin content comes largely from the milk used.

What else does chocolate contain? Interestingly enough it contains a substance called oxalic acid which is also present in some of the green leafy vegetables that grow in our gardens. Beet greens, rhubarb, spinach and swiss chard are especially rich in oxalic acid. Oxalic acid has one very undesirable quality. It combines with whatever calcium is in the plant and by this combination, renders the calcium useless for assimilation by human bodies. Furthermore, after it gets in the digestive tract it combines with whatever calcium is there, too, and wastes it, so far as human nutrition is concerned.

Not so many years ago spinach was widely promoted as the ideal, if much detested, food for youngsters. Popeye and other comic strip characters beat the drum for spinach as *the* food which would put hair on the chest and strength in the arms of puny kids. Spinach is rich in iron and calcium, vitamins A, B and C. But, its oxalic acid content nullifies the calcium and also destroys a considerable amount of the calcium in any other food eaten at the same time. So gradually we came to be much more cautious about spinach, and the related greens that are also high in oxalic acid. Eat them in moderation, we say now, for they contain much that is nutritious. But do not depend on them for calcium. And, if you eat lots of spinach, make certain that you double or triple the amount of calcium you are getting in other foods, for this precious mineral is essential to most body functions and you dare not be deficient in it.

Oxalic Acid in Cocoa

Where does this leave us, so far as chocolate and cocoa are concerned? In a list of common foods high in oxalic acid, cocoa is eighth, coming right after spinach, swiss chard and rhubarb. Spinach contains .89 per cent of oxalic acid, rhubarb .50 per cent and chocolate .45 to .49 per cent. *Bridges' Dietetics For the Clinician* (Lea and Febiger, 1949) states: "If a food contains enough oxalic acid to combine with all of its calcium to form calcium oxalate, the indication seems to be that the calcium is of little or no use to the body."

Adelle Davis, in *Vitality Through Planned Nutrition* (Macmillan, 1949), says that a recent investigation showed that 90 per cent of the milk sold in school cafeterias is chocolate milk, so studies were made of the amount of milk calcium used by the body when the milk was taken in the form of chocolate milk. Two groups of laboratory animals were given the same diet but one group received plain milk and the other chocolate milk. Those drinking the chocolate milk absorbed less calcium and phosphorus from their food. Their growth was retarded, their bones small and fragile, a result surely to be expected if they were not absorbing calcium and phosphorus from the main source available. Miss Davis concludes, "Both chocolate and cocoa interfere with absorption of calcium to such an extent that it is valueless to attempt to obtain this mineral by taking cocoa or chocolate."

Now if the American diet were overflowing with calcium so that all of us had more than we could use, eating chocolate or drinking chocolate milk or cocoa would be harmless. But we are, as a nation, notoriously deficient in calcium. *The Englishman's Food* by J. C. Drummond and Anne Wilbraham (Jonathan Cape, 1939) tells us that the average fifteenth century diet contained 1.3 grams of calcium per day. The average middle class diet today contains but .6 grams of calcium. The officially recommended daily minimum for children is from 1 to 1.4 grams of calcium daily. So we are already far short of what we need of this tremendously important mineral.

Part of the reason for this is that we have removed the minerals from many of our foods in processing them. Part of the reason is that we throw away the bones from our meat, rather than eating them. Earlier civilizations got much of their calcium from bones, and many primitive peoples still do. Part of the reason is that we eat so many unnecessary and harmful foods in the way of desserts, soft drinks, candy and so forth that we simply do not have room for the valuable, protective, mineral-rich foods. For modern children milk is about the only reliable, day by day source of calcium except, of course, bone meal.

But if we are going to insist on doctoring up milk with chocolate it is easy to see that even this not so satisfactory source of calcium is lost to us. For the oxalic acid in chocolate milk or cocoa will destroy the calcium in the milk (so far as our body's use of it is concerned) and, if we drink it at the same time we are eating cheese or green vegetables, these other good sources of calcium will also be rendered useless.

Is Cocoa Partly Responsible For Our Deficiency In Calcium?

As we went further in our research on chocolate and oxalic acid, we became convinced that chocolate products must be held responsible for much of the calcium deficiency so evident today in decayed teeth, bones that break easily, nervousness, heart trouble and all the other symptoms that indicate clearly a serious lack of calcium.

You may argue that the amount of chocolate used in cocoa or chocolate milk is very small. You do not, for instance, eat cocoa in the quantity you eat spinach. But on the other hand *you do not eat spinach every day!* And many, many Americans—especially children—eat considerable quantities of chocolate milk, cocoa, chocolate candy, sodas, milkshakes or desserts *every single day of their lives!* How many lunches go to school that do not contain a chocolate bar? It gives energy. Of course, because it contains so many calories. But it is a temporary form of energy. How many youngsters do not stop for a chocolate drink, a piece of candy or a soda fountain concoction after school or after a basketball or football game? Sit down some day and figure out—if you can get the facts—just how much chocolate your own young ones have had during any given week and we think you will probably be amazed.

To sum up, we have in cocoa and chocolate (in a little less quantity) exactly the same caffeine we have pinned so many crimes on in relation to coffee-drinking. Caffeine stimulates the heart, raises the blood pressure, lowers the blood sugar, creates a false sense of security in that it appears to relax and rest tired nerves. In addition, we have in cocoa and chocolate another substance like caffeine (theobromine) which also produces these same undesirable results in body metabolism. And, as if this were not enough, we also have in cocoa and chocolate, oxalic acid which wipes out the body's most valuable mineral, vitally concerned with teeth and bone health, nerves, heart functions, resistance to infection and so forth.

Cocoa and Chocolate Are Not For Children!

Perhaps we might find excuses for chocolate if it were exclusively food for adults. In past eras it was considered just that. But in present-day America we use chocolate almost exclusively as a treat for the children—a harmless flavoring substance which induces them to drink milk and eat their pudding. We hope we have convinced you that it is not harmless at all, but may in fact be an important source of one of our most troublesome nation-wide deficiencies.

Your doctor may tell you that chocolate products are harmless for the small fry, unless of course he is dealing with a child afflicted with acne, in which case chocolate is generally the first food forbidden, probably because of its high fat content. But the Committee on Foods of the American Medical Association has this to say on the subject: "Special recommendations for children are not permissible for foods consisting largely of chocolate or cocoa; no objection will be taken however to such recommendations in the case of foods that are merely flavored with chocolate or cocoa and which in the quantities likely to be consumed are free from any probable effects due to theobromine or caffeine." As we have shown, the amounts of chocolate being consumed by present day American children cannot by any stretch of the imagination come under the heading of "flavoring."

And still, although all these facts are well known to nutritionists, school lunch counters go right on serving chocolate milk, cocoa, chocolate pudding and candy bars. And we go right on importing enormous quantities of chocolate. The booklet *Golden Harvest* tells us that even very inferior grades of cocoa are eagerly sought after *for the present world demand for cocoa far exceeds the supply.*

Chocolate and Pruritus Ani

A most interesting article in *The American Journal of Surgery* for November, 1951, presents a paper in which Laurence G. Bodkin, M. D., of Brooklyn, discussed the possible causes of pruritis ani (an itching anus). In the discussion that followed Dr. Bodkin's presentation of his paper, Dr. F. B. Bowman of Hamilton, Ontario, Canada, contributed the following: "Allergy has been mentioned. I have found that three or four foods are frequently the culprits. . . . The question is always asked

Are you a coca cola drinker?' I think of a doctor who consulted me in such a state (of pruritus ani) that he was considering giving up a practice. On questioning him I found that he was a confirmed chocolate eater. The condition was as bad or worse than any discussed by the speaker. In a very short time he was perfectly well after stopping his chocolate. If he takes an ABS and C coated laxative tablet (we assume this is chocolate-coated) it will throw him into a spasm of pruritus ani. A young lady with pruritus ani was cancelling her arrangements for entering a training school. When she stopped drinking coca cola the condition disappeared." Dr. Bodkin, in closing the discussion, said, "Chocolate is one of the greatest offenders in the whole group."

What Can You Do About Giving Up Chocolate?

Our suggestions are, first, that you conduct a real educational program, especially among the children of your family. Children admire good health and good appearance. Explain to them what continued eating of chocolate may do in the way of poor teeth, soft bones, bad hearts and nervousness. Second, keep on hand a plentiful supply of healthful snack-foods: peanuts, popcorn, sunflower seeds, apples, raisins, and other dried fruits such as dates and figs, bananas, almonds, fruit juice, cheese wedges, radishes, celery, carrots. Third, if your children refuse any drinks unless they are flavored, either hot or cold, with chocolate, start now to change over to carob flour as a substitute. Carob flour is a nutritious food which tastes very much like chocolate. It goes without saying that any sensible adult will be easily persuaded to drop chocolate items from his menu, once he knows in full the harm they may be doing him.

Finally, until you can cut down on your family's consumption of cocoa and chocolate, or if they have been eating large quantities of it in the past, by all means make certain that they get enough calcium by taking bone meal, the richest and best natural source of this supremely important mineral.

Citrus

We feel that just a word is in order on the subject of drinking citrus fruit juice. There is considerable evidence in work done by various researchers that the consumption of large amounts of citrus fruit juice may be harmful, especially to the tissues of the mouth and the enamel of the teeth. Henry Hicks, D.D.S., writing in *Oral Surgery, Oral Medicine and Oral Pathology* for July, 1951, described five cases from his own practice in which the drinking of large amounts of citrus juice had resulted in bleeding gums, tooth cavities, anemia, stomach pains, acne, fatigue, sinusitis and so forth. When these patients stopped drinking so much citrus juice and took only three whole oranges a week, their symptoms were relieved.

In the *Journal of the American Dental Association* for July, 1950, Dr. Hicks reported on seven cases from the files he has been keeping for fifteen years—seven cases with symptoms similar to those described above. In all cases, eliminating citrus juices relieved the symptoms. Dr. Hicks believes that citrus juices can cause tooth erosion (because of their citric acid content) and can, as well, cause harmful side effects to the deep and connective tissues of the mouth.

Edward Stafne, D.D.S., and Stanley A. Lovestedt, D.D.S., writing in the *Proceedings of the Staff Meetings of the Mayo Clinic,* March 5, 1947, discuss the dental health of 50 patients at the clinic who customarily drank lemon juice as soon as they got up every morning. Tooth cavities were common. The researchers earnestly advised discontinuing the practice. A study on fruit juice for ulcer patients was made by John D. Yeagley, M.D., and David Cayer, M.D., and reported in the *North Carolina Medical Journal* for November, 1948. They found that the drinking of orange juice by 19 actively ulcerated patients increased their discomfort by bringing on pains and burning sensations. In 32 less active cases the intake of orange juice caused an increase in stomach acidity without causing pain. They suggested that, if citrus juice is to be given to ulcer patients it should be in combination with other foods, or at regular mealtime.

In the now famous experiment at Cornell where rats were given various beverages, it was found that orange juice caused some erosion in the teeth of the rats who drank it, and at the end of the six months experiment there was considerably more erosion. The erosion caused by orange juice was graded as being midway between that caused by phosphoric acid (such as appears in cola drinks), which caused the most erosion, and tomato juice, which caused the least.

Other Symptoms From Citrus Juice Drinking

We have also accumulated evidence from readers that drinking citrus juice may cause pruitus ani (itching anus). Other readers have written us of such symptoms as rash, bleeding gums, infected fingernails, and so forth, which were apparently caused by drinking large amounts of citrus juice, since they disappeared after the juice was omitted. On the other hand, we have received evidence from readers who use only organically grown oranges and who tell us that they have no ill effects from drinking juice made from these oranges.

Apparently there are several reasons why citrus juice may be inadvisable. Squeezing the orange to extract the juice seems to result in some of the oil from the rind entering the juice. Perhaps this is the harmful substance. Then, too, it has been shown in animal experiments that eating the fruit does not produce the erosive effect produced when we drink the juice. No one knows why, but apparently something in the fruit juice or in the way it circulates around the teeth as we drink it causes erosion to take place, which does not occur when the fruit is eaten. It has also been suggested that we would not ordinarily eat two or three oranges or grapefruit at one sitting. But we may drink the juice of two or three at one time without even thinking about it. And it is possible that the citric acid contained in the citrus juice is too acid for us, in such large quantities.

We do not advise doing without citrus fruit entirely, but we do advise *eating* the fruit rather than juicing it and we advise cutting down to several oranges or grapefruit a week. We especially deplore the use of canned or frozen citrus juice in which there may be added sugar, synthetic coloring matter or even added synthetic flavoring.

Of course, we do not need to add that rose hips are far higher in vitamin C than citrus fruit is. Whether you grow your own roses and make syrup or puree from the rose hips, or whether you buy rose hip preparations as a food supplement, you need have no fear of lacking vitamin C so long as you are taking rose hips in some form.

Coffee and Blood Sugar

Day by day scientists are coming to an increased appreciation of the importance of proper blood sugar levels to good health. All of us know that the one sure symptom of diabetes is a high blood sugar—that is, the mechanism in the body which controls the use of sugar goes awry and the veins and arteries are flooded with sugar which eventually shows up in large quantities in the urine. Not so many of us know about low blood sugar—the opposite of diabetes which also involves a defect in the mechanism that controls the use of sugar.

According to E. M. Abrahamson, M.D. and A. W. Pezet writing in *Body, Mind and Sugar* (Henry Holt, 1951) low blood sugar is far more common among Americans than high blood sugar or diabetes. Its symptoms are perhaps not so dramatic, but it, too, can lead to poor health. And because it has just recently come to the foreground as a cause of all kinds of disorders, ranging from asthma and epilepsy to fatigue, gnawing hunger and dizziness, many doctors do not give patients tests to determine whether or not their blood sugar is too low.

The way low blood sugar (hypoglycemia or hyperinsulinism are the scientific names for it) comes about is this. When sugar is eaten, it goes almost immediately to the blood because it does not need to be digested. This raises the blood sugar to an abnormal height. But instead of staying at this height, the blood sugar level plunges almost immediately to far below what it should be. Then the individual feels uncomfortable, tired or hungry and eats something else that is sugary or starchy. His blood sugar level soars again, only to drop far below what it should be a half hour or an hour later. You can see that such a condition produces a vicious cycle, in which the blood sugar level is not continually high, as in diabetes, but instead rises precipitately, then drops just as fast. A graph of the blood sugar level goes up and down in peaks and valleys. The ideal blood sugar level is one which rises a little after a meal, when the body is busy digesting the food just eaten, then falls gradually just a little and levels off in a plateau, falling down just a little again before it is time for the next meal.

White sugar and products made from it are among the worst offenders in producing low blood sugar. A second criminal in the low blood sugar case is tobacco, for puffing on a cigarette has the same effect of lifting the blood sugar level, only to plunge it to dangerous depths within a half hour or so. The third offender is—you've guessed it—coffee. We do not know whether it is the caffeine in coffee that produces this effect, but we rather imagine it is, for blood sugar responds in this way to any poisonous substance taken in. At any rate we know that this is one reason for the "lift" you get from a cup of coffee.

Quite apart from its effect on heart, breathing, blood pressure and so forth, coffee causes the blood sugar to rise rapidly, then fall just as rapidly. So, if you suffer from low blood sugar, the effects of those three cups of breakfast coffee will wear off in an hour or so, and you will find your efficiency decreasing. Your head may begin to ache, you may get grumpy and irritable, you may have an "all-gone" feeling in the pit of your stomach, you may be just plain hungry. Obviously it's time for you to have another cup of coffee. You do and the cycle begins all over again.

Folks who take their morning cup of coffee and don't run into any of these difficulties apparently have a sugar-regulating mechanism strong enough to bring up the blood sugar level after the drop occurs. These are the folks who work vigorously and well straight through the morning and feel just pleasantly hungry by lunch time. Nine chances out of ten they won't feel the need for coffee at lunch. With their blood sugar level holding steady throughout the afternoon they won't need a "coffee break" at the office around three o'clock. By dinner time, once again they are just pleasantly hungry and while they may or may not have a cup of coffee with dinner, they don't feel a violent craving for it, as many of the rest of us do.

Coffee Addiction Must Be Broken If You Would Be Healthy

What about the coffee-addict, who has three or more cups for breakfast, another at 10:00 A.M., several more for lunch and dinner and tops off the day with a midnight snack and several more cups of coffee? His blood sugar level must be zigging and zagging all day, from depths to heights. The main reason for the low blood sugar is the coffee he drinks and the lower the blood sugar goes, the more coffee he must have to bring it up again! Truly a vicious cycle!

About coffee Dr. Abrahamson says in *Body, Mind and Sugar* "Caffeine stimulates the adrenal cortex to produce more of its hormones which in turn induce the liver to break down glycogen into glucose which flows into the blood stream. This is why a cup of coffee 'gives you a lift.' Trouble develops because the islands of Langerhans (that part of the pancreas which is disordered in diabetes and in low blood sugar) cannot distinguish between the effects of drinking coffee and eating food. They don't know and don't care whether the sugar has come from the food that is being digested or from previously stored glycogen, broken down by the action of the caffeine's stimulus to the adrenal cortex. To the islands of Langerhans sugar is sugar. They go to work to force the blood sugar to its normal level. In the course of time, because of their repeated stimulation, the islands become so sensitive that they overrespond to a normal stimulus.

"Anyone trying to lose weight who drinks black coffee to still the pangs of hunger is only making matters worse for himself. The repeated stimulus to the islands of Langerhans makes them more sensitive, and the resultant low blood sugar only makes the onerous diet more onerous. Dieting to reduce is much easier if coffee, as well as caffeine in other forms (such as strong tea, chocolate and soft drinks containing that alkaloid) is excluded."

Dr. Abrahamson in his book gives a case history of one patient whose addiction to coffee was nearly her undoing. At the age of thirty-six, she was nervous and irritable. She had trouble taking care of her home and never had enough energy to go out in the evenings. Her test for blood sugar level showed that it was low. She responded very well to the recommended diet and expressed her amazement that she got along without barbiturates which she had been taking, on her doctor's advice, for her "nervousness." But she missed her breakfast coffee—three cups! She was advised to omit the coffee and she did and got along nicely. But she kept inquiring how soon she might drink coffee again. She was then told that she would never be able to drink it. "Moderate use of caffeine is perfectly harmless to the average person; once the insulin apparatus has been sensitized by overindulgence, however, coffee must be avoided. In a way this is similar to the alcohol problem. Moderate use of alcohol is not only relatively harmless but actually of help in withstanding the stress of civilized life. If a person has been an alcoholic and conquered his craving, he must not take another drop."

Our patient could not believe that "just one" cup of coffee would hurt her. So she tried it for a few months and her symptoms returned—butterflies in her stomach, indigestion and nervousness. As soon as she returned to the diet once again, the symptoms disappeared. This is but one of the case histories related in Dr. Abrahamson's book. They are all equally revealing. And we believe that every reader should have the book for the wealth of splendid information it contains. You can buy it at your local bookshop or order it from the publishers, Henry Holt and Company, Inc., 383 Madison Avenue, New York, New York.

The Diet for Attaining a Normal Blood Sugar Level

The cure for low blood sugar is a diet high in protein and fat and low in starches, sugars, and coffee with as few cigarettes as possible. Dr. Abrahamson lists the following foods as permissible on the diet to raise blood sugar levels: Vegetables: asparagus, avocado, beets, broccoli, Brussels sprouts, cabbage, cauliflower, carrots, celery, corn, cucumbers, eggplant, Lima beans, onions, peas, radishes, sauerkraut, squash, string beans, tomatoes, turnips. Meats, fish, cheese, milk and eggs. Apples apricots, berries, grapefruit, melons, oranges, peaches, pears, pineapple, tangerines. Salads, mushrooms, nuts. Any unsweetened fruit juice except grape juice or prune juice. Weak tea, decaffeinated coffee, coffee substitutes.

These foods are forbidden: sugar, candy and other sweets such as pie, cake, pastries, sweet custards, puddings and ice cream. Caffeine—ordinary coffee, strong brewed tea, beverages containing caffeine, potatoes, rice, grapes, raisins, plums, figs, dates and bananas, spaghetti, noodles, macaroni, wines, cordials, cocktails and beer.

By this second list we mean *that you should not eat any of these foods,* even if it means changing your meal habits entirely, getting up early enough to eat a hearty high protein breakfast, carrying lunch instead of eating at restaurants, and declining evening invitations when you know that coffee and forbidden sweets will be involved when refreshment time comes. It should take you only a short time to revise your blood sugar level readings so that you can ease up on the restrictions. But by this time if you have really been concentrating on a high protein diet, you may be surprised at your own reluctance to go back to the diet you were eating before.

You may be delighted to find that you simply don't crave dessert, that a piece of pie or a doughnut looks repulsive at ten in the morning, that the evening meal leaves you feeling satisfied and content without any dessert other than fresh raw fruit. What a happy state of affairs for someone trying to reduce! Quite apart from the beneficial effects on blood sugar levels, such a diet is just about all that one could wish for as a permanent diet. We're sure we don't need to point out to interested readers that, after your blood sugar level has risen to normal and you feel you can begin to add some of the forbidden foods, you should add only the fruits and vegetables, *never* the pastries, cakes, pies, candy and so forth. Those should be on your permanently forbidden list.

Brewer's yeast, meat flour, wheat germ, sunflower seeds, amino acids, desiccated liver and many other health-giving food supplements are rich in high-quality protein and of course can be added with great success to Dr. Abrahamson's diet.

Coffee and Evidence Against Coffee

We made a very significant observation in our research on the scientific proof of the harmfulness of coffee-drinking. From 1900 to 1915 medical and scientific journals were full of articles on experiments done. From 1915 to 1925 there were far fewer articles. From 1925 to 1945 the number declined still more. And from 1945 on there has been, practically speaking, little or no investigation of the effect of coffee on human health. We do not know what this may mean. Does it mean, perhaps, that medical men are discounting the facts discovered earlier and hence do not think it worth while to pursue the investigation further? Does it mean that new drugs, chemicals and poisons now demand so much time that we cannot spare time to investigate older substances? Or does it mean simply that physicians and researchers alike have decided that the fragrant brown beverage most of them drink all day long can't possibly need any further investigation?

As far back as 1746, a treatise was published on *Tobacco, Tea and Coffee* by Simon Pauli, an Italian writer. Pauli appears to be a writer of some substance, for his works were accepted widely among the learned of his day. We know there were many misconceptions about physiology in those days and of course present-day methods of investigation were not available. Yet it is startling that Pauli believes "it (coffee) is esteemed a great cooler (thirst quencher) for which reason it is drank by most, but if it is used to excess, it extinguishes the inclination to venery and induces sterility." He tells us further that in ancient times women of the East used coffee brewed extra strong as a purgative to prevent conception. Perhaps this is the reason why its use was forbidden to women for many centuries by the early caliphs. He advances the theory that coffee induces sterility because it gradually dries up the body's procreative powers on account of the large amount of sulfur it contains.

Later in our own country a writer on health, Dr. William Alexander Alcott, wrote that coffee is essentially and properly a medicine—a narcotic. He quotes authorities of that day (his book was published in 1844) as saying that coffee possesses nervine and astringent qualities, is suspected of producing palsies, has a powerful effect on the nervous system, a pernicious effect on the stomach and bowels, exhausts the sensibilities of the part on which it acts, induces weakness, produces debility, alters the gastric juice, disorders digestion and often produces convulsions and vertigo, feverish heat, anxiety, palpitations, tremblings, weakness of sight and predispositions to apoplexy.

He quotes Dr. Hahnemann, founder of homeopathic medicine, as saying that "coffee is strictly a medicinal substance. All medicines in strong doses have a disagreeable effect on the feelings of a healthy person." He also quotes Hahnemann as saying that coffee drinking produces the following diseases: nervous or sick headaches, toothache, darting pains in the body, spasms in the chest, stomach and abdomen, costiveness (constipation), erysipelas, disease of the liver, uterus and bones, inflammation of the eyes, difficulty in breathing and bowel affections. He compares the action of caffeine to that of arsenic, lead or prussic acid, asking "will anyone attempt to say that these substances are not poisonous because they poison slowly?"

Dr. Alcott is a cousin and associate of Amos Bronson Alcott, who was a famous educator and the father of Louisa May Alcott of *Little Women* fame.

It Is An Established Fact That Caffeine Is a Poison

Now perhaps these older writers may have jumped to conclusions when they laid down the unqualified statement that coffee was responsible for all the ills mentioned. Undoubtedly they did not use present-day laboratory methods to prove their statements. But they must have questioned their patients as to whether or not they used coffee and based conclusions on the answers. So while it does not follow that coffee-drinking was the sole and only cause of the symptoms their patients described, it does seem quite possible that coffee-drinking may have played a part in them. And it does seem significant that so much was written in times past about the possible harm of coffee-drinking. We do not find treatises attacking the use of apples, potatoes, carrots, bread or cheese. So we know, that, from way back, physicians have been concerned with the medicinal and narcotic aspects of coffee. And we cannot discount this concern as an old wives' tale.

We know that caffeine, the substance in coffee which apparently is responsible for its effects on the human body, is a powerful poison. A drop of caffeine injected into the skin of an animal will produce death within a few minutes. An infinitely small amount injected into the brain will bring convulsions. The amount of caffeine in a cup of coffee is quite small. Yet we drink coffee because of the effect of the caffeine, just as we smoke because of the effect of the nicotine. Both are drugs, both are habit-forming. We uncovered some interesting accounts of headaches produced as "withdrawal symptoms" when coffee-drinking was abruptly stopped. We also know that efficiency of work performance decreases when a confirmed coffee-drinker stops taking his daily dose of coffee. These are symptoms typical of addiction. When any drug is taken away from a drug addict, he suffers "withdrawal symptoms."

Habitual Coffee-Drinking and Stomach Ulcers

What do some of the modern researchers have to say about the effect of coffee on the human body? There are two modern disorders that the general public usually associates with coffee drinking—ulcers and heart trouble. This may be mostly because physicians frequently forbid coffee to their heart and ulcer patients. There seems to be no doubt that coffee is bad for the ulcer patient, although we do not find any researcher who has proved that coffee actually produces ulcers in human beings. J. A. Roth and A. C. Ivy whose animal experiments on coffee are famous, tell us in *Gastroenterology* for November, 1948, that 1. Caffeine produces gastro-duodenal ulcers in animals to whom the drug is given in a beeswax container so that their stomachs are absorbing caffeine continually. 2. Caffeine moderately stimulates the flow of gastric juices. 3. Caffeine produces very definite changes in the blood vessels of animals which are similar to changes produced by prolonged resentment, hostility and anxiety. 4. As we know, one difficulty involved in ulcers is an excessive flow of hydrochloric acid into the stomach. Most peptic ulcer patients, say Drs. Roth and Ivy, respond to caffeine with a prolonged and sustained stimulation of the output of free hydrochloric acid. In other words, coffee causes more and more hydrochloric acid to pour into the stomach of the ulcer patient for quite a long time after the coffee has been taken. So, say these authors, although they cannot prove that caffeine causes ulcers, still it does seem that taking fairly large amounts of coffee may contribute to the development of ulcers and may aggravate the condition of an ulcer that exists already.

An investigation carried on at the University of Oklahoma by Vern H. Musick, M. D., Howard C. Hopps, M. D., Harry Avey, M. D., and Arthur A. Hellbaum, M. D., and reported in the *Southern Medical Journal* for August 1946 involved a total of 39 patients—10 of them with no symptoms of digestive tract trouble of any kind, 25 of them patients with duodenal ulcers and four patients with gastric ulcers. The researchers found that the flow of digestive juice is considerably increased in the normal person when caffeine comes into contact with the lining of the stomach. In the patient with duodenal ulcer the flow of digestive juice is "prolonged and excessive." Dr. Musick, in discussing the subject before a meeting of the Southern Medical Association concluded, "I think it is all right for the normal person to drink caffeine-containing beverages but an ulcer patient or a patient who has a high secretory curve (that is, someone with a generally high level of hydrochloric acid in the stomach, which might predispose him to ulcers) should not drink coffee. He should not drink alcohol and by all means he should not drink black coffee the next morning after alcohol.

Now you will notice that, in all of these researches, caffeine was used —not coffee. This might lead someone to say "Well, of course straight caffeine is bad for you, but there is so little caffeine in coffee that surely coffee can't hurt me." On the same basis one could say there is so little nicotine in cigarettes, so little preservative in processed foods, so little arsenic on the outside of a sprayed apple, so little fluorine in fluoridated water, that there is no harm in taking any of these either. Once you begin to add up all these "small doses of poison" that you are taking every day, the sum total gets to be quite frightening.

Dr. R. Wood, M. A., B. M., B. Ch., B. Sc., writing in the *British Medical Journal* for August 7, 1948, tells us of experiments with cats in which he found that caffeine in the stomach has a powerful action on histamine, a substance which regulates gastric secretion He also found that theobromine and theophylline (substances that occur in cocoa and tea) also have a similar action in some animals. "Our results support the Roth and Ivy conclusions," he says, "that ulcer patients should restrict their intake of beverages containing caffeine and also that it is desirable to limit their consumption of foods and drinks containing theobromine and theophylline."

Coffee, Heart Disorders and Blood Pressure

Concerning heart trouble and coffee-drinking, most nutritionists and books on health state that coffee has a definite effect on the heart and blood pressure. According to James S. McLester, M. D., in his book *Nutrition and Diet in Health and Disease* (W. B. Saunders, 1927) coffee raises the blood pressure slightly, slows and strengthens the heart, stimulates renal activity and prevents fatigue and depression. It also gives mild brain stimulation. He goes on to say that its excessive use is harmful, for stimulation and irritation are closely related. In cases of insomnia, cardiac irritability and rapid heart beat, even one cup a day will cause trouble when the heart is already irritated. More than one cup is especially harmful.

H. M. Marvin, M. D., in his book *You and Your Heart* (Random House, 1950) states that the effect of alcohol, tobacco and coffee all vary among different individuals. Some find that their heart beats faster after a few drinks of alcohol or cups of coffee. Others find that their hearts beat just a little faster, or not at all faster. He says that no one knows why this should be so. Perhaps some people develop a "tolerance" for coffee and others do not.

That word "tolerance" keeps recurring in all the literature about coffee. Our medical dictionary defines "tolerance" as "the ability of enduring the influence of a drug or poison, particularly when acquired by a continued use of the substance." It seems peculiar that the word should be used in speaking of coffee if indeed coffee has no harmful effects on the body. And, is it possible that those of us who suffer no apparent ill effects from coffee have simply accustomed ourselves to it over a period of time, so that we can throw off the ill effects?

Kathryn Horst, Rex E. Burton and Wm. Dodd Robinson, writing in *The Journal of Pharmacology and Experimental Therapeutics,* Volume 52, 1934, tell of an experience involving a number of young men whose blood pressure was tested before and after they began to drink coffee habitually. The maximum rise in blood pressure occurred during the first week they were drinking coffee. Later on, the article explains, a "tolerance" was developed, and the blood pressure remained at the same level.

When the coffee was withdrawn, the blood pressure returned to "normal." We don't know how you interpret this experiment, but to us it seems to show definitely that some substance in the coffee does have an unhealthful effect on the blood pressure. For those who can, after a time, build up a "tolerance" to this effect, the blood pressure does not go higher. But what of those who do not build up this tolerance? Might not coffee be a very important factor in continued high blood pressure which, of course, is one of the most widespread disorders in our country today?

Leafing on through our notes on coffee and heart ailments we find that Jean Bogert in *Nutrition and Physical Fitness* (W. B. Saunders, 1949) states that coffee quickens the respiration (that is, makes you breathe faster), strengthens the pulse, raises the blood pressure, stimulates the kidneys, excites the functions of the brain and temporarily relieves fatigue or depression. Max M. Rosenberg, M. D. in *Encyclopedia of Medical Self Help* (Scholastic Book Press, 1950) tells us that coffee should be avoided by individuals who have heart disease, angina, high blood pressure, stomach trouble, skin affections, arthritis, liver trouble. Garfield G. Duncan, M. D. in *Diseases of Metabolism* (W. B. Saunders, 1952) tells us that caffeine causes an increase of 3 to 10 per cent in the basal metabolic rate within the first hour after the coffee is taken. (So, incidentally, does the smoking of one cigarette!) Basal metabolism is the rate at which your body makes use of the food you eat.

Does a Tired Body Need Stimulation or Rest?

We want to elaborate a little on the whole business of coffee stimulating the heart. For someone whose heart needs a momentary stimulation you might use coffee as you would use a hypodermic injection—for that occasion only. But what happens, do you suppose, when the heart, sick or well, is constantly stimulated, day after day, while all the time it is protesting that it is tired and wants to rest? One writer on the subject compares coffee to a whip used on a tired horse. Of course the horse will move faster when he is whipped, but how long can you keep up this form of stimulation before the horse drops from exhaustion? The main danger, it seems to us, in the use of coffee by people who may have heart trouble (as well as the rest of us) is that instead of resting as they should when they are tired, they whip themselves to more effort by a cup of coffee and eventually—sooner or later—they are going to have to pay for the rest they are not getting.

Many people use the excuse that they drink coffee only in the morning, so it doesn't matter if they over-stimulate their bodies. They are not trying to go to sleep! Instead they have to gird themselves to meet the day's problems, responsibilities and hard work, so they need to be stimulated. There is a serious fallacy in this kind of reasoning. If they are indeed so tired and run-down that each morning they cannot face the day without a cup of stimulation, then certainly there is something wrong somewhere. Either they do not get the right food, enough sleep, enough relaxation, or enough freedom from worry. Over-stimulation even at breakfast time, means that an already tired body is "hopped up" to carry on when it should be resting.

Coffee Tars and Cancer

Does the use of coffee have any relation to cancer incidence? There is at least one researcher who believes that it does. We know well that certain kinds of tar produce cancer. Coal tar is cancer-producing. The tar from tobacco products produces cancer in laboratory animals. A. H. Roffo in an article published in *Boletin del Instituto de Medicina Experimental,* volume 15, 1939, describes obtaining tar from coffee. He found that this tar has the same physical characteristics as that obtained from tobacco. He treated laboratory animals with this tar and 73 per cent of them developed tumors which ended as cancerous growths. In a later experiment he fed coffee tar to rats in non-toxic doses. That is, they did not receive enough of the tar to make them ill at any one time, for he was trying to discover what the long-continued effect of the tar would be. Definite sores in the stomachs and digestive tracts soon became ulcers which eventually developed into cancers.

Roffo believes that it is the roasting of coffee that produces these tars. He also says that they are not soluble in water, so perhaps they are not present in coffee as we drink it. Still, in chemical tests such as spectography and fluorescence, the coffee tars show the same characteristic as coal tar. This is the only scientific evidence we could find of a possible relationship between coffee-drinking and cancer. It seems strange that no one has done any further investigating to find out, for instance, how much, if any, of the offending tar we drink in a cup of coffee. Or, perhaps, is the tar that ugly black scum that settles on the bottom of the coffee pot and is so hard to wash off, if the coffee has been standing for any length of time? Come to think of it, that black scum looks and acts very much like the black deposit on the bottom of a very dirty ash tray.

Should Pregnant Women and Nursing Mothers Drink Coffee?

A German scientist, Heinz Fischer, has done research on the effect of caffeine on the placenta and embryo of pregnant rabbits. The rabbits were given caffeine daily in water solution. In an article in the German medical publication, *Zeitchrift fur Mikro-Anatomischer Forschungen,* volume 47, 1940, Dr. Fischer describes the results.

The growth and development of the embryo were slowed down. In the liver and kidneys of the embryo as well as in the blood vessels, there was obstruction of the passage of blood, resulting in edema or unhealthful swelling. The skin of the embryo was damaged and the cells of its liver showed definite disease. When all of these harmful symptoms became serious enough, the embryo died and was re-absorbed, becoming just a crumbled mass in the mother's womb. The placenta (the sac covering the unborn child) became swollen and diseased.

It is interesting to note that these results were reported for rabbits to whom caffeine was given first when they became pregnant. Other rabbits were given small amounts of caffeine over a period of time until they established a tolerance to it. (There's that word "tolerance" again!) Then, when they became pregnant, the placenta and embryo suffered no damage. Once again, we remind you that caffeine (the concentrated poison that exists in coffee) was given to these animals—not coffee. But, even so, does it sound like such a good idea for an expectant mother in these days to drink coffee, taking into account the already considerable amount of various poisons she is getting in food, in air pollution, in chemicalized water and perhaps in cigarettes?

Does Coffee Affect Brain and Nerve Tissue?

The Department of Agriculture published a booklet in 1917 called *The Toxicity of Caffeine.* Their experiments involved animals. They tell us that the reaction of human beings and animals to caffeine may be quite different. Yet most scientific research these days (on chemicals, insecticides, cosmetics and so forth) is done with animals and it is taken for granted that any substance that shows up as poisonous to animals is quite likely to be not very good for men.

The authors tell us, too, that the effect of caffeine on individual animals is different in its intensity and the effect varies with the dose. On the same basis, undoubtedly some human beings are less resistant to poisons than others. William Salant and J. B. Rieger, authors of the booklet, tell us that only one rabbit in ten survived injected doses of caffeine. Those that survived generally succumbed to a second or third dose. The effect of caffeine on guinea pigs was even more drastic, although dogs and cats reacted differently. All showed symptoms of poisoning, which resembled poisoning from strychnine. In relation to its harmful action on tissues (chiefly brain and nerve tissue) caffeine is far more destructive than morphine. They conclude that the continued use of caffeine-containing beverages over a long period of time seems bound to be harmful.

Well, would you consider giving your family—children and old folks included—ever so small a dose of morphine every morning as part of breakfast, no matter how much they might like the taste? Keep in mind that caffeine showed up as being far more destructive than morphine.

This is the bulk of our evidence on the possible harm that may result from habitual, prolonged and excessive coffee drinking. It does not seem to us that someone who drinks one cup of coffee a day should go to a lot of trouble to give it up. But probably he will be the person who could give it up most easily. The person who is in danger from coffee, we believe, is the person who simply can't get along without it and who, if he stops and soberly counts up how many cups of coffee he has in any one day, may find that coffee is indeed a drug to him and that the habit of throwing off weariness and worry with a cup of coffee has brought him nothing but sorrow and ill health. These are the people who should be persuaded to give up coffee entirely.

If this should prove to be impossible, we have one last suggestion. According to our standards, we should eat and drink nothing that does not contribute in some way to nutrition. Any food or drink that contains neither vitamins, minerals, enzymes or protein should automatically be crossed off the list, for it is crowding out in our diets those beneficial protective foods we all need so desperately. If you must continue to drink coffee, then at least make certain that the rest of your diet is as healthful as possible. This means plenty of fresh raw fruits and vegetables every day along with plenty of good meat, eggs, fish and nuts. This means only completely whole grain cereals. This means no food at all that contains white flour or white sugar in any form, even including chewing gum and soft drinks. This means taking food supplements: fish liver oil for vitamins A and D, brewer's yeast or desiccated liver for the B vitamins, rose hips for vitamin C and wheat germ oil for vitamin E.

Colds-Personal History of Colds

As a boy I was not the hale and robust physical type. I was already taking bromo-seltzer at the age of seven, and can recall violent headaches as long back as I can remember. I was never laid up with any serious illness but was continually plagued with those little recurring situations that had mostly nuisance value. There were dizzy spells at times, my swimming endurance was limited to about eight strokes, there was a condition of almost continuous semi-catarrh, and whenever the wind blew the wrong way I caught a cold. From about October to April I could expect to have them one after another.

When I look back now I can see clearly why I was not stronger and able to resist colds, headaches, etc. It was mostly wrong diet—too much starch and sugar. I was imbibing sodas, candy, pastries, ice cream, bread, etc., in enormous doses. In those days (I was born in 1898) only the faintest glimmerings of nutrition were known. Had I known then what I know now the story would have been entirely different.

At about twenty-one I began a systematic quest to discover ways and means to eradicate these colds. I took up tennis and went at it like a demon, but all it did was to give me a heart murmur. I then became a vegetarian, but that did not accomplish the task. Over the next twenty years I experimented with M.D.'s, osteopaths, chiropractors, Turkish baths, Swedish massage, diathermy, and everything else on the popular health agenda, but the colds continued to come with clock-like regularity. I will venture to say that I must have read 500 articles describing how to dodge catching a cold. In the main the theme was—be sure to wear your rubbers when it rains and stay away from drafts. How ridiculous this now sounds! We shall see later how I mastered the cold bogey, but now I want to show you how important it is not to take any of the popular health concepts for granted. We must question every generally accepted health tenet or dogma, as rooted as it may be in the public's mind. You must observe the effect on your own bodily processes of your basic daily actions. Make your own interpretations.

This was beautifully expressed seven hundred years ago by Roger Bacon, who in *Of Regimen of Health* said, "A man's own observation, what he finds good of and what he finds hurt of, is the best physic to preserve health."

Colds Were Frequent and Certain

When I was about 40, I can remember that all I had to do was to take the two and one-half hour railroad trip from Allentown to New York in the winter and invariably a cold would come out of it. To sit at a football game meant a sure cold, and the same thing would occur after a Thanksgiving gorging. I distinctly recall that colds would occur after emotional upsets. At this time I was beginning to make speeches in favor of the organic method of farming and gardening, and was so fearful of being on a platform that the first three or four experiences resulted in a cold the next morning. I always had had an inferiority complex, but I am glad to admit that today I am more the extrovert, having given hundreds of talks, and recently even held an audience for about ten minutes with a purely humorous speech, which, if I may be pardoned for my vanity, had them rolling in the aisles for the entire time. It is possible that the same thing that finally gave me an immunity to colds also chased away my inferiority complex.

Dr. E. W. Braithwaite, consulting psychiatrist to the Ministry of Health of England, has the following to say about colds in the October 2, 1944, issue of the *British Medical Journal:*

> "The following facts may be of interest to either sufferers from, or investigators of, the common cold. During the course of 25 years' practice of psycho-analysis for the treatment of psychoneurotics, I have observed that in them (1) a cold invariably occurred in a particular emotional state (2) the occurrence of a cold could be prognosticated whenever this state developed (3) the cold could be aborted if a different emotional state could be produced in the course of treatment or could be shortened if it had started (4) cold, wet, hunger, exhaustion and a source of infection do not result in the development of a cold in the absence of the appropriate emotional state (5) cold 'proneness' disappears completely as a result of successful treatment and does not recur.
>
> "Though these observations have little immediate practical value, my experience demonstrates to me, at least, that the solution of the problem of the common cold lies in the sphere of preventive psychological medicine. The specific factor is psychological; the microbic one secondary."

While this is interesting, I believe that the proper nutritional preparation will enable the mind to get into all kinds of emotional states without causing colds. What Dr. Braithwaite says is true of persons who are eating a devitalized diet and not fortifying it the way it should be.

Importance of Calcium in Cold Prevention

I would like to mention that the first relief in the reduction of the incidence of colds was given me by a New York City osteopath, Lucius Bush. Dr. Bush had developed a technique by which he placed his finger into the patient's nose, and gradually enlarged the passageways in it. He called it finger surgery, I believe. Dr. Bush claims that the habits of civilization are gradually reducing interior spaces of the nose, preventing oxygen from circulating, and creating a wonderful breeding ground for cold-causing organisms. By a series of treatments Dr. Bush gradually opened up the passageways in my nose and I experienced immediate benefits in having less colds, and milder ones. But I did not go long enough. It required 15 treatments, whereas I stopped at number four. It is possible that by Dr. Bush's method one can get practically complete immunity to colds.

In this respect may I mention another factor that may be responsible for the recent sharp increase in the number of colds experienced by the general public. In the nose there are little, almost microscopic hair-like things called cilia, which cover the mucous membrane and which move back and forth like a field of wheat in a wind. They are as close together as the "hair" on a rug. They move the secretions of the nose into proper channels. They are easily affected and then either function poorly or not at all. One thing that can do this is medication, and secondly a lack of calcium in the system. The cilia need calcium for "back bone," to stand up to their job, and since a terrific percentage of the public is calcium deficient, we can see one place which courts trouble as far as colds are concerned. This shows one advantage of taking bone meal, and staying away from nose drops.

At this period, namely about 1942, my condition had progressed to such a point that my colds were turning into asthma. The last phases of each cold, after about two weeks of severe suffering, would cause asthmatic wheezing, and when I would sneeze it felt as if the top of my head was coming off. Thus I was in deathly fear of an oncoming sneeze. I recall terribly sleepless nights, saturated with agonized worryings, and the future looked quite dark.

New Or Badly Designed Houses Can Be Responsible

I would like to mention an experience we had that winter which carries a valuable lesson. We moved into a new house on the organic experimental farm, and within a few days the entire family, the five of us, were in bed with a bad case of the grippe. I attribute it to the fact that the new plaster of the walls was not yet dry. There was too much moisture in the house, and sleeping with our heads near a "wet" wall, was, I am sure, the causative factor which had brought about our condition. It is best not to be too anxious to move into a new house. Make sure first that the plaster is thoroughly dry. I wonder if this is why people hold "house warmings" in connection with moving into a new house. Incidentally, I once noted that when we built an addition to our printing plant, a linotype machine standing close to a brick wall suffered a bad case of rusting, due I am sure to the water still in the mortar.

Another thing I would like to mention is that we had a duct system of heating in our old house, the kind of ducts used for air conditioning, and many of the ducts were at floor level. In that house we all had had bad colds. In fact this was where I began to get the attacks of asthma. An engineer friend of mine told me later that ducts should not be at floor level because from there they can set up currents of air or drafts which might bring on colds. He maintained that the ducts should be as high up on the wall as possible. This is a matter that should be discussed with heating engineers if you are in the process of building a house.

Investigations on Nasal Temperature

About this time I read of some medical researches which changed my entire thinking along the lines of securing immunity from colds. The work, which took three years, was done by Doctors Irwin Spiesman and Lloyd Arnold of the University of Illinois. Sixty-three persons were used and they were of all types. Some of them rarely or never caught colds, while others were of that group that suffers one cold after another. It seems astonishing that the findings of Drs. Spiesman and Arnold have not received continuing publicity, since the project was done in cooperation with the research laboratories of the Illinois State Department of Public Health.

The scientists caused their sixty-three subjects to be seated, bare to the waist, for half hour periods, in a room eight feet square, free of draughts and at a constant temperature. Ice-cups were clapped to their backs, and at the same time the temperature inside their noses was measured. Another portion of the experiments included the application of hot water to the bare backs of the subjects, along with the taking of their nasal temperature.

Drs. Spiesman and Arnold discovered that when the body was suddenly chilled by application of the ice-caps, the temperature of the mucous membrane of the nose dropped as a result of the nasal veins becoming constricted. However, in normal persons the nasal temperature soon rose to normal again even though ice-cups were held continuously to the back. On the other hand, the nose temperature of chronic cold victims remained for a fairly long period at a low level.

The experimenters discovered that these differences in nose temperature were more important in causing colds than infection from one person to another. It was while the nasal temperature was below normal that the bacteria always present in the mucous membrane of the nose and throat were able to become active and bring about the congested and inflamed condition we know as a common head cold.

Having discovered this, Drs. Spiesman and Arnold sought some means of causing the membranes of the nose to react normally when the individual was exposed to sudden changes of temperature. The doctors experimented with cold injections. These injections were given subcutaneously (under the skin) every other day over a period of three months. However, according to Drs. Spiesman and Arnold's report, "The frequency of colds was not affected by this treatment, nor was there any effect produced upon the temperature reaction in the nasal veins of the subjects treated."

However, the doctors did discover a means of causing the membranes of the nose to react normally when the individual was exposed to sudden changes of temperature. The solution to the problem lay in giving the subject a treatment of baths and in having him follow a system of dieting.

A hot bath followed by a cold one in the morning, and repeated in the evening, before dinner, was decidedly beneficial in tuning up the circulation responses in the nose so the arteries did not react too radically to sudden chill. Without sudden changes in nose temperature cold germs were unable to gain a foothold. Drs. Spiesman and Arnold found that a few of the subjects showed marked improvement in ability to resist colds, as a result of these baths, but most of the individuals studied showed little benefit from bathing alone.

Wheat Products and Immunity to Colds

Far better than baths in keeping the nose temperature normal was the exclusion from the diet of bread and other carbohydrates, especially of the wheat-cereal variety. Time and again the doctors noticed that after subjects were freed from the nuisance of head colds, because wheat foods and bread had been dropped from their diet, they returned to their former weakness in regard to colds the moment they started eating bread and other wheat products.

Regarding the diet used by Drs. Spiesman and Arnold for their subjects, the Spiesman-Arnold report says:

"All products made from wheat, i.e., white flour breads, pastries, pies, cookies, etc., were eliminated from the diet. The patients in this group were requested to abstain from the use of tea, coffee or alcoholic beverages, and to smoke sparingly. They were instructed to eat two large vegetable portions, or a vegetable and fruit salad each day, and to make the salad the main course of the meal. They were also asked to eat as much fresh fruit as they could daily . . . and to drink six ounces of tomato juice per adult per day. Eight glasses of water were prescribed a day. Fried foods were prohibited. No condiments. Butter was to be added very freely to all cooked vegetables and eaten generally very freely; two to four egg yolks for each adult and one to two for a child per day. The patient was not to hurry while eating, nor be tired or worried. He was to take a short rest after every meal.

* * * * *

"The patients on this regime improved clinically. We found, in our experience with dieting of these patients, that an overindulgence of carbohydrates, especially of the wheat-cereal variety, was most to be guarded against. Time and again we observed, after excellent results were obtained, that a return of the patient to an excess carbohydrate diet caused a recurrence of symptoms."

Drs. Spiesman and Arnold observed that persons unusually sensitive in regard to cold-catching benefited most of all when they followed both the bathing and the dieting systems. During the three years the patients were under observation, the hypersensitive individuals were placed on the elimination-of-bread diet alone, then given the bathing treatments without the dieting, and finally given both dieting and bathing at the same time. It was found that they benefited more from the bread elimination than from the bathing, but showed most improvement of all when dieting and bathing were used together.

Drs. Spiesman and Arnold discovered that, curiously enough, the benefits in avoiding colds brought about by wheat and cereal elimination, as well as by the taking of baths, were completely offset by worry and apprehension in the individuals studied. No matter how faithfully they dieted or followed the rules in regard to bathing, if these subjects worried about such things as the loss of job, the illness or death of a relative, etc., they immediately became susceptible to colds.

As long as a subject remained in a state of mental uneasiness he failed to benefit from either dieting or bathing. Drs. Spiesman and Arnold noted specific cases of individuals who suffered great mental distress for one reason or another; one suffered death in his family; another experienced the harrowing ordeals of bankruptcy; another lost his job.

Drs. Spiesman and Arnold, in their report, mention physical exercise as an important element in setting up resistance to colds. Twenty minutes of setting up exercises, in the nude, in a cool room, prior to taking a hot and cold shower, are advocated. A brisk walk for one hour a day, either in divided time or for an hour continuously, never hurrying, breathing deeply, is excellent. A rest, even a brief one, after each meal, is recommended.

This experiment made sense to me, and the whole family decided to cut out the grain foods. We noticed an immediate effect, a great reduction in the number of colds that were "caught," but what was very important also, a reduction in the severity and duration in the fewer colds that did come. This family diet went on for about a year but was then abandoned as it seemed to be giving the lady of the house too much trouble in preparing school lunches for the children. As far as I am concerned I went on and off a breadless diet over the last ten years or so and I find it excellent for keeping weight down. I will never forget the way my head catarrh vanished when first I began to cut out bread, and anyone so afflicted should give this diet a "try," but one should take wheat germ and vitamin E to replace those elements that are usually secured from the grain foods.

An interesting thing occurred in the case of my son Robert during the year we went off the grain foods. He had always been extremely sensitive to poison ivy, and was attacked by it even if he did not come in direct physical contact with the plant. But he seemed to become completely immune to it during our breadless year. The only reason I can ascribe for this astonishing happening is that children usually stuff themselves with bread and cookies and therefore have little room or desire for vegetables. Lacking in the greenstuffs, he must have developed a subclinical case of scurvy, and it is possible that the ivy will easily burn a scorbutic skin. When Robert could not eat bread and cake he had to eat the vegetables or go hungry.

This might be a good place to mention my own experience with poison ivy. When we moved out to the farm I began to learn the ways of this plant, much to my own physical discomfort. Every summer I could expect to have it poison me once or twice. About seven or eight years later I received a letter from one of our readers, in which the writer related that he had suddenly become immune to poison ivy and believed it was due to cutting out sugar and taking bone meal as well as a few vitamins. Since I was on the same dietary program I felt that the same thing must have happened to me also, as I suddenly came to a realization that for a year or two I could not remember being afflicted with poison ivy trouble. As I related the contents of this letter to the family at the evening meal I announced that I was going outside immediately, would find some poison ivy and rub it on my arms. To their horror I did it, Nina, Ruth, Bob and Anna following me, thinking I was fooling. I rubbed the leaves on my arms vigorously and then washed my hands only, as I did not want to rub the stuff into my eyes. To my gratification nothing happened. The vaccination did not take, which convinced me that the vitamins and minerals I was taking, and the cutting out of sugar, had fabricated a new healthier skin for me, and I have not been bothered with poison ivy since.

Diet and Colds

Today I am practically immune from colds and will get one perhaps only when I try some nutritional experiment. For example, a few years ago I cut eggs completely from my diet. Within a month I had a cold. At another time I decided to eliminate all fruits, just to see if anything would happen. This was the first time I ever caught a cold in the middle of July. Of course, at the time I was not taking halibut liver oil perles (vitamins A and D) and rose hips (vitamin C).

I must not forget to give credit to my organically-produced diet, which began about 1941. On our 60-acre farm, beginning in that year, we began to grow crops without the aid of chemical fertilizers, and tests later showed that they had higher vitamin and mineral content than average. Slowly I noticed a resistance developing against colds, and especially the complete disappearance of all asthmatic symptoms. It is difficult, however, to pin this down to any one thing as a complete and specific preventive. However, we know that the eating of organically-grown foods has made the whole family healthier.

I must remark that in the old days, once I began to get the first sniffles of a cold, the cold always developed fully. Today I will sometimes experience a few sniffles, but rarely do they go further.

I believe one of the greatest aids in my preventive history of colds is the taking of vitamins A, D and C (halibut liver oil perles and rose hips). The advisability of this supplementation is covered thoroughly elsewhere in this book. But there can also be no question that my taking of bone meal, wheat germ and vitamin E, and cutting out the grain foods, sugar and salt, are also contributing factors. The body can be like a machine which does not get the proper fuels and other supplies required to run it. Then it may not function properly. I suppose that machines develop afflictions that may be compared to colds in human beings.

Good Nourishment Prevents Colds

Just a few words about the various fallacies that fly about regarding colds. Don't sit in a draft, they say. Keep your feet dry and warm. Gargle with x-brand of antiseptic—etc., etc., etc. These are all well and good for the badly nourished person, but one who is in top form from our point of view need not fear a draft or getting the feet wet. This is illustrated by an experience I had last January 1st. I called upon a friend who was suffering from an unusually severe cold, and when I proffered my hand in greeting he said, "You had better not shake my hand. I have a very bad cold and you might catch it."

I surprised him by insisting that I shake his hand anyhow, and not only did I make sure to give it a thorough shake but I amazed him by saying, "Now watch what I'm going to do!"

I took my hand and rubbed it into my nostrils!

His eyes bulged!

"Why do you want to have a cold?" he asked.

"I don't want to have a cold,'" I replied.

"Then why did you do this?"

"Because I have built my body up to the point where it does not catch colds from anyone, and I want to prove to you what good nutrition can do in warding off colds."

But the next morning I had a cold, albeit a mild one which left in about four days.

Now, why did I catch my friend's germs? If you will recall, I stated above that the visit was on January 1st. The night before was New Year's Eve and I had been out celebrating. It is easy to follow diets and rules under ordinary conditions but it is much more difficult when you are out New Year's Eve'ing until three in the morning, and then get up at six o'clock the same morning to work on an article you are writing. It was too stiff a test. I had also been cutting down somewhat on my eggs at that time

On my farm I have developed a flock of chickens that are practically disease-resistant. We feed them only on food we raise ourselves, without benefit of chemical fertilizers. Ordinarily a conservative farmer will not permit another farmer to enter into the chicken house for fear that on the bottom of his shoes he may be carrying disease germs from his own flock. A few years ago a group of about 20 farmers visited my chicken house, and I asked them to rub their feet vigorously in the litter. They thought I was crazy, but I told them that my chickens were so healthy that no germ could do a thing to them. And I was right. Nothing happened, because my chickens do not go out New Year's Eve'ing.

Taxi drivers get fewer colds than any other segment of our population. The next time you take a taxi, check up on this. It is due to the fact that the taxi driver sits in so many drafts that even with his characteristically poor diet, he gains practical immunity. But your average taxi driver is more susceptible to kidney trouble. This organ cannot take the year-in-year-out shaking up that it gets in the course of a taxi driver's daily work. If I were a taxi driver I would wear a kind of high belt worn by motorcyclists, and if necessary would spend my own money to equip the car with an extra set of, or stronger, springs or shock absorbers.

Benjamin Franklin, as part of his daily physical regimen designed to condition himself, sat at an open window in the nude for considerable lengths of time, every day, but, although he lived to be in his eighties, he finally succumbed to pneumonia which arose due to one of these window sitting sessions. Or so the legend goes! Franklin should have quit when he was ahead.

Dancing and Colds

About 20 years ago I had a severe head cold which had settled in my throat. My vocal cords were on a sit-down strike and I could talk only in a whisper, and even then only with difficulty. Bob was only two years old then and he lay on a couch, the picture of melancholy gloom, for he also had a cold. A lively number was playing on the phonograph and before I knew it my feet began to move in rhythm with it. Since Bobby began to smile at what was passing for eccentric dancing my feet gathered momentum. My body went into more active motion, contorting itself weirdly and defying the rules of gravity. I had to laugh myself and Bobby shrieked with delight. After all, he was only a baby and thus could not distinguish between his father and Fred Astaire. But the more he shrieked the crazier I contorted my body, and after awhile I practically collapsed in a corner.

I noticed that now my voice came a hundred per cent easier. A complete transformation had occurred. The soreness had miraculously disappeared. I could talk with ease. The physical exertion had stimulated my breathing, and my uncontrolled laughter must have driven the accumulation of months of stale air out of my lungs. The quick change from the depths of melancholy to the pinnacle of joyous exhilaration accomplished in about ten minutes what would otherwise have required days of suffering.

Gustave Doré, the gifted Alsatian artist who illustrated the works of so many famous authors, was so fond of dancing that he could not go to sleep unless he first danced for his aged mother who accompanied him on the piano. He was skilled in the hornpipe and Highland fling. He was especially adept in boleros, cracoviennes and cachuchas, but his specialty was the cancan. Those who had seen the sumptuous profusion of statues, pictures, busts and models which filled his apartments, and the fact that he never smashed a thing, marveled at his astonishing agility in executing these Terpsichorean antics.

He claimed that this dancing animated his spirits and put him into the exciting moods that stimulated his creative genius. On going to bed after such a riotous orgy of prancing, he found that his aroused mind was enabled to plan the pictures which made him famous. Of course, this might be bad for insomniacs.

Dancing has a health-giving value and also acts as a stimulant to the mind. Since the beginning of time man has danced. He has cast out devils in this manner. He danced to get rain, to make seeds germinate, to bring bountiful harvests, to have good luck in the chase, to increase fecundity and to praise God. He danced on joyous as well as sad occasions. He lived practically every aspect of his daily life through dancing. Primitive man did not dance for enjoyment but as a means to master his daily problems, as a means to attain power. He may not have realized it, but it kept him in good health and spirits.

More than half the world today dances the traditional folk dances that have been handed down without change for thousands of years. This includes the American Indian, African savage tribes, Mexicans, Central and South Americans and practically all people of Asia. Dancing must have great value, otherwise it would have died out in these places. Wherever urban civilization develops, it seems to disappear automatically, to be replaced by our modern jazz dancing which has a purely sensual basis. In such cities many never dance. Our cities seem to breed tired people.

I believe that Henry Ford in bringing back the square dances was giving grim warning to the country of the dangers of going all-out in the direction of machine-age culture. It was his way of showing that people were not moving in the right direction in the ways of their daily life, that they had better keep one eye on the machine and the other on Old Mother Nature—that somewhere in between lies the happy medium.

Colds and Vitamin C

Cold weather may mean you need more vitamin C! Yes, it's true, at any rate for guinea pigs who are the only creatures, aside from apes and human beings who cannot manufacture their own vitamin C inside their bodies. Jolliffe, Tisdall and Cannon in their monumental book *Clinical Nutrition* (Paul B. Hoeber, Inc., 1950) tell us that rats exposed to cold weather, develop more vitamin C, inside their bodies, to protect them from this stress of cold. Those rats who, for some reason, cannot produce the required amount of vitamin C, may begin to show a decrease of vitamin C in their tissues which may indicate that the cold actually uses up their store of vitamin C. Guinea pigs, who, like man, cannot make their own vitamin C, must depend on an increased intake in their food if they are to be able to survive cold weather. The lower the temperature the more vitamin C is required.

An amount of vitamin C that is perfectly adequate for a guinea pig at room temperature is reported to be completely inadequate at a temperature of freezing or 32 degrees Fahrenheit. The small animals can adapt themselves to cold and manage to live healthfully only if their supply of vitamin C is increased. In studying the guinea pigs it was found that this vitamin C supply was in the tissues of the bodies, especially the adrenal glands, of those which managed to survive. And when their supply of vitamin C was discontinued, those who had taken a large supply of the vitamin previously were found to survive longer than those who had not.

In our file on colds we found a letter from the *British Medical Journal* for April 21, 1951, written by John M. Fletcher and Isabel C. Fletcher, expressing surprise that more material does not appear in medical journals on the potency of vitamin C in protecting against cold germs. These two physicians state that in their own practice they have found vitamin C an excellent preventive of colds. Perhaps, they say, the general disregard of the vitamin as a cold preventive results from the difficulty among the experts in reaching agreement as to what actually is the daily requirement of vitamin C. With adults, they say, the disease of scurvy will occur when the adult is getting less than 10 milligrams of vitamin C daily. But, they continue, this represents far, far less than "saturation level." By this they mean that to soak all the tissues of the body in vitamin C a much larger amount than 10 milligrams a day is necessary. In cases of fever or hard physical exertion, the body uses up vitamin C much faster than usual. So it is not ever possible to set one figure as the absolute daily requirement for all people under all circumstances.

We agree wholeheartedly with the Fletchers only, as usual, we would carry their argument a little farther. Aside from fever and exertion, modern adults are subjected to countless other hazards that deplete their vitamin C—sleeping pills, for instance, tobacco-smoking, exposure to lead, benzene and other industrial poisons. And since no one has ever suffered from too much natural vitamin C, why in the world should we limit ourselves to a daily minimum when, apparently, the more we take the better we will feel in every way? We know from laboratory experiments that animals suffering from infections have a very small amount of vitamin C in their bloodstreams. We know, too, that animals deliberately kept on diets low in vitamin C develop more infections than those who are getting enough. These two facts alone are sufficient indication that vitamin C in large quantities is necessary in the fight against any infection —including, of course, cold infections.

Preventing Infections With Vitamin C

The Fletchers go on to tell of a number of experiments in Holland, Germany and Australia in which colds were prevented by the administration of vitamin C. In the German experiment there was a marked fall in the amount of illness over a period of eight months among factory workers given 100 to 300 milligrams of vitamin C a day, a benefit not found when they were given 20 or 50 milligrams. N. W. Markwell, writing in the *Medical Journal of Australia,* volume 2, page 777, 1947, descibes the technique of giving vitamin C in cases where cold symptoms have just begun to appear. The colds were frequently but not always dispersed within a few hours and the after effects and complications which often accompany common colds were nonexistent. The Fletchers conclude: "We believe that, unlike the outcome of the antihistamine trials, the results may show considerable benefits can arise from ascorbic acid (vitamin C) treatment given in sufficient quantities at the right time."

In the *British Medical Journal* volume II, page 617, 1942, Doctors A. J. Glazebrook and S. J. Thompson report an experiment in an institution in England caring for boys. At this institution the handling of food —that is, the way it was stored, prepared, served and so forth—had resulted in a vitamin C intake of 15 milligrams per boy per day—just barely enough to prevent symptoms of scurvy. Part of the boys were given vitamin C for six months. The other boys went on eating their regular diet. During the brief period of six months there was no appreciable difference in the incidence of colds in the two groups, *but* the boys who had the vitamin spent only an average of two and one-half days in the infirmary whereas those who had received no vitamin C spent an average of five days being sick. So the additional vitamin C, even for this brief period, apparently strengthened the children's resistance to germs so much that they were able to throw off the effects in half the time it took the untreated children.

H. W. Holmes, M.D., writing in *Science,* volume 96, page 497, 1942, describes his own experiences in relieving hay fever, food allergies and asthma with vitamin C. He gave it in large doses—200 to 500 milligrams every day for a week. Does this perhaps demonstrate that the usual daily minimum we casually accept as correct for adults (about 75 milligrams per day) may be far too low?

We have shown the power of vitamin C against infections, when it is used in large doses. For instance, discussing vitamin C in relation to infections, Rhinehart, Connor and Mettier in *International Clinician,* volume 2, 1937, and *The Journal of Experimental Medicine,* volume 59, 1934, tell us they found that guinea pigs suffering from scurvy (vitamin C deficiency) who were infected with a streptococcus germ, developed a condition similar to rheumatic fever and rheumatoid arthritis in human beings. They suggest that a "sub-clinical" degree of scurvy may make up the rheumatic tendency which, with an added factor of infection, causes the development of rheumatic fever. This means simply that infections develop more readily in animals (and why not also in persons?) who lack vitamin C—not to the extent of producing scurvy, but just to the extent that most of us lack it—a "sub-clinical deficiency."

It has been found that diphtheria susceptibility is greater in guinea pigs who lack vitamin C. And children with scurvy are more susceptible to diphtheria. Lawrynowicz in the *Journal de Physiologie et de Pathologie Génerale,* volume 29, 1931, suggests that scurvy may so reduce the resistance that a diphtheria carrier may become the victim of the bacteria which it previously carried without any ill effects. Three investigators showed that added amounts of vitamin C assist animals on normal diets in their reactions against tuberculosis.

Vitamin C—A "Super Antibiotic"

An experiment in a tuberculosis sanitarium showed the potency of even small amounts of the vitamin against tuberculosis symptoms. The patients were grouped in pairs. One patient was given a daily orange, while his control, in the other group, received a pastry. It seemed that the addition of vitamin C even in such small amounts assisted in healing the tuberculosis symptoms.

S. W. Clausen writing in the *Physiological Review,* volume 14, 1934, throws light on the subject from the point of view of natural products supplying the vitamin. In testing guinea pigs, several researchers have found that an abundance of fresh green fodder which contains, of course, natural vitamin C, has protected against infections. In a study of 400 animals, one scientist (Wamoscher in *Zeitschrift für Hygiene und Infektionskrankheiten,* volume CVII, 1937) showed that sub-acute scurvy—that is just a slight case of scurvy—predisposes to spontaneous pneumonia. Cure sometimes followed the administration of vitamin C in orange juice.

W. J. McCormick, M.D., of Canada uses vitamin C in enormous doses for curing disease. He tells us in an article in *The Archives of Pediatrics* for April, 1952, that vitamin C is important for the healing of wounds, the prevention of hemorrhaging and the building of a barrier against germ invasion. It contributes to building up disease fighters or antibodies in the bloodstream; it neutralizes toxins in the blood—that is, it helps to build a natural immunity to infectious diseases and poisons. In the rapidity with which it stops the course of some diseases it compares favorably with the sulfa drugs, says Dr. McCormick, and it does not have after effects that may be unpleasant or dangerous. Dr. McCormick uses injections of vitamin C to saturate completely his patient's tissues. Any excess is carried away by the kidneys. Dr. McCormick has used vitamin C successfully in treating tuberculosis, scarlet fever, pelvic infection, septicemia and so forth.

F. R. Klenner, M.D., of Reidsville, N. C., has used vitamin C successfully in the treatment of many serious diseases. He describes his point of view in a paper presented before the 52nd Annual Meeting of the Tri-State Medical Association of the Carolinas and Virginia, February 19 and 20, 1951. He compares the action of vitamin C with the antibiotics. "It has been reported," he says, "that one of the mold-derived drugs (antibiotics) is a super-vitamin. Conversely we argue that vitamin C, besides being an essential vitamin, is a super-antibiotic." Dr. Klenner believes that it is the capacity of the vitamin as an aid to oxidation that makes it valuable against germs. Apparently it unites with the toxin or virus and helps to destroy it.

He describes the case of a patient with chills, fever and head cold for 14 days and severe headache for three days. She had been given sulfa, penicillin and streptomycin without effect. Vitamin C injections were given. Within 72 hours she was "clinically well of her pneumonia." In three other cases of pulmonary virus infection, results were equally good, using vitamin C injections.

In a person suffering from a virus infection, says Dr. Klenner, vitamin C is not only absent from the urine, but is also missing from the blood. So it seems that as the infection gets worse the patient's need for vitamin C becomes greater, for his body tissues are depleted and what vitamin C he obtains from his food is rapidly used up in fighting against the virus. This is why Dr. Klenner gives massive doses of the vitamin in cases of serious illness. "Hippocrates declared the highest duty of medicine to be to get the patient well." He further declared that, of several remedies, physicians should choose the least sensational. "Vitamin C would seem to meet both these requirements," says Dr. Klenner.

Perhaps many of us suffer from frequent colds for two reasons: first we are not careful enough to choose foods that contain vitamin C and second, we may not know how to preserve the vitamin C in foods until the time we eat them. Vitamin C is the most perishable vitamin there is. It is lost when foods are stored or cooked. It seeps away into the water when foods are soaked.

So choose vitamin-C rich foods the year 'round. In general this means fresh fruits and vegetables. Frozen foods generally contain more vitamins than canned. Buy your fruits and vegetables as fresh as you can get them, never buy wilted or soggy produce. Wash it quickly as soon as you get home and put it immediately in the refrigerator. Prepare it just before you eat it, as quickly as possible; most of the vitamin C will be lost if you leave fruits or vegetables for even a half hour at room temperature. Eat as many fruits and vegetables raw as possible. Those you must cook place directly into a very small amount of boiling water. As soon as the water boils again, turn down the heat and cook slowly just until tender—no longer. Save the liquid left in the pot for soup.

And finally in the wintertime especially, make sure of enough vitamin C by taking rose hips or one of the other natural vitamin C food supplements. If you should feel the symptoms of a cold coming on, double or triple the amount of natural vitamin C you take daily. It can't possibly harm you. Any excess which your body does not need will be excreted harmlessly.

Colds and Vitamin B

Vitamin B has been shown to be effective against invading germs. Dr. A. E. Axelrod of Western Reserve University, speaking at a meeting of the National Vitamin Foundation on April 4, 1952, described an experiment in which he deprived rats of three of the B vitamins and found that the animals were severely impaired in their ability to build up antibodies with which to fight disease. Another experiment reported at the same meeting involved human beings.

Young men, on an ordinary diet, were immersed in cold water for eight minutes and this stress, although brief, produced chemical changes in the blood and urine, as well as in the temperature, blood pressure and heart rate. There was a significant increase in two substances in the blood—the granular red blood cells and the circulating white blood cells, which are the disease-germ fighters of the body.

Then for six weeks the men were built up with large doses of a member of the vitamin B group and again given the cold-water experience. Tests identical with the former showed that the changes in the blood and urinary components were less than before and that this occurred because the vitamins had strengthened the effectiveness with which the adrenal glands produced various hormones, possibly including cortisone. These adrenal outpourings help the body to overcome physical strains and thus the B vitamins increase the body capacity for resistance.

Two articles from the *Proceedings of the Society of Experimental Biology and Medicine* (Volume 67, 1948 and volume 62, 1946), describe experiments on animals made deficient in pyridoxine, thiamin and biotin—all B vitamins. In all cases, the rats who were deficient in the vitamins were able to produce fewer antibodies in their blood, for fighting off germs.

Experiments With Multiple Deficiencies

Finally let us examine an article in the *Journal of Laboratory and Clinical Medicine,* volume 30, 1945, in which L. J. Berry, J. Davis and T. D. Spies discuss the influence of the B vitamins on the resistance of rats to infection. We were glad to find the name of Dr. Spies listed as an author on this article, for we have come to expect from him most unusual and very practical experiments which add greatly to our knowledge of how human beings manage to get along. He did not disappoint us in this article. These researchers tell us that "single vitamin deficiency studies are important in elucidating the metabolic function of the vitamins, but single deficiencies seldom occur naturally." That is, in terms of human nutrition, a person who suffers from a lack of one B vitamin is certain to lack the others too, for they occur mostly in the same foods. And they react with one another in the body. Someone who lacks vitamin B will probably lack vitamin C as well. If a person does not get enough vitamin A in his food, he almost certainly will not get enough of the other fat soluble vitamins—D and E, for they occur in many of the same foods.

In their experiment these nutritionists decided to place one group of rats on the diet commonly eaten by many of the patients who visit their clinic in Birmingham, Alabama. They divided the rats into ten groups—two of which received only the basic diet as eaten by families in the neighborhood. Two other groups received the basic diet plus casein (a protein). Two other groups received the basic diet plus casein and minerals. Two other groups ate the basic diet plus casein, and B vitamins. The final two groups received the basic diet plus casein, minerals and B vitamins.

The basic diet consisted of corn meal, white flour, pork fat and cane sugar. Yes, this was the diet the researchers had discovered their clinic patients were eating every day. The animals were permitted to remain on the diets for two months before they were checked. The pictures taken at that time indicate more clearly than any words what condition the rats were in by then. Those on the basic diet were small, scrawny, weak. Their coats were rough and ugly. As the various elements were added to diets, the appearance of the rats improved. The final picture shows a handsome, sleek, healthy-looking rat who was of course eating the minerals, vitamins and proteins as well as the basic diet.

Laboratory tests showed that the leucocytes (disease-fighting blood corpuscles) *decreased steadily in the rats on the deficient diets.* As the diets became progressively better, the number of leucocytes increased and the total number of leucocytes was normal only in the rats on the best diets. "These studies support the working hypothesis that resistance to bacterial invasion may be depressed by inadequate nutrition," say these investigators. "Their importance is enhanced by the fact that the animals were eating the same diet that gives rise to the mixed deficiencies seen in patients in the clinic. . . . Therefore in mixed deficiencies, the importance of restoring the organism to a balanced nutritional regime becomes apparent if that organism is to be able to defend itself against the onslaughts of bacterial invasion."

Now how can we use the information from these experiments to prevent colds? To us they seem to indicate that an abundance of vitamin B in the diet, as well as vitamins A and C, will help the body's defenses against germs. So, when you feel a cold coming on, what should you do—go to your doctor and ask for an injection? We think not. We believe you should use vitamin B, along with other vitamins, every day, as protection, so that you simply do not contract colds.

Our recommendations would go something like this: Meat or fish in your diet every day (organ meats like liver at least once a week), fresh vegetables and fruits in abundance especially during the winter (and be sure to include green leafy vegetables and yellow vegetables every day) and nuts. Omit all foods made from white flour or white sugar, for they rob your body of B vitamins. When you are preparing food to eat, observe carefully the suggestions we make in the article on vitamin C in this book. And finally, just to make certain, take desiccated liver and/or brewer's yeast every day for B vitamins. It's simple, really, to adjust your diet along these lines—and less expensive, too.

Colon

Let's say you're just sitting down to a large holiday meal—including some foods that are good for you and some that are not. What happens to each bite of food after you've swallowed it? A small part of the carbohydrate food is digested in your mouth by saliva (a good reason for chewing starchy foods well). Then the food goes to your stomach where digestive juices work on the proteins and fats for a considerable time, while the partly digested carbohydrates pass along into the intestines.

But somehow, some way, all this partly digested food must be absorbed into your blood. How and where does it occur? The absorption or assimilation of food occurs in your small and large intestines. The small intestine joins the stomach through a proficient little valve, the pylorus, which opens automatically to let a given amount of food pass, then closes again until the food has passed along down the intestine, then opens to admit more. Your small intestine, if it were spread out full length on the ground, would be something like twenty feet long and the food must pass through this entire length. Of course your body would never be able to contain such a lengthy piece of equipment if it were not folded and re-folded into many tiny sacs and pockets.

When the food enters the small intestine, a series of rhythmic waves begins—first the segmenting waves in which the walls of the intestine are squeezed into little pouches. The muscles relax again and then squeeze themselves into another series of pouches. All this causes the food to be ground into smaller and smaller particles. Then along comes a big wave —a peristaltic wave—in which the walls of the intestine contract to push the food downward. While this is taking place, all the various juices of the small intestine are at work breaking down the proteins and carbohydrates even further. The proteins become amino acids. The carbohydrates become simple sugars, through the chemical action of these juices or enzymes.

But how are these amino acids and sugars absorbed through the wall of the intestine into the blood stream? We do not know exactly. We learned in physiology class that food was absorbed by a process called osmosis. That is, the watery solution containing the food would, we learned, pass right through the porous walls of the intestine, as a thick soup might be strained through a cloth. But today's biologists realize that the process of assimilation is much more complex than this. They know, for instance, that different kinds of substances are absorbed at different rates of speed. They know that the walls of the intestine are composed of living cells and that somehow the food enters these cells and from there enters the blood.

Just stop to think a moment of what we've said above. While you are relaxing after your holiday meal, hundreds of chemical processes are going on in your small intestine—processes that are not as yet understood and cannot be duplicated in a chemical laboratory. The good, nutritious, natural food you've just eaten probably won't cause your small intestine much trouble. It's equipped to handle that speedily and well. But what about those crusty white rolls, that ice cream full of synthetic sugar, that pie made from shortening so highly processed that it resembles no natural fats? Is it any wonder we, as a nation, suffer from countless ailments that begin right here in the small intestine?

The colon is the large intestine which is attached to the small one. It has three functions. First, it is the storage place for waste accumulation. All the food that has not been absorbed passes into the colon. Secondly, this waste material moves quite slowly along the colon, so that water may be absorbed from it through the colon's walls. Otherwise the body would be losing this moisture constantly. The last function of the colon is to carry the waste material (called feces) away from the small intestine toward the rectum where it is excreted. Not all of the waste matter is excreted at any one time. Some is always retained in the colon. And the time for excretion is meticulously controlled by muscles and nerves, so that waste material does not actually enter the rectum until it is time for a bowel movement.

Many and varied are the diseases of the colon and small intestine—ranging all the way from constipation (when the feces become hard and packed inside the colon) to dysentery, when there may be an almost constant discharge of watery feces. Colitis, enteritis, regional ileitis, diarrhea, sprue, celiac disease—all these and many more are disorders of the intestinal tract. Some are caused by harmful bacteria which create inflammation; some are caused by lack of beneficial bacteria which normally live in the intestines; some are caused by deficiency in vitamins and minerals which are absolutely necessary to this whole complicated process of assimilation. In colitis, for example, there is a notable lack of vitamins A and C in the blood serum. Vitamin A is destroyed in the intestinal tract by mineral oil. Perhaps this is the reason for its deficiency in many cases of colitis. The B vitamins must be present in the intestine for carbohydrates to be assimilated. The white roll and the ice cream you had for dinner cannot be absorbed into your blood stream unless you are getting ample B vitamins. The important minerals—calcium, phosphorus and so forth—are also necessary to this process. So your best plan for avoiding any and all diseases of the colon is to eat nothing at all that will not add to your body's nutrition, and to eat plentifully of all the wholesome, nutritious foods.

Constipation

From the variety and quantity of laxatives sold today one would assume that constipation is widespread among Americans. But just how widespread it is becomes frighteningly apparent with a glance through the medical literature. In one series of 3000 patients studied and reported on, 55 per cent were constipated. The disorder was 50 per cent more common among women than men. It was also found in studying 500 patients with hemorrhoids, 250 patients with anal ulcers, 100 with perianal abscess and 125 with fistula, that these condtions are far more common among individuals who are not constipated. These findings were reported in the *Southern Medical Journal,* for July 1950.

In healthy animals and in many primitive people, the bowels move after every meal, almost as automatically as breathing. It is believed that taking food and chewing it brings about a reflex which stimulates bowel action. That is, as soon as the food enters the mouth and chewing begins, a message is sent by the nerves to the muscles of the digestive tract so that they are prepared to start the work of elimination. Mechanically speaking, it seems like good engineering for the incoming food to push out the residue of what is left from the last meal. But undoubtedly there is more to the story than mere mechanics. Else why would constipation be spoken of as a disease of civilization? Surely we have more regular mealtimes than wild animals or primitive people who may not know where their next meal will come from or when!

Constipation begins in the colon—the large intestine. This part of you is nothing more or less than a storage tube. Very little actual digestion takes place there. The digestion occurs in the stomach and small intestine. Into the colon, then, after a meal, come the residues of food that cannot be digested, many of the bacteria which took part in digestion in the small intestine and mucous that has sloughed off from the intestinal wall. About one-third of the entire mass of feces consists of bacteria. This liquid mass moves along in the colon and water is absorbed from it so that, as it passes along, it gradually becomes drier and firmer. As the mass approaches the lower end of the colon—the rectum—movements of the colon called peristaltic waves propel the mass along into the rectum. Nothing enters the rectum until just before defecation. As the fecal mass is pushed into the rectum the individual feels the urge to defecate.

So much for the way the whole mechanism works. Now what exactly is constipation? The simplest definition seems to be: infrequent or difficult bowel movements. There is wide variation in individual habits in regard to "regularity" of bowel movements. Many people have a bowel movement after every meal. Others have one a day, regular as clockwork. For many more, a bowel movement every second, or even third day is "regularity." There are instances on record of individuals who may remain perfectly healthy a week or ten days without a bowel movement.

Psychological Aspects of Constipation

One of the main causes of constipation seems to be psychological. In the case of children, toilet training plays a large part. The child's parents, when they give him food, are answering his most urgent need and gratifying his senses. But when they try to teach him cleanliness (in this case toilet training) they are trying to get him to accept adult ideas of a way of life which is not natural to him, so he may have severe emotional difficulties over this problem.

Dr. Milton Senn, in his book *All About Feeding Children* (published by Blakiston) says "An appalling proportion of juvenile constipation is the direct result of an indiscriminate use of suppositories, enemas and laxatives administered by over-zealous mothers in the fanatical effort to force a daily bowel movement."

"Many children are constipated as a result of faulty habits of elimination attributable either to premature or too rigid toilet training. A child old enough to sit unsupported may be placed upon a toilet as needed, but he should never be forced to sit there for long periods or under circumstances which he will consider frightening."

In general, the rules for discouraging constipation in children hold for adults as well. Intense concentration on bodily functions, worry about a day gone by without a bowel movement, recourse to laxatives and enemas will, in many cases, produce constipation rather than preventing it. We have explained above the reflex or impulse that gives us the urge to defecate. If this impulse is thwarted time after time, as it is when you take laxatives or enemas, it will cease to function. The muscles of the colon have the job of contracting in wavelike movements. A laxative bombards the fecal mass along so fast that these muscles get no chance to do their work. Like the muscles of an arm in a sling they degenerate.

According to all the medical articles, the chief cause of constipation is probably simply that we ignore nature's call too many times. Whether or not the bowels move at approximately the same time every day, we are too busy with work or social engagements to take the time necessary for a bowel movement, when the call comes. The child whose normal time for evacuation may be just after breakfast has to hurry to school instead. Many children who feel the need of a bowel movement at school are afraid to risk the teacher's displeasure by asking to leave the room. These habits pursue us into adult life. Working conditions and after-work social obligations force us into the position of simply not having enough time for personal hygiene.

The first and cardinal rule, then, for preventing constipation is to have a regular time at which to move your bowels every day. Give yourself plenty of time. If this means getting up and having breakfast half an hour earlier, that is how you must arrange things. If it means postponing evening activity for an added half hour, then that is the only answer for you.

Here are several suggestions for making the physical mechanics of bowel movements easier. We were not made to sit on a stool while defecating. Primitive people squat on the ground and this, of course, is the natural position to take. Assuming as near this position as possible will give the best results. It may mean having a stool on which to raise your feet, or even two stools, one on each side of the toilet bowl, on which to squat.

Pulling in on the abdominal muscles and relaxing the muscles around the anus will help. If you can relax better while reading, then read by all means. Some people believe that lighting a cigarette or drinking a cup of coffee or chewing a stick of gum will produce the urge to defecate. Researchers say that perhaps these things will do just this, but it is not because of any special value in the activities themselves. It is simply that they represent a ceremony to which one is accustomed, so they call up a kind of automatic response from the body.

Your Meals and Constipation

Does food have anything to do with constipation? It certainly does. And we are of the opinion that the food primitive man ate had as much to do with his lack of constipation as did his more lenient social customs. In refining, processing and cooking food we remove much of the bulky, fibrous material which primitive men ate. It appears that mechanically speaking, these substances are necessary for the process of pushing the food along through the colon. Nutritionally, they carry many of the food elements that are necessary to prevent constipation.

The intestines are muscles. Healthy intestines are capable of doing their job of working the food along at the proper rate of speed. To keep them healthy means eating all the food elements you need to keep the rest of the body healthy. Vitamins are necessary in order for the body to use the proteins, carbohydrates and fats you eat. If you do not get enough of the B vitamins, the body simply cannot handle the carbohydrates in your food. From the moment you chew them until they finally end up in a body cell somewhere, everything goes wrong. None of the body processes, including digestion, can possibly go smoothly.

Experiments have shown that inositol and niacin, to mention only two of the B vitamins, prevent constipation in animals. Laboratory volunteers on diets short in thiamin, another B vitamin, become constipated. A deficiency of vitamin K produces constipation in animals. Calcium, phosphorus and the other minerals are necessary for preventing constipation. A diet too high in fat may prevent you from using calcium properly. The fat tends to combine with the calcium to form soapy-looking curds in your intestines which carry the calcium out along with them before your body has the chance to use it. Finally, vitamin E is most important for the health of muscles. The intestine is a muscle. Could the nation-wide deficiency in vitamin E be responsible for our widespread constipation?

Sir Adolphe Abrahams, O.B.E., M.D., F.R.C.P., writing in *The Practitioner* for March, 1953, says, "When chronic constipation is termed a disease of civilization one has in mind the revolt of the alimentary canal against the alterations in dietetic habits and the character of modern foodstuffs." He goes on to say, "The aperient (laxative) action of certain foodstuffs is well known. The cellulose and pulpy constituents of fruit and vegetables provide a stimulus to peristalsis (the movement of the intestines); mechanically by distension or irritation of the mucosa; chemically by the content of sugar and neutral salts. The chief foodstuffs, some of which have an exaggerated reputation, are spinach, cabbage, asparagus, onions, parsnips, lettuce and most fresh and dried fruits." He mentions, in addition, that the astringent quality of some foods, like tea when taken in excess, may tend to constipate.

Drugs and Fluid Intake Affect Constipation

Special diets, and drugs may constipate. A. Littman, M.D. and A. C. Ivy, Ph.D., M.D., writing in *Gastroenterology* for December 1950 review the cases of 31 patients with peptic ulcer. During their observation, 79 per cent of the patients had definite constipation. They found that ulcer disease itself and the use of ulcer diets (with practically no "roughage") caused constipation in only a few cases. But the antacid medicines given were solely responsible for the constipation in 14 of the cases and in an additional 35 per cent the medicines undoubtedly contributed to the condition.

Persons who are reducing may claim that they are simply not getting enough food in bulk to encourage the proper activity of the bowels. But reducers have an excellent opportunity to prevent constipation while they are on the very diets they complain about. Raw fruits and vegetables contain more bulk and fewer calories than any other kind of food. On any and every reducing diet you are, or should be, allowed to eat as much as you want of these foods.

The amount of liquids you drink apparently has a lot to do with preventing constipation, too. According to an article in *College and University Business,* for July, 1950, the incidence of constipation in patients seen by a specialist was 55 per cent. Constipation usually occurs in normal persons whose dietary bulk is far less than it should be, and whose fluid intake is not adequate. The constipated individuals studied had a daily fluid intake of 2½ pints. An equal number of non-constipated patients used an average of 3½ pints of fluid daily. These investigators believe that a diet for preventing constipation should include fresh or stewed fruits for breakfast rather than juice. Lunch should include a fresh fruit or a bulky salad (both, we would suggest). Dinner should include a large salad and generous servings of two such vegetables as cabbage, sprouts, sauerkraut, green beans, peas, asparagus, corn, spinach, okra or baked squash. Raw carrots, celery, lettuce, water cress and tomatoes should be used freely. Fresh fruits should be taken daily, especially before going to bed. And patients should drink a full eight ounce glass of water every waking hour.

Suggestions for Preventing Constipation

To summarize: keep yourself and your family free from constipation by following these suggestions:

1. Establish a regular time for defecation which can be observed without strain, hurry or anxiety every day.

2. Don't take a laxative because you missed a bowel movement one day. Give yourself a chance to come back to normal without artificial means.

3. Omit all processed and refined foods from your meals, especially those containing white sugar and white flour. Eat as little bread and cereal as possible, and make that little completely whole grain. A friend of ours cured himself of constipation by omitting bread entirely from his diet. That was the only change he made.

4. Eat more than you think you can possibly need of fresh fruits and vegetables, especially the ones that have bulk—the green leafy vegetables and the fruits with lots of fiber

5. Drink plenty of fluids—water if you prefer that. If not, make your fluids vegetable and fruit juices, unsugared and unsalted. Or herb teas, or drinks made with carob flour. Don't of course try to make up your daily fluid intake from tea, coffee, soft drinks or cocoa.

6. Devote yourself to getting plenty of vitamins and minerals in your meals and in your food supplements. The B vitamins are probably the most important from the point of view of preventing constipation. But if you are already short on B vitamins (and most of us are) you probably need lots more than you are getting of all the other vitamins too. Take brewer's yeast and/or desiccated liver for B vitamins, fish liver oils for vitamins A and D, bone meal for calcium and other minerals, rose hips for vitamin C and vitamin E made from pure vegetable or cereal sources. And incidentally, sunflower seeds are an excellent and delightful source of many minerals and vitamins, as well as the fibrous bulky food material you need. Eat them for between meal snacks.

Copper

In studying copper you meet often, perhaps more often than with any other food element, with the baffling but intriguing words, "It is not known . . . it has not been discovered . . . it is still a mystery." We don't actually know very much about the ways in which the body uses copper. We know that it is essential—no one can live without it. Yet it is so widespread in foods that it is difficult to design a diet which contains no copper.

We know too that copper works with iron in the body, just as it accompanies iron in many foods. Copper is a "trace mineral"—that is, it appears in extremely small amounts and we require it in very small amounts. It appears to take some part in the formation of chlorophyll, the green coloring matter of plants. It occurs quite abundantly in some kinds of sea food. And the inky discharge of an octopus contains large amounts of copper. Just as small amounts of copper are known to be indispensable, so large amounts are known to be poisonous. We do not know exactly how copper poisons, but it appears to act on protein substance, disorganizing it and precipitating the protein so that it is useless.

Apparently the most important function of copper in the human body has to do with hemoglobin—the red coloring matter of blood. In this case, copper works with iron to produce this substance. You can be anemic because of lack of iron, but even though you start to take plenty of iron you may still be anemic if there is not enough copper in your diet to work with the iron to form hemoglobin. These facts were discovered by studying animals living on a milk diet. Milk contains very little iron, so the animals became anemic. But addition of iron to the diet did not improve their condition. It was not until copper was added too that their red blood count came back to normal. It has been found also that in some kinds of human anemia copper added to iron will give results, while iron alone will not. When there is no copper in the diet, iron will be stored by animals, but it will not be made into hemoglobin until the copper is added. If an animal is provided with plenty of copper but no iron, the copper in the blood increases, as if it were collecting deliberately to be ready for action as soon as the iron is available.

Copper is also involved in some obscure way with the body's use of vitamin C. Although they are not certain, researchers believe that copper helps in the oxidation of vitamin C in the body. We know that copper oxidizes vitamin C in vegetables and fruits when it comes in contact with them during food preparation; perhaps the same thing takes place in the body, so that we can use the vitamin C we eat. At any rate, we know that animals on diets so low in vitamin C that they would otherwise get scurvy do not get this disease if copper is added to the diet. So perhaps the additional copper helps the body to make use of whatever vitamin C there is.

In two sections of the world—parts of Australia and England— a very peculiar disease has appeared among lambs which investigators believe to be caused by lack of copper in the soil, resulting in very little copper in the grass which these lambs eat. The disease is cured by giving the lambs copper supplements in their diets. It is generally agreed, however, that it is not healthful to continue treatment with inorganic copper compounds for very long.

Babies of all animals are born with quite a large supply of copper stored in their livers, supposedly to tide them over the period when they will live on milk, which is poor in copper. This is one reason why calves liver is more valuable in nutrition than beef liver because it will provide you with eight times more copper, in addition to its considerable content of iron.

One of the most tantalizing pieces of information we have about copper is that a certain kind of rat turns gray-haired when its diet lacks copper. Right away we are eager to apply this finding to human nutrition and suggest that perhaps lack of copper may be partly responsible for prematurely gray hair in human beings. But it's not that simple apparently. For increasing the copper content of human diets does not seem to make any difference to human gray hair. However it is something to keep in mind, if you are concerned with graying hair, and it certainly won't hurt to make certain your meals contain plenty of copper-rich foods. In general they are foods that are good for you for other reasons as well.

Nutritionists agree that copper deficiency in a human being is unknown. And they have no very definite recommendations as to how much you should get in daily meals. The National Research Council has officially stated that from one to two milligrams per day should be the safe amount for adults. They also believe that most adults get about two milligrams in ordinary diet, so there seems no reason to worry about deficiencies.

Foods Contaminated By Copper

We ran across one fact about copper in food that disturbed us considerably—that is the open acknowledgment that much of the food we eat is contaminated with copper somewhere along the line before it reaches our tables. In *Foundations of Nutrition* by Mary Swartz Rose (The Macmillan Co.), a standard book on nutrition, we are told that milk frequently contains copper which it accumulates passing over heated copper rollers while it is being pasteurized, or being transported in copper containers. Jacobs in *Food and Food Products* (Interscience Publishers, 1951), tells us that the copper in plants is closely related to the copper content of the soil, especially where copper fertilizers or insect sprays have been added. In Bridges' *Dietetics for the Clinician* (Lea and Febiger, 1949), we read that foods held in copper containers or "treated with copper sulfate to retain the green color when they are canned" may provide toxic doses of copper. Alice Hamilton in her book, *Industrial Toxicology* (Harper and Brothers, 1934), tells us: "In 1921 Mallory and his colleagues published a paper on the relation of chronic copper poisoning to a disease known as hemochromatosis or bronzed diabetes. . . . The cause is unknown. . . . Mallory believes that the disease is much more common than is usually supposed and that it is caused by chronic copper poisoning, the source of the copper being in most cases alcoholic drinks contaminated with copper from the stills . . ."

Now it is generally well known that copper contaminates liquids or foods with which it comes in contact. It seems to us that alcoholic beverages would be even more subject to contamination than other things. So it was difficult for us to believe that brewers used copper in their breweries. What was our surprise, then, to find in a brewery magazine a double-page ad for copper piping and copper brew kettles with the slogan "Copper brews beer best." The ad went on: "Schaefer trusts to copper for its great beers." Under these circumstances, we will not trust to Schaefer for our beer, thank you.

As readers know we do not advise drinking alcoholic beverages, beer included. But if you must drink beer, at least do make an effort to find out whether your brand is made in copper brewery equipment. Write to the manufacturers and ask them. Ask them too what tests they have done to prove that the copper does not contaminate their product. And in choosing foods, where there is the slightest doubt in your mind, don't take a chance on anything that may be contaminated with copper. Commercially-made cider, for instance, may contain copper from insecticides.

This warning holds good for your kitchen utensils as well. Copper utensils are beautiful to look at and they glow brightly on kitchen shelves. Keep them on the shelves and admire their beauty, but under no circumstances use them in any way where they will come in contact with food! Many stainless steel utensils are made with copper bottoms which distribute the heat more evenly. In this case, the copper should be only on the *outside of the bottom;* it should not ever appear on the inside of the kettle where it will touch the food. Dispose of old paring knives or kitchen spoons whose tin coating has worn thin. Copper may be exposed. Use stainless steel. When you are preparing vegetables or fruits, especially, make sure that no copper comes into contact with them, for it destroys vitamin C instantly.

Don't Drink Water From Copper Pipes

Many readers have written us about copper piping in their homes. Our advice is—shun it. One young housewife wrote that she had just moved to a new home where the pipes were copper. If she left clothes soaking under the water faucet they were soon coated with a green color—a sure indication of the presence of copper. On our advice she began to buy bottled spring water for drinking and cooking and uses the piped water only for washing and cleaning. Even if the pipes are not copper, don't use water from your hot water faucet for cooking. An answer to an inquiry in the *British Medical Journal* for November 17, 1951, tells us "The parts of an instantaneous-type gas water-heater in contact with the water are copper or brass, and may be bare, tinned or lacquered. Any toxic hazard would therefore only arise from the presence of copper in the water. . . . The permitted limit in drinking water in the United States is .2 parts per million." Since, as we have already shown, most of us are already getting some food that has been contaminated with copper, we repeat our recommendation—don't take a chance on copper pipes or water from the hot water faucet.

At this point you are probably wondering "if copper is necessary for health, why can't we get it just as well from drinking water as from plants? How come the one is toxic and the other is healthful?" We have never heard of anyone being poisoned from eating plants in which copper occurs naturally. But when copper is added artificially in an insecticide, or to drinking water or food through contamination, this is another matter entirely. Our bodies simply cannot deal with this copper and, if we eat it in large amounts, it is bound to be poisonous.

So we would suggest that, instead of being concerned over whether you are getting enough natural copper in your food, you should worry instead over whether you may be getting too much copper contamination by accident. The following table shows the approximate amounts of copper in some copper-rich foods. A glance over it will probably show you that you are getting an average of 2 to 2½ milligrams daily.

Food	*Copper Content in Milligrams*
Apricots	.37 in 3 apricots
Almonds	1.21 in about 50 nuts
Avocados	.69 in ½ avocado
Beans, navy	.86 in ½ cup
Beans, kidney	.65 in ½ cup
Beef liver	2.15 in 1 piece
Bran, wheat	1.17 in about 5 cups
Brazil nuts	1.39 in 12 nuts
Broccoli	1.37 in one cup
Calves liver	4.41 in 1 piece
Chocolate, bitter	2.67 in 5 squares
Codfish	.47 in one piece
Corn	.44 in ½ cup
Currants, dried	1.12 in 1 cup
Figs, dried	.35 in 6 figs
Filberts	1.35 in 12 nuts
Graham flour	.49 in 100 grams
Lamb chops	.42 in 2 chops
Lima beans, dried	.86 in ½ cup
Molasses	1.93 in 5 tablespoons
Mushrooms	1.79 in 7 mushrooms
Oatmeal, raw	.50 in ½ cup
Peanut butter	.55 in 5 tablespoons
Peanuts	.96 in 50 peanuts
Peas, dried	1.40 in 1½ cups
Pecans	1.36 in about 50 nuts
Prunes, dried	.41 in 12 medium prunes
Rye flour	.42 in 100 grams
Walnuts, English	1.00 in about 50 nuts
Wheat, whole	.72 in 100 grams

Corn

"I tell thee, 'tis a goodlie country, not wanting in victuals. On the banks of those rivers are divers fruits good to eat, and game aplenty. Besides, the natives in those parts have a corne, which yields them bread; and this with little labor and in abundance. 'Tis called in the Spanish tongue 'mahiz'." Sir Walter Raleigh was speaking of corn which, even today throughout the world except America, is called "maize."

Corn is today by far the most valuable annual food crop in the country. Only six to eight per cent of the total crop is used for food and industrial purposes. About one-half of this is used for the "wet milling" process in which corn starch, corn oil and feed by-products are made.

Of the rest about one-third is used for corn meal, and breakfast cereal and the remainder goes for distilled liquors. Of the total world supply of corn only about 21 per cent is used for human food. The rest becomes food for animals.

In earlier days corn was "water-ground" meaning that it was ground between stones in a mill powered by water. This produced a meal that had the full value of the original grain—germ and all—with the result that the meal was highly perishable. Today, we have "improved" all that. Nowadays we mill corn as we mill flour, by removing all of the vital, alive food elements in it, so that the meal will keep in storehouses and on grocery shelves practically indefinitely. Then we "enrich" some of the meal by attempting to put back (in synthetic form) some of the natural vitamins and minerals we have removed. Enriching corn products presents a lot of problems, for the vitamins are water-soluble and likely to drain away during the various washing processes through which the corn products go. At present the enriching is done by combining the vitamins with a "harmless" substance which renders them insoluble in water, but supposedly leaves them assimilable to the human stomach. Our advice is to buy corn products ground by the "old process," if you can get them. The commercially processed kind available in grocery stores contains no more of the original food value of the corn than white flour contains of the original value of the wheat.

The protein of corn is called "zein." In general it is thought that it is slightly less well digested than the protein of wheat or rice. Most of the vegetable and cereal proteins are not as complete as the animal proteins—that is, they lack some of the essential amino acids or building blocks of protein. In corn, the amino acid lysine is lacking entirely and the amino acid tryptophane is scarce. When the whole grain is eaten, this lack may not cause any trouble, for the other amino acids tend to make up for this deficiency. But when refined, processed corn forms the basis for most meals, as it does in many parts of the world, we run into trouble, for then the lack of these two amino acids assumes serious proportions.

The history of the disease pellagra is a perfect instance of what can happen when we tamper with foods. Tryptophane, the amino acid, changes into niacin (one of the B vitamins) in the body. When processed corn products are eaten as the main part of the diet, especially among poorer populations where other foods containing niacin are lacking, niacin deficiency is almost certain to result. This produces the disease pellagra which for many years raged unchecked in the southern part of our country, after the new milling process began to be used. Now we know that eating processed corn as the mainstay of the diet produces pellagra—not because of any poison in the corn, but because what we have done to the corn has resulted in niacin deficiency among our corn-eating population. Yet we still go right on milling corn and trying to doctor it up with synthetic vitamins, instead of going back to the oldtime milling process.

Corn is about 10 per cent protein of which the germ contains about one-fifth. Seventy-three per cent of the corn kernel is carbohydrate and 4.5 per cent is fat, of which more than 80 per cent is in the germ—which is of course removed in the milling. Corn oil is made from the corn germ, and corn oil is a rich source of the unsaturated fatty acid, linoleic acid—a substance essential to good health. Like other cereals corn is quite poor in calcium and rich in phosphorus. The calcium, phosphorus and all other minerals are contained chiefly in the germ which is removed during milling. Most of the vitamins are also in the germ. So when you consult the table (following) for vitamin and mineral content of corn, keep in mind that we are talking about whole grain corn that has not had its valuable food elements removed by milling. Don't make the mistake of buying corn products from your local grocery and expecting them to provide you with this quantity of vitamins and minerals.

One final word about corn. The best way to eat it is, of course, in the ear, right from the stalks. If you have your own garden or if you can persuade a friend to sell you sweet corn from his garden, keep in mind some basic facts about the best way to prepare fresh corn. Eat it raw if you can. You will enjoy the wonderful sweetness of the natural sugar in the kernels. If you plan to cook your corn, don't waste a minute in getting it from the stalks into the kettle. Someone we know once suggested building a fire right in the cornfield and dousing the ears into hot water while they are still attached to the stalks! You needn't be quite that fussy, but do remember that every moment away from the stalk means freshness, sweetness, vitamins and minerals lost from the corn. If you must buy your corn at the market, keep it, husks still on, in the refrigerator until you are ready to cook it. Plunge the ears into rapidly boiling water and cook only until they are heated through—the longer you cook corn the tougher it is likely to become.

Here are the vitamins and minerals in about one-half cup of steamed corn:

Calcium	9 milligrams
Phosphorus	120 milligrams
Iron	5 milligrams
Vitamin A	390 Int. Units
Vitamin B—	
Thiamin	.15 milligrams
Riboflavin	.14 milligrams
Niacin	1.4 milligrams
Pantothenic acid	310 micrograms
Biotin	32 micrograms
Vitamin C	12 milligrams

Cortisone

This is the century of the miracle drugs. And what an astounding parade of cure-alls and near-cure-alls it has become! Hardly a month goes by that the popular magazines do not headline an article on a new antibiotic, a new pain-killer, a new reducer of blood pressure, a new heart trouble cure, a new medicine for controlling mental disease, or something of the sort. Almost always a cautious note is sounded at the end of the article—specialists are not sure whether this is the cure-all for *all types* of a particular disorder, or they warn that there may be after-effects. Or they announce that the new discovery is merely in the "experimental stage." Meanwhile the dreadful march of degenerative diseases goes right on, side by side with all these new discoveries.

A friend of ours got a sore muscle one day last spring doing some particularly heavy job in the garden. When we saw her a few days later she said everything was fine; the doctor had given her something for it. We asked what he gave her and she said cortisone. A couple of months later she (a very healthy person) developed a complicated ear infection which almost necessitated an operation. Was there any relation between the ear infection and the dose of cortisone the doctor had given her for a sore muscle? Possibly not, but it set us to thinking. An article in the *Journal of the American Medical Association* (October 2, 1954) gave us more food for thought.

In this article, Paul H. Curtiss, Jr. M.D., William S. Clark, M.D. and Charles H. Herndon, M.D., describe four male patients with rheumatoid arthritis "in whom severe compression fractures of the vertebrae have developed during the administration of cortisone or corticotropin or both." The authors go on to say, "Although demineralization of the skeleton is a recognized complication of cortisone therapy, these cases have prompted the authors to emphasize the importance of possible pathological fractures when prolonged treatment of this nature is used."

In other words, it is quite well known among physicians that giving cortisone may result in drawing the minerals out of the bones of patients so that the bones fracture or break. In one of the cases described, a 57-year-old man was given cortisone and corticotropin for arthritis. After six months on cortisone, the doctors stopped giving it and the patient's temperature shot up. So they gave him corticotropin. When he came back to the hospital about two years later (we assume he had been taking the drugs all this time) he had the "moonface" and the "buffalo hump" that seem to accompany long dosage with cortisone, also a hemorrhaging disorder of his skin. An x-ray showed that there was "partial collapse" of five vertebrae.

A 67-year-old patient who had also been taking cortisone for arthritis had a fracture of one vertebrae and "extensive generalized demineralization" of all the vertebrae. The third patient was a nine-year-old boy suffering from arthritis, (and isn't it a shocking thing to hear of a child of this age suffering from what is believed to be a degenerative disease—a disease of old age when bones and muscles have worn out!) In this case, too, there were fractures of the vertebrae and "demineralization" of the vertebrae. The fourth case was that of a 65-year-old man whose x-rays showed fractures of two vertebrae and two ribs and osteoporosis (a softening of the bone) in his thigh bones.

Cortisone Is Being Used Indiscriminately

The authors explain that such conditions are apparently the result of excessive loss of calcium, phosphorus and nitrogen, presumably caused by the cortisone. A little farther along they say "It is not known how effectively diet can prevent the disturbances of nitrogen and mineral balance induced by cortisone." For goodness' sake, why isn't it known? And, considering the careless and widespread way in which cortisone is being prescribed by physicians, isn't there ample opportunity to find out what effect diet might have?

For instance, since it is well known that cortisone causes loss of body minerals, why were not mineral supplements given to these patients to replace the calcium and phosphorus they were losing so rapidly? We have no answer to this question, just as we have no answer to the question constantly staring us in the face—why do not medical practitioners in general realize that the human body can keep itself healthy only on whatever food, air and water is taken in!

But quite apart from this question, let's consider for a moment which you or I would prefer to have—arthritis or a broken back? We are told that practically everyone in this country over the age of 45 suffers to some degree from arthritis. Are we solving anything by giving them medication which is quite likely to cause their bones to break?

So much for one aspect of cortisone treatment. Here is another. *Nature* for September 18, 1954, reported on studies conducted by Drs. T. Nicol and R. S. Snell which indicated that cortisone may depress the activity of a certain system in the body which is believed to protect against the growth of cancer. Well, "you pays your money and you takes your choice"—which will you have—arthritis or a drug that may alleviate your arthritis symptoms and make you susceptible to cancer?

Side Effects of Cortisone

Articles from the *Journal of the American Medical Association,* the *Cambria County Medical Society Bulletin,* the *British Medical Journal, The Lancet* and the *International Medical Digest* have pointed out, respectively, that:

1. Cortisone paralyzes the body's natural defenses against infection.

2. Cortisone may produce harmful symptoms in tuberculosis, schizophrenia, diabetes and peptic ulcer.

3. Cortisone masks the symptoms by which doctors recognize the progress of diseases in patients, so that the disease may go right on its deadly way while the patient feels good enough to go back to work. If the cortisone is withdrawn, symptoms will probably return and may be even worse. Or the patient may contract some infectious disease since his defenses against infection have been lowered.

4. We described the case of a patient who committed suicide after being given cortisone for arthritis.

5. We quoted the Council on Pharmacy and Chemistry of the American Medical Association which said "We have repeatedly called attention to the fact that the time is definitely overdue when their use (cortisone and ACTH) in 'practically every disease process encountered by the practicing physician' must now yield to some measure of common sense and conservative thinking."

Now, almost three years later, we find an article indicating that patients nine years old are being given such large and lengthy doses of cortisone that their bones are snapping. We have the evidence of our friend that doctors are prescribing cortisone for such everyday ailments as overworked muscles. And, finally, we have the theory that cortisone may make one susceptible to cancer.

How Cortisone Works

We cannot explain how cortisone works. Even the specialists in this field are still debating all the possibilities. We do know some things about it. It is a hormone—that is, a substance produced by a gland of the body. In this case, the adrenal gland. We know, too, that any meddling with the powerful substances our glands secrete as hormones can throw out of balance many functions of the body. Under normal conditions the hormones given off by the adrenal glands protect the individual against shock, stress, infection, intense heat or cold.

If we place in the body of a patient a gland product, there is every reason to believe that the gland itself will stop making this product. For the glands are very delicately adjusted mechanisms. There is always some reason, some stimulation that causes a gland to manufacture a hormone. If the hormone is already there (put there by pills or injections) the mechanism warning the gland to produce does not work. The gland stops secreting its hormones. And eventually, since it is not working, it atrophies or wastes away, just as one would lose his sight if he wore a bandage over his eyes all the time, or the use of his arm if he kept it in a cast.

Sure enough, an article by Dr. Walter C. Alvarez in his column *Your Health,* September 6, 1953, indicates that autopsies of many patients who had taken cortisone *(for only five days in some cases)* showed atrophy of the adrenal glands. What do you suppose has become of these glands by the time the patient has taken cortisone over a period of several years? There seems to be no possible chance that they could be coaxed back to normal functioning again. In addition, administration of cortisone may bring about severe reactions on such varied parts of you as the skin, the kidneys, the blood, the sex organs, the hair, the stomach, the mind and personality, the nerves, the heart and blood vessels. That's how powerful the adrenal glands are. Their influence is felt all over the body.

Vitamin C and Cortisone

One last note from the German medical magazine *Munchener medizinsche Wochenschrift* for February 22, 1952. H. Schroeder, the author of the article, says it has been found that vitamin C is lost rapidly when cortisone is given. Vitamin C is stored in the adrenal glands which are the glands that make the hormone cortisone. The author goes on to say that a deficiency in vitamin C may impair the function of a certain organ, even though the individual does not have any apparent signs of vitamin deficiency. Different organs in the body may have different sensitivity to vitamin deficiency. He concludes by saying that a diet high in vitamin C is advisable in all conditions that may produce a vitamin C deficiency in the adrenal glands. And in addition, vitamin C should always be given whenever cortisone is given.

"All conditions that might produce a deficiency of vitamin C in the adrenal glands"—let's see, vitamin C is an enemy of poisons and germs. But in fighting the poisons and the germs, vitamin C itself is destroyed. You use up more vitamin C under conditions of stress—strong emotion, fatigue, shock, severe cold or heat. Maybe even lack of sleep, overwork and worry. Consider for a moment all the poisons and germs to which you are subjected every day of your life in air, water and food. Consider for a moment all the stresses to which you are subjected. Does it not seem possible that all of us are suffering from a mighty nation-wide overwhelming deficiency in vitamin C which may be at the root of many of our troubles? Does it not seem wise to get as much vitamin C as possible in every day meals (fresh raw fruits and vegetables) and to take in addition a natural vitamin C food supplement? Does it not seem possible that when we finally discover, unravel and understand all the complexities of physiology and nutrition, we may find that plenty of vitamin C may give us such good adjustment to emergencies, stress and strain that we may not any longer suffer from the diseases for which drugs like cortisone are given?

Cosmetics

We were especially glad to find an article in the *Eye, Ear, Nose and Throat Monthly* for June, 1952, dealing with the subject of the dangers of careless and indiscriminate use of cosmetics and—what is perhaps best of all—written by a woman physician, Dorothy Niederman Bogdanow of Chicago, who has apparently specialized in treating the kind of disorder that may arise from using cosmetics.

Dr. Bogdanow tells us that the skin disorders caused by cosmetics are, generally speaking, not brought about by something that irritates when it is first applied, but by something that sensitizes the skin. A sensitizing agent is some substance in a cosmetic that does no harm when it is first applied. But after several days, weeks, or months it may bring about skin trouble. The difficulty in diagnosing the trouble lies in the fact that most of us use cosmetics all the time without thinking very much about them, so when we break out in an unexpected rash we would never think of blaming it on the lipstick we have been using for years or the shampoo we bought from a salesman several months ago.

Freckle creams, bleaching creams and cleansing creams are the worst offenders for producing unpleasant reactions on the skin, says Dr. Bogdanow. Acids and oxidizing agents such as perborates, hydrogen peroxide, and zinc peroxide are the ingredients most likely to cause trouble. Vanishing creams may produce reactions due to the stearic acid, the alcohol, fats, lanolin or synthetic preparations they contain. In addition, vanishing creams leave the skin alkaline whereas the natural condition of the skin is acid. Then too, she says, the perfume in the vanishing cream may be responsible for skin trouble.

Cleansing creams contain mineral oil, petrolatum, parrafin, beeswax, borax, lanolin or vegetable oils. The substances that cause the most trouble are the petroleum oils, the detergents and the perfume they contain. Don't forget for a moment, when the names of these ingredients hit your consciousness, that practically all of them are made from coal tar—most specifically the petroleum oils, detergents and perfumes. We believe that coal tar preparations are suspect—whether you take them inside or outside. Many of them have been shown to be cancer-causing.

We have no proof to offer showing that the coal tar products in cosmetics produce cancer—but why take a chance, when we know that certain other coal tar products are regularly used in laboratory experiments to produce cancer?

Astringent creams contain salts of zinc sulfate, aluminum sulfate or bismuth sulfate, resorcinol or salicylic acid (which is also used in aspirin). None of these should ever be applied to the skin, in our opinion. And Dr. Bogdanow indicates that they quite frequently produce dermatitis (or skin trouble). Depilatories may contain sulfides or sulfhydrates, carboxylic acid or calcium thioglycolate. All of such preparations should be strictly avoided by the health-conscious person, we believe.

Hair Preparations Most Dangerous

The cosmetics that most often cause dermatitis are those used as hair preparations—dyes, bleaches, lacquers, tonics, straighteners or wave lotions. The complicated names of the substances in these preparations are not important. It *is* important to know that numerous eye injuries have been caused by their use, including extremely serious disorders which in some cases have proved to be fatal. One of these substances is forbidden today in eye make-up, but is apparently still being used in preparations for the hair. Beauticians are required today to make a patch test of any dye they use—that is, they must paint some of it on a skin surface, cover it and examine it 24 hours later for evidence of irritation. Such a test is good, but not nearly conclusive enough, for the sensitivity to the substance may not develop for several days and the surface painted with the dye is very small indeed compared to the whole scalp which is exposed to the dye when the hair is dyed.

Listen to the list of substances that may be in the hair lotion some honey-tongued salesman has talked you into buying—resorcinol, arsenic, tar, sulfonamides, glycerine and quinine! Any or all of these substances can cause dermatitis. Permanent wave solutions—many readers have written us inquiring about one or another of these! Skin disorders may result, says Dr. Bogdanow, from either the reducing agents used with cold wave permanents, or from the gums that are added to hold the curl. Wave setting solutions, used for finger waves, very rarely cause dermatitis. According to *U. S. Public Health Reports, Reprint No. 2523,* there has been a recent outbreak of skin trouble from hair lacquers in which a resin of maleic anhydrid was used. Bleaching preparations made from chlorine or oxalic acid can cause dermatitis. Those containing hydrogen peroxide or sodium carbonate seldom do.

The perfumes, dyes, oils, waxes, fats and flavors of lipsticks—chiefly the indelible lipsticks—can cause serious trouble mostly about the corners of the mouth. Nail polish dermatitis may mislead the person searching for the source of the trouble, for the eruptions may occur around the eyes, ears, face or chest where the fingers have touched. Several years ago a member of the Rodale Press staff was miserable for a couple of weeks with a dermatitis about her eyes and eyelids which proved to be the result of the nail polish she was wearing. Non-allergic nail polishes are available in many drug stores—but why not avoid the problem once and for all by doing without nail polish entirely? A fine set of nails, well-trimmed and well-cared for, with the cuticle carefully pushed back to avoid harming it, is every bit as handsome as a set of blood red ones.

Perfume and Powders

Do you know what perfumes are made from? Alcohol, a natural flower oil and a fixative such as musk or ambergris are the main ingredients and these may cause not only dermatitis but sinusitis and "runny nose" as well. Sensitivity to perfumes is common and it is extremely hard to locate which ingredient of the complex perfume recipe is responsible. Liquid, cream or cake face powders may be responsible for dermatitis—regular face powder rarely is. Soap, as readers know, is very hard on one's skin, because, in order to remove dirt, it must contain alkalis and the normal condition of the skin is acid. So next time you read a magazine ad which counsels you to scrub your face well with such-and-such a soap as a "beauty treatment," take it with a grain of salt. Scrub your face *without* the soap, if you would have beautiful skin. It's perfectly possible for other ingredients of soap, aside from the alkalis, to cause skin reactions—the dyes, perfumes, solvents, fatty acids and so forth. Shaving soaps, shampoos and after-shave lotions are just as likely to cause dermatitis as soap is.

Now how are you to know whether that annoying, itching, burning or runny blotch on your face is the result of some cosmetic you have been using? Says Dr. Bogdanow, it's hard for even a professional dermatologist to find out. The time-honored method is the patch test. A small amount of the suspected substance is put on a piece of muslin, covered with cellophane and taped to the upper part of the back or the arms—cellophane side out, of course. After forty-eight hours, take off the patch and examine the spot of skin. If no redness or irritation is present you may feel pretty safe, although of course there is such a thing as a delayed reaction. If you find your skin irritated, you must go through the long and often costly process of having a doctor break down the cosmetic into its various ingredients and then test each of these to find out which you are sensitive to. In some instances you may fail, for, in the case of lipstick, for instance, the kind of skin on which you use lipstick is different in texture from the skin where you have the patch test. If you cannot solve the problem with a patch test, perhaps you can with a usage test. Stop using all cosmetics until the eruption has cleared. Then begin using just one at a time until one or another of them brings the dermatitis back again. From then on, that is the cosmetic to avoid assiduously.

We think there are two far better solutions than either of these for avoiding reactions from cosmetics. First, stop using them, if you can. Secondly, if you must use them, make certain that you are in such a robust state of health that they won't cause you any trouble. Most of us have certain cosmetics we are slaves to. Suppose you simply can't get along without lipstick. Wear it, then, but eliminate those sixty other cosmetics that clutter up the top of your dressing table. Perhaps you don't feel well-dressed without face powder. Use it, then, but eliminate as many as possible of the rest. Did you honestly every try cleansing your face with plain water—soft water, even if you have to put out a bucket and catch it as it falls from the sky? Try it sometime for a month and see if your skin is not just as attractive and soft as it was when you were using a dozen different kinds of creams and lotions. Remember too that the largest part of the price you pay for cosmetics goes for the perfume, the color, the packaging and the advertising that surround this so-called dainty and alluring product which may bring you nothing but grief.

Of course there are available in health stores cosmetics made from vegetable and herb substances with none of the possibly damaging ingredients. Many of them have been especially designed to be really good for your skin. Use them if you feel you just aren't properly turned out without cosmetics.

Incidentally, we can't advise you whether or not the cosmetics you are using may be dangerous. Aside from information such as appears in this article we do not know any more about what may be contained in any product than you do. If you have pretty definite evidence that one or another of your cosmetics is causing you trouble, stop using it at once. Then write to the manufacturer to find out, (if he will tell you) what this particular cosmetic contains. This will be a great help to your doctor when he attempts to treat you.

Cranberries

The holiday season and a golden brown turkey or chicken on the table almost automatically mean cranberry sauce or jelly as a side dish. Cranberries are natives of the western hemisphere. In Europe they are not produced commercially. For some reason or other these bright red berries like dampness while they are growing. They grow in bogs where the weather is cool and moist. New Jersey and Cape Cod are famous on the east coast for their cranberry crops.

Like other fruits cranberries are at their best when they are allowed to ripen on the vine. Indeed their total sugar content does not develop properly until they have ripened on the vine. Furthermore, they lose sugar when they are stored. However, they can be stored fairly well at about 32 degrees Fahrenheit. They should not be kept in airtight boxes with no ventilation whatsoever, for the berries soon die from "smothering." So when you store them, let them breathe.

Cranberries are good food, fairly rich in vitamins and minerals. Our objection to them is that they are generally prepared with sugar. Indeed if you plan to make cranberry jelly, you must add sugar if you want it to "jell." We recommend instead eating the berries raw (you can grind them in your food grinder very successfully). Mixing them with whatever vegetables you enjoy you can make a fine raw cranberry relish which has all the good flavor of cranberries but does not need sugar. If you need to sweeten the relish, you can use raw honey.

We don't advise buying canned cranberry jelly. Part of the reason, of course, is that we don't recommend canned foods at all. Then too, the cranberry jelly has had sugar added to it. But in addition, listen to this comment from Jacob's *Food and Food Products* (Interscience Publishers), "The discoloration of canned cranberry sauce was found to be due to the formation of soluble iron from the inner surface of the can and to the reaction of the iron with the coloring matter and to a less extent with the tannin in the fruit."

One other fact to keep in mind about cranberries—they have an acid reaction in the body. All other fruits and vegetables except cranberries, plums and prunes eventually add to the body's alkaline store. But these three fruits, for some reason, contribute instead to acidity. When you are planning meals you should try to balance alkalinity and acidity. Meats and other animal products, cereals, some nuts and the three fruits mentioned above are acid in reaction. All the other fruits and vegetables, milk and other nuts are alkaline in reaction. Starches, sugars and fats are neutral. So don't count on cranberries as an alkaline fruit when you are planning meals.

Here is a listing of the vitamin and mineral content of cranberries:

Vitamin A	40 I. U. in every cup
Vitamin B—	
Thiamin	.03 milligrams
Riboflavin	.02 milligrams
Niacin	.9 milligrams
Vitamin C	15 milligrams
Iron	.6 milligrams
Sodium	1 milligram
Calcium	14 milligrams
Phosphorus	11 milligrams

Dates

A food of great antiquity, dates are mentioned frequently in ancient writings. One researcher says they must have been utilized as food in the Near East and India before the Bronze Age.

At some time or other back in prehistoric days someone must have noticed that any fruits left on the tree dried in the sun and were thus preserved. They probably tasted good, too, and so we got our idea of drying fruit in the sun.

The date grows on the date palm, a graceful, long-lived tree which may grow to 80 or 100 feet in height. The trees are uni-sexual—that is, there are male and female trees. The female trees are the only ones that bear fruit. The date-grower must fertilize the fruit artificially, using pollen from the male trees. When harvest time comes, all the fruit does not ripen at once, so that each tree may have to be picked as many as eight times. The harvesting season in Southern California may last from September into early January. Picking fruit from a tree a hundred feet high present problems which those of us who have apple and peach orchards are unaware of. Each tree produces from 200 to 350 pounds of dates a year. They require large amounts of water and a warm climate that makes southern California about the only spot in this country where they can be grown.

For readers who are looking for a substitute for desserts and sugar there is no better answer than the date, unless you happen to be reducing, in which case we strongly advise you to avoid dates. Their sugar content is too high, and they taste so good that they tempt one to go on eating after he has eaten one. And the calories mount up.

As the date ripens, the amount of sugar it contains increases steadily until, when fully ripe, its sugar content may be from 35 to 75 per cent of the whole fruit. We are sure that no one could possibly finish off a meal with two or three dates for dessert and claim that his sweet tooth was not satisfied. In fact, many people find dates too sweet for their taste. They are fairly rich in calcium, phosphorus, iron and copper and good sources, too, of chlorine, potassium, manganese and magnesium. In addition, they contain some vitamins B and A.

The vitamin and mineral content of 15 medium-sized dates is as follows:

Calcium	72	milligrams
Phosphorus	60	milligrams
Iron	2.1	milligrams
Sodium	1	milligram
Potassium	790	milligrams
Vitamin A	60	International Units
Vitamin B		
Thiamin	.09	milligram
Riboflavin	.10	milligram
Niacin	2.2	milligrams

DDT

DDT has made the headlines recently all over the country. We have received from just about every state clippings on the press release of Dr. W. Coda Martin of New York City and Dr. Morton S. Biskind of Connecticut concerning their findings of DDT residues in the tissues of their patients.

Dr. Biskind, author of the article that appeared in the November, 1953, issue of the *American Journal of Digestive Diseases,* does not pull his punches. He states clearly, authoritatively and forcefully that there is ample evidence of the harm being done by the new insecticides to individuals who have never knowingly been exposed to them. He leaves not an argument unturned of the facile, superficial and irresponsible statements that have been made by those who, for some reason or other, keep on pretending that we can continue to take in incredible amounts of deadly, cumulative poisons and not eventually suffer for it.

Dr. Biskind quotes the U. S. Public Health Service as saying, in 1950: "The finding of hepatic (liver) cell alteration at dietary levels as low as 5 parts per million of DDT and the considerable storage of the chemical at levels that might well occur in some human diets, makes it extremely likely that the potential hazard of DDT has been underestimated." In 1951 they pointed out that DDT is a delayed action poison, that it is excreted in the milk of cows and nursing mothers and that children and infants are especially susceptible to it. The Department of Agriculture has announced that the chlorinated naphthalene insecticides (of which DDT is one) are implicated as a cause of X disease in cattle which has caused millions of dollars of loss to cattle growers.

Now, in 1957, more and more DDT is being used, and to make matters worse, every so often an article appears announcing that Dr. so-and-so has declared that the insecticides are completely harmless and "he knows of no ill effects from their use." This is a very tricky way of putting things. It is the same demagogic choice of words that the profluoridators use when they are asked about the possible toxicity of artificially fluoridated water, "We know of no ill effects," they say. In other words, although the medical and scientific magazines are full of documented information about the toxicity of the new insecticides, so long as this particular physician has not bothered to read this information, he can rush into print claiming the insecticides are safe because "he knows of no ill effects."

Here is a typical sample clipped from the *Journal of Commerce,* for December 4, 1953. Says Dr. Paul J. Chapman, Cornell entomologist, "No one denies that most spray materials are toxic. . . . But fortunately many of them are much more toxic to insects than to man." Now what kind of a statement is that? "Many of them are more toxic to insects than to man." How many and which? And how about the others which are, we assume, more toxic to man than to insects? After such a brilliant stroke of double-talk, Dr. Chapman concludes with this reassuring statement: "To my knowledge no one has ever been killed or made definitely ill by eating foods that may have traces of spray residues. Claims to the contrary have been made. But we are concerned with facts rather than supposition and rumor." In this way, Dr. Chapman, having stated no facts himself, dismisses as "rumor and supposition" the cold, sober facts presented in such excellent articles as Dr. Biskind's.

Dr. Biskind tells us that apparently a new principle of toxicology has become entrenched in medical literature—"No matter how lethal a poison may be for all other forms of animal life, if it doesn't kill human beings *instantly,* it is safe. When nevertheless it unmistakably does kill a human, this was the victim's own fault—either he was 'allergic' to it (the uncompensable sin!) or he didn't use it properly."

Symptoms of DDT Poisoning

Dr. Biskind began as early as 1949 to publish reports implicating DDT in that set of diseases called "virus X" because no one knew what caused them. He showed at that time that exposure to DDT brought about a strange set of symptoms whose combined aspect was unknown before the introduction of these insecticides. Some of the symptoms Dr. Biskind mentions are: acute disturbance of the gastrointestinal system, with vomiting, diarrhea and abdominal pain. Respiratory symptoms with a cough and persistent sore throat, joint pain, muscle weakness, sometimes dizziness, faintness, headache, and a peculiar emotional disturbance which Dr. Biskind describes in great detail—"one of unbearable emotional turbulence. . . . Perhaps the one common phenomenon is extreme apprehensiveness." Rapid beating of the heart, a fear of losing consciousness, pain in one part of the body or another, disorders of taste, vision, smell, extreme fatigue and so forth. Dr. Biskind mentions twelve other physicians in medical literature who have reported these same symptoms in patients.

Now, of course, even a layman can see that just outlining the symptoms and ascribing them to exposure to DDT is not enough. How can one prove that DDT brought on the symptoms? As long ago as 1950 Dr. Biskind reported to the Delaney Committee on many, many cases in his own practice where removal from exposure to DDT brought the symptoms to an end. Furthermore, when the cured patient was inadvertently exposed to DDT again, the symptoms returned, and disappeared after the patient was removed from the room, or food or piece of clothing that was contaminated with DDT.

As Dr. Biskind points out, it is extremely difficult these days to eliminate DDT completely from one's surroundings. Exposure to it is almost universal, he says, and any food which by chance was not treated with DDT by the farmer is almost certain to have been exposed to it before it reaches our tables. DDT is in practically every mouthful of food we eat, it has been used in sprays for the house, the yard, the neighborhood, the clothes closet, the screens, the swimming pool, the restaurant, the amusement park, the food market. If you were an M.D. just how would you go about telling a patient to avoid exposure to DDT? Rooms sprayed with it must be painted or varnished, floors waxed, clothes dry-cleaned, and so forth. Since DDT accumulates in body fat, diets low in fat meat, butter fat and other dairy products are necessary. Fruits and vegetables must be peeled. With all these precautions taken, the DDT poisoned patients recovered. Why is this not proof enough of the fact that DDT is slowly but surely poisoning every one of us, especially when we know from laboratory experiments that DDT is poisonous to every form of life?

Polio, Hepatitis and DDT

Dr. Biskind discusses the very significant facts in regard to DDT and the rise of polio. In the United States, he says, polio had been increasing at a rather steady rate up until 1945. Beginning in 1946 the rate of increase had more than doubled. DDT was released for general use in 1945. The same has happened in other countries where the insecticide has been introduced. In Israel, for instance, there were only two or three isolated cases a month, before 1950, when DDT was introduced. During 1950, 1,600 cases were listed—about one case per thousand population.

He also describes the rise of hepatitis in the American population. We know from laboratory work that DDT is a liver poison. Hepatitis is a disease of the liver and its increase in the general population, young and old, since 1945, is without parallel in health history. Hepatitis is now one of the major medical problems. And at the same time that it has appeared with such frequency among human beings, it has also suddenly appeared in dogs, cattle and other domestic animals, which are, of course, exposed to the insecticides too. Without exception, everyone of the chlorinated cycle hydrocarbons is a liver poison, says Dr. Biskind. In speaking of chlordane, another related insecticide, he says, "In a hospital in which technical chlordane is applied routinely in the kitchen and food storeroom, and less regularly elsewhere in the institution, for roach control, an epidemic of hepatitis has persisted among the resident nursing staff for three years. This disorder was considered 'infectious' yet despite adequate . . . precautions the cases continue to appear. The chlordane is still in use."

DDT, chlordane and other insecticides of this same family are stored in body fat. Hence their action is cumulative. It is not as if you might eat or breathe a little chlordane or DDT one day, excrete it within the next few days and then be free of it until you eat some more. No ! These insecticides lodge in body fat and stay there, so the more you eat, the more of the insecticide accumulates in your body. If you are reducing your diet will cause you to use up body fat rapidly. And you may well be exposed to all this accumulated DDT. If you are ill in bed, you may lose weight, and once again the accumulated poison in your body fat will be released to do you harm.

The paragraphs in Dr. Biskind's report which caused the most stir among newspaper men who wrote about them were the ones dealing with the amounts of DDT found in the body tissues of persons who had not been exposed to DDT. In 60 out of 75 cases in one series of tests. In seven out of seven cases and 30 out of 32 cases of mother's milk. The highest concentration found in any individual in another series was in an infant—a concentration of 34 parts per million! In a recent study by the Public Health Service, specimens of body tissue were obtained from 113 volunteers from all of the country. In 111 of these, the range of DDT content was as high as 68 parts per million, with an average of 6.41 p.p.m. (As little as 3 parts per million has been found to interfere with an important enzyme necessary for healthy heart action!) Two individuals who handled DDT as part of their job showed concentrations of 91 and 291 parts per million. Recently a New York physician, W. Coda Martin, reported that he had found traces of DDT in 23 out of 25 patients who had never knowingly been exposed to the insecticide.

Year After Year the Situation Grows Worse

Dr. Biskind quotes the Council on Pharmacy and Chemistry of the American Medical Association as saying: "It is not reasonable to expect that human beings can avoid injury if they are exposed . . . year after year to a toxic agent in atmospheric concentrations that kill insects in a few hours . . . the resultant injury may be cumulative or delayed, or simulate a chronic disease of other origin, thereby making identification and statistical comparison difficult or impossible." Vaporizers containing DDT or chlordane are commonly used in restaurants and food markets to kill flies. Dr. Biskind tells us that in an eight hour period an average of from 1.3 to 13 milligrams of DDT or .9 to 2 milligrams of chlordane might be inhaled by the ordinary person in a room where one of these devices is operating. And this is in addition to all the insecticide that clings to food, food utensils, clothing and so forth! The California State Board of Health, the Federal Interdepartmental Committee on Pest Control and the American Medical Association have all issued warnings on insecticide vaporizers, especially condemning their use in homes or in any place where food is exposed.

On December 12, 1950, Dr. Biskind made an impressive report to the Delaney Committee on DDT and the other new insecticides. Three years later, with the appearance of this present article in the *Journal of Digestive Diseases,* we might look for some improvement of the situation. Instead it has grown steadily worse. More and more insecticides are used each year—and in 1950 more than 200 million pounds were used in agriculture alone!

Now why is it, do you suppose, that the papers are not full of this kind of news every day—why is it that insecticide makers go right on making, advertising and selling these poisons year after year without anyone being permitted to know what a terrible chance we are taking with the health of Americans ten or fifteen years from now? We do not believe the fault lies with the doctors. Certainly many of them are aware of the dangers. Those who write articles or release statements to the press, such as Dr. Biskind, Dr. Martin of New York, Dr. Mobbs of North Carolina, Dr. Krohn and Dr. Pottenger of California and many more, call down on themselves all kinds of vitriolic condemnation from people who certainly should know better. An article in *Newsweek* for September 29, 1952, announces that research at the Savannah (Georgia) Public Health Service's Communicable Disease Center shows that there is "No Harm in DDT." However, this same spokesman warns against the use of a still newer group of insecticides—the organic phosphate group. These, he declares, are really deadly, but it's all right because we have a blood test that will show when somebody has had too much of them.

Here is another piece of calculated idiocy which any reader should certainly have spotted if he read the article in his local paper. A popular physician who writes a widely syndicated daily column on health had this to say one day about DDT: "The consumer never should take chances. Fresh fruits and vegetables must be washed thoroughly before they are eaten. DDT is insoluble in water. . . ." Now if DDT is insoluble in water, what earthly good will it do to scrub the fruits and vegetables for a couple of hours? The DDT will remain. Yet so confused have we become in our thinking about poisons that a widely read physician tells us to wash produce thoroughly in order to get rid of a poison which, as he tells us in the next sentence, water will not wash away!

What Can We Do About It?

Who then is to blame for the insidious but certain poisoning of our nation that is steadily and tragically taking place? Not the physicians, not the chemical manufacturers who are simply trying to supply enough of their poisonous products to keep up with the demand. We are responsible—you and I. We are responsible because we know the facts and we do not protest; we do not speak out. We do not storm into our grocery store and tell the grocer that we will not buy food that has been poisoned. We do not write letters to our newspapers protesting the DDT spraying for mosquitoes that goes on year after year, while the mosquitoes go right on increasing. We do not write to our legislators in Washington demanding that we be protected by federal law from this wholesale poisoning. We do not even tell our friends and relatives what is happening to the food they eat before they eat it. Let's get to work and wipe out this disgraceful menace!

You will be told that there will be famine if we give up the new insecticides. In this great wide country of ours we cannot raise enough food unless we cover the food with poison. That's what they will tell you. Dr. Biskind reminds us that before the introduction of DDT and the newer insecticides we had enough food. How did we manage then? He also reminds us that "the use of the newer insecticides is not only not helpful, but in the long run actually detrimental, both for the growth of crops and the prevention of disease carried by insect vectors. Everywhere that DDT has been used for any length of time strains of insects have become resistant not only to DDT but to related compounds as well. This has been shown to be caused by the long persistence of the toxicity of these compounds. The phenomenon never occurred so long as only short-acting insecticides like pyrethrum and rotenone were employed.

Send 80 cents for a copy of the November, 1953, issue of the *Journal of Digestive Diseases,* published at 229 W. Berry St., Fort Wayne, Indiana. This carries Dr. Biskind's article, whose bibliography lists 119 references in medical and scientific literature. Show it to your friends, your doctor, and the editor of your local paper. This is one of the oldest and most conservative medical publications in the country. Can Dr. Biskind possibly be dismissed as a "crank?" You might also send to Dr. Biskind at Otter Pond, Westport, Connecticut, for a copy of his splendid statement before the Delaney Committee in 1950. These two pieces of literature contain all the arguments you need in a discussion about insecticides.

Meanwhile, to make certain you do not fall prey to poisoning yourself, watch your diet like a hawk. Make every piece of food count for good nutrition. If you possibly can, buy only organically-raised fruits and vegetables, free from poison sprays. Persuade friends and relatives living in the country to garden organically so that you can buy your fruits and vegetables from them. If you must buy produce at a market, peel everything before you eat it; avoid any markets where there are insecticide vaporizers. And protest, protest, protest!

Detergents

In the days before detergents, we used to speak of the curse of "dishpan hands." Now, with the onslaught of the "miracle" cleaners, the curse has become a menace. Not only do our hands have that tell-tale roughness, but cases of real skin disease are cropping up which can definitely be traced to constant contact with the new "grease cutters."

Though the advertisers can rightly claim that the new soapless detergents are the joy of the housewife—time-savers that eliminate unnecessary scrubbing, labor-savers that eliminate rinsing, beautifiers that make clothes dazzle, that make dishes fairly sparkle, there is of course no mention of the possible loss of time, beauty, and even health that results from the bad effects on the poor old human hands.

After the day's chores are done, how much time do we spend rubbing and softening our hands with lotions—often to no avail. More important, how much discomfort do we undergo from the chips and cracks in our skin; how much concern do we feel when we want to look our best and have to display ugly, crinkled, dry hands alongside our best bib-and-tucker; and, perhaps, how much more time (and money) do we lose by our visit to the skin doctor to cure our condition?

One wonders, in this day of high gloss, whether we are more concerned with the appearance of our things than of ourselves. Of course, as one ad so cleverly put it: "the choice, dear lady, is up to you."

Why all this harsh talk about detergents? Do they really have such a bad effect on our hands? Perhaps you are the lucky one who has had no reaction—perhaps the certain detergent you use happily doesn't cause the same irritation that others do, in your particular case, or you have skin with the resistance of iron. If so, you are one in a million. But there is no question about it, detergents do dry up the skin and cause irritation.

We think the standard tests of two well-known detergent-makers to demonstrate the effectiveness of their products prove the point. The manufacturers fix up a solution of detergents and put a duck on the surface of it. A duck has a small gland in the top part of his back that secretes oil, which keeps his feathers oily enough so that he can stay afloat in water. When placed on the detergent solution, the natural oil of the feathers is reduced so greatly by the detergent that much of the duck's buoyancy is lost and he must struggle to keep afloat. Not very nice for the duck. But it shows what happens to the natural oils. So how about your hands?

If we are concerned with our appearance, we are concerned with our hands. When we meet someone for the first time, we shake hands—an impression starts then, almost before we have had a chance to take a good look at our acquaintance's face. Are we offering a harsh piece of sandpaper or the smooth-as-silk hand that we would like to have represent us?

Fortune tellers are said to be able to determine a great deal from hands. And it's not a lot of hocus-pocus. They can look at the condition of the skin, the dryness of the nails, the cuts and bruises, calluses and what not, and know a great deal about the way of life, occupation, financial status and health, and from there hazard a good guess about character. You yourself can do the same with people you meet for the first time. Your hands betray you.

What Are Detergents?

We should not commit such slander, without first knowing a little about detergents. What are they? Why do they do harm? Detergents are a substance like soap, but their molecules are arranged differently. This is what gives them their miraculous cleansing power. So far, no obvious harm. But detergents are made from petroleum or coal. They are coal tar products which are, one by one, being proved to be highly toxic to living organisms. In some of the earlier brands of detergents you could smell a strong odor of petroleum when you poured them from the bottles. Detergents are hydrocarbons—chemical substances made of hydrogen and carbon. In our opinion, coal-tar hydrocarbons are not good substances to be taken into your body regularly.

In October 1951, the *Chicago Tribune* carried the story of a man who was suing a detergent manufacturer for the death of his baby. Three other infants had died and many more had become seriously ill in a Chicago hospital. The Board of Health said that a detergent used to clean formula bottles was believed responsible. The detergent was kept in a room near the nursery and it had not been determined whether some of the detergent got into the formulas by mistake or whether the babies were poisoned by what remnants of it clung to the inside of the bottles after they were washed.

You will say, "But we do not *eat* detergents, so what harm is there?" One answer to this is the illustration of a firm manufacturing an antiseptic detergent for the use of surgeons and operating room personnel. Its advertising says that the substances in the detergent "adhere to the skin *and resist rinsing.*" The anti-bacterial effect is prolonged and absorbed by the skin, and provides protection from germs in its deeper layers. The more often you use it, the deeper it goes.

One of the most frequent advertising claims of all detergents is their ability to penetrate and cling to the surface of whatever they are used on. After they have dissolved the dirt and grease, they needn't be rinsed off. "Glasses sparkle *without rinsing or drying.*" Just so. The detergent stays on—and you drink or eat a bit of it with every meal—to say nothing of the quantities your hands absorb washing dishes three times a day, every day, plus laundry, plus perhaps washing the windows, plus any number of other detergent-and-water activities.

As we mentioned earlier, skin diseases can result from excessive contact with detergents, as well as with plain soap and water. According to an article in the *American Practitioner and Digest of Treatment* for June, 1954, by Dr. Martin F. Engman, Jr., of St. Louis, Mo., "Since the advent of the new soapless detergents, the number of cases of housewives' eczema has increased many times." He says that though "the cause of housewives' eczema cannot be given simply," as there is never a single cause, "housewives' eczema of the hands is the most prevalent industrial skin disease"—considering housewivery as the largest industry in the world.

According to an article in *Time Magazine* for November 9, 1953, "Skin eruptions on the hands are responsible for much misery, and for a big share of a dermatologist's practice nowadays. . . . An eczema-like eruption of the hands is often caused by the defatting and drying effects of soap and detergents used in dish washing, especially during cold weather. In the *American Medical Association's Archives of Dermatology and Syphilology,* Drs. Richard L. Sutton, Jr. and Samuel Ayres, Jr. report that this condition may be aggravated by many common household irritants such as bleaches, waxes, polishes, or even hand lotions and cold creams, as these create a breeding ground for germs."

How to Avoid Skin Trouble

The solution is not easy. When the main aim of washing appears to be to get it over with in the best, quickest, and easiest fashion, it is hard not to use the product that achieves this end. But, in spite of what may seem like inconveniences, we, along with skin specialists, advise cutting out detergents.

If you live where water is particularly hard, and you feel you must use a detergent to combat this, it would be wise to cut the use to a minimum, and wear rubber gloves. Also water should be lukewarm rather than hot, as hot water tends to defat the skin.

Skin doctors advise against the excessive use of lotions to soothe irritation, as often this tends to increase rather than decrease the problem.

Weather also plays a part in the condition of the skin. Irritation is usually greatest during the winter, and skin diseases most frequently improve during the summer months. So another answer may be to follow your weather man and act accordingly.

And, for those who insist on continuing to use a detergent without gloves, our last advice is to build up a large reserve fund of good health, by eating a diet rich in minerals and vitamins which will help your body to withstand chemical poisons of all kinds.

Diarrhea

By **CARL L. THENEBE, M.D., West Hartford, Conn.**

You perhaps would not remember the days of the not too distant past when the term "Cholera Infantum" in the urban, or perhaps the expression the "Take Off" in the rural districts, could strike terror into one's very being, but I do, most vividly. Not only was it most alarming to the parents, but it was often much more so to the physician who had no specific approach in treating this condition. In other words, thousands of these infants and children did not survive, nor do they all live today. Before the hydration-electrolyte-transfusion-carrot era, I have, personally, observed over one hundred twenty-five of these pitiable infants and children pass away. Our national figures are most delayed in coming through, but the death rate in the United States, alone, for the year of 1949 revealed that 5,012 infants had died, under the age of one year, with diarrhea (enteritis). *According to the statistics, there still remains an appalling number of needless deaths which could be avoided each year with certainty!*

Mrs. Smith brought her infant into my office at the behest of my nurse, who has an intuitive sense for determining the urgency of the many phone calls which are cleared each day.

Mrs. Smith started the history of his present illness. Wee Jim, we call him, for the reason that he appears so tiny alongside of his big father who is also a James.

Wee Jim was just two weeks old. He had diarrhea since returning from the hospital, eight days before. His stools were never right and were becoming worse, despite what the doctor had prescribed to remedy the situation. Wee Jim's mother stated that the feedings seemed to go right through him. Now he was having sixteen watery, green stools daily; in fact, there were so many that she had lost count of them. For the past eighteen hours, Wee Jim had been vomiting all of his formula. He had lost one and one-half pounds during the past four days.

Mrs. Smith mentioned that she and her husband had hoped and prayed seven years for Wee Jim, who was her first born, to arrive. *"We do so want you to save him."*

Wee Jim was truly a very sick child. Even his hunger cry was strained and weak. The skin and the mucous membranes of his mouth and throat were very dry. He was one of those "Must Hospitalize at Once Cases" for emergency measures were in order.

And then there was Little Mary whose age was one year. She had been "out of sorts" as her mother explained, for the past three days and she had lost her appetite. She had also become irritable and pale in appearance. But it had only been during the past twelve hours that she had thirteen watery, green stools, with cramps in her "stomach." There was a slight temperature rise to 100.4 degrees. There was no vomiting present.

Little Mary did not appear too ill. Her mother was given the carrot soup instructions to be used at home. Within twenty-four hours the abnormal stool frequency had ceased. These had taken on the usual carrot, non-watery consistency and were yellow in color. Her temperature had fallen to normal. Mary's mother stated that she was like herself and she was even playful. Wee Jim and Little Mary are typical examples of the usual cases that the physician is called upon to treat successfully.

Carrot Soup Used in Europe

In the June issue, *Journal of Pediatrics,* 1950, there appeared an article entitled "Carrot Soup in the Treatment of Infantile Diarrhea" by P. Selander, M.D., of Sweden. He stated that the use of carrots for this purpose had received many very favorable reports from Germany, France, Belgium and his own country, Sweden. Judging from the paucity of medical reports upon the use of carrot soup in our own land, it could be definitely stated that little attention has been given to Dr. Selander's paper.

In order for the pediatricians, the general practitioners and the internists to become aware of the value of carrot soup, some one of this group, in a given community, must take the initiative to prove its worth.

Those who do not care for the flavor of carrots might believe that the carrot soup could be quite horrible. To me, the carrot savor is quite agreeable. The young infant cannot determine the flavor of carrot, for the reason that the sense of taste has not developed as yet. For the older infants and children wherein the sense of taste has been acquired, sucaryl, a foodless sweetener, may be added for a sweet, or a beef bouillon cube may be added for a tastier dish.

Why not try a harmless, foolproof measure which could even be started by the parents, especially in the rural districts where physicians were not readily available, or at least until their doctor could be contacted? To treat diarrhea (enteritis) as early as possible after its inception, before the rapid loss of weight occurs, could be life saving in itself!

It is most important to know just what does take place when a severe diarrhea (enteritis) strikes. When the circulating body fluids, the blood particularly, become depleted of water, the cells of the body are called upon to make up the deficit. When these cells become dry, a state of dehydration exists. Coincidentally with the water loss, there is an outpouring of the electrolytes,* which are so essential in the sustained life of the cells—potassium, phosphorus, sodium, chlorine, calcium, sulphur and magnesium. Finally, there is an outgoing of the cellular protein. The depletion varies from slight to severe; the latter is manifested in acidosis (the reserve base has been expended) and in shock (the state of collapse caused by acute peripheral circulatory failure). These life-giving elements are poured out actually in the watery stools (bowel movements), into the vomitus should vomiting be present, in the expired air and also in the ever present perspiration. (The urinary loss is minimal.)

Now the question arises: "What would carrot soup do that could be indispensable to the emergency welfare of the diarrheal sufferer?"

Why Carrot Soup Is Effective

Carrot soup supplies water to combat dehydration. It replenishes potassium (its potassium content is high), phosphorus, sodium and chlorine especially with the added table salt, also calcium, sulphur and magnesium. Pectin, a proven antidiarrheal remedy, is provided in abundance. Carrot soup renders the secondary effect of mechanically coating the inflamed small bowel, which not only soothes and enhances healing, but it prevents further extension of the process. It reduces the abnormally increased peristalsis (movements of the intestine) to normalcy. It has a slowing effect upon the increased growth of the undesirable intestinal bacteria which have been favored by the diarrheal state. It prevents vomiting, if this has not already started, by impeding the toxic intestinal products and the detrimental bacteria from entering the duodenum and stomach.

Doctor Selander reported a mortality of two per cent in the four hundred and fifty cases of infantile diarrhea treated with carrot soup. This would have been less if the four moribund diarrheal cases, who lasted only a few hours after hospital admission, had not been included in his statistics.

I have used the carrot soup treatment in the hospitals and the homes of over six hundred sufferers of enteritis, without a known mortality. These cases included premature infants, epidemic diarrhea of the new born, infantile diarrhea and diarrhea of older children. Many of these were treated and received follow up treatment via the telephone route. I have also observed adults with acute enteritis and children suffering with acute colitis who were truly benefited with the use of carrot soup.

Fortunately none of the patients treated by me had a fatal ending. It could be tomorrow, however, that I would be less favored.

The carrot soup ingredients described in Doctor Selander's article are as follows: 500 grams (one pound) of fresh, washed, well scraped and finely chopped carrots were placed in a pressure cooker (which is

* mineralolytes.

essential) * with 150 grams (5 ounces) of water for fifteen minutes at fifteen pounds. The entire pulp is passed through a fine strainer and diluted with sterile, hot water to make 1000 grams (1 quart); table salt (sodium chloride) is also added, 3 grams (three-fourths level teaspoon). For the bottle and tube feedings, this may be further diluted with sterile tea or Ringer's lactate solution (a solution of calcium, potassium, phosphorus and so forth) by one-third more of the total quantity.

I have modified the above, frequently, to make the dilution with sterile water to one pint, instead of one quart, in the early hydrated patients. The thicker formulas are more difficult to vomit and give twice the concentration of the needed electrolytes. Sterile tea was offered between feedings. The hospital patients, with an appreciable anemia, were given blood transfusions.

Carrot soup is usually spooned in, but it may be bottled in (the entire top of the nipple may be removed) or it may be tubed in. A small plastic catheter is passed through the nose into the stomach and retained in place by anchoring the nasal end down by taping it to the cheek. The diluted carrot soup is injected at regular intervals through the tube into the stomach. (This method of feeding is used, of course, only in a hospital under expert supervision.)

Other Foods To Take With Carrot Soup

At the beginning of the treatment, usually for the first twenty-four hours, the carrot soup is given at very frequent intervals, often one-half hourly, in small amounts not to exceed one ounce to start.

There is definite improvement within twenty-four hours after starting the carrot soup treatment in the average child. I usually start boiled, skimmed milk in small, but in daily increasing amounts, after the first forty-eight hours of the carrot regime. The adding of skimmed milk depends entirely upon the character of the stool; in other words, is the patient ready for additional food? Mello-ripe or Kanana dried bananas, or very ripe black skinned bananas, or Appella (dried apple) are added next, in order, when the child is ravenously hungry, because of the pectin content. These are discontinued, if not tolerated, and other foods have to be substituted. The carrot soup is continued for about eight days, or it may be prolonged indefinitely. When the milk and new foods are increased, the carrot soup is gradually decreased. Occasionally, a child may be allergic to cows milk and substitutions have to be tried, the most popular, at present, being the soybean preparations. Pertaining to the child's sensitivity to carrot, to date I have not encountered one instance.

Doctor Selander stated that he did not use extra fluids parenterally, (outside of the digestive tract), for instance, these fluids administered under the skin or into a vein, nor did he use the preliminary starvation treatment of twenty-four or more hours. For the average patient, the early hydrated one, I have found that starvation and extra fluids are not necessary. (Little Mary's classification.) But, with the border line or

---

* The editor does not advocate pressure cookers in the preparation of foods as a routine measure, because vitamins and enzymes are destroyed by the high heat, nor does he approve of artificial sweeteners, the use of which Dr. Thenebe suggested earlier in this article. But so long as carrot soup is used as an emergency measure and for a short period of time, and since there is no safe alternative at this time, we have permitted the author to recommend them.

the more severely ill patient, the administering of extra fluids cannot be passed over lightly. The decision becomes an immediate *must*. *The giving of extra water to relieve the dehydration, the electrolytes to replenish the depleted body cells and the combating of acidosis and shock by administering solutions directly into a vein (intravenously) or under the skin (subcutaneously) will depend upon the status of each individual.*

The person suffering with impending shock or the one who is in actual shock, the truly far gone one, demands immediate emergency measures (Wee Jim's physical status). A solution called Ringer's lactate is started at once followed by blood transfusions. These procedures are necessary for the preservation of life.

In summation, I am gratified in being able to report to you that carrot is a tried and proven life-saving measure in the defeat of the number two killer (infectious) of infants and children which is acute diarrhea (enteritis). It should be used more extensively.

Diet for Good Health

Most fruits and vegetables these days are grown with chemical fertilizers and insecticides which do immense damage to the natural vitamins and minerals in the soil. This results in food lacking in these important elements. Commercial fertilizers, unbalanced so far as minerals are concerned, and too easily soluble for the gradual kind of nutrition needed by growing things, are not the healthful answer for soil that is depleted and lacking in the live food provided by organic fertilizer.

We recommend, if possible, raising your own food organically—that is, with natural fertilizers (leaves, grass, manure, etc.) using no insecticides or chemical fertilizers. If you cannot have your own garden, buy food raised organically. The hundreds of deadly poisonous insecticides (DDT, parathion, chlordane, etc.) with which our commercially grown food is sprayed may have far-reaching and serious effects on our health.

Recently an order was signed at the Food and Drug Administration permitting the use of a systemic insecticide in foods—a substance that is injected into the plant, making the entire plant so poisonous that insects will die if they take so much as a single bite of it. This insecticide will be in the food we eat from now on. Which foods? There is no way of knowing which foods you buy at the grocery store have been treated with this or other insecticides. The best answer, of course, is to raise as much of your own food as you can.

White Sugar and White Flour

Refined white sugar is not only worthless as food, but extremely dangerous to health in the quantities in which we consume it. About 50 per cent of the average American diet today consists of products made of white sugar and refined, chemicalized flour. In milling white flour, practically all of the vitamins, minerals, enzymes and proteins are removed and nothing much but starch is left. Then enormous quantities of chemicals are added to make the bread easier to prepare. Preservatives are added so that it won't mold.

In the case of both white sugar and white flour and all other refined carbohydrates, such as "cold" cereals, the B vitamins have been removed. The body cannot handle carbohydrate substances without these vitamins, so they are stolen from the body and a B-vitamin shortage is certain to result. Minerals, too, are lacking in both these foods. So people who eat quantities of these foods are bound to be short in minerals. We believe all this may be an important reason for the enormous increase in degenerative diseases. We urge you to eliminate from your diet sugar and all products made from it (fresh raw fruits and vegetables contain all the sugar you need!) and all refined cereal products. This means no candy, no cake, pie, ice cream, desserts, soft drinks, chewing gum or any of the other goodies that are ever-present in our society. Don't eat any food that has been in a factory.

The Place of Salt in the Diet

It is common medical practice to limit salt consumption in cases of kidney disease, dropsy or high blood pressure. We have found evidence indicating that table salt may be an important factor in cancer, heart disease, sinus trouble, obesity, hives—to mention just a few disorders. A salt-free diet in pregnancy means an easier delivery. Cases of cancer have been reported which improved within two weeks on a salt-poor diet. Completely deaf persons have regained their hearing just by giving up salt. We believe that most of us eat far, far too much salt and would do well to eliminate it entirely from our tables and cooking. You obtain ample salt (sodium chloride) in the natural foods of a good diet.

Citrus Fruits in Moderation

We have discussed the harm that excess citric acid does to human teeth. We suggest that not more than one or two oranges, grapefruit halves or tangerines a week be eaten—not juiced. By juicing fruits you throw away the pulpy part which is by far the richest part nutritionally speaking and drink the juice from which much of the vitamin and mineral content has been strained. We deplore the use of canned and frozen juices.

Processed and Canned Foods

Processed and canned foods, almost without exception, contain preservatives, coloring matter or other objectionable substances in small amounts. The effect of these is cumulative—they accumulate in the body. In addition many vitamins and minerals are lost during the canning process when high temperatures are used. Buy fresh foods, as newly picked as possible. If you must buy canned foods, read the label. Buy the brand that contains no preservative, even if it is more expensive. Frozen foods are generally safer this way, but there too chemicals are sometimes being added.

Vegetarianism Versus Meat Eating

We are not vegetarians, for our research indicates that a high protein diet is healthiest and we believe we must include animal protein because it is more complete than plant protein. It contains all of the essential amino acids, or building blocks of protein, whereas plant protein contains only some of them. We recommend eating lean meat (except ham, pork and bacon) eggs and fish for protein. If you can get your meat and eggs from an organic farmer you will notice an improved flavor and a better state of health. Eat ocean fish, which has not been swimming in polluted waters, as many of our rivers and lake fish do these days. We believe that milk is not the perfect food, and that it should be drunk sparingly by adults.

Fruits and Vegetables

We believe you should eat lots of fruits and vegetables They are certainly the best foods for you. If you can't possibly get organically-grown, unsprayed fruits, peel them before eating them. Pineapples, bananas, coconuts and so forth are recommended because their skins are so thick the insecticide sprays cannot penetrate. Vegetables not organically-grown are certain to contain spray residues. Peel them. Taking bone meal will make up for the loss of minerals when you peel fruits and vegetables. Eat as many fruits and vegetables raw as possible—eat some raw with every meal. Raw food is far better for you than cooked food.

Cook vegetables in as little water as possible just until they are tender, in a tightly covered utensil. Not aluminum, please! Use glass, enamelware or stainless steel Store foods, covered, in the refrigerator.

Tobacco and Alcohol

We take for granted that readers of a health book know that tobacco in any form and alcohol in any form are harmful. Tobacco leaves have been sprayed with many poisonous chemicals adding to the toxic effect of the nicotine. Smoking and alcohol use up some of the body's vitamins—smoking uses up vitamin C; alcohol uses up the B vitamins.

The Necessity for Taking Vitamin and Mineral Supplements

Even though you eat the best possible diet, you do not obtain enough vitamins and minerals for robust health from today's refined and chemically fertilized foods. Much of the fresh food you eat has lost most of its vitamin content during the long shipping process before it reaches your grocery. We advise you to supplement your diet with vitamins and minerals from natural sources.

Vitamins A and D—most plentiful in fish liver oil. Make certain the product you buy is natural, not synthetic.

Vitamin B—Take brewer's yeast and/or desiccated liver for all the vitamins of the B complex. It is much better for you to get your B vitamins from a natural source like this than to take just one or several in a synthetic vitamin preparation.

Vitamin C—Rose hips contain more vitamin C per gram than any other food. You must have vitamin C every day. Your body cannot store it. Take a rose hip preparation for vitamin C.

Vitamin E—Get this from natural vegetable sources. It is a most important vitamin which has been almost entirely removed from our foods by processing. It benefits muscles and blood vessels, including the heart. Children as well as grown-ups should take vitamin E. It is present in wheat germ but in small quantities. Other food elements are present in wheat germ, too. We believe you should take both vitamin E and wheat germ daily.

Lecithin—is a fatty substance occurring with cholesterol in foods. It is believed that lecithin renders the cholesterol harmless. Anyone fearing hardening of the arteries or high blood pressure should get plenty of lecithin.

Rutin—a substance that occurs with vitamin C in foods. It is used in treatment of high blood pressure.

Bone Meal—Lack of calcium, phosphorus and other minerals is one of our most serious diet deficiencies, resulting in tooth decay and scores of other ailments. Inorganic fluorine added to drinking water is no answer. We need minerals in an easily assimilated form. Bone meal provides them in completely natural form. Take bone meal every day—either in tablets or powdered.

Sunflower Seeds—Eat some of these tasty snacks every day. They're full of vitamins and minerals. Finally, to summarize, eat lots of meat, fish and eggs. Lots of fresh fruits and vegetables And nothing much else, if you would be healthy.

Digestion and Absorption

Absorption is the process by which all the things we eat and drink are passed into the bloodstream. Any student of nutrition knows that the study of absorption is almost as important as the study of what the various foods contribute to the body's health. For no matter how much attention you pay to your diet, no matter how much trouble you take to eat exactly what is best for you, unless it is absorbed properly, most of its nutritional value will be wasted.

The list of all the varied aspects of absorption is almost endless. There are anatomical, physical and chemical reasons why food elements are not absorbed. Perhaps the best way to pass this information along to you is simply to list the different facts about absorption as they relate to the different vitamins and minerals.

Vitamin A is absorbed from 3 to 5 hours after it is eaten. By this we mean the vitamin A found in fish liver oil or other animal products. Carotene, which occurs in vegetables and fruits is changed into vitamin A in the body, so its absorption takes six to seven hours. Only about 1 per cent of the carotene in raw carrots is absorbed, because it is bound up in starchy cells which are very difficult for the body to break down. Of cooked carrots, about 5 to 19 per cent of the carotene is absorbed, for the cooking has softened the starchy cells. Apparently liquefying or juicing the carrots results in all the carotene being absorbed, for this, too, breaks down the cells.

Vitamin C is absorbed better when it is taken along with food. That is, your vitamin C supplements, whether they are made of rose hips, green peppers, or what-not, will do you more good if you take them along with meals, so that they can mix with the other food.

The B vitamins are extremely important both for digestion and absorption. Carbohydrates will not be digested or absorbed properly unless you are taking plenty of the B complex of vitamins. There is some evidence showing that vitamin A is not absorbed properly if you have a shortage of B vitamins. In an experiment, pantothenic acid, one of the B vitamins, was added to the diet. It was found that it increased digestion 51 per cent and increased absorption 37 per cent.

A deficiency in B vitamins also means that you will lack hydrochloric acid in your stomach. Without hydrochloric acid, protein and minerals will not be absorbed. What do we mean by this? Do we mean that, if you are short of hydrochloric acid, every single ounce of protein or tiny bit of iron and calcium you eat will simply pass through you without doing you any good at all? No, but we do mean that you will undoubtedly show the bad results of a great shortage of protein and minerals which can have very serious consequences. So in order to assure proper absorption of protein and minerals you must have plenty of vitamin B in your diet.

Mineral oil hinders the absorption of all the fat-soluble vitamins—that is, vitamins A, D, E and K. If you know anyone who has taken mineral oil over a considerable period of time, you will almost certainly find that he has serious symptoms of deficiency in all these important vitamins. Doctors are concerned over what may happen to a patient going under surgery, if he has been taking mineral oil. For vitamin K, which the mineral oil destroys, is vitally important for proper blood coagulation.

Bile salts are necessary for the proper absorption of all the fat soluble vitamins. This substance is manufactured by the liver, so if your liver is not working properly, you may have considerable trouble using the fat soluble vitamins you are getting in your food.

Vitamin B12 is given in cases of certain kinds of anemia. Sometimes this vitamin is not absorbed by anemic patients. This may be because the right amount of digestive juice is missing, so these patients must take a preparation which includes some material from the lining of an animal's stomach, which will help absorb the vitamin B12.

So much for vitamin absorption. With the minerals, we find that calcium and phosphorus must be accompanied by vitamin D for proper absorption. The vitamin D can come from sunshine or from food, preferably fish liver oils, since other foods contain so little. Similarly, vitamin D does not do much good in the absence of calcium and phosphorus. Calcium that is bound chemically to protein is more available to our bodies than calcium in plant material. Phosphorus, too, from meat, eggs, and so forth, is more readily absorbed than phosphorus from cereal where a substance called "phytin" may interfere. In the case of all minerals, there must be plenty of hydrochloric acid in the stomach or they will not be wholly absorbed.

Protein digests slowly; carbohydrates rapidly. So a diet high in protein keeps the food long enough in the digestive tract for the precious vitamins and minerals to be thoroughly absorbed. Any disorder that hurries food through the intestines too fast may result in little or no absorption. Diarrhea and colitis are examples. Harsh laxatives, too, result in little absorption of food. Eating when you are emotionally upset, hurried or angry causes such a turmoil in your digestive system that little food is absorbed.

Is the situation beginning to sound completely hopeless? It needn't. The main principle by which to guide your eating for good absorption is very simple: shotgun therapy simply doesn't work. Taking one vitamin and ignoring the others doesn't work. Taking vitamins and ignoring minerals doesn't work. The functions of all of them are so closely intertwined that you cannot be healthy unless you have enough or more than enough of all of them.

Dirt

By J. I. Rodale
Editor of *Prevention*

Is everyday dirt a menace from the health angle, or should we take for granted our traditional "peck of dirt"?

Some day I am going to write an essay entitled *In Defense of Dirt,* because I think that too much dependence is attached, as far as health is concerned, to cleanliness. Cleanliness in itself, like Old Mother Hubbard's Cupboard, is a bare, empty thing. It is sterile. I can see the cleanest person in the world coming down with tuberculosis, or rheumatism, or cancer. It is not cleanliness that gives health. As I said in my book *The Healthy Hunzas,* if I were in the act of taking a vitamin and it dropped upon the floor I would not hesitate to pick it up and put it in my mouth without any further ado. If a knife or a spoon falls on the floor I don't make a federal case of it, even in a restaurant. I will pick it up and use it, for I am a devout believer in the old adage that we must eat a peck of dirt before we die.

The Hunzas of northern India, one of the healthiest people in the world, make a kind of butter which they call *maltash,* which is buried in the dirt of the earth until it stinks to high heaven. Then they eat it! But European visitors cannot go near the vile stuff. Yet the Hunzas have never had a case of cancer among them. We have heard of the long-living Bulgarians putting a moistened piece of bread over an open jar of pickles, permitting it to become putrid and mouldy, then they mix it with the pickle juice and consume it along with the pickles.

It is a known fact that your average slum boy who wallows in the dirt of the gutter is a healthier specimen usually than the hygienized equivalent of the wealthier families. There is even a theory held by some that germs do not cause disease but that they multiply when disease comes into the body. Most of us harbor the polio virus but it becomes active only in some of us and under certain conditions.

There is an amazing article in *This Week* of August 8, 1954. Dr. Eugene H. Payne, a member of the medical research staff of the pharmaceutical firm of Parke, Davis and Co. on an expedition to South America observed that in the town of Cruzeiro in Brazil, a place of poverty and unbelievable filth there is no cancer—not a case in the experience of the local health officer.

Dirt is an involved subject, and I have accumulated a great deal of evidence which shows that under certain conditions and in certain cases it is not as harmful as we imagine; in fact, sometimes it may conduce to good health. Of course, I would not want to drink polluted water, nor wear a shirt more than one day, but I brush my teeth, not to clean them, but only because it gives my mouth a pleasant tasting feeling. I am not ready to go into the general subject of dirt at this time and please don't go out and start wallowing in the gutter, but I would like to reproduce here an item which would be part of my essay on dirt. It is a translation of a chapter from a French book I came across the other day which describes what was done in France with the crusts of bread that the average French housewife threw out. The book is termed *The Rag-pickers' Basket* and was published in 1885. It seems that nothing that was thrown out in Paris in those days eluded the skilled hand of the rag picker. If it had no value he blew the breath of value into it. Let us see how they handled thrown out bread crusts in the Paris of the eighteen eighties:

Bread Crusts

You remember well the answer given me by a rag-picker whom I asked what he did with the crusts of bread he gathered in the gutter.

"When they are clean," he said, "I eat them, but when they are dirty I make you eat them."

The bread crusts are gathered almost exclusively by travelling rag-pickers. Almost any home, even the most modest, throws away some bread. When the bread is not too dirty, the cooks give it to the rag-pickers. When it is too dirty they throw it in the garbage can, to the very bottom of which the rag-picker will dig to find it.

When he returns to the city, the rag-picker sorts out his bread just as he sorts out rags or bones. First he puts aside what is on top of the basket—that is, the cleanest, the most appetizing crusts—those are for him. That is the bread he and his family dunk in their soup. If the harvest is good (and for the travelling rag-pickers the bread harvest is very important) he resells the crusts to his colleagues who have no home—the rovers and the outriders; he sells them too to all those poor friends who live near the city, who never eat and whose children never eat any other bread except what they buy from the rag-pickers.

There are in Paris small shopkeepers who cannot keep their children with them and who, not wishing to farm them out in the country where it would be hard to go to see them, give them over to the fine characters of Clichy or Puteaux who undertake to care for them. The poor parents never know that the only thing their children have to eat at the homes of these honest burghers is pap made from the crusts of bread bought from the rag-pickers. Wander around the Boulevard de la Révolte any morning between seven and nine and you will see in every corner of the street and in the miserable shops enormous sacks full of bread crusts. Housewives arrive and demand 'two cents for my foster child.' For their two cents they get more than a pound of bread. Thanks to this system the foster parents are able to raise a little Parisian child and realize a good profit over their modest pensions.

When the bread crusts are dirty, they sell for a penny and sometimes a half a penny a pound. They use them to fatten poultry, rabbits and pigs. With these bread crusts the travelling rag-picker feeds his horse. The poor beast never tastes oats. They give him every day six or seven pounds of bread crusts. If this is not enough it is up to the horse to get himself some grass browsing around.

But sometimes it happens that the bread crusts are all dirty. They have been trampled in the gutter, they give off a nauseating odor. The rabbits refuse to eat them. The chickens (which are not especially fastidious) sneer at them. The ducks themselves scorn them. What to do? The rag-pickers have sought and they have found out. Since the animals won't eat them, they say to themselves, well, then we'll give them to the good middle class families to eat. And, in fact, all these dreadfully dirty bread crusts are eaten by just such families The process is very simple. They treat the crusts just as if they were coffee. They place them in a broiler and roast them. When they are toasted to the point where they are crisp, they powder them in a coffee mill. This powder is then sifted. The coarsest part which will not go through the holes of the sieve is sold as bread crumbs. With these bread crumbs the restaurant keepers of the Latin Quarter sprinkle their hams from Reims, and bread their cutlets *à la milanaise*.

What can you expect when for 18 cents they give you soup, two platters, a dessert and a bottle of wine, they've got to be economical somewhere! Even so the students don't complain much. They know full well that what passes for butter is margarine; they know that what is listed on the menu as rabbit is really cat; they know too that the filet of beef was cut from the flank of a horse; and that the wine they are drinking contains more red dye than the juice of the grape. But they know too that their meal complete costs only 18 cents and for them that is the main thing. Perhaps they ignore the fact that under the guise of soup with croutons and breaded cutlets, they eat bread crusts that no one could get animals to eat.

One day at the Sorbonne I attended a conference on the rag-picking industry. At the moment when I was speaking of how these bread crusts are used, one listener who could no longer restrain his indignation, turned to his neighbor and cried "Here is a fellow who wants to ruin commerce!" The gentleman was Mr. . . . Mr. X I'll call him, one of the restaurant owners of the Latin Quarter who for 18 cents gives you a complete meal.

The commerce in bread crusts must be pretty important if this honorable man of industry could no longer contain his indignation but had to blurt out all the mysteries of his kitchen.

However, for bread crumbs, the rag pickers can use only the crusts that are not too fine or too brown. What then of the powder—absolutely black and hard—the crusts that were burned in the toasting? You think perhaps our friends, the rag-pickers, are at a loss as to what to do with these? I guess you don't know them very well. Out of this powder made of burnt toast, they make tooth powder and chicory which your grocer sells you with the label "extra chicory." In this case the "extra" is an abbreviation for "extraordinary."

* * END * *

You would imagine that with such an unsanitary conception underlying the preparation of restaurant food at least half of Paris should have died out in a plague. Now, while the death rate was high in the Paris of the eighties, I wonder if the eating of such bread had much to do with it? I am merely wondering! We must not jump to conclusions. Let us leave this point unsettled until some future date when I can go into the subject more thoroughly. In the meantime, I resort again to wondering. Which would you rather eat—the rag-pickers' bread, or our modern staff of life with polyoxyethylenemonosterate, sodium propionate, coal tar enrichments and the host of other chemicals that it is treated with down the line of processing? I am just wondering!

Dizziness

"How do you describe this dizzy feeling of yours?" asks the doctor of the many patients who come to him complaining of dizziness. "It's a terrible sensation of spinning and whirling," one patient may say. And another, "I feel as if I were going to faint and I become anxious and perspire." Another patient may say, "I feel dizzy only when I'm walking or standing," or "It's only in the early morning when I first get up that I feel dizzy," or "I'm dizzy only when I have my eyes open" or "When I get up suddenly from a lying-down position, everything whirls around me." Some patients describe a plunging sensation, as if they were falling from a great height. Others tell of blacking out soon after the dizzy spell has passed.

Medical men agree that getting an accurate description of the sensation of dizziness is difficult. The doctor, you see, has no way of knowing how you feel. He cannot see, or hear, feel or test your dizziness. You have to describe it to him. And you may do so with great hesitancy because your friends and family may have been scoffing at your "dizzy spells" and calling them imaginary or psychosomatic.

Apparently a large number of patients over middle age go to their doctors complaining of dizziness. In fact some medical men speak of dizziness as one of the commonest symptoms in their older patients. In articles on the subject, printed in medical magazines, all the possible physical reasons for dizziness are explained. These have to do mostly with eye and ear ailments and disorders of the heart and blood vessels. In general, doctors can locate the cause of the trouble in these cases and can relieve the dizziness whether or not they cure the thing that was causing it.

There is a disease called Ménière's Disease (after the physician who first described it) which involves vertigo (or spinning, whirling sensations) and generally deafness, too. It is believed that the disease comes about as a result of a hemorrhage into the semi-circular canals—those small, delicate parts of the inner ear. Other ear troubles can cause dizziness, too. Among young people, dizziness is frequently the result of eye disorders and new glasses will often clear it up entirely Anemia can cause dizziness, because in anemic individuals less oxygen is being carried to the brain. Acute infectious diseases may bring on dizziness, too. Or a sudden attack of labyrinthitis, which is an infection of the inner ear, generally resulting from a bad cold.

The dizzy sensations associated with blood vessel disorders can be relieved by bringing the pressure down, or up in the cases of too low blood pressure. As we grow older many of us begin to develop "hardening of the arteries" which means that there are deposits on the inside walls of the blood vessels, narrowing them so that there is much less room for the blood to flow freely. Someone with high blood pressure may find that getting up from a lying down position brings on an attack of dizziness. Older arteries cannot so easily adjust themselves to a sudden demand for extra blood in one part of the body or another. So as you swing your feet to the floor and stand up, especially if you do it hastily, the blood may be drained out of your head too fast, bringing on a feeling of dizziness.

On the other hand, the person whose blood pressure is quite low may have the same experience. In this case the pressure under which the blood is flowing through the arteries may not be enough to raise a sufficient amount of blood to the head, when the position is changed suddenly. This is spoken of as "postural hypotension," for the sudden demand for blood lowers the blood pressure rapidly and it takes a few minutes to adjust to the new position.

Of course, readers should know that we believe blood pressure that is too high or too low can be controlled very satisfactorily by proper diet. It is important, too, not to subject yourself to these sudden changes in position. If you are lying down when the telephone rings, take your time about getting to your feet. Move slowly and let your blood vessels adjust gradually to the changed posture. If the telephone has stopped ringing by the time you get there, never mind. They will call back if it's important.

Much Dizziness Seems to Have no Organic Basis

But what about those cases of dizziness that have no basis in anything being physically wrong? Suppose you have been suffering from dizziness, or vertigo, or giddiness or whatever you want to call it, and the ear and eye doctor can find nothing wrong. Your own doctor tells you that your blood pressure is not responsible. Where do you turn then? Judging from medical magazines, there must be a vast number of bewildered folks walking around with just such a problem and no answer as to what to do for it Are you imagining the dizziness? Are you becoming dizzy in order to avoid something unpleasant that you don't want to face? Should you see a psychiatrist?

First of all, we must remember that dizziness may be a symptom of vitamin deficiency. It has been found even in mild cases of niacin and thiamin deficiency. These are two of the B vitamins. And, as we have stated many times, it is impossible to be deficient in just one or two of the B vitamins. They occur together in many foods. If you have not been getting enough of those foods, you will lack all of the B vitamins, not just one or two. It is also true that these same healthful foods are rich in other vitamins as well, so you may be suffering from a case of what the doctors call "multiple deficiency" if you are well enough to get around and carry on your activities, but are suffering from dizzy spells.

One more very good reason why you might suspect B vitamin deficiency, is that modern American diets are glutted with refined carbohydrates which can cause deficiency in B vitamins even in someone who does eat some healthful foods as well. By "refined carbohydrates" we mean those foods that have been processed to such an extent that few if any vitamins remain in them—white bread and anything else made from white flour like cake, macaroni, crackers, and so forth. White sugar has been refined, so that anything containing white sugar is quite likely to bring about a vitamin B deficiency for this reason: carbohydrates must be accompanied by B vitamins or your body cannot digest and assimilate them. Every mouthful of refined carbohydrates you eat robs your body of B vitamins which are essential for good digestion, healthy nerves, skin, tissues and scores of other body functions. Perhaps your dizziness is the result of a diet that regularly contains such items as soft drinks, pastries, candy, ice cream and so forth, and not enough of the protective foods.

Breathlessness, Dizziness and Palpitation

An article by Lawrence C. Kolb of the Mayo Clinic in Minnesota appears in the October, 1950, issue of the *North Carolina Medical Journal.* Dr. Kolb tells of patients who complain of breathlessness, dizziness and heart palpitations. Before we get into a description of his observations, we want to remind you that lack of B vitamins, especially thiamin which is vitamin B_1, can result in breathlessness. By this we mean a feeling of not being able to take a good deep breath, with the result that you are always puffing and panting and sighing without ever having the feeling of getting enough breath. A friend of ours suffered from this feeling for several years; no doctor gave her any relief and she had resigned herself to seeing a psychiatrist when someone suggested that she switch to whole grain cereals and whole grain bread, and take brewer's yeast. Her breathlessness disappeared in a matter of weeks.

Dr. Kolb believes that breathlessness, palpitation and dizziness may be caused by what he calls "over-breathing"—that is, breathing too deeply and too rapidly. The first symptom is light-headedness or giddiness, he says. Then the individual may feel that he is going to faint, he may perspire profusely and his gait may become unsteady. Then he feels suffocated and begins to breathe even more deeply and rapidly to gulp in as much air as possible. This, of course, makes matters worse. His fingers and toes may begin to tingle and contract in cramps. As he gets more panicky, the symptoms may become worse and worse until he finally becomes unconscious.

What is happening, of course, is simply that he is taking in air too fast for his lungs and blood to adjust their carbon dioxide-oxygen ratio. He is getting too much oxygen for the amount of carbon dioxide in his body. "Hyperventilation" is another word for it. Anxiety may bring on the attack. The anxious person tends to sigh, pant and yawn. This brings in too much air for his lungs to handle properly, so he feels he must take even deeper breaths. (And let us remind you again at this point, even though Dr. Kolb does not mention it, that B vitamin deficiency can produce exactly this same state of affairs.)

Dr. Kolb goes on to discuss what a medical doctor can do to relieve his patients of the anxiety that causes them to "over-breathe." He describes several interesting cases. In one case a girl who was taking flying lessons developed giddiness, tingling and cramps in her hands just as she was bringing her plane down to earth. In another case, a very energetic and capable woman had attacks of breathlessness every morning. It turned out that the anxiety which brought on the attacks resulted from an unsympathetic husband and the woman's own repressed desire to be doing some useful and creative work. Her children had married and left home and all her energy and ability were being wasted, she believed. Dr. Kolb always explains to his patients what is meant by over-breathing and then tells them to practice it, right there in his office. By breathing deeply and rapidly they can often reproduce exactly the symptoms they have been trying to describe. The surest way to bring the whole business to a happy conclusion is, first, to learn to breathe slowly and naturally. It may be necessary to hold one's breath or breathe into a paper bag to stop attacks resulting from "over-breathing." (The reason for the paper bag is that by breathing into it, you re-breathe some of the needed carbon dioxide.)

Low Blood Sugar and Insecticides May Be Responsible

Low blood sugar is frequently mentioned in medical literature as a cause of dizziness. This would, it seems to us, explain the many people who complain of dizziness when they first get out of bed in the morning. For blood sugar tends to be lowest just before breakfast. Low blood sugar is the opposite of diabetes and involves a blood sugar mechanism that does not manage to keep the blood sugar high enough all day long so that the individual feels well. Other symptoms are fatigue, abnormal hunger, irritability and so forth. The low blood sugar patient generally feels fine (and not dizzy at all) just after meals, for eating raises the blood sugar up to where it should be. But long before his next meal he may feel tired, hungry or dizzy and, in extreme cases, may actually black out.

The cure is very simple—a diet high in protein and low in starches and sugars, a diet that includes none of the refined carbohydrates we were speaking about earlier. Coffee, alcohol and cigarettes are far worse for the low blood sugar patient than for ordinary people, for each of these raises the blood sugar too high, then plunges it far below what it should be. The persons bothered with low blood sugar (and one prominent physician estimates that they are far more numerous than diabetics) should eat frequently. But all between-meal snacks should be protein (meat, fish, eggs, nuts, etc.) or fruit. Never, never starchy or sugary snacks.

One last, but very important, comment on dizziness. It is one of the early symptoms of poisoning by insecticides. We do not mean to imply that everybody who feels dizzy from time to time has been fatally poisoned with DDT, chlordane, lindane or one of the other new and powerful insecticides. But we do believe (and there is ample proof in medical journals) that people who continually eat sprayed fruits without washing and peeling them, eventually store up enough of these cumulative substances to bring on the early symptoms of poisoning.

Editor Rodale has told of his experience eating cherries that had been sprayed and the persistent attacks of dizziness that tormented him for days until he analyzed the probable cause and stopped his cherry-eating binge. Cherries, grapes, berries and other fruits that cannot be peeled are not recommended, unless you can get organically grown ones. With other fruits, buy those that have been sprayed the least, scrub them thoroughly (though this does not accomplish a great deal) and then peel them before eating them. The same goes for vegetables. If you possibly can, buy your produce organically grown. If not, take the utmost care in preparing it. And protest to your local farm agent and to the people from whom you buy produce. Tell them you much prefer fruits and vegetables that have a few worms or bugs to fruits and vegetables thoroughly poisoned by insecticides.

Drugs—Doctor Chooses Milder Drugs

By J. I. Rodale

In my capacity as editor of *Prevention* magazine, it is necessary to read a certain number of medical journals each month, in search of new developments in the field of preventive medicine. Occasionally in such reading I encounter an item which falls in two categories. It deals with some health or medical subject and at the same time illustrates something of interest to agriculturists. Being also editor of our gardening magazine, I do not have to tell you that when I find such an item my blood courses a little faster through my veins. In this respect I am extremely fortunate in not only being interested in these two fields of knowledge, but in having the opportunity of being so close to both of them. It is as if I am sitting comfortably atop a broad wall which cleaves two large fields. In one of them the doctors are working. On the other side are the people who are producing our food. One group seldom sees the other, but fortunate *me* in sitting on top with the wonderful privilege of seeing into both. It is my hope that in the not too distant future, this wall will be demolished, so that food will be produced with the cooperation of the medical profession, and that medical research will be combined with agricultural research.

I came across the particular item which made me write this article a few months ago in the *Archives of Pediatrics* for July, 1952. It was in an article entitled "Light Magnesium Carbonate in the Treatment of Acute Glomerular Nephritis," which gives you an idea of the stuff I have to read in order to keep up with my activities. But whether it is glomerular nephritis, or some other kind, you don't have to worry. All you have to know is that nephritis is an inflammation or disease of the kidneys, and let the doctors take care of the rest.

The article is based on the observations of, and was written by C. L. Thenebe, M.D., of West Hartford, Connecticut, and I can say that he is a man after my own heart. He doesn't take things for granted. Just because it has become the custom to use a certain medicine for a certain condition does not mean that Dr. Thenebe blindly keeps on using that medicine. He is not afraid to experiment towards finding a milder and safer one, and herein lies our lesson.

Part of the usual treatment for glomerular nephritis is magnesium sulphate, but in the case of his patients, Dr. Thenebe began to use the simpler magnesium *carbonate* form of this medication which was recently developed by Merck and Company.

Before I go any further, it would be best if I explain the difference between two forms of fertilizer, which also illustrate the difference between two methods of using the same substance. Then you will the better see what I am driving at in comparing the two forms of magnesium medication. Organic farmers and gardeners use the raw ground-up phosphate rock for their phosphate. It is a product made with a minimum of manufacturing processing. The rock is merely ground up, and this is done as fine as possible so that the small particles will disintegrate in the earth with the proper conditions of moisture, warmth, the presence of the necessary organic matter and soil organisms. And the smaller the ground-up article, the quicker its decomposition.

But it is the belief of those who advocate the use of chemical fertilizers that this decomposition is not quick enough—that there is not enough release of phosphate for the needs of the plant. This may be true in soil which has been treated with chemical fertilizers for a long time and which is low in organic matter, but organic practitioners have had no trouble getting sufficient phosphate from the raw phosphate rock. Their harvesting results prove it. The companies that manufacture superphosphate take this raw, ground-up phosphate rock powder and mix it with an equal amount of sulphuric acid—fifty-fifty. The resulting compound is a very soluble one, making the phosphorus more available to the plant's nutritional requirements. While this may be true, it is the feeling of the organic school that too much solubility is harmful. The plant absorbs too much of some elements, other needed items being left out of the plant's feeding, and imbalances occur. It is similar to the way some persons eat a lot of candy, coca-cola and highly refined foods. It peps them up for the moment, but what is the ultimate effect on their bodies? In the case of the product we have been discussing, namely, superphosphate, the plant can use much phosphate but little of the sulphur, which, therefore, piles up in the soil cumulatively each year, to give it a far too high sulphur content.

There are many kinds of bacteria in the soil—each with its own function to perform, and among them are the sulphur-reducing organisms whose sole work is to reduce sulphur compounds. If sulphur keeps on piling up, these bacteria keep on multiplying and a strange thing happens. This sulphur-reducing bacteria feeds on a certain mold which itself has an extremely important role in the soil fertility processes. This mold aids in the decay of organic matter, so that the more superphosphate is used, the more sulphur piles up in the soil, the more sulphur-reducing bacteria are brought into existence, the more they feed on the organic-matter-decaying molds, and eventually the crop residues that are plowed under will take much too long to decay for lack of the necessary organisms which do this work.

Lady Eve Balfour in her book *The Living Soil* (Devin-Adair Co., New York) describes an experiment in which a quantity of cotton was placed in a soil treated organically and a similar quantity in soil where chemical fertilizers had been used. The cotton decayed much faster in the organic soil, and the theory described above was probably one of the reasons for it.

Experiments and actual farming practice indicate that where there is sufficient organic matter in the soil, the raw rock will equal, if not exceed, the effect of the superphosphate. The organic matter also reduces the alkalinity of some soils which (alkalinity) prevents the raw phosphate rock from working. The raw rock is not only much cheaper, but it is also much healthier for the soil.

It is this same thing that I would like to indicate as between the doctor's use of the plain magnesium carbonate and the more dangerous magnesium sulphate. But in order to get more information on the difference between magnesium carbonate and magnesium sulphate, let us consider limestone. Practically 90 per cent of the average limestone is calcium carbonate. Carbon, in the form it occurs in rocks, is not a dangerous substance for the soil. In fact, carbon sometimes makes up 40 per cent of the content of plants. But in gypsum, which is found in the form of a powder, we find that the formula is—calcium sulphate—which means a very large amount of sulphur. In the organic method we shun the use of gypsum on account of its high sulphur content, and because, while it gives good results the first few years, it depresses the crop yields later. There is an old saying that the use of gypsum enriches the father but impoverishes the son. We see, therefore, a difference between the use of limestone (calcium carbonate) and gypsum (calcium sulphate), which is so similar to the doctor's use of magnesium—that is, magnesium carbonate instead of magnesium sulphate.

But chemistry is quite a tricky thing and I must describe a product which seems to indict the *carbonate* form of a substance, for I do not wish to be accused of picking out only those parts of the subject which suit my convenience. A commonly used chemical fertilizer is nitrate of soda. However, a plant can use much of the nitrate but little of the soda. With a yearly application of this fertilizer, therefore, the soda keeps piling up in the soil, combining with carbon to form sodium carbonate, more usually referred to as carbonate of soda, which is nothing but washing soda, and which destroys the soil's structure, causing a severe hardening.

I know, in this case, that the carbon in the carbonate of soda must take some share of the blame, but that it is the soda that is the principal mischief-maker. As between the magnesium carbonate and the magnesium sulphate, of the doctor's experiment, we know from actual experience that the carbonate form is a very mild substance compared to the sulphate form. It is the same with the calcium carbonate, or limestone, which is fed to babies in the form of limewater and which is a mild form indeed. Many of us get much calcium carbonate in our drinking water. That is what makes it "hard."

According to the article in the *Archives of Pediatrics,* Dr. Thenebe states that he used the magnesium carbonate on eight patients. He says, "Comparably, magnesium carbonate tastes much better and it is not at all nauseating. It is harmless in large doses."

Using sulphur in the soil is one thing. We believe it to be very bad farming practice. But putting it into one's own stomach is a hundred times worse. In agriculture, the plant screens out a good part of the effect of the sulphur, but to subject the human organism directly to the poisonous effect of this chemical is to be flirting with great danger.

Let us talk a little about sulphur. In 1949 and 1950 I wrote thirteen articles in *Organic Gardening* magazine, under the title "Cancer; Can it be Prevented?" Unfortunately this book is out of print and unavailable. In this booklet I describe a theory based on the work of C. E. Green, discussed in his book called *The Cancer Problem,* that sulphur ingested by the human system is one of the causes of cancer. Green, who, by the way, is not a physician, builds such a remarkable case against sulphur, that I don't see how anyone who reads his book can fail to be influenced by it. He gives detailed statistics for England showing that where much coal smoke is breathed in, there is more cancer. There is much sulphur in coal smoke. His book is out of print and is available only in a few large libraries (the New York library is one).

I think that in view of Mr. Green's work, the medical profession should be conscious of the danger of using drugs in the sulphate form in their medications. A whole series of experiments should be made to find substitutes. I note that many valuable mineral preparations which are given to people to prevent disease are in the sulphate form. *Prevention* will not accept advertisements of such products. In an emergency, where it is a case of life and death, sometimes the sulphate form of a drug might be advisable, but it should be avoided in treatments that extend over a period of time.

We recall grandma's old panacea of sulphur and molasses as a springtime tonic. I have never taken it for such a purpose and certainly do not recommend it to anyone. It is a shot-in-the-arm method, resulting in a temporary quickening of the system. Rather take vitamins and minerals which do not contain dangerous amounts of sulphur. We know that some sulphur is needed by the human body, but we can get a sufficient amount of it from a well-balanced diet.

Incidentally, the magnesium sulphate which Dr. Thenebe is trying to get away from is commonly called epsom salts, which the dictionary will tell you is "a white crystalline substance used in medicine as a cathartic or commercially in dyeing or finishing cotton goods, etc." If they would take *my* advice, they would strictly limit its use to dyeing and such things.

Dr. Thenebe has done an excellent piece of thinking. He just didn't blindly accept what he found listed in the *Materia Medica.* He was considerate of the general welfare of his patients' bodies, while at the same time being cognizant of their condition of disease which he must cure. Dr. Thenebe, you should be highly complimented.

Drugs

Here is a casual letter to the editor that appeared in the *British Medical Journal* for February 13, 1954. The physician inquires what can be done for the deafness that is caused by therapy with streptomycin, how long it is likely to last and whether a hearing aid will be useful in such cases. Just as casually the editor replies that prolonged therapy with streptomycin (one of the antibiotics) may result in deafness, especially if more than one gram daily is given for at least three weeks. If there is to be any improvement in this drug-induced deafness, it will likely take place within a few weeks after the patient has stopped taking the drug. It is unlikely, says the *Journal,* that any further improvement will occur after six months. A hearing aid may help, but again it may not, depending on the amount of destruction that has been done.

We might assume from this correspondence that the physician in question has given streptomycin for some condition (possibly even a minor one) and has discovered that his patient has developed a much more serious condition which may turn out to be incurable—deafness. Many pages of many issues of medical journals are given over to warnings about the indiscriminate use of the antibiotics and the possible dangerous results. Yet in many other articles there are reports of antibiotics like streptomycin being given casually without an inkling as to whether or not they ever have been or will be useful in such conditions. And the risk the patient unknowingly runs is permanent deafness! In other pages of the same medical journals we have found accounts of disorders for which antibiotics are frequently prescribed being cured with vitamin and mineral therapy where there is no possible, conceivable after-effect except improved health.

Why is it? Are all patients today looking for a one-shot cure, regardless of side-effects? Are all doctors too busy to spend any time at all talking nutrition to their patients? Or do they simply ignore the wealth of information in their own medical journals having to do with nutrition in its relation to good health? We do not know.

Unhappy Results From Drugs

A second article comes from *Consumers' Research Bulletin* for January, 1954, quoting Dr. William Boyd, Professor of Pathology, University of British Columbia, in an address before a medical meeting. Dr. Boyd pointed out that in many cases the treatment of disease—even with all our modern knowledge of the action of drugs—brings about unhappy results. For example, he said, a patient suffering from pain may be given barbiturates only to die of agranulocytosis (a decrease in the number of blood cells); burns relieved with tannic acid may be followed by necrosis of the liver (destruction of liver cells); blood transfusions may save countless lives, but may also be responsible for cases of hemoglobinuric nephrosis and anuria (kidney disease and suppression of the urine), no matter how carefully the blood may have been grouped and matched.

Dr. Boyd goes on to say that changes in diet and habits bring new perils; excessive use of tobacco, consumption of over-refined foods and the stress of modern living are likely to produce new disease symptoms. Does anyone warn us day by day of these hazards? Does your daily paper ever point out the perils of barbiturates, blood transfusions, over-refined foods? If not, why not?

Absorption of Ink Nearly Fatal

Here is shocking news that appeared in *Time* magazine for February 15, 1954. Thirty newborn infants in a Uruguay Hospital turned blue from a hemoglobin disorder. Fifteen of the babies seemed to be near death. Oxygen tents were brought in and the blood of all of the infants was completely changed by transfusion—that is, all of each baby's own blood was drained out while other blood from the blood bank was poured into his veins. (What did we just find out about possible danger from blood transfusions?)

The cause of this almost tragic incident was the ink used for marking the hospital's name on the babies' diapers. Aniline oil from the ink had seeped through the skin into the babies' blood. How is it possible, with our present scientific knowledge, for such an accident to occur? It is possible because we have become so accustomed to treating poisonous substances casually that we simply do not take proper precautions. We do not know whether such marking ink is used in hospitals in this country. If it is, we suppose there will have to be some similar incident here before orders will be issued to check carefully that all diapers have been boiled before being used.

Arthritis From Blood Pressure Drug

An article in *Science News Letter* for March 6, 1954, tells us that one of the new remedies for reducing blood pressure has been found to produce arthritis and other diseases of the joints in 17 of 211 patients who were taking the drug. It goes by the name of hydralazine hydrochloride combined with hexamethnium chloride—the whole treatment being called "hyphex therapy." The arthritis disappears when the drug is stopped, we understand, but then the high blood pressure returns. "Meanwhile" says *Science News Letter,* "because the arthritis and other reactions are reversible and do not develop in all patients and because the hazard of service and malignant high blood pressure is real, doctors may have to take the 'calculated risk' of continuing to use hydralazine in some patients whose high blood pressure endangers their health."

Why? Medical literature mentions many completely harmless remedies for high blood-pressure in the way of diet. In many other lands than ours high blood pressure is unknown. Have we devoted as much time and money to studying the reason for this as we have spent developing the drug that causes arthritis? Which of us is being unreasonable and far-fetched—the researcher who says, "I have here a drug that will bring down your blood pressure but will give you arthritis instead" or the so-called food-faddist who says "I have here a diet that will prevent your getting high blood pressure and will cure you if you have it?"

Our main concentration in modern medicine appears to be to remove the symptoms of disease. High blood pressure is a symptom of disorder. What use is there to remove the symptom and let the disorder go on unchecked? Especially, if removing the symptom means bringing on other equally bad, or worse, symptoms.

Synthetic Blood Plasma

Dextran is the newest and most famous blood plasma substitute. Plasma is the fluid part of the blood, as separate from the corpuscles and other bodies that float in the fluid. In our modern preoccupation with synthetics, we have decided that we can manufacture blood plasma every bit as good as that nature gave us. Then instead of giving transfusions of real blood plasma we can save money by transfusing a synthetic substance into the live veins. According to an article in *The Medical Journal of Australia* for December 19, 1953, dextran has not produced any dangerous reactions in patients who had lost a great deal of their own plasma. However, more recently it seems there have been quite serious effects produced in normal healthy people given dextran as an experiment. In the case reported, five volunteers, with the normal amount of plasma, had injections of dextran. Reactions were produced in each of the five. They began with a sudden case of hives which lasted up to two hours or more after the injection was over. Then there were serious vasomotor disturbances—that is, disorders of blood pressure. Finally there was pain around the heart, a feeling of fullness in the head, breathlessness and a reduced capacity for exertion.

Now you might decide that these manifestations of something wrong were just the result of the volunteers having too much blood plasma altogether, with the synthetic added to their own. But you might discover, on the other hand, that the dextran itself, in its synthetic purity, had brought about these alarming symptoms. If this is indeed the case, why go on infusing dextran into the blood vessels of people suffering from wounds, shock or illness?

Our hat is off to those medical men mentioned so often in these pages who treat well patients in order to keep them well, to those medical men who prescribe good nourishing food and food supplements for their patients who are ailing, thus preventing any more serious illness. And finally we salute those medical men who have steadfastly held to the belief that the substances placed by nature in food are the true preventives and cures for disease and who use carefully prescribed diets and vitamins and minerals in massive doses if need be, to cure illness, rather than using drugs and taking the well-known "calculated risk" so popular these days.

Drugs and Headaches

At a hospital in France a 31-year-old woman was recently treated for a severe headache. Her symptoms indicated that there might be something as serious as brain tumor involved. An operation revealed that her brain was extensively swollen. Later it was discovered that she had been taking pills for a boil. She had taken 29 of these in six days. The pills contained an organic stannous salt—that is, a salt made from tin. According to the report from France, given in the *Journal of the American Medical Association* for September 11, 1954, many deaths have been reported in that country from symptoms suggesting brain abscesses or tumors and in many cases the board of health has discovered that these patients, too, were taking pills containing the tin solution.

Arthritis Drug Produces Liver Disease

A drug called phenylbutazone is the villain in a horrifying story in the *Journal of the American Medical Association* for September 11, 1954. The author, Ephraim P. Engleman, M.D. and his associates relate the stories of six women who had been taking this drug for bursitis or arthritic pains. All the women developed hepatitis or liver disease. Two of them died, the others recovered in from 3 to 15 weeks. It is well known that hepatitis can result from blood transfusions or other injections in which the needle may not have been properly sterilized. But none of these patients had had injections. The authors conclude that it was the phenylbutazone which brought on the hepatitis and they add "hepatitis is another possible hazard in the therapeutic use of this drug." They do not state what the other hazards are, but we assume from this that there are many others as well. There always are in the use of drugs. No matter how hard we try, we are never going to find a drug that cures a disorder in one part of the body without throwing something else out of kilter. Good health is the result of natural foods and a healthful way of life. It cannot be induced by drugs.

Anesthesia Victims

A study of spinal anesthesia reported in the *Illinois Medical Journal* for April, 1954, reveals the fact that of more than 10,000 consecutive cases studied, there were complications in 18 which could probably be traced to the anesthesia. In all cases these were nerve disorders. In five of the cases it was found the conditions had existed prior to the operation which indicated that this kind of anesthesia should not have been given. The authors, M. S. Sadove and M. J. Levin, stress the fact that complete neurological examinations should be made before the type of anesthesia to be used is decided upon. The other 13 patients had strokes, cardiac arrest, persistent headaches, chronic backaches and so forth, resulting from the anesthesia. The authors do not believe that these eighteen cases should constitute an indictment of spinal anesthesia, for, they say, this compares favorably with the record for other kinds of anesthesia. They *do* indicate that there are apparently quite a number of physicians who oppose the use of spinal anesthesia altogether.

Epilepsy Drug Harms Gums

A drug given for epilepsy has been found to cause a serious gum disease, according to *The Medical Press* for June 30, 1954. That *epanutin,* or *sodium diphenyl dydantoinate,* can produce these results has recently been shown by Dr. W. J. King's article in the *British Dental Journal* for May 18, 1954. King studied closely the characteristic gum symptoms that occurred in human beings who had taken the drug. Then, by feeding the drug to laboratory animals, he brought about the same conditions in the animals' mouths. Do you suppose it has occurred to any of these investigators that the drug, being poisonous, may use up the body's supply of vitamin C—the vitamin that fights valiantly against body poisons? And surely if you are trying to get along on too little vitamin C, your gums will suffer, probably first of all. If doctors have to give poisonous drugs, why not give something at the same time to help counteract their poisonous effect?

Boric Acid Poisoning

Another warning on boric acid is sounded by the *Medical Journal of Australia* for July 24, 1954. Recently our American newspapers have carried articles purporting to show that there is no danger at all from using boric acid. We rather suspect these articles owe their origin to the press agents of some of the many firms that sell boric acid products. The Australian *Journal* begins its article with this statement: "That boric acid is potentially a poison which may have fatal results has been known for a long time, but it continues to be used particularly for infants from the traditional belief that it is a mild antiseptic and being mild must also have low toxicity." Reviewing two articles which discuss 105 cases of boric acid poisoning, 60 per cent of which were fatal, the *Journal* tells us that poisoning is most likely to occur on spots where the skin is broken. We are also told that probably many milder cases of poisoning have often occurred without being reported. The article ends, "It is incredible that a drug with such toxic propensities and doubtful therapeutic value should continue to enjoy such popularity in the armamentarium of so many physicians and occupy such a prominent place in the home medicine cabinets . . . boric acid should be replaced in medical practice with more efficient and safer medication."

Drug Addiction and the Medical Profession

From *The Journal of the American Medical Association,* volume 157, page 654, we learn that there is an alarming increase in addiction to a drug called demerol which is used in the treatment of chronic psychiatric and physical ailments. According to two physicians, a total of 144 persons were admitted yearly to the Public Health Service Hospital at Lexington, Kentucky, during 1950-1953, as compared with only six such patients during 1946-1947. Nearly one-half of the addicts admitted were physicians, nurses, or other individuals closely associated with the medical profession.

There is no reason, of course, why just the mere fact of being part of the medical profession should make one less susceptible to drug addiction. It does seem, though, that people who see illness and drug addiction constantly around them should be a little more wary of taking that first or second pill. And it does seem, too, that, with all the information available in medical journals on good nutrition that will make drugs unnecessary, there is less excuse for medical personnel to become addicts.

Pneumonia from Oily Nose Drops

Oily nose drops for colds not only give no relief, but may be the source of dangerous complications later on. In a study conducted by a group of Washington, D. C., physicians and reported in *Newsweek* for December 26, 1949, Dr. Theodore Winship of Garfield Memorial Hospital disclosed that lipoid pneumonia occurs most frequently in patients who have used nose drops or sprays over a long period of time, and also, incidentally, in persons who regularly use mineral oil as a laxative.

Such medicines are not poisonous in themselves, but they can get into the windpipe and so into the lungs. Death from lipoid pneumonia results from asphyxiation. It is especially important to avoid using nose drops on children who can easily inhale oily fragments of these preparations.

Miracle Drugs

According to a recent issue of a national magazine, the profits from the sale of "miracle" drugs have zoomed from $157,000,000 in 1939 to $1,100,000,000 in 1952. As noted by our informant, the A-V published by the American Anti-Vivisection Society, Philadelphia, Pa., "This is truly the 'miracle' drug industry since no one, not even pharmacists, will believe that sickness and disease have increased 700 per cent in the same period."

Drugs and Artists Don't Mix

The old idea that drugs can inspire artists to better creative work gets some confirmation from a study reported at the American Neurological Association, according to a Science Service release in the *New York Times* for August 10, 1955. But the study also confirms another idea scientists have had for some time—that nothing much comes of this drug-stimulated inspiration because the effect of the drug on the artist is to make him lack initiative, so that he won't start on new work.

In the tests four painters of national prominence were given two drugs—one of which is extracted from the Mexican plant peyote. Visions of color and music are supposed to be produced by using this drug. The painters duly reported that they saw wonderful pictures in their minds. But only one of them took to painting. The others just wanted to sit and enjoy the visions they saw. When somebody finally drove them to painting they did, according to judges, somewhat better painting than they ordinarily did.

Writers did not have the same experience. Only one was tested—a playwright. He had hallucinations and delusions as a result of taking the drug, but when he sat down to his typewriter he did not have much success and what he turned out did not come up to his usual level of literary performance.

How Drugs Affect You

An enlightening article in the *Illinois Medical Journal* for May, 1955, describes some of the toxic reactions you can expect to get from some of the drugs now being prescribed. Most of them can be alleviated by giving, says this author, "epinephrine, ephedrine, anti-histaminic agents, cortisone acetate or corticotropin." When you get into trouble giving drugs, you see, the way to get out is to give more drugs. Allergy is not the term to be applied to all such reactions as these, says the editor. Many times it is simply the original toxic or cumulative action of the drug that is showing itself. "Some drugs are so toxic they prove dangerous unless the patient is cooperative and reports frequently. Digitalis, curare, dicumarol and the thiocynates are in this group."

Then of course there are the reactions that are not deadly, but can be annoying—the drowsiness produced by some of the anti-histamines, the palpitation, jitters and shaking associated with the use of benzedrine. So long as we announce in loud tones that there is nothing harmful about symptoms such as these, other drug manufacturers can make good use of the drugs that cause them. For instance, anti-histamines are now being sold as sedatives! Amphetamines produce the disagreeable symptom of "no appetite." So we fix it up in a fancy box and sell it to people who want to reduce!

Then there are what the doctors call "secondary" effects of drugs. The best examples are the symptoms accompanying changes in bacterial flora of the intestines when you take certain of the antibiotics. To say it a little more plainly, the antibiotics kill bacteria—the good and the harmful bacteria alike.

Then there are idiosyncrasies—did you know that a sedative causes some people to become excited rather than sleepy? Intolerance to drugs is evidenced by the patients' developing symptoms of overdosage when he has had just a tiny amount of the drug. With all the trouble they have with drugs you'd think they'd find it easier to treat patients with vitamins. Vitamins never give anybody any kind of harmful reaction, except in a few isolated cases where tremendous doses of synthetic vitamins have been given. A better idea yet—since the drugs produce such pesky reactions, why not stay so healthy you'll never have to take them at all!

Eggs

Treasure houses wherein lie
Locked by nature's alchemy
Flesh and blood and brain and bones.

So goes an old rhyme on the subject of eggs. And, as we often find in folk sayings, the singer knew whereof he spoke. Eggs are in truth one of our best foods, especially to satisfy individual needs for protein which are heightened under certain circumstances. Children and infants, for instance, need protein for building new cells during growth. Prospective mothers need protein. Invalids recovering from sickness need protein for rebuilding broken down tissues. And for those of us who are healthy, the need for protein is also great, since body cells and tissues are constantly breaking down and wearing out and must be replaced.

Eggs are high quality protein—that is, they contain the essential amino acids, or building blocks of protein, in the correct quantity and proportion. This is not surprising when you stop to think that the actual substance of eggs, which we eat, has been carefully supplied by nature to nourish the unborn chick. So naturally just the proper food elements are there in just the right proportion. One egg contains about six grams of protein. The white of an egg is almost pure protein even to its jelly-like consistency. Aside from protein, eggs are rich in all the protective and essential vitamins and minerals, with the exception of vitamin C.

The shell makes up about 10 per cent of the weight of an egg, the white about 60 per cent and the yolk 30 per cent. The shell consists mostly of minerals—calcium, magnesium and phosphorus. The old practice of eating ground egg shells is a sensible one, as we now know, for it is one of the easiest and cheapest ways of securing minerals. If the shells can be ground finely enough the resulting powder will not be gritty. The egg white of a fresh egg should be a thick opalescent jelly. We sometimes try to judge the freshness of an egg by observing whether the white keeps its shape after the egg is broken rather than "running." But it has been discovered that some hens lay eggs whose whites are naturally "runny" even when they are fresh. The yolk of the egg is inside a protective membrane and we have not as yet discovered all the substances contained in egg yolk—they are many. And all of them apparently are important for human nutrition, as well as chick nutrition.

From the point of view of nutritive value, the fresher the egg the better it is for you, quite apart from the fact that its taste is better. Some slight amount of value is lost with every day the egg is in storage. Aside from fresh eggs, we can buy frozen or dried eggs. The whole egg does not freeze well, for the yolk becomes leathery, due to the content of the membranes in which it is enclosed. But eggs which have been separated and beaten may be frozen, either as whites, yolks or whole eggs. The resulting product will keep almost indefinitely in a deep freeze and, after thawing, can be used for cooking just as a fresh egg is. Since about half the "lay" for the entire year takes place on poultry farms between March and June, these good quality eggs may be frozen for use during the rest of the year when eggs are scarce and expensive.

Eggs are dried commercially by spraying them into heated air. During World War II the dried egg business grew into a major industry in this country. In the year 1941 alone 42 million pounds of dried eggs were processed. Dried eggs do not keep very well when stored at room temperature, for they have a tendency to develop "off flavors" and to absorb odors from other foods stored about them.

Handling and Storing Eggs

Candling is the process whereby eggs are inspected so that they may be graded as AA, A, B, or C quality eggs. The egg is held against a strong light in a darkened room and the experienced egg-candler can thus determine from a glance at the egg what it will look like after it is broken. If the embryo chick has already started to develop blood vessels the egg is discarded. If the white of the egg is bloody, indicating a possible hemorrhage in the egg-duct of the hen, the egg is discarded. Small flecks of blood in the egg yolk are not considered to be defects important enough for condemning the egg for human food. The government sets specifications for eggs which must be strictly followed by egg dealers. Incidentally so far as we have been able to determine, there is no difference nutritionally between white and brown eggs. In some localities white eggs are preferred and hence are more expensive. But there is no reason for this aside from customer preference.

You might think, looking at eggs, that the shell forms an impermeable coating capable of keeping out all bacteria. But egg shell is covered with microscopic air holes, making the egg liable to infection from germs unless it is handled correctly. Using water to wash eggs makes it even more likely that germs will pass through the air holes into the eggs. And of course by washing dirty eggs you will be certain to wash some of the dirt into the inside of the egg. So experts tell us that eggs should not be washed until they are ready for use. If they are to be stored they should be stored dry. They should always be kept at a cool temperature. Even a few hours at room temperature in the summer may render an egg useless for marketing. For of course heat encourages the growth of bacteria which cause spoiled or rotten eggs. So put your eggs into the refrigerator as soon as you bring them into the house—just as you do milk or butter.

In scientific literature we find only two cautions about eggs in human dietaries. It has been discovered that large amounts of raw egg white given every day produce illness. A substance in the raw egg white (called avidin) destroys the B vitamin biotin in the intestinal tract. So if you like raw eggs, as is or in fruit juice, we suggest having them that way not oftener than once or twice a week. Cooking destroys the avidin, so cook your eggs on the other days. Egg yolk contains cholesterol, the substance that has recently come into the limelight as a factor in hardening of the arteries. Some physicians forbid eggs to their high blood pressure patients. It is our belief that the formation of cholesterol on blood vessel walls indicate a disorder of body functioning and does not mean that too much cholesterol is being eaten. In natural foods, such as eggs, we believe that the substances (B vitamins) protect against hardening of the arteries and are present in ample quantity to safeguard health.

Down through the ages eggs have been the symbol of happiness, fertility and rebirth. In almost every culture—eggs are used ceremonially at holiday time, as we use them at Easter. The roundness of the egg indicates wholeness; the fact that it is the forerunner of the chick signifies rebirth, including all the hope and gladness of spring when the earth is renewed and reborn.

Eggs are rich in vitamins and minerals. They assume great importance as infant food because the human baby is naturally very short on iron. Eggs contain lots of iron and in addition copper which is necessary for the body to use iron properly. Eggs are one of the very few foods that contain vitamin D. They are rich in vitamin A and all the B vitamins.

Here is the vitamin and mineral content of 100 grams of eggs—which is about two medium sized ones:

Vitamin A	1140 International units
Vitamin D	50 units
Vitamin E	3 milligrams
Vitamin B	
Thiamin	120-150 micrograms
Riboflavin	340 micrograms
Niacin	.1 milligram
Pyridoxine	22 micrograms
Pantothenic acid	800-4800 micrograms
Biotin	9 micrograms
Calcium	68 milligrams
Phosphorus	224 milligrams
Iron	2.52 milligrams
Copper	.23 milligrams
Magnesium	.03 milligrams
Chlorine	106 milligrams

Eggs and Rheumatic Fever

Is it possible that eating or not eating eggs may have something to do with the occurrence of rheumatic fever? An editorial in the April 17, 1954, issue of the *British Medical Journal* discusses this theory at some length. It seems that one researcher, Wallis, first began to study the question of eggs in the diet of rheumatic fever patients. May G. Wilson, in her book, *Rheumatic Fever* (published by Oxford University Press, 1940), theorizes on the fact that cases of rheumatic fever reach their height in April and then decline during the summer months. Could this be because of the fact that eggs are plentiful during the spring and summer and not so plentiful (hence more expensive) during fall and winter months?

The scientific argument goes like this: Eggs contain choline, a B vitamin, which is essential for the health of the liver. Further facts about choline—it is necessary for all animals, especially the young. It must be present in the diet for the normal nutrition of baby chicks and for egg production in the hen. Choline is necessary for the manufacture of a certain substance in the blood—phospholipid. This substance, phospholipid, is one of the elements in normal blood that fights against streptococcus infection. Rheumatic fever is associated with streptococcal infection. Therefore, the reasoning goes, rheumatic fever might be conditioned partly by egg intake.

The editor of the *Journal* states that this is a long and tenuous chain of reasoning, but it can be tested to a certain extent. Wallis, writing in the *American Journal of Medical Science,* Vol. 227, page 167, 1954, relates how he did a survey among 184 adult and adolescent patients with rheumatic heart disease and a group of normal subjects. Forty-one per cent of the rheumatic heart patients said they thought they ate few eggs in childhood. Only 16 per cent of the normal people claimed they did not eat eggs. Ten per cent of the rheumatic heart patients declared they did not like eggs, as compared to five per cent of the other group.

How dependable can such figures be, since they are based on the patients' memories of their childhood? Perhaps we cannot call them infallible, but all precautions were taken during the survey to eliminate bias from the answers. Two other researchers, Coburn and Moore, reporting in the *American Journal of the Diseases of Children,* Vol. 65, page 744, 1943, state that the former diet of rheumatic heart children appeared to be lacking in eggs as well as other valuable nutritional elements. So they supplemented the diet of thirty convalescent children with the equivalent of four egg yolks a day. (The yolk of the egg is the part highest in choline.) The rheumatic fever recurred in only seven per cent of these children compared with a recurrence of 38 per cent in children whose diets were not so supplemented. Later in 1950 Coburn reported in the *Journal of the American Dietetic Association,* Vol. 26, page 345, that eight to ten egg yolks daily given to children who had previously had rheumatic fever prevented relapses when the children were later subjected to streptococcal infection.

What Does This Theory Mean To Us?

The editor of the *British Medical Journal* frankly admits that this whole theory about egg yolks is only a theory, but, says he, "we should welcome theories if they are founded on fact and lead to the discovery of more facts. The egg theory might be described as 'good in parts'."

By telling our readers this story from one of the leading medical journals of our day, we do not mean to imply that stuffing children with egg yolks to the exclusion of other foods will positively prevent or cure rheumatic fever. We think the theory is interesting from an entirely different point of view. What if a close examination of the diet of children who contract rheumatic fever should indicate that, through some quirk of circumstance or appetite, their diets were completely lacking in choline—the B vitamin that is apparently so important for preventing the disease? This would certainly mean that other B vitamins were lacking as well, for they appear in most of the same foods as choline. The lesson to be learned, we believe, is simply that the rules of good diet cannot be disregarded by any conscientious mother. And how and where are mothers expected to learn these vitally important facts about the proper foods for their children? Certainly not from the women's magazines.

Every mouthful of candy, soda pop, white bread, cake or dessert robs a child of a mouthful of good wholesome nutritious food which will protect him from many diseases, not just rheumatic fever. Every egg, piece of fruit, meat or cheese, every vegetable, every salad, every serving of real honest-to-goodness whole grain cereal means just so much more protection from the menace of poor health. And for the mother whose child refuses to eat foods that contain choline and the other B vitamins, the answer is just as simple as buying a package of powdered brewer's yeast (higher than any other food in most of the B vitamins) and using it liberally in preparing food in the kitchen. For suggestions on using brewer's yeast every day in your kitchen, we recommend our favorite general cook book, *Let's Cook it Right* by Adelle Davis, published by Harcourt, Brace and Company, New York, N. Y.

Epilepsy

From biblical times individuals have been afflicted with "seizures"—mysterious fits during which they fell to the ground and foamed at the mouth. Perfectly normal, happy, intelligent people the rest of the time, they suddenly appeared to have been bewitched when a seizure overtook them. Seizures, being unpredictable, often occurred in public, to the horror and fear of onlookers. Thus, during past ages a whole tradition of the supernatural grew up around epilepsy. Plainly these sufferers were possessed of demons. Why else would they froth at the mouth, twitch convulsively and be unaware of what had transpired after they awoke from the sleep that follows epileptic seizures?

As superstition waned and people ceased to believe overtly in witchcraft some other notions grew up to explain the phenomenon of epilepsy. Perhaps, since this disease seemed to be hereditary, it was caused by sins of the parents. It led to insanity, people said, or it led to feeblemindedness. It was caused by masturbation, they said. Epileptics became criminals, they said, they should not marry or have children. In fact, laws were passed in many states forbidding the marriage of epileptics.

Today medical learning has wiped out once and for all every single one of these misconceptions of epilepsy. However, much of the old superstition remains in those dark, unexplored corners of peoples' minds where are hidden all the silly fallacies we hate so much to give up, because giving up the fallacies means that we have to make an effort to think our way through to the truth. So today the families of epileptics still conceal the disorder from their friends and neighbors. Epileptics themselves feel shame as though there were some terrible disgrace attached to epilepsy which does not apply to diabetes, arthritis or tuberculosis, for example. Yes, incredible as it seems, there are still individuals in our enlightened 20th century who whisper dark shameful gossip about those unfortunates who suffer from one of the most mysterious and dread disorders—epilepsy.

Lewis J. Pollock, M.D., writing in *Today's Health* for May, 1951, tells us that epilepsy is not a disease; it is not related to feeblemindedness; it is not, nor does it lead to insanity; it does not lead to delinquency, vice, crime or mental deterioration. In most instances it should not interfere with good health, education, technical or professional training, or commercial, manufacturing or professional pursuits. It is compatible with courtship, marriage, bearing and rearing children, the pursuit of happiness and normal social life and good citizenship. It bears no shame.

Beyond the mouldy vestiges of superstition, why do we persist in talking and thinking of epilepsy as something shameful, which should be hidden from others? It may be because of the violence of the epileptic convulsions. A teacher in a classroom may have an exaggerated fear of the possible disruption caused by an epileptic student. Yet diabetics in coma or insulin shock exhibit frightening symptoms, too, and there is no shame attached to diabetes. Only recently we heard of a splendid student who was asked to leave one of the women's colleges after the college physician discovered that she was epileptic. Surely such treatment is monstrously unfair and can only be the result of ignorance. True, an epileptic may be injured in a convulsion, and the question of responsibility arises in the mind of his employer or school principal. But there are thousands of ways for people to injure themselves and we do not refuse education or employment to anyone else on the basis of possible injury on the premises. It seems that a lot more educational work must be done before the epileptic will be accepted as a person *who is sometimes ill,* just as most of us are. Readers can help to spread the true facts about epilepsy.

Epilepsy Is Commoner Than You Think

Almost anyone to whom you mention epilepsy will tell you that it is an uncommon disease. So it is surprising to find that there are as many epileptics in this country as there are sufferers from diabetes, or from active tuberculosis. One American out of every 300 or 400 people has epilepsy. Measured in money—and not counting lost man hours, epilepsy accounts for more than 60 million dollars annually. Yet 80 out of 100 epileptics can at present lead almost normal lives.

What is epilepsy? In our research we studied about five learned medical articles debating the question. In many aspects of the problem of defining epilepsy, the authorities were not agreed. We have found out many things that epilepsy is *not*. But we still know little of what it *is*. We do know that it is not, in itself, a disease. It is rather a symptom of some kind of disorder in the body. Says Dennis Williams, M.D., D.Sc., F.R.C.P., Physician in charge of Neurology at St. George's Hospital, England, in the January 24, 1953, issue of the *British Medical Journal:* Every ordinary doctor sees many patients with symptoms of loss of memory or consciousness, muscle-twitching, feeling of faintness or unreality, disturbances of vision and so forth. Since the patients are usually quite well when they come to see him, he can diagnose the illness only from their descriptions of their feelings. How many of these are epileptics and where does the physician draw the dividing line between epileptics and non-epileptics? "We know that epilepsy can occur without loss of consciousness, without amnesia, without involuntary movement and without any of the simple features which would enable us to make a certain diagnosis of epilepsy. None of the definitions will do, for they are all too narrow," says Dr. Williams.

We do have an instrument which will diagnose epilepsy—the electro-encephalograph. "Encephalo" means "brain" and "graph" means "writing," so this jawbreaker of a name refers simply to an instrument which records the electrical workings of the brain in writing. The brain, like the heart, gives off electrical currents. In using the electro-encephalograph, the patient merely sits while electrodes are attached to his head through which his brain's electrical currents are recorded. The brain of an epileptic records a different kind of pattern from that of a non-epileptic.

There is pretty general agreement on the different kinds of epilepsy. *Petit mal* (meaning *little sickness* in French) is a form of disorder which is much more common in children than in adults. Seizures generally are quite frequent—in fact there may be hundreds in one day. They last only a few seconds and may be overlooked, because they may give no indication except for a slight hesitation or confusion. The child may drop whatever he is holding, or he may fall and immediately get up. There may be rhythmic twitching of the eyelids or eyebrows. *Petit mal* attacks are usually worse in the morning hours and they usually grow less frequent and serious as the sufferer grows older.

Grand mal (big sickness) is what most of us mean when we think of epilepsy. The patient becomes unconscious and falls. Saliva may appear on his lips, he may cry out (although he is not feeling any pain), his muscles tighten into a spasm or convulsion and he twitches violently for a minute or two. Actually the seizure does not last long although it may seem long to the helpless observer. During an attack of *grand mal* the patient may mimic normal movements. He may appear to be beckoning with his fingers, his eyes or head may turn to one side or another as if he were actually looking to that side. He may get up after the attack and feel dull and drowsy for a time, or he may go into a deep sleep and sleep for hours.

Psychomotor epilepsy is the most difficult to diagnose because symptoms vary from patient to patient. This is the kind of disorder that may cause individuals to do things which they later do not remember, such as suddenly going to a strange city, unreasonably beginning to push the furniture around or throw things. Jacksonian epilepsy involves twitching of muscles on one side while the patient remains conscious. Many epileptics have a warning when they are going to have an attack. It is called an "aura" by physicians. It may be a strange feeling in the stomach, a dizzy feeling, or it may involve an unpleasant odor that the patient believes he smells.

Not many, but some, cases of epilepsy are caused by damage to the brain either at birth or later in life. In the other cases, the disorder is called "functional" or "idiopathic," meaning that a physical examination reveals nothing wrong with any organ. However, it is possible that functional epilepsy may result eventually in injury to the brain or other parts of the body, if seizures are frequent.

The difference between an epileptic seizure and a "faint" is that the first is a disturbance in the brain, the second involves a sudden lowering of the blood pressure, which causes the patient to become unconscious. A faint generally has some outside immediate cause—the sight of blood, bad news, etc. But an epileptic convulsion comes without any such circumstances, Dr. Williams, concluding his definition of epilepsy, says

"It might be said in criticism of this didactic and rigid distinction between epilepsy and other states that the borderland between epilepsy and psychopathy is a narrow one, hardly explored and that the basis of neither state is understood."

At present drugs are given which are effective in relieving epileptic convulsions. Dilantin and mesantoin for *Grand mal* and triodone for *Petit mal* have proved to be effective in many cases. However, as with all drugs, there are side effects and sometimes very serious ones, which necessitate the closest supervision by the physician and constant testing to make certain that these side effects are not fatal.

Can We Prevent Epilepsy?

What about prevention of epilepsy? We began our research on the subject with an article in the *Quarterly Review of Allergy and Applied Immunology,* June, 1952, by Hal. M. Davison, M.D., of Atlanta, Georgia. Dr. Davison presents and discusses evidence that allergies cause symptoms and disease conditions in the nervous system. Many of these symptoms are the same that are encountered in multiple sclerosis and epilepsy. Drawing from an enormous amount of reference material (192 articles and personal communications are listed in the bibliography) , Dr. Davison describes many patients whose convulsions disappeared when the food to which they were allergic was removed from their diet. For instance, in one patient with *Petit mal* and *Grand mal,* attacks were produced five times by the ingestion of cauliflower and were relieved by the omission of this food. . . . One child aged four with asthma, headache, mental and emotional symptoms, and convulsive attacks all relieved by injections of extracts of pollen to which the patient was sensitive. . . . Four patients were definitely proven to have epileptic attacks due to specific foods, one to eggs, one to milk, one to mushrooms, and one to cereals. . . . Patients had convulsions beginning in infancy with the first real change in their diet. Some of these attacks persisted for years and were still present; some had been relieved by removing certain foods from their diet. . . . Eastlake reported one patient with epilepsy shown to be due to beef, in whom the injection of four drops of sterile beef broth produced an attack of great intensity. The woman's eldest daughter also had epilepsy proven to be due to certain meats. . . . Eighteen allergists reported thirty-three patients with *Grand mal,* two with *Petit mal* and three with both *Grand* and *Petit mal,* all relieved by allergic treatment alone. . . ." We could go on and on giving most convincing case histories from this article.

"The fact," says Dr. Davison, "that some of these patients with allergy and other symptoms involving the nervous system suffered from periods of unconsciousness without convulsions, some had convulsions, and some had twitchings and spasmodic contractions of muscles over various parts of the body without unconsciousness, led us to believe that epilepsy itself could be a manifestation of allergy." He goes on to tell of sending a letter to 1494 specialists in allergy, asking for their opinion of allergy as a possible cause of epilepsy. Of the 207 answers he received, typical ones were: "not suspected, never occurred to me, overlooked," and so forth. This in spite of the fact that articles on allergy and epilepsy have appeared frequently in medical magazines throughout the past 30 years, as Dr. Davison's list of references testifies.

Dr. Davison tells us how epileptic attacks frequently begin with some manifestation of allergy—a six year old boy who developed epileptic symptoms along with eczema, digestive disturbances, hives, hay fever, asthma and finally convulsions. A 32-year old woman who had digestive upsets, then hay fever, hives and migraine, followed some years later by convulsions. He also says that precipitating factors which often bring about convulsions are: fear, anxiety, fatigue, chilling, sexual excess, or overindulgence in alcohol or some unusual food.

In spite of the splendid array of evidence, Dr. Davison concludes, "No one believes that allergy is a causative factor in all cases of idiopathic epilepsy. It is evident and already proven that epilepsy is a symptom complex produced by many different causes. In some individuals the epileptic attacks may have several causes cooperating to produce them." He pleads for a greater realization of the part that allergies may play in this tragic disorder and outlines the steps that doctors should take to check *first* on allergy as a possible cause.

Further Evidence of Allergy as a Cause

Dr. Foster Kennedy writing in the *Archives of Neurology and Psychiatry* for June, 1938, adds some astounding evidence, including the case of a 21 year old nurse who had an epileptic attack every time she ate chocolate. Dr. A. H. Rowe in the *Journal of Nervous and Mental Diseases,* May, 1944, tells us of allergies to eggs, tomatoes, cereals, milk, veal, pepper, pollen and animal hair which brought on symptoms of dizziness, fatigue, headache, depression, confusion, spots before the eyes, tinnitus (ringing in the ears), tingling in hands and feet and so forth, in addition to convulsions. In every case the symptoms disappeared on Dr. Rowe's "elimination" diet by which various foods were omitted one at a time, until the villain was found.

In *Modern Medicine* for December 1, 1951, Susan C. Dees, M.D., and Hans Lowenbach, M.D., report on 37 children under the age of 14 with *Petit* and *Grand mal* who also had a wide range of allergic symptoms —asthma, eczema, colds, etc. In 24 of the children all symptoms were controlled by finding the offending allergen and eliminating it from the diet. The brain patterns of these children improved steadily. However, as soon as the program was stopped and full freedom was allowed to eat anything they wished, all symptoms returned again.

Now, tracking down an allergy is a tedious and expensive business. It involves going back to the specialist week after week for tests which may go on for months or even years until the allergen is found. A friend of ours turned out to be allergic to everything! After weeks of frantic testing his doctor finally gave up, then he made one last try in which he discovered that our friend was allergic to the serum in which the various tests were being administered. Then they started all over again and finally tracked down the villain.

An elimination diet would seem to be an easy enough solution for discovering whether you have any food allergies. We suppose any physician can make up such a diet. Of course, it must be adhered to without fail if you really want to uncover a food to which you are allergic. And possibly you might make up your own elimination diet by simply omitting one certain food every week and seeing whether the allergic symptoms may disappear. Of course, such things as alcohol and tobacco, coffee, tea and so forth should be suspect, too.

Now finally we come to our last suggestion which appears to us to be the most sensible of all. We have referred many times in these pages to a book by E. M. Abrahamson, M.D., *Body, Mind and Sugar,* published by Henry Holt and Co. Dr. Abrahamson writes in this book about low blood sugar, which, he says, is far more prevalent in America than its opposite, which is diabetes. He tells almost unbelievable stories about curing allergies with a diet which keeps the blood sugar at its normal level and does not let it fall below. Asthma, hay fever, alcoholism, depression, neurosis (so-called), fatigue, dizziness, headache, migraine, weakness, and many more common ailments take flight never to return, sometimes after only three weeks on the prescribed diet.

Allergies and Low Blood Sugar

Dr. Abrahamson believes that it is not necessary to have allergies at all. In fact, he claims that no one who adheres rigidly to the prescribed diet *can* have allergies. In speaking of epilepsy he says "at a meeting (Dr. Myerson) attended, some psychiatrist advanced the hypothesis that epileptics are men who hate their fathers. Myerson commented that he knew a lot of epileptic cats who had never met their fathers." He continues, "Among the signs and symptoms behind which hyperinsulinism (low blood sugar) masquerades, Seale Harris included those of *Petit mal.* It is significant that some women who suffered from epilepsy appeared to improve during pregnancy, as rheumatoid arthritis and peptic ulcer patients did—when the blood glucose (sugar) tends to be higher. Other pregnant epileptics, however, seemed to suffer more severely. A number of persons subject to epileptic seizures were given the glucose tolerance test which indicated low blood sugar curves. *It has also been found that the brain wave tracings of persons afflicted with Petit mal were similar to those of hyperinsulinism victims (that is, people who had low blood sugar).* (Italics ours.) While these facts are insufficient in themselves to indicate that epilepsy is a manifestation of hyperinsulinism, they provide enough evidence to warrant further investigation of the relationship between the two diseases."

We do not know how long it may take for the medical profession to get around to this "further investigation." Research is expensive and, we suppose, some people actually prefer drugs rather than adhering to a diet. However, those of us who believe in the effectiveness of diet in preventing disease can surely do ourselves a big favor by trying out Dr. Abrahamson's diet which, incidentally has a lot to recommend it whether or not you suffer from allergies, headaches, epilepsy or any other disorder. It is an extremely simple and inexpensive diet to follow and we can just about guarantee that anybody will feel better on it, no matter how good they felt to begin with.

Here is the diet for bringing up blood sugar levels and keeping them normal. It must be followed exactly and *no meals are to be missed.* Skipping breakfast or lunch may mean the difference between success and failure.

On arising—medium orange, half grapefruit or four ounces of fruit juice.

BREAKFAST—Fruit or four ounces of juice, one egg with or without two slices of ham or bacon; only one slice of bread or toast with plenty of butter, beverage.

Two hours after breakfast—four ounces of juice.

LUNCH—Meat, fish, cheese or eggs; salad (large serving of lettuce, tomato or Waldorf salad with mayonnaise or French dressing) vegetables if desired; only one slice of bread or toast with plenty of butter; dessert; beverage.

Three hours after lunch—8 ounces of milk.

One hour before dinner—4 ounces of juice.

DINNER—Soup if desired (not thickened with flour); vegetables; liberal portion of meat, fish or poultry; only one slice of bread if desired; dessert; beverage.

Two to three hours after dinner—8 ounces of milk.

Every two hours until bedtime—4 ounces of milk or a small handful of nuts.

Allowable vegetables: Asparagus, avocado, beets, broccoli, Brussels sprouts, cabbage, cauliflower, carrots, celery, cucumbers, corn, egg-plant, lima beans, onions, peas, radishes, sauerkraut, squash, string beans, tomatoes, turnips.

Allowable fruits: Apples, apricots, berries, grapefruit, pears, melons, oranges, peaches, pineapple, tangerines. May be cooked or raw with or without cream but without sugar. Canned fruits should be packed in water not syrup.

Lettuce, mushrooms and nuts may be taken as freely as desired.

Juice: Any unsweetened fruit or vegetable juice except grape juice or prune juice.

Beverages: Weak tea (tea ball, not brewed); decaffeinated coffee, coffee substitutes.

Desserts: Fruit, unsweetened gelatin, junket (made from tablets, not mixed).

Alcoholic and soft drinks: Club soda, dry gingerale, whiskey and other distilled liquors.

Avoid Absolutely

Sugar, candy and other sweets such as cake, pie, pastries, sweet custards, puddings and ice cream.

Caffeine: Ordinary coffee, strong brewed tea, beverages containing caffeine. (Your doctor will tell you what these are.)

Potatoes, rice, grapes, raisins, plums, figs, dates and bananas.

Spaghetti, macaroni and noodles.

Wines, cordials, cocktails and beer.

(We have included bacon, ham, soft drinks and distilled liquors in this list, as Dr. Abrahamson does, but we assume that readers will have crossed these off automatically as they read the list. Then, too, we do not recommend using citrus fruits as freely as Dr. Abrahamson suggests and we do not approve of drinking citrus juice.)

Is Epilepsy Inherited?

There is a lively controversy in scientific circles over whether or not epilepsy is inherited. Incredible amounts of investigation have been done to prove one side or the other. In one article we read, 20,000 relatives of 4000 epileptics were interviewed, and the conclusion drawn was that "the genetic factor in epilepsy is probably no greater than it is in many other common diseases. Assets that are transmissible such as sound vital organs, good intelligence, personality and social responsibility may outweigh the liability of a tendency to seizures. Hence, advice regarding marriage and children must be individualized." Other researches show us that the inheritance factor in epilepsy is 1/10 of that in diabetes, and 1/25 of that in migraine. Surely no one would question the advisability of marriage for someone who suffers from migraine headaches, and is worried for fear he or she might transmit the disorder to children. Yet migraine headaches "run" in 25 times as many families as epilepsy does! And speaking of inheritance we can't fail to come back to a favorite question of ours—how much is inherited and how much is due to food patterns?

Very early in life you are conditioned to the foods you like and those you don't like. It comes about largely through your family's ideas about food. If no one ever eats lamb in your family, chances are you won't eat it after you are grown. If your family has spaghetti once a week, you'll probably serve spaghetti often in your own home, while the family that lives next door may never have tasted spaghetti and so are convinced they wouldn't like it. If epilepsy is indeed related to allergies, and allergies are unquestionably related to food patterns, then, without studying the daily menus of everyone involved, how can we be sure that any predisposition to epilepsy is "inherited"? And what about those members of an epileptically-inclined family who break away from the established food pattern and free themselves from prejudices where food is concerned? Might they not be the very ones who do not "inherit" the epilepsy?

One last statistic. It has been found that one person in every ten has some irregularity in brain wave patterns when being tested by the electro-encephalograph. Only one person in every 200 has epileptic seizures. How many of us then can say that we do not have a tendency toward epilepsy if we are the one person in 10? Robust health is our best safeguard against such a tendency. This means—whether you follow the Abrahamson diet or not—no foods that contain white sugar or white flour. No soft drinks. Only whole grain cereals. Plenty of fresh vegetables and fruits, as many raw as possible. And enough of the protective foods—meat, eggs, cheese, nuts. In addition, because all of our food has been robbed of vitamins and minerals before it reaches our tables, take natural food supplements: brewer's yeast or desiccated liver for vitamin B, fish liver oil for vitamins A and D, rose hips for vitamin C, wheat germ oil for vitamin E, and bone meal for minerals.

Enzymes

Physiology teaches us that man lives by the process of converting some of his food into building blocks of protein which replace his cells as they wear out, and by burning other food as energy which enables him to play, work and enjoy life. We all learned in school that the various substances of which food is made (carbohydrates, proteins and fats) are "changed" by the digestive process and in this "change" they become useful to our bodies. Now obviously considerable change must take place. Look at a plate of steak, potatoes, vegetables, salad and fruit. It certainly does not look like the flesh of a human being. Yet that is what a large part of it becomes. It certainly does not seem possible that by burning that plateful of food in a fire, one could obtain enough energy to carry a working man through a day of strenuous ditch-digging or hard mental work. Yet the energy released by that plate of food does just that, once it has been exposed to the chemical magic of digestion and assimilation.

We know in a general sort of way that our body is equipped with digestive juices. We know that, during a meal, the saliva pours out a substance that partly digests starchy foods; the stomach pours out another substance that digests protein; the pancreas and the intestine exude some substance that finishes up the digestion of protein and starch. So right here—during and immediately after a meal—this process of "changing" food into human substance begins. But what is it in the digestive juices that works this magic? Finding the answer to this question leads us into the complex and largely unexplored, but very fascinating story of enzymes.

Scientists have known for many years that there are substances present in tiny quantities in every living cell that possess marvelous properties. It all began with a study of yeasts and fungi. The active living organism that causes fruit juices to ferment and bread to rise is yeast. As the tiny yeast plant grows, changes take place in the medium in which it is growing. The fruit juice becomes alcoholic; the bread dough rapidly expands to many times its former volume. But early scientists discovered that after the yeast plants had been killed, something remained that was not a living plant as the yeast is. This something was called a "ferment" because it brought about a state of fermentation. Not until many years later was it named an "enzyme."

What are enzymes and where do they exist? Are they alive? Are they necessary to life? How can they best be preserved and how are they destroyed? What do they do in the body? What do they do in plants? Can we make them synthetically in a laboratory? These are some of the questions that have occupied researchers in the intriguing study of enzymes. Out of all this study have come many observations that have greatly increased our knowledge of how human beings live and also what and how human beings should eat. We will try to answer these questions, so that you can understand the immense importance of enzymes. Some of the answers are not completely understood as yet even by the most learned scientists, for enzymes still involve much that cannot be answered with our present means of exploration. Perhaps in the enzyme we have the secret of life itself.

Enzymes Cause Chemical Changes

As you know, many physical things take place in this world because of chemical changes. If you drop some sugar into a teacup of water the sugar changes. It dissolves. During this process many chemical changes take place in the mixture you have in your teacup. If you let the teacup stand for several weeks other changes will take place gradually and slowly.

But if you heat the mixture, changes begin to take place right away. The sugar and water turn into syrup. Now imagine that you have in your kitchen some substance which, if you dropped it into the cold cup of sugar-water, would immediately change it into syrup, without any cooking. Such a substance is called in chemistry a "catalyst." It brings about a chemical change immediately, without heat.

A catalyst is further defined as a substance which will perform this job of bringing about a chemical change without itself becoming involved in the change. In other words, you could, with proper chemical procedure, remove all the catalyst from your syrup and it would still be syrup. The catalyst needs to be present in extremely small amounts—one part of a catalyst can act chemically to change substances whose volume is millions of times greater than its own. For instance, one part of catalyst to millions of parts of sugar-water would still produce the same effect. And the catalyst would remain unchanged in the middle of all this chemical activity.

An enzyme is a catalyst. So enzymes are present wherever chemical changes take place rapidly without the added stimulus of heat. Since everything that takes place in physiology involves chemical change, enzymes must be present everywhere. They are. They are present in great abundance in every living cell—plant and animal. Are they alive? James S. McLester, M.D., in his book *Nutrition and Diet in Health and Disease* (W. B. Saunders, 1949), says "As crystalline organic compounds these materials are lifeless; as substances which have the property of increasing in the presence of living cells, they assume a property characteristic of living things."

The antiseptics that kill living organisms like germs and yeasts do not inactivate enzymes. You could drop formaldehyde or iodine or lysol into your teacup, destroying all germs that might be there, but the chemical process brought about by the enzyme you have in the cup would go right on, proving that the disinfectant has not disturbed it.

However, there are two circumstances that disturb the activity of enzymes very much—cold and heat. Cold inactivates them. That is, if you put your teacup into the refrigerator, no chemical change would take place. The enzyme would stay there in the cup, but the sugar would remain sugar and the water would remain water. You would have no syrup. But when you take the cup out into the warm air again and the temperature of the mixture goes up to room temperature, the enzymes would become active again and would make syrup. So they haven't been destroyed. They have only ceased activity for a short time.

A small increase in heat causes the enzymes to work more rapidly. But more heat destroys them entirely and, even after the mixture has cooled down, they will not become active again. Between 32 degrees and 104 degrees Fahrenheit—that is, anywhere from freezing up to the temperature of a hot summer day—enzymes are very active. But when you heat them to a point above 122 degrees Fahrenheit, enzymes are permanently destroyed. The boiling point of water is 212 degrees Fahrenheit. So when you boil vegetables or fruit all enzymes in the food are destroyed. When you roast meat at a temperature of 200 or 300 degrees of course all enzymes in the meat are destroyed.

What does this mean so far as preparing food and cooking are concerned? Well, it means first that refrigeration is one of the greatest inventions of modern times, for foods can be kept with their enzymes intact but inactive so long as you keep them in the refrigerator or freezer. While a plant is growing and ripening, the enzymes are busy inside forming vitamins and bringing about other changes that make the fruit or vegetable tasty and nutritious. But as soon as the food is picked it should be refrigerated, for otherwise the enzymes go right on working and this time their activity is destructive. Lettuce and radishes wilt and fruit skins wither when they are kept at room temperature, for the enzymes go on working. On the other hand, when you cook food at high temperatures you destroy immediately all enzymes. Is this good or bad? Healthful or unhealthful? To have the answer we must know what enzymes do in the body.

How Enzymes Act in the Body

Actually they must be present (in very small amounts) for any process that takes place in the body. They are present in every cell (and don't forget that your body contains many billions of cells) and they are the cell's only connection with the outer world. That steak on your plate is some day going to form part of a certain number of cells of your body, but it can't possibly do that unless there are the correct enzymes in the right places at every single moment during that transformation.

The salivary glands, the pancreas, the wall of the stomach and of the intestines contain the chief digestive enzymes (there are nine of them). But even after the food has been changed by these enzymes into a form that can be transported to all the cells of the body, there must be other enzymes in those cells that continue the process of changing this substance even more, according to what use the body will make of it.

We talk a lot about vitamins and we know that vitamins are essential for good health. But vitamins can do their work only in the presence of enzymes, for they form part of complicated "enzyme systems." For instance, thiamin, a B vitamin, is necessary to good health. Thiamin forms part of an enzyme system that digests sugar and starches. The thiamin must be present if these carbohydrates are to be converted into energy, but the enzymes must be present too. Every vitamin whose use in the body is known has been discovered to be a part of an enzyme system. There are (so far discovered) five enzymes which contain riboflavin, a B vitamin. "It has been claimed for some time that vitamin C is also an essential constituent in enzymatic reactions in the cell" says Morris Jacobs in his book, *Food and Food Products.* (Interscience Publishers, 1951.)

Enzymes are named in accordance with the food substance they "work on" chemically. So an enzyme that brings about a chemical change in the presence of phosphorus is called phosphatase, an enzyme that works to break down sugar (sucrose) is called sucrase and so forth.

Now, of course, the temperature of the body will never rise high enough to destroy the body's enzymes. But there is another characteristic of enzymes that makes them subject to destruction in the body. They are fussy about the acidity of substances in which they are working. Some enzymes can work only in a quite acid medium. Others need to have more alkalinity. Pepsin, for instance, which is the enzyme that breaks down protein in the stomach, functions at a pH (or acidity) of about

1.2 to 1.8. Trypsin, the enzyme in pancreatic juice, must have much more alkaline surroundings—about 8.2. Now if, because of some condition of ill health, there is not enough hydrochloric acid in your stomach to keep the pepsin working properly, you will not be able to digest proteins. As people grow older the hydrochloric acid in their stomachs tends to decrease, so they may have trouble digesting proteins because their supply of the enzyme pepsin simply cannot function in an alkaline stomach. Taking bicarbonate of soda also makes your stomach alkaline and stops the activity of pepsin.

How does it happen, then, if the stomach is acid enough, and there is plenty of pepsin that the walls of the stomach are not digested? They are made of protein. There is disagreement among scientists as to why we do not digest our own stomachs. One school believes that there may be anti-enzymes secreted by the cells of the stomach wall which prevent the digestive enzymes from working on them. Others say that the thick mucous coating on the lining of the stomach protects it from coming into contact with the digestive enzymes. How does it happen that tapeworms can live in a human intestine? Apparently, say the scientists, there is something present in living cells that prevents the enzymes from breaking them down and digesting them.

Can We Obtain Enzymes From Food?

Where does the body get the material from which it manufactures enzymes? Just stop and think for a moment of the enormity of this chemical factory that is humming away inside you day and night. Think of all the complicated processes in which these enzymes take part. While you are eating, all the digestive organs are pouring out juices rich in enzymes. In every tiny cell, from your brain right down to your little toe, enzymes are fermenting furiously, combining and recombining into the thousands of different enzyme systems that move your muscles, stimulate your nerves, keep you breathing, thinking and feeling. The body manufactures enzymes out of food, water and air—those are the only ingredients available. So what you eat becomes many times more important when you consider it from the point of view of manufacturing enzymes.

In the days before fire was invented, man ate his food raw, just as wild animals do. Raw food contains enzymes, as we know. Aside from other chemical changes that take place, cooking food destroys enzymes. It seems logical that enzymes from raw food could be transformed into useful enzymes for one body system or another, after they have been eaten. They consist of the same chemical substance—that is, a plant enzyme contains the same elements in the same proportions as the enzymes of a human body contains. Is it possible that the raw food our ancestors ate, far back in history, contributed vast stores of enzymes to their bodies, so that they themselves did not have to manufacture so many enzymes? Might not such an arrangement have a very beneficial effect on the body? After all, manufacturing enzymes is a difficult job, especially when the only materials available are present-day denatured, diluted, processed foods.

Yet our bodies must go on manufacturing enzymes in enormous quantity every day if we are to go on living. After an enzyme has completed its work, the next process that takes place generally destroys the enzyme so we must be replenishing the supply all the time. For instance, salivary enzymes function only in an alkaline medium. When we swallow our food, all the salivary enzymes which are busy breaking down starch and sugar are thrown into the stomach where the high acidity destroys them within a half hour or so. So our salivary glands must immediately manufacture more.

Might it not be that this continual loss from the body of enzymes that are not replaced in our food is one of the main causes of aging and disease? In the Bible we read of men who lived many times longer than we do today. The mythology of other religions also contains stories of men who lived to a great age. In those early days men lived on fruits, nuts, berries, raw meat and unheated milk. What cooking was done was very primitive and the heat could not penetrate to the very interior to destroy enzymes. Perhaps this kind of nourishment was so full of enzymes that bodies were not worn out so soon by the incessant need for producing more.

Wild animals, who have no contact with man, do not become diseased in their wild state, unless of course they must exist under conditions of starvation or drouth. Wild animals brought to the zoos of civilized cities used to show a high mortality from the diseases to which man is subject—pneumonia, tuberculosis, cancer and so forth. Because these animals were so very valuable, zoo keepers experimented and found that diets of completely raw food kept the zoo animals healthy. Morbidity rates have dropped almost to zero in zoos where all animals are fed only raw food. We know of course that many of the chemical changes brought about by cooking destroy vitamins and otherwise decrease the nutritional value of the food. *But perhaps the destruction of enzymes is much the most disastrous result of cooking.*

We know that those primitive Eskimos who eat practically all their food raw do not suffer from the diseases of modern man; in fact they have so little sickness that there is no tradition of medicinal remedies or medicine men among them. On the other hand, the American Indians, who cooked their food, have an enormous array of medicines and remedies and their medicine men were the most important persons in the tribe.

Another interesting observation is that an herbiverous animal who lives entirely on uncooked plants, has a pancreas which is extremely small compared to man's. Apparently its pancreas does not need to produce nearly so many enzymes as a human pancreas, because a large part of the necessary enzymes are already present in its uncooked food. It is true too that Oriental peoples whose diet consists largely of cooked starch have pancreas glands much heavier than Americans. This seems to indicate that the amount of enzymes needed to deal with this cooked starch necessitates an overworked pancreas which continually increases in size trying to become more efficient. Herbiverous animals have inactive salivary glands. The salivary glands do a big part of the job of digesting starches. But even so, the cow can get along with the small amount of starch-splitting enzymes turned out by a tiny pancreas, while man, with his efficient salivary glands, must have a large pancreas, and the more cooked starch he eats, the larger his pancreas becomes.

We have shown in other articles some almost miraculous cures performed by raw fruit and vegetable diets. We have related the experiments of Kouchakoff who found that the pathological condition present in the intestine after meals (with many white corpuscles present) did not take place when raw food was eaten. It does not seem possible that at our present stage of civilization, we could obtain almost all the necessary enzymes from our food as the cow apparently does. But we do believe that eating raw food day after day, in as great a quantity as possible will, over the years, greatly increase one's body store of enzymes and so will greatly benefit health, for there will be much less strain on enzyme producing organs if they do not have to work overtime supplying enzymes which should logically be supplied by food.

What about the possibility of taking synthetic enzymes? We know enough about the structure of enzymes that we can make them synthetically. Quite a number have been synthesized. Jacobs, in *Food and Food Products* says that our synthesis of enzymes has not contributed greatly to our knowledge of them. We know only that they are proteins and we still have to solve the problem of protein structure. Jacobs also says "In their normal environment, enzymes are partially protected against inactivation attributable to heat or other energy factors and to inhibition by metals. As they are progressively purified, these protective factors such as proteins, carbohydrates and the like are removed, leaving the enzymes open to attack by chemical and physical agents which inactivate them."

As you know, we do not recommend taking synthetic vitamins. It seems to us that a synthetic ("pure") enzyme would be an even worse gamble, because there is not a chance that any of the natural substances protecting the activity of the enzyme would be present. And Dr. Jacobs substantiates this theory of ours. How then can you add to your enzyme supply, if you are interested in what we have said above and if you agree with us that we moderns probably age earlier than we should and contract needless diseases simply from lack of enzymes?

How To Get Enough Enzymes

First of all, make it your business to eat as much raw food as possible and by this we mean that if half your diet is raw, that certainly won't be too much! Never cook fruits. There is no excuse nutritionally for destroying most of the food value of this excellent food, especially when fruits taste so much better raw! If your family and friends insist on serving stewed, baked or broiled fruits, simply refuse to eat them and ask for your portion raw. In the winter when fresh fruits are scarce, eat frozen rather than canned fruits. Having your own freezer is by far the best idea, for you can hurry the luscious beauties straight from the trees and bushes right into the freezer with a very minimum food value wasted. And remember, frozen food retains its enzymes! They disappear rapidly as the fruit thaws, however, so eat frozen fruit just as soon as it has thawed.

If you must eat often in restaurants you probably suffer more than the rest of us from lack of enzymes, for the preparation and the wait before serving take just about all the food value from any restaurant food. But even here you can get fresh raw food, if you insist on it. A piece of fruit or a raw fruit or vegetable drink at the beginning of a meal, celery, salad, radishes during the meal and some other fresh fruit for dessert—these raw foods are available in most restaurants. And if you patronize one establishment, they will be glad to have raw foods on hand for you.

Eat as many vegetables raw as possible. Never cook carrots, cabbage, Swiss chard, spinach, broccoli stalks, onions, celery, turnips. Sure, it's rabbit food, but did you ever know a rabbit who died of heart disease or cancer?

Become an expert in fixing delicious raw vegetable dishes. Use a grater, a food mill, a blender, a chopping board. Use salad dressings for garnish if your family objects to plain raw vegetables. Try raisins, dates, fruit and nuts as "fixings." And remember, keep all raw foods chilled all the time.

Then too it seems quite possible that organically-raised fruits and vegetables are richer in enzymes than commercially-raised produce. It has been shown time and time again that animals raised on organic food do not contract the diseases to which other animals are subject. Sir Albert Howard in his splendid book, *The Agricultural Testament* (Oxford University Press, 1949), recounts the story of his cattle raised on organic food who were pastured alongside cattle with hoof and mouth disease. Even rubbing noses with these diseased animals, Sir Albert's cattle remained completely free from the epidemic malady. Now undoubtedly there is much more food value in food that has been raised organically—that is, without the use of chemical fertilizer and insecticide. Perhaps the most important of these food elements may turn out to be enzymes.

So our second recommendation is to buy and eat organically-raised food if you possibly can. Unless you live in an apartment there is probably a small plot of ground somewhere near the house where you can put in a garden of your own, even if it means spading up lawn to do it. Or you can find through our *Organic Food Directory* (available from Rodale Press, for 25 cents) a list of farmers throughout the country who sell organically-raised produce. Perhaps there are some organic farmers who live near you. Or you can persuade some farmer (or gardener) friend or relative who lives nearby to begin gardening organically so that you can buy produce from him. It isn't really too difficult or expensive to make certain that at least a part of your food is organically-grown. Perhaps a large measure of the increased good health you will experience will be due to the supply of enzymes in this most healthful kind of food.

Enzymes In Daily Life

By

Joseph J. Martin, D.D.S.

and

Albert Schatz, Ph.D.

Dr. Martin, a dentist in Rochelle Park, N. J. is an enthusiastic gardener and Dr. Schatz is Director of Research at the National Agricultural College. They are well qualified to deal with the subject of enzymes.

You may be surprised to learn that without enzymes plants would not grow, seeds would not germinate, organic matter would remain unchanged on a compost pile, microbes would not function, and there would be no soil. Enzymes are therefore among the most important things in our world, and so it would pay us to learn about them. You already know a lot about enzymes since you've lived with them all your life. You could not have been born without enzymes. They help you grow and keep healthy.

If they stopped functioning for one single minute, the chances are that you would stop living. As a matter of fact, you are already quite familiar with many things that enzymes do. When hydrogen peroxide is poured in an open wound to kill germs, it froths and hisses. This is caused by an enzyme, in our cells, that changes hydrogen peroxide to water and oxygen gas. Other enzymes are involved when blood clots, and when milk sours. It is by means of enzyme action that yeast can raise dough. For the same reason, the freshly cut surface of raw apples, bananas, pears, and potatoes turns brown in the air. Digestion, which is one of the processes that keeps us going, could not occur without enzymes.

Let's do some simple experiments to understand this important process. We know some foods contain starch. Which ones are they? To find out, just add a drop of tincture of iodine from your medicine cabinet to different foods. Try bread, cream, butter, rice, raw egg white and yolk, olive oil, sugar, cake, tapioca, the inside flesh of fresh fruits and vegetables, milk, meat, gelatin, nuts, honey, cornmeal, buckwheat, and other cereals. Do the same thing with corn starch or potato starch. Notice that iodine colors certain foods blue or violet. This is a chemical test for starch. Foods that contain starch turn blue or purple when stained with iodine. If starch is not present, the color will not form.

Would you like to make starch disappear? Don't be surprised to learn how easy this is. You've already done it thousands of times without realizing what was happening. There's no trick involved. Suspend just enough corn starch in half a glass of cold water to get a slight cloudiness. Then make absolutely sure that starch is there to begin with by testing a few drops separately with iodine as you did in the food tests.

Now mix a teaspoonful of the starch suspension with the same amount of saliva. Stir with a toothpick for 10 to 15 minutes. By this time the original cloudiness will have disappeared and the solution will be perfectly clear. Examine it closely and see for yourself. Now try the iodine test for starch once again. This time you will get no blue or purple color because starch is not there any more. Where did it go? What happened is that something in the saliva changed the starch chemically into sugar. The sugar dissolves in water but does not give a color with iodine. Test some sugar with iodine and prove this for yourself.

Enzymes in Digestion

Whenever you eat starchy foods, the starch disappears in this way. It begins to change to sugar in your mouth as soon as you chew food and mix it with saliva. In the stomach and intestine, a similar change takes place with meat, cheese, fat, oil, and other foods that do not dissolve in water. The body changes them chemically into forms that do dissolve in water. To do this, the body digests these foods. Digestion is therefore a way of changing foods so that they can dissolve in water.

Now you may ask, "Why does the body do this?" or "Does the body have to do this?" The answer is that all foods must first be dissolved in water before they can pass through the wall of the intestine. After they are absorbed in this way, digested foods are taken up by the blood and carried to all parts of the body. Unless foods are first digested and dissolved they cannot get from the intestine into our bodies and reach the tissues and cells where they are used. In plants, too, starch and other foods must be digested so they can be transported from one part of a plant to another.

You can see how this works by pouring salt over dry soil. Imagine that the soil is our body and the hard, dry, crusted surface is the wall of the intestine. The dry salt obviously does not pass through the surface and go down into the soil. Now pour a little water over the salt. As it dissolves, see how it is washed into the soil. In living organisms, digestion does the same thing to foods. In our bodies, for example, it dissolves foods so they pass through the wall of the intestine into the body.

You may say, "Very well, I understand that now, but exactly how do animals, plants, and microbes actually carry out the digestive process? What is that mysterious something in saliva that changed the starch to sugar?"

Well, it's all very simple, as you will see. There is absolutely nothing mysterious about digestion or about anything else, as far as that's concerned. To understand how we digest food, we must learn a little about enzymes. Saliva, plant juices, and many microbes contain an enzyme called amylase. This name comes from the Latin words meaning "starch-splitting." The enzyme amylase splits starch or changes it chemically into sugar. This splitting or changing is the digestion of starch. The end product is sugar which easily dissolves in water but does not give the iodine test that starch does. Now you understand how the starch disappears.

Enzymes Need Proper Environment

Enzymes are the chemical tools with which living cells work. We use hammers, saws, and pliers over and over again. Living cells also use their enzyme tools repeatedly. For example, after some enzyme has been used to bring about a chemical change such as the digestion of a microscopic starch granule, it is then freed to digest more starch. From this, you can see how a small amount of enzyme "goes a long way." This is like our doing a lot of work with a few tools, *provided they are the right ones.* This raises another very important point about enzymes. We cannot saw with a hammer, nor do we drive nails with a paintbrush. In a similar manner, each enzyme is a specific chemical tool and has a particular function of its own. A starch-digesting enzyme will not digest protein. Nor will a protein-digesting enzyme produce a chemical change in fat.

Many of our tools are made of metal. A good many enzymes also contain metals. Iron, calcium, magnesium, zinc, cobalt, copper, manganese and other metals are necessary for the normal functioning and the very life of living cells. Some of these metals are part of enzymes. This is one reason why we require iron in our diet and why plants require trace elements.

Tools are ruined if heated because the metal loses its temper. Likewise enzyme tools cannot stand heating. All enzymes consist of protein in part or entirely. Because of their protein nature, they are easily destroyed by heat since proteins are changed when heated. For example, the common protein egg white coagulates when fried or boiled and cannot be changed back to its original form. It is easy to show how heat affects enzymes. If you carry out the starch experiment with saliva that has been boiled it will not work because the protein enzyme amylase has been destroyed by heating. The amylase has been chemically changed to another form of protein which does not act as an enzyme.

We use wall-papering tools inside our homes and gardening implements outdoors. In a similar manner, there are enzyme tools for use inside and outside of cells. The enzymes that digest insoluble food are secreted or given off by living cells into the environment outside the cells where the undissolved foods are present. These enzymes digest the foods or change them to products that dissolve in water. In this form, the digested foods diffuse or pass into the cells where they are then handled by different enzymes that are present only inside cells.

Enzymes Have Other Uses, Too

This is what happens in our own bodies. Like a hose, our intestine is a long folded tube with open ends. The intestinal contents are as much "outside" of the body as is a coin in a clenched fist or food in one's mouth. Digestive enzymes pass out into the intestine and there digest the food. This takes place completely "outside" of the body cells in which these enzymes were formed. After digestion, the changed and soluble food passes through the wall of the intestine. Then the blood carries it to all parts of the body. Inside of our body cells, it is handled in different ways by many enzymes that never function outside the cells.

Living cells use their enzyme tools for many purposes besides digestion. After food is digested, some of it is oxidized in the body by certain enzymes in order to provide the energy which all living things must have. Oxidation is a process of combustion or burning that goes on within our cells and elsewhere. It is similar to the burning of leaves in the fall, the burning of coal, oil, and wood in a furnace, and the burning of gasoline in an automobile engine.

When we breathe we take up oxygen from the air and give off carbon dioxide. With enzymes as chemical tools, the cells in our bodies are able to use oxygen to burn sugar and other digested food. In this process, they produce the energy required by our bodies and the waste product carbon dioxide. This gas is given off in the air we exhale.

Oxidation by a burning fire and biological oxidation in living cells both yield energy. But there is one very important difference between the two. A fire is an uncontrolled combustion. In a short period of time it releases most of the chemical energy of the fuel in the form of heat. Biological burning, inside of living cells, is controlled so that the energy is liberated slowly and at a rate regulated to satisfy the needs of the body. Certain hormones in our bodies are the thermostats that regulate our temperature. It is believed that these hormones may do this by speeding up or slowing down enzyme action. Plants also have hormones which control their growth and function.

This temperature control in animals is very important. Can you imagine the explosion that would occur if a tank full of gasoline in an automobile were to burn up all at once within a fraction of a second! Just about the same thing would happen in our bodies if a stomach full of food were to be oxidized all at once. We would really burn up in the full sense of the word. That is why it is so important that oxidation inside our bodies be regulated so that the energy is liberated as slowly as it can be handled.

This story about enzymes began with such things as sour milk and bananas. It ended up with the energy all living things need to remain alive. Only a very few enzymes have been mentioned. Many other enzymes are important in the production of antibiotics, and to remove dead tissue in the treatment of wounds. They are also used in the textile, leather, and food industries. Enzymes therefore affect our lives in many ways which we do not usually realize.

Exercise and Constipation

Will exercise help prevent constipation? Of course it will, if you are exercising correctly. A reader once wrote us that she does a great deal of work in libraries and is always annoyed by the fact that she almost always feels the need of having a bowel movement after she has been in the library only a short time. She tried to track down the reason for this, studied all the food she ate and the things she did and finally came to the conclusion that the whole thing is the result of squatting, then standing erect again as she looks for books in the low and high shelves at the library. This is indeed a form of exercise—and a very beneficial exercise—for the person who fears constipation. Squatting, knees bent, back held straight, then rising to an erect posture again is one of the best possible exercises for the abdominal muscles. And those concern us most in preventing constipation.

Many of us think we don't have time to exercise. It's easier to take a laxative, we figure. But those of us who have found that we can easily work exercises into our daily routine have found increased benefits from doing so. Any time of day, no matter where you are, you can exercise your abdominal muscles. Simply straighten your back, tuck in your buttocks and pull in on those tummy muscles! You can do it sitting down as well as standing up. Press your back against the back of your chair, pushing hard against that hollow place where you probably curve in too far. If your muscles are lax and droopy it will take some time to get them to respond. But once you do, you can be sure that you can easily keep them firm and tight from then on, which will mean a great improvement in posture and appearance as well as health.

Here are some more exercises for health. You can try these just before you crawl under the covers at night. Lie flat on your back and raise yourself to a sitting position without using hands or arms. You will immediately feel the pull on those abdominal muscles that means they are getting in trim. Or, to reverse the process, lie flat on your back and lift your feet high in the air, without bending your knees. The same abdominal muscles will tense and then relax, as you gradually lower your feet again. The slower you do this one, the harder it is, for keeping your legs raised just a little from the floor or bed is more difficult than raising them all at once to a 90 degree angle. Don't overdo this one right at the start or you may be stiff the next day.

More Exercises for You

Another good lying-down exercise is to bend your knees, bringing your thighs back against your chest, or as far as you can get them. Keep in mind about all exercising that it isn't really important whether or not you accomplish the final position of the exercise. You derive the benefit from *trying* to do it. While you're lying there so cozily in your bed, just before you go to sleep, you might try this one too: lie flat, with hands behind your head, elbows out and flat against the bed. Now, not lifting your shoulders from the bed, bend your right knee and bring it over and touch the bed on the left side. Bring it back to position, bend the left knee and touch the bed on the right side.

Just after you've had your bath is a good time for these next exercises. Hold both arms straight out at right angles to the body and walk on tiptoe back and forth. It is almost impossible to do this comfortably without pulling in on your abdominal muscles. If you have a full length mirror you might study your posture while you do this exercise. The minute you pull those abdominal muscles in, you'll suddenly look as graceful as a ballet dancer preparing for a difficult step. Here's another exercise: keeping your abdominal muscles in tight, place your hands on your shoulders, elbows up, then bend forward from the waist, then back, then to the right and then to the left, slowly. Exercising rapidly only wears you out and gets you to puffing without actually flexing your muscles, which is the main purpose of exercise. Now stand tall. Then, holding your back straight, squat down on your haunches, slowly, then rise erect again.

If you get any opportunity during the day to sit on the floor or the grass, you can make a fine exercise out of getting on your feet again. Instead of muddling around in a graceless way and pushing yourself up with your hands, fold your legs under you, as the Chinese Buddhas do, then just straighten your legs and stand up, without using your hands at all. This one is hard and you will need to give yourself a boost with your hands when you first try it. But gradually you will be able to get to your feet gracefully without any support.

Walking is wonderful exercise, if you watch your posture while you walk. Gardening is perhaps the best exercise of all, if you keep your back straight, head high and bend your legs rather than your waist, when you are weeding or digging with a trowel.

Exercise and Heart Disorders

In pursuit of opinions about the relation of exercise to heart symptoms and to pulse rate, Editor Rodale recently wrote to a number of physician friends, asking their opinion on this subject. He explained to them that he has been taking a long walk every morning and has noticed an improvement in his pulse rate. But, he asked, how might such exercise work out for other kinds and degrees of heart trouble? The answers he got are so entertaining and worthwhile that we are printing them here just as they came to us.

All of the doctors queried are M.D.'s, all of them in agreement with our program of good food, raised organically, several devoting their time and thought to treatment and prevention of disease by the use of various vitamins and minerals.

Doctor Number One writes as follows:

"Each 'heart case is different and I cannot give you exact directions concerning the amount of exercise you should have. In general, a person with any type heart disease should do as much exercise as is possible without serious fatigue or shortness of breath. We had a symposium in Detroit several years ago with five heart specialists discussing various types of heart diseases. I particularly remember the man from the east, I believe Boston, who stated that he recommended gradually increasing amounts of exercise for his patients who had coronary thrombosis. As you know, coronary thrombosis is the end result of coronary sclerosis. His patients, even with a fairly extensive thrombosis, usually worked up to a golf game of 18 holes each day. This will give you an idea of the amount of exercise tolerated with even fairly serious heart diseases. In my opinion, it is the sudden burst of extreme exercise which does the harm.

"There is a lot of disagreement among physicians as to the amount of exercise any particular patient should have. My feeling is that every patient should have as much exercise as he can reasonably tolerate, but the exercise should be regular and, if possible, daily. Sudden bursts of extreme exercise should be avoided.

"I trust this answers your question."

Moderate Exercise Appears to Help

From doctor Number Two we received the following very full and helpful advice:

"The question of exercise is a very controversial one. For many years doctors have thought that exertion played a part in the onset of coronary occlusions and have restricted the activity of the patients who had had one, at first completely so that, when they were put to bed after the occlusion, they were not allowed to do anything for themselves. Very often, the bowels were constipated on purpose, then large doses of laxatives were given so that along with enemas the bowels could empty without any effort on the part of the patient. This extreme care is still given by most specialists in the United States and one of my patients told me that they even had a nurse to grunt for him at the first bowel movement. After the patient was up and around, he was not allowed to do anything for himself or even to walk very far for over 6 weeks so that it was 3 months before he was allowed to do anything, by which time he had no muscles left and it was suggested not to climb stairs, to sell his business and take it easy for the rest of his life.

"Two or three years ago, Dr. Samuel Levine shocked the world by suggesting that such patients did much better if they were not confined to bed except for sleeping, but placed instead in an easy chair by the side of the bed, allowed to use a commode or the bathroom on the same floor. Of course, this suggestion has met with all sorts of opposition; but more and more people are finding that he is right, the complications of lying in bed are so great that the danger of being up is much less. Of course, he would have had no chance at all with this suggestion if it had not been that for the last 10 years doctors have learned that to prevent clots in the vessels of the legs and to keep the patient from becoming so weak that convalescence is prolonged, the answer is to get them up within 24 hours after major surgery or child birth, if it is possible at all. For example, my wife had been in bed 10 days after her first child and was months regaining her strength, but she had the second baby at noon and got up and walked over to the window with me at 7 p.m. the same day and felt that apart from a little regional tenderness she had never had a baby at all. The contrast was most striking. So, heart patients getting up is one more example of this principle.

"In the last 2 or 3 years also, there have been several reprints from doctors investigating the relationship of exertion or exercise and the onset of a coronary occlusion, and most agree that there is nothing but the most casual relationship in most instances. All this is sheer apostacy and the old timers are fighting back; e. g. one of the current English medical journals very strongly points out that coronary patients must get absolute bedrest.

"The first man to suggest that patients after a coronary be given graded exercises and return to full activity, was a Philadelphia cardiologist, once the president of the American Heart Association and a great raconteur. He knows more really funny jokes than any doctor in America; so he is in great demand as an after dinner speaker. He has long advocated graded exercise and return to normal activity for his post-coronary patients, but also suggests that the way they should live, is with a glass of alcohol in one hand and a cigar in the other, the former dilating the vessels, the latter constricting them, so that very few people listened to the scientific point of his talks. However, a year or two ago, Dr. Paul White, who is a very respected cardiologist, also a past president of the American Heart Association, wrote an article suggesting a return to normal living for those patients who had coronary thrombosis, and the normal living to include consistent exercise. He has gone so far as to suggest to people growing older that they should take regular exercise. This is of course pure heresy, and it has not been listened to either, because of Dr. White's pursuit of the whale in Greenland's waters to obtain an electrocardiogram on it. This is considered a little eccentric.

Vitamin E to Prevent Blood Clots

"We believe that exertion and the stress of living have nothing to do whatever with the onset of a coronary occlusion. The reason for an occlusion is most probably a total lack of the necessary antithrombin in the blood stream. The authority on anticoagulant therapy, Dr. Irving S. Wright, just published a report showing that Vitamin E given by mouth does cause a rise of the Vitamin E in the blood stream. Zierler and Ochsner, you know, have said that alphatocopherol (Vitamin E) is an active antithrombin, perhaps all or most of the human antithrombin. You yourself, published very recently a quotation from *Time,* on Oct. 19, 1953 on the subject quoting Dr. Arthur M. Master. I cut it out and keep it in the frame of a picture behind me to show to patients when we discuss this problem.

"On the other hand, we also think that a heart which is badly damaged by an attack, is evermore somewhat in danger of trouble, just as is the tube of a tire that is patched. It is never as good as a new tube, may last quite a while yet or may suddenly give out and some of these hearts have lost a lot of muscle and have a wall fairly well replaced by scar tissue. These patients, we think, should walk and play golf and do anything which is moderate activity, but should never try to show how fast they can run or how strong they are.

"Your question, however, actually is what types of heart disease should *not* have exercise. The answer is, too badly damaged coronary hearts in which there is already failure of circulation evidenced by swollen ankles, etc., chronic rheumatic hearts in which there is evidence of failure, and these only. Even these can exert themselves up to the point of increasing shortness of breath and increasing failure with beneficial results, even if this exercise only means walking a little from chair to chair around the house. Rheumatic hearts can exercise up to the point of difficulty and we tell them to find out what that point is; the same is true with patients who have angina pectoris. They should walk until they have the beginning of trouble, and then, having found that point, should stay well short of it for at least a month or two, until they try again where the point of difficulty is. This, of course, varies from day to day with the climate and other conditions, just as a normal person varies from day to day, but they should stay clear of trouble. Up to trouble at this point, it is just as safe as doing nothing and more beneficial."

The third physician preferred to discuss the matter fully, in person. He wrote:

"In your last letter you asked me to express my opinion about exercise and heart disease. This is a very interesting question and I would prefer to discuss it personally when you come to New York. In general, I favor exercise, slowly increasing in some cases of heart disease to a certain extent. Overdosage is extremely dangerous and I would suggest to be very careful because the limit between overdosage and helpful exercise is hard to determine. Mistakes may be fatal."

Vitamins and Good Diet in Circulatory Disorders

From a long-time friend who has done outstanding work in vitamin therapy for different diseases came this reply:

"Replying to your letter of the 31st (August), graduated exercises for ambulatory heart cases have long been recognized as helpful. Dr. Schott, of Nauheim, Germany, pioneered in this method of therapy which he combined with a system of carbonated baths, employing the naturally carbonated waters of the Nauheim springs. I understand that Schott used a series of graded walks in the grounds of his institution in which the inclines were gradually increased. However, very little was known in Schott's time about coronary disease. He used his system of exercises and baths in the treatment of organic or valvular heart disease and consequent cardiac hypertrophy.

"In coronary sclerosis there is a constriction of the coronary blood supply to the heart muscle due to thickening and hardening (sclerosis) of the blood vessels. The severe pain (angina pectoris) develops whenever the working demand exceeds the supply of oxygen to the heart. For this reason pain is the urgent indication to slow down or stop the activity until an equilibrium is re-established. High blood pressure generally is a concomitant of coronary sclerosis.

"I recently had a case of very high blood pressure in a middle-aged man. The systolic pressure was 260. I persuaded him to stop tobacco and alcohol and put him on an antitoxic diet, stressing fruit and vegetable juices and reducing his intake of red meats. In three months on this regimen, supplemented by high-potency vitamin-B-complex tablets and vitamin C tablets (100 mg.), six of each daily, his blood pressure was reduced to 200. He was so improved generally that he was able to resume his occupation. A further check a month later showed a further reduction of blood pressure to 180.

"You perhaps know that the prognosis in coronary sclerosis is much more favorable than in coronary thrombosis. In both of these diseases it is imperative to limit physical activity to comply with the lessened capacity of the coronary arteries to deliver oxygenated blood to the heart muscle. Activity or emotional stress in the slightest excess of this limitation precipitate acute precordial pain (angina pectoris), for the quick relief of which amyl nitrite or nitro-glycerine is usually employed."

Exercise, Importance of

A friend of ours decided to mow his big lawn one hot Saturday afternoon and went at it with vigor and determination. He wouldn't stop until he had finished slicing off the last tuft of crabgrass. That night he went to the hospital with a heart attack. He had overestimated his own capacity for violent exercise. Every fall the newspapers carry stories of businessmen who have heart attacks while they are out scouring the hills on all-day hunting trips.

Medical authorities are pretty well agreed on the fact that exercise, especially in competitive games, can be quite dangerous after you've reached middle age. *The Journal of the American Medical Association* for June 21, 1952, carried an editorial headed "Exercise is Good—For What?" They call it a medieval therapy and comment: "Abundant medical evidence shows that with few exceptions strenuous exercise does not give increased resistance to disease, does not promote longer life, does not improve 'health'; rather it may damage the heart, cause temporary anemia and avitaminosis, produce strains, sprains and fractures and make a person better able to do only one thing—exercise."

We have shown in other articles the harm that can come from competitive athletics; we have related cases of heart attack and other serious disorders brought on by unaccustomed vigorous exercise which seems to become more hazardous if there is competition involved, which make the panting, exhausted participant struggle on in spite of his fatigue, so that the "team" will come out ahead. Such exercise is harmful. It is harmful too to overdo exercise that comes under the heading of work. An office worker who spends Saturday in the unaccustomed pastime of mowing a large lawn or getting an overdose of gardening or carpentering in the hot sun is courting trouble.

However, we believe that mild exercise has a place in the annals of good health, especially for those of us who lead a completely sedentary life, and get our only exercise swinging from the strap of a bus or subway, or pressing our feet to accelerator pedals or brakes. Exercise does increase the body's intake of oxygen which is especially important for someone who works inside all day. It does stimulate the circulation of blood. It brings about healthful changes in the bone marrow. It rests certain parts of the body that have been in positions of strain or tension, and, most important of all, the correct exercises improve posture.

There are almost as many systems of exercise for good posture as there are people who teach exercising. For everyone has developed his own system which, he claims, is better than any other. But if you study these exercises carefully you will find that they all aid in doing one job—strengthening those muscles which support the body in an upright, well-balanced position. Your body has a set of muscles which hold it upright, carefully matched, so that the muscles which pull you forward are teamed with those which pull you back. When one or another of these muscles becomes weakened, the pull is stronger from the opposing muscle and bad posture results.

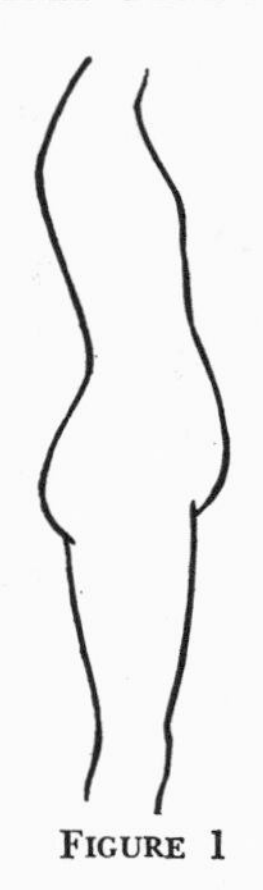
FIGURE 1

There are few of us that can boast of perfect posture. Among younger folks there is a tendency for shoulders to droop and chests to become flat and hollow. Among older people a tendency toward sway-back complicates things still further. As the muscles of your abdomen are weakened, there is more of a drag on the back muscles, pulling the spine down into an ugly, exaggerated curve. The pelvic structure tilts forward. If the stomach muscles are allowed to sag, the buttocks are bound to protrude, to keep your center of balance undisturbed. So you find more and more older people developing into a peculiar S shape (Figure 1). In the body's effort to preserve good balance, the knees turn in, the feet turn out. And gradually the curve in the back becomes more pronounced.

Exercise For Good Posture

Most posture exercises are designed to correct these faults. And most of us need these exercises. They should be done slowly, as slowly as possible. Lie on the floor (or, if you prefer, on a bed), and put a hand behind the small of your back. You will probably find that although your shoulders and buttocks touch the floor, there is a hollow large enough for your fist right beneath the small of your back. Bend your knees, keeping your feet on the floor. This should enable you to flatten your entire spine along the floor, so that there is no hollow place left (Fig. 2). Now, lower your feet gradually, trying to keep your back flat on the floor. This will strengthen the back and abdominal muscles. A very few minutes of this exercise every day for several months should enable you to hold your abdominal muscles in when you stand erect, so that the "sway-back" will gradually disappear.

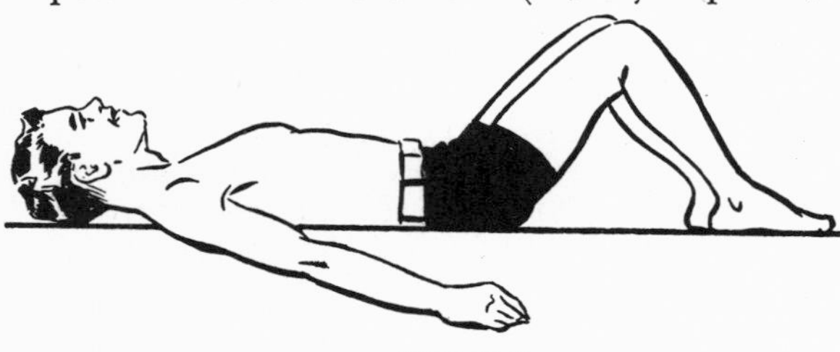
FIGURE 2

Here is a more difficult exercise. Lie flat on the floor—the bed is too soft for this one. Raise your feet a little off the floor and you will feel a strong pull on your abdominal muscles (Fig. 3). Lower your feet and the next time try to raise them a little farther. Don't hurry. You must exercise slowly if you want it to be effective.

If you don't have time to go through these muscle-strengtheners every day, you

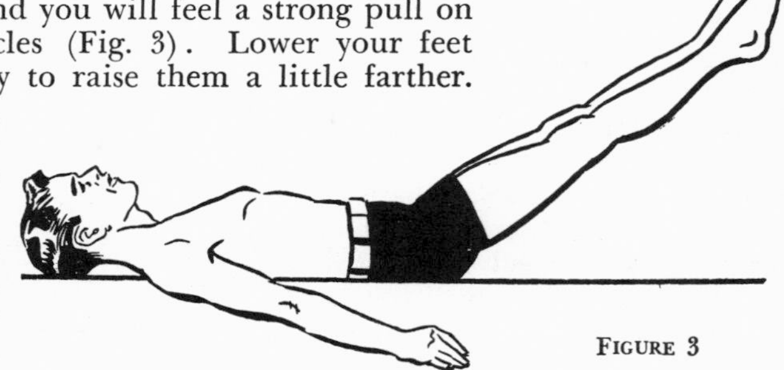
FIGURE 3

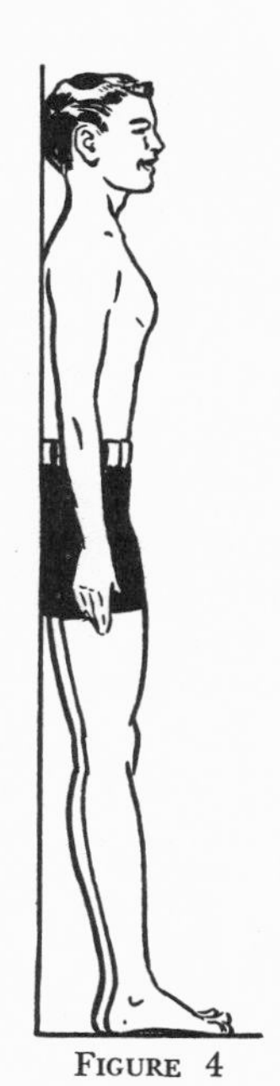

FIGURE 4

can accomplish the same thing while you are standing waiting for someone, talking on the phone, riding in an elevator and so forth. Stand against a wall, with your feet about four inches out from the wall. Push your back against the wall as hard as you can. Reach back with your hand. You'll probably find that ornery hollow still there, right at the small of your back. Pulling in on your abdominal muscles, try to straighten your whole back flat against the wall (Fig. 4). Moving your feet out from the wall will make it easier, but as you become more expert you should slide your feet closer to the wall.

Now, after you have managed to strengthen the abdominal muscles enough that the hollow in your back disappears when you stand against the wall, try your best to remember to pull those muscles in all day long wherever you are, whatever you are doing. You will find it is almost impossible to pull in your stomach muscles while your chest droops. So while you are pulling in below, watch how your chest rises. Soon you will be standing straight and well-balanced.

If your main trouble is drooping shoulders and hollow chest, it is necessary to strengthen the shoulder and chest muscles. Sit on the floor, with your legs straight in front of you, or, if it is more comfortable, cross your legs, or put your feet on the floor and bend your knees. Rest your fingers on your shoulders, lift your arms up, forward, backward and down again (Fig. 5). Can you feel the pull on those shoulder and chest muscles?

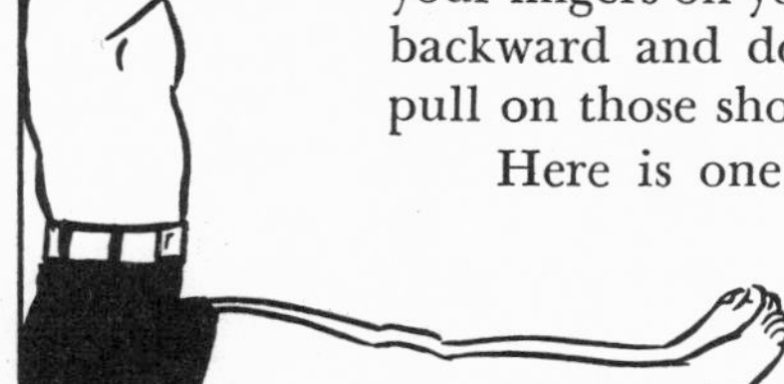

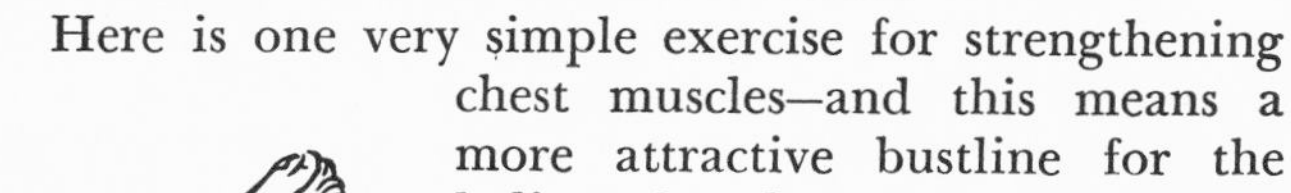

FIGURE 5

Here is one very simple exercise for strengthening chest muscles—and this means a more attractive bustline for the ladies. Stand up straight and tall, pulling in your abdominal muscles. Pick up a quite heavy book. A telephone directory or a desk dictionary will do nicely. Bend your arms and raise your elbows up level with your chin. This will bring your hands directly in front of your face. Hold the book between the fingertips of both hands and press as hard as you can (with your fingers and thumbs) as if you were trying to push right through the book on both sides. Do not use the flat part of your hand—only your

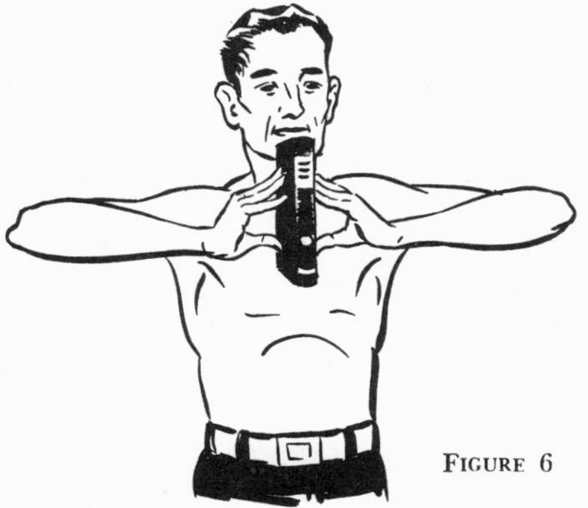

FIGURE 6

fingers (Fig. 6). And don't overdo this exercise the first day or you'll have sore muscles.

Most of us could do with some toning up when we get out of bed in the morning. Editor Rodale suggests one exercise which he performs every morning, first thing, to wake him up, get his blood to circulating freely, and dispose of the lazy feeling across arms, shoulders, neck and head. He stands straight and tall, and raises his arms at the sides to shoulder height. Then, keeping his elbows stiff, he rotates his arms in small circles, first clockwise, then counter-clockwise (Fig. 7). In fact, any firm, regular movements of the arms from the shoulders, keeping the elbows stiff, will be a handy aid in preventing stiff shoulders and loosening up joints.

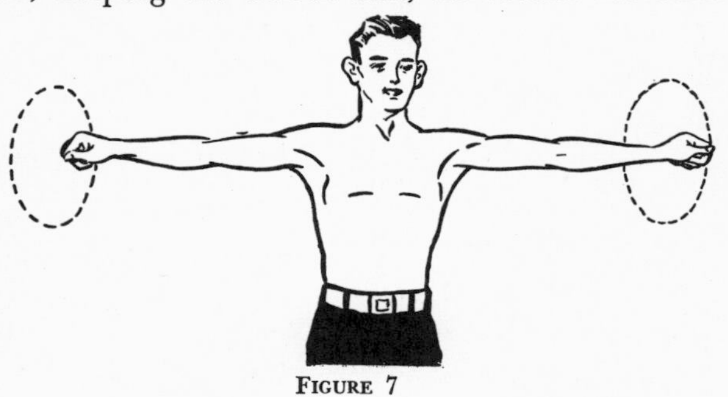

FIGURE 7

Exercising Under Water

We recently ran across a series of exercises that we feel have much to recommend them, especially for folks suffering from high blood pressure or some other disorder that precludes strenuous exercise. They are based on the fact that the body weighs less underwater! A 140-pound person weighs only about ten pounds when he is submerged in water. So doing exercises under water is much easier. With a very small amount of exertion the muscles can get a good workout and all the benefits of exercise can be had without any strain on the heart. It just involves filling up your bathtub with water at body temperature and exercising in the bath tub.

The 76-year-old Englishman who invented this method of exercise became quite famous in the pages of the conservative *British Medical Journal* and *The Lancet,* when a number of British physicians began to realize what a boon such exercises would be to their heart patients and patients who were partially bedfast. T. R. Togna, the inventor of the exercises, did careful experiments to prove how blood pressure, plus rate of oxygen intake varied during the process of exercising in a bathtub full of water.

He found that the pulse rate increased only slightly above normal during 15 or 20 minutes of bathtub exercise, whereas a similar amount of regular exercise might increase it a great deal.

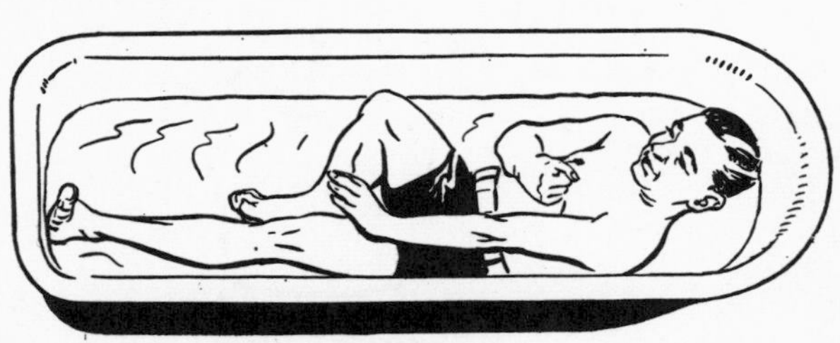

FIGURE 8

He found that blood pressure is generally reduced. There is no increase when the blood pressure is normal. If it is high, the exercise reduces it. If it is low, it is raised toward normal. He also found that the amount of oxygen intake for each pulse beat is high, with, of course, excellent results from a health standpoint because plenty of oxygen is an essential for health.

He suggests massaging the body while you are exercising so that the by-products of metabolism will be swept away rapidly in the bloodstream. Here are some of Mr. Togna's exercises you might want to try tomorrow morning when you are bathing. Water in the bathtub should be about six inches from the top after you are in the tub. Lie down with your head resting on the end of the tub. Stretch your legs out full length. Double your right hand into a fist in front of your chest while you bend your right knee and bring it up out of the water (Fig. 8). Then lower the right leg and stretch the right arm out on top of the water, while you bring up the left leg. And so forth. It is pretty much like bicycling, with your arms moving in unison with your legs except of course that your body has little weight so there is very little exertion.

Then for a second exercise, as you bend your knees, massage them and your thighs just before you lower them into the water again. Another excellent bathtub exercise involves lying with your hands below you, bracing the buttocks. Raise the trunk so that it is suspended in the water. Then, do the exercise once again with the hands resting on the abdomen. Massage the abdomen while you are raising and lowering the trunk in the water.

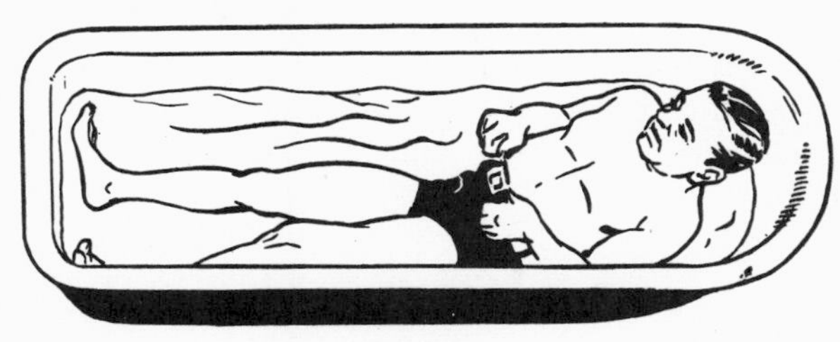

FIGURE 9

Waist twisting is done in the same position by pivoting on the toes and swinging the body from side to side while the head and feet remain stationary (Fig. 9). As you become more

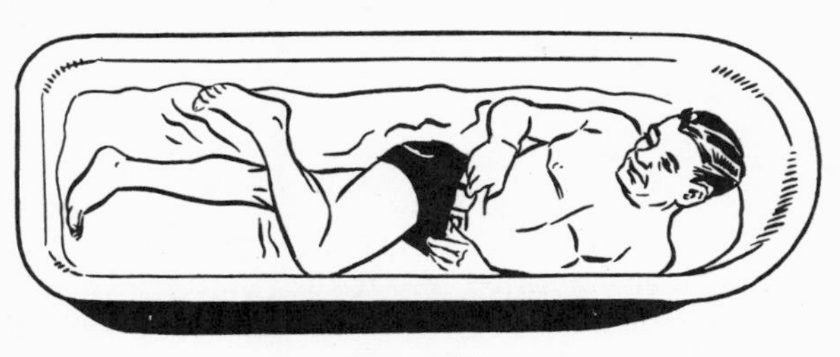

FIGURE 10

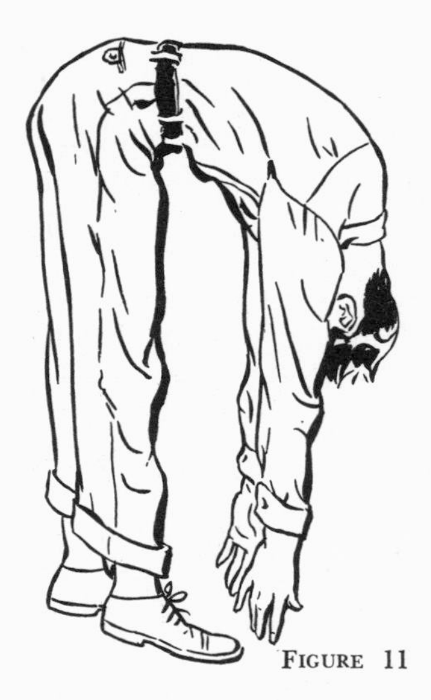

FIGURE 11

adept at twisting from side to side, vary the exercise by bending one knee at a time and crossing it over the other knee (Fig. 10). If you find the twisting exercises too difficult, lay a straight rod across the bathtub and support yourself with it as you twist and turn.

Finally let us remind you of perhaps the most elementary principle of exercise, which is that almost any form of gentle and slow movement will rest muscles that are tired from being in one position too long. If you bend over your work all day, whether your work be reading, writing, typing, drawing, cooking or what not —stop frequently and turn your head from side to side, slowly and gently. Or stand up and bend over from the waist. Let your whole upper body hang as limp as possible. Let your arms dangle as though they belonged to a rag doll. When you straighten up, you will be surprised at the relaxed feeling in those tired muscles.

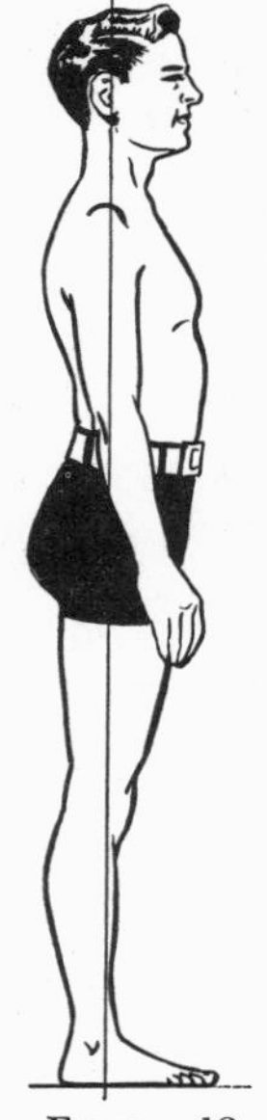

FIGURE 12

In general, keep in mind that violent rapid exercise which makes you puff and pant and get red in the face, not only brings you no benefit, but can actually do you harm. Simple, slow, stretching exercises are beneficial, especially if they rest some tired, cramped muscle, or if they improve posture. And improving posture nearly always boils down to pulling in on abdominal muscles, tucking your buttocks underneath you and raising your chest, until you have achieved really superb posture.

Eyes—Bates System of Eye Training

Not so long ago a new system for training eyesight which would make glasses unnecessary became popular. Later, enthusiasm died down considerably and we have not seen anything about the "Bates Method" for quite a long time. We feel the time is ripe to revive interest in this very sensible and successful method of treating eyes and preventing eye disorders.

To Dr. W. H. Bates, a New York oculist, came the idea that the great majority of visual defects are functional and due to faulty habits of use. These habits develop from strain and tension. By teaching his patients how to relax and how to use their eyes in a relaxed way, Dr. Bates found that vision was improved and errors in their sight were corrected.

Actually when you stop to think of it, why should any of us be content to wear glasses? If the defect were in the knee instead, would we be as content to go on a crutch? Of course not! We would try every doctor and every known technique that might bring our knee back to usefulness so that we could discard the crutch. But we seem to take it for granted that eventually, if not at once, we will have to be fitted with glasses and once we have been, we will always have to wear them, while our eyes, depending on the glasses as our legs would on a crutch, get progressively worse, needing stronger glasses from time to time.

On the other hand, if we did not use our legs correctly, we would probably feel the need of a crutch in time. And so with our eyes. At any rate, this is the basis of Dr. Bates' theory which is explained in his own book, *Better Eyesight Without Glasses* (Published by Henry Holt and Co., 383 Madison Ave., New York 17) and another book *The Art of Seeing,* written by the famous English author, Aldous Huxley. Mr. Huxley, who very nearly lost his sight at the age of sixteen, attributes to the Bates system his recovery of sight in one eye and a great improvement of sight in the other.

According to Mr. Huxley, ophthalmologists are interested in the physiological aspects of seeing. Artificial lenses in spectacles work mechanically to correct physiological sight defects. But what of the mental, the psychological aspect of seeing? What of the right and the wrong ways of using the eyes? Isn't it possible that by learning to use the eyes correctly one may correct defects that have probably been caused by using the eyes incorrectly?

In his book Mr. Huxley describes many of the Bates exercises. We have time for only a few here. Perhaps the most important is "palming" whose purpose is to relax the eyes. Bates students are requested to "palm" often. Resting the elbows on a table, cover the eyes with the hands, one hand to each eye. Rest the palm of the hand on the cheek, the fingers on the forehead so that the hand does not touch the eye itself. You should see nothing but black. If there are spots, flashes of light or other disturbances, keep palming, relaxed and effortless, until you see nothing but black. It will help to think of the color black or to think of some pleasant happening in the past, "seeing" the incident in your mind's eye, with your physical eyes closed.

A second helpful exercise from the Bates method is blinking. According to Mr. Huxley, one outstanding fault of the person with poor eyesight is his tendency to stare. He is so eager to see well, he wants so desperately not to miss a thing, he know his eyes are bad and so he makes a great effort and strains hard to see better. All that he actually does is to make himself see worse.

"Movement," says Mr. Huxley . . . "is one of the indispensable conditions of sensing and perceiving. But so long as the eyelids are kept tense and relatively immobile, the eyes themselves will remain tense and relatively immobile. Hence anyone who wishes to acquire the art of seeing well must cultivate the habit of frequent and effortless blinking . . ."

He suggests a "blinking drill" every hour or so, followed by a few seconds of relaxing the eyes by closing them. Half a dozen light butterfly-blinks, then closing, another half-dozen blinks, then closing, and so on for about a minute. This kind of exercise is especially important for those engaged in close work where the eyes can be harmed by straining and staring.

Some Eye Exercises That Are Fun To Try

Another good habit is to squeeze the eyes shut every so often—wrinkling up all the other face muscles at the same time. Do this when you are tempted to rub your eyes, for you should never, never rub your eyes for any reason at all. Nor should you massage them, but you can rub the temples which will relax and soothe the eyes, and you can rub and knead the muscles in the upper part of the nape of the neck which will help.

"Flashing" is another exercise recommended in the Bates method—important for making the eye more mobile and increasing these powers of the mind that perceive and interpret what one sees. Flashing is the opposite of staring. Rather than straining to see all parts of an object, glance at it quickly, almost casually, then close your eyes and remember what the object looked like. You will be surprised to find that your physical eye "saw" more than you knew it saw. For, with your eyes closed, you will be able to remember far more about the object than you were conscious of seeing.

Children who are re-learning how to use their eyes have no trouble with "flashing" for they are much less self-conscious that adults. "A child is shown some object, say a domino, or a printed letter or word, from a distance at which he cannot normally see. He is told to take a flashing glance at it, then close his eyes and 'reach up into the air for it.' The child obeys the order quite literally, raises a hand, closes it on emptiness, then lowers it, opens it, looks into his palm and gives the correct answer, as though he were reading from notes."

"Shifting" is another exercise, for, says Mr. Huxley, "people with normal vision keep their eyes and attention shifting unconsciously in a series of almost imperceptibly small movements from point to point. People with defective vision, on the contrary, greatly reduce the number of such movements and tend to stare. It is, therefore, necessary for them to build up consciously the habit of small-scale shifting which they acquired unconsciously in childhood and subsequently lost."

When you are "shifting" you don't try to see the whole thing at which you are looking. Make yourself look at it piece by piece, studying first this portion, then that. If it is as large a thing as a house, look first at the windows, then the roof, then the door and so forth. If it is as small as a printed letter M, look first at the straight line, then at the slanting down line, then at the line that slants up and finally at the last upright line. In this way your eye, instead of staring at the letter, will move over it, bit by bit. This is good training for good sight.

Imagination is Important in Eye Exercises

One very amusing exercise which apparently Mr. Huxley often uses is "nose writing." Sit comfortably in an easy chair and imagine you have a pencil attached to the end of your nose. In fact, everything you do in this exercise involves your imagination. Using the imaginary pencil attached to your nose, begin to write, moving your shoulders and head as you need to. Imagine that you are drawing a large circle. If it looks uneven to your "inner eye," draw over and over it until you have a fairly presentable circle. Then draw a line through the center, and another at right angles to it, and so forth. The object of this exercise is to relax and rest the eyes. Of course you must be using your imagination in a lively fashion throughout. And this, too, teaches you how to use your imagination later on in some of the more difficult eye exercises which, according to Dr. Bates, will improve your eyesight greatly.

It is impossible to sum up in a sentence the full meaning of the Bates treatment. But it is, generally speaking, a treatment designed to correct eyesight by teaching the individual to use his eyes correctly. This means that he will see correctly.

Dr. Bates' book describes some astonishing cures of eye disorders all the way from myopia to glaucoma. He tells of cases among his own patients where the prescribed treatment (without glasses) brought relief from pains of neuralgia, headaches, and other physical symptoms aside from cases of improvement in actual sight that sound well nigh unbelievable. During his lifetime Dr. Bates suffered from the persecution that is universally visited upon those who discover something new in the way of treatment and use it successfully. He was called quack and charlatan. "It is quite true," says Mr. Huxley, "that oculists and optometrists have never observed such phenomena as are described by Bates and his followers. But this is because they have never had any dealings with patients who had learned to use their organs of vision in a relaxed, unrestrained way."

We would suggest that you get Dr. Bates' book out of your local library. If they do not have it, perhaps they will order it for you. Or you can order the revised edition from Henry Holt and Co., 383 Madison Ave., New York 17, N. Y. We are quite sure the book by Huxley from which we have quoted will be in your library. It is published by Harper Brothers, 49 E. 33rd St., New York, N. Y.

Eyes—Bloodshot Eyes

A Cincinnati physician writes to the editor of the *Journal of the American Medical Association,* July 24, 1954, commenting on chronic bloodshot eyes. If no weakening chronic disease is present to account for the bleary-looking orbs, says he, it is very possible that the patient has not been getting enough of the right kind of nutrition. Omitting alcohol and putting the patient on a diet high in vitamins, *with particular attention to the B vitamins,* may correct the condition entirely. So before you decide that your neighbor with the bloodshot eyes probably spends most of his time bending an elbow at the local bar, why not suggest helpfully to his wife that she begin to serve more liver and get into the habit of using brewer's yeast in some way or other in the family's meals. Any good book on nutrition at the local library will tell her what other foods are rich in the B vitamins.

Eyes—Cataract

What is Cataract?

Cataract is a disorder of the lens of the eye, generally spoken of as a "degenerative disorder"—that is, it results from things wearing out and breaking down, rather than "catching something" or being injured.

In the eye with cataract, the lens becomes opaque, like a misty or fogged windowglass. The lens is that part of the eye which gathers the rays of light and focuses them on the nerve endings behind it. Apparently what happens in cataract is that cells die or become damaged, turning white in the process. Clusters of these white cells are what you see in the eye with the fully advanced cataract. Cataract is not a "growth" —that is, it is not in the same class with tumors. It does not represent cells growing abnormally. It appears to represent rather cells dying off and becoming useless.

Is There More Than One Kind of Cataract?

Yes, there are several. Senile cataract is the commonest—the one most people mean when they speak of cataract. The word "senile" is used here because this kind of cataract usually afflicts people who are advanced in age, although, just like gray hair and wrinkles, it can occur in quite young persons as well.

Congenital cataract occurs in babies at birth. Diabetic cataract sometimes afflicts diabetics of any age. It is believed to go along with degenerative changes in blood vessels that also occur in diabetics.

Does Cataract Cause Blindness?

It does. It is the first and most important cause of blindness in this country today. It is estimated that 49,000 Americans are sightless because of cataract. This does not mean, of course, that everyone who gets cataract will become blind; quite the contrary is true. Modern surgery can remove the lens of the eye on which the cataract is spread, replacing it with a powerful lens in spectacles. The patient then can see so long as he has his glasses on. When the cataract is fully developed, light cannot pass through the opacity, so there is no way for an individual with a fully developed cataract to see, so long as the cataract remains on his lens.

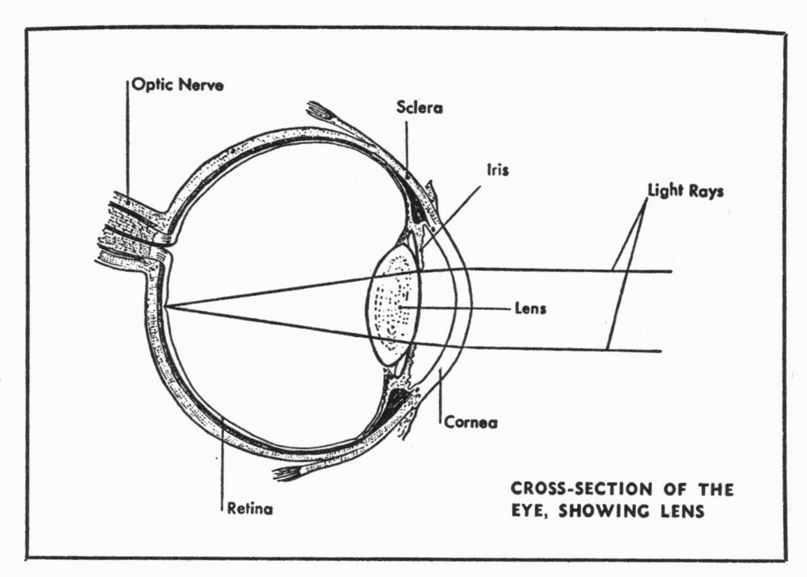

CROSS-SECTION OF THE EYE, SHOWING LENS

Is the Operation for Cataract Painful and Risky?

No. It seems that the biggest hazard is the patient's frame of mind. He may have worked himself into such a state of dread and anxiety that it takes him a long time to recover his peace of mind after the operation. But the time in the hospital is, it seems, far pleasanter than for most operations. Generally a local anesthesia is given so that the discomforts of general anesthesia are avoided. The percentage of failures is apparently very low. If there are not other complications there is every chance that the patient will be able to see quite well after the operation is over and the new lenses have been made.

We are not, of course, enthusiastic about surgery. We believe that cataracts can be prevented by proper diet and care of the eyes. But, if one has *not* prevented the cataract and is in imminent danger of losing his sight, it does seem sensible to think calmly and reasonably about an operation.

What Causes Cataract?

We do not know. Oh of course, we do know of some circumstances that appear to be related to the formation of cataracts. Men who work in extremely high temperatures, exposed to the blasting heat of great furnaces, are especially susceptible to cataracts and it is assumed that these cataracts are occupational diseases. Dinitrophenol is a drug taken as a reducing aid. It increases the basal metabolism rate so that the patient can lose weight. Cataracts are quite common, we are told, among women past forty who have taken this drug to reduce. And cataracts can be produced in animals by giving them this drug. (Isn't it amazing that women would take such a dangerous drug and risk blindness rather than reducing sensibly?)

We know, too, that smoke may have a lot to do with causing cataracts —cigarette smoke and smoke from fires. The Hunzas, for instance, a perfectly healthy nation otherwise, suffer from eye disorders because of the arrangement of their houses where there is not much room for the smoke from their fires to escape. When one considers the thick pall of tobacco smoke in which many of us pass our days (whether we smoke ourselves or just spend our time with those who do) it is not surprising that cataracts are so common, for the tobacco smoke is highly irritating to the eyes.

It has been suggested that long-exposure to bright sunlight may have something to do with producing cataracts, for people living in India are especially susceptible to them. And rural folks who work outside a lot seem to have more than those who work indoors. However, we must not forget that other things may be responsible as well. One researcher tells us that the average cataract patient in India is suffering from a number of different deficiency diseases. Perhaps the cataract is just one of these.

The tendency in old age is to harden, according to one authority. Cataract is another manifestation of this tendency, he says. The blood vessels harden, the muscles become stiff, the skin becomes horny. And the lens of the eye becomes opaque says he. It's just another indication of old age and nothing can be done about it. This does not, of course, explain the many young people with cataracts, nor yet the babies who are born with cataracts.

We believe that the cause of cataracts is faulty nutrition. We have a lot more to say in support of this theory in the next article. In doing research for this article we were astonished to find that many, many scientists and physicians admit that cataract is a result of poor nutrition, but very few of them suggest correcting or preventing it by diet!

Before birth, blood is brought to the human lens by a blood vessel which withers away before the baby is born. So the lens, which is bathed in the fluid of the eye, has no way of getting nourishment except from that fluid. Hence it cannot rebuild itself as well as tissues in other parts of the body can, well nourished as they are with food brought by the blood. It gradually becomes brittle and inelastic. The center of the lens gets less nourishment than the edges, so generally the cataract starts in the center and spreads out gradually.

How Can I Tell Whether or not I have a Cataract?

You can't actually. Many cataracts are undetected by the individuals who have then until they begin to interfere with vision. If you notice any peculiarity of vision it would be best to have your eye doctor check your eyes. Sometimes cataracts produce foggy vision which gradually becomes dimmer. Sometimes bright light is painful. There may seem to be bright-colored rings around lights at night. If you want to be reasonably sure you don't develop any of these symptoms, regardless of your age, we'd suggest that you start now to improve your nutrition, which will automatically improve the nutrition of the lens of your eye which must certainly remove you farther and farther from the danger of cataract.

Why Are Cataracts Called This Peculiar Name?

Cataracts have been known for thousands of years. The ancient Greeks "had a word for it." They thought that a cataract was a flow of cloudy fluid in front of the lens. So they named it just that—a waterfall. We have kept the name, even though we know there is no actual flow of water involved.

Eyes—Preventing Cataract

It is impossible to say categorically that this or that vitamin, mineral or food is "good for the eyes." The eyes, like other parts of the body, must be nourished by all the various parts of food that make it nutritious. Vitamin A is extremely important for good eyesight. Deficiency in vitamin A can cause night blindness which means that you have difficulty in adjusting to light after darkness, or darkness after light. The B vitamins (especially riboflavin) are extremely important for healthy eyes. A kind of twilight blindness and a very definite fear of bright light result from not getting enough riboflavin. Vitamin C is important for good eyesight, as it is important for every other function of the body. Calcium is needed in the fluids of the eye. Protein is needed to replace eye tissues that have been broken down. And so it goes.

Are any of these important for the prevention of cataract? All of them are, for they are all necessary to good eye health. You cannot imagine a wonderfully healthy eye, strong, efficient, never giving any trouble, with a cataract beginning to cover the lens! Of course not! What is good for the rest of the eye is also good for the lens. And vice versa.

But we know that certain vitamins may have a somewhat greater importance than others in preventing cataract. For instance, vitamin C is concentrated in the lens of the healthy eyes. Why? We do not know. It is also concentrated in certain tissues in other parts of the body—the adrenal glands, for instance. We cannot help but believe that this concentration of the vitamin must mean that it is needed in that spot especially for some good purpose. Now when we find out that the lens that has a cataract contains very little or no vitamin C, this seems to indicate something very important. Is the lack of vitamin C responsible for the cataract or is the cataract responsible for the lack of vitamin C? If cataract were a contagious disease spread by germs we would certainly think that the vitamin C had been used up fighting the germs. That's what vitamin C does, you know. But there is no germ involved.

How then can we explain this peculiar lack of vitamin C in the lens with cataract? One function of vitamin C is to keep repairing the cement between the cells. Could it be that lack of vitamin C has caused these cells to degenerate and form the cataract? It seems likely. And sure enough, we find that in laboratories, researchers have produced cataracts in laboratory animals and then slowed down their growth by giving vitamin C at the same time.

Rats fed large amounts of *dinitrophenol* (the reducing drug that produces cataract, you will remember) responded very rapidly when they were given vitamin C. Other rats developed cataract when they were fed enormous doses of galactose, a form of sugar. If the vitamin C was given along with the sugar the appearance of the cataracts was delayed. We have this information from a book called *The Newer Knowledge of Nutrition* by McCollum, Orent-Keiles and Day. (Published by Macmillan Co. New York, N. Y.)

Riboflavin, Too, Is Important for Eye Health

We also know that when scurvy (the disease of vitamin C deficiency) is produced in guinea pigs, there is a marked decrease in the vitamin C of the lens. And it is sometimes possible to produce cataracts in guinea pigs on what is called a scorbutic diet—that is, a diet containing little or no vitamin C. We rather suspect, however, that the reason this is difficult is because cataracts may result from deficiency in several different vitamins—not just vitamin C. And so the guinea pigs whose diet contains plenty of other vitamins may not get cataract.

McCollum and his associates also tell us that they have a report from a Dr. Josephson indicating that he gave from 15 to 300 milligrams of vitamin C daily to patients with cataract with marked improvement. Within a week mature cataracts became transparent enough to allow some vision.

Vitamin B_2—riboflavin—is extremely important for eye health. The eye is one of the most sensitive organs in the body to a deficiency in riboflavin. In fact, if you are suffering from any peculiar eye symptom we'd suggest taking many times the minimum amount of riboflavin each day, no matter what medical treatment you are getting for your eyes. The riboflavin is bound to help. And it's very scarce in most of our diets, so there's a good chance that we may be short.

In one experiment rats kept on a diet containing no riboflavin got cataracts—almost one hundred per cent of them! It occurred only in rats who were deprived of the vitamin at an early age, not those who got the deficient diet after they were mature. Could it be that the very widespread incidence of cataracts today is the direct result of lack of riboflavin in the diet of folks who were growing up fifty, sixty, or seventy years ago? In other experiments these clear-cut results have not been secured. It is believed that possibly these laboratory diets were not as deficient in riboflavin as the investigators thought. However, nutrition books in general relate deficiency in riboflavin with cataract.

Could then the reason for cataracts in newborn babies be caused by lack of riboflavin and vitamin C in the mother's diet? There seems to be no reason why not. The mineral calcium is also related to the formation of cataract. Cantarow in his book *Calcium Metabolism and Calcium Therapy* (Lea and Febiger 1931) says that a lack of calcium in the diet allows the cataract to form. He also says that calcium seems to be necessary for the body to use vitamin C correctly. Remember what we said about not just one but many, many elements being important for any body function?

Finally we have abundant evidence that a diet low in protein is likely to make one susceptible to cataract. Researchers have been able to produce cataracts in animals by feeding them diets in which one or another of the important amino acids (forms of protein) is lacking. The essential amino acids work together—one cannot function without all of them. Adding the missing amino acids to the diet delayed the appearance of the cataracts.

Treating Incipient Cataract with Diet

Now listen to what one practicing M.D. has to say about preventing and treating cataracts, for this gentleman has been doing wonderful work among cataract patients. Dr. Donald T. Atkinson of San Antonio, Texas, wrote in the February, 1952, issue of *The Eye, Ear, Nose and Throat Monthly* an article entitled "Malnutrition as an Etiological (causative) Factor in Senile Cataract."

He tells us first that there has been a lot of discussion about the possibility of cataract resulting from dehydration of the lens—that is, perhaps the water has been extracted from it. Cholera patients, it seems, go blind in the last stages of their illness because the lenses of their eyes dry out. A frog placed in salt water soon develops cataract because the salt extracts the water from the lens of the eye. Put the frog back into fresh water and the cataract disappears. Dr. Atkinson does not mention the danger of too much salt in the diet of human beings, but his story about the frog makes us wonder whether the vast amount of over-salting we do has anything to do with cataract.

Dr. Atkinson became intensely interested in the relationship of diet to cataract when he was treating the wife of a young physician for cataract. At about the same time, he says, there were numerous other cases of cataract among young people in that part of the country. He remarked to himself that all these young people seemed to be remarkably badly nourished, including the physician's wife.

All of them lived mainly on corn products and salt pork. Their principal beverage was coffee; they drank little water. Fresh foods were almost non-existent in their diets. As for bread, they ate refined wheat and corn bread raised with bicarbonate of soda—not yeast. The soda rapidly destroyed whatever vitamins might have remained in their bread. And the lack of yeast removed the one last source of B vitamins that might have remained to them.

So Dr. Atkinson began to suggest to his patients who were just beginning to get cataracts that they adopt diets rich in some of the vitamins, especially vitamin C—cabbage, oranges, carrots, tomatoes, rutabagas, turnips and so forth. Result? Several patients who really followed the diet found that their cataracts were getting no bigger; in some cases they improved.

The other food factor that Dr. Atkinson used in treating his cataract patients was chlorophyll. He reminds us that green plants are more nutritious than dried ones; that animals do better on green pasture than dried hay, as evidenced by their half-starved looks in early spring, and the rapidity with which they recover once they begin to eat green grass again. The chemical properties of chlorophyll, the green coloring matter of plants, are almost the same as the properties of hemoglobin, the red coloring matter in the blood. The chemical formula differs only in the fact that in the hemoglobin molecule an atom of iron corresponds to the atom of magnesium in the chlorophyll.

"It is a very engrossing fact," says he, "as it now appears, in the retardation of cataract that the formula of chlorophyll and hemoglobin are so nearly alike. Willstatter found carotin, a type of chlorophyll in the body of fresh carrots, and he suspected that its administration had a wholesome effect on vision. So far as I know I was the first to prescribe a diet of green tops of garden vegetables to cataract patients and I still find that this diet has its advantages in incipient cataract cases."

Will Not Such a Diet Prevent Cataract?

This is the kind of diet Dr. Atkinson uses in cases of cataracts: a greatly increased intake of water—from 8 to 10 glasses a day in addition to the tea, coffee and whatever other beverages the patient is drinking. From a list of the green tops of 6 selected garden vegetables he has them add one as "greens" to the diet daily. We suppose they can choose whichever they like best. Then in addition he gives them chlorophyll tablets, large doses of vitamin C—we mean as much as 1000 milligrams a day. Then he gives them 200,000 units of vitamin A every day. Each patient is required to have a pint of milk* and two eggs daily. (Look over this diet if you are worried about cataract and see whether *your* daily diet is this good.)

At the time he wrote this article, 1952, Dr. Atkinson had 450 patients with elementary cataract. Over a period of eleven years in a number of these the cataract had shown no progress. Formerly his patients went through the regular routine with cataract—letting it mature, then having an operation. Now, he tells us, only a limited number have had to have operations.

We think we know another reason for the success of Dr. Atkinson's diet, quite apart from the amount of chlorophyll in it. It contains plenty of vitamins A and C. The green things from the garden are rich in vitamins A and C as well as riboflavin—the B vitamin we found in our research to be important for the prevention of cataract. There is calcium, too, in those green leafy vegetables—lots of it. Then, too, when one is eating plenty of fresh vegetables and fruits, he just can't water his diet down with a lot of white bread and rich desserts. He just hasn't the room. And this is bound to be helpful, too.

We would add to Dr. Atkinson's diet for preventing cataract brewer's yeast, which is the richest possible source of riboflavin and all the other B vitamins. We would certainly add bone meal for additional calcium and other naturally occurring minerals. And we would add vitamin E, to preserve the health of blood vessels, thus assuring better nutrition for all the tissues of the body.

---

* We suggest bone meal and brewer's yeast. Rather than milk.

Eyes—Crossed Eyes

Crossed eyes can be corrected at any age, but the best results are obtained before school age is reached, according to A. L. Morgan, M.D. in the *Canadian Journal of Public Health,* for February, 1955. There is of course the psychological reason—the child doesn't want to be different from his friends and classmates. Then too, chances of developing good coordinated vision in both eyes are better if the correction is undertaken early. It is particularly dangerous to neglect crossed eyes in a baby, for this may be the first sign of a tumor in the turned eye. Most babies do not coordinate their eyes in the first few months, but they should be using their eyes together by the age of six months. It is well to keep in mind, too, that eyes can be crossed without appearing to have anything the matter with them. Perhaps they cross only when the child is tired or sick.

A visit to the doctor will establish the fact that the child's eyes are not normal, if this is indeed the case. Don't forget, when you are considering treatment, that a number of books have been written dealing with exercises for eye health.

Eyecups

A note in the New Hampshire *Health News* points out that the eyecup is in the same category as the family toothbrush—a menace to health. Dr. Cogwell, author of the article, reminds us that infection of one kind or another can be easily transferred by using a common eye cup, so the gadget should always be boiled or sterilized before using.

But, perhaps more important is the fact that there doesn't seem to be much sense to using an eye cup at all—even a sterilized one. The eye secretes a liquid called lysozyme. This enzyme is a powerful antiseptic against most bacteria. Left to itself, it will probably take care of whatever is bothering the eye. Why wash it away?

Eyes—Overuse

From the *British Medical Journal* for August 15, 1953, comes a comment on eye-damage, made by J. H. Doggart, M. D. Says he: "It is almost impossible to damage the eyes by long hours of reading and sewing, even if great fatigue is experienced at the time."

It has always seemed to us that using your eyes is good for them and especially if you use your eyes properly in a relaxed fashion, as Dr. Bates taught in his books on the subject, you can use them just about indefinitely without doing them harm.

Don't forget, too, that what you eat influences eye health. Vitamins A, B and C are especially important where eye tissue is concerned.

Eyes, Spots Before the

A question to the editor of the *British Medical Journal* (April 17, 1954) inquires "What are the causes of 'spots before the eyes'? What are their significance and treatment?" The editor answers that spots before the eyes may be an indication of something generally wrong, such as a disorder of the blood vessels or the liver. Or it may be the result simply of opaque spots in the vitreous or transparent part of the eye, in which case they are completely harmless and nothing to worry about.

There is a possibility, of course, that they may come from quite serious eye diseases, such as choroidoretinitis (inflammation of the retina) or a detached retina. In these cases they do not generally seem to be just plain "spots," but there are shimmering lights, haloes around things at night and other manifestations of something wrong with the eyes.

The editor tells us that there is no treatment for spots before the eyes. First, of course, one should have an eye examination. If nothing is amiss with the eyes, a general examination should reveal whether there is a disorder of the blood vessels, the liver and so forth. If all the tests are negative, then it seems best to ignore the spots, for they do not signify anything important, says the editor.

A friend of ours who had vivid, flashing spots of light before her eyes, went to an oculist who could find nothing wrong with her eyes, and said goodby to her in these words, "If you find out what causes it, let me know. I've had just such spots for the past five years." A general examination showed that she had an abscessed tooth which had spread infection throughout her body and resulted in anemia, as well as deficiency in all the vitamins and minerals. After the tooth came out, a good diet with supplements of vitamins A, B, C and D and bone meal dissolved the spots in a few weeks.

Eyes and Vitamin Deficiency

There are many parts of your body which act as sentinels—that is, they will give danger signals when things are not going well. We all know that a doctor looks at your tongue when he is diagnosing your ailment. He may also examine your fingernails and lips. But if he is a good doctor and, especially if he is very conscious of the importance of good nutrition to health, he will probably also examine your eyes for symptoms that will indicate clear as a bell what may be causing your difficulty.

Deficiency in any of the major vitamins results in eye symptoms. In one way this is good, for those of us who study nutrition can be aware of these symptoms and if we find them in ourselves or in members of our family, we can hazard a pretty sound guess that vitamin deficiency may be responsible. For instance, burning, itching eyes that are frequently bloodshot may indicate eyestrain. True, this may mean that you are using your eyes too much or that you may need glasses. But if you get the glasses and use your eyes a lot less, and the symptoms still continue, we would suggest sitting down and going over a week's menu with a certain vitamin in mind. If you find, as you are likely to, that you have been steadily skipping this important vitamin without even being aware of it, then is the time to become very conscious of it, reorganize your menus to include it and then watch for improvement in the eyes.

An interesting article in the *Medical Press* for June 4, 1952, summarizes the effects of the deficiency of various vitamins on the eyes and indicates how to remedy these conditions. The author of the article is A. J. Cameron, M.D., Ch.B., D.O.M.S., FRCS, a surgeon at the Royal Eye Hospital in London, England. Dr. Cameron tells us that for the last 50 years amblyopia has been reported which seemed to be due to nutritional deficiency. Amblyopia means simply dimness of vision that is not caused by an organic disease of the eye or some defect in the eye mechanism. In England, before the war, says Dr. Cameron, nutritional deficiency was unusual. But after the war it became quite common to find the symptoms of a partial vitamin deficiency which showed itself in delayed healing of wounds, tardy return to health after an illness, and extension of the time an infection might be expected to run its course.

In these cases of more or less slight vitamin deficiency it is not unusual to find definite changes in the cornea, lens and retina of the eye. Of course this does not always indicate simply that the necessary vitamin or vitamins are lacking in the diet. It may mean instead that the person is unable to assimilate them, no matter whether he has plenty of them at hand. Pregnant women and nursing mothers are more liable to this kind of deficiency because of the drain on their own body resources. Usually deficiency of one vitamin alone does not occur. An individual deficient in one is almost certain to be deficient in others as well. This is one reason why we, at the risk of being repetitive, stress a wide variety of diet. It is also one very good reason for never taking synthetic vitamins. It is hardly possible, for instance, to be deficient in just one of the B vitamins. Taking a synthetic B vitamin is quite likely to lead to a deficiency in another of the B vitamins. Dr. Cameron tells us that the vitamins most important from the point of view of eye health are: A, the B vitamins, C and D.

Vitamin A Deficiency and Eye Health

Most of us know that lack of vitamin A causes definite eye symptoms. These are night blindness, xerophthalmia and keratomalacia. Xerophthalmia is a dry and thickened condition of the conjunctiva or eye tissues which sometimes follows conjunctivitis or a disease of the tear glands. Keratomalacia is a softening of the cornea.

It is known that the normal retina and the choroid (an eye membrane) contain enormous amounts of vitamin A. Apparently, vitamin A is necessary for the process that goes on inside the eye when your body moves from darkness to light, or from light to darkness. So a lack of vitamin A would hinder this process.

It has been found that night blindness resulting from vitamin deficiency may be accompanied by scotomata—that is, dark spots in the field of vision. We know that both these conditions are caused directly by too little vitamin A and can be cured by increasing the amount of vitamin A available for the use of the body.

Often night blindness is accompanied by dryness of the cornea and the eye tissues, with triangular spots, silver gray and shiny which are called Bitot's spots, after the physician who first studied them. The area that is affected by this dryness feels gritty, as if there were grains of sand on the eyeball. Then too, as if there were a film of oil over it, it cannot be "wetted."

Keratomalacia is an advanced and much more serious state than either or both of these first two conditions. Dryness is first noticed, followed by a softening of the cornea which becomes gray, dull and cloudy. Since this condition is an indication of severe vitamin A deficiency, other tissues in the body also suffer and may finally be so starved for vitamin A that the patient dies.

Vitamin B is Important Too

It seems that most of the B vitamins, as well, are necessary for eye health, and that even partial deficiency in one or more of them results in symptoms that can be recognized by physicians. Serious lack of thiamin (one of the B vitamins) may bring on beriberi or neuritis. In the eyes, this takes the form of retrobulbar neuritis, or pains behind the eyeball. There may also be many dark spots on the field of vision, probably near the center of this field.

In describing cases of repatriated prisoners of war from the far East, Dr. Cameron tells us that he found three different kinds of symptoms: 1. Dark spots in the center of the field of vision; 2. General lack of clear vision in the entire visual field; and 3. Psychogenic symptoms—that is, examination could discover nothing wrong with the eyes, but the patients complained of sight disorders. These soldiers who had been imprisoned, eating completely inadequate diets, found that their symptoms persisted for as long as 8 to 12 months, and when they returned to a good diet they very often found that for a while the symptoms grew worse. Then, of course, the addition of the necessary B vitamins in large enough amounts brought about a cure of all symptoms.

Riboflavin, niacin, pyridoxine, pantothenic acid and folic acid, other B vitamins, are also concerned in eye health. In certain forms of pellagra, for instance, giving just niacin will not cure the disease. These other members of the B family of vitamins are necessary as well. In pellagra there is inflammation of the eyelids and loss of eyelashes, erosion of the eye tissues and clouding of the cornea. When riboflavin is lacking in the diet, the eyelids may smart and itch, the eyes grow tired, vision may be poor and cannot be improved by glasses, it may be difficult for the individual to see in dim light and there may be extreme sensitivity to light. This does not mean that the patient cannot stand any light at all, but rather that he suffers actual physical discomfort in the presence of bright light.

Adelle Davis in her book, *Vitality Through Planned Nutrition* gives more details about eye conditions that result from lack of riboflavin. Dr. Day at Columbia University produced cataract in rats who were deficient in riboflavin. If they were not given riboflavin, they eventually became completely blind. Dr. Sydenstricker of the University of Georgia, studied 47 patients all of whom lacked riboflavin. They suffered from a variety of visual disturbances. They were sensitive to light, suffered from eyestrain that was not relieved by wearing glasses, they had burning sensations in their eyes and visual fatigue. They were sensitive to light and their eyes watered easily. Six of them had cataract. Within 24 hours after the administration of riboflavin, symptoms began to improve. After two days, the burning sensations and the other symptoms began to disappear. Gradually all disorders were cured. When the riboflavin was taken away from them, the symptoms gradually appeared again and once again were cured by riboflavin.

Vitamin C is All-Important For Eye Health

Vitamin C, also called ascorbic acid, is one of the most important elements in a diet for good eye health, and one of the most difficult to obtain in abundance. Vitamin C is not stored in the body, so you must eat foods containing vitamin C every day. In scurvy which is the disease indicating severe vitamin C deficiency, there are hemorrhages of the eyelids and eye tissues. The eyes have a tendency to water, the conjunctival membranes grow dry and there may be softening or ulceration of the cornea.

There are large amounts of vitamin C in the lens and other parts of the normal eye. In cases of cataract the amount of vitamin C is diminished. We do not know, says Dr. Cameron, whether it is lack of vitamin C that brings on the cataract or the cataract that results in lack of vitamin C. Adelle Davis tells us that the blood and urine of individuals suffering from cataract contain far less vitamin C than that of people the same age who do not have cataract. She also tells us that large doses of vitamin C have brought about improvement in cataract patients.

Vitamin D is that vitamin which our body manufactures from the ultraviolet rays of the sun. It is necessary for the proper use of calcium and phosphorus by our bodies. Rickets is the disease resulting when there is not enough calcium, phosphorus or vitamin D. In some kinds of rickets, a cataract of a certain kind develops. Ample vitamin D in the form of fish liver oils or sunshine will forestall rickets and also this kind of cataract, if there is also enough calcium and phosphorus. Adelle Davis tells us that myopia or near-sightedness has been developed in puppies by depriving them of vitamin D and calcium. Vitamin D has also been used successfully in preventing and curing nearsightedness in children.

Dr. Cameron mentions that vitamin E as used by Dr. Shute and his co-workers in their treatment for heart disease and high blood pressure results in improvement of the inflammation of the retina that may accompany hypertension. Vitamins K and P are frequently used with vitamin C to prevent or improve hemorrhages in various parts of the eye. In fact, Dr. Cameron tells us that two European surgeons are in the habit of giving vitamin C for two or three days before and ten days after an operation for cataract.

Dr. Cameron's observations and conclusions on the subject of vitamin deficiency in relation to eye health are that treatment for these various symptoms should be begun within two months of the time they first appear. Although there may be great improvement in vision, he says, small dark spots in the field of vision may persist indefinitely.

Planning Your Diet For Eye Health

It is not easy, of course, for a lay person to recognize these eye symptoms in himself. And there is no reason to become alarmed and decide one is suffering from severe deficiency if one's eyes get tired and irritated after a day of reading in a library, for instance. On the other hand, eye symptoms may come gradually, so gradually that you are hardly aware of them and by the time you have a fully developed case of night blindness or spots before your eyes, the deficiency may have reached such proportions that it will take a long time of concentrated attention to diet to bring you back to normal. So the wise precaution is to prevent any of these symptoms from ever appearing. A fully adequate diet will do it. This means ample protective foods—meats, eggs, green leafy vegetables, yellow vegetables and fruits (for Vitamin A), all kinds of fresh vegetables and fruits for vitamins B and C. And we can't stress too strongly how necessary it is to eat fruits and vegetables raw whenever possible. Heat and exposure to light and air are not friendly to B vitamins and vitamin C. So the more cooking, shredding and storing you put your foods through before eating them, the less of these two vitamins you will have. If you live in the north, it is hardly possible to get enough vitamin D in the winter, unless you supplement your diet with fish liver oils. Never take synthetic vitamin D.

Fish liver oils contain larger amounts of vitamin A than any other food, so they are, we think, an absolute necessity for eye health, especially if you aren't willing to make a conscious effort to eat lots of yellow vegetables such as carrots and sweet potatoes. The B vitamins are those neglected orphans, so scarce in our present-day diets which include so much of white bread, cake, refined cereals and white sugar. You must eat completely whole grain cereals, lots of fresh vegetables and fruits and organ meats, such as liver and kidney, if you want to get even a smattering of the B vitamins you need. In addition, we strongly suggest supplementing your diet with desiccated liver or brewer's yeast for those extra B vitamins. Don't take synthetics, which may contain only one or only a few of the B vitamins. You must have them all, for they work together in your body's chemistry and if you are short of one, you are almost bound to be deficient in others, too. Brewer's yeast and desiccated liver contain them all.

Finally just a few extra cautions on vitamin C. Over and over again it has been brought to our attention that aging goes hand in hand with vitamin C deficiency. Maybe we need more vitamin C as we grow older. Perhaps we just gradually stop eating vitamin C rich foods after middle age. At any rate, cataract, along with so many other diseases of old age, is closely related to vitamin C deficiency. Is there any logical reason why we should look forward to an old age clouded by cataract, when all kinds of vitamin C rich foods are available to us the year 'round? We think not. And this is why we dwell so persistently on the importance of vitamin C in our diets. Don't shove aside that decorative bit of parsley on your plate. Parsley is rich in vitamin C. Eat it by the handful every day. Buy watercress whenever you can find it, or grow your own if you live in the country, and get used to the idea of whopping big tossed salads that are green with watercress, endive, raw spinach and any other greens you can find. Bleached vegetables have few vitamins. Shun them. And finally, because we are sure you are not getting enough vitamin C every day of your life, take rose hips as a food supplement. They contain more vitamin C than any other food and are rich in vitamins A, E, K and B as well. For nibbling between meals, you won't find anything more delicious or better for your eyes than sunflower seeds. . . . Here's health to your eyes!

Fatigue

"There isn't anything the matter with me except that I'm tired all the time." How many people do you know with this complaint? What exactly are they complaining of? What is this fatigue? W. B. Spaulding, writing in the *Canadian Medical Journal* for December, 1953, says in defining fatigue that it may be "lassitude or weariness resulting from either bodily or mental exertion," "loss of power due to continued work but removable by rest." Actually, says Dr. Spaulding, fatigue is a "*feeling* of difficulty in doing things. This may vary all the way from the mild aversion to activity experienced by one patient, to the overwhelming feeling of exhaustion rendering another patient incapable of exertion despite a strong desire to be active."

It seems that there are two general kinds of fatigue—the healthy kind and the kind you should worry about. A good hard day of work or play makes you tired. If rest refreshes you so that you no longer feel tired, there's nothing to worry about. That's the healthy kind of fatigue. This article is concerned with the other kind—the dragging, nagging chronic fatigue that wears on, day after day, no matter how much sleep or relaxation you get.

A study of disease shows that almost all of the diseases produce fatigue, either when the patient is contracting the disease, during the disease or during convalescence. Anemia and tuberculosis are perhaps the first diseases that come to mind, for the fatigue experienced by these sufferers is excessive. But heart disease, cancer, diabetes and other metabolic diseases, disorders of the glands and infectious diseases, nervous and mental disorders—all these mean fatigue for their victims. If you are feeling tired all the time, it is best to have a physical examination just to set your mind at rest and know for certain that you do not have a serious disease.

Surprisingly enough, worrying about whether or not you are ill may cause you to feel tired. Dr. Spaulding gives several instances of this in his own practice. In one case a tuberculosis patient, discharged from the sanitarium, was certain that her symptoms would return. So she stayed in bed and finally became bedfast, suffering from insomnia, tension and inability to walk. After it had been explained to her at a psychiatric clinic that her fears were groundless and she was in no danger, the fatigue, insomnia and nervousness disappeared.

If your fatigue stems from some organic or functional disorder, in all probability it will increase with exertion. That is, if you stay in bed it will improve; but the harder you work the more fatigued you will be. Fatigue that springs from neurosis may vary from hour to hour without any reference to work or exertion. It is true too, that the neurotic generally wakes up in the morning feeling tired and his fatigue decreases as the day goes on until he may be feeling quite chipper by midnight. The person who is physically ill generally grows more tired right up to bedtime.

Everyday Contributions to Fatigue

If you are healthy and still feel "tired all the time" here are some further suggestions for preventing fatigue. First, check carefully on your physical surroundings. They may be responsible for more fatigue than you know. It has been found, for instance, that noisy surroundings cause fatigue, regardless of how light the work may be. An article in the *Journal of Education* tells us that experiments at Colgate University showed that mental work in a noisy environment demanded 19 per cent more energy than the same work done in reasonable quiet. Noise causes greater fatigue and more errors. Students given reading tests and subjected to loud noises lost over seven per cent of the ability to comprehend the material read. Now if you work in a boiler factory, running a drill, or even typing in a large office, it's quite possible that you cannot avoid noise while you work. But employers are coming to realize more and more that their workers are more efficient in a quiet atmosphere so it is possible that the situation in general may improve. If you do have a lot of noise while you work, as least you can chalk up some of your fatigue to this circumstance. And you can take precautions to avoid noisy places after work.

There are undoubtedly some kinds of people who tire you more than others. Indeed there are probably people who exhaust you completely after an hour or so in their presence. Talking loudly or arguing is exhausting. Too much or too little light can be a constant source of annoyance and result in fatigue. Too little light of course necessitates putting in a strong bulb (and make sure it does not make a glare on your work). The sun shining in your eyes while you are trying to work may necessitate changing the position of the furniture or making some arrangement at the window.

High humidity and high temperature result in more fatigue. This does not mean you have to be in the tropics. Canning day in the kitchen or washing day in the laundry bring increases in both temperature and humidity. Working too long at one kind of job, especially if it is very monotonous, can produce not only fatigue, but inefficiency in the job. It pays in the long run, to take rest periods—short ones at frequent intervals rather than one long one. You will find that the work moves along faster and your fatigue is less.

A study done at Tufts College and reported on during the General Electric Science Forum on March 29, 1950, indicated that actual fatigue is not necessarily the reason for decreased efficiency. Volunteers were put through all kinds of hardships—such as no sleep for several days, a thirty mile hike and so forth. At the end of this time the subjects were *able* to perform as well as when they were rested, but they were *"either unable or unwilling* to exert themselves to maintain their level of performance." The author concludes "So the next time you feel the lethargy and drag of fatigue, particularly if your previous living routines have been fairly normal, ask yourself if you really feel this way or whether you are not just trying to escape the duties of the moment."

The Psychology of Fatigue

This brings us to a consideration of the psychological aspect of fatigue. It seems that nothing can exhaust you sooner and nothing can be a quicker and more effective cause of day-by-day fatigue than one's emotions. *Today's Woman* for October, 1953, carried an article on the very common fatigue experienced by young married women. George E. Paley, M.D., tells us that in a study of 300 adults who were always tired, Dr. Frank N. Allen of the Lahey Clinic in Boston discovered symptoms of illness in only one-fifth of the group. Eighty per cent of the group were suffering from emotional fatigue. "As his study showed and other research has confirmed, most perennially tired people are neither overworked nor physically sick, but are troubled by frustration, insecurity, hostility and other conflicts." This condition is called "civilized fatigue." The fact that this fatigue springs from emotion does not mean that you exhaust yourself staging scenes (although a 15 minute fit of anger or "scene" can tire you as much as a full day of work). But this "civilized fatigue" may also arise because you don't blow your top often enough! If you are living under circumstances that you resent or conditions that cause you frustration, your fatigue may come just from the pent-up feelings inside you that are never released and taken out for a good airing.

One physician tried an experiment with a patient who was always tired. He asked her to keep a diary, noting especially those things that bothered her every day—the little annoying, pesky things about which she didn't complain. She was instructed to put down exactly what her husband did or said on any given day that annoyed her, what household duties she resented doing, how the children got on her nerves. And, sure enough, she found that on days when she felt "put upon" and kept her resentment to herself, she grew fatigued. Days when everything went smoothly and she had some diversion to break the monotony, she felt rested and serene, no matter how much work she did.

When you stop to think of it, it's amazing how a series of little annoyances can mount up into a feeling of complete frustration that leaves you limp and weary at the day's end. The faucet drips, the washing machine collapses in the middle of the day's washing, a favorite plate slides out of your hands and breaks, or your secretary gets an important message wrong, a client breaks an appointment that means a big order for you and you just miss the bus coming home. If your trouble is fatigue, why not try keeping a diary for a few weeks just to see how much of your fatigue is due to daily frustration and resentment. Deeper personal problems, involving family relationships, may require the help of a therapist, if you want to iron out the difficulties and do away with the fatigue.

How much does the way you work have to do with your feeling of fatigue? Perhaps your clothes are not comfortable, your shoes are tight, your working tools are not in good order, or they are arranged at such a height that you must bend or reach in order to work. Good posture plays an important part in a rested feeling. Check on yours. Slumping over your work—stomach hanging forward, back curved in, shoulders drooped and head forward—will tire even the strongest man after an hour or so of light work. Do you arrange your work to involve the least possible amount of walking, reaching and standing? One further caution: aimlessness is tiring. Don't begin one job, then drop it and start another. Plan to work in an organized way while you are working and relax completely after work is over.

The amount of restful sleep you get is important too, in preventing fatigue. If you must be out late one night or two nights a week, see to it that you get to bed in plenty of time the other nights to make up for lost sleep. No one can tell you how much sleep you should have, for it is an individual matter. But you should wake up feeling rested, at about the time you must get up—that's what we mean by plenty of sleep. Naps in the afternoon are a wonderful idea, if you can manage them. But if you are napping out of sheer boredom, for lack of anything interesting to do, you won't derive much benefit. A hobby or an interest outside your regular work is stimulating and restful. A man who does office work all day can actually rest while he is carpentering at night in his home workshop. A woman, tired out with the monotony of housework, can rest very satisfyingly while she is pursuing some hobby that takes her out of the house.

Low Blood Sugar and Fatigue

There is one aspect of chronic fatigue that has been discussed more and more of late in the lay magazines. It has been known for years to physicians. This is low blood sugar—the opposite of diabetes—a condition which seems to arise from a diet that is too high in carbohydrates and too low in protein and fats. Chronic fatigue may be simply the result of a high carbohydrate breakfast (toast or hot cakes) and a sandwich and pie for lunch. The curve of blood sugar raises sharply just after such a meal, then drops swiftly to dangerous levels. A piece of candy or a soda will give a quick pick-up, so the tendency is to nibble sweet and starchy snacks all day long to prevent that "all-gone" feeling.

The answer is not more carbohydrates. The answer is more protein, with carbohydrates sharply restricted. If your feeling of unhealthy fatigue does not yield to any of the suggestions above, try changing your diet radically for several weeks. A breakfast and lunch high in meat, eggs, fish, cheese or nuts will probably set you right again. And during those mid-morning and mid-afternoon slumps, chew some peanuts, eat a piece of cheese, drink a glass of fruit juice. But stay away from foods high in starch and sugar! Countless scientific experiments have shown the value of high protein meals in combatting fatigue and the very definite role played by sugar in causing fatigue.

Vitamins and Minerals Versus Fatigue

Finally we come to a consideration of the part played by vitamins and minerals in preventing fatigue. We combed our textbooks—fat and heavy ones—to see if we could find a single vitamin mentioned whose lack did not cause fatigue. We could not. One of the first symptoms of deficiency of any vitamin is bound to be fatigue. It may go as far as the devastating prostration of beriberi, scurvy or pernicious anemia. It may be simply the general tiredness, lack of energy and lack of interest shown even by laboratory animals when they are not getting quite enough of one or another of the B vitamins. But do not think for a minute that you can get along on a borderline diet and not feel fatigue. Vitamins are needed, along with minerals and enzymes, to activate the whole process of digestion and assimilation of food. If you do not have all three of these food elements in abundance, your food will not be broken down into substances that will create the energy and initiative you need to carry on your daily life.

To prevent fatigue, you need food supplements in addition to your meals. But don't be taken in by the ads for synthetic vitamins. These are put together by chemists and may contain one, or several vitamins of any given group, such as the group of B vitamins. But you need all of the vitamins in the exact proportions in which they occur in foods.

Here is an example to prove the effectiveness of natural food supplements in preventing fatigue. Drs. Jolliffe, Tisdall and Cannon in the volume *Clinical Nutrition* (published by Paul B. Hoeber, Inc.) tell the story of an experiment in which two groups of men were put to doing hard physical work on a diet that was deficient in thiamin, one of the B vitamins. The first group was then given a supplement of thiamin—enough to make up their daily requirement. The second group was given none. Throughout the experiment, the performance of the first group was a little superior to that of the second, but their performance also deteriorated. Later on, both groups were given brewer's yeast as a food supplement and the performance and energy of both groups went back to normal. This demonstrates clearly that taking just one or several of the B vitamins will not do the trick. They are combined in foods and they should be eaten in this combination—as in brewer's yeast or desiccated liver.

Another experiment worthy of note is that of three groups of rats eating three different diets which were tested for endurance in a swimming test. The first group, eating a basic diet fortified mostly with synthetic vitamins, performed reasonably well in the swimming test, staying afloat for 13.3 minutes. The second group, who had this same diet, further fortified with B vitamins, did just a little better. The third group had been getting 10 per cent desiccated liver in addition to their original diet. Three of these rats swam for 63, 83 and 87 minutes respectively and nine others were still swimming and showed no signs of giving up at the end of two hours.

It would seem there are two lessons to be learned here: for rats at least, natural food substances, rich in natural vitamins, give far better results than synthetic vitamins. Secondly, there must be some as yet undiscovered substance in liver, quite apart from the B vitamins, which makes it a very valuable food indeed if it can have this amazing effect on endurance performance.

Dr. Max Gerson who has done remarkable work in New York City treating diseases with a special diet, tells us in an article in *The Medical Record* for June, 1943, that a diet high in the K or potassium group of minerals is necessary to defeat fatigue. The reason for this is that the potassium group and the sodium group are antagonistic to one another. When foods high in sodium, chlorine and so forth are taken, the potassium, calcium, phosphorus and magnesium are displaced in the cells, resulting in fatigue. Therefore, say Dr. Gerson, "there is increasing evidence that fatigue is a problem of metabolism, the basis of which is a loss of potassium, phosphorus and other minerals, and penetration into the cell of sodium and other elements. To avoid these pathological unhealthful changes as far as possible, I worked out the fundamental principle of salt free diets. . . ." He also says "the mineral salts of the K group (potassium, phosphorus, calcium, magnesium, etc.) which are able to neutralize the waste products (of fatigue) must be so abundant in the food that the amounts taken in will always be in excess of those used up."

It is well known that the average American eats far more salt (sodium chloride) than he needs and makes this situation worse by not eating enough foods that contain the other group of minerals—calcium, potassium and magnesium especially—fresh raw vegetables and fruits, dairy products, nuts and the various elements in bone. For this reason, then, we recommend bone meal as a food supplement—for it contains these latter minerals in quantity and in exactly the proper proportions. In addition, of course, fresh garden and orchard products should form a far larger part of our diet than they do.

We want to close with an unsolicited letter from a reader on the subject of fatigue. Says Mrs. Harvey S. Lawrence of Mulberry, Indiana: "*Prevention* is a wonderful magazine. And do not be disturbed by the people who object to the advertising. There is nothing more exasperating than to learn of something which sounds as though it would be a great help and then not be able to buy any of it to try. I have been taking the various vitamin products for about two years now and find the effect accumulative, for I feel stronger and better and more alert and alive the longer I take them. I felt draggy and exhausted all the time for years. Now I am ready for the day and not especially tired in the evening. It has been a great blessing to me and I want others to share it."

May we all soon be able to feel "ready for the day and not especially tired in the evening."

Fats In the Diet, Unsaturated Fatty Acids

In determining what food factors constitute a vitamin, certain general principles have been laid down by researchers. If the food factor is essential to good health and if a deficiency in this factor causes a deficiency disease, then the factor is a vitamin. This in general is the criterion by which we designate or do not designate certain substances as vitamins.

When a new substance is discovered which seems to have the properties of a vitamin, much research is done with animals. The animals are put on carefully prepared diets which include all necessary elements except the one being tested. If some disorder results, the substance in question is then administered to see whether it will cure the disorder. If it does, then we are fairly sure that such-and-such a food element is necessary for health—at least in the case of animals. With some substances, it seems that animal tests do not prove out in the case of human beings. We then assume that such-and-such an animal needs such-and-such a substance, but human beings do not. This has always seemed to us like a most unsatisfactory way of doing things. Animal physiology is very much like our own. If it were not, there would be no reason at all for using animals in diet experiments.

It has always seemed to us that the very strict controls employed in animal experimentation may be the reason why some of these experiments do not prove out in regard to human beings. When a diet is decided upon for an animal experiment, nothing can be left to chance. There is no possibility for this rat or guinea pig to get out of his cage and go on a binge of eating forbidden foods. Temperature, rest, bedding, possible psychological irritants, family life, emotions, water, air, light—all these factors are most rigorously controlled, so that the animals' health cannot possibly be influenced either negatively or positively by any of these things. In planning diets for the experiments, the utmost care is taken to feed only those foods which have been shown to produce the ultimate in good health; vitamins and minerals, proteins and enzymes are supplied in ample quantities. Only the substance being tested is left out of the food for the first part of the experiment, then put back into the food for the latter part. And it is perfectly true that we know a lot more about what constitutes a healthful diet for a laboratory animal than for a human being. So, safe to say, these animals get the very best of everything that can be had.

Human beings do not live this way. No single human being lives this way. On this troubled planet, it is impossible to conceive of a human being who can live in the safe, unhurried, unstressful, relaxed, healthful atmosphere of one of these animals. Our human diets are full of all kinds of errors, no matter how careful we may be. The air we breathe is full of pollution from industry. Our water is loaded with chemicals. Our lives are subject to stress, insecurity, frustrations, hurry, lack of proper rest, lack of exercise or possibly work that is too heavy and exacting. We try to keep up with the Joneses. Early in life we are endowed with a set of ideals that glimmers before us constantly from then on, inspiring us to try to achieve many things that may be far beyond our reach. Surely we need much more of the important food elements to carry us through this kind of life than a laboratory rat needs to live healthfully in his hygienically controlled environment.

The subject of this article is a set of food factors that were once spoken of as a vitamin. Animal experiments show that they are essential to the good health of animals. But we still do not classify them as vitamins in speaking of human nutrition. We want readers to know of these food factors and then to decide for themselves whether or not they should be included in a healthful diet for human beings. These food factors are the unsaturated fatty acids, once called vitamin F. Specifically they are linolenic acid, linoleic acid and arachidonic acid. The names need not frighten you. The chemical names of most of our familiar vitamins are equally long and unpronounceable.

Unsaturated Fatty Acids in Animal Health

There is a disease which occurs in laboratory rats called "fat deficiency disease." By breaking down the different fatty elements of the diet, researchers have found that the disease occurs not from lack of fat—any kind of fat. It results only from lack of the unsaturated fatty acids. The rats show arrested or retarded growth, a raised metabolic rate (that is, they burn their food up very rapidly), changes in skin and hair, kidney disorders and impairment of reproductive function. Rats who received no unsaturated fatty acids in their food ate just as much as the control rats, but they did not grow or put on weight so apparently the food was simply burning rapidly without contributing anything to building the body. First over the paws, then over the face and gradually over the rest of the body a dryness and scurfiness (dandruff) spread. Cold weather—the kind that chaps hands—accentuated this condition. The rats developed kidney stones and many difficulties in reproducing. In the case of the female rats there was disturbance of the whole reproductive cycle. In many cases litters were not born but were re-absorbed. Or, if the mother rat finally had the litter, she had prolonged labor and hemorrhage and the litters were underweight and sickly. Male rats deprived of unsaturated fatty acids refused to mate and were sterile. It was found, too, that there was some relationship between deficiency of unsaturated fatty acids and pyridoxine and pantothenic acid, two of the B vitamins. A deficiency of any two of these factors caused a much worse condition than a deficiency of just one.

Now in regard to human beings, there are two extremely important aspects to this problem. First of all, human milk is rich in unsaturated fatty acids—far, far richer than cow's milk. If these acids are not vitally important to human nutrition, how could Mother Nature have made the mistake of including them in such quantity in mother's milk where every drop must count towards the nourishment of the child? Furthermore, it has been found that stores of fatty acids are built up in the heart, liver, kidney, brain, blood and muscle and the body holds on to them tenaciously. In rats who were deprived of fatty acids for a long time, it was found that there was still some remaining when 76 per cent of the body fat of the rat had been used up. As soon as the unsaturated fatty acids were completely gone, the animal became very seriously ill. The body stores food factors it will need. And in cases of deficiency or starvation, it relinquishes first those factors which are not so important and until the very end hangs on to those things that are essential to life. So on this basis, too, we believe we are justified in assuming that the unsaturated fatty acids are important enough to be called a vitamin.

We are told that nothing is known about human requirements for the unsaturated fatty acids. Yet the National Research Council which sets the standards and makes the decisions on matters of this kind in this country, says "in spite of the paucity of information . . . it is desirable that the fat intake include essential unsaturated fatty acids to the extent of at least one per cent of the total calories." Bicknell and Prescott, writing in *Vitamins in Medicine* (Grune and Stratton, 1953) tell us that only about one half this amount has been available in England since 1945. In this country there is no shortage of foods that contain unsaturated fatty acids, but do we realize how important they are and do we make every effort to include them in every day's menu?

Human Diseases That May Be Related To Deficiency

A number of human disorders appear to be related to deficiency of unsaturated fatty acids. Medical literature contains many instances of infant eczema that has been cured by including the unsaturated fatty acids in the infants' food. As a matter of fact we recently found an ad in *The Practitioner,* a British medical publication, for a substance called F99 to be used in the treatment of eczema. It consists of unsaturated fatty acids to be used, says the ad, "in cases of infantile eczema, adult eczema, furunculosis (boils) and other skin disorders associated with a deficiency of essential fatty acids. It is also successful in cases of varicose leg ulcers of long standing." So the physicians are already using these food elements to cure disease. But we are not allowed to speak of them as a vitamin. And apparently the amount of research that has been done on them in recent years is sparse indeed, for we could find very few references to them in medical literature throughout the past 15 years.

Bicknell and Prescott (in *Vitamins and Medicine*) suggest that the acids may be very important in any disease where fat absorption is impaired. This includes diarrheal conditions of many kinds. It may include many cases of underweight. Much of the research we did some time ago on acne seemed to show that acne patients are unable to use fat properly. Could a deficiency of unsaturated fatty acids be one of the causes of acne? Could it be one cause of the dandruff that appears almost universally on American scalps? Bicknell and Prescott tell us that the fact that the unsaturated fatty acids are so carefully stored and husbanded by the body may be why symptoms of deficiency are not more marked and severe. In other words, many of us may be suffering from a subclinical deficiency—not enough to make us definitely ill, but enough to prevent our being completely healthy.

The Lee Foundation for Nutritional Research, 2023 West Wisconsin Avenue, Milwaukee 3, Wisconsin, has contributed perhaps the most to the study of unsaturated fatty acids in this country. They have booklets available on the subject: *A Survey of Vitamin F* and *Vitamin F in the Treatment of Prostatic Hypertrophy* which present startling evidence of the importance of these substances in human nutrition. Harold H. Perlenfein, who wrote the first booklet, tells us that the unsaturated fatty acids reduce the incidence and duration of colds. He says that deficiency may be responsible for dry skin, brittle, lustreless, falling hair, dandruff, brittle nails and kidney disease. He states that the acids function in the body by cooperating with vitamin D in making calcium available to the tissues, assist in assimilation of organic phosphorus, aid in the reproductive process, nourish the skin and appear to be related to the proper functioning of the thyroid gland.

James Pirie Hart and William DeGrande Cooper, writing on prostate treatment (Lee Report No. 1) describe nineteen cases of prostate gland disorder which were treated with unsaturated fatty acids. In all cases there was a lessening of the residual urine—that is, the urine which cannot be released from the bladder due to pressure from the enlarged prostate gland. In 12 of the cases there was no residual urine at the end of the treatment. There was a decrease in leg pains, fatigue, kidney disorders, and nocturia (excessive urination at night). In all cases the size of the prostate rapidly decreased. Chemical blood tests which were made showed a great improvement in mineral content of the blood at the end of the treatment. We have been able to find no further work that has been done along these lines, but we believe that the findings are significant and we want to share them with our readers.

Processed Foods Cause the Deficiency

Why should any of us be deficient in the unsaturated fatty acids? For the same reason we are deficient in so many other necessary food elements—food processing. Bicknell and Prescott tell us that in processed and stale foods, these acids have deliberately been destroyed to improve the keeping qualities of the food. Unsaturated fatty acids occur in vegetable and seed fats—such as corn oil, cottonseed oil, wheat germ oil, peanut oil and so forth. They may occur in animal fats, such as butter, depending on what the animal has been fed. They are destroyed very easily by exposure to air, and they then become rancid. This rancidity can be responsible for destroying other vitamins as well—vitamins A, D and K are destroyed in the presence of rancid fat. When fats are hydrogenated much of the unsaturated fatty acid is changed into saturated fatty acids. This means that certain chemical actions take place which completely change the character of the fat and render it almost useless for the various conditions we have described. Hydrogenizing gives the fat a solid form, rather than a liquid form.

At present, much of the fat we use has been hydrogenized. Shortening such as we use for making pastry or for frying has been hydrogenized, margarine has been hydrogenized—little or no unsaturated fatty acids are left. In a family where the meal-planner depends on fried foods and pastries for fats and where margarine is consistently used in place of butter, there is every possibility that such a family will be deficient in unsaturated fatty acids, unless a lot of salad oil is used, unheated, in salads. This is one reason why we feel certain that Americans in general may have a serious sub-clinical deficiency along these lines.

Here is the unsaturated fatty acid (or vitamin F) content of some of the common fats:

	Per cent of essential unsaturated fatty acids
Butter	4.0 to 6.0
Beef fat	1.1 to 5.0
Lard	5.0 to 11.1
Mutton fat	3.0 to 5.0
Liver fat	3.0 to 7.0
Milk	.15 to .23
Fish oils	Traces
Margarine	2.0 to 5.0
Barley germ oil	63
Cocoa butter	2.0
Coconut oil	6.0 to 9.2
Corn salad oil	70
Cottonseed oil	35 to 50
Linseed oil	72 to 83
Maize germ oil	42
Oat germ oil	31
Olive oil	4.0 to 13.7
Palm oil	2.0 to 11.3
Peanut oil	20 to 25
Rice bran oil	29 to 42
Rye germ oil	48
Soybean oil	56 to 63
Sunflower seed oil	52 to 64
Wheat germ oil	44 to 52

Some of these foods sound exotic to us and, so far as we know, are not at present available to American consumers—such as oat germ oil, barley germ oil and so forth. But surely we have all heard enough about wheat germ oil during past years to realize anew that this extremely important substance (rich in vitamin E as well) should be a part of our diet. Corn oil, cottonseed oil, peanut oil, soya bean oil are sold as salad oils in every grocery. So far as we can determine, nothing has been done to these oils in preparing them for the market that would destroy their content of unsaturated fatty acids. But we would advise crossing off your shopping list all hydrogenated fats, such as the shortening that comes in a can, and margarine.

See to it that your family eats plenty of vegetable or seed oils—in salads, as that is by far the best way of taking them. If you must fry something—and we take a dim view of frying anything—use liquid vegetable oils for the process. But keep in mind that the less heat you apply to any oils or fats, the better they are for you. In addition we firmly believe that all present day Americans (and especially those who cannot bake their own real whole grain bread) should take wheat germ oil as a daily food supplement. This contains not only the unsaturated fatty acids we have been talking about, but vitamin E as well as the other fractions and elements of the wheat germ that may be vitally important for health, even though researchers have not as yet gotten around to isolating and defining them.

Fatty Acids, Sources of

We hear a lot these days about the large amount of fat in the national diet of Americans and we are frequently warned by health-conscious researchers that too much fat is not good for us. In general, the whole subject of fats has been investigated less in scientific laboratories than almost any other aspect of nutrition. It's a most complicated subject, for it presents a number of seeming contradictions and we just don't have all the information we would like to have about it.

However, we do know certain things that have been established without question. We know that we must get some fats in the diet, for fats are built into the structure of every cell and fats are burned to make energy. We know, too, that the fat-soluble vitamins—A, D, E and K—are absolutely essential to good health. No one can possibly get along without an ample supply of these vitamins which occur in fatty foods. In addition we know that there are certain substances called fatty acids, many of which can be manufactured inside the body from sugar. But three of these fatty acids cannot be manufactured in the body. Therefore, they must be included in the diet. One of these is linolenic acid, another linoleic acid, the third arachidonic acid.

Now of course you can't walk into a grocery store and find foods labelled with these names, so how are you going to make certain you get enough of these three necessary parts of food? It is our aim in this article to clear up any confusion about these acids and tell you everything we could find out about them.

Fatty substances are made up of various atoms of carbon, hydrogen and oxygen, linked together like chains. Some are long, meaning they have many atoms linked together; others are short. Some kinds of fats have open links, you might say, where other atoms can be attached to them. These are called the "unsaturated fatty acids." By "unsaturated" we mean that these open links in the chain are there, ready to be filled or "saturated" with an atom of some other substance.

Linolenic, linoleic and arachidonic acids are just such "unsaturated" fatty acids. That is why they are so extremely valuable to good health. What do we mean by that? Well, you see, since they have open links in their chain of atoms, they are ready, willing and able to combine with other substances in the big chemical laboratory that is the body. So they take part in all kinds of different things that go on. They can combine with other parts of food; they can help to carry these other parts of food through the miles of blood vessels and they are used in building cell structure. They can do all this because—and only because—the open links in their chains of atoms invite other substances to join with them in various chemical combinations.

Well and good, you may say, so all we have to do is eat plenty of fat and we'll get enough unsaturated fatty acids to be healthful. Of course it's not that simple. First of all, certain things can happen to these *unsaturated* fatty acids that change them to *saturated* fatty acids before we eat them. In this case, the open chains have already been filled with some other substance and there is no chance that this kind of fat can take the active part it should take in the body's laboratory.

When oxygen is combined with the unsaturated fatty acids, an atom of oxygen moves into the empty link, joins itself chemically with the other atoms and what happens? The fat becomes rancid. When hydrogen is added, it moves into the empty link, joins itself to the other atoms and we have what is known as "hydrogenated fat"—a thick, almost solid, substance like lard. In both cases, of course, since the empty links have been filled, the fat can no longer fulfill its duties inside the body, because it is now "saturated"—there is no place for body substances to join with it and help in the work of the body.

Naturally nobody ever purposely makes fats rancid, for the taste is unpleasant and, as we have discovered, rancid fat in the diet is responsible for the destruction of fat-soluble vitamins. So rancid fats should be carefully avoided. Natural fats in their natural state, such as those in sunflower seeds, for instance, carry along with them substances called anti-oxidants which prevent oxygen from turning the fat rancid. But in many of the processes to which our table and cooking oils are subjected today, the anti-oxidants are destroyed.

Do you know what difficulties people who sell potato chips and roasted nuts get into, trying to keep their products from turning rancid? Next time you read on the label of some fat product the name of some complicated chemical preservative that has been added, you can be sure that this was put there to "prolong the shelf life" of this product, as the food processors like to say. In other words, they first destroy the things in the fat that keep it from turning rancid, then they have to add something, a preservative, to keep it from turning rancid, so that it can stay on the grocer's shelf until it is bought.

Hydrogenated Fats Are the Worst Offenders

What about hydrogenated fats? We have just shown you how the "unsaturated fats" are changed into "saturated" fats in this process by the addition of hydrogen. Margarine is hydrogenated—most of the unsaturated fatty acids in it are destroyed. Cooking fats—the solid white ones—have been hydrogenated. Processed cheeses are hydrogenated and peanut butter. It is our opinion that this process of adding hydrogen to so many otherwise healthful foods may eventually have to bear the responsibility for a lot of our present-day ills.

For, people who depend on processed foods for their unsaturated fatty acids are just not going to get them. And people who are told by their doctors to eat a fat-free diet are not going to get them. People who eat diets high in animal fats are not going to get them for they are most abundant in vegetable and cereal fats, and not at all plentiful in animal fats, such as butter, eggs, milk and meat fats.

How then are you going to be sure you get enough unsaturated fatty acids? And a look at another article in this book on the same subject will convince you further of how important they are. Well, there is a lot of the unsaturated fatty acids in seeds—plain, unprocessed seeds like sunflower seeds and sesame seeds. Nuts and avocados are two other excellent sources. Also, whole grain cereals, but be sure they are fresh for they become rancid rapidly.

What about salad oils? The richest sources of all are corn oil, soybean oil and cottonseed oil, which are composed of from 35 to 70 per cent unsaturated fatty acids. Wheat germ oil (which you don't generally think of as a salad oil) is rich in these fatty acids, as well as, of course vitamin E.

Readers frequently ask us about salad oils such as you buy in the grocery store. Do they contain the unsaturated fatty acids? Or has almost everything nutritious in them been destroyed by the various processing they go through?

We have written to a number of producers of salad oils—peanut oil, corn oil, cottonseed oil and so forth. They have told us that the processing of the oils has little effect on the unsaturated fatty acid content of their products and they have, in some instances, sent us reports on tests indicating that the unsaturated fatty acid content of their products compares favorably with the amounts on the chart below. So far as these important fats are concerned, then, there seems to be no reason for not using plenty of salad oil—the kind you buy at the grocery store.

Unsaturated fatty acids are the building blocks of lecithin. If you keep in mind that lecithin plays an important part in transporting fat efficiently in your body and in utilizing oxygen to best advantage, then you'll understand the nature of the fatty acids.

The chief sources for the essential fatty acids (linoleic and linolenic acid) are the oils of the cereal germ and various seed oils. Here is a table from European sources giving the average content of fatty acids in several foods:

Source of oil	*% Linoleic Acid*	*% Linolenic Acid*
Walnut	51-73	4-10
Rye Germ	52-72	2-11
Wheat Germ	57-66	1.6-5.5
Corn	38-61	1.5-8.5
Poppy Seed	58-65	...
Hemp Seed	50-65	16
Linseed	17-62	21-50
Sunflower Seed	46-58.5	...

Source of oil	*% Linoleic Acide*	*% Linolenic Acid*
Soybean	50-57	2-5.8
Rose Hip Seed	54.2	32
Squash Seed	44-45	...
Peanut	18-27.4	...
Almond	15-19	...
Hazelnut	3-10.6	...
Olive	7-15.7	...

Fatty Acids, Using for Health

We know that certain of the unsaturated fatty acids are absolutely essential for human health and we know that they cannot be produced by the body so they must be included in the diet.

Now listen to the facts about some cheering new research that has come to our attention from a couple of medical scientists who have been trying unsaturated fatty acids in cases of various disorders.

We know that millions of Americans are asthmatic. It seems pretty obvious that diet has a lot to do with causing asthma. Here is new evidence that the addition of a few simple items in the diet may mean all the difference in the world to people who are now wheezing and suffocating in the clutches of this prevalent disease.

In one experiment reported in *Medical Times* for July, 1955, N. E. Silbert, M.D. and H. E. Worne, Ph.D. gave unsaturated fatty acids to thirty infants with asthma. They were also receiving a vitamin supplement containing plentiful amounts of vitamins A, B, C, D and E. An additional ten infants got only the vitamin supplement along with their daily diet. No unsaturated fatty acids. And another ten babies got no special treatment. The two doctors report that at the end of ninety days those who got the vitamin supplements *plus the fatty acids* "showed some clinical evidence of cessation of their symptoms." Some of the infants had suffered from eczema, too. This seemed to improve. The children who got only the vitamin supplements did not have as favorable results as the first group. And of course those who got no special treatment showed no improvement. The two researchers conclude that the fatty acids and the other vitamin elements in which the child may be deficient are important factors in the treatment of asthma and eczema and should be studied further.

Using These Fats for Asthma

In another study reported in *The Journal of Applied Nutrition* for Spring, 1955, these same two doctors observed the effects of a diet supplement plus the fatty acids and found that forty per cent of their asthma patients either were entirely relieved of their symptoms or else noticed that they improved greatly. The other sixty per cent did not respond. As a further test, the researchers gave another group the same supplements minus pyridoxine, one of the B vitamins. Their results were not nearly so good. Drs. Worne and Silbert believe this shows that this particular B vitamin is most necessary in the diet if the body is going to use the unsaturated fatty acids to their best advantage.

Another aspect of the place of unsaturated fatty acids in the diet arises when we ask what happens to someone on a fat-free or low-fat diet. Obviously, if one is watching carefully to see that he does not get any foods at all that contain visible fat and is also avoiding foods that contain "hidden fat" (like nuts, avocados and so forth), he is surely going to be short on the unsaturated fatty acids, for they occur only in fats.

What may be the result? Dr. Worne and J. Schneider, M.D., Ph.D., writing in the *Archives of Research,* August, 1954, describe the state of 24 gall bladder patients who had been on a fat-free diet for a year or longer. This means, they tell us, that less than one per cent of their daily calories was in the form of fat. The two researchers did tests on the blood of these patients to determine its fatty acid content. It was well below normal. All of the subjects suffered from "a dry, flaky skin, threaded with fine lines and wrinkles." There was also a slight to moderate itching in most cases.

They were given a cream containing unsaturated fatty acids which they were to apply every night and morning. Results were excellent. And most of the patients had a rapid response. No one seemed to have any unpleasant side effects. We don't know the name of the product used in this experiment and we doubt that it is available for anyone not a physician to buy. If you suffer from the conditions mentioned here, we suggest that you ask your doctor to get a cream or salve containing unsaturated fatty acids, if you want to try it out.

In another experiment (*Archives of Research,* August, 1954) Drs. Worne and L. A. Scinta, M.D., and S. W. Hausman, M.D. tried both salve and preparations to be taken by mouth in cases of various skin diseases. In all, there were fifty cases, some having allergic breaking-out, some having eczema and some having psoriasis. The investigators first tested the amounts of unsaturated fatty acids in the blood of these patients. The normal concentration is 180 to 265 milligrams per 100 cubic centimeters, an average of about 225 milligrams. The level in the blood of these skin disease patients fell as low as 92, and the highest was only 152.

Was this deficiency in blood related by any chance to the skin diseases? To find out, fourteen of the 28 patients were given four grams of unsaturated fatty acids and, in addition, a cream made of the acids for putting on night and morning. The rest of the patients did not get the four grams to take orally, but did get the cream for applying to their skin.

What were the results? Within eight days all of the cases of eczema were completely cured; eight of the dermatitis ones were cured in nine days and the ten cases of psoriasis showed great improvement and, within two weeks, complete absence of scaling. In the case of those patients who got only the salve, their troubles began gradually anew (in all but six cases of the eczema) when the salve was withdrawn. Those who had, in addition, received the unsaturated fatty acids to take in a food supplement, did not have a recurrence of the breaking out after the salve was discontinued. So it seems that getting the fatty acids in your diet is far superior to using them in creams for the skin.

Arthritis and Mongolism May Be Caused by Deficiencies

Two final experiments—one dealing with rheumatoid arthritis and the other with mongolism. Using thirty-one patients and giving them four grams of unsaturated fatty acids daily along with a general vitamin supplement for three months, Dr. Worne and Dr. Schneider found that the fatty acids are "of major importance as adjuncts in the treatment of rheumatoid arthritis." They admit that they do not know why. But they present a theory having to do with intricate chemical changes that go on in the body which they think may explain the results they got.

Before starting their treatment they tested the blood of the patients for vitamin C and the fatty acids. Before the treatment began the levels of these two important food elements ranged from .30 to .80 for vitamin C and 108 to 183 for the unsaturated fatty acids. At the end of the experiment the blood was tested again and the range was from .63 to 1.30 for vitamin C and from 171 to 329 for the fats. Quite a difference! We do not know why the vitamin C level was checked in this instance, nor do the authors mention what part vitamin C may have played in this story. We believe that vitamin C is of great importance for individuals suffering from rheumatism or arthritis.

What were the exact results of the treatment described above? The three cases of children involved were completely cured. Their blood chemistries were normal, joint swelling and all tenderness and swelling were eliminated and all gained weight and were able to return to normal activity. The rest of the cases, with the exception of four, were classified as completely relieved as far as arthritis symptoms were concerned. They, too, returned to their usual activities.

Mongolism is a condition present at birth which results in mental deficiency and other serious symptoms. The Mongoloid child does not live long. It seems to most observers that the child is born with these handicaps because of some deficiency in the mother. Many theories have been advanced as to exactly what is responsible. In general, medical science believes at present that the mother's age may have a lot to do with it. However, Dr. Worne while he was studying the effects of lack of oxygen on animals found a number of cases where deficiencies of the mother resulted in brain damage for the child.

He tested and reported in *Archives of Research,* August, 1954, on 25 cases of Mongolism. He found that 40 per cent of these children were deficient in vitamin A, 36 per cent were deficient in vitamin B_1 or thiamin, 100 per cent were deficient in vitamin B_2, riboflavin, 91.8 per cent deficient in vitamin C, 84.1 per cent were deficient in vitamin E and 100 per cent were deficient in the unsaturated fatty acids.

The children were given a nutritional supplement containing all of the important vitamins and the unsaturated fatty acids. To give you an idea of how rich this supplement was in vitamins, it contained 200 milligrams of vitamin C—the amount contained in about 10 oranges—and comparatively high amounts of the other vitamins. At the end of three months tests were again made of the children's blood. The increase in all of the vitamins was of course, great. But, in addition, the dryness and roughness of the skin were eliminated, the nails were far less brittle. In several of the cases the shape of the face changed so that the Mongoloid appearance was lessened. All the mouth and tongue disorders cleared up as if by magic. And, perhaps most amazing of all, there was a marked improvement in the way these children could do things, as well as improvement in their mental capacity. In two cases where mental tests had been given previously, new tests showed considerable improvement. Dr. Worne tells us that more studies are now being conducted to see what more can be done nutritionally for these children, heretofore considered hopelessly handicapped.

Getting Enough of All the Vitamins is Important!

We think that the stories above are remarkable. We think they will interest our readers especially, because in every case the researchers *gave a vitamin supplement along with the treatment they were testing.* We will never know, possibly, how much of their success is due to this fact. But we do think that, when other investigators claim that giving vitamins has no effect on conditions such as this, a large part of the reason may be that they are *not* giving all the other vitamins at the same time—and that is of the utmost importance!

Dr. Worne showed in these experiments that pyridoxine (part of the vitamin B complex) and vitamin C are both important in order for one to use the unsaturated fatty acids properly. The other vitamins undoubtedly play some part in it, too.

How can you avail yourself of these facts to prevent such conditions of ill-health developing? Eat the very best possible diet including whole grain cereals, (we prefer barley, rice, oats and so forth, rather than wheat) natural seeds such as sunflower seeds, and vegetable oils, and take food supplements—fish liver oil for vitamins A and D, rose hip preparations for vitamin C, wheat germ oil for unsaturated fatty acids and vitamin E in addition. And then, to make certain that mineral deficiency won't defeat your purpose, take bone meal for all the important minerals and kelp tablets for iodine. How can you best get unsaturated fatty acids in your diet? Eat seeds. Sunflower seeds are especially rich in these acids, but all seeds contain large amounts of them. Don't eat refined cereals from which all the unsaturated fatty acids have been removed.

Fats, Importance of

The essential unsaturated fatty acids which Dr. Sinclair discusses in the April 7, 1956, issue of *The Lancet* may be necessary for the prevention of many conditions of ill health as well as heart and vascular troubles. Dr. Sinclair believes, and we think with good reason, that lack of the essential fatty acids may be responsible for leukemia, lung cancer, seborrhea and nervous and mental trouble.

Let's see what his reasoning is. First of all, he tells us, men need five times more of these fatty acids than women need. We do not know why this is so. However, in a family where much the same foods are eaten by all, the men of the family are likely to show symptoms of deficiency in these fatty substances far sooner than the ladies will.

Lung cancer, we have been told many times, is far more prevalent among men than among women. It has been suggested that the reason for this may be the widespread tobacco-smoking among men which has only within recent years become popular among women. Deaths from leukemia (cancer of the blood) are somewhat more common among men than among women. Cholesterol deposits in the important heart arteries of people dying of lung cancer are very common. So it is not far-fetched to relate the three diseases to a common cause which might well be lack of essential fatty acids.

Dr. Sinclair tells us that it has also been proved that animals who lack the essential fatty acids are far more susceptible to radiation and perhaps also to its cancer-causing effects, as well as to the cancer-causing nature of certain chemicals. Now, if deficiency leaves one more susceptible to cancer, would it not follow that men, who might be far more deficient than women in the fatty acids, would naturally suffer most from any cancer-causing substance in tobacco smoke?

In the case of leukemia, deaths have increased rapidly during the past 20 years. They are commoner in countries where X-ray is used widely and are nine times more frequent among USA radiologists than among other physicians. X-ray may cause cancer. Lack of essential fatty acids makes one more susceptible to damage done by X-ray and possibly cancer-causing drugs. Could a combination of the two not be largely responsible for widespread leukemia deaths?

And what about cancer-causing chemicals in food? Would it not be reasonable to expect them to produce cancer of the stomach in persons especially susceptible to it? And who would be more susceptible than modern men who may be five times more deficient in essential fatty acids than women? As we know, cancer of the stomach is far more prevalent among men than among women.

Other Disorders Possibly Caused by Lack of the Right Fats

Seborrhea is a skin disease also more common among men. *It resembles the sores that can be produced in laboratory animals by depriving them of essential fatty acids.* Dr. Sinclair believes that some cases of seborrhea may be due to deficiency of these fats. In laboratory animals researchers can make the skin far more permeable by taking these fats out of the diet. So perhaps the rashes caused by modern detergents may come about because these extract the fatty acids from the skin, leaving it far more susceptible to damage.

Finally what of the nervous system? We know that it is rich in fatty substances. The presence of abnormal fatty substances would probably make it function badly. We do not know what effect processed fats and oils may have on nerve structure. But disseminated sclerosis, a disease of the nerves, is prevalent only in so-called civilized countries where processed fats are eaten and is unknown in more primitive cultures.

Finally, in laboratory animals, we can produce stomach ulcers by feeding the animals saturated (that is, processed) fats. Dr. Sinclair does not say this means all human stomach ulcers come from eating homogenized shortenings or foods fried in deep fat. But if this kind of food can and does produce stomach ulcers in animals, doesn't it seem wise to restrict its use sharply in your own diet if you would avoid ulcers?

We have one final comment to make, about a subject that Dr. Sinclair does not discuss but which we think is related to his theory. We publish in this book an account of an M.D. who treated prostate gland disorders with the essential fatty acids. Prostate gland "trouble" is a modern disease, from all that we can learn about it. Is it possible that one of the reasons why men need so much more essential fatty acids than women is because of this gland which occurs only in the male—a gland where the sperm fluid is manufactured. And could it be, therefore, that a deficiency in the fatty acids is responsible for the modern curse of prostate gland disorders which are very widespread, especially after middle age.

One final note—lack of essential fatty acids produces baldness in animals.

We hope we have set you to thinking in a new way about fats in your diet. They are important. You must have them. *But you must have the right kind.* The wrong kind will not only do nothing beneficial for you but in all probability will do you serious harm. Don't let yourself or your family become a victim to one of the degenerative diseases that may be simply the result of not enough of the essential fatty acids.

Feet

Imagine, if you can, going about your work every day wearing a pair of gloves so tight that your fingers are cramped and bent into a crippled position. How much work could you get done and how much pain would you endure from these twisted, deformed fingers! Yet this is what most of us do to our feet every day and our feet perform harder work than our hands, for they must support our weight and carry us every place we go, over hard sidewalks and floors.

We are told that more than 75 per cent of us suffer from foot trouble, mostly we suppose because we do not know or we ignore the basic facts about foot physiology. Your feet are made of 52 bones and 214 ligaments, put together in a mechanism that is the marvel of any engineer who studies it. These slight bones and trim ligaments form an arch whose curve supports your foot in comfort, gives your step elasticity, permits you to run, jump, stand, ride a bicycle, swim or do ballet dancing.

The arch is the most important part of your foot and the part that can give you most trouble. It can function well only when you have trained yourself to walk correctly so that the weight of your body is borne on your heel and the outer part of your foot. Just as soon as you turn your toes out—"point" them—your weight shifts to the inner part of your foot which is composed of muscles and ligaments. In time this part gives way and you are left in the painful and ugly condition of fallen arches. Walking correctly comes hard to us moderns because we must spend so much time on hard surfaces and because our shoes generally encourage incorrect walking posture.

A good exercise for training children to walk properly is to make, from wrapping paper, a chart of two footprints walking parallel to a straight line as well-mannered feet should. Spread the chart out on the floor and let the children walk on it, placing their feet in the footprints on the chart. Encourage them at all times to point their feet straight ahead. And see to it that their shoes and socks are large enough—a half to three-fourths of an inch longer than their feet.

Study your feet as you walk barefoot on a beach or a lawn and you will easily see what a burden shoes and hard pavements lay on your feet. Your toes should be able to curl into the surface you are walking on, so that they can perform their function of speeding your next step. Your heels should be level with the rest of your foot so that your weight is not tilted forward onto your toes, as high heels force it to be.

Walking is easier on your feet than standing, so when you have to wait for the bus you will be less tired if you pace back and forth rather than trying to stand in one position. Standing for long hours is perhaps the hardest torment your feet must endure. If your job entails standing, make a change in jobs if you can. If not, take advantage of every allowable rest period. Rest your feet on a chair, slip off your shoes and exercise your feet. Laying a handkerchief on the floor and picking it up with your toes is a good exercise. Picking up a marble or a small ball with your toes is restful.

How you sit is also important for your feet. When it is impossible for you to prop your feet up on something, try to sit with your feet flat on the floor, rather than crossing your legs. Crossing legs or ankles throws your whole body off balance so that your spine is out of line. In addition it hinders circulation.

Some years ago Editor Rodale discovered firsthand the close connection between cold, wet feet and trouble in the nose and throat. He was soaking his feet each night in icy cold water as treatment for athlete's foot and he ended by developing a "strep" throat. For some reason we have never seen discussed in medical journals there seems to be a very definite tie-up between cold, wet feet and respiratory disorders. So keep your feet dry if you would be healthy.

The kind of shoes you wear is of utmost importance to foot health and this is especially true of children. Whereas a toothache calls instant and painful attention to tooth ill-health, feet may be deformed almost past remedy before one is aware that something has gone wrong. Growing children should have new shoes every three or four months regardless of whether the old ones are worn out. Shoes should be heavy enough to give support to feet and protect them from stones or other rough surfaces. They should not be stiff. They should provide for ventilation. You should change shoes and stockings several times a day. Socks and stockings should be large enough so that feet are never cramped. You should never wear worn-out shoes, down at the heels and otherwise out of shape. For further information on foot health and rules for the daily care of feet, write to the National Foot Health council of Rockland, Massachusetts.

Feet and General Health

Human hands appear to be marvels of fine workmanship and design. What miracles may not be accomplished by a human hand, trained in some delicate skill or made powerful by practice for anything from violin playing to carpentry! But it seems that our hands are mere slabs of insensitive flesh compared to our feet. Dr. Frederick Wood Jones of the University of Manchester says that man's hand is a "ridiculously simple and primitive appendage . . . (but) man's foot is all his own. It is the most distinctive human part of his whole anatomical makeup." He adds that the foot is man's crowning achievement, his finest piece of adaptation.

The 52 bones and 214 ligaments composing our two feet are small, delicate and finely balanced. Yet they carry our weight over the eight miles or so that most of us walk in a day, they endure, for the most part uncomplainingly, hours of standing on hard floors or walking on hard sidewalks. No human engineer could construct so efficient a machine for weight bearing and motion.

Yet we esteem our feet so little, treat them so badly and neglect them in such a wholesale fashion that something like 75 per cent of us suffer from some foot disorder, of which we may or may not be conscious. For evidence of foot troubles does not necessarily appear first in the feet. Pain in your legs, your back, your neck or your head may be coming from your feet. Poor posture may be the result of faulty foot function and likewise painful feet may result just from poor posture. Your weight is important, too, for it goes without saying that every extra pound adds to the work your feet must do. And if your overweight results in your getting little or no exercise, then your feet suffer even more, for their muscles must be exercised or they degenerate, just as muscles in other parts of the body do.

Consider for a moment how feet were made to be used. Primitive man walked barefoot. His feet were adjusted to soft earth which he could grasp with his toes as he walked. Today even those of us who live in the country spend much of our time walking on hard level floors. City-dwellers pound the hard sidewalks every time they step outdoors. Practically none of us who are adult ever go barefoot, preferring to wear slippers even for that short walk from our evening bath to the bedroom. From the time we are toddlers our feet have been shod in shoes—usually badly fitted shoes. The women of modern times have earned (and we believe they deserve them) countless foot disorders because of their vanity in selecting shoes that look small and flattering regardless of what they do to feet. There is no engineer, physician or chiropodist who could find any excuse for high heels except vanity.

The way we stand and walk has more to do with the health of our feet than any other one factor. The weight of your body should be borne on the outside arch of the foot which is made of bone for the express purpose of bearing weight. The inside arch is made mostly of ligaments and muscles. When we walk incorrectly and stand with an incorrect posture, the weight is thrown instead on the inside arch. Muscles and ligaments endure all they can, and then give way, resulting in fallen arches which is one of the most painful conditions known, and may involve all kinds of dreadful apparatus necessary to bring relief. The purpose of these contraptions is, of course, to take the place of the muscles that have collapsed. Exercise is important, too, in curing fallen arches, as well as specially designed shoes. All of them very expensive and very painful.

Good Posture Helps Prevent Foot Trouble

What can we do to prevent foot trouble? As you might expect, we should concentrate our preventive efforts in childhood and much of the literature dealing with foot health concerns training and proper shoeing of children. We must be aware of the fact that foot disorders are very often not apparent for years and a child's foot may become deformed so gradually that he experiences no pain and his parents may not suspect that anything is wrong. Posture is of utmost importance. One's feet should at all times be straight—that is, parallel to one another, rather than turned out or turned in. Pigeon-toes suggest immediately that something is wrong and the pigeon-toed child will usually be taken to the doctor. But until quite recently it was considered genteel to turn the toes out in walking and many of us suffer today as a result of this fad. When the toes turn out in walking or standing, the weight of the body is thrown on the inner arch which sooner or later is bound to give way. So the first and most important exercise for healthy feet is learning to walk and stand with feet parallel. When we take a step the weight should be first on the heel, then as we go forward, it is transferred to the outer arch and finally to the great toe.

But it is, you will agree, impossible to walk correctly unless you have comfortable shoes. We will not even discuss trying to walk in high heels, for this comes under the heading of "hobbling" rather than walking. It is impossible to walk correctly in high heels. Regardless of whether you are holding your feet correctly parallel, they must slip forward in your shoes due to the height of the heel. And many of the foot troubles of modern women are concentrated in the forepart of the foot which is, of course, that part which is twisted and deformed by high heels.

High heels aside, there is considerable controversy as to what constitutes correct shoes. They should, of course, be big enough and right here is where so many foot troubles have their start in childhood when little feet are growing rapidly, getting too big for shoes long before the shoes wear out. In a recent school survey in England, reported in *The Medical Press,* June 18, 1952, we learn that 61 per cent of the boys and 83 per cent of the girls were wearing shoes that were too short for them. Corns and calluses were practically universal on all children over the age of ten. A foot health program examining school children in Massachusetts in 1943-44 discovered that 75 per cent of the children were wearing improperly fitted shoes. The number of incorrectly styled shoes increased with age, as did the foot defects. Eighty per cent of the stockings or socks were too short, resulting in just as much discomfort and deformation as too-short shoes; and children five to ten years of age were 40 to 50 per cent foot defective, while high school children were 80 per cent defective, for they had corns, calluses, ingrown toenails, hammer-toes, bunions, etc.

Children Outgrow Shoes Rapidly

An active youngster takes 30,000 steps in one day. If his shoes do not fit properly, is it any wonder that his feet soon suffer from all kinds of ailments? Children's shoes should be replaced as soon as there is any indication they are too small. The fitting should be carefully made, with the child standing, so that the full weight is on the feet. There should be the width of an adult's thumb between the toes and the end of the shoe. And since you never know how fast your child may be growing during any given time, you should make frequent examinations between shopping trips, just to make sure that junior's feet still have enough room inside his shoes. In general, it appears that shoes should be firm enough to give support, yet should not be made of stiff unyielding leather which might be appealing because of its durability. Nor should sneakers be worn a great deal of the time. If your child finds that sneakers are comfortable during the summer, make sure that he wears leather shoes part of the time, for sneakers or tennis shoes do not give enough support for constant wear.

Until the age of 16 or so, children's shoes should be renewed every three or four months, if you want to be certain their shoes are not too small. Hand-me-downs are an excellent way to save money on clothes, but poor economy in shoes. No one, child or adult, should ever wear shoes that someone else has been wearing. Heels should be straightened whenever they seem to be run over. And, incidentally, heels worn down either on the outside or the inside are an indication that posture is poor and feet are not functioning as they should.

The first evidence of badly fitted shoes appears on the skin—redness or blisters anywhere on the foot indicate friction or pressure, which mean poor fit. Corns and calluses may develop in a person with foot deformity who wears perfectly fitting shoes and also in a person with perfect feet who wears badly fitting shoes. However, in general, preventing corns and calluses is simply a matter of making sure your foot-gear is not causing friction or pressure at any one point and throwing away any pair of shoes that cause trouble. One of the major causes of foot trouble in housewives is wearing old shoes to do housework and saving the comfortable good ones for going out. Any housewife knows that she walks miles during the average work day using her feet constantly. So she should make certain that everyday shoes are the most comfortable ones she has—of course, with low heels. And always remember that properly fitting stockings and socks are just as important as properly fitting shoes.

A New Kind of Shoes

We received some time ago a most interesting book on the subject of shoes which presented so revolutionary a view of what proper shoes should be that we want to share it with you. Written by a professional skater who decided to make his own shoes when he could not find any that were comfortable, *Shoes and Feet to Boot* by Alan E. Murray tells the story of his search for correct footwear. Suffering tortures from painful feet which were also his only means of livelihood, Mr. Murray set out to make his own shoes and, after years of experimenting, designed what he calls the "Space Shoe." It is a shoe that apparently meets all requirements in that it lets you walk as primitive man walked. That is, the shoe fits your foot almost as tightly as your own skin; each toe is outlined. And you walk on a soft platform. Your toes can sink in as they do when you are walking on the sand of a beach.

As you might expect, such revolutionary shoes do not look like ordinary shoes. One commentator tells us they look more like a catcher's mitt. Yet these shoes are being worn today by countless people who have formerly suffered agonies from painful feet. They are worn by dancers and actors, by waiters and nurses, by salesgirls and barbers and other people who must stand or walk the greater part of the day. Arthur Godfrey and Robert Cummings wear Space Shoes. Each shoe is made individually from a plaster cast of your individual foot. After you get used to the strange sensation of "walking on air" which the shoes give you, you find that your foot defects begin to disappear and gradually your feet are remolded into the perfect shape which hard sidewalks and floors have so cruelly deformed. The testimonials in the book tell almost unbelievable stories of pain relieved and many varied ailments cured—ailments that at first glance seem to have nothing to do with feet.

If you are interested, the book is published by The Orange Printshop, Chapel Hill, North Carolina. Mr. Murray's shop where he designs and makes the shoes is at 130 West 10th St., New York, N. Y. The shoes are expensive, as you would expect, but at the time this book was published, 1950, Mr. Murray also had for sale a shoe kit containing material and instructions for making shoes yourself at home—two pairs of adults size shoes and as many as four pairs for young children or very small feet.

Now, if you plan to write Mr. Murray and inquire about his Space Shoes, we'll leave you to the years of peace and comfort these amazing clodhoppers will bring. But if you plan to struggle along with the shoes you can buy at your regular shoe store, here are some rules for foot health as outlined by the United States Public Health Service:

1. Select shoes and hose that fit properly. Tight shoes cause pressure and shoes that are too large cause friction. The heels of shoes should be kept straight.

2. Shoes should be well supported through the arch of the foot, particularly of children, whose feet tend to flatten when they stand up.

3. The growing child should be taught the importance of foot cleanliness and how to protect the feet against ill-effects of what may seem to him to be minor injuries.

4. During adult life, foot trouble may be a part of a general bodily condition where attention should be directed toward the improvement of general health.

5. When standing for long periods, place the feet 2 to 4 inches apart, point them straight ahead and support the weight on the outside of the feet. (When walking, keep the feet parallel and pointed straight ahead.)

6. In stepping forward, the weight should fall first on the heel, whereupon the body is carried forward over the foot, weight being applied along the outside of the foot from the heel to the small toe and finally across the forward part to the great toe.

7. The toenails should be cut straight across and not too short.

8. Frequent cleansing, and careful drying of the feet, together with frequent changes to dry hose and shoes may aid in relieving excessive perspiration.

9. Prompt care of all wounds and blisters on the feet may prevent serious consequences.

10. Fallen arches are the result of weakened leg muscles which allow the main or lengthwise arch in the foot to sag. An orthopedic surgeon should be consulted about this condition, as special treatment is indicated.

11. The feet should be bathed at least once a day with soap and warm water and then thoroughly dried. (We say: Omit the soap. Your skin is naturally acid and soap makes it alkaline, resulting in an unhealthy condition where all kinds of germs can take hold.)

12. Exercise the feet. The arches may be strengthened by bending the toes—best accomplished by picking up small objects such as marbles, with the toes.

We would add three last suggestions: Take off your shoes whenever you can and walk around in your bare feet, especially if you can walk in a yard or on a sandy beach. When you are tired, rest with your feet up. Or lie for a half hour or so with your feet higher than your head, on a slanting board or with pillows beneath your legs. The shop where you buy shoes may have a fluoroscope for fitting shoes. Many warnings have appeared in medical journals about the dangers of these machines if they are used too frequently. They are powerful machines and children, who enjoy the novelty of looking at their foot bones inside their shoes, may want to try the fluoroscope again and again, with quite serious results. Once or twice a year is often enough to use a fluoroscope in fitting shoes—don't let your children overdo it.

Feet, Congestion of

J. I. Rodale
Editor of *Prevention*

Mrs. Paul E. Barber of Empire, Michigan wrote me about an exercise she figured out for herself which she claims helped her lame knee a great deal. She suggests standing with the feet about twelve inches apart, then alternately lifting the right and left heel, bringing them immediately back to the flat position. The front part of the foot remains stationary while the rear part keeps moving up and down.

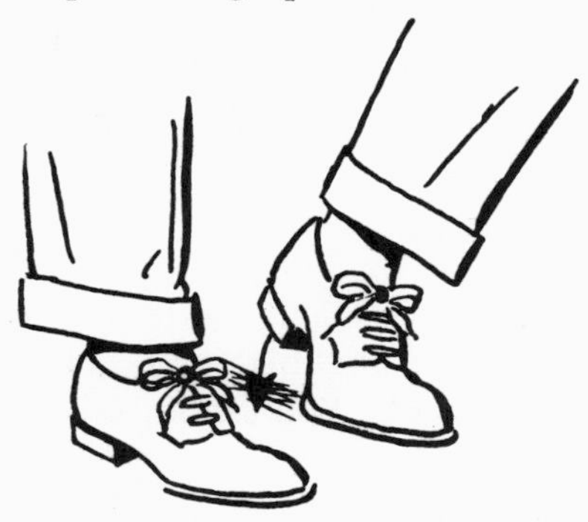

Mrs. Barber soon noticed that her thighs began to loosen up and the skin areas feel soft. She states that the exercise actually reduced the fat by shaking it up. She has tried other exercises to reduce certain areas, but states that results just seemed too slow. Her exercise can be done while doing dishes or any time the urge comes on to do it, she advises.

I began to do this exercise but soon came up with an exciting variation of it which I think has tremendous possibilities as an exercise, and I have never seen that movement mentioned in exercise books. In the case of Mrs. Barber's idea it is a motion that one does in walking—in doing that you have to lift your heel with each step. Her exercise then can be characterized as *walking while standing still.*

Now here is my idea, and it has two variations. One—instead of alternately bringing the heels up, bring the toe or front part of the foot up, as shown in the following picture:

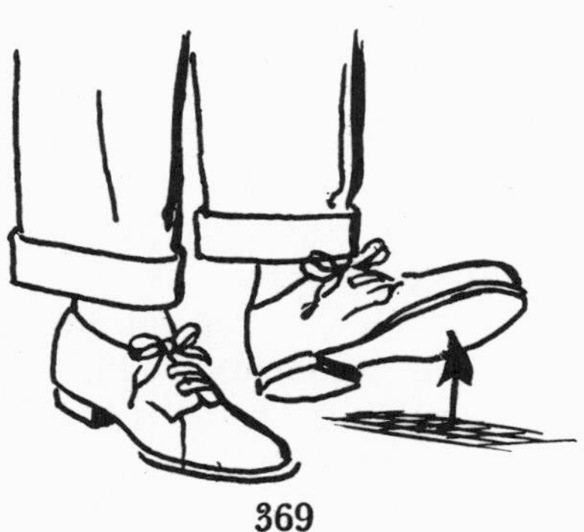

The toe portion is brought as far back as possible until a sort of tension is felt. In the second variation one sits on a chair as in the following pictures:

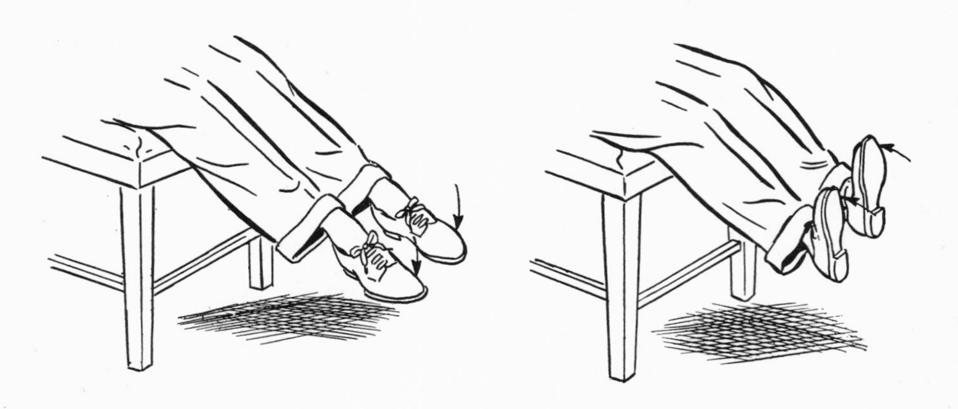

First one brings both feet as far forward as possible and then as far towards the leg as possible. I like this way best because in standing you cannot bring your feet forward. You can do this exercise for reasonable periods of time. Always moderation in everything.

Now, if you will do my exercise barefoot, that is the one where you stand up, you will notice several things. As you bring the toe part back you will see that the front bone, the *tibia,* between the ankle and the knee, moves out. Secondly, you will notice that as the toes come back, the five metatarsal bones in the foot spread out, thus opening up the toes, and that as you bring the foot back, to the flat position, the toes will come together. This shows that this exercise can greatly stir up the blood circulation in the feet, which usually is a place where stirring up is badly needed. The foot is the point farthest away from the heart and it takes a lot of pumping to get the blood there and all the way back. The demand on the pump is greater while standing up. That is why so much trouble and stagnation occurs there, and why there is a real need for a good exercise to keep the blood "moving" at that spot. It is also a reason why persons who have jobs that demand a lot of standing have trouble with their feet.

I noticed that when I do the exercise my breathing seems to improve. It appears to make me want to breathe. So perhaps the effect of this simple exercise is felt through the entire body.

While you are in your bare feet you can do the following exercise: Holding the feet forward, but stationary, while sitting, you merely move your toes as far forward, then as far backward as possible, doing it 12 to 15 times. This will stir things up right into the toes. You can even do this exercise with your shoes on, although you probably will not get the maximum possible movement that way.

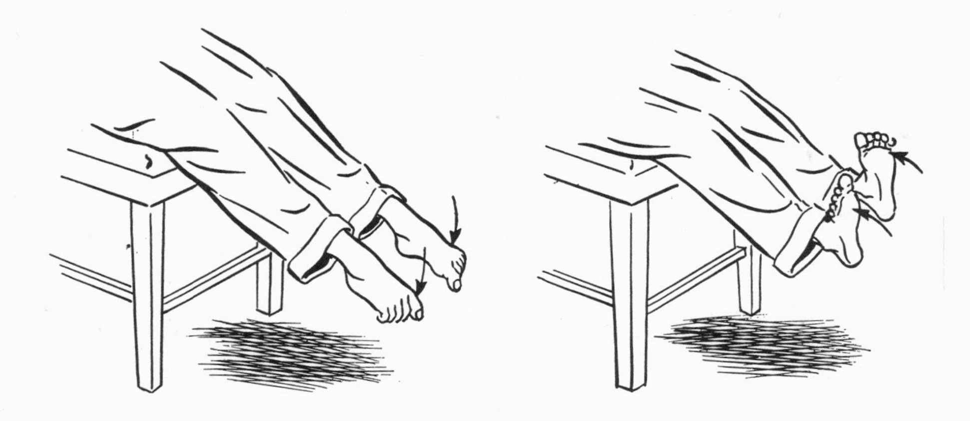

A combined exercise can be done while standing. You rock backward and forward on your feet, alternately bringing up the front and the back portions of the foot. This is a combination of Mrs. Barber's and my own ideas.

A friend of mine began to do my exercise and in about a week I began to notice things. The skin in the whole foot region became as soft to the touch as that of a baby, and an occasional touch of itching feet, the last vestige of athlete's foot, completely vanished. Incidentally one of these days I must go into the subject of athlete's foot, because it is not known generally, that in many cases the offender is not a fungi or germ, but a stagnation of the blood circulation. The exercise, then, is highly recommended for all cases of athlete's foot. It is possible also that the fungi of athlete's foot prefers a sick skin and will die or depart if the skin becomes real healthy. This is true with regard to many insects in gardening.

Now comes result number three. He tells me that there used to be a slight odor coming from his feet. After a month of doing this exercise it is entirely gone. His skin now is really and in every way like that of a new-born baby. One swallow of course does not make a summer, and I am not offering this in the way of scientific evidence, but I am doing it so that some of my readers may try it and report to me if they get similar results. *Prevention* magazine is a great laboratory with friendly readers as technicians. How fortunate we are!

This exercise can be done when sitting at the dining room table or at one's desk with no one being aware of it. It would also loosen up tired feet on a long automobile trip.

There is much trouble in this world in the human foot and leg. There are athlete's foot, phlebitis, varicose veins, gout, Buerger's disease and diabetic conditions. These exercises, both Mrs. Barber's and my own, could be effective as a protective, preventive measure, and also to ameliorate conditions that may already exist.

Who knows but that these exercises may accomplish another effect. If they can do what has been described above why couldn't they also exert a wholesome effect over the sweat glands, and permit the pores of the feet to "breathe" more effectively. All in all it would seem that everyone should add these foot exercises to the others that they do. There will be an entirely new feeling in the foot region, you will see.

Incidentally, another very effective foot exercise is done by walking up and down on one of these rubber mats with hundreds of little upward protruding knobs on it. Between this and the exercises described above the foot is in for a new life.

A word about these foot exercises and the heart. In a water system, if there is a collection of dirt or some other solid matter that is clogging the pipes at some point, there will be extra work for the pump, and it will take more fuel. The same should apply to the heart. If there is congestion at such a distant point from the heart as the foot, there can be no question that it has to pump harder. Now how would this affect a heart case? I would imagine that with such a person, it would be quite important to clear up all points of congestion in the body. This idea may open up a new thought in connection with heart cases. Should not an attempt be made in such cases to clear up congestions everywhere in the body? But I would not do it with drugs.

Dr. Edward Matthew of Weymouth, Massachusetts, one of the foremost specialists in diseases of the muscles, said, in reference to wearing tight shoes—that it could cut off the circulation of the blood in the foot, and that when the circulation is cut off in any part of the body, an added strain is placed on the heart which has to pump frantically in order to force the blood into the constricted area.

The taking of vitamin E would be another way to clear up congestions because it oxygenates the tissues in the entire body. I know a man who had the beginning of Buerger's disease, a dreadful condition which attacks mostly cigarette smokers, and in which the toes become gangrenous. He was greatly helped by taking vitamin E.

Another means would be massage and manipulation of the various parts of the body where congestions could occur. I am still speaking of people with heart trouble. Something should be done for them to insure that the blood is sailing as free as a song through every part of the body, thus not putting extra loads on the heart. Chiropractic and osteopathy could be of help here.

The exercises I have outlined and vitamin E are extremely important for smokers, because experiment have shown that every puff a smoker takes causes a constriction of the arteries in the foot. In such cases congestions are bound to occur.

I would like to suggest another foot exercise which can be done only while one is seated. First both feet are turned outward as much as possible, until the feet feel tense. Then they are turned as far inward as possible, again until a tenseness is felt. These positions are illustrated in the following pictures:

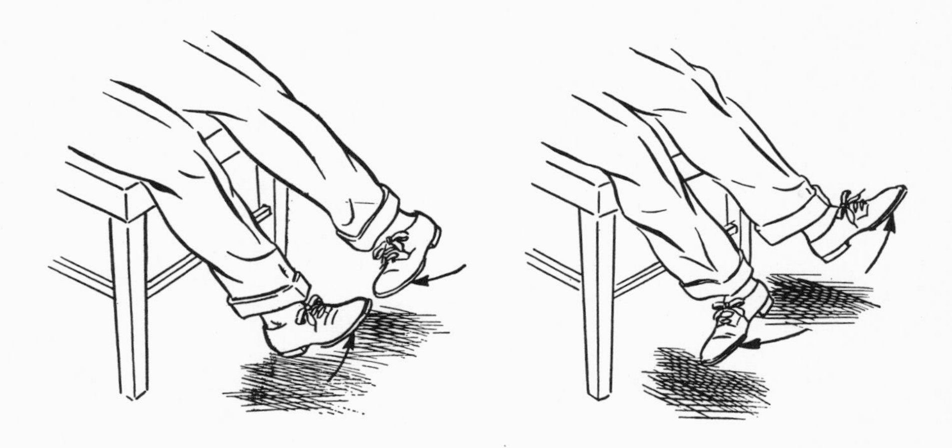

It could be another important influence in completely eradicating all congestion in the foot.

These exercises might be helpful in cases of ingrown toenail. I have had a black toenail since that day some years ago when something heavy fell on my foot. Cutting and re-cutting the nail had no effect on it. When I began to take a walk every morning, the black nail began to turn white again, from the base of the nail out. This certainly seemed to show that more blood was getting to the toe and rejuvenating it.

In the winter I stopped my walks until spring. Within a month the nail began to turn a darker shade. Then I began the foot exercises described above. Now, starting from the middle of the nail and going towards the right side, the nail is once again taking on its natural color.

Figs

Pliny, the Roman naturalist of the first century A.D., wrote:

"Figs are restorative, and the best food that can be taken by those who are brought low by long sickness, and are on the way to recovery. They increase the strength of young people, preserve the elderly in better health, and make them look younger, and with fewer wrinkles. They are so nutritive as to cause corpulency and strength; for this cause, professed wrestlers and champions were in times past fed with figs."

We know from history that figs are indeed a superlatively good food, for there are nations of people who live healthfully and almost exclusively on them. They probably originated in South Arabia; were known in Greece as early as the ninth century B.C. They were probably planted in England by the Romans. An Egyptian papyrus dated 1552 B.C. mentions figs as a tonic. Mithrydates, the ancient king who was an expert on poisoning, honored figs as one of the three ingredients of his "universal antidote."

There are many accounts in the Bible and various histories of figs being used medicinally, for respiratory illnesses, measles, smallpox, as a poultice on boils and so forth. We even have a record of Aaron Burr once using a fig poultice on a swollen jaw. The swelling was gone by morning. There seems to be nothing about the chemical composition of figs that gives any clue to their reported effectiveness against disease. True, they are rich in minerals, but so are many other fruits which do not have half this reputation. Perhaps the fact that figs have been plentiful and cheap down through the years has accounted for some of their popularity with the early doctors.

Figs are most noted for their effectiveness as a laxative. To this day, in spite of all the research that has been done on figs, we do not know why this should be. Some researchers believe it is simply the bulk fiber and seeds of the fig that give it its laxative properties. Others believe that the acids and minerals in the fruit are responsible. Syrup of Figs, incidentally, contains very little fig juice. It depends for its results on its content of senna.

Figs are not shipped raw to any great extent because of their extreme perishability. They are dried or canned. They are also made into preserves, syrup, jam, paste, coffee substitute; they are spiced, pickled and candied. In countries around the Mediterranean they are distilled into alcohol and made into wine. The fig newton is a product of America. No one knows exactly why it is called a "newton" except that it was originally manufactured in the town of Newton, Massachusetts. It appeared first on a price list in 1892.

Figs are dried in a drying yard where they are fumigated and stored in gas-tight houses. Then they are dumped and spread on trays for drying in the sun. Or they can be dried in a dehydrator in which hot air circulates. They are then washed, cooked in boiling water and packed in bricks or bulk.

Like papaya and pineapple, figs contain a protein-dissolving enzyme, called *ficin* or *cradein.* This enzyme could be used for tenderizing meat. On the island of Majorca housewives prepare curdled milk by beating the milk, then stirring it with split fig branches which cause it to coagulate rapidly. There is apparently so much of the enzyme in the branch of the fig that it brings about the desired reaction.

The total mineral content of figs is two to four times that of most fresh foods. Only cheese and one or two nuts have higher calcium content. Figs are also richer in iron and copper than most foods. Figs are a fair source of riboflavin, a B vitamin, and a good source of thiamin, another B.

Here is the vitamin and mineral content of 100 grams of dried figs (about six small figs):

Vitamin A	80 International Units
B Vitamins	
Thiamin	.16 milligrams
Riboflavin	.12 "
Niacin	1.7 "
Calcium	186 "
Phosphorus	111 "
Iron	3 "
Sodium	34 "
Potassium	780 "

A recent news story tells us that a French scientist believes that figs contain an anti-cancer factor. Dr. L. F. Bordas says that the anti-cancer factor appears to be related to the infinitesimal radioactive bodies which have been shown to be present in figs both from this country and the Mediterranean. These are also present in some other food products—pollen grains and royal jelly. There have been reports that cancer is rare in regions where lots of figs are eaten. Dr. Bordas thinks they can prevent the formation of pre-cancerous conditions in the body.

Fingernails

In about the third or fourth month of life in the mother's womb the unborn child begins to develop fingernails. Cuticle is a remnant of the fetal skin from which the nail developed. We do not know very much about fingernails, but apparently they are formed by the skin cells in the cuticle, which have the special function of manufacturing the horny substance of which the nails are made.

The cuticle is a very tender and valuable substance which should be treated with great respect when you are manicuring your nails. It should not ever be cut with nail scissors. Instead, push it back about once a month or so, with an orange stick. When you are washing your hands use the towel to push the cuticle back very gently and you can avoid hangnails and infections of the cuticle.

The matrix is the part of the nail from which it grows. The part of this that can be seen is the whitish "half-moon" at the base of the nail. Several studies have been done on the growth of fingernails. William Bennett Bean, M.D., tells us in an article in the *Journal of Investigative Dermatology,* January, 1953, that he checked on the growth of his own fingernails over a period of ten years. He found that they grow at about the same rate of speed the year 'round, but that they appear to grow more slowly as one grows older. The average rate of growth, he found, is about .119 millimeters daily. Another writer tells us that nails grow about one-eighth of an inch every month. Dr. Bean found that climate, occupation and emotional stress had nothing to do with the rate of nail growth. But he also found that his nails stopped growing while he had the mumps. He tells us that the nails of malnourished children have a rate of growth considerably slower than that of well nourished ones. Also, it seems that paralysis of the hand may stop the growth of nails. Nail-biters have nails that grow about 20 per cent faster than normal nails, perhaps because the body is trying to keep up with the rapid rate at which the nails are being destroyed.

The most common disorders of fingernails involve dryness and brittleness, white disfiguring spots, splitting, and ridges, either lengthwise or crosswise. From the research we did, it appears that dryness, splitting and brittleness of nails result from lack of certain food elements. They also may come about because of exposing the hands excessively to water, especially water in which there is soap or detergents. The nails are almost pure protein, so a lack of good grade protein in the diet can affect them. Meat, eggs, cheese and nuts should form a considerable part of the diet every day.

Brittle nails also occur sometimes in cases of iron deficiency anemia which should of course be treated by a doctor. Lack of calcium, vitamin A, vitamin D or vitamin B may cause brittle nails. One physician counsels full vitamin therapy with calcium and doses of gelatin in cases of brittle nails. Infections of the cuticle may be caused by exposure to water or by injuring the cuticle while manicuring it. They may also result from anemia, chronic fatigue, worry or malnutrition. One physician stated that 300 milligrams of vitamin C daily would be useful in infections of the cuticle. (An orange contains about 25 milligrams—we suggest rose hips as a richer source.)

The little white spots that sometimes appear on nails are a mystery to the medical profession. They occur most frequently in children and may run in families. Usually they appear only on one finger or two and they may be the result of injury to the base of the nail. Or they may indicate simply that a certain spot on the nail did not build up its horny structure as it should have. Lengthwise ridges of the nails are just an indication of old age, say the medical men. To us this suggests that if your nails are ridged and you are not yet middle-aged, you would do well to get plenty of the anti-old-age vitamins and minerals—vitamin A and calcium are perhaps the two most important. A crosswise ridge on the nail may mark the incidence of a disease or a period of malnutrition. We are told they have sometimes appeared after such a slight illness as a cold or a bout of seasickness.

Finally the nail disorders that plague a lot of us may be due entirely to various chemical substances we use, either externally or internally. There is a substance called phenolphthaline which is used in laxatives, chewing gum and toothpaste, that has been known to cause purplish lines on the nails. Nail cosmetics can be especially dangerous, mostly because they are worn consistently and the nail has no "breathing space" in which to throw off possible bad effects. In the *Journal of the American Medical Association* for June 28, 1952, we found an article on a very troublesome disorder caused by wearing false fingernails. Even though this patient wore the nails for only 24 hours, it was five months until she was completely cured. Apparently the adhesive substance used to fasten the nails on was the offender in this case. An inquiring letter from the physician to the company which manufactured the adhesive went unanswered.

For nail health in general we propose the following suggestions: use as few cosmetics as possible—polish, polish remover, etc. Keep the hands dry; wear rubber gloves when you are working in water, and gardening or working gloves when you are working outside. Remove stains with lemon juice, which is generally good for the hands because it restores them to their natural acid condition. Soaps and detergents are alkaline and so are bound to be harmful to the skin of the hands. Finally, a diet rich in protein, vitamins and minerals, especially calcium (bone meal), vitamins A, B, C and D will be the best tonic for ailing nails.

Fish

One of the complaints most commonly leveled against our diet suggestions and those of leading nutritionists is that a high-protein diet is too expensive. This is a sample of the very justifiable wail we hear when we mention high protein diet: "It's all right for you to talk about how healthy we and our children would be on a diet high in proteins and low in carbohydrates, but just compare for a minute the price of meat and the price of processed cereal, the price of cheese and the price of baked goods, the price of eggs and the price of macaroni."

We agree that protein foods are inexcusably high in price. We remind our readers why this is so. Carbohydrate foods are harvested, processed and sold with a minimum of difficulty. Protein foods are produced chiefly from animals which are fed on carbohydrate foods. The number of cattle that can be raised on a field is very small compared to the amount of wheat that can be raised on that same field. So, sure, the wheat products can be sold for 16 cents a package with a space cadet uniform thrown in. And meat may be anywhere from sixty cents to a dollar and half a pound.

However, the fact that carbohydrate foods are cheaper does not mean that they are healthier. You need carbohydrate foods, but, nine chances out of ten, you need more protein and less carbohydrate foods than you are now getting. That is why we are proud to present an excellent source of protein which is also cheap, and which is a good food from many other points of view as well—fish.

No one has to plant or harvest fish, or worry over the proper proportion of elements in their diet. There's no loss from contagious diseases. You don't have to buy a farm and a lot of expensive machinery, you don't have to give a hoot for the fluctuations of the grain market or the political fortunes of subsidies; you're not even bothered by the weather—if you're a fisherman. All you need is a boat, and a line or a net and you're in business. These, we suppose are some of the reasons why fish can be inexpensive, even in spite of the fact that they are as good a protein as meat.

Fish weren't always inexpensive. J. C. Drummond and Anne Wilbraham in their book *The Englishman's Food* (Jonathan Cape, London), tell of days in 18th century England when the price of fish was exorbitant.

This was because there was no refrigeration and in order to have the fish edible by the time it reached inland towns the most expensive methods of transportation had to be used. One enterprising gentleman set up a system of speedy "land carriages" for bringing fish to inland markets and even succeeded in having a bill passed to exempt these carriages from the customary road tolls. By 1820 fish was being transported packed in ice, but this was expensive, too.

Earlier, way back in the 16th century, the English church established two "fisshe dayes" per week, to encourage ship building and because meat was so expensive. There was a fine of three pounds or three months imprisonment for anyone eating meat on the two prescribed "fisshe dayes." Of course this was long before industrialization had concentrated people in cities, so transportation problems were not so pressing. And even so there were laws to prevent the selling of decomposing fish "lest the air might become infected through the stench arising therefrom." The fishmongers' companies enforced these laws. It was at this time that salt became such an important item of trade, for much of the fish was salted to preserve it.

Today fish is an eleven million dollar business. The Boston pier alone handles 300 million pounds of fish annually. And yet the average American eats only about 15 pounds per year of all fishery products. Compare this to the 100 pounds of white sugar per year per American, and you may arrive at some conclusions as to why many of us are sick much of the time.

Eat Ocean Fish—Not Inland Fish

For, make no mistake about it, fish, especially ocean fish, is good food. First of all there has been no tampering with it. Commercial fertilizers and insecticides play no part in the fish business. Preservatives, artificial flavorings and colorings cannot be used on fish. Ocean fish cannot be doped, chemicalized or processed.

We do want to inject at this point just a hint of some of the things that are happening to inland fish. A recent clipping from *Chemical Week* (August 1, 1953), tells us that trout breeders have found that brook trout can be more easily transported alive from place to place if they are given sleeping pills before they are placed in their containers. This prevents them from moving about so much. What it may do to people who eat the fish over a long period of time has, of course, not been investigated. We also have in our files a horror story about methods now being used to "clear" lakes before trout are released. The other "inferior" fish are killed off, it seems, by scattering rotenone, says *Chemical Week* for August 29, 1953. Then, too, inland fish are subjected constantly to the tons of poisons dumped each day into our rivers and streams by industrial firms. No one gets very excited about this (even though residents are drinking the water) until fish begin to die by the thousands, as happened recently in the Buffalo, New York area. Then the newspapers take up the hue and cry, the pollution ceases for a while and everyone forgets the entire incident.

So we would advise against eating fish from inland waters, unless you yourself have caught the fish in a mountain stream or lake which you know is far enough away from "civilization" that no contamination can have reached the waters. But ocean fish—taken from the great fishing banks far out to sea—come to us unpolluted. And most of the fish sold in inland markets comes from either the Atlantic or Pacific.

For a long time there has been a prejudice in the American mind against eating commercially frozen fish, says Morris B. Jacobs in his book, *Food and Food Products* (Interscience Publishers, New York City). This is apparently because, in the early days, only those fish that seemed too far gone to be marketed were frozen, and of course their quality was very low. But today with the quick freezing methods that are available frozen fish is every bit as good, or perhaps even better, than fresh fish for inland folks. The marketing of fish is a race against time, for the whole metabolic system of fish is set up on a very rapid scale, because of the cold temperature in which they live. So deterioration sets in much faster than it does in meat. Actually the meat of a fish begins to deteriorate the moment it is taken from the water. Quick freezing halts this process immediately.

So if you live far inland, the frozen fish, packed in airtight containers very shortly after the fish is caught, has probably more food value than a whole fresh fish which has been frozen or packed in ice for the long trip from the ocean to your market. You cannot determine, says Jacobs, by the brightness of the eye or the color of the gills how fresh a fish actually is. Your only criterion for judging is the keeping quality of the fish after you buy it, its appearance and odor while you are preparing it and its palatability. Small pieces like fillets freeze more quickly than whole fish, so less food value is lost in freezing. In addition, when you buy frozen fillets there is no waste and the waste matter in a whole fish may be as high as 70 per cent, as they are sold. Any housewife who has ever struggled to prepare a trout or bass brought in by her ever-loving provider knows well what a pile of fish trimmings accumulates in the garbage can compared to the tiny morsels that find their way to the table. So it's economical to buy frozen fillets.

Amino Acids In Fish

Now, why do we claim that fish is a healthful food, aside from the fact that it is not tampered with? Fish is chiefly protein, as good a protein as meat. By this we mean that it supplies all the differtn kinds of protein that are needed for health. Some proteins contain all the known building blocks that are needed for building and repairing tissues, while other proteins lack some of these essential building blocks. The building blocks are called "amino acids." About ten of these are absolutely essential for health—that is, they are required in the diet of man. Comparing the amino acids of fish with those of chicken and beef, we find that they are as good or better.

Other Valuable Constituents of Fish

Fish contains valuable minerals, too. And here we run headlong into a discussion that is at present occupying many Americans who are arguing about the advisability of artificially fluoridating their water supply. Fish contain fluorine in considerably higher quantities than do most foodstuffs. Says Jacobs, "It might appear that the presence of five parts per million of fluorine in sea foods would have a harmful effect.

However, Lee and Nilson have shown that this is not the case. (U.S. Bureau of Fisheries, Investigational Report 44, 1939.) Apparently, the fluorine is present in some form such that assimilation is much less than is the case with added inorganic fluorides." This seems to us another overwhelming evidence against water fluoridation. Organic fluorine in food is not harmful. It is only when we begin to concoct fluoride compounds in a laboratory with no regard for what form the compound takes or what may accompany it in the solution we end with, that anyone suffers any difficulties from ingesting fluorine.

Fish contain, too, relatively large amounts of calcium, copper, iron, magnesium, phosphorus, potassium, sodium and strontium. It is the high phosphorus content of fish that has made it famous as a "brain food," for phosphorus is one of the important constituents of brain matter.

Fishmeal is manufactured from the wastes of fish and is used in animal food. Nutritionally it is one of the richest of foods, for it contains all the vitamins and minerals in concentrated form. This being the case, we "civilized" Americans feed it to our animals, of course, rather than eating it ourselves. In New England fisheries, the whole carcass of the fish, including the bones, is ground up, along with the head, fins and other waste material. After it is dried it will keep well without refrigeration and has been found to be an excellent source of the rare vitamin B_{12}, along with the other B vitamins.

A recent news release from the World Health Organization announced that they planned to send fishmeal to remote parts of the world where famine stalks, for it would provide all the protein necessary to sustain life. We corresponded earnestly for a long time with embassies and commerce departments in foreign countries but could not locate in this country a source of fishmeal for human consumption. Perhaps some day someone in this country will begin to sell fishmeal as a food supplement for human beings.

In our research on fish we ran across several reports of sensitivity to fish among folks inclined to be allergic. As you know, we believe that a correct diet will protect against allergies. We also believe that those who choose their fish with care and eat it along with other foods should not have difficulty with it. A member of our staff recalls that a neighbor's child broke out with hives whenever she ate fish but the investigating physician discovered that the child ate *only* fish whenever fish was served, so his instructions were to try eating other foods along with it. And there were no more hives. If you happen to be sensitive to fish, here's a hint. Be sure you never lick the sticky side of labels, for the glue on the back is often made from fish gelatin. As a matter of fact, it's just as well never to lick any adhesive substance. A little gadget from the dime store will do it for you much better.

Shellfish and Canned Fish Are Not For You

We have not discussed canned fish for, as readers know, we take a very dim view of any canned food. We believe you should eat fresh foods, no matter how convenient it is to open a can. But in the case of canned salmon we're inclined to draw the line not quite so sharply. For salmon is canned with the bones intact and perhaps the health value of eating these softened bones outweighs the negative health angle of the can. Let's put it this way: If, because of circumstances beyond your control, you have to eat your protein food for dinner tonight out of a can, let it be canned salmon rather than canned meat. You'll be getting a good start on your daily calcium requirements that way. And you won't be filling up on the preservatives that most canned meats contain.

Only three words about shellfish—don't eat 'em. True, they are richer in some food elements than other fish. But there is a very sound reason why the "Oysters R in Season" sign does not appear on restaurant windows until September. We believe—and we have ample evidence in our files—that present-day Americans are taking too great a chance on pollution when they eat shellfish. Too many of our shellfish are taken from beds near where rivers empty into the sea and untold poisonous matter is released. You do not know where the shellfish you buy have been caught. You could not possibly track down this information. So, from where we sit, Shellfish R Never In Season.

We want to emphasize just one more aspect of the healthfulness of fish menus before we list for you the various vitamins and minerals present in fish. One of the recognized deficiencies in diet occurring in many parts of America is lack of iodine which in many cases is related to disorders of the thyroid, or goiter. Iodized salt is not the answer, we believe, for here again, as in the case of fluoridated water, the mineral has been added by chemists. But ocean fish (not inland fish) contain large amounts of iodine. So it seems likely that at least one fish meal a week would supply enough iodine to prevent any deficiency in your family. And this is important, for iodine is mighty scarce in other foods, in many parts of the country.

Here is how fish stacks up in the vital matter of minerals and vitamins. These figures must be approximate for the content of fish is extremely variable depending on when and where they were caught. We have chosen halibut as a popular and typical fish.

	Amount in 1 serving (about ¼ pound) of Halibut
Calcium	20 milligrams
Phosphorus	200 milligrams
Iron	1 milligram
Copper	.23 milligrams
Magnesium	.01 milligrams
Iodine	250 parts per billion
Vitamin B	
Thiamin	90-120 micrograms
Riboflavin	222 micrograms
Niacin	6 milligrams
Pyridoxine	100 micrograms
Pantothenic acid	150 micrograms
Biotin	8 micrograms
Calories	121

Fish Liver Oil

In the 18th century the physicians of England discovered that fish liver oil could cure rickets. Fish liver oil had been eaten in Iceland and Norway for centuries before that. In those days, this is how they made oil, because there was no other method known for extracting it from the fish livers. The livers were allowed to putrefy, to rot, until the oil came to the surface and could be skimmed off. The imagination is staggered at the thought of the aroma that must have clung to the walls of the buildings in which this process took place, the clothes worn by the fishermen, the containers in which the fish liver oil was collected.

And yet, hundreds and hundreds of years ago, human beings knew so much about the potency of fish liver oils that determined mothers in northern countries pinned down their squalling youngsters and poured into their protesting gullets quantities of this putrid, offensive oil. And watched them grow tall and straight and healthy as a result. It was not suspected until quite recently why fish liver oil is so important to growth and good health. From the Manchester, England, Infirmary, Dr. Robert Darbey wrote to a friend in 1782: "For several years after I came to the infirmary I observed that many poor patients, who were received into the infirmary for the chronic rheumatism, after several weeks trial of a variety of remedies, were discharged with little or no relief. . . . About ten years since, an accidental circumstance discovered to us a remedy, which has been used with the greatest success, for the above complaint, but is very little known, in any county, except Lancashire; it is the cod, or ling liver oil." Drummond and Wilbraham go on to tell in *The Englishman's Food* that the infirmary doctors were so pleased with the results they obtained that no less than 50 or 60 gallons were prescribed annually in spite of the fact that the smell and taste were so repulsive that many patients could not stomach it.

In those days almost any disorder of the bones or joints was called "rheumatism" so of course rickets, tuberculous joint diseases and so forth were among those cases of "rheumatism" cured by the new remedy. About the middle of the nineteenth century, an incident in the London Zoo confirmed the potency of the new medicine. The curators had always been unable to raise lion and bear cubs, for they developed rickets easily and early and soon died. The animals were fed on a raw meat diet. On the advice of a prominent British physician of the time, crushed bone, milk and cod liver oil were added to the meat. From then on, there were no further casualties among the 200 animals. Looking for the reason for such wonderful properties, one investigator of the early 19th century decided it was the iodine in the fish liver oil that performed the miracles. And indeed up until the time of Sir Edward Mellanby and his famous experiments with rachitic puppies only about 30 years ago no one knew that the precious ingredients of fish liver oils are the concentrated vitamins A and D they contain. Nor does anyone know up to the present time why these vitamins occur in such abundance in fish livers. Presumably they are stored there by the fish, but why in such quantity?

"It is not surprising," say Drummond and Wilbraham, "that the possibility of other fish liver oil possessing therapeutic value aroused interest after cod liver oil re-established its reputation in England. *The Lancet* drew attention to the possibilities of using shark liver oil in 1855, but the extraordinary potency of the liver oils of such fish as the halibut and tunny was unsuspected until quite recently. Perhaps this is understandable. Cod liver is exceedingly rich in fat (30-50 per cent) whereas most of the livers which yield the very potent oils contain a much smaller proportion (2.8 per cent). When substitutes for cod liver oil were sought it was natural to turn to those like the shark, which also have a large amount of oil stored in the liver."

H. C. Sherman, Columbia University's world-famous nutritionist, in his book *Food Products* (The Macmillan Company, 1941) has this to say about fish liver oils as food: "Hitherto in this country, the fish liver oils have been commonly considered as medicines rather than food. But cod liver oil has been a stable article of food in some fishing communities; moreover its clinical value seems to lie in its contribution of two dietary essentials, vitamin A and vitamin D. For these reasons, there is justification in thinking of these fish liver oils as vitamin-rich foods."

Why Fish Liver Oils Are Important

Vitamin A can be obtained from animal and vegetable food. Vitamin D is available only in animal products and in the ultra-violet rays of the sun. That is, some substance in your skin can manufacture vitamin D from sunlight. And the amount of vitamin D in animal products (cream and butter, for example) is infinitesimal compared with the wealth of vitamin D in fish liver oil.

Vitamin A is necessary for a healthy skin. It is important, too, for the eyes. Its deficiency results in "night blindness" which means inability to adapt to light after darkness, or darkness after light. Research has indicated that vitamin A is important for the prevention of infections, such as colds. It has been found that plenty of vitamin A in the diet helps the condition of people with goiter or other thyroid trouble. Vitamin A deficiency results in inability to store fat. For children, the vitamin is an absolute essential if bones and teeth are to be healthy and if the child is to grow strong and tall. Bladder stones are caused in laboratory animals by lack of vitamin A.

Vitamin D is essential for the proper use by the body of calcium and phosphorus—perhaps the two minerals most important for good health. No matter how much of these two minerals you get in your diet, you cannot use them unless you also have plenty of vitamin D. So rickets, a deforming bone disease, can be caused in children by lack of any one or more of these three—calcium, phosphorus or vitamin D. Animals manufacture their vitamin D from sunlight. And it has been found that hibernating animals do not hibernate when they have been given enough vitamin D. They know, you see, that the sun's rays in winter time are not strong enough to provide the amount of vitamin D they need. Osteomalacia is the adult disease corresponding to rickets in children, when the bones become decalcified from lack of one of the two important minerals, or vitamin D.

For many years it has been accepted practice to give babies in this country fish liver oil to prevent rickets. And the incidence of rickets has greatly decreased as a result. But why should we stop giving this vitamin-rich food when children reach adolescence? At that time they are growing very rapidly and need all the calcium and phosphorus they can get for making bones and permanent teeth. Calcium is one mineral that, all nutritionists agree, is deficient in the American diet. We do not eat enough leafy green vegetables, eggs and cheese to supply anything like the amount of calcium we need. Why not, then, just to be on the safe side, get plenty of vitamin D so that we can use effectively all the calcium we get?

We believe that everyone, children and adults alike, should take fish liver oils to be assured of getting plenty of both vitamin A and vitamin D. In case you live in the south and spend a lot of time out in the sunshine, take one of those oils which is richer in vitamin A and has less vitamin D. If you live in the north you are well aware how puny and how brief are the rays of the winter sun, especially when they are filtered through the smog and smoke of a large city. Do you think you can afford to take a chance on too little of either of these necessary vitamins?

How To Take Fish Liver Oils

Here is a table taken from *The Englishman's Food* showing the variety of vitamin D content of the different fish liver oils:

	International Units of Vitamin D per gram
Cod	50-200
Halibut	1,000-4,000
Sea Bass	4,000-5,000
Swordfish	4,000-10,000
Yellow Fin Tunny	13,000-45,000
Striped Tunny	220,000-250,000

Compare this, please, with the vitamin D contained in butter (1 unit per gram) or egg yolk (1.5 to 5 units per gram). Halibut liver oil has largely displaced cod liver oil as a food supplement today because it is also extremely rich in vitamin A, so that a small amount of it provides much more vitamin A than cod liver oil does.

Because of the high concentration of vitamins in fish liver oil, don't make the mistake of deciding that, if a little is good, a lot will be better, for fish liver oil taken in enormous quantities is dangerous. Read the directions on the container in which you get your oil. The minimum daily requirement of vitamin A is 5000 units per day for adults and from 1500 to 6000 units per day for children, according to age. The vitamin D requirements are 400-800 units for children. The National Research Council, which sets these minimums, does not suggest any minimum requirements of vitamin D for adults. More than 400,000 units of vitamin D daily is considered toxic for adults and more than 30,000 units daily is toxic for children. This is easily understandable when you think of the vitamins in terms of food. Eating five times as much as you should have of almost any food would be bound to make you sick, no matter how healthful the food may be. So be guided by the suggested daily dose on the container.

One word more. There are food supplement manufacturers who do all kinds of things to vitamin preparations. They may use synthetic vitamins—that is, they make up the vitamins in a chemical laboratory putting together the chemical elements (oxygen, hydrogen, nitrogen and so forth) as they occur in the natural vitamin. These are not for you, if you would be healthy. Then some processors take natural fish liver oil and add different substances to it, to increase the potency. These are also not for you. When you buy fish liver oils, for yourself or your children, make certain that they contain nothing—but nothing—except the fish liver oil. The label will tell you what the contents are, and the potency. That is, the label will indicate that one perle contains 5000 units of vitamin A and 200 units of vitamin D or whatever it may happen to be. Take the fish liver oil according to the suggested dosage.

And—lucky you!—to be alive today when fish liver oils have been shorn of their taste and smell!

Fluoridation and Goiter

From South Africa comes a letter to the editor of the *Rand Daily Mail* in Johannesburg, written by Dr. Douw G. Steyn, Professor in the Department of Pharmacology of the Institute for Pathology, Pretoria. Says Dr. Steyn: "Fluorine is probably the most dangerous of all poisons as far as chronic poisoning is concerned, as it has a very marked tendency to accumulate in the body. This tendency of a substance is of the utmost importance when its addition to food or domestic water supplies is contemplated, as under such conditions there is hardly any time for detoxification in the system or excretion, with the result that the risk of chronic poisoning is very great. The (medical) literature on fluorine poisoning is voluminous and it is obvious that I cannot go into detail here. Suffice it to say that the symptoms of chronic fluorine poisoning may appear up to periods of 30 to 40 years after the inception of ingestion of minute quantities of this element.

"It is common knowledge that the most prominent symptoms of chronic fluorine poisoning are disease and destruction of the teeth and bones. What is not so well known is that the long-continued ingestion of minute quantities of fluorine may also cause disease of the thyroid gland (goitre). This was brought home to us very forcibly in the course of recent investigations into endemic goiter in the Northwestern Cape Province conducted by the South African Goitre Research Committee which functioned under the auspices of the Medical Faculty of the University of Pretoria. Also this malady may appear five, ten, twenty or thirty years after commencement of the drinking of water containing minute quantities of fluorine. We saw goitre in children, adolescents and adults drinking water which contains only 1.6 parts per million of fluorine.

". . . Of great importance is the fact that fluorine induces goitre in spite of the fact that the water contains many times more iodine than the normal requirement of man. Of further interest and importance is the fact that iodized salt, which is a most effective preventive of endemic goitre caused by iodine deficiency in food and water has no effect on fluorine-induced goitre. The soundness of these observations and facts has been confirmed by animal experiments.

"I would strongly urge that before it is contemplated to take steps to add fluorine to our domestic water supplies, a committee be appointed to consider the advantages, disadvantages and inherent dangers of such a step from all angles."

Fluoridation, One Part Per Million

By J. I. Rodale

Editor of *Prevention*

In applying fluorides to drinking water, in order to reduce the number of tooth cavities in children, only a very small amount of the chemical is used—an infinitesimal quantity—namely, only one part of fluorine to a million parts of water. But, to anyone who has even a rudimentary knowledge of chemistry, the fact that an amount is small is not the only factor to be guided by. The important thing is—how chemically *active* is that small amount?

It depends on the chemical with which you are dealing. For example, you can put a thousand times more calcium in the water than fluorine without any harm being done at all, because calcium is *not* too active chemically. But with fluorine, you are dealing with a powerful substance which is used as the base of many commercial poisons for destroying cockroaches, rats, and such ilk. A compound as death-dealing as that must be under strict, continuous control.

To the ordinary lay-mind, one part in a million parts seems like a negligible quantity. But when we realize that this tiny fraction can reduce the amount of cavities in some children's teeth, we must admit that, however infinitesimal it may be, THAT tiny amount has had an effect in the human body. Now—if only one part per million can accomplish one effect—there is no earthly reason why it could not accomplish another one, elsewhere in the body—an effect we did not bargain for—namely, a harmful one.

Sodium fluoride is an extremely powerful protoplasmic poison, and is very soluble. It is this factor of solubility that gives it the power to enter the blood-stream, at once, and in full force—to stream through to every part of the body in a matter of moments, and to get into its every cell—teeth and all.

The body contains billions of cells. Yet this practically invisible quantity of one part per million of fluorine has the property of being able to divide itself so that some of it is apportioned to every one of those cells of the body. We must strain our imagination to conceive a degree of smallness, a microscopic diminution—a transmutation that enables part of this one part per million to be portioned out—to penetrate into the body's billions of cells. However, some of this fluorine penetrates into cells of sensitive organs where its presence may become a cumulative detriment.

The ability of the body to reduce things to minuteness, is utterly fantastic. The cell, as microscopic as it is, is complete—self-contained—a microcosm—a world in miniature. Within it there are thousands of chemical compounds with their millions of molecules weaving in and out, exchanging atoms, and operating under scientific law. But man is only on a primitive threshold with regard to it. He is only first beginning to become aware of the merest elementals that make the cell an operating entity and much of what it does is a closed book to him. When, therefore, we intrude by force, a tiny amount of fluorine into that cell, however tiny that amount may be, we must be sure that we know exactly what it will do there, or take the consequences of a very unscientific action. The cell does not *want* this kind of forced fluorine. It does not *need* it. But it has to take it—willy-nilly.

Cells Affected by One Part in a Hundred Million

To give you an idea of how effective smallness can be in connection with its effect on living matter, let us consider an announcement that has just come out of the University of Wisconsin, in connection with a cancer study that has been going on there. In that institution a team of botanists and biochemists have isolated a chemical called *kinetin* which has the power to make a cell divide into two parts. But the thing that should be interesting to us in this discussion of smallness is that it takes only one part in a *hundred million* to do it. This is only one one-hundredth of the amount, as compared with the quantity of fluorine used in water fluoridation. This extremely tiny amount of *kinetin,* when applied to plant tissue, causes it to multiply by division. In other words, it produces cancer of that tissue. When this small amount of *kinetin* is applied to plant tissues, cancerous tumors are formed. This unusual phenomenon was announced in *The Cancer News,* published by the American Cancer Society in April, 1955. Now, I do not say that fluorine will do this, but we do not know exactly what it *will do.*

And if you think that one part in a hundred million is small let us look at an example of the miniature that will really astonish you. Let us consider the science of homeopathy, a method of medical curing that resorts to such incalculable degrees of infinitesimality that the mind just cannot conceive or measure it. The word homeopathic itself has actually become an adjective in our language, meaning extreme smallness.

In homeopathy, substances are diluted to such an extent that they get down to next to nothing. The homeopaths use drugs in which the quantity of them have been so diluted that it can be measured by a fraction having one as the numerator, and *one* followed by 20,000 noughts as the denominator. This is more than a million billion times smaller quantity than the amount of fluorine used in water fluoridation. And yet homeopaths who are accredited M.D.'s achieve definite effects with such smallness. Otherwise there would not be the thousands of homeopathic physicians practicing their profession every day.

The idea of smallness is not a new concept in science, and if you wish an additional example, think of bacteria, millions of which can occupy the space of a pin-head. Yet, only one of them, if it is of the right species, can start an epidemic which could kill out thousands of people.

But, if you think bacteria are small, then turn your attention to the virus, an example of smallness which baffles even the microscope, and defies all measurement. So you can see that it is *not* smallness of itself which is the prime factor in the consideration and evaluation of a substance, but what properties it hides within its interior.

In chemistry there are effects brought about by reduction of quantities which science cannot explain, but which are encountered time and time again. In a book called *Selective Toxicity,* written by Dr. Adrien Albert, there are related the interesting details of an experiment throwing further light on this principle. In this experiment a certain solution was applied to a culture of bacteria called *staphilococcus* and they were able to live with it. *But* when the amount of this self-same solution was reduced beyond a certain point, it acted as a poison and killed out all the bacteria. The experiment was carried out repeatedly and the results were always the same. A passing below a certain point of smallness of the quantity caused it to become a killer.

Small Amounts in Agriculture

A most astounding example of the effects of smallness was shown in an unusual series of experiments performed in 1920 at the Biologic Institute at Stuttgart, Germany, which was part of a project to develop a remedy for hoof and mouth disease. At this institute they were working by the homeopathic method to potentize a substance, that is, to make it more powerful-acting. But they attempted to do it by reducing its quantity. They were not interested in mere matter as such, but in the force that lay behind it. In other words, they said, "What do we want in reality—the substance itself, or the inner quality of that substance?"

For example, they began to reason, a farmer may feel that a certain field needs some calcium as a fertilizer. To supply this requirement he usually digs a large amount of lime into the soil. But at the Stuttgart Biologic Institute they felt differently. It was *their* opinion that it was merely the *effect* of the calcium that the soil needed and not its quantity. Their problem was to see to it that each molecule of soil and soil compounds should come in contact with *some* calcium, however small that amount might be; and not to approach it by the sledge-hammer method of putting in a huge quantity of calcium, figuring that only in that way would some calcium reach every molecule.

They studied the influence of smallest entities by using lime as the calcium-giving substance on the germination of wheat seed. They did this by a method of reducing the potency of a mixture of calcium hydroxide in water. They produced eight successive dilutions, retaining some of each dilution down to the last or eighth one which was down to one part of calcium hydroxide to a hundred million parts of water. This is a hundred times smaller in amount than that of fluorides used by the water people. The results were nothing short of fantastic!

I wish you could see the pictures of each group of wheat seedlings, going from the first on down to the eighth, showing how they were influenced by the gradually reducing amounts of calcium. With the gradually lessening quantities, the size of the wheat seedlings increased, the eighth one being by far the biggest of them all—yet having had the least amount of calcium.

This principle of the influence of smallest entities was repeated in growing hyacinths, measuring the effect of silver nitrate upon it—in growing *gladioli,* studying the effect of slaked lime upon it—on sunflower seeds and a solution of cow manure upon it, and dozens of other plants and substances that act upon them. In every case they established firmly the principle of the effect of smallness and did it so thoroughly that no scientific mind that sees the German thoroughness of these experiments, the multiplicity of its charts and photographs, can doubt their validity.

In the growth of plants there are trace mineral elements such as zinc, manganese, copper, boron, molybdenum, etc., which, for optimum plant growth conditions, should be present in "trace" quantities only. For example, in the case of zinc, only up to 1/20 of one part per million in the soil is required for healthy plant growth. Larger quantities act as a poison, and will prevent the proper germination of the seed and growth of plant. The same holds true in the human body where certain minerals must be present in "trace" quantities only. Unfortunately, less is known about the effect of the trace minerals there, because not enough research has been done on that subject by the medical profession. This subject is a sleeper, a dark horse, and may very well become the white-haired boy of medicine of the coming decades. It may hold the solution to cancer and polio.

In agriculture the trace mineral research was done (and there is a vast literature on the subject) because it is a matter of dollars and cents to the farmer. It involves economic values—a sort of industrial medical economics. But human beings are not valued at amounts in financial statements. They are not rushed off to market to be sold, so the heat is not on. The philosophy is, if we don't conquer cancer in this age, we will do it in the next one. The doctors are just about beginning to brush the edges of the subject of trace mineral elements. That is why so little is known about the effect of fluorine (a trace mineral) on the human body. But the U. S. Department of Agriculture by means of researches has found that fluoridated water is harmful to pregnant pigs, and has warned the farmer about it.

A curious example showing the disastrous effect of failure to take into consideration an element of minuteness, occurred at the London Aquarium a few years ago. A consignment of salt water fish had been brought in, but there was not enough sea water for them. It was decided therefore to make some sea water based on its known formula. The curators assembled the minerals and other compounds, and made the water, but when they placed a fish in it, it soon died. The process was repeated several times, but in each case the fish could not live in the artificially made sea water.

Then one curator at the aquarium had a bright idea. He said, "In the next batch of sea water we make, let us put in a tiny pinch of the real stuff. Perhaps it might contain a gleam of something which science has been unable to measure as yet, but which is essential to the life of a fish." And they did just that! In the next batch of sea water made, there was added the merest trace of real sea water—the slightest pinch of it—and lo and behold—miracle of miracles—the fish could live in it. It seems, therefore, that only God knows the whole formula of matter, and we are mere children playing in the complicated mazes of chemical science. But, and this is extremely significant, here is a microscopic gleam of something—a something which probably must be measured perhaps by the millionth millionth of a part, as far as fractions go, and yet that small millionth millionth of a part, or the lack of it, could mean life or death to a fish.

Dilution in Sea Water

While we are on the subject of sea water, let us consider another aspect of smallness in the life of a fish. The sea itself contains all the elements found in the human body. But, says the *Encyclopedia Britannica,* "One can look on sea water as a mixture of very dilute solutions of particular salts (or minerals), each of which after the lapse of sufficient time fills the whole space as if the other constituents did not exist." (End of quotation.)

What this means is that the total of a certain space in the sea may be filled with an unusually small amount of some minerals, but when it is so diluted that some of it fills the whole space as if the other constituents did not exist, then it truly exists in fantastically small proportions. And in such small quantity it is a tonic to the fish. But should something happen to cause some of these minerals to accumulate in one spot to an extent that makes them poisonous, it could spell death to any fish that may come into that area. That this sometimes happens is evidenced by the millions of dead fish that are occasionally found floating on the water, with no satisfactory explanation for it.

Now the blood stream of the body is a sea, and the same thing could happen there with regard to fluorine taken in through drinking water. Should some emergency condition arise which distorts the body's chemical processes, it might accumulate fluorine in some weak organ which could begin a process of disease or pathology that could begin the death process. And there are millions of people today in hospitals whose body chemistry is distorted. Dare we give them fluorine?

In review, we saw how the substance *kinetin* in a dilution of only one part in a hundred million, can cause cells to divide. This is a bad effect. On the other hand, we saw a good effect through smallness in homeopathy where their drug dilutions are as low as one part in a million billion. We saw how microscopic bacteria and viruses can kill thousands. We saw staphilococcus bacteria killed out by smaller amounts of a substance, where a larger amount permitted them to live. We reviewed the work at the Biologic Institute at Stuttgart where the smaller was the amount of calcium applied the larger grew the wheat seeds, and the London Aquarium experience where the overlooking of the need for a tiny gleam of substance caused death in fish. In other words, we have seen that smallness can be harnessed both ways—for good and for bad.

What About Fluoridation?

With all this evidence before us, we must not lull ourselves into a submissive attitude, favoring fluoridation, merely because the amount of fluorine used is only one part in a million. One cannot go by our everyday experience and attitudes with numbers and amounts. This is further illustrated by the case of the man who began to work for one cent the first day, with a doubling of the amount of pay every succeeding day, for 30 days. On the thirtieth day he was receiving a salary of over $5,000,000. Numbers and amounts are illusive things. So again we caution an antagonistic attitude towards this philosophy of there being no danger merely because the amount of fluoride used is only one part in a million parts of water. We must resist the attempt of the vested interests of medical science to browbeat an entire country into an untested, dangerous experiment where only a millionth part of a very potent poison might accomplish unforeseeable but hazardous consequences in the human body. As the old proverb goes—a small hatchet fells a great oak.

In closing may I cite a paragraph from a book called *The Failure of Technology,* written in 1939 by Dr. Frederich Georg Juenger: "We can reasonably assume, for example, that an apple contains a number of substances that so far have eluded the chemist and the biologist. It is likewise quite certain that even if all these substances *could* be synthetically reproduced in a pill, they could not replace the apple. For the apple embodies a principle that is higher than the sum of its parts. It is not a lifeless preparation, like the substances that have been, or could be extracted from it, but an expression of life that grows and smells and ripens and has fragrance."

It is the same thing with a child's teeth. They can retain their wholeness by feeding them wholeness, but it is our fragmented devitalized diet which is giving them holes. The basis for good teeth is not in fluoridation.

Fluoridation and Mottled Enamel

"To one who is familiar with the disfiguring dental defect known as mottled enamel which affects the teeth of every person who drinks water containing as little as one ppm of fluorine in the years of tooth formation this recommendation seems, to put it mildly, unsafe. There is ample evidence that mottled teeth, though they may be somewhat more resistant to the onset of decay, are structurally weak, and that unfortunately when decay does set in, the result is often disastrous.

"A survey of the mottled teeth of the inhabitants of St. David, Arizona, showed caries once started evidently spreads rapidly. Steps taken to repair the cavities in many cases were unsuccessful, the tooth breaking away when attempts were made to anchor the fillings, so that extraction was the only course. That decay was widespread is shown by an incidence of more than 50 per cent of false teeth in the age group of 24 to 26 years."

Bulletin of the University of Arizona

Fluoridation, Reaction of Fluoride In Body

Supporters of fluoridation assure us that no knowledge of harmful effects of fluoridation has come to their attention. Do they deliberately ignore material in scientific and lay journals such as the following? These are only a few of the many articles in our files.

"When sodium fluoride (the chemical used in fluoridating water) is brought into intimate contact with powdered teeth and bone, fluorine is deposited in the form of a salt progressively and phosphate is displaced also progressively. If, therefore, fluorine ions reach the bloodstream in excess of calcium ions present, the fluorine will react with bone and the result will be a serious disturbance of both calcium and phosphate metabolism. This condition is likely to be met with in many cases in natural water supplies containing fluorine, and where these conditions are fulfilled mottling of teeth and bone will be a common feature and of clinical significance.

"Sodium fluoride reacts with bone, displacing phosphate progressively while still in concentrations low enough to be completely ionized, while calcium fluoride does not react but is progressively absorbed. . . . If a water supply containing calcium ions is fluoridated with sodium fluoride, then, depending on the amount of calcium ions present, the fluorine may reach the bloodstream in balanced proportions and behave towards bone as calcium fluoride, but if there are not sufficient calcium ions present in the water to balance the amount of sodium fluoride added, then the toxic effects attributable to sodium fluoride will be present to a degree."

Charles Dillon, DDS, LDS, *The Dental Practioner*, November, 1952, Bristol, England

Fluoridation, Fluorine In Toothpaste

Biggest news in fluorine toothpaste, announced by Procter and Gamble, says *Science News Letter* for February 12, 1955, "Whether the fluoride tooth paste would provide too much fluoride for persons living in regions where the water has fluorine in it naturally or by controlled addition is a question still to be decided." It seems that the Food and Drug Administration may demand a special labelling on the toothpaste.

According to *Chemical Week,* February 12, 1955, the American Dental Association hopes that "commercial interests will not jump the gun as they have done so frequently in the past." In other words, now that we have heralded the new tooth paste with all the superlatives at our command, we are going to "hope" that commercial interests will wait patiently until exhaustive tests have been done to prove the complete safety of the toothpaste.

And sure enough, a clipping from *The Cincinnati Inquirer* for February 15, 1955, announces that the toothpaste has been put on sale there. The article, written by James T. Golden, Jr., is incredible in its naivete and gullibility. He says (and obviously he has this information straight from Procter and Gamble) "unlike fluoride in drinking water the fluoride in *Crest* (the toothpaste) acts directly on the exterior enamel of the tooth, chemically combining with it to form a barrier against acid damage and bacterial invasion . . ."

No one has the slightest idea of how fluorine acts in the body. This is one of the main reasons why conservative scientists advise so sharply against the use of fluorides. We simply do not know anything about how the body handles them! Scientists have no idea whether the fluoride in drinking water is absorbed and goes to the teeth through regular channels, or whether the contact of the teeth with the water during drinking causes the enamel to harden. Scientists who have spent their lifetime studying fluorine do not have the answers to these questions!

But a soap company (!) has now announced to the public that the fluoride in their toothpaste acts directly on the exterior enamel, forming a barrier against acid damage and bacteria! This statement is just as phoney as all the impassioned talk about "acid stomach" among the patent medicine boys, just as ridiculous as the ads for salves to grow hair on bald spots, just as evasive as saying that aspirin cures colds. Except that it is far more dangerous. For fluorine is the deadliest poison known to man, and no one knows what the symptoms of slight chronic fluorine poisoning are!

A letter to *Chemical Week* for February 26, 1955, asks, "Who knows what trouble we may get into by fluoridizing toothpaste? Fluoridized toothpaste might be satisfactory for regions where water is not treated, but what agency is going to restrict its use to them? The Salt Producers Association has turned down a movement to add fluorides to salt because of the danger of over-fluoridization and disapproval of the Federal Food and Drug Administration. (Signed) C. D. Looker, Director, Advisory Service, International Salt Co., Inc., Watkins Glen, N. Y."

Fluoridation, Toxic Possibilities and Preventive Medicine

By **W. J. McCORMICK, M.D., Toronto, Canada**

This article is reprinted in its entirety from *Archives of Pediatrics,* April, 1953, by permission of the editors. We have included Dr. McCormick's references at the end of the article purposely, for we hear so often from fluoridation advocates that those of us who oppose fluoridation do not have ample scientific evidence for our statements. Where footnotes appear, these are in all cases comments of the editors of *Prevention.*

For many years the dental condition known as "mottled teeth," or "Texas teeth," has been recognized in both mankind and in domestic animals in many parts of the American Southwest; but not until the research of Professors H. V. and Margaret Smith, biochemists of the University of Arizona, in 1930, was it discovered that fluorine in the natural waters of these regions was the culpable agent. For a decade, following this discovery, public health researchers and industrial engineers sought by physical or chemical means to devise methods for the removal of fluorine or mitigation of its toxic effects in domestic water supplies. A summary of such methods may be found in the April, 1935, number of the *American Journal of Public Health.*

Shortly before the last world war, when Hereford, a town in Deaf Smith County, Texas, was heralded as the "Town Without a Toothache," a new angle was projected into the problem. The unusually good condition of the teeth of children in this locality was studied by dentists and public health workers, and the assumption that the natural fluorine content of the local water supply was the beneficient agent was quickly made. It was noted that even in the cases where the teeth were mottled, the incidence of decay was apparently minimized. In seeking the cause of this anomaly little attention was given to the possible favorable effects of sunlight in producing natural vitamin D, or to the possible superior mineral content of the foods grown in that region, or to the fact that these same regions were prolific in production of citrus fruit with its high content of vitamin C, although all these factors may have contributed.

Such an alternative explanation is supported by the work of Dr. R. S. Harris, Director of the Nutritional Biochemistry Laboratories of the Massachusetts Institute of Technology. He fed two groups of hamsters milk and corn from Texas and New England. The animals receiving the Texas food developed only half as much tooth decay as those fed the New England food, although the amount of fluorine in the Texas food was so little different from that of the New England food that it could not appreciably affect the result of the experiment. Dr. Harris also found that riboflavin, a non-toxic B-vitamin nutrient, was almost as effective as fluorine in preventing caries.

Further evidence of the role of nutrition in dental health is provided by the work of Dr. M. T. Hanke and an associate group of physicians and dentists, who, in 1933, conducted an unusual experiment in the town of Mooseheart, Indiana. In this community, privately owned by the Order of the Moose, some 1300 orphans were housed and cared for by a competent staff of teachers, dieticians, recreational directors, etc. For the purpose of the experiment some 200 of these children were given a daily dietary supplement of twenty ounces of orange juice, while the remainder, who were fed otherwise in the same manner on a good average diet, were used as controls. The experiment was continued for three years, during which time the dental and general health status of all the children was carefully charted. It was found that the group receiving the extra-citrus-fruit supplement had a very much lower incidence of new dental cavities and a marked freedom from gingivitis and pyorrhea, as well as a greatly lowered incidence of colds and acute infectious disease, as compared to the control group. It was thus shown that malnutrition, with special emphasis on vitamin C deficiency, provides the background for bad dental health and the usual infectious diseases of childhood. On this basis dental caries should not be considered a separate disease entity, but rather as an index of nutritional status and constitutional resistance to infectious disease.

The precipitous conclusion regarding the relation of fluorine to dental health has quickly led to agitation for mass application of artificial sodium fluoride to domestic water supplies in an effort to duplicate the supposed favorable effect of the fluorine found in natural waters, and already some twenty million freedom-loving Americans are compelled to partake of this medicated beverage irrespective of its possible long-term deleterious effects.

History and Chemistry of Fluorine

The historical background of fluorine may provide related interest. Fluorine was discovered by Scheele in 1771, but because of its intense affinities for so many other elements, it was not produced in gaseous elemental purity until 1886 by Moissan. Because of its most active affinity it has been regarded as the wildcat or villain of the chemical world, being also the most poisonous. The inhalation of the pure gas is invariably lethal. The soluble forms, as in sodium fluoride,* are extremely poisonous, being used commercially for rat and roach extermination. The non-soluble forms, as in calcium fluoride, are much less toxic. Sodium fluoride is the form proposed for general use in domestic water supplies. It is an artificial chemical, specially prepared from mineral fluor spar for use in the production of aluminum. Otherwise heretofore it has been a well-nigh useless product, having limited commercial use because of its extreme toxicity. Among its few industrial uses are the following: vermin extermination, laundry bleach, rubber coagulant, fixer in dye works, flux in metallurgy, glass etching, optical grinding paste, glue manufacture, emery wheel binder and concrete hardener. Its value in the last two items

*This is the form used to fluoridate water, whereas calcium fluoride appears in bone meal.

is due to its strong affinity for calcium—the same property which makes it unite with the calcium of teeth and bones.

The geographical source of fluorine is related to volcanic activity. For this reason it is found in highest concentration in the southwestern mountainous regions of New Mexico and Arizona. There are many extinct volcanoes in these parts. The spread of fluorine eastward extends only as far as the Alleghenies. The continued ingestion of vegetable and animal food from these areas has resulted in the cumulative deposition of this element in the bones and teeth of man and animals in combination with the calcium of these structures. For this reason fluorine should not be considered a biological requisite. The bones of cattle on the western prairies have been found to be so hard and stony from high fluorine content that the U. S. Department of Agriculture has forbidden the use of such bones in the production of bone meal for human consumption except from animals under 2½ years of age.* Dr. E. V. McCollum, the great nutritionist, says fluorine serves no useful purpose in the animal organism.

Possible Harmful Effects of Fluoridated Water

It is the strong affinity of fluorine for calcium which results in its deposition in dental and osseous tissues, and which, when present below a certain critical level, builds into the calcifying dental enamel in increased density and hardness which gives apparent resistance to dental decay. This is essentially a chemical reaction, analogous to the industrial use of fluorine in the hardening of cement and concrete. It is nevertheless a pathogenic process, as is also the deposition of calculus (tartar) on the teeth, which also is known to give a certain degree of immunity to caries, while at the same time it is conducive to periodontal disease—gingivitis and pyorrhea. Fluorine likewise may be concurrently conducive to periodontal disease. Dr. H. K. Box, a periodontist of international repute, on the Dental Faculty of the University of Toronto informs the writer that he has checked the dental status of a number of subjects who have been using naturally fluoridated water for several decades and has found appalling periodontal (gum) disease, with marked morphological changes (changes in structure) such as enlargement of the roots and narrowing or closure of root canals and pulp chambers, indicating premature aging of the tooth structure, making extraction very difficult and prone to root fracture. Many of these cases had severe gingivitis and pyorrhea and premature need for dentures.

When the long continued ingestion of a foreign substance (fluorine) results in such marked local changes in the teeth, it is only logical to assume the possibility of remote systemic effects. Such findings have been reported by a group of Danish researchers among workers in cryolite mining who were inhaling fluorine in dust. Not only did these subjects exhibit the above-mentioned dental defects (thickened roots and nar-

*We wish to point out that all bone meal used for human consumption must contain only a given amount of fluorine, so there is no chance of your getting too much fluorine from bone meal. As you will see, later on in this article Dr. McCormick recommends the use of bone meal to counteract the possible harmful effects of fluoridated water

rowed pulp chambers), but supercalcification was also manifested in osteophyte (bony outgrowth) formations on bones, osteosclerosis, calcification of tendons, "poker backs" and fixation of thoracic wall. These same effects have been noted also in parts of Africa and India where the natives have long been using naturally fluoridated water. Associated malnutrition seemed to accentuate the defects.

In England, in 1948, bone defects in three groups of school boys were studied. Two groups were from districts where the water supply was practically free from fluorine. The third group was from the town of Launton, where the natural water supply contains one part per million of fluorine. X-ray examination revealed that 20 per cent of the first two groups had mild nonspecific spinal irregularities. In the third group, 64 per cent were found to have spinal defects and lesions were more severe.

Brandl and Tappeiner fed very small amounts of sodium fluoride to young growing dogs for 21 months and examined their bones microscopically. Deposited in the bones were found vivid crystals of calcium fluoride. They believed that soluble fluorine salts combine with the calcium of the bones, causing increased brittleness. The bones of fluorine-fed animals are always chalky and fragile as are the teeth.

Recently, in Switzerland, cattle grazing in the vicinity of aluminum smelters were found to be suffering from a fatal disease which veterinarians diagnosed as fluorosis, a form of osteomalacia producing spontaneous fracturing of bones. The cattle had acquired the disease from eating the grass upon which were deposited fluorine emanations from the aluminum plant.

More recently (1952), Udall and Keller have reported an outbreak of fluorosis in cattle on farms about five miles distant from an aluminum plant near Vancouver, Washington. The animals were subjected to increased intake of fluorine from the fumes of smoke stacks. In rainy or foggy weather the toxic effects were greatly increased, due to moisture taking up the fluorine and depositing same on the cattle fodder. The younger animals seemed to be affected mostly in stunted growth and marked disturbances in reproduction, lactation and alimentation. The leg joints were noticeably enlarged, inhibiting locomotion. The hooves were soft and spreading, with grotesque distortions. The teeth were increasingly blackened. These lesions were obviously due to extreme depletion of calcium, the latter being taken up from the food in the alimentary tract to form the insoluble calcium fluoride, thus preventing assimilation. The alimentary and reproductive disturbances were related to the toxic action of the fluorine. A surplus of calcium in the diet apparently compensates for the fluorine-calcium loss and to some extent saves bone deficiencies, but it has little effect in retarding tooth damage, owing perhaps to the more direct exposure of the teeth to the fluorine intake in addition to the internal systemic effect. This may explain why children of low-income families, with minimal milk intake, are found to be more sensitive to fluorine.

Reaction of Human Body to Fluorine

The Smiths, of Arizona, previously referred to as co-discoverers of fluorine as a cause of dental mottling, report studies in the naturally fluoridated areas indicating that while the incidence of caries was low in young children the degree of decay increased sharply after 21 years of age (or after 21 years exposure to fluorine), and furthermore that the decay and weakening of tooth structure was so severe that repair was more difficult, resulting in a high percentage of extractions. Even in communities where the fluorine content of water is only one part to 1,000,000, they report fluorosis (mottling) in 10 to 12 per cent of the inhabitants.

Regarding the effect of fluoride on body enzymes: Sodium fluoride is known to be particularly harmful to the action of lipase (a fat-splitting enzyme) in fat metabolism. Solutions with a fluorine content as low as one part in 15,000,000 may inhibit the activity of lipase as much as 50 per cent. The enzymatic breakdown of carbohydrates is also very sensitive to fluorine. It has been found that the normal catabolic transition to lactic acid and pyruvic acid is greatly disturbed, thus nullifying to some extent the catalytic action of thiamine.

Regarding the effect of fluorine on blood coagulation: Stuber and Lang report a high blood level of fluorine in a number of cases of hemophilia (delayed clotting of blood). There seemed to be a direct correlation between the blood-fluorine level and the prolongation of the blood coagulation time. Knowing that goose blood and rabbit blood clot slowly, they found on investigation a high blood-fluorine content in these animals. Cat and dog blood, which is known to clot rapidly, was found to be free from fluorine. (This last finding may be due to the fact that carnivorous animals eat bones, the calcium of which would take up the fluorine in the alimentary tract and prevent absorption—W.J.M.) Continuing their observations they found that human subjects, using drinking water with varying content of natural fluorine, had a blood coagulation time 6 to 20 times that of subjects using fluorine-free water.

Smith and Leverton report studies regarding the relative toxicity of various fluorides in the experimental feeding of rats. They found, for instance, that sodium fluoride is 85 times more toxic than calcium fluoride, as determined by lethal dosage. The obvious reason for this disparity is the fact that sodium fluoride is very-soluble, whereas calcium fluoride is practically insoluble. (Sodium fluoride is the form used in artificial fluoridation, while calcium fluoride is found in natural waters.)

Carnot, a French scientist, who studied the fluorine content of bones, was the first to suggest a method for removing fluorine from drinking water (1893) by treating it with pulverized bone or bone ash. By this means the fluorine was taken up by the calcium of bones outside the body before it could gain access to the bones within the body.

From the foregoing it must be evident that domestic water fluoridation at best is a poor substitute for better nutrition. When major dependence is placed on such measures, public interest in food reform and oral hygiene is sure to suffer.

In conclusion I wish to offer suggestions, based on laboratory experiments, for protection against the toxic effects of fluorine for those who find themselves unwilling subjects of this latest experiment in mass medication.

1. The daily ingestion of small doses (5 to 10 grains) of certain innocuous salts of calcium, notably calcium lactate, citrate, gluconate or

ascorbate, which should provide a surplus of calcium for reaction with the sodium fluoride of the drinking water, thereby producing an insoluble precipitate (calcium fluoride) which is then mostly eliminated without absorption from the alimentary tract. Calcium ascorbate is particularly valuable in this respect, since it at the same time releases vitamin C, the antitoxic action of which should help to counteract the toxic effect of that portion of the sodium fluoride which may be absorbed. Vitamin C has been used successfully as an antidote in lead poisoning, also for rattlesnake and scorpion venom, and it should be equally effective in counteracting rat poison.

2. An optimal intake of foods rich in calcium is desirable, such as milk products and green salad vegetables. A surplus of these in the diet provides the calcium necessary for neutralizing the fluoride as previously explained. Bone meal, as a dietary supplement should have similar effect.

3. Last, but not least, make sure of an optimal intake of citrus fruits to provide the natural vitamin C to help counteract the toxic fluoride.*

Summary

The literature regarding fluorosis in men and animals is reviewed, with special reference to dental and systemic effects.

The writer admits the apparent immunity to dental caries conferred in young children by either topical application or ingestion of fluorine in dilution of one part or less per million, but regards the local dental reaction as a pathogenic (disease) process analogous to the deposition of calculus (tartar), resulting in severe periodontal disease in later life, as well as possible deleterious systemic effects.

Suggestions regarding prophylactic medicinal and dietary measures to counter the toxic effect of fluorine in drinking water are offered for those who find themselves unwilling subjects of experimentation.

References

1. Smith, H. V. and Smith. M. C.; *Arizona Experimental Station Tech. Bull. No.* 43, 1932.
2. Hanke, M. T., et al; *Nutrition and Dental Health,* Chicago University Press. 1933.
3. Box, H. K.; Dental Faculty, University of Toronto, personal communication, Feb., 1953.
4. Brandl, J. and Tappeiner; *H. Ztschr. f. Biol.,* 28:518, 1891.
5. Udall, D. H. and Keller, K. P.; *Report on Fluorosis in Cattle in the Columbia River Valley,* Cornell, Vet., Vol. XLII, April, 1952.
6. Stuber, B. and Lang, K.; *Fluorine in Relation to Blood Coagulation,* Biochem. Ztschr., 212:96, 1929.
7. Smith, M. C. and Leverton, R. M.; *Comparative Toxicity of Fluorine Compounds,* Indust. & Engin. Chem., 7:791, 1934.
8. Carnot, A.; *Recherches sur la composition generale et la teneur en fluor des os modernes et des os fossiles des differents ages,* Ann. Mines, 9:155, 1893.

*We advise the use of rose hips for their high vitamin C content, especially for those who find citrus fruits difficult to take.

Fluoridation, Review of a Medical Article

It is reported that there are some 5,000 medical and scientific articles bearing more or less directly on the subject of fluoridation. It is claimed that, without exception, they support the thesis that addition of fluorides to community water is safe and will reduce tooth decay by about 65 per cent. Few things are that simple. So says F. B. Exner, M.D. of Seattle, Washington, in a series of three articles which appeared in *Northwest Medicine* for 1955. Dr. Exner's approach is so convincing, his arguments so sound, his integrity so unimpeachable, that we have decided to condense these three articles for *Health Finder* readers. Incidentally the original articles are available in reprint form from Dr. Exner, Medical and Dental Bldg., Seattle 1, Washington. We will in time cover more of what Dr. Exner says in the articles in *Northwest Medicine.*

Is the public water supply a suitable medium for fluoridation? Of course not, says Dr. Exner. Chlorine is added to many water supplies to purify the water. Fluorides are added for the express purpose of acting on the bodies of consumers and altering their structure and function. Thus, fluorides are a drug given indiscriminately to everyone in the community. Fluorides do not produce their effect by contact with the teeth. They must be swallowed, absorbed into the blood and taken to the teeth, while the teeth are in the process of calcifying and before they erupt into the mouth.

The cells which make use of the fluorides have no way of knowing, of course, how much water was mixed with the fluorine; they are influenced only by the concentration of the fluorides in the blood. This depends on the amount of fluoride absorbed, *not on the amount in the water drunk.* Now it is perfectly obvious that an individual who drinks ten glasses a day of water which contains 1 part per million of fluoride is getting just as much fluorides as if he drank one glass of water containing 10 parts per million of fluoride.

No one knows how much water any individual is going to drink and it is certainly true that one person may drink ten times as much as another. So how can the United States Public Health Service advocate one part or one and a half parts per million of fluorides in drinking water as the proper amount for all of us? Will it indeed give the "correct dosage" of fluorine? They tell us it will. For whom? The person who drinks one glass of water a day? Or the one who drinks ten or more? For the person who drinks many cups of coffee or tea made from fluoridated water, eats soups in which the fluorides have been concentrated by long boiling, and vegetables which have taken up fluorides while they were cooking? Or the one who drinks only milk and eats canned or frozen foods in which the fluorides of his water supply do not enter? Questions like these show the complete idiocy of declaring that one part per million of fluorides in drinking water will provide the "right" dose for all children.

Says Dr. Exner, "When fluoride is put in the drinking water, no child gets the right dose of fluoride (whatever that may be) except the child who happens to drink the *right* amount of water. All others get more or less than intended and often far more or far less." This is one reason why the Public Health Service fully expects from 15 to 20 per cent of children in such areas to have teeth permanently disfigured by fluorides —indicating an overdosage, while others—those who got too little fluorides —will show no benefit at all in reduced decay.

What other hazards accompany water fluoridation? When fluorides are prescribed as drugs, a pure, drug-grade fluoride is used. The commercial grade (clearly marked "For Industrial Use Only") is used for water fluoridation. Fluoride is a cumulative poison. Some of its effects may not be known for as long as twenty years. So, even though certain results are attained in the mouths of children drinking fluoridated water during the period from birth to eight years of age, we cannot possibly predict what dangerous symptoms may begin to show up years from now in these same children.

And what of adults who are unusually susceptible to damage from the fluorides? We mean those who drink excessive amounts of water— diabetics, for instance, or those who work under hot, dry conditions; those with defective kidney function; allergic persons; undernourished and malnourished persons and especially those who do not get enough calcium in their food, for fluoride attaches itself to calcium in the body and inactivates it. What about those who are exposed to fluorides in industries in which they work, and those who live near industrial plants that pollute the air for miles around with fluorides? Many lawsuits have been won in this country by individuals who have suffered damage from such pollution—even without any additional fluorides in their water supply!

The downright foolishness of fluoridating an entire water supply becomes immediately apparent when we remember that of each ten thousand dollars used for fluoridation, some $9,975 goes for things other than drinking. Then, too, plumbing and whole city water departments may suffer continual damage from the fluoride crusts in the pipes. Morristown, New Jersey, attempting to distribute 1.2 parts per million of fluorides after four years of fluoridation, found that water from different taps might contain anywhere from zero, .26 p.p.m., .39 p.p.m., .41 p.p.m, or .05 p.p.m. In Bauxite, Arkansas, three years after switching from water with a high fluoride content to a fluoride-free system, there was still enough fluoride in the water system to cause mottled tooth enamel in some who drank the water. This was supposedly because of the incrusted fluorides in the pipes!

Is Water Fluoridation Morally Justifiable?

"No," says Dr. Exner. In scientific circles it is always up to the group which wants to add a poison, to prove that the poison is not harmful, rather than for those opposing it to prove that it is harmful. Where are the proofs in this case? The Public Health Service fully expects fifteen to twenty per cent of the children who drink fluoridated water to get mottled teeth. Does this indicate the harmlessness of fluorides?

When the fluoridation experiments were started at Newburgh, New York and elsewhere, the amount of fluorides added to the water supply exceeded the allowable limit for a public water supply as set forth at that time by Federal law. Also, of course, such experimentation on human beings without their consent is quite illegal and indefensible. But even if fluoridation could be proved to be absolutely safe for every individual (which of course it never could be) even then, adding fluorides to the drinking water is unconstitutional, for it violates the basic right guaranteed by the constitution—the right to determine what shall be done to one's own body.

There are other ways of getting fluorides, if one wants to take them. A gallon of water in which the proper amount of (drug-grade) fluoride has been mixed by a druggist would cost about two cents and would last for about two years.

Dr. Exner next takes up and dissects some of the 7,000 articles which prove supposedly that fluoridated water is safe to drink. We cannot go into all of the detail with which he demolishes the arguments of the profluoridators based on the experiments by McClure, of the National Institute of Dental Research, which are the "classic" experiments upon which the whole idea of water fluoridation is based. His analysis of McClure's work is brilliant. For instance, in regard to the amount of water that any of us might drink in a day, he quotes McClure as saying that a reasonable estimate seems to be about 2.5 to 3.4 pints daily. Yet in McClure's own published experiments, he describes one case in which the young men he was working with, who kept strict account of their water intake, drank from 3.5 to 16.2 pints of water in a day! The higher figures were in a hot, moist environment, without any activity. Had the air been dry or had the young men been active they would probably have drunk even more than that.

Dr. Exner quotes another experiment of McClure's in which he used water from Galesburg, Illinois (with 1.8 p.p.m. of fluoride) to prove his point. "But when his subjects drank as much Galesburg water as they wanted, it spoiled his experiment and failed to prove what he wanted to prove." The boys began to drink enormous quantities of water because the weather was hot, so he restricted them to only a certain amount of Galesburg water every day; the rest of the time they had to drink Urbana water with a fluoride content of .3 p.p.m. This is the kind of double-cross that went on in scientific (!) experiments which we are asked to believe prove beyond a shadow of a doubt that water fluoridation cannot possibly be harmful.

In addition, a recent experiment done at the University of California for the Atomic Energy Commission has proved almost exactly the opposite of what McClure supposedly proved by his experiments. Using radio-active fluoride which could be traced in its course through the body, this investigator, Dr. Wallace-Durbin found that no matter how little fluorine was ingested, some of it was always stored in the body. In no instance was it all rapidly excreted, as McClure claimed.

Where Is the Proof That Fluoridation Is Harmless?

For those of us who are not experts in medical terminology and scientific procedures, what Dr. Exner says about the McClure experiments may seem complex and much too difficult to explain to a city editor or a group of pro-fluoridationists. Briefly, the important thing which Dr. Exner points out is that the experiments which all the professional organizations endorsing fluoridation point to as solemn proof that fluoridation is safe do not prove that at all, and are in fact open to devastating criticisms of their scientific validity. McClure is *the* expert, called in by all the other experts, to repeat over and over again his so-called evidence of the harmlessness of fluoridation. His evidence does not prove its harmlessness, says Dr. Exner.

He goes on to say that the reason he spent so much time on McClure's work is that "there are quite reliable reports, over a period of more than 40 years and from all over the world, of serious, cumulative, chronic fluoride poisoning, especially of the teeth and skeletal structures. All these are lightly brushed aside as having no applicability where there is only one part per million of fluoride in the water."

Dr. Exner then takes apart with consummate skill the oft-quoted pronouncements of Dr. John W. Knutson of the Public Health Service, who ridicules the possibility of fluorides causing "any number of dire ailments ranging from cancer and nephritis to discolored teeth." That quote indicates the degree of concern with which Dr. Knutson admits that fluorides in the water can cause certain ailments, but where they do occur it is always in communities where the water contains at least 12 or 15 times the quantity recommended for fluoridation. He gives references to six other scientific articles to prove this point. "You would reasonably expect that they would support it," says Dr. Exner, "you would be wrong." in one of the articles which Dr. Knutson uses to prove that no harm can come from water fluoridation, serious chronic poisoning was found in 12 per cent of the adults where the water contained only 1.2 parts per million of fluoride! At present, the Public Health Service is recommending up to 1.5 parts per million for drinking water in this country!

In the second part of his treatise, Dr. Exner discusses mottled enamel, describing the complete confusion that exists about this dental defect in the statements of the pro-fluoridators. Mottled enamel has been known for many years. Less than fifty years ago water supplies were being abandoned and new ones found in areas where the natural fluorine in the water caused mottled enamel. "In the light of present knowledge, however, even the slightest mottling must be considered a sign of probable damage elsewhere," says Dr. Exner. He goes on to analyze the findings of the fluoridationists themselves, turning their very words and statistics against them, for what the actual facts and figures show is that tooth mottling is in truth a very serious result of drinking fluoridated water and it must be expected that large numbers of children who drink this water will suffer from this dental defect. The Public Health Service declares that not more than ten per cent of all children will suffer from mottling

—and that mottling not severe enough to matter at all. Exner proves, using their own statistics, that the reverse is true.

Says he, "McKay forgot to tell APHA that in every place he investigated in Colorado, where there was as much as 1 p.p.m. of fluoride, from 85 to 100 per cent of the children had mottled teeth. He did not mention that wherever there was as much as .2 p.p.m., more than 15 per cent of the children had mottling. Neither did he say that he and John Frisch found 91 per cent of children to have mottled teeth at Salida, where the fluoride content was reported to be the same as Joliet, Illinois where only 25 per cent mottling is reported."

Furthermore, Dr. Exner uses a report of the Public Health Service on two Texas cities, Bartlett and Cameron, to show that, among other things, 40 per cent of the people in Bartlett (the fluoride city) had lost *all* their teeth, whereas only 20 per cent had done so in Cameron (the non-fluoride city). "At the end of the study period, 47 per cent of the tooth loss in Bartlett and 25 per cent in Cameron was attributed by the individuals themselves to periodontal disease"—that is, disease of the gums. "It is interesting that, having thus used periodontal disease to explain away the differences in tooth loss, the authors (of the report) tell us in their conclusions that there was no more periodontal disease in Bartlett than in Cameron . . . We are now told that the Bartlett-Cameron studies have disproved the absurd charges that waterborne fluoride causes periodontal disease!"

The Effect of Fluorine on Calcium is Important

Dr. Exner goes on to describe the great importance of calcium in the diet of those who drink fluoridated water. Dillon, in England, showed that in a laboratory test tube sodium fluoride reacts with powdered bone displacing phosphorus in the bone. Sodium fluoride is the substance used for fluoridating water. Calcium fluoride, on the other hand, is the form in which fluorine exists in food, in bone meal, in vegetables and so forth. Calcium fluoride is merely absorbed by tooth and bone and the effect is reversible, for the calcium can be absorbed or released depending on the amount of calcium fluoride in the solution.

A number of experiments have shown that fluoridated water is better tolerated by those whose diets are good, especially so far as calcium is concerned and is far more destructive to those whose diets are deficient in calcium. We know full well—for every good nutrition book written in the last fifty years points it out with alarm—that deficiency in calcium is one of our major problems.

This, then, is the answer—or one answer—to the statement often made by the pro-fluoridators that artificially fluoridated water is exactly the same thing as naturally fluoridated water. The calcium existing along with the fluorine in the water or the calcium in the diets of the local residents may make all the difference in the world as to exactly how toxic fluoridated water will be!

"This difference is highly significant," says Dr. Exner. "Joliet, Illinois, was said to have 11 times as much calcium, and half as much fluorine, in its water as Colorado Springs. We have every reason to believe that the eleven-fold difference in calcium has far more influence than the two-fold difference in fluorine in producing the dramatic difference in the incidence and severity of mottling which is reported in the two places."

What effect does fluoridation actually have on tooth decay, asks Dr. Exner. His answer could well be *your* answer to the next Public Health orator who tries to sell fluoridation to your city on the basis of the tests just concluded at Newburgh and Kingston, N. Y. This orator will tell you that tooth decay was reduced by about 60 per cent in Newburgh, which was fluoridated.

"When we come to the subject of fluorine and tooth decay, we enter Never-Never Land, with no reliable landmarks," says Dr. Exner. "It seems fairly clear that decay behaves differently and has different consequences in fluorosed than in non-fluorosed teeth. Beyond that, all bets are off." How is the rate of decay determined in such tests? By recording what is called the DMF rate—that is, the number of teeth that are decayed, missing or filled.

In this total, says Dr. Exner, the tiniest cavity counts the same as a tooth completely destroyed and a cavity filled 50 years ago counts the same as active disease. It is just as silly and pointless as when children count their coins without regard to denomination, to see who has the most money. The problem "when is decay" is not important in daily life. If the dentist can't tell whether you have a cavity, you can wait and see. If, however, you must decide right now for statistical purposes whether someone does or does not have tooth decay, the margin of error is unbelievable, he tells us.

What About the Newburgh "Test"?

This aspect of the matter is most beautifully illustrated in the recent release of a document by the Board of Education Health Department of New York State, showing that the Newburgh children had about 45 per cent more "dental defects" than the Kingston children. When an explanation was demanded of these figures, everyone was hastily assured that the difference came about because of differences in methods of examination! Besides, the authorities said, this included *all* dental defects, not just decay! So, according to this very explanation, the Newburgh children are in far, far worse shape than the Kingston children for, even subtracting their 60 per cent less tooth decay, they still have about 45 per cent *more dental defects* than the Kingston children! And once you have accepted the fluoridators' explanation that a difference in the examining method caused this tremendous difference in statistics, then you are forced to the conclusion that such examinations are completely meaningless and can easily be tailored to fit the examiner's preconceived idea of what he wanted to find.

We have a copy of *The Newburgh News* for December 14, 1955—2 days after the triumphant announcement of the successful test was made. Here are some quotes:

"Despite the reports favoring fluoridation as a means to cut tooth decay in children, there was nevertheless at least a definite undercurrent of lukewarm or even unfavorable comment among three of the dentists questioned.

"One prominent member of the Newburgh Dental Society dismissed the effects of fluoridation with this comment: 'What little effect it might have had was not apparent.' He suggested that 'those fellows' who had participated in the study were 'biased and they set out to prove what they wanted to find.'

"He offered from his own personal experience that one of his five children had been born when the study was just underway. Presumably this eight-year-old boy had been exposed to a lifetime of fluoridated water.

" 'Yet he has the worst decay of all my five kids," said the dentist. Another dentist is quoted as saying "I'm still seeing a lot of children with decay . . . and the amazing thing is the number of children in the ages of 2 to 3 years who have nothing but shells left when they come in." "At least one dentist" said he could see a distinct difference in the rate of decay, according to the *News*. *One dentist could notice a difference!*

And what about Kingston—the unfluoridated city in the test? Shouldn't they be crying, screaming, protesting so that *they* might have the benefits of fluoridation, too? Dr. Dudley Hargrave, health officer in Kingston, says, according to *The News,* that there has not been much expression among the Kingston people generally about fluoridation. And what he has heard has been generally in opposition.

Peculiar, isn't it?

Whether or not fluoridation is a burning question in your locality, we think you should send for a copy of Dr. Exner's articles as they appeared in *Northwest Medicine,* a fully accredited and conservative medical journal. You will receive quite a thick booklet which will give you just about all the answers you need on water fluoridation, stated clearly, understandably and forcefully. Send one dollar to Dr. Frederick Exner, Dental and Medical Bldg., Seattle 1, Washington.

And incidentally, here are some other sources of excellent material:
National Fluoridation News, 2920 W. Grand Boulevard, Detroit, Mich.
N. J. Dental Research Association, 250 Broadway, Passaic, N. J.
Mrs. Aileen Robinson, 5217 E. 43rd St., Seattle, Wash.
Harper's Magazine (February 1953 issue), 49 E. 33rd St., New York, N. Y.
Citizens Committee on Fluoridation, 1311 G St., N.W., Room 210, Washington 5, D. C.
Rodale Press, Emmaus, Penna.
(Booklet—Facts About Water Fluoridation—50¢)

Dr. Exner, in his final article goes into some of the motives that are behind water fluoridation. First he mentions the prospect of direct profit from the sale of chemicals and equipment. This does not mean just fluorides. The fates of aluminum cooking utensils and phosphate fertilizer (two most profitable businesses) are also involved. Both these contain fluorine. To lay once and for all the very active ghost of the dangers of aluminum cooking utensils it was necessary to show that fluorine is not only harmless but positively desirable. The terrible pollution of air and water in the vicinity of aluminum plants has already cost millions in damages. The fluorides washed down by the rain from the fertilized fields and the polluted air, eventually make their way into drinking water. How pleasant for all the commercial interests concerned to prove that fluorides are as necessary as calcium or potassium to human welfare!

Dr. Exner then proceeds to dissect argument after argument of the fluoridation "experts" with a careful and objective scalpel. He takes up in detail the careers of several of the first-rank promoters and shows how one thing leads to another once the basic premise of the correctness of fluoridation has been firmly established.

Perhaps most valuable to readers will be his section on "weasel words." For instance, the Surgeon General of the United States, at the time when the fluoridation promotion was just getting started, said, "scientific evidence indicates overwhelmingly the safety to the population." Exner goes on to explain, "He will, of course, be quoted as saying fluoridation is 'safe' but if he is challenged he can say 'I did not say it was safe for any individual. I merely said it is safe for the population!' As we have seen that merely means that he does not expect more than about 20 per cent of the people to be injured," says Exner.

Weasel words must be watched for, recognized and nailed down for what they are. They are used to confuse and to convince the unthinking. But perhaps even more dangerous is the new concept of public health, of which fluoridation appears to be the opening wedge. Says Dr. Exner, "Except as pertaining to troops, the idea that government may sacrifice individuals to the public good is something new in American political philosophy." In this case, 21-57 per cent of the population is destined to get "questionable" or "definite" mottling of the teeth, (according to the plans of the fluoridators) with the associated chronic poisoning (about which we know little) so that 20 per cent of the population can be "protected" from dental decay up to the age of 14. That is what the situation boils down to.

The Legality of Fluoridation

Under our constitution every American has the right to decide for himself what is to be done to his own body. Public health departments have the power to protect us from conditions that might endanger our health (such as germs in the water supply that might cause epidemics). But the idea that they also have the right to promote our health by doing things to us without our consent is a new and different idea. We agree with Dr. Exner that such a suggestion is of course completely unconstitutional. And it is the opening wedge for a long series of "treatments by drinking water."

"In this grandiose new concept of public health, there is only one major obstacle. We shrink from compulsory medication even in communicable disease, while for non-contagious disease it has been considered unthinkable. That is where fluoridation comes in. It is to serve as the first legal precedent for compulsory medication in non-communicable disease. That is its sole purpose, and so far it has done all right," says Dr. Exner. He then quotes F. J. Maier of the Public Health Service who wrote in 1950 that water fluoridation has "led to the concept that the treatment of drinking water might include addition of specific substances to prevent disease."

So all the local writers of "letters to the editor" who suggested with heavy sarcasm that the city government dose the water with aspirin (lots of folks have headaches) and digitalis (for all the heart patients) and cascara (for everybody that was constipated) never realized how little they had to be sarcastic about! *That is actually what the public health service seems to have in mind!* And what a field day for the drug companies when *that* day comes! For of course only the tiniest fraction of the water supply is used for drinking. But all of it will be treated!

Dr. Exner goes on, in the rest of his very concise and thoughtful article, to discuss science by edict whereby the Salk vaccine is "declared safe" as of ten o'clock one morning, water fluoridation is "declared safe" as of April 24, 1951, and so forth. He reminds us that, even in the case of polio, a supposedly contagious disease, there is as yet no compulsory vaccination. Why then should everyone be forced to drink fluoridated water for preventing a disease that is certainly not contagious?

Gall Bladder

One adult in every five may eventually have gallstones. At least half of the women living into their sixties will have them. And any woman has eight times as much chance as a man to hear a surgeon say "Better take it out." For operations seem to be the prized answer of medical science to problems of the gall bladder.

This tendency is apparent in medical books and journals. Descriptions of gall bladder trouble are lengthy, talk about operations and possible complications of surgery is ever-present. But when you look under "Gall Bladder Disease, Therapy" you find only a few half-hearted suggestions on diet, on which there is considerable disagreement, and nothing much else.

Tucked under the right lobe of the liver, the gall bladder is, we think, quite an important organ, although one of the authorities we consulted referred to it as a "side pocket" for which the body has no use, like an appendix. This hardly seems reasonable to us since all of us come equipped with such a gadget and since it has a definite function to perform which is certainly done much less effectively should the gall bladder be removed. The gall bladder stores bile, a substance manufactured by the liver to help digestion. The liver makes bile all the time, but it is needed only when there is some fat in the intestine to be digested, so the reserve stocks of bile are sent to the gall bladder which concentrates them and keeps them until they are needed.

Bile does not actually digest fat. But it encourages the digestive action of pancreatic juice, stimulates intestinal action and aids in emulsifying fat so that it can be used by the body. How, then, do all the folks whose gall bladders have been removed get along? The bile ducts or tubes that lead from the liver to the gall bladder and then into the intestine enlarge so that more bile can flow through them, and some of this is apparently stored there. But, of course, this is not as efficient a system as the original one. So naturally it is best to keep your gall bladder if at all possible, and to keep it in the best possible health.

Cholecystitis (from *chole,* the Greek for bladder) is the word meaning inflammation of the gall bladder. Formerly it was thought that this condition resulted from "germs" in the gall bladder. At present this theory is out of date. But inflammation of the gall bladder can be and is dangerous and painful. With or without gallstones.

Cholelithiasis is the medical name for gallstones. What causes them? Many possible causes have been mentioned down through the years. There seems to be no doubt, however, that the formation of gallstones is intimately related to diet. Those who have trouble with their gall bladders are usually overweight. This means, of course, that they overeat. Or at any rate, that they eat more than they should of certain foods. Usually, too, they are over forty, although recently more and more cases of gall bladder trouble are occurring in younger people.

The flow of bile may be obstructed in cases of overweight people and pregnant women, where the actual weight of the fleshy tissue stops off the flow of bile in the little ducts. This causes it to back up into the gall bladder, and trouble ensues. Then, too, it seems that gallstones may be caused by what is called "disturbed metabolism" of cholesterol. Cholesterol is a fatty substance that exists in fatty foods of animal origin —eggs, butter, fat meat and so forth. Most gallstones contain cholesterol and it seems obvious that the stones would not have formed in the first place had not something gone wrong with the way the body is supposed to use cholesterol. Apparently the amount of cholesterol in the diet has little to do with the formation of stones. Yet the favorite diet given to gall bladder patients for relieving gallstones is a cholesterol-free one.

An article in *Today's Health* for March, 1956, explains the formation of gallstones like this: "The materials which go to produce gallstones are made when your body burns fat. The way your body burns fat depends on your glands. The amount of fat it has to burn depends on your diet. If anything is wrong with either, gallstones are much more likely."

Risk Appraisal, a book for the insurance companies and their doctors, has this to say, "Coronary disease affects many individuals with gall bladder disease." The author, Harry Dingman, thinks this may be because the individual with heart trouble becomes sedentary and often fat and this makes it more likely that his gall bladder ducts would become sluggish and stones would result.

True. And we constantly point out the wisdom of daily exercise for everyone and especially for those who fear heart trouble. But isn't it also true that the very same inadequate diet that brings on the heart complications may be responsible, too, for the gall bladder trouble? So mightn't the same diet that prevents heart and blood vessel diseases also prevent gall bladder disorders? We think that it may.

You Must Have Certain Foods in Your Diet to Use Fat Properly

What are the various elements in the diet that are most involved in the way the body uses fat? Almost everything in the way of vitamins, so it becomes perfectly obvious that the vitamins in one's diet are of utmost importance—far more than the amount of fat or cholesterol one eats.

For instance, choline, a B vitamin, is used in the body to transport digested fats from the liver to the various fat deposits in the body. A complete deficiency in choline produces high blood pressure in laboratory animals within a week. Replacing choline in the diet reduces the blood pressure. Removing all choline from the diet of rats (from a cancer-susceptible line of rats) causes the death of the rats within a short time. Putting back just enough choline to keep the rats alive results in 50 times more cancer than would normally have occurred on a diet rich in choline. How can we possibly overlook choline as one of the most important single items in the diet so far as fat metabolism is concerned? Yet it was not mentioned once in all the material we read on gall bladder disease.

Inositol, another B vitamin, is intimately involved with the way the body uses cholesterol, this dangerous fatty substance from which gallstones are chiefly made. Here is one experiment showing the relationship. Rats fed a regular diet and large amounts of cholesterol were divided into two groups. One group got, in addition, added inositol. At the end of the experiment, the rats who got just regular diet and the cholesterol had a cholesterol increase of 337 per cent in their blood. The rats which got the inositol (along with just as much cholesterol) had an increase of only 181 per cent. Would you say, therefore, that inositol is important if you are going to be sure that the body uses fats, and especially cholesterol correctly? We have never seen it mentioned in connection with gall bladder trouble.

Biotin, another B vitamin, is directly involved in the assimilation of fat by the body. It must be present in the intestine in ample quantity or fat cannot be digested. Would you say that it is important for the prevention of gall bladder trouble?

Please don't write in and ask where you can get choline, inositol and biotin. You can't get them, so far as we are concerned, except in food, for we believe that taking these three B vitamins apart from the other B vitamins is a serious mistake. In food you can get them most abundantly in egg, liver, wheat germ, beef heart and brewers' yeast. They have been carefully removed from all processed foods, such as white flour and white sugar.

The fat soluble vitamins, (A, D, E and K) must be considered when you are planning a diet to prevent gall bladder trouble. First of all, they are present in fatty foods, and if you should decide to go on a low-fat diet to prevent gall bladder trouble, you are likely to run into serious difficulty because you will simply not get enough of the fat soluble vitamins. And vitamin K is directly affected by anything that goes wrong with the gall bladder. Bile must be present in the intestine or vitamin K cannot be absorbed by the body. Vitamin K is responsible for the proper coagulation of the blood. Could a lack of vitamin K caused by gall bladder disorder be partly responsible for today's tragic incidence of cerebral hemorrhages or "strokes"? We think it might be.

We are also told that a lack of vitamin A may affect the lining of the gall bladder. This seems likely since vitamin A is important to the health of all the membranes of the body, but especially the linings of organs and passageways.

Vitamin C and Gallstones

Now we come to the theory of a great friend of ours, W. J. McCormick, M. D. of Canada whose work with vitamin therapy we mention many times in this book. Dr. McCormick, in *The Medical Record* for July, 1946, presented the theory that lack of vitamin C may be responsible for the formation of "stones" of various kinds in the body. He tells us that more than a hundred years ago "stones," especially kidney stones, were much more prevalent than they are today. He reminds us that more than a hundred years ago, vitamin C was in very short supply in the diet, especially in the wintertime. Scurvy, which is the disease that comes when vitamin C is completely lacking, was a common disease then. People died of it. Today it is almost unknown. Why? Because these days we have fresh raw fruits and vegetables throughout the winter months and we know, at least most of us know, that we must eat a certain amount of such foods to be healthy. Still we have gallstones and kidney stones and tartar on the teeth, which, according to Dr. McCormick, is another evidence of lack of enough vitamin C.

Dr. McCormick, giving massive doses of vitamin C along with a liberal amount of vitamin B, found that, among his own patients, he could clear up evidence of deposits in the urine and at the same time his patients remarked on their freedom from tartar.

There are two ways, he says, in which lack of vitamin C may bring about the formation of stones. Vitamin C is absolutely necessary for the health of tissues. It must be present to form the cement that holds cells together. When there is not enough of it, cell material flakes off and forms a kind of garbage which has no place to go. In the genitourinary tract these provide the nucleus for kidney stones which bring a certain amount of infection and begin to collect layers of other materials around them.

In support of his theory, Dr. McCormick describes one country after another where "stones" are almost universal—and vitamin C is almost completely lacking in the diet. Among Tibetans and Szechwanese, he says, almost everyone has gallstones and inflammation of the gall bladder. The diet of these people consists of butter, tea, barley flour and rice, with little or no fresh fruits or vegetables. The high fat content of the diet, with practically no vitamin C to counteract it, may well be responsible for the fact that gallstones rather than kidney stones are the common ailment.

Dr. McCormick's theory is only a theory. We have yet to hear of a doctor putting his patients on a diet high in vitamin C to prevent or cure gallstones. We long for the day when we will read of such a doctor. But meanwhile, and especially since vitamin C is just about the most important single item in anybody's diet, regardless of his health, why not give the theory a try? There is nothing to prevent you, and a world of good health to gain.

And what of the other vitamins we have mentioned? They are all necessary and highly important. Where do you get them? First, in a well-planned diet, high in protein (meat, fish, eggs, nuts) and fresh fruits and vegetables—a diet that has no room at all for foods made from white flour and white sugar, a diet that is not watered down to little more than calories by the inclusion of candy, soft drinks, doughnuts, and all the other treacherous sweets that spell disaster. Isn't it significant that the chief common characteristic of gall bladder sufferers is obesity? The very same foods that made them fat give them the gall bladder trouble.

In addition to a good diet (*every day—no exceptions for weekends or holidays!*) you need food supplements for vitamins and minerals—fish liver oil for vitamins A and D, brewer's yeast, and/or desiccated liver for vitamin B, rose hip preparations for vitamin C, natural vitamin E and wheat germ oil, bone meal and kelp for minerals. If you fear gall bladder trouble, or if you want to reduce safely and surely, this is the diet and these are the diet supplements for you!

Garlic

The Dutch herbal *Kruydeboeck,* written by Rembert Dodoens some four hundred years ago contains some delightful information on garlic. As one commentator puts it, the virtues of many of Dodoens' recipes are now known to be more or less exaggerated. Regardless of this actual value, they are interesting because they represent herbal medicines in one of the most brilliant periods of world history.

Here is what Master Dodoens had to say about garlic: (The spelling of the ancient translation is preserved.)

"It is good against all venome and poison, taken in meates or boiled in wine and dronken, for of his owne nature it withstandeth all poison; insomuch that it driveth away all venemous beast from the place where it is. Therefore, Galen, prince of physitions, called it poore men's Treacle.

"The same eaten rawe or boiled cleareth the voice, cureth the old cough. It is very good against the toothache, for it staketh the same, pounde with vinegar and laid to the teeth; or boiled in water with a little incence, and the mouth washed therewith, or put into the hollowes of the corrupt teeth. It is of the same vertue mixt with goose grease and powed into the eares.

"The same brused betwixt the handes and laide to the temples, staketh the old headache. The same burned into ashes and mingled with hony, healeth the wild scab, and scurffe of the head and the falling of the heare, being laide thereupon. Laid to in the same manner, it healeth black and blew scarres, that remaine after bruses and stripes.

"The Danger: Garlicke is hurtfull and nought for cholerique people and such as be of a hot complexion, it hureth the eies and sight, the head and kidneies. It is also nought for women with child and such as give sucke to children."

It is not surprising that authors of old herbalists thought that garlic was not for the "hot complexioned" folks. Garlic itself is so "hot" that one would be better advised to give it to mild, gentle people. And of course the suckling child would probably not relish the taste of garlic in its mother's milk and we do not doubt for a moment that the taste would be there if the mother were an inveterate garlic-eater.

We are told that from Dioscorides (first century A.D.) to Hippocrates and Pliny the Elder, from ancient Hindu medical literature to St. Hildegard, Paracelsus and the medieval herbals, one can follow through medical literature the mention of garlic and its powers for good health. It is poison resistant, purgative and diuretic, and it also enjoyed a reputation as a means of diminishing susceptibility in times of great epidemics. During the fury of the Great Plague in the 14th century, the graves of the dead could be kept from becoming breeding places of contagion only by being cauterized daily with tips of garlic. This favorable effect could also be observed during the first World War in places in which epidemics of dysentery and typhus sprang up.

Probably the reputation of garlic for warding off evil was mainly responsible for its honored place as a magical charm against the forces of darkness. In folklore garlic plays a prominent part. It is almost as efficacious as holly or mistletoe for hanging over the door to secure the protection of all within the house. Even today in many parts of the world people wear chains of garlic to protect them from witches and the evil eye.

Why Did the Old Herbalists Recommend Garlic?

Undoubtedly much of its reputation must have come from its strength. Anything that smelled so bad and smelled so strong must be powerful against a lot of things! But we cannot be too disparaging of the old herb doctor's knowledge. He had nothing but herbs to use as medicine, remember. There were no antiseptics, no antibiotics, no laxatives, no analgesics, no tonics, no vitamin supplements! So the herb doctor had to observe keenly and dose wisely. Once he had discovered that his potions would not kill the patient, he had to experiment until he found which herbs seemed to be valuable in which conditions. We cannot brush aside as worthless his estimate of garlic as a germ-killer, even though he did not know the word "germ." Experiments in today's laboratories have showed that garlic indeed does have anti-bacterial power.

Today's physician might say that he does not need to use garlic—he has more potent and pleasanter tasting germ-killers. But we would put this question to him—does he have germicides that destroy only the harmful germs, leaving the beneficial ones untouched? This is what we would expect garlic to do.

A modern investigator, Roos, who has worked with garlic, does not attribute its effect on the harmful intestinal bacteria to any ability it may have to kill germs, however. He believes that garlic brings about a change in the general reaction of the intestinal membrane as a result of which the harmful bacteria are crowded out and normal intestinal activity is restored. We know that sulfur compounds are released during digestion. Do these have some part to play in the relief that garlic is said to bring to numerous digestive disorders?

There is an article in the *Medical Record* for January 15, 1941 in which E. E. Marcovici of New York tells of his experiments in garlic therapy of the digestive tract. He found that garlic does indeed exert a curative and prophylactic action on various disorders of the digestive tract, and the complaints of the elderly patient with chronic hypertension or high blood pressure. Dr. Marcovici pleads in his article for wider use of garlic which he calls "harmless and effective."

If indeed garlic restores the normal action of the intestinal bacteria then its importance in modern times is even greater than in olden times. For today we may kill off the beneficial bacteria in our digestive tracts every time we take an antibiotic by mouth, for drugs like the antibiotics, sulfa drugs and so forth do not distinguish between helpful and destructive bacteria—they kill them all. And many a pneumonia or virus patient has shaken off his infection only to be left with a condition perhaps much worse—indigestion of the most uncomfortable kind, with gas, constipation or diarrhea, loss of appetite and a gloomy outlook on life.

Garlic in Digestive Disorders

I. S. Klieger, M.D. of New York wrote in *The Medical Record* for April 5, 1939, of how he used a preparation containing garlic on underprivileged children in a New York hospital. They ranged in age from one to fifteen years. All were below par in appetite, blood count and weight. There seemed to be no reason for any of this. And the children failed utterly to respond to any other kind of treatment. Of fifty children given the compound, twenty-five gained in weight and appetite, nine gained weight only, thirteen showed no change and three lost weight. Of the twenty-five who improved when taking the compound, almost all reverted to their original condition when the medicine was stopped.

Dr. Klieger goes on to say that among his own private patients to whom he gave the compound and who could be depended on to take it, the percentage of weight and appetite gains was even higher. He concludes that because of the excellent gains obtained from these experiments, he believes this compound merits the consideration of other physicians who may be having trouble trying to conquer lack of appetite and he intends to go on using the medicine.

In the *Review of Gastroenterology* for January-February, 1944, Harry Barowsky and Linn J. Boyd, both physicians, tell of using garlic on fifty patients who suffered from "various disorders commonly associated with gastro-intestinal symptoms." Flatulence (gas) was relieved in the vast majority of cases. The effects were not spectacular, they say, but the relief from nausea, vomiting, gas, abdominal distention and after-meal discomfort was sufficiently regular and marked for this remedy (garlic) to merit consideration as a treatment when these symptoms are present.

McDuffie treated tuberculosis with garlic and found it to be the most effective among fifty-six various treatments with which he experimented.

In the *Review of Gastroenterolgy* for May 1949 F. Daran and E. A. Ferguson report on the therapeutic value of garlic in digestive disorders. They found that gas and nervous dyspepsia were improved, the garlic had a sedative action on the stomach and intestines; belching, nausea and after-meal discomfort were all relieved. They tell us that the garlic tablets are perfectly safe for long continued use and may be prescribed for a wide variety of disturbances of the stomach and intestines. We are told that Dr. Albert Schweitzer has used garlic in cholera and typhus.

In an article in a European publication, *Praxis* for July 1, 1948, G. Piotrowski, visiting lecturer and member of the faculty of medicine at the University of Geneva, writes of his experiences with the use of garlic on "about a hundred patients." Dr. Piotrowski contends that garlic lowers the blood pressure by dilating the blood vessels. He administered oil of garlic for three weeks and blood pressure dropped 2 cm. in 40 per cent of the patients. In addition "subjective symptoms" were alleviated—backache, headache, dizziness, angina-like pains. Dizziness was cleared up in 80 per cent of the patients, incidentally.

From the *German Pharmaceutical Magazine* for February 1, 1950, we learn that "modern physicians have found and have reported that patients placed on garlic dosage speak of a feeling of general well-being and increased vitality after a short time. This possibly may result from the ability of garlic to reduce blood pressure as well as to effect dilation of the blood vessels and detoxification of the entire organism. Patients also report themselves freed from apprehensions and neuroses they previously felt. Garlic, the evidence shows, is definitely a blood pressure regulator. It also favorably influences nervous cardiac manifestations and good results have been obtained in the female climacteric (menopause) especially in those cases with accentuated pulse, hot flashes, irritability and insomnia.

"The entire digestive tract is acted upon favorably by garlic . . . It tends to detoxify the entire organism, with special influence upon the heart, blood vessels and blood pressure, especially in the aged. This attribute may be responsible for its successful use on excessive tobacco users in chronic nicotine poisoning. The good effects of garlic also extend to the microorganisms, including intestinal worms."

We do not know what substance in garlic brings about the health benefits in which we simply must believe. We know that garlic contains some of the B vitamins and vitamin C. But it seems unlikely that these could be responsible for such almost miraculous benefits, for they occur in relatively small amounts, considering how much garlic one can eat at a time.

We think garlic is an absolutely necessary part of diet. You can improve almost any meat, vegetable or salad dish with garlic. Many people write us that they love the taste so much they eat garlic sandwiches. Today, in a society where garlic-eating is not general and the subject of halitosis has been widely treated in the press, it is almost mandatory to find some form of non-odorous garlic if one wants to be accepted socially. Of course the smidgeon you use at mealtime should not bother you or those with whom you associate. And you can always top off the meal with a bit of parsley; parsley positively disperses any garlic smell. (It's rich in vitamin C, too!)

If you want to take garlic in larger doses, garlic perles are available which contain everything in the original bulb—but which do not begin to dissolve until they have progressed to the lower reaches of the digestive tract, so there is little danger of any odor on your breath.

Alex Schneider of Boulder, Colorado writes us: "Eight other men and I went to Florida for deep sea fishing. The water was rough. We had planned to stay out for three days, but all the other men were so seasick that we had to come back. We were out two days and two nights.

"The day before I left home, I read the article in *Prevention* about using garlic perles and desiccated liver. I started to use it right away and I never felt sick or dizzy at any time, as the others did. Thanks for the information."

From P. P. Pleasants of Honolulu comes this information: "I have eaten garlic for the past several years and often wonder if one can eat too much. I eat three or four little sections a week and usually eat it just before retiring. No odor is noticeable by morning. I am bothered with soreness and pains through my back about the hips, which are commonly referred to as lumbago pains. Eating garlic sure knocks them for a curve! This soreness occurs only in the morning about getting up time."

Caroline Gook of Los Angeles writes us that she uses garlic perles for colds, also raw crushed garlic in a cup of warm milk with good results.

Alice S. Cutler, M. D. of Los Angeles writes: "I was interested in your article on garlic. I personally know of several cases of exophthalmic goiter cured by using garlic. These patients were treated by a Hungarian physician in this country. Of course they were not cured in several weeks, but at the end of a year they had no goiters. There is no limit to what garlic can do for a person, that I am sure of."

Nellie Varner writes us: "I do not believe there needs to be a social hazard from eating garlic. Eat a clove of raw garlic, then after your meal eat a sprig of fresh parsley and I believe you will find that no one who has not eaten garlic will know that you have eaten it."

Two more letters from readers who take garlic supplements regularly. From Denver, Colorado comes a grateful letter: "As of now I am taking regularly the following: desiccated liver, garlic and natural vitamin E in wheat germ oil. I am not in any sense sick. But I find that the supplements benefit me greatly. I will not describe fully my past symptoms, but I will mention only one. I was subject to blackouts. Dizzy spells. Only momentary, but a source of much worry to me. Through editorials or articles in *Prevention* I got the idea that garlic and vitamin E would help. They have. All the dizzy spells disappeared entirely. I now have no worries that a heart condition has a hold on me. I am sure I haven't high blood pressure."

From California a woman writes: "I wish to express my appreciation for the work you are doing for your country and for your generation by helping so many to live happier lives.

"Through reading your article on garlic a friend of mine got rid of a chronic cough that produced as much as a third of a cup of phlegm. She was living in a foggy, rainy climate. I was calling on her when she said, 'Now I am going to have a coughing spell. Every evening about five I cough for about twenty minutes.' So I said, 'Why don't you take garlic this winter? Surely you have nothing to lose by giving it a trial.' The following March she wrote me that the cough was all gone and was she ever thankful! She said garlic did it. She took two cloves a day."

Gelatin

The substance from which gelatin is made occurs in bones and cartilage. To obtain gelatin, bones are treated for several days in cold dilute hydrochloric acid. The residue is then soaked in water to remove the acid. Then it is boiled in water and gelatin results.

Gelatin is chiefly valuable to the food industry because it is soluble in hot water and creates a jelly when it is cooled. So food manufacturers use it extensively in making candies, ice cream and so forth. Drug manufacturers use it for pills and capsules.

You may have had gelatin recommended to you as an excellent health food because of its protein content. Actually this is our only concern with gelatin—the fact that it does contain considerable protein. However, we must report that the protein of gelatin is not complete and hence gelatin cannot be relied on to produce good health, if it is your only or main source of protein.

What do we mean by "complete" protein? There are many different amino acids or forms of protein that occur in food. Some of these are made in the human body, so we do not need to get them in our food. But others cannot be manufactured by the body, so we must get them in food, and fairly regularly too. There are ten essential amino acids—arginine, histidine, isoleucine, leucine, lysine, methionine, phenylalanine, threonine, tryptophan and valine.

In proteins such as meat and eggs all these amino acids appear in abundance. But gelatin is low in nearly all of them except arginine. Tryptophan is completely absent. Now if you plan to get a large amount of your protein requirement from gelatin, you can see that it simply won't work out. For you are likely to throw something completely out of balance by not having the proper balance among the essential amino acids. It's not enough, you see, to have just one or just two or even more of the essential amino acids in your diet. You must have them all every day.

Does this mean you should not eat gelatin at all? Of course not. There are many excellent recipes for vegetable salads and fruit desserts which contain gelatin. By using the gelatin rather than serving just plain vegetable or fruit salad, you are increasing your family's daily intake of protein, so, from this point of view, it's a good idea to use gelatin. But the next time anyone tells you enthusiastically that you can reduce successfully by going on a diet in which gelatin is your main source of protein, steer clear of any diet like that. It can produce serious deficiency.

When you are planning to use gelatin in your menus, use always the plain gelatin, uncolored and unflavored. The other kinds have artificial color and flavor which of course make them taboo for anyone concerned about his health. You will notice that cook books tell you not to use raw pineapple or papaya in gelatin dishes. This is because these two fruits contain enzymes that quickly digest protein, so they will make your gelatin completely ineffective for "jelling" purposes. By cooking the fruits to destroy enzymes, you can use them successfully with gelatin. Of course other fruits and vegetables should be used raw.

Glands—Adrenal

Did you ever watch the hair on a dog's back stand up when a stranger comes to the door and the dog is fearful and ready to attack the stranger? Did you ever feel goose pimples yourself when something has frightened you? Did you ever notice that your food doesn't digest if you are angry or frightened or in pain at mealtime?

The mechanism behind all these reactions is a small set of glands located just in front of the kidneys—the adrenal glands. They consist of two parts, the medulla or central portion and the cortex or covering. The medulla is partly a gland and partly an extension of the nervous system. This is the alarm box that prepares you to fight or run away when you encounter danger. You have often heard of people performing almost inhuman feats under the stress of great danger. They can do this because the adrenal medulla is rushing all kinds of extra stimulation to all parts of their bodies.

When you are frightened, angry or in pain, the adrenals release into the body a hormone called adrenalin or epinephrine which immediately raises the blood pressure, constricts the arteries, causes the heart to beat faster, raises the blood sugar level, brings the blood from the visceral organs and the skin into the muscles (to prepare you for a quick getaway) and causes the contraction of certain muscles—the dog's hair stands on end and the goose pimples rise on your skin. The release of adrenaline also increases the rate of metabolism, that is, transforms your food more quickly into energy and gives you an increase in muscular power and resistance to fatigue. It brings about the release of some substance in the blood which causes it to clot more quickly. In other words, adrenalin prepares you for an emergency. You can run faster, fight harder and longer, perform feats of endurance, and, in case you are wounded, your blood will clot more quickly so that you will not bleed to death.

However, these days not many of us are required to fight or run when we are frightened or angry. What happens inside us when we become angry at a reckless driver who nicks the fender, or frightened at some news story we happen to read? We may yell at the driver and go to the movies to forget the newspaper article. Neither of these will use up all the extra equipment with which our adrenalin has provided us. It seems to us that this situation may be the answer to many of our difficulties today—both physical and psychological. We cannot use the forthright means of action our body prepares for us—escape or battle. Have you ever noticed what a fine sense of relief you get from scrubbing a floor, pulling weeds, or hammering nails when you are good and angry about something? You're working off the adrenalin!

We were interested to find that the graying of hair is apparently related to disorder of the adrenals. It might be possible, then, for someone's hair to turn white overnight under conditions of great stress, as the old stories and legends tell us. We also found that a deficiency of pantothenic acid (one of the B vitamins) can bring on a strain that will result in increased activity of the adrenal cortex which may result in the exhaustion of the gland's secretion. We have learned that graying hair has been produced in animals by deficiency of pantothenic acid.

We also find that there is abundant vitamin C in healthy adrenal glands—a great deal more proportionately than in other parts of the body.

Is it stored there? Is it a necessary substance for the proper functioning of the gland? We do not know. But it seems to us that, if you would have healthy adrenal glands, you should by all means make certain you are getting lots of vitamin C in your diet every day. We found, too, that the amount of vitamin C in the adrenals regulates our resistance to cold—another good reason for getting plenty of vitamin C every day during the cold weather.

When something goes wrong with the adrenals—tuberculosis or some other disorder that causes the glands to stop functioning or to function less efficiently, Addison's Disease may result. This was first described as a disease in 1855 by the physician whose name it bears. In Addison's Disease some of the symptoms are these: there is an increased excretion of sodium which releases water into the body. So this is one condition in which it is necessary to increase one's intake of table salt, or sodium chloride. In addition, the potassium of the blood increases, perhaps up to 100 per cent more than its former level, the blood pressure is lowered and the body can no longer deal efficiently with carbohydrates. Low blood sugar results. The metabolism of proteins and minerals is also upset in Addison's Disease, there is great muscular weakness, vomiting and a peculiar brown pigmentation of skin and mucus membranes.

An article in *Newsweek* for February 4, 1952 tells us there may be a relationship between adrenal function and schizophrenia, the most dreaded form of insanity. In a series of experiments conducted over many years researchers at the Worcester Foundation for Experimental Biology found that schizophrenics did not respond in the same way as normal people to tests designed especially to stimulate adrenalin. Under conditions that called forth an increase of adrenalin in normal men, the adrenalin level of the schizophrenics remained the same. Is this because of their mental condition? Or is the mental condition caused at least partly by a disorder of the adrenals? We do not know, but this report seems to indicate that we are closer to understanding schizophrenia.

The adrenals are involved, in some way, in diabetes. They also have a definite influence on the sex life of an individual, for disorders of the adrenals, especially in unborn children or very small children, may result in faulty development of the sex organs. Since they are so importantly involved in so many functions, we'd suggest taking very good care of your adrenal glands. An all-'round good diet is undoubtedly essential and the two vitamins B and C seem to be of paramount importance.

Glands—Breast

The human breast is part of the reproductive system of the female whose function is carefully regulated by the various sex hormones or gland substances. Although the breast itself consists mostly of gland tissue, its size depends usually on the amount of fat surrounding the gland tissue. So, in general, individuals who tend to accumulate fat will have large breasts while those who are thin or bony will have small ones. Of course there are many exceptions.

The breast contains lobules or sections and about 15 ducts or small tubes which, in the mother who is nursing a child, collect the milk from the lobules and conduct it into the nipples. The nipple, which projects from the surface of the breast, has openings through which the milk ducts run. Surrounding the nipple is the areola, a more heavily pigmented section. It is believed that, during pregnancy, the sex hormone progestin, which is produced by the ovaries, causes the breasts to enlarge.

Soon after the birth of the child the breasts begin to secrete milk. It is believed that this process is begun by the hormone prolactin which is produced by the pituitary gland. As the child continues to nurse, the production of milk is stimulated by the emptying of the milk ducts. As the child is weaned, less and less milk is drawn from the gland so the milk-producing cells gradually degenerate and disappear.

During pregnancy and lactation, the care of the breast is most important, whether or not the mother nurses her child.

Breast feeding is infinitely better for both mother and child than bottle feeding. Many present-day mothers do not nurse their children, partly because of the inconvenience and the feeling that it may destroy the appearance of the breasts. However it has been shown that the mother who nurses her child invariably "gets her figure back" much more quickly after childbirth. This is undoubtedly due to some physiological mechanism that is put into activity by the hormones connected with the flow of milk.

In addition some modern women are unable to nurse their children due, we believe, to our modern devitalized diets which do not provide enough sound nutrition for the mother to have milk for her child. It seems that a well-nourished mother who actually wants to nurse her child has little or no difficulty in doing it.

For the woman who is not pregnant or nursing a child, breast cancer is the chief concern where breast-health is involved. Causing more deaths among women than any other form of cancer, breast cancer is the almost ever-present dread of many modern American women. Readers know that we believe cancer can be prevented chiefly by following a diet rich in natural, unrefined foods, hence rich in vitamins, minerals and enzymes. It is also advisable, of course, to avoid injury or irritation to the breast. Modern brassieres which give the breast good support without confining it too closely are the best protection against the sagging condition which produces fatigue and ill-health as well as unsightly appearance.

All our muscles tend to sag as we become older, and the muscles that support the breast are no exception. Here, too, the results of years of poor posture and poor diet show clearly in broken down tissues which ruin appearance as well as health. There is nothing you can do to change the structure or improve the tone of the actual gland tissue of the breast. But you can do something about the muscles that surround and support it and in many cases, simply by improving posture, you can improve the appearance of the bustline. Remember always to carry your head high, chest high, back straight, chin in. Exercises to improve posture will help. Good diet will help even more, for muscle tone depends on the quality of the food you eat. Plenty of good protein with lots of vitamin—and mineral—rich foods are your best assurance against flabby muscles.

An excellent exercise for conditioning the muscles around the breast, which will be of value whether you want to increase or decrease the apparent size of your bustline, is this: stand tall and straight, the end of your spine tucked in, your shoulders back, chest high, chin in. Pick up a heavy book—a dictionary or encyclopedia volume would be best. Hold it in front of you with your elbows widespread like wings, arms parallel to the floor. Now, using only the tips of your fingers, press hard on the book, as if you were trying to make your fingertips push right through the book and meet. Don't do the exercise too many times at first, for you will notice a strong pull on all the muscles of your chest and under your arms. This easy exercise can be done any time at home or at the office.

Glands—Pancreas

Diabetes and hyperinsulinism. High and low blood sugar. How do they happen and what can you do about them? The answers are hidden in a little-known organ of your body called the pancreas. Located near the stomach, the pancreas is part of the digestive system, for it secretes pancreatic juice, which, as we all learned in school, is released into the intestines where it helps the other digestive juices to break down our food for assimilation. In this case, protein.

Fairly recently, relatively speaking, it was discovered that another important function of the pancreas is the regulation of blood sugar. One small section of the pancreas, called the Islands of Langerhans, is in charge of this procedure. If we understand fully just how and why this regulation takes place, we would know the secret of what causes diabetes and low blood sugar.

In addition to its digestive juice, the pancreas produces a hormone called insulin. A hormone is a substance produced by one gland and remaining within the body to influence the activity of other organs and glands. Insulin is the spark that ignites the fire for burning sugars and starches and turning them into energy and heat. If the pancreas is diseased or does not function, the sugar is not burned and instead flows into the urine, after the blood has become saturated with it. This is the condition we call diabetes. The treatment for it is injection of insulin to replace the insulin that the pancreas is not producing. And a special diet. There are many different diets prescribed for diabetes, depending on how serious the condition is and what the ideas of the attending physician are. But in general, they involve a curtailing of sugar and starch—in other words, carbohydrates. It seems that obesity may have a lot to do with diabetes, for layers of fat accumulated on any organ or gland certainly upset the functioning of that particular organ or gland.

Although diabetic patients can, with insulin and special diet, live almost normal lives, there are hazards involved. For instance, acidosis resulting in death can be brought about by neglect of the prescribed diet. Insulin shock can result in coma and death, if an overdose of insulin is taken or if a moderate dose of it is taken without enough carbohydrates.

The actual chemical nature of insulin has not been determined—that is, we do not know exactly of what chemical substance it is made. We know that it must be injected rather than taken by mouth for it is destroyed in the digestive tract.

Recently we have come to realize that the condition opposite to diabetes may have just as serious results—that is, hyperinsulinism or low blood sugar. In this condition, too much insulin is secreted by the pancreas and conditions similar to insulin shock may be produced. More commonly, however, low blood sugar results in fatigue, hunger, a "letdown" feeling and, as several specialists have recently shown, may bring on such serious disorders as asthma, polio and epilepsy. Low blood sugar, too, seems to be caused by a diet high in carbohydrates, for its remedy is a high-protein diet with frequent meals and between-meal snacks, to keep the blood sugar at a consistent level. Drinks containing caffeine are also forbidden on the diet for low blood sugar patients, for caffeine, along with tobacco, has a tendency to raise the blood sugar precipitately and then cause it to fall just as sharply.

Although we do not know exactly what mechanism causes the pancreas to get into such bad shape that diabetes or hyperinsulinism result, it seems pretty obvious that, if a high-protein diet will cure these conditions, a high-protein diet might very well prevent them. Our recommendation—if you are afraid of diabetes or low blood sugar—would be that diet which we mention so often in these pages—plenty of the protective foods—meat, fish, eggs, cheese, nuts, fresh vegetables and fruits—nothing at all that contains white flour or white sugar and, for starches, only completely whole grain cereals and vegetables such as potatoes and beans. Yes, by this we mean no candy, no pastries, no cake, no chewing gum, no soft drinks, no white bread, no dumplings, noodles, spaghetti or macaroni. And no white sugar added to fruits or vegetables. Whether or not you think you may have symptoms of a badly functioning pancreas, try the diet for a couple of months. You will be surprised at the encouraging improvement in your health!

In the case of a doctor large doses of high potency vitamin E, taken under the supervision of the Shute Institute of Canada, completely cured a case of diabetes, which had progressed to such a stage that his gangrenous leg had been amputated.

Glands—Parathyroid

It seems impossible that four tiny glands so small they can barely be seen can have such an important effect on one's health as the parathyroids do. We are not at all sure yet just how these glands work or what different mechanisms they control. But we do know that they are vitally concerned with what happens to calcium and phosphorus in our bodies.

The parathyroids are four minute glands located back of the thyroid gland in the neck. If the parathyroids of an animal are removed during the period of growth, the animal soon shows signs of rickets—that is, his bones do not have enough calcium; they become bent and distorted. In an adult animal, removal of the parathyroids results in tetany—that is, cramps and convulsions which may eventually bring about death. Other symptoms of calcium deficiency occur, too—the heart beats erratically, for calcium controls the heart beat, and the nerves beome irritable. If not quite all of the glands are removed, the animals acquire latent or chronic tetany. That is, they may live apparently free from disease until some upsetting circumstance, such as an infection or pregnancy, brings on the symptoms of cramps and convulsions. They may also get cataracts, suffer from deafness, loss of appetite and loss of hair.

All of these symptoms suggest that plenty of calcium and a smoothly-running machine to handle the calcium are most important for the health of the eyes, hair, heart, muscles and nerves.

The kidneys are also affected when something goes wrong with calcium metabolism, for too much calcium may be excreted in the urine, resulting in kidney stones. Recklinghausen's Disease and Paget's Disease are believed to be caused by hyperfunction of the parathyroids—that is, the glands are excreting too much hormone. This is generally caused by a tumor in the parathyroid glands. It causes pains in the bones, an increase of the calcium of the blood and a decrease in the phosphorus, kidney stones, shortness of breath, heart palpitations and fatigue. In case one's diet is high in calcium, the kidney stones are almost unavoidable. If one's diet is low in calcium, the mineral will be withdrawn from the bones and serious bone disease will result. Of course, kidney stones are caused by other things than a disorder of the parathyroid.

Just as parathyroid tumors can bring about a complete upsetting of the calcium mechanism of the body, so can a disorder of the calcium-phosphorous metabolism bring about a disease of the parathyroids. So it seems wise to assure oneself of ample minerals, especially calcium and phosphorous in the right proportions so that this whole complex mechanism will function normally. We believe that taking bone meal as a food supplement is the best possible way to assure yourself of enough calcium and phosphorus in a natural form in which it is easily handled by the body.

Glands—Pituitary

Circus sideshows present the best opportunity for observing what happens when the pituitary gland goes awry. A dwarf or a giant may result from an under-or-over-secretion of the growth hormone which is produced by the pituitary gland. Important as this growth hormone is, its production is only one of the many functions of the pituitary, which is called the master gland because it controls so many other glands in the body.

Apparently from the time a child is born, the pituitary is sending its growth hormone out into the bloodstream, so that day by day the child increases in stature and weight. If there is some disorder in the pituitary gland, he may suddenly stop growing. He will develop in proportion as he grows older, but he will never attain normal height. Or he may suddenly begin to grow at a rapid rate and shoot up far beyond the other children of his age and eventually develop into a giant whose height and all other measurements will be far greater than those of other children. Nowadays many such growth difficulties can be controlled by giving pituitary extract.

The growth hormone is arranged for by the anterior or front part of the pituitary. This section also controls the gonadotrophic or sex-regulating hormone. When a youngster arrives at the age of puberty, it is this part of the pituitary gland which sets in motion the various changes that take place—the development of sex organs, the voice changes in a boy, and all those other manifestations of adolescence. Then too the front part of the pituitary secretes the lactogenic hormone which is essential for lactation. Without it no milk would form in the mammary glands of a new mother.

Then, as another of its complex functions the pituitary regulates the output of the adrenal glands—by secreting the adrenocorticotropic hormone. This hormone has become familiar to us recently in its capitalized abbreviation ACTH—the now famous substance which is used so much in modern medicine, for treating a wide variety of diseases. If you are beginning to have some idea of the tremendous importance and complexity of the pituitary gland, you can have some appreciation for all the difficulties doctors have in administering ACTH to their patients. Actually we know very little as yet about the functions of any glands. So a substance that involves both the pituitary and the adrenal glands may have widespread and devastating results on other parts of the body and we are not equipped as yet to say in advance just what all these results may be.

Finally the anterior part of the pituitary is occupied in stimulating the thyroid gland by its thyrotropic hormone. Now the thyroid gland in itself is a most complicated affair so the whole relationship between the pituitary and the thyroid is also complicated. It is believed, too, that the anterior pituitary has a lot to do with the way carbohydrates (sugars and starches) are used in the body. In other words, if the pituitary is not functioning properly the body may not handle these foods correctly and disease may result. The calcium and protein in our food seem also to be managed directly or indirectly by the pituitary.

Glucose

From the super market shelves, rows of glistening, jewel-colored jellies and jams beckon invitingly. Brightly colored candies, newly baked cakes, sparkling fruit juices shine in every aisle. Some of these delicacies contain natural food products in small quantities. But the foods we have mentioned, as well as catsup, cocktail sauces, canned vegetables and many more, contain a substance that, it seems to us, is more dangerous to health than white sugar. This is commercial glucose, or corn syrup, made by treating corn starch with sulfuric or hydrochloric acid. The resulting syrup is then neutralized with sodium carbonate and decolorized with carbon or boneblack.

According to Royal Lee, D.D.S., President of the Lee Foundation for Nutritional Research, commercial glucose is the only known sugar to cause diabetes when it is fed to test animals. He gives as his reference for this fact Dohan and Yukens, *Endocrinology,* Volume 42, page 244. Furthermore, says Dr. Lee, Dr. Joslin of Boston, our leading diabetic authority, has said that at the present trend of increase in diabetes, in another fifty years the American people will *all* be diabetic. How much of the responsibility for this frightening prediction can be laid at the door of glucose or corn syrup?

According to Daniel T. Quigley, M.D., of Omaha, synthetic glucose must be suspected as being a cause of cancer, for he has found that it is impossible to treat successfully some types of cancer until all traces of glucose have been eliminated from his patient's diet. Dr. Quigley made this statement in the *American Journal of Roentgenology and Radium Therapy,* Volume 34, No. 1, page 83. Since the preparation and processing of glucose actually make it a synthetic food there seems to be ample reason why it should produce all kinds of serious disorders, for, let the chemists say what they like, our bodies simply are not adapted to synthetic foods. As Dr. Lee says, when you feed your body synthetic foods, your cells adapt more appropriate forms for making use of the new situation. "What better definition can you frame for cancer? Feed your cells rubbish and they will lose their identity and revert into forms that can better live upon the rubbish."

Dr. Lee tells us also that glucose blocks the assimilation of calcium. Calcium is the single most important element necessary to strengthen us against many different kinds of disease. Is it possible that our tremendous national deficit in body calcium is due to the amounts of glucose we have been eating over the years? Look at your neighbor's grocery order and you will be horrified to see the quantities of processed, canned, preserved, pickled and prepared foods she buys, even when fresh foods are available and cheap!

Finally, Dr. Lee tells us that glucose destroys amino acids in the body. Amino acids are forms of protein. Protein is our most important category of food for health. The fruits, grains and vegetables we buy are declining each year in protein content, due to chemical fertilizer. Now, in addition, the prepared food we eat destroys more protein in our bodies. Says Dr. Lee "Lack of lysine (an amino acid) causes fatigability and nervousness. Lack of methionine, another amino acid, brings about toxic symptoms, liver disease and obesity. Yet glucose held at blood heat in the body along with protein, destroys 90 per cent of the lysine and 50 per cent of the methionine in this protein within 30 days."

We do not know how to advise you of the best methods for avoiding glucose, except to counsel you quite simply: No matter how rushed you are, no matter how meager the food budget may be, *don't buy foods that have been processed in any way!* You have no way of knowing which foods contain glucose and which do not. The addition of glucose need not be stated on the label. Canned fruits, canned vegetables, canned juices, preserves, jams, jellies, sweetened condensed milk, catsup, candy, syrups, sauces, ice creams, bakery products, cereals—all these and many other kinds of food may contain glucose. They will be appealing because they will be cheap. That is the reason why glucose is used—so that the food can be sold more cheaply. In more expensive brands of foods perhaps less glucose is used.

Practically, how can you avoid glucose? Use fresh fruits and vegetables *always* rather than canned ones. When fresh foods are not available, buy frozen ones which are much less likely to contain synthetic material like glucose. For mayonnaise, catsup, chili sauce and so forth, we advise making your own at home, so that you will know what the ingredients are. We don't advise using condensed milk for any purpose and we believe you should eat only unprocessed whole grain cereals.

Readers will undoubtedly think of many foods we have forgotten to list that probably contain glucose. Look with a suspicious eye on all commercially prepared foods. Before you pull out that attractive can or bottle from the grocery shelf, remember once again all the evidence against glucose. Do you want your family to eat this synthetic food?

Grapes

America produces more grapes than any other fruit except apples and oranges. Flame Tokay, Malaga, Emperor, Cornichon and Thompson Seedless are grown in the western states and Concord, Catawba, Moore Early, Worden, Niagara and Delaware in the eastern part of the country. The state of California heads the list, with 90 per cent of all the country's grape production.

Though grapes have been used by man since earliest days, we rather suspect that their chief popularity was due to their very satisfying taste and their adaptability to wine-making, rather than any wealth of health-giving qualities they might possess. For a number of years the European "Grape Cure" has attracted devotees who claim marvelous benefits from having lived on a diet of grapes alone for several weeks. Undoubtedly the very simplicity of the diet and the invigorating living conditions under which it is carried out do much to correct the effects of heavy diets of rich food.

As in the case of other fruits, sugar develops in grapes as they ripen and they should be eaten only after they are fully ripe, a condition that cannot always be observed just by judging the color of the grapes. Grapes shipped from California are generally fumigated with sulfur dioxide before shipping to reduce the browning of stems and to delay the growth of decay organisms.

Grape juice is prepared in this country by heating the grapes and extracting the juice by hydraulic pressure. In Europe a cold process is used, which is superior to ours. Grapes are easily digested, except for the skins and seeds which cause trouble to some folks. Grape juice then is quite easily digested, and we would recommend it heartily except for the fact that commercially bottled juice contains sugar or some form of synthetic sugar of which we disapprove. Raisins are made by drying grapes. In California they are sun-dried with no pre-treatment. Sulfur bleached grapes are prepared by dipping seedless grapes in alkali to check the skin, then sulfuring them, then exposing them to the sun for three or four hours, then drying them in the shade.

A pound of grapes contains about 400 calories. The minerals and vitamins contained in about 20 Malaga grapes are as follows:

Calcium	17	milligrams
Phosphorus	21	milligrams
Iron	.6	milligrams
Copper	.06	milligrams
Vitamin A	80	Int'l Units
Vitamin B		
Thiamin	.05	milligrams
Riboflavin	.03	milligrams
Niacin	.4	milligrams
Vitamin C	4	milligrams

Growth

What makes us grow? How does it happen that, within the space of a very few years, a tiny human being becomes a man or woman, not just in temperament, tastes and maturity, but also in actual weight, height and size? We do not know the full story of growth, but much of it has been studied. We know that growth is a progressive increase in the number and size of cells, the material they produce and deposit between them.

Growth is partly governed by the laws of heredity. That is, a baby who has inherited small bone structure from his parents can grow fairly tall if he has good nutrition. But his growth is limited by his inheritance. No amount of feeding will make him as tall as another baby who has inherited potentially long bones. On the other hand, a boy whose parents bequeathed him great height can be stunted by poor nutrition, gland disorders or illness.

The four circumstances that are most likely to stunt growth are: 1. a restriction in the quantity of food eaten. This is what happens during wars and famines, when the actual quantity of food—any food—is low. 2. Inadequate intake in the essential food elements. This is likely to occur among poor or ignorant families who are not supplied with the vitamins, minerals and proteins necessary for growth. Or it may happen among whole nations of people where the climate or the economy is such that the essentials are not available.

3. Interference with utilization of food or elimination of waste. Diseases such as diarrhea or dysentery for instance, can greatly influence the

growth by making inaccessible even those growth-promoting elements the child does eat.

4. Endocrine deficiencies. The endocrine glands, especially the anterior pituitary, the thyroid and the gonads have a great deal to do with stimulating or retarding growth.

This is the aspect of growth of which we know little. We do know that the pituitary gland—the "master gland" produces hormones that control the extent of growth. A deficiency in this hormone may cause the individual to become a dwarf. Too much may produce a giant. The thyroid and parathyroid glands also regulate growth, for they control the rate at which calcium and other minerals are deposited to make bones. No matter how much of these minerals may be in the diet, if the thyroid gland is not functioning correctly, the bones will not grow properly.

The gonads also regulate growth. These are the glands located in the reproductive organs. Growth proceeds, normally, until the animal is mature. This means that the sexual organs have developed and the animal is full grown. Then the growth process is shut off and the individual does not grow any more. This shutting-off process is believed to be arranged by the gonads. This function of the sex glands is important from another angle, too. Some disorders of childhood, especially glandular disorders, are accompanied by very early or very late development of the sex organs. This provides an indication that something is seriously wrong.

Many studies have been done on the nutriments needed for proper growth. In one experiment two groups of orphanage children were used. One group received the usual diet of the institution which, in this case, was remarkably good. The other group of children received, in addition to the diet, some extra vitamin B from brewer's yeast and wheat germ. They grew much faster than the first group of children. Records of school children over the years show that today's youngsters are taller and heavier than those of fifty or even thirty years ago. We assume the reason for this is the better diet of today. That is, in general, our children are getting more fresh fruits and vegetables, more milk, cheese, eggs and so forth.

In laboratories, we can discover exactly what food elements are necessary for growth. Leave them out of the chow and the animals do not grow. Put them back in and growth begins again immediately. All of the minerals are important, of course, for the skeleton of the body is composed of these. Iron is especially important during growth because the amount of blood is increasing, too, and blood must contain plenty of iron. Proteins are needed for growth, for most of our body structure consists of proteins. The B vitamins are tremendously important, especially pantothenic acid, riboflavin, niacin and pyridoxine. It has recently been discovered that vitamin B_{12} is a growth factor, too.

Vitamin A and vitamin C are both important for growth. Iodine is necessary for the health of the thyroid gland which helps to regulate growth. We do not know exactly how all these various food elements work to produce growth, but we do know they are essential. Even if they were all included in a good diet, it is possible that growth still might be disturbed if the glands were not functioning properly. But it also is true that a good diet would probably assure the proper functioning of the glands, as well as providing the basic essentials for growth.

Hair

Probably the loudest hue and cry about "good looks" comes from the womenfolk—and understandably. But noise or no noise, the men also have their share of concern when it comes to hair, particularly the loss of it.

Baldness

Though there are cases of women losing their hair, they are rare, and the problem of baldness usually confines itself pretty much to men. Specialists, over a long period of time, have tried to find the cause of the general pattern of loss of hair in middle age, and have come up with an amusingly large and varied number of answers. Some say it is purely hereditary; others attribute it to disease of the scalp or some vitamin deficiency, or dandruff. But to most of these reasons, the question can usually be asked: "Why does it not happen to women?" Women may have poor circulation, they wear hats more frequently than men, often, and their scalps are not always models of health or free from dandruff.

We, unfortunately, cannot supply the answer, but probably, as Dr. James B. Hamilton of the Long Island College of Medicines, states, the basic reasons are due to three principal factors: genetic inheritance, age and the presence of a plentiful supply of male hormones. Perhaps, as Dr. Marion Sulzberger (who is bald), of the New York University Post-graduate Medical School, humorously reasons: "Perhaps hair, like tails, is something left over from man's early ancestry. Perhaps we baldheaded men are a step higher on the evolution ladder than our wives." In any case, it seems right to assume that it is a natural phenomenon, which, unless a method is found to prevent it, is bound to occur in many a male.

However, in this matter of prevention, we should not scoff too heartily at all the theories and reasons for its existence as they can give us clues as to possible cures, and eventually prevention itself. In an article in *Science News Letter,* for November 10, 1951, an account is given of the findings of Dr. Peter Flesch and associates at the University of Pennsylvania in Philadelphia, which state: "Men get bald because the male sex hormone stimulates oil-producing glands in the skin to change the amount or quality of the oil they produce. . . . The skin oil is technically termed sebum. When painted on the skin of rabbits and mice, all the rabbits and many of the mice lost their hair in 10 days." In his experiments, Dr. Flesch also found that excessive amounts of vitamin A taken over a long period of time may lead to loss of hair, particularly in children. As with his experiments with sebum, Dr. Flesch and his staff painted vitamin A on the skins of their laboratory animals, with the result that the animals lost their hair. Next, the doctors hope to be able to find a way to check baldness in humans.

Since there is evidence that few Americans get enough vitamin A, there seems little chance that too much vitamin A would be causing the widespread baldness among American men, especially since baldness is unknown among many people whose vitamin A intake is far greater than ours.

In the matter of circulation nothing has actually been proved, but it is generally believed that regrowth can occur through massage, frequent brushing, and methods of bringing the blood into the hair region. Charles V. Ferrante, in his book *Baldness—Its Cause—Its Prevention,* published by the author, after examining many theories for baldness, arrives at the simple conclusion that lack of exercise of the scalp is the sole cause of men's loss of hair on the crown of the head. He states that women do not lose their hair because they have always had to "exercise" it from earliest childhood, while men's hair needs no such tending, for appearance's sake. The reason men do not lose their hair on the sides and in the back is that these regions receive friction from the pillow at night, while the crown does not. He discredits the male hormone theory, citing the lack of baldness in male Indians.

We have two more suggestions—just suggestions—as to why men may become bald while women do not. Could one reason be the tight collars men wear, which women do not? Or could it be the fact that women, in general, have wider arteries than men? We have heard that this is so and it occurs to us that this may result in better circulation in general among women.

Graying

Graying is another hair problem which men share with women. Is gray hair a necessary part of growing old? Can it be prevented, and what about the cases of gray, or even snow white hair which occur at a much earlier age? Though the experiments have dealt mainly with animals, diet has been found to be the key to the problem. Animals have been fed diets in which one or another of the vitamins is lacking. Then they have been observed to see whether there is a loss of hair color. If so, the vitamin is then replaced in the diet to see whether the color will return.

Dr. James Hundley, of the National Institutes of Health at Bethesda, Md., found significant results when he experimented with rats a few years ago. Reporting to the International Physiological Congress in Copenhagen, Denmark (*Newsweek,* August 28, 1950), he stated that in his studies of some 200 black rats he had found copper to be a necessary element in the diet for normal hair growth and color in rats. When Dr. Hundley increased the amount of copper in the diets of rats whose hair had turned gray from inadequate diets, the hair suddenly started darkening in five days, and complete change back to black hair occurred in three months.

In experiments by Dr. Douglas V. Frost and F. Pierce Dann, reported in the *Journal of Nutrition,* for May, 1944, laboratory animals were fed good diets which contained also synthetic B vitamins—thiamin, riboflavin, niacin, pantothenic acid and pyridoxine. Within two to eleven months the animals' hair began to gray. Weight decreases, anemia, and other indications of ill health accompanied the grayness. None of the female animals came in heat or could be bred successfully during this time. No change took place even when three other B vitamins were added—inositol, para-amino-benzoic acid, and choline. Then the experimenters took whole liver and, by chemical means, separated out those vitamins mentioned above, and fed the animals the remaining part of the liver, the "filtrate factor." Others they fed whole brewer's yeast. Almost immediately rejuvenation of the hair began, as well as improvement in hair growth, weight, appetite and muscle tone. So it was found that something in liver and yeast, aside from the known vitamins, brought about the change.

There are many other theories about the cause of loss of color in the hair, for example the effect of sulfa drugs. It is believed they rob the body of its store of pantothenic acid, another B vitamin. This is discussed by Harold D. West and Raven Rivera Elliott in *Archives of Biochemistry* for January, 1948. Dr. E. Geiringer, of Edinburgh, suggests in the *Revue Medical de Liège,* October 15, 1950, that vitamin C may play an important role in the preservation of hair pigment.

When all the evidence is in, the major guilt seems to lie in diet. We cannot say, after hearing all the testimony, that we can be sure of any one vitamin or food factor as being the single cause of grayness. But we do believe it is obvious that when grayness occurs some one or variety of the valuable food elements is missing. We recommend the following food supplements if there is a suspicion of deficiency in your diet: Fish liver oil perles for vitamins A and D; desiccated liver and/or brewer's yeast for all the B vitamins; vitamin C from natural food supplements and minerals from bone meal.

Care of the Hair

The question has often been asked as to the damage done by hair dyes and permanent wave lotions and chemicals. We believe that nothing should be put on the scalp—creams, lotions, soaps, even water—as they tend to alkalize a normally acid scalp and destroy the natural oils. But medical verdicts have proclaimed that no serious harm is *normally* done when these substances are cautiously used. Though beauty-parlor treatments and home permanent-wave sets have been thoroughly tested for the *average* effect, they do not claim to avoid causing a harmful reaction in certain cases of sensitivity.

Some enlightening remarks are given by John Goodwin Downing, A.M.A. of Boston University School of Medicine and Tufts College Medical School, Boston, Mass. Writing in the *Archives of Dermatology and Syphilology,* volume 63: page 561, May, 1951, he says that there are both mechanical and chemical dangers to scalp health. Metals used in connection with the hair may cause trouble. In the case of the chemicals, most of the dangerous and irritating ones have been removed by the industry, but they cannot of course remove all the substances to which individual persons may be sensitive.

He states further that there are many chemicals used that may cause trouble—the oils in bay rum, the synthetic perfumes in brilliantine, the various oils and resins in creams and wave preparations. The scalp lotions and tonics contain irritants and other substances that may sensitize individuals. Shampoos contain perfume and various sulfur mixtures, coconut oil shampoos are perfumed with several synthetic oils, any one of which may be harmful to individual users. "Hair dyes and rinses are the oldest but still the most dangerous hazard of the hairdressers' trade," he says.

Reporting on the ultra-fashionable fashions in 1950 (November 13), *Time* magazine had an article on the latest hair style—the "chignon," or false buns, braids or curls. Speaking of the hair used for such glamorous creations, Joseph Fleischer & Co., in Manhattan, made this interesting comment: "Only hair bought from European women has the quality necessary for good chignons . . . the hair of American women is damaged by too much pampering, tinting and shampooing (all the things the beauty shops do to it). The hair of European women is like a well-manured garden. The quality is good, but sometimes it doesn't smell too well."

We believe that the hair will keep its health and natural lustre, and hence its beauty, if it is allowed to grow unmolested by any solution or process, letting the natural oils do the work, along with frequent brushing and exercising of the scalp. Editor Rodale does not wash his hair, but cleans it with vigorous brushing. His barber has remarked that he has a very clean and healthy scalp.

Combined with this, as a "beauty prescription" we heartily advise a well-balanced diet, rich in the essential vitamins and minerals. The hair, like the rest of our bodies, must be fed, and, similarly, it responds best to those elements of food which are vital to its life and health.

Headaches

A common ailment, common in fact to about 65 per cent of Americans, an ailment for which individuals seldom seek medical help, but an ailment that afflicts perhaps one per cent of us every single day of our lives—this is headache. Our figures come from a carefully conceived and supervised survey done by Henry D. Ogden, M.D., of New Orleans and presented at the annual meeting of the American Academy of Allergy in New York, February 5, 1951. In his survey Dr. Ogden studied 4634 individuals whose answers to his questionnaire appear in an article in the *Journal of Allergy* for January, 1952.

These were not patients of the doctor's. They were farmers, housewives, students, laborers, salespeople, clerical workers and so forth, selected at random and given a questionnaire to fill in or interviewed by a professional interviewer. The questionnaire included almost every conceivable question that might be asked about headaches, including the subject's own opinion as to what might be causing his headaches.

This is quite a large group of people to be interviewed on one subject and we feel that the answers give a representative picture of what the situation nationally is in regard to headaches. The results showed that 64.8 of all the 4634 subjects suffer from headaches. People with headaches have a higher incidence of various respiratory symptoms than people who don't have headaches. There is also quite extensive history of family complaints of allergy of one kind or another among people who have the most headaches. Only 18 per cent of headache sufferers go to a doctor for their headaches. Pain in the front of the head is the commonest kind of headache. There is more headache among women, younger adults, single people, educated individuals, executives, students and professional people. Dr. Ogden also concludes from his survey that along with emotional and occupational problems allergy should be investigated by physicians dealing with headache patients.

We found several other significant things in the results of the survey. Over one per cent of the people interviewed said that they have daily headaches! 13.3 per cent of the headaches were present when the individual wakes from sleep in the morning and 10.2 per cent reported that their headaches appear in the afternoon. Headaches are not so frequent among older people. Of the women answering the questionnaire, 71 per cent had headaches, whereas only 50.7 per cent of the men did. Manual laborers have a very low incidence of headaches. Fatigue and eyestrain are the two most common causes of headache in the opinion of the individuals themselves.

Using figures in a much smaller survey we find that one doctor questioned 400 adults as to when their migraine headaches began and found that 34 per cent of them reported that they had migraine headaches before the age of 15.

Drugs Are Not the Answer

We have an enormous file of medical articles and articles that have appeared in general magazines on the subject of headache. Most of them consist of discussions of the different kinds of headaches—and there are many—the possible causes—and there are at least 30 of these, and cures ranging all the way from neck stretching to drugs to high protein diet.

We will not discuss the subject of drugs at all in this article. We believe that drugs do not cure and do not prevent headaches. They may of course relieve pain, but they surely do not remove the cause, and in killing the pain, they may well bring about aftereffects or side effects that are as bad as or worse than the headaches. It is pretty generally agreed among members of the medical profession that the worst way to treat a headache is to dose yourself with the advertised headache remedies, without going to a doctor or trying to discover what is causing the headaches. There are many reasons for this. The patent medicine remedy may relieve the pain of your headache and you may postpone indefinitely finding out what causes it . . . a serious mistake. The headache remedy, as in the case of salicylic acid, which is in aspirin and other remedies, may do you serious harm. And, by the constant use of headache remedies, you may develop a genuine drug addiction that will be harder to cure than the headaches.

There May Be An Emotional Basis For Headaches

Most writers on headaches pay some attention to the possible emotional causes. In this of course we are not speaking of headaches that have a definite organic cause. Migraine headaches in 15 children studied by three physicians of the Headache Clinic of the New York Montefiore Hospital and reported in the *New York State Journal of Medicine* for October 1, 1950, showed that nine of these children demonstrated definite neurotic tendencies which were apparent just on questioning by the doctors, without the aid of any psychological tests. Only three of the remaining six children appeared to be well adjusted to their environments. A sample case history is given of a 13-year-old girl whose headaches started at the age of 18 months. In this case the obvious difficulty was the child's relationship with her mother which was tempestuous and violent. They battled constantly, and yet the child was so dependent on her mother that she had few friends, stayed home with her mother whenever she was not at school and went out of the house only in her mother's company. It is easy to see how such a situation could result in chronic headaches with nausea, vomiting and severe prostration, which occurred every ten weeks with such regularity that future headaches were marked on the calendar for months in advance.

Other observations made during the study indicated that various conflicts in the children resulted also in temper tantrums, unreasonable fears, frequent nightmares, bed-wetting, nail-biting, thumb-sucking and other personality difficulties that go with maladjustment. It seems quite possible to us that when these children grow up they may learn to control the outward manifestations of neurosis such as we have just mentioned, but would not this very suppression of emotion probably bring about even more violent headaches? In other words, the adult cannot fling himself on the floor in a temper tantrum, so, holding in his rage and frustration, may he not develop even worse symptoms?

A physician who writes in the *Medical Journal of Australia* says yes, and he speaks from his own experience in trying to cure his own headaches. J. Bostock, M.D., first experimented on his eyes, purchasing glasses to correct his astigmatism. This had no effect on his headaches. He believed that focal infection might be causing them and had his tonsils removed, with no effect on the headaches. He had read that constipation, resulting in "autointoxication" could cause headaches. Keeping his digestive tract completely unobstructed with laxatives made no difference to the headaches. Then it occurred to him that headaches might be caused by "repressed hate" as he calls it. There is a war in the mind between what you want and what you can obtain. In the ensuing frustration, the victim feels that he is in a trap and the headache appears. Dr. Bostock feels that the term "migraine" should be re-defined to include a consideration of this psychological factor.

What About Eyestrain?

It is noteworthy that fatigue and eyestrain are the principal reasons for headaches, according to the people interviewed in our original survey. Some medical opinion agrees with this, other doctors disagree. Francis M. Walsh, M.D., of the University of Minnesota, and Leon D. Harris, M.D., of the Lutheran Deaconess Hospital, Minneapolis, writing in *Modern Medicine* for March 1, 1952, say that actual eye disorders are quite infrequent among children brought to them. Studying 100 young patients from 4 to 17 years of age, they found that 46 had "depressed" vision, but were free from any other symptoms. The remaining 54 had normal vision without glasses, but were brought to the doctor complaining of headaches, eyes that hurt, being slow readers and holding books close to their eyes while reading.

"Children with good vision may complain of headaches or eye pain to gain parental attention," say these physicians, "the first born whose place is usurped by a new baby . . . may feel neglected and sometimes resorts to this stratagem." In the opinion of these doctors, slow reading and holding books close to the eyes are caused by other things entirely and they seem to feel that getting glasses for the child will not affect cures. "Emotional origin" is a far more common cause for headaches.

On the other hand, Dr. Albert D. Ruedmann, Professor of Ophthalmology at Wayne University School of Medicine declared in the October 14, 1952, issue of the *Journal of the American Medical Association* that 25 per cent of all headaches are caused by eye difficulty. He said that eyes are overworked, overused and used under poor working conditions (bad light, etc.). He gave as examples the child who is inattentive, the business man who has a headache at noon which is relieved by lunch and then has a recurrence about 3 or 4 o'clock in the afternoon, the convalescent patient who reads in bed and so forth.

They may require, he said, medical exercises, surgical treatment, glasses, or all three. He also believes that pains in the neck which may lead to headache are caused by imbalance in the muscles of the eyes. The neck muscles function chiefly to move the head so that the eyes are in a good position to see. If there is a disorder in the balance of the eye muscles, the neck muscles must be strained to get good sight.

Low Blood Sugar and Headaches

We are interested in that businessman mentioned by Dr. Ruedmann —the man who gets a headache around noon which stops when he has his lunch and begins again around 3 or 4 p.m. We are interested in him mostly because of another clipping in our file in which J. A. Harrill, M.D., writing in the *Laryngoscope* for February, 1951, gives the case histories of 72 patients whose headache and dizziness were caused by low blood sugar and completely relieved by a high protein diet. The headache was described as dull and throbbing, often present at night and often related to meals.

Dr. Wilkinson of the University of Michigan Medical School cured 11 cases of migraine headaches with a high-protein diet. One of his patients had suffered from migraine for 35 years. Another got his headache regularly every Sunday morning when he changed his regular high-protein breakfast of bacon and eggs to waffles and syrup (carbohydrate) Dr. Wilkinson suggested that he try eating his regular high-protein breakfast on Sundays, too, and the headaches disappeared immediately.

There is a fascinating and provocative book on the subject of blood sugar by E. M. Abrahamson, M.D., and A. W. Pezet, *Body, Mind and Sugar,* published by Henry Holt and Company. In this book we find that the patient with low blood sugar is apt to feel worse in the early morning hours, (3 or 4 a.m.) or after he gets up in the morning. This is because he has not had any food for so long that his blood sugar is especially low. If he eats little or no breakfast and especially if he eats carbohydrates for breakfast (cereals, toast, waffles, coffee) his blood sugar drops again before lunch and again in the late afternoon. Now in our original survey on headaches we found that the two commonest times for headaches to appear are upon arising in the morning and again in the afternoon. It seems seldom that anyone gets a headache in the evening, unless it is the direct result of eyestrain or a particularly fatiguing day. In the evening, after a big dinner, with plenty of protein, blood sugar level is high.

We do not say or imply that all unexplained headaches are caused by low blood sugar, but we do earnestly suggest that if you suffer from headaches, and especially if they occur in relation to the time you get up and the time you eat meals, you should certainly get Dr. Abrahamson's book and try the high protein diet which he recommends. It is not a difficult diet to follow and it may produce startling results.

Just two further comments on the subject of high protein diets in relation to headache. Dr. Abrahamson found that so-called "allergic" conditions responded very well to his diet. He regularly cured asthma and hay fever patients with it. We saw in our initial survey that people who suffer most from headaches also have a higher incidence of respiratory disturbances and a family history of allergy. Can these disorders also be caused by the same low blood sugar that is causing their headaches?

Then, too, we constantly encountered mention of neurosis in connection with headaches—especially migraine headaches. We know that a high carbohydrate diet (which is also an inexpensive diet) requires lots of B vitamins for its proper digestion. We know, too, that all of the B vitamins have been removed from our popular processed carbohydrates such as breakfast cereals, white sugar and white flour. In addition we know that the B vitamins are responsible for morale.

Refined Carbohydrates Guilty Again!

Anyone who does not get enough B vitamins suffers from "nerves," depression, and even neurotic symptoms. Can it be that a diet high in refined carbohydrates is responsible for both the migraine headaches and the nervous, tense, hypersensitive personalities that go with them?

In defense of this theory we present a letter from a reader which speaks for itself:

> "I am a migraine. It's a long story but to make it short—I got so I figured I'd most rather not live than go through another long vomiting attack so, shall we say, I prayed to find a way so I'd no longer have those terrible weakening vomiting spells which occurred at least once a month. An advertisement came, advertising your splendid magazine, *Prevention*. I subscribed immediately. Not immediately was I able to carry out the suggestions in it, but when we could, we sent clear to California for naturally milled flour. We have been using no bleached flour or bakery bread since then. We avoid all canned foods with preservatives. I make whole wheat bread regularly. *And I don't have vomiting spells any more!*
>
> "During the time I cut Christmas trees last fall I went without whole wheat bread made from naturally milled flour for about two weeks, I believe, and the vomiting came back, so it is plain it is the bread made from the natural wheat with nothing added or taken out that helps me the most.
>
> "You can guess that after the one vomiting spell, when I had been off the brown bread, I have made it regularly. . . .
>
> Phyllis B. Crockett, Evans, Washington."

Other Possible Causes For Headaches

Other physicians have developed theories on the relation of muscles to headache. In *Munchener Medizinische Wochenschrift,* a German medical publication, we find C. Baeckmann writing of what he calls "myogenic headaches" which occur most frequently in women of middle age, with pain at the base of the skull leading to a stiffening of the neck. Dr. Baeckmann believes that the various household chores that women perform in cramped positions such as sewing, knitting, peeling potatoes and so forth may well result in "an unnoticed and lasting" elevation of the shoulders, caving in of the chest, and sway-back, which lead to stiff neck muscles and so to headache. He suggests massage of these neck muscles and relaxing exercises, application of heat, and of course postural exercises to correct the various postural defects the years have brought. R. J. Dittrich, writing in *The Journal Lancet* for February, 1951, describes a lower back pain that frequently leads to headaches. The lower back pain resulted from "abnormalities of subfascial (under the muscles) fat in the lower back," and although it is not clear just how the headache could result from low back pain, Dr. Dittrich says that apparently it did.

The New York State Journal of Medicine for March, 1953, claims that neck-stretching is the cure for "most headaches." Two surgeons who have treated more than 500 chronic headache cases report that they cured 60 per cent, achieved real improvement in 30 per cent and failed in only 10 per cent by using "traction" on the patients' necks. They continue their treatment for several months, even if the headache has disappeared meanwhile. It is not a remedy you could try at home, for it involves stretching the patient's neck with a series of weights varying from 5 to 60 pounds.

Aniseikonia, A Recently Discovered Eye Disorder

We cannot leave the subject of headaches without telling one story from our own experience. A friend of ours had headaches for 20 years—blinding, searing, nauseating headaches that put her to bed at least three or four days out of every month. She had taken thirty or forty different treatments all to no avail. Her glasses (for astigmatism) were changed regularly and each time her glasses were changed her headaches grew worse. Her friends began to believe the headaches must be a sign of neurosis. She herself was at the point of complete desperation and had made arrangements to have an examination for brain tumor.

A neighbor who was an optometrist asked if she would stop in at his office before she went out of town for her examination. Figuring that she had nothing to lose, she did. With a series of curious and very complicated machinery, Dr. Benton Freeman of Allentown, tested her eyes and told her she had aniseikonia, a maladjustment of eyesight. Over a period of six months he adjusted and re-adjusted a set of curved lenses. When they were perfectly adjusted for the degree of aniseikonia that she had, he made permanent lenses for her. This all took place five years ago. From the time the first aniseikonic lens was placed in the frame of her glasses, she has not had a headache. What is perhaps even more surprising, she continually bit her fingernails down to the quick during the years when she had headaches. A month after the headaches stopped, she found to her amazement that she had stopped biting her nails.

Aniseikonia is an eye disorder in which each eye sees objects at a different distance and different position in space. The effort made by her brain in trying constantly to adjust these two images was the cause of our friend's headaches. The aniseikonic lenses cannot cure this maladjustment of her eyes, but so long as she wears them she is free from all symptoms. In her case, each time her lenses were adjusted for astigmatism, her aniseikonia became worse, because then she saw each of the two images even more clearly.

Aniseikonia was discovered at Dartmouth a number of years ago and research and experimentation were done on a grant from John D. Rockefeller whose headaches were cured by aniseikonic lenses. It is estimated that more than one per cent of our population may have aniseikonia. There are only about 25 doctors in the country who have the equipment to test for it. They can tell you in a half hour whether you have aniseikonia or not and if you have they can, without fail, prescribe lenses to correct it. It is a lengthy procedure, but certainly well worth the time and money.

Dr. Freeman has patients from all over eastern United States, some of whom must be brought to his office in an ambulance, if they happen to break their lenses, for their symptoms are so violent without their glasses. Many ophthalmologists refuse to believe in the existence of such a disorder, even after they have interviewed these same patients, some of whom cannot stand on their feet or sit in a chair without falling, once they take off their glasses. If you believe aniseikonia may be causing your headaches, we'd suggest that you write to Dartmouth and ask for the name of the doctor nearest to you who can test you for it. Address Dr. Robert E. Bannon, Dartmouth Eye Institute, Hanover, New Hampshire.

There are several other aspects of headache that we should mention, although they seem to be quite obvious. If you suffer from sinus trouble, this can be a cause of headache. Impacted teeth may press against a nerve and cause agonizing headaches which have no apparent cause, if the impacted tooth is undiscovered. Eye strain is something we should all avoid. And this means simply: don't read or do close work over too long a period or in a light which is not adequate.

Allergy can cause headaches. One of the articles in our file relates the story of a man who always got a headache when he went to New York. His trips to New York were the only times he ever ate lobster. He was allergic to it. Bright's Disease, uremic poisoning, tuberculosis, malaria, fevers and infections may cause headaches. There is a headache called the "hypertension" headache suffered by patients with high blood pressure. "Nervous" headache may be just the result of a busy, busy day when you are trying to accomplish more than is humanly possible and this in the midst of strain, noise and hurry. The obvious preventive is relaxation and a reorganization or change of work to eliminate the strain.

Our Suggestions

If you still have headaches and have eliminated any of the above as possible causes, we'd suggest:

1. Check on your emotional state. See if you can discover whether some actual frustration or repressed "hate" or intolerable personal dilemma is responsible. If so, either resign yourself to chronic headaches, or change the mental attitude or situation, no matter how impossible

it may seem at first glance. You may need the help of a psychiatric counsellor.

2. Correct your posture. There are many good books on this subject available at your local library. Check on your posture often while you are working, and guard against working in a position that cramps or tires you.

3. Take better care of your eyes. During an evening of television rest your eyes frequently and be sure you are sitting far enough away from the screen. Don't read or work in inadequate light. Get plenty of vitamin A and vitamin C in your diet—two food elements that are mighty important for eye health.

4. If you have violent headaches that resist all diagnosis, write to Dartmouth for information about aniseikonia.

5. Read up on blood sugar. Ask your library to get a copy of Dr. Abrahamson's book on the subject.

Heart Disease—Coronary Thrombosis Causes

By W. J. McCORMICK, M.D., Toronto, Canada

(This article appeared originally in *Clinical Medicine* for July, 1952. In some places where medical terminology was used, we interpreted Dr. McCormick's remarks so that they would be understandable to the lay reader. Dr. McCormick has done outstanding work on vitamins C and B in the treatment and prevention of many different diseases.)

Since the beginning of the present century diseases of the heart and blood vessels have been steadily assuming a more prominent place in our vital statistics, and in this group we find coronary thrombosis in the lead. (Coronary thrombosis is the formation of a blood clot in the coronary artery leading to the heart. We sometimes call it a "stroke.") So rapidly has the mortality from this disease risen in recent years that it is now the principal cause of death for all past fifty years of age.

For some time the increasing toll taken by heart disease has been attributed to the increasing tempo and stress of modern life. Recently, however, a more attractive explanation has attained general acceptance—the theory that our aging population, due to the average increase in life span, results in more people reaching the age in which diseases due to senility take their toll. Both these theories are conducive to medical complacency. A striking example of this tendency was manifested in a public lecture in Toronto recently by a leading health authority in the statement that "there are few more creditable things for a city to have than a high cardiac death rate." In further explanation the speaker said,

"The city with the best public health always has the highest cardiac death rate, because the one-hoss-shay has to give out sometime and it is the most natural way to pass out between 60 and 70," the implication being that in such a city a larger number of people must have lived to the age of 60 or more.

Unfortunately, however, this specious theory does not harmonize with the facts for the following reasons: 1. Coronary thrombosis, the form of heart disease chiefly reponsible for the rising mortality, is not a senile disease, since it takes most of its victims between the ages of 45 and 55 and not a few below the age of 40. In the case of the "one-hoss-shay" it "went to pieces all at once and nothing first." 2. This theory does not explain the unprecedented increase in heart disease relative to pneumonia and cancer, both of which it has superseded as cause of death in recent years. Neither does it explain the higher female incidence relative to that of the male, which will be referred to later. 3. While it is true that the average span of life has doubled in the last half century, this has been accomplished mainly by reduction in infant and child mortality. The toll of degenerative diseases of middle life, however, has not beeen reduced or postponed. Accordingly, post-65 life expectancy has only slightly increased. 4. The rate of increase in heart disease, particularly coronary thrombosis, has been disproportionately greater than the rate of aging of our population. Vital statistics of deaths of American physicians from 1933 to 1940 inclusive, indicate a rise in cardiac deaths from 33 per cent to 41 per cent of total deaths. Obviously the aging of the medical profession in this short time could not possibly account for such an increase, particularly the relatively higher increase in coronary deaths from three per cent to 19 per cent in this same period. Neither is it reasonable to believe that improved methods in diagnosis could have brought about such a change in so short a time, since the electrocardiographic method of diagnosis has now been in use for fully forty years and physicians as a rule have consultations with leading specialists in their own illnesses.

Study of Coronary Thrombosis Group

In an effort to discover the nature of this insidious causal factor I have made a survey by means of a questionnaire mailed to the widows or next of kin of middle-aged males who have recently died suddenly in the Toronto district, assuming that many of these would be coronary thrombosis cases. It was thought that the widows of these men would be best qualified to supply detailed information regarding their personal living habits—diet, exercise, use of narcotics, age, height, weight, etc. After ruling out deaths due to accidents and infectious diseases there were 269 replies suitable for tabulation. Of this number 151 were found to be cases in which a definite diagnosis of coronary thrombosis had been made by the attending physician or coroner. The remaining 118 cases included non-coronary heart disease, cerebral hemorrhage, cancer, anemia, nephritis, diabetes, etc.

In the coronary thrombosis group (151 cases) the average age at death was found to be 52 years, the average weight was 168 pounds. Sixteen were 200 pounds and over, one being 295. Ninety-four per cent were reported as tobacco smokers and six per cent as non-smokers at the time of death. A further check on the latter elicited the fact that a number of them had discontinued smoking a month or so before death, either on their own volition or on medical advice. Fifty-eight per cent of the smokers were rated as "heavy smokers" and 42 per cent as moderate or light smokers. Fifty-five per cent were addicted to alcohol as well. The average age of the heavy smokers at death was 47 years, that of the moderate and light smokers was 58½ years, that of those addicted to tobacco and alcohol was 47½ years (apparently the addition of alcohol, as advised by some writers to counteract the vasoconstrictor effect of nicotine, did not prolong life in these cases). The two youngest in this group, who died at 27 and 29 years, were heavy users of both tobacco and alcohol.

In the non-coronary group as a whole (118 cases) the average age at death was 60½ years. Sixty-six per cent of this group were addicted to tobacco and 29 per cent to alcohol as well.

Nutritional Habits of These Thrombosis Cases

Regarding the nutritional habits of the coronary-thrombosis group, it was found that as a whole there was a marked tendency to deficient intake of the B and C vitamins, in that nearly all were predominantly white-bread users and low in their use of fresh fruits and salads. The ingestion of milk was also sub-optimal, the principal liquids being tea, coffee, alcoholic and soft drinks.

The most striking feature in the above findings and that providing the most obvious etiological clue (that is, clue as to its cause) is the higher incidence of tobacco smoking and the use of alcohol in the coronary-thrombosis group, 94 per cent and 55 per cent respectively, as compared to the combined non-coronary group, 66 per cent and 29 per cent respectively. The breakdown of the age figures in the coronary-thrombosis group also provides evidence of the precipitating effect of narcotic addiction in this disease, the average ages at death being as follows: Forty-seven and one-half years for those addicted to both tobacco and alcohol, 52 years for those addicted to tobacco only and 59½ years for those not addicted to either. The definite correlation of the life span and the degree of narcotic addiction is also most significant, the heavier addiction being associated with a corresponding drop in average age at death.

The Role of Tobacco in Thrombotic Diseases

A correlated study of other thrombotic disease processes may help to clarify the possible . . . role of tobacco. Another form of arterial thrombosis, known as . . . Buerger's disease, has long been recognized as being . . . related to tobacco smoking. Silbert says, "The importance of tobacco as the exciting cause of this disease must be stressed. The evidence in support of this contention is overwhelming. In over a thousand cases of this disease studied by the writer a typical case in a non-smoker has never been seen. Cessation of smoking regularly arrests the disease, while continued use of tobacco is coincident with progression."

(Dr. McCormick then explains exactly what happens in the human being who has just raised a cigarette to his lips. When the nicotine encounters the sympathetic nervous system the adrenal glands release a substance into the body, which in turn produces a release of blood sugar from the liver, resulting in temporary hyperglycemia—or too much sugar in the blood. What happens then? The sudden increase in blood sugar is a warning to other organs that a poison is present and must be dealt with. Digestion, and stomach and intestinal movement are slowed down, blood shifts from abdominal organs to heart and lungs, causing increased heart action and respiration. The spleen discharges extra red blood corpuscles and platelets which increase the oxygen-carrying ability and the coagulability of the blood—as an emergency protection in case of hemorrhage. This increase in the blood-coagulation rate may have a great deal to do with the development of thromboses, especially considering how often this reaction is repeated in an individual who smokes steadily, day after day and year after year. Dr. McCormick tells us that a similar reaction occurs in post-operative conditions, as a result of the shock, loss of blood and effect of the anesthetic. This reaction would explain the frequency of thrombosis after operations.)

Effect of Tobacco on Nutrition

There is still another approach to this problem—the indirect effect of tobacco and narcotics in general upon the nutritional status, particularly the vitamin reserve and the possible influence of such effect upon the development of thrombosis. Quastel and Wheatley have shown that narcotics (which would include tobacco and alcohol) greatly increase the bodily requirement of vitamin B1, thus increasing the tendency to deficiency of same. The tissue concentration of vitamin C is also known to be rapidly depleted in toxic conditions (whether their source is within or without the body). When thus utilized, less of the vitamin remains for physiological needs, thus accentuating the (unhealthy) effect. To illustrate, I have found in clinical research that the smoking of one cigarette increases the bodily requirement of vitamin C by 25 milligrams, or the vitamin C content of one orange, thus precluding the likelihood of any heavy smoker ever attaining an optimal tissue level of this vitamin. Recently Patterson has called attention to the low vitamin C status of coronary thrombosis cases. He found that 81 per cent of such cases in hospital practice had a subnormal blood-plasma level as compared to 55.8 per cent in a corresponding group of general public-ward patients. He . . . suggests that patients with this disease be assured of an adequate intake of this vitamin (C).

Cholesterol and Hardening of the Arteries

(Dr. McCormick reminds us that a discussion of hardening of the arteries and heart disease would not be complete without some mention of cholesterol, since recent research has shown a definite relationship between this substance and the disease. It is quite true that a high level of cholesterol in the blood is generally associated with heart disease, but it seems quite possible, says Dr. McCormick, that this condition may be caused by an inability to assimilate this substance in the body rather than too much of it in one's food.

A deficiency of the B and C vitamins may result in liver damage so that the cholesterol cannot be assimilated by the body. Patients afflicted with high cholesterol blood content are usually advised not to eat liver, eggs and other cholesterol-rich foods. On the other hand, when patients are given a diet that contains ample vitamin B and C, and then are given desiccated or cooked whole liver, there is usually a dramatic decrease in the blood cholesterol, in spite of this much larger intake.)

Sex Distribution of Coronary Thrombosis

Relative to the predominant male-sex incidence of coronary thrombosis Levine says: "The sex distribution of this disease is most striking—a ratio of three and one-half males to one female. It is difficult to explain the great frequency of coronary disease in the male. One may ascribe it to the greater amount of work that men do, although some might question this and maintain that the humble housewife does just as much work in her home. . . . Another factor that may be mentioned is the possible role of tobacco. . . . Certainly the consumption of tobacco has been in the past almost entirely confined to men, and has been one of the few acquired differences in habit between the sexes. It is therefore logical to suspect this habit of playing some possible role in producing such a male preponderance of susceptibility to this disease. A more definite answer may be apparent before long if the coming generation of women continue the smoking habit that seems to have become so general." This forecast was made in 1929 and already the anticipated answer seems to be in evidence. Prior to 1929 the sex ratio of incidence of coronary thrombosis has been estimated as high as five males to one female. However, recent figures supplied by the Toronto Health Department indicate that the present ratio in this disease is two males to one female. Apparently the rising tide of tobacco addiction in women is exercising a leveling action on the sex ratio of incidence of this form of heart disease.

Tobacco Consumption in Relation to Coronary Thrombosis

It should further be noted that the rising incidence of coronary and other forms of thrombotic disease has been closely concurrent with the increase in tobacco consumption. Cigarette consumption in Canada has risen from approximately five billion in 1935 to 18 billion in 1951, an increase of over 350 per cent while in the same time the population has increased about 50 per cent. During this same period the incidence of coronary thrombosis, Buerger's disease and post-operative thrombosis has shown a closely proportionate increase. A closely parallel situation prevails in United States where the tobacco per capita consumption is about double that of Canada. One thing is certain, there has been no such increase in the consumption of cholesterol-rich foods by the populace at large during the same period, as would be expected if the cholesterol-ingestion—cause of this disease is sustained. On the contrary, statistics indicate a noticeable drop in the per capita consumption of such foods (milk, butter, eggs and meat) during the period in question.

In recent years much stress has been given to the deleterious effects of involuntary inhalation of toxic elements in industrial smoke and fumes ("smog"), tetra-ethyl lead in gasoline, DDT, etc. These are all undoubtedly pathogenic, but with the redeeming feature that they are usually taken in a high degree of atmospheric dilution. On the contrary, little or no attention is given to the voluntary inhalation of toxic fumes in concentrated form in the smoking of over 400 billion cigarettes annually by the people of America. We "strain at a gnat and swallow a 'camel'."

Heart Disease and Diet

By ERNEST KLEIN, M.D.

It is early in the morning and I have just had one of those tragic cases of coronary thrombosis. The man was 46 years old and his wife called me up because her husband, who had always been in perfect health, did not feel well. It was about 5 a.m. When I arrived, the patient was dead. He had had a periodic check-up once a year in his place of employment. I tried to find out what had happened. The periodic check-up did not reveal any heart disease.

It happened that the man, a clerk in the Stock Exchange, bought a new home a few weeks before. Since his new house was just around the corner from the old one, he carried most of their belongings himself to the new house. Last night, after dinner, still in perfect health, he went bowling.

To start at the beginning, let us describe just what happened inside this patient's body before he died. A blood clot closed up the heart artery —that is, the artery that supplies the heart with blood. Fifty per cent of the victims of a "heart attack" (the common name for coronary thrombosis or infarction) survive the attack. Those who survive have a damaged heart muscle. Many people blame the heart itself in cases of "heart attack." This is a wrong conception. The heart is usually in good condition. Generally the blood is at fault. The blood normally flows easily and steadily through all the arteries and veins, carrying nourishment to all parts of the body. If this flow of nourishment stops for some reason, the tissues starve. If the flow stops entirely, they die. In most parts of the body, if the flow of blood stops, another blood vessel tries to replace the disordered one, so that the blood can continue to flow to the starving part.

There is no replacement for the artery that flows into the heart. If this is closed by a blood clot, the heart tissue starves. There are, however, many branches of the coronary (or heart) artery. If a blood clot slips into the coronary artery the result depends on whether it blocks the main artery or one of the many branches. If it blocks the main artery partially, the attack is not fatal. If it blocks it completely, it is. If it blocks a small branch artery, then the part of the heart that receives nourishment from this branch dies. The name for this is "occlusion of the coronary artery" or "coronary occlusion." Another name for it is "infarction."

One of the unsolved mysteries of the whole process is why the blood clots or coagulates inside the veins. And one of the common treatments for a patient surviving a heart attack is to give him anti-coagulants—that is, drugs that will prevent his blood from clotting too readily.

Now going back in my own personal history, let me tell you of my first observations concerning the blood, which resulted in my conclusions as to how to prevent thromboses or blood clots.

As an admitting physician during the last war I had the chance to observe many coronary occlusion cases. It was routine to take a sample of the patient's blood and examine it. When I took samples of the blood from coronary thrombosis patients, I found that it coagulated so rapidly that I could not get it out of the little glass instrument I was using—a pipette. It stuck to the walls of the pipette so closely that I could not remove it even with peroxide. The pipettes were ruined and I had to discard them all. I made this observation on about 60 or 70 patients. When I eventually found a way to push the blood out of the pipette so that I could examine it, I was surprised to find that the hemoglobin was in all cases up to 150 Sahli. And the coagulation time was only a few seconds, whereas normally it is about two minutes.

To explain the above, Sahli is the name of a physician who discovered a way of measuring the hemoglobin. Hemoglobin is the red coloring matter in the blood—a very complex substance containing iron. Because it readily holds oxygen, the greater part of the oxygen in the blood is combined with the hemoglobin. This oxygen is distributed to the various organs of the body and is re-supplied to the blood as it passes through the lungs.

The simple apparatus needed to make the Sahli test can be handled by any physician or lab technician. In normal individuals the Sahli test is about 85. But in these coronary thrombosis cases it was up to 150! And, in addition, the time it took the blood of these patients to clot was only a few seconds, compared to the normal two minutes. My conclusion was that the high hemoglobin number together with the short clotting time may be important factors in coronary thrombosis. I believe that my observation could be used to prevent coronary thrombosis, if you can discover the abnormal thickness of the blood before the clotting starts.

Among patients having coronary thrombosis, there are, of course, exceptions. Those suffering from severe changes of the inside walls of the blood vessels may not have a high hemoglobin number and may suffer from a clot anyway caused by the condition of the blood vessel walls. Then, too, patients who have been given anti-coagulant drugs for a former heart attack will not have the high Sahli hemoglobin number and the short coagulation time, for the drugs will have prevented this.

In order to work further on my theory, I went to the blood donation center of the famous Post-Graduate (now University) Hospital in New

York where I was put in charge of testing the hemoglobin, the condition of the heart and so forth, of all donors. For three years I had the opportunity of examining the blood of perhaps several hundred people a day. And I had the chance to get their cooperation in testing out various diets to find which diet would reduce a high Sahli number and lengthen a short coagulation time. At the end of a few days or weeks I could once again test their blood and determine whether or not the diet had accomplished what I wanted.

I came to the conclusion that ⅓ natural fruit juice, ⅔ water, some sugar (according to the taste of the individual) and a small amount of salt (to retain the fluid in the body) are the most suitable liquid foods to drop the hemoglobin number as quickly as possible to the normal level. (*Editor's Note:* It goes without saying that we do not believe in adding sugar to anything least of all fruit juice, or salt, which we believe is harmful in the amounts in which we usually eat it.)

At the same time, everything that is dry, like bread, potatoes, cake and so forth should be restricted, because this kind of food seems to use up body fluid. The proportion of fruit juice and water can be changed to ¼ juice and ¾ water or ½ juice and ½ water, according to the taste of the patient. Pure fruit juice or plain water seem not to be of any help. Water is not retained by the body for a longer period and concentrated fruit juice seems not to agree with most of the test persons if it is taken in the amount necessary to "thin-down" the blood.

All the foods that build up the blood in anemic patients should be restricted or eliminated if we want to get the opposite effect—that of reducing hemoglobin. Then, too, meals with too much steak, liver and eggs push the hemoglobin number still higher.

In January of 1949 I decided to present my observations to the staff of the Post-Graduate Hospital, but I found out that there was no way for me to do this. I might either publish my findings without any support or approval, or forget about everything I had done in the past years to fight coronary occlusion and to find a way to prevent the most dreadful disease of our times. I decided to write a short article and take the risk of being fired from the hospital. I believed that it was more important to attract the attention of progressive physicians who could help me finish the work I considered so important than to keep my discovery a secret and keep my job at the hospital.

After four months the committee of physicians of the Medical Society of New York accepted a very short version of my article and published it in *New York Medicine* for May 20, 1949. This is a reputable medical journal of the highest standing. On May 21, 1949, I was fired from my position at the hospital. My daughter, who also worked there, was fired, too. This is the story of my contribution, or let me say attempted contribution, to the fight against the most successful killer—heart disease.

How to recognize the danger and prevent the clotting of the blood by thinning it down to the normal concentration (85 Sahli) is the important thing for the prevention of coronary thrombosis. Diagnostic laboratories should be located all over the country and periodic tests of the "thickness" of the blood will reveal the danger of clotting before it is too late. The hemoglobin number (Sahli) is one of the most important parts of this laboratory test, the prothrombin (coagulation) time is the other. Either test can give us a warning signal that clotting of the blood may occur. Loss of body fluid may occur in many different ways. Two of these are perspiration (many heart attacks in the hot weather) and too little intake of fluids to replace the loss. If the blood concentration is high, the chance of being a victim of coronary thrombosis is greater.

To return to the patient whose story opened this article—in all probability his blood concentration was high. The heavy activity of moving his furniture from one house to the other caused him to perspire freely, depriving his body of fluid. Later when he went bowling, he lost more fluid and the hemoglobin of his blood probably shot up to 135 or 145 Sahli—the danger point at which one may develop thrombosis. It need not be in the heart artery. A clot in a brain artery causes sudden paralysis of an arm or leg or loss of speech, depending on which part of the brain is supplied with blood by the affected artery.

Had this patient been given laboratory examinations showing the two factors I have mentioned—hemoglobin and clotting time of the blood, he might have "thinned" his blood to such an extent that he would not have had the thrombosis. The proper diet for him then would have been vegetarian without any starch or with very little starch and an additional eight to ten glasses of the water-fruit-juice mixture. You may ask why water or tea would not fill the bill in a person whose hemoglobin level is high. Water quenches the thirst but is eliminated into the bladder within 20 to 60 minutes and does not "thin down" the blood for a longer period. The blood holds the fruit-juice-water mixture as a liquid food and keeps it to thin down the blood. The volume of blood increases. This can be shown by determining the blood volume, by taking the hemoglobin number or by observing the weight of the patient. A drop from the dangerous 140-150 to the normal 85 in hemoglobin may take place in some patients within a few days or weeks or it may take years. Even if all or nearly all starches are eliminated from the diet, even if all meats and eggs are strictly avoided, the weight increases 2 to 6 pounds. This weight increase must be due to the increase of blood volume caused by the intake of plenty of fruits, plenty of salads and plenty of water-fruit-juice mixture.

In the individuals at the blood donation center who tried out my vegetarian-fruit diet I found that there was a drop of 30-40 points in the hemoglobin. Another group was asked to eat nothing but steak, liver and eggs. Liquids were mostly eliminated. Small sips of water were permitted. The hemoglobin number went up quickly and the coagulation time was rapidly shortened. If persons of this group were sent to a Turkish bath, the perspiration robbed the circulatory system of body fluid and the hemoglobin number went sky-high within a short period. Frequent heart attacks while in Turkish baths or while engaged in strenuous exertion could thus be explained.

I also discovered that starchy foods like bread, cake, cereal, cookies, pretzels and so forth take away body fluid and are to be considered harmful unless the intake of this kind of food is compensated for by the intake of plenty of liquids. The more cake, cookies, etc. you eat, the more fruit-juice-water mixture you have to drink to prevent dryness in your circulation. This dryness causes an increased concentration of the blood thereby raising the hemoglobin number and causing a decrease in the blood volume. The decrease in blood volume causes the blood cells to move closer together and this increased concentration of the blood cells causes the high hemoglobin number and the shortened coagulation time of the blood. This favors clotting of the blood.

To summarize, coronary occlusion or thrombosis is preventable. The thickness of the blood may be measured with the hemoglobinometer (the Sahli test) and so be discovered before the heart attack. It may be prevented by using liquid food (natural fruit juices plus water) for the purpose of thinning down the blood.

This mixture must be taken six to ten times a day. Fruits and salads should form the largest part of the solid food. Meat and eggs should be reduced. Starches of any kind take away body fluid when they are digested, thereby causing further concentration of the blood. They should, therefore, be restricted or temporarily eliminated.

(Editor's Note): We have presented Dr. Klein's article as an instance of the kind of observations and deductions that many and many a physician has probably made throughout a long and busy practice. We presented it to show the difficulties faced by such physicians when they try to get help for continuing their research, even when the subject under investigation is as important as coronary thrombosis. We do not believe these conclusions are final—and we are sure Dr. Klein would be the first to agree with us on this. Surely a subject as new and startling as this needs a great deal more laboratory work and closely-controlled experimentation before we know the final answer. But the point is that Dr. Klein apparently cannot get this kind of research help. How many other would-be researchers are in the same fix? And what can be done about it?

We have suggested to Dr. Klein that he try vitamin E therapy in conjunction with his diet for patients whose tests indicate that they may have too high a Sahli number and too short a coagulation time, and hence may be heading for coronary occlusion. The effectiveness of vitamin E therapy in heart cases has been demonstrated in many thousands of heart patients. Recently we reviewed a book on this subject—*Vitamin E in Cardiovascular Therapy* by Evan and Wilfrid Shute of the Shute Clinic in London, Ontario, Canada. The book, which is "must-reading" for your physician, is available from the Ryerson Press, Toronto, Canada.

Heart Disease and International Uses of Vitamin E

Every time we mention in these pages the use of vitamin E in the treatment and prevention of heart disease, we receive more mail from readers than any other articles bring us. This is certainly understandable, for heart disease is today's number one killer and any one of us has very good reason to fear it. Formerly thought of as a degenerative disease attacking only those well past middle age, heart disease now claims for its victims many persons in their thirties and forties, as well as a frightening number of teen-agers and persons in their twenties.

The Bulletin from the Vitamin E Society of Canada brings us news of cures worked by the powerful alphatocopherol (vitamin E) in other countries. It is an impressive story, well worth carrying with you to show to dubious friends, who may doubt the potency of vitamin E because it sounds too easy. "What," they may say, "a mere vitamin given in its natural form, can cure phlebitis, Buerger's disease, heart disease, thrombosis? Impossible. You are being taken in."

Well, folks, here is the record. And at the risk of cluttering up our pages with a series of long, academic-looking words and foreign words, we are giving you the full names of authors, periodicals, volume numbers, dates and countries from which this information comes. If your own physician should tell you he doubts that vitamin E can really be of any benefit in heart and vascular conditions, perhaps he is sincerely unaware that so much research has been done. Perhaps he does not really know what wonders have been worked in recent years with vitamin E. Physicians are busy men with little time to study. But they are receptive to new ideas if they come from dependable sources. If he is doubtful, show your physician these references. Ask him to write to the Shute brothers in Canada (pioneers in vitamin E therapy) and obtain even more information.

In the *American Journal of Physiology,* volume 153, page 127, 1948, K. L. Zierler, D. Grob and J. L. Lilienthal describe laboratory experiments in which they discovered that vitamin E has a profound effect on the blood, especially the clotting of the blood. It has a strong anti-clotting effect both in laboratory experiments and in the veins and arteries of human beings. Now there is a special natural substance in the blood called heparin which is made in the liver, whose job it is to prevent the coagulation of blood. In their tests these scientists found that all action of vitamin E on the blood takes place regardless of how much or how little heparin is present in the blood stream of the patients. So there can be no doubt but that the anti-coagulating action is the result of the vitamin E and nothing else.

In an Italian journal, *Bollettino Societa Chirurgia* volume 18, page 155 (1948) R. Castagna and G. Impallomeni report on seven patients with phlebitis (inflammation of a vein) and one 71 year old woman who had had an ulcer measuring five by three inches on her lower leg. The phlebitis responded dramatically to the use of vitamin E alone. The woman patient's ulcer healed in 26 days. The authors have also used vitamin E in treatment of vascular disease (any disease of the blood vessels) and for "strokes." They tell us that in thrombophlebitis (inflammation of the vein in which a blood clot is involved) the improvement by using vitamin E is extremely rapid. In addition, they say, treatment with vitamin E does not require a rigid blood control as do other medications.

Reports From Brazil, Norway, Germany and France

From Brazil (Publication of the O Hospital for July 1949) D. de Olivera describes two cases of phlebitis, one during a pregnancy and one following childbirth. In both cases fever fell rapidly and there was no recurrence of the disease when the first patient had her child. The conservative British medical publication, *The Lancet* volume 2, page 132, 1949, carries an article by A. M. Boyd, A. H. James, G. W. H. and R. P. Jepson saying that clinical results with vitamin E are far better than any obtained with any other treatment in cases of obliterative diseases of the blood vessels. It can be used most successfully for the relief of cramps in the calves of the legs. "May we repeat," say these authors, "that it is our considered opinion that the clinical observations so far made warrant the continued use of vitamin E therapy."

O. Mantero, B. Rindi and L. Trozzi, writing in the Italian magazine *Attivita Congresso degli Cardiologia,* Stresa, May, 1948, discuss five cases of acute and subacute phlebitis which were rapidly healed by vitamin E therapy. J. H. Kay, S. B. Weiss, G. H. and A. Ochsner mention in *Surgery,* volume 28, page 124, 1950, four cases of phlebitis treated only with vitamin E given orally in which "inflammation subsided and the swelling disappeared."

A Norwegian physician, H. Sturup, writing in *Nordisk Medicin,* vol. 43, page 721, 1950, tells us he has seen a number of cases of thrombosis helped by vitamin E therapy. He discusses in detail the case of a 33-year old patient who had chronic phlebitis of the left leg, five years after an operation. This patient was not even confined to bed, but took vitamin E daily and within six days the pain and swelling disappeared.

The Annals of Surgery, vol. 131, page 652, 1950, reports that vitamin E and calcium appear to be helpful in the treatment of vascular diseases. Dr. A. W. Allen of Boston, commenting on this article tells us that he has used vitamin E on a number of patients and can report that 50 of these who were "vulnerable"—that is susceptible—to thrombosis escaped this serious condition. This seems to us particularly important, for in these cases vitamin E was used to prevent rather than to cure, and fifty lucky patients continued in good health. Dr. J. C. Owings of Baltimore comments that he has treated many leg ulcers due to phlebitis with a combination of rutin and vitamin E, all of which stayed healed, so long as the patient continued to take the medication.

Postgraduate Medicine, volume 10, page 794, 1951, carries a report by A. Ochsner who believes that vitamin E is the best preventive of a blood clot, because it is a natural substance, so there is no hazard involved in its use. The use of other anti-coagulants is dangerous and tying off veins should not be practiced because it will not protect against the detachment of clots. He states that he does not know whether vitamin E combined with calcium is the final answer, but adds that it seems to be best, because it is perfectly safe and does not bring any danger of producing bleeding.

Medical Thesis, published in Paris, Number 471, 1951, quotes a physician as saying he has found vitamin E and calcium useful for preventing blood clots after surgery. R. Bauer, writing in *Wiene Klinisch Wochenschrift* a German publication, volume 31, page 552, 1951, says Dr. Ochsner's method can be used successfully in reducing one tenth of the usual incidence of thrombosis and should perhaps be used to decrease the danger of clot in coronary thrombosis. M. Reifferscheid and P. Matis writing in *Medizinische Welt* Germany, volume 20, page 1168, 1951, announce they have found vitamin E to be definitely protective against vascular clotting. They found that large daily doses were necessary. They describe five cases of diabetic gangrene, nine cases of Raynauds disease (a gangrenous condition) seven cases of Dupuytren's contracture (contraction of tissues under the skin of the palm) and 14 cases of hemorrhagic (bleeding) diseases all yielded to treatment with vitamin E.

Dr. W. E. Crump and E. F. Heiskell, writing in the *Texas State Journal of Medicine,* Volume 11, 1952, agree that the use of the regular anti-coagulants for routine prevention of clotting diseases in patients after operations is too dangerous for general use. In most cases where these medicines are used, as many patients die of hemorrhage as might have died of clots and 16 per cent of other cases develop non-fatal bleeding complications. When vitamin E was used as treatment by these physicians no bleeding occurred and only minor side reactions were noticed. When cases of phlebitis occurred during treatment, they were mild and had no complications. There were no lung clots, fatal or non-fatal, in patients being treated with vitamin E. Dr. Terrel Speed, commenting on these statements, says "considerable evidence is accumulating to substantiate the value of this therapy. However I have gradually expanded its use and now it is used routinely in essentially the same group of cases mentioned by the authors. If the promising preliminary results are borne out, relative protection against one of the most feared complications of surgery will have been obtained."

Two German physicians, S. Schmid writing in *Wiene Klinisch Wochenschrift* volume 64 and H. Wagner writing in *Aertzliche Wochenschrift* volume 7, page 248, 1952, say they have achieved good results in treating thrombosis with vitamin E.

The Shute Brothers Ask for Fair Consideration for Vitamin E

In spite of this kind of evidence that has accumulated in increasing quantity over the years, some medical journals are still taking pot shots at vitamin E therapy and spreading doubt as to its effectiveness. Such an article appeared in the *British Medical Journal* for December, 1952. It was answered promptly by Dr. Evan S. and Wilfrid E. Shute, the two Canadian doctors who have specialized in the use of vitamin E in the treatment of vascular cases. Say these two doctors: "The leading article on 'The Therapeutic Uses of Vitamin E' (December 20, 1952) certainly calls for comment by us, the proponents of the use of alpha-tocopherol in cardiovascular disease.

"Such an article might conceivably have been written in 1948 or 1949. However, the picture has changed so rapidly since that time that your leading article now simply does not reflect the findings of investigators in this field. This is best illustrated perhaps by the current issue of our medical journal, *The Summary,* which contains the abstracts of 122 reports which have appeared in the medical literature supporting our original contentions. It seems that alphatocopherol shares with

Christianity both its beneficence and the observation that those who say it has failed have rarely tried it. Since the American Aristotles first condemned it, too many doctors have dropped a pebble from their own towers to make that condemnation stick.

"Briefly, our current *Summary* records that 17 reports have supported us in the use of alphatocopherol for the menopause; 5 in its use for nephritis; 6 for kraurosis vulvae; 4 for capillary permeability; 4 for purpura; 5 for vascular dilatation; 11 for Buerger's disease; 10 for vascular sclerosis; 15 for thrombosis; 3 for muscular power; 20 for indolent ulcers; 14 for diabetes; 4 for Roentgen tissue damage; 4 for incipient gangrene; 2 for wound healing. Finally 46 reports have supported us in the use of alphatocopherol for heart disease.

"It is difficult to believe that all these investigators have duplicated an error. Certainly it is cavalier to dismiss such work in one paragraph. Fortunately, our forthcoming book should help to keep the record straight and we will recommend it to your perusal. Also, as Auden, one of your poets, has said,

'One notices, if one will trust one's eyes,
The shadow cast by language upon truth.'

Wilfrid E. Shute
Evan V. Shute"

In order not to cast any further "shadows upon truth" in our language about vitamin E and to clear up confusion in the minds of some readers about the proper use of vitamin E, let us review some of what we have said in previous chapters. In cases of actual heart or vascular disease, vitamin E is used in large doses as medicine.

If you have no difficulty with your heart or circulation, we suggest that you take vitamin E and/or wheat germ oil so that you will at all times have an abundance of vitamin E and will run no risk of suffering a deficiency. A minimum daily requirement of vitamin E has not been set in this country, so no one can tell you officially how much you should take every day. Follow the dosage recommended on the bottle in which your wheat germ oil or vitamin E comes to you. Considering that heart patients in a weakened condition take enormous doses of pure vitamin E, there is little chance that you can get too much. And if you habitually eat products made from white flour from which the germ has been removed, if your diet is short on vegetable oils and green leafy vegetables, there's every reason to believe that you are not now getting enough vitamin E for full protection.

A *Prevention* Reader Gives Her Experiences With Vitamin E

Finally, here is a completely unsolicited letter from a *Prevention* reader who did just what we suggested above, when she discovered that she was beginning to have trouble with her heart. Please note that this is not a miraculous, overnight cure. Mrs. Paetz is still taking vitamin E and will for perhaps a long time to come. But note, too, the wonderful change from despair to hope, note the improvement, the confidence, the well being.

"Dear Mr. Rodale:

"I had always thought I was pretty healthy because the only times I had ever the occasion to see a doctor was for physicals for positions I held, my pre-marital examination and my pre- and post-natal care when I carried my one and only baby, now a doll of eight years.

"Then about two years ago I began having some pretty gruesome symptoms: chest pains, extreme heaviness in the chest, difficulty in taking a deep breath, extreme weakness and undefined fear, such as I'd never known. I was so afraid—of what I don't know—that I would not go twenty feet from my door unless my mother (who lives on the first floor) or some member of my family went with me. All this from a gal who used to take her baby miles from home both in the baby carriage and in a bus or taxi!

"At first, although I was very ill, I procrastinated—didn't want my husband to know how really bad I felt, and passed most of it off as 'nerves.' I took Nervine by the bottleful and of course, since it deadened some of my senses, I did get a little relief. Then when that didn't work any more, I attributed my aches, pains, feelings of pressure and suffocation, etc., to fifteen pounds I had put on since marriage. But the day came when I couldn't procrastinate any longer. I went to a doctor who had been highly recommended. After hearing all my symptoms, he immediately put me under the fluoroscope. Fortunately for me he found my lungs and heart of normal size and seemingly normal in their functions. But, when he examined my heart under the stethoscope, his very expression changed and he asked 'Did you ever know that you have a very loud heart murmur? It's probably something you carried over from childhood.' A loud heart murmur! And it accounted for my awful symptoms. Then I remembered my mother telling me that my brothers and I had had only one childhood disease, but it was a bad one—scarlet fever! (And just a year ago my little girl had scarlet fever too.) When I told the doctor what my mother had told me, he said, 'I'm sure your heart was damaged then, but now you'll just have to live with it. I'm going to give you some medication and some medicine to help you take off 15 pounds.'

"When I got home I took the mail from the mail box and one of the items was the August *Prevention*. Imagine my delight when I read the article titled 'Vitamin E, Cure for Heart Disease.' It wasn't till October of 1952 that I contacted Dr. Wilfrid E. Shute and on October 15, 1952, under his personal supervision began taking 90 milligrams of vitamin E daily, to be increased to 120 milligrams daily and later up to 300 milligrams. Of course, I had to be certain that my E came from entirely natural and not synthetic sources. During these first early weeks there were no dramatic results—but there certainly were about Thanksgiving. With extra guests, stress and strain, lots more work (especially for one in my condition) I should have been feeling it, as it were. Instead I was actually feeling swell! I was breathing normally and not gasping every time I did more than walk straight! I suddenly realized that I didn't have that terrible heavy feeling on my chest and that those vague aches and pains in my chest were gone. My heart had quieted down to the point where I was no longer conscious of my own heart beats, flutters and palpitations, simply because my heart was beating normally and I no longer had those other abnormal sensations. This I definitely attribute to taking vitamin E on Dr. Wilfrid E. Shute's advice.

"Also after having *Prevention* as a welcome guest in my home for over a year now, I realize the truths of the statements that our so-called 'wholesome good food' is not what it's cracked up to be, but filled with poisons and so forth to keep the color good, to improve the keeping qualities and to enrich those things that have been tampered with and contaminated in the first place. As a result, I bought wheat germ, wheat germ oil capsules, natural sea kelp for iodine, vitamin A and D capsules, fresh garlic and garlic perles, desiccated liver tablets and, because our water is heavily chlorinated, I now buy mineral water by the case. Of course it's expensive, but it all enabled me to throw the doctor's prescription down the drain and for me, it enabled me to regain a semblance of my former self, with vigor and vitality in spite of a 'heart' ailment. My little girl, too, has enjoyed a year of perfect health because of these natural food supplements, and, God willing, we'll go on this way.

"All I wish to add in conclusion is, I think you are doing a wonderful job, Mr. Rodale, in your *Prevention* and I thank God for men like you and Dr. Wilfrid E. Shute and his brother Dr. Evan Shute. I hope their days are without number. Yours very truly, Mrs. Robert J. Paetz, 1007 North 20th Avenue, Melrose Park, Illinois."

Heart Disease—More on Vitamin E

"'A dose of alpha tocopherol calculated by Skelton on the basis of his dog experiments and much higher than had ever been used in clinical medicine before, viz., 200 milligrams per day, was given to the patient, whose myocardial failure quickly vanished. . . . Encouraged by this I next treated my barber, who was dying from a recurrent coronary thrombosis and was in the terminal stages of heart failure with status antinosus. In three weeks' time he was playing the tympana in the local theatre. Next my mother's severe angina pectoris disappeared on alpha tocopherol therapy. Then Dr. Wilfrid Shute and I recalled our first successful angina patient of 1936 and the four other patients treated at that time. Accordingly, we began, with the assistance of Dr. Vogelsang, to collect the series of observations on cardiovascular patients that we may presume to say have changed the face of cardiology." So begins the saga of alpha tocopherol, vitamin E, as related by Dr. Evan Shute in the new book on the subject, *Alpha Tocopherol in Cardiovascular Disease,* published by the Shute Foundation for Medical Research, London, Ontario, Canada.

It is an amazing story—the story told in this book—exciting, inspiring, at times heroic, but also completely scientific and objective. The Shute brothers take the reader on a tour of their file of case histories—well over 10,000 patients treated for heart and vascular disorders with vitamin E. Of particular interest is a chapter by Dr. Wilfrid Shute on classical cardiac therapy—that is, the treatment other than vitamin E that has been used up to now for heart trouble. He discusses digitalis, quinidine, mercurial diuretics, and other drugs.

He quotes the President of the Texas Heart Association who said in the *Texas State Journal of Medicine* in 1951, "More than 637,000 deaths annually in the United States from cardiovascular disease account for about 44 per cent of all deaths. . . . When a physician makes a diagnosis of organic heart disease, he realizes that in the care of the patient he has begun a losing fight. In the earliest stages he offers general advice: 'Avoid strenuous activities; live sensibly; watch your weight; don't worry; the heart is a wonderful organ.' Before too long symptoms develop and the doctor braces the patient with digitalis or other drugs, restriction of usual activities, more rest and more encouragement. Again, before long, more urgent symptoms force a retreat. Bed rest, low sodium diet, diuretics and other well known measures are brought to the front and the line is stabilized. But not for long. All too soon increasing pressure bends the line and retreat begins again. Now there are left no more reserves—no more in the heart and no more in the hands of the one trying to help the heart. Then only surrender remains. Not infrequently the enemy strikes suddenly with overwhelming power, and surrender occurs before the doctor can mobilize his forces." How indeed could one better describe the usual case of heart disease treated by the usual methods?

This is, this *has to be,* the point of view of doctors using the time-honored prescriptions against this mysterious and deadly disease. How heart-warming and encouraging, then, to turn the page and find cheering, confident and convincing evidence of the marvelous effectiveness of vitamin E in heart and vascular cases! There are chapters in this book on the use of vitamin E in coronary sclerosis, coronary occlusion, rheumatic heart disease and hypertension. In the chapter "Tailoring the Dose" full instructions are given for using vitamin E in heart therapy, with descriptions of the various categories of patients and the characteristic problems they present in treatment.

Vitamin E to Prevent Heart Disorders

Furthermore, there are chapters on the cardiovascular aspects of diabetes, indolent ulcer, arteriosclerosis, thromboangitis, peripheral thrombosis, geriatrics (the study of old age) and finally a chapter on the use of vitamin E in veterinary medicine.

In the last chapter called "Hopeful Margins," Dr. Evan Shute lets his hopes and his dreams envisage the thoughts of the other benefits that may in time come to be proven from the use of vitamin E in ophthalmology, diabetes, peptic ulcer, varicose veins, intracranial birth damage, dermatology, hypertension. He also discusses the use of vitamin E as a prophylactic measure for preventing cardiovascular disease long before it rears its lethal head. He says, "We have long urged the prophylactic use of alpha tocopherol (vitamin E) rather than its administration only to people already showing cardiovascular disease. Habitually, food factors such as the vitamins prevent what they relieve. With that in mind the Profession has long urged the prevention of beriberi, peripheral neuritis, pellagra, scurvy, rickets and hemorrhagic disease of the newborn by the timely use of the appropriate vitamin—long before any frank evidence of scurvy or rickets or the rest could possibly appear. . . .

"Now one of the outstanding characteristics of the cardiovascular diseases . . . is that they are long-term degenerations or that chronic degenerations lay the groundwork for their appearance. . . . The average person in this country is exposed to a slow though much less pronounced deprivation of alpha tocopherol than is developed in the laboratory. . . . Whatever harmful results are thus produced may not reveal their existence for years—perhaps for decades. But just as these degenerations come on so slowly and insidiously as to escape recognition until well advanced, so appropriate preventative measures have years in which to get under way, and need never be radical or extensive if undertaken in time. It should demand but little in the way of substitution to remedy a food deficiency which is only partial.

". . . Why need alpha tocopherol be added to diets from which it first has been carefully extracted by modern milling processes? Why should the latter not be revised until foods are no longer alpha-tocopherol-deficient? This would seem to be the logical approach to the question and one in which the aid of such governmental agencies as the Pure Food and Drug Administration of the United States should be enlisted.

"It is commonly said that the average diet in this country contains adequate amounts of tocopherols. This is misleading. Such observations are based upon total tocopherol content, much of this consisting of the relatively inert gamma form (a second part of vitamin E as opposed to *alpha* tocopherol). But if one investigates alpha tocopherol values in the average diet, as two groups of workers have, the results are much different. It then appears that the average diet in Europe or America contains only 10 to 90 per cent of the normal requirement. This, too, is vitiated by intakes of rancid and unsaturated fats. It is obvious that slow alpha tocopherol starvation is the rule, not the exception, and is found among the wealthy quite as often as among the poor."

Buy This Book For Your Doctor

We are going to recommend whole heartedly that readers buy this book and, strangely enough, we do not care especially whether or not you read it. We have something else in mind. It is written for doctors in medical terminology. You will enjoy, as we did, reading the case histories it contains, reading the Introduction and the Historical Note at the beginning, and the last chapter which holds out such wonderful hope for future therapy with vitamin E. But your doctor is the person who should be reading this book. And we are going to recommend that you buy a copy for him. Yes, buy it and march in to his office with it in your hand.

It is a handsome book, well bound and illustrated in color. It cannot possibly be dismissed by your doctor with a wave of the hand and the pronouncement that vitamin E has been tried and has failed. This book shows that it has not failed. And if your doctor is actually interested in curing his heart patients, he will read this book. He has no choice. For, as the book itself points out, and as the Texas physician points out, there is no other therapy for heart patients. Vitamin E is the *only* treatment holding any promise of cure, the only treatment that can be given without the slightest fear of harmful side effects, and perhaps, best of all, the only treatment that can be used as a preventive measure.

For, as the Shute brothers show so eloquently in this book, heart disease can be prevented; worries about heart disease never need trouble you if you use vitamin E along with your food as your preventive.

If every reader who has heart disease and every reader who has a relative or friend with heart disease buys a copy of this book, presents it to his physician or heart specialist and insists that he uses this information at least in treating *him,* we are certain that no more powerful blow could be struck against the greatest killer of our time—heart disease.

Alpha Tocopherol (Vitamin E) in Cardiovascular Disease may be ordered from the Ryerson Press, 299 Queen Street West, Toronto, Canada. The price is seven dollars in Canadian money. But Dr. Shute tells us "There is one unfortunate thing that Americans should remember —their dollar is worth less than the current Canadian dollar. There is an amount of exchange which fluctuates, which might amount to about twenty cents per book; sometimes a little more, sometimes a little less." We suggest that you call your bank or post office and check on the current rate of exchange before making out your check.

Heart Disease and Views on the Shute System

Readers who bought the last book on this subject *Alpha Tocopherol (Vitamin E) in Cardiovascular Disease,* will be glad to know that there is another. The last book was directed to physicians.

The new book, *Your Heart and Vitamin E* (available from Devin-Adair, 25 E. 26th Street, New York City) is written for lay people—you and me. It explains carefully and in language that you can easily understand just what vitamin E is and how it works in your body. It takes up the various kinds of heart disease and disorders of the blood vessels—hypertension, rheumatic heart disease, angina pectoris, coronary heart disease, Buerger's Disease, kidney disease, hardening of the arteries, etc., and tells in every case just what vitamin E may be expected to do to prevent or to relieve such conditions.

Then the authors, Dr. Evan and Dr. Wilfrid Shute of the Shute Institute, London, Ontario, Canada, talk about the use of vitamin E in other disorders, not apparently related to heart trouble: sterility and miscarriages (Dr. Evan has specialized in this field) menstrual problems, pregnancy, eye diseases, old age, burns, scar tissue, diabetes and so on. In some cases the news is wonderfully encouraging. In others, vitamin E did not perform miracles, but it seemed to help, more than anything else had helped, at least. The Shute brothers are remarkably sane and objective about their enthusiasm for vitamin E, as true scientists should be. They do not promise miracles; they do not believe that vitamin E is a cure-all for everything. On the other hand, they base their enthusiasm on years of work with the vitamin and thousands of patients they have treated with it. So they have every right to enthuse. For they have seen patients for whom no other remedy could do anything come back to good health while taking vitamin E.

In addition to all the valuable information in *Your Heart and Vitamin E,* the book is written clearly and well. It is a real pleasure to read a book dealing with such a difficult subject and find it so entertaining and satisfying. If you happen to suffer from any of the complaints the authors discuss in the book, of course your interest will be heightened, for then they will be talking very directly about you and your problems.

How Should You Take Vitamin E?

We are truly sorry that we must take issue with several statements in the book, but we believe that readers should know that our point of view differs from that of the Shutes on several rather important questions. Not on the effectiveness of vitamin E therapy. We are in perfect agreement with that. But we find that we cannot go along with them in their suggestions *as to how each of us should benefit most from their discoveries.*

They say early in their book "We understand that there are hundreds if not thousands of people using vitamin E on their own, without the advice and guidance of their physicians. This we deplore." We have been urging readers to take vitamin E on their own and we shall continue to do so.

The Drs. Shute believe that only doctors can prescribe vitamin E and unless your doctor can and will prescribe it for you, you should not take it. This, we believe, leaves most of us just where we were before we read the book. For the vast majority of doctors, in the United States at least, will not or cannot prescribe vitamin E. Either they do not know enough about it or they believe that it is not effective. And the American Medical Association itself has taken the very conservative position that there is not sufficient evidence that vitamin E is of any help in heart and vascular conditions.

Has any reader managed to interest his family doctor in prescribing vitamin E? We hope so, for we agree that the ideal situation is for doctors everywhere to make use of this excellent remedy. But if they can't or won't, what are the rest of us to do—just read about vitamin E and know that such a remedy exists, but also know that we cannot possibly take advantage of it? Or should we journey to Canada and be treated by the Shutes? Many readers have, of course, but certainly everyone in this country suffering from the many disorders described in the book cannot possibly do likewise. So readers who follow the advice of the Shutes against "self-medication" as they call it, are doomed to dreadful frustration, we believe.

We appreciate the concern of the Drs. Shute in this matter. For if we—all of us—begin to take vitamin E for our heart conditions and take the wrong amount and get no results, then of course we are not going to believe that vitamin E is any good. And it is true that the dosage of vitamin E is important. But we still cannot go along with the philosophy of "get your doctor to give you the vitamin or don't take it" for most doctors today just won't give it to you. And the Shutes know this as well or better than anyone, for they always fight valiantly for recognition of Vitamin E as a therapeutic agent.

Then we disagree with our authors in their sentiments about wheat germ oil. That is, we partly disagree. They say (page 14) "We no longer use it (wheat germ oil) and heartily decry its commercial eixstence." Now if they are talking about using wheat germ oil as a source of vitamin E, we agree with them. The amount of wheat germ oil one can take in daily doses does not give you enough vitamin E to matter especially. But it does give you all those things which come along with vitamin E in foods —and if you eat mostly today's refined and devitalized food, this is extremely important. You get in wheat germ oil the other parts of the vitamin E "complex" aside from alpha tocopherol; you get unsaturated fatty acids, you get a certain natural hormone substance that is extremely beneficial apparently. For any one who does not get the whole, natural, unspoiled parts of cereal seeds in his daily diet (and this means most of us) wheat germ oil or flakes are an essential.

Furthermore, on page 117, the Shutes give glowing accounts of experiments that were performed showing that wheat germ oil increased the endurance of athletes. Wheat germ oil—not vitamin E. It seems to us that these experiments contradict their earlier assertion that they wish wheat germ oil were not available.

What Kind of Vitamin E Should You Take?

Now finally we come to the question of what kind of vitamin E you should take. The book covers this in the final chapter—"The Preparations of Vitamin E on the Market." The authors tell us that no preparation sold in the United States should be taken. The only ones that are of any account are those that they themselves recommend which they know are reliable. They tell us that in European countries and Canada very careful regulations govern the sale of vitamin E preparations which must conform to the International system of labelling. But in the United States, they say, "The situation has been chaotic to put it benevolently."

They then list ten American preparations, giving the label claim of 100 milligrams of vitamin E and then giving the actual content of the supplements. In one case the content was as low as 46 milligrams. In another as high as 136 milligrams. Then they go on to tell us that there are two or at the most three industrial firms that make all of these products. The wholesalers buy a given amount of oil, have it put in capsules by "one or two great encapsulating firms" and then sell it. So, they say, price bargains are really impossible. "If a cheap alpha tocopherol is put on the market," they tell us, "it is either less potent or mislabelled or it is marketed by some tiny firm with little or no overhead and no assay laboratories or detail men going about the country to interview doctors and druggists—or all these difficulties are present."

We have tried, over a period of years, to clear up in our own minds what is meant by this kind of talk. We have written repeatedly to the Cardiac Society about it and have had either no answer at all, or unsatisfactory ones. Vitamin E is manufactured by only two or three firms. And it is put into capsules by only one or two firms. Then it is sent out to wholesalers. And we are to believe that the vitamin E which goes into the capsules sold to the sources of which the Shutes approve, and the vitamin E that goes into the capsules sold by American firms, are two entirely different products, even though they are all made by the same two or three firms. We cannot believe this and we will not.

We have checked closely with *Prevention* advertisers to see if they have any explanation of this point of view. They have none. At our request they have had their products analyzed and of course they come out exactly as represented on the label. Food and Drug restrictions are extremely well enforced in matters of this kind. Any food supplement seller who puts out a product that is mislabelled is flirting with a heavy fine and imprisonment. Why should anyone take such a chance?

And furthermore, unless he were an avowed crook, deliberately bent on cheating his customers, how in the world could he sell a product that did not measure up to the standard? The product is prepared for him at the main source; it is put in capsules at a central place. Unless he has a written agreement that either or both of these firms conspire with him to defraud customers, how could his product be inferior to any of the other products that are produced and encapsulated in the same way and at the same establishments?

Our advice to readers, therefore:

1. By all means, if you can get your doctor or any doctor to prescribe vitamin E for you, do so. Talk about vitamin E to doctors and to friends, neighbors and relatives. Show doubters your copy of *Your Heart and Vitamin E.*

2. If you cannot take vitamin E under a doctor's prescription, then we say take vitamin E on your own. If you are healthy and have no problem with heart or blood vessels, how much should you take? It has been estimated that, before our foods were refined, we human beings probably got fifty milligrams of vitamin E a day. It would seem reasonable, therefore, to add that to your diet unless you are convinced that you already get that much from your food and food supplements. Do you take wheat germ or wheat germ oil? Do you eat your own home-made whole grain bread? How does your diet stand on the other good sources of vitamin E—chiefly seeds and seed oils?

3. If you suffer from heart and blood vessel conditions and cannot find any doctor who will treat you with vitamin E, we see no reason why you should continue to suffer when perhaps your own intelligence can tell you how much or how little you should take to improve your condition. It seems logical—and the Shutes have advised this in their book directed to physicians—to start with a small dose, say 50 milligrams, and

increase the dosage very gradually until you arrive at what seems most satisfactory. If you have any unpleasant symptoms, this would seem to indicate that you may be getting too much. Cut it down to the former dose and keep it at that.

One very important caution—Taking a considerable amount of vitamin E may have a tendency to raise blood pressure sharply right at the beginning. If you have high blood pressure, then, you should use extreme caution in determining the dosage. Start with a small dose and raise it very, very gradually!

We know from past experience that many readers have used vitamin E with marked success. And we think other readers will be a lot happier and healthier, too, if they do the same, experimentally and carefully, than if they resign themselves to suffering the rest of their lives, knowing that there is a possible remedy in vitamin E but that it is unavailable to them.

4. What vitamin E should you take? Should you take only alpha tocopherol or should you take mixed tocopherols—all the tocopherol family—delta, gamma and the rest?

There is a difference of opinion on all of these matters. The Shutes believe that only alpha tocopherol should be taken in the treatment of the various disorders they discuss in their book. They believe that the other parts of the tocopherol family do not contribute nearly so much and so should not be used.

Other authorities believe that all the tocopherols should be used, even though alpha tocopherol is the most potent. Editor Rodale takes mixed tocopherols, believing that, as in the case of the B vitamins, one should not break up the family to which the nutrient belongs, but should take it along with the things that occur with it in nature. For his heart condition he takes the mixed tocopherols.

We will have to leave it up to readers to make up their own minds on this question, until some further research provides us with a final answer. So we have only one recommendation to make, which is this: get your vitamin E from a natural source. Don't take synthetic vitamin E. If the label on the bottle you buy does not say whether it is from natural sources, write to the producer and ask him. If you are not satisfied with the results you get with one product, shop around. Perhaps individual differences in reactions may be responsible for all the controversy over vitamin E. Try different brands and kinds, until you find the ideal one for you. And, too, get all the vitamin E possible in your diet—that is most important!

Heart Disease and Vitamin C

Many reasons have been offered for the modern incidence of heart and vascular disease which has become the number one killer of our times. More and more we are finding medical men coming to the conclusion that the dire condition of the heart and circulatory system of most of us may be due almost entirely to what we do and do not eat. In Editor Rodale's book, *How to Eat for a Healthy Heart* (Rodale Press,

$1.00) he deals with this subject in detail, mentioning the importance of vitamin E, calcium, vitamin B, wheat germ oil and vitamin C.

It is reasonable to assume that vitamin C is especially important for the health of the blood vessels and also of the heart. It is an established scientific fact that lack of vitamin C weakens blood vessel walls, making them fragile. This means that any disturbance in the flow of blood which causes an extra amount of blood to accumulate in any given place is likely to cause the blood vessel to rupture at that point, if the individual does not get enough vitamin C in his food. Perhaps the vast majority of cases of hemorrhage—and that includes "stroke"—could have been prevented by building up the individual's store of vitamin C which would in turn strengthen his blood vessels to the point where they would not rupture or hemorrhage.

In addition we now have evidence that plenty of vitamin C prevents the formation of cholesterol in places where it does not belong. Cholesterol is a fatty substance which, as we grow older, tends to collect inside the walls of the blood vessels, narrowing them so that the blood has a hard time making its way through. This is one of the causes of high blood pressure. If you think of the circulatory system in terms of a hose and a pump, you can easily understand what damage the cholesterol would do. While the pump (the heart) continues to push the blood along with the same amount of pressure, any narrowing of the hose (the blood vessels) will of course cause higher pressure because the blood has to flow through a space so much narrower. Then too, cholesterol helps to bring about the process of "hardening of the arteries" which is the dread of all those of us past middle age.

How could vitamin C which is soluble in water possibly be related to cholesterol which is a fatty substance? No one knows exactly how, but one thing is certain. The amount of vitamin C in the diet certainly seems to have a great deal to do with the formation of excessive cholesterol in the body. Willis and Fishman, writing in the *Canadian Medical Journal* for April 1, 1955, tell us of studying the vitamin C content of the arteries of patients who had died in their hospital. They found that the vitamin C content of the arteries of patients dying from the routine diseases was very low. In seven of 20 cases there was none at all. In the older age groups the level of the vitamin was lower than in the younger patients. In two cases of thrombosis (a clot of blood closing off the artery) there was no vitamin C at all in the arteries. These authors feel that the lack of the vitamin was probably due to the stress of the fatal illness, in most of these cases—not to any lack in diet. *But isn't it possible to give sick people enough vitamin C so that they will not become deficient, no matter how much the stress of their illness might drain from them?*

Where Cholesterol Collects in the Blood Vessels

These authors also found, interestingly enough, that the arteries which, because of their location, were subject to the most mechanical stress, showed most evidence of hardening of the arteries and complete lack of vitamin C. Those arteries on which the strain was not so great showed less "hardening" and more vitamin C! This finding certainly seems to indicate that lack of vitamin C and hardening of the arteries go hand in hand. Dr. Willis and Fishman tell us that guinea pigs who have contracted scurvy from lack of vitamin C are always easy prey to rapid hardening of the arteries. It has also been found that the process of manufacturing cholesterol in the body is several times more rapid in tissues that are depleted of vitamin C.

In an earlier experiment performed by Dr. Willis, he studied the incidence of hardening of the arteries in guinea pigs whose diet contained no vitamin C. This is reported in the *Canadian Medical Association Journal* for July, 1953. Dr. Willis tells us that deficiency in vitamin C produces hardening of the arteries in scorbutic guinea pigs whether their scurvy is acute or chronic. The condition of the arteries resembles very closely that of the blood vessels of human beings suffering from hardening of the arteries. Injecting vitamin C prevents the cholesterol from forming on the artery walls.

In *The Lancet,* an English medical journal, there is a report (June 20, 1953) by Dr. King of the Nutrition Foundation, New York, who, in experiments with rats, found that in a deficiency of vitamin C there is an increased formation of cholesterol. *The Lancet* goes on to caution "Although he is a champion of high human allowances of ascorbic acid (vitamin C) he was careful not to claim that ingestion of the vitamin would decrease atherosclerosis (hardening of the arteries)."

We suppose scientists must be cautious. But vitamin C even in massive doses year after year has never been known to harm anyone. So what possible harm could be done by giving a large number of heart and vascular patients massive doses of vitamin C to see whether or not hardening of the arteries could be prevented or even slowed down? They might be disappointed, the doctors will answer, perhaps we'll raise their hopes and then not get the results we were looking for. Granted. But what, good masters of medicine, are you doing for such patients today that *does* get results? Can you show us any one treatment that does prevent the formation of cholesterol on the inside walls of blood vessels? There is none. So why not at least *try* vitamin C?

Treating Hardening of the Arteries With Vitamin C

In an article in *Drug and Cosmetic Industry,* May and June, 1954, we find mention of researchers who have used vitamin C in treatment of heart and vascular pttients. Gale and Thewlis (*Geriatrics,* February, 1953) said: "Because of the role of (vitamin C and vitamin P) in maintaining vascular integrity, it is believed that many instances of hemorrhage and thrombosis in the heart and brain may be avoided if adequate amounts of vitamins C and P are given. These views have been confirmed clinically: vascular disturbances relieved by these agents include dizziness, nose bleed, and chronic heart failure with intermittent dyspnea (breathlessness). It is also pointed out that vascular disturbances of the aged suggests that latent scurvy may be fairly frequent and that large amounts of supplementary vitamin C are necessary."

The same article tells us, too, that "mention should be made of studies that point out the role of vitamin C as a regulator of the rate at which cholesterol is formed in the body; deficiency of the vitamin speeding the formation of this substance. In experimental work, guinea pigs fed a diet free of ascorbic acid showed a 600 per cent acceleration in cholesterol formation in the adrenal glands."

Dr. W. J. McCormick in *Clinical Medicine* for July, 1952, says that when patients are given a diet ample in vitamins B and C there is usually a dramatic decrease in the blood cholesterol, even in cases where there is a much larger intake of cholesterol in the food they eat. Dr. McCormick says that patients afflicted with high cholesterol in their blood are sometimes advised by their doctors not to eat liver, eggs and other foods rich in cholesterol. But when they are given a diet that contains ample vitamins B and C and then are given desiccated or cooked liver, there is usually a dramatic decrease in the blood cholesterol, *in spite of the fact that this kind of diet has increased the cholesterol they are eating.*

So it seems, according to Dr. McCormick, that the answer to hardening of the arteries is not to cut out all foods rich in cholesterol, but to find out what mechanism in the body is not functioning properly when cholesterol collects dangerously and then correct that mechanism. Could it be that vitamin C controls that mechanism? Could it be that our modern troubles with high blood pressure, heart trouble, strokes, etc. are caused at least in part because we do not have access to fresh raw foods, brimming over with vitamin C and all the elements that go with this vitamin in foods?

Vitamin C also reduces blood pressure. In the *Canadian Journal of the Medical Sciences* for August, 1951, Doctors Heroux, Dugal and Paul describe investigations which showed that vitamin C given in large doses reduced high blood pressure. At the same time they give an account of their own investigation which led to the same result.

In *Clinical Medicine,* volume 50, 1943, page 152, Doctors Davis and Poser describe the results in four cases in which high blood pressure was greatly reduced by giving vitamin C.

What assurance can we offer to readers suffering from heart and blood vessel diseases that they can secure relief by taking vitamin C? We have presented our evidence above. We would suggest that you show it to your physician and ask him to look further into the various articles we quote in the medical magazines.

For the rest of us, we believe that we should be getting every day far, far more vitamin C than the recommended daily allowance if we would keep our hearts and circulatory system healthy and prevent any disorder in this department. How much vitamin C should one take to prevent circulatory disease? We discuss in another article in this book the question of how much vitamin C you should take to be healthy.

Heart Disease and Vitamin E

As Seen By A Famous Magazine

An article in the Canadian magazine, *Macleans,* for June 15, 1953, gives the facts about vitamin E therapy for a number of diseases, chief among which is heart trouble.

Eric Hutton who wrote the article traces the story of the Shute brothers (medical men of Canada) who became interested in vitamin E when they discovered that it was useful in treating complications of pregnancy. Their mother was their first heart patient. Mrs. Shute, so ill that she could not walk across the room, was gardening four weeks after she began to take vitamin E.

Here is other testimony from Shute patients cured by taking vitamin E: "Phlebitis in my legs made me a bed case. The Shutes treated me with vitamin E and now I find that I can do a day's work comfortably." "Coronary thrombosis put me on my back for four months and I was told never to work again. After vitamin E treatment I've been back at my job in a Toronto carpet plant for five years."

Why does organized medicine officially oppose the use of vitamin E in the treatment of disease? We do not know, but Mr. Hutton tells some astounding stories of this opposition. When the Shutes submitted a report on their experience with the vitamin, the governing body of all physicians and surgeons in Canada, after studying the report for several hours, announced that "on evidence submitted, the committee is convinced that vitamin E has no place in the treatment of heart and blood vessel disease." They implied that the people cured had been wrongly diagnosed as having heart disease. This in spite of the fact that some of the patients whose cases were described in their report were diagnosed as heart patients by the very physicians who gave out this announcement.

The Shutes themselves say, "Some of our loudest critics are taking vitamin E themselves. Many dispense vitamin E but will not sign a prescription for it. Many doctors returned to practice on vitamin E, after coronaries disabled them, are ashamed to admit the source of their help, even to their closest friends"

Enough vitamin E being shipped to a certain Canadian hospital to treat about 16 patients daily came to the attention of the Shute brothers. They inquired and were told that no tests were underway and no patients were getting vitamin E. It was all being used by staff physicians to treat their own disorders. The Shutes say that about 180 doctors and their families are among the 10,000 patients they have treated for heart and circulatory disease.

Mr. Hutton tells of person after person to whom he spoke who had been cured by vitamin E but refused to let his name be used in the article, saying that he chose not to expose himself to the possible cries of "crank" and "faddist" that would be hurled at him. Mr. Hutton did a survey among pharmacists in Toronto and was told that 28 per cent of the doctors use vitamin E and approve of it as a therapeutic measure, even though they will not indicate openly their approval. In a survey made by one company among 800 doctor customers, 228 made enthusiastic comments on the effectiveness of vitamin E in treating heart disease.

The Shutes' explanation of how vitamin E works is this: they say it has no special affinity for the heart as insulin does for the pancreas. But what vitamin E does is to decrease the amount of oxygen needed by the body cells. In other words, taking vitamin E does not "cure" a damaged heart or circulatory system by rebuilding or regenerating them. It does enable the heart and circulation to get along quite well on the lesser supply of oxygen which a damaged heart or circulation may necessitate. The actual cells are enabled, when plenty of vitamin E is present, to exist on a much smaller supply of oxygen than a cell deprived of vitamin E.

The Shutes are practicing at present at The Shute Clinic, London, Ontario, Canada. They have published many, many medical articles on vitamin E. They are known the world over and regularly appear at learned gatherings where vitamin E therapy is discussed. It is difficult indeed for even the most perverse medical man to pretend they are quacks. Yet while deaths from heart disease continue to soar into tragic figures, vitamin E therapy is ignored by official medicine as if it did not exist.

Heart Disease—Heat for Heart Emergency

A heating pad, hot wash cloth or handkerchief applied to the heart region can do much to relieve quickly an attack of angina, of the heart, according to a letter from P. Pickerill, M.D. of New Zealand writing in *The Lancet* for January 15, 1955. In fact, if the local heat is applied quickly enough, it may completely abort the attack. A wash cloth or handkerchief could be used while the pad is heating up. They should be about 110 degrees fahrenheit—just a little hotter than can be comfortably tolerated on one's bare arm. Sipping hot tea or hot water at the same time is helpful.

There seems to be no doubt, too, that cold can precipitate an attack. During the recovery from extreme cold, it seems that the brain and the heart compete for oxygen to such an extent that warming the body all over may have no good results at all, for the oxygen is spread out to such an extent that there is not enough for the heart to "make a comeback." But heating just the area around the heart will assure the heart of enough oxygen. Cooling the head at the same time might be helpful.

In answer to Dr. Pickerill's suggestion, a letter in a later issue of *The Lancet* (January 22, 1955) recommends the use of an infra-red lamp. This physician, W. Annandale Troup, uses infra-red irradiation for a half hour or so over the heart region for the purpose of lessening the incidence of angina attacks.

Hemorrhage

"He died of hemorrhage," "He was a bleeder, so of course the operation finished him," How many times have you heard comments like these about someone who was ill? Did you know what they meant when they said "hemorrhage?" Why is it that some people in accidents die of hemorrhage while others, just as seriously wounded, recover? What is a hemorrhage anyway?

Hemorrhage is bleeding—any bleeding. Yet the term is generally applied only when the bleeding is excessive or dangerous. The seriousness of loss of blood depends on the length of time the individual bleeds, the proportion of blood lost and how effective are the compensatory arrangements made by the body to get along without this lost blood. Blood pressure goes down when blood is lost. It is easy to see why this should be, for when there is less blood the arteries are not so full and the blood flow does not have the force it normally would.

It is of course dangerous for the blood pressure to drop rapidly. On the other hand, the person who is bleeding dangerously may be thankful that his blood pressure has dropped, for this slows down the rate of flow of the blood to such an extent that there may be just a small trickle even from a large artery by the time the blood pressure is fairly low. It is unusual for anyone to die of loss of blood. Usually coagulation takes place in time, so that there is still sufficient blood for the body's functions to go on by the time the bleeding stops. If the blood lost does not exceed 30 to 40 per cent of the natural circulating volume of blood, then the blood pressure will rise again, once the bleeding is stopped. This will usually take place within thirty minutes.

How does the body make up for the loss of blood? Eventually, of course, new blood is manufactured. But in an emergency the small blood vessels in distant parts of the body, such as hands and feet, empty and remain empty so that whatever blood is available may go to the heart and brain. At the same time, tissue fluids that are always circulating through the body pass through the blood vessel walls and increase the volume of blood. This whole procedure may take about a half hour. Of course the sooner the full volume of blood is restored the better, for the parts of the body where the small blood vessels emptied are bound to suffer. No part of you can go safely without blood for very long. This is where modern blood transfusion practices have saved countless lives.

Any hemorrhage except that from a large blood vessel has a tendency to be checked by coagulation of the blood before the loss of blood becomes dangerous. Blood begins to coagulate at a distance from the wound or break in the blood vessel, gets a firm hold on the tissue there and gradually builds up a blood clot which soon covers the bleeding wound. Surfaces that are moving or are too smooth hinder coagulation. For instance, it would be hard to form a blood clot on the wall of the heart or intestine, for both are constantly in motion.

Slow internal hemorrhaging over a long period of time is a little different. In this case, the individual may be unaware of the fact that he is losing blood. Finally he becomes anemic, his circulation is poor, he is pale and listless, has a rapid heart beat. When he stands up suddenly he gets a ringing in his ears, spots or flashes before his eyes, or he is suddenly dizzy. These symptoms are generally indications of too little blood and a thorough physical examination is in order.

The actual clotting of blood is brought about by a substance called prothrombin which begins the process. In those who do not have enough prothrombin in the blood, a hemorrhage could be serious, for the blood cannot coagulate properly. Vitamin K is given to such patients, for the vitamin, which got its name from the Danish "Koagulation" helps in this important function. Then, too, for those whose blood coagulates too easily, there is danger of blood clots. For these patients anti-coagulant drugs are given. Hemorrhaging may occur in any part of the body. Nose bleeds, bloody vomit or bloody stool are indications that something serious is wrong. But the fatal accidents in the line of hemorrhaging are in the brain or the abdomen. Then the symptoms are alarming indeed. A "stroke" is a hemorrhage in the brain blood vessels.

Best insurance against hemorrhage anywhere is a network of capillaries so healthy and strong that they do not burst easily so hemorrhages are impossible. Plenty of vitamin C is a necessity for this kind of healthy vascular system.

Honey

Since the earliest days of recorded history, men have been using honey, as a food, a preservative, a medicine. A cave stone-painting from the neolithic age shows that about 15,000 years ago men gathered honeycombs for food, even as we do today. In the Egyptian pyramids, some 3000-year-old honey has been found—dry and dark, but still pure honey. In Greek and Roman civilization honey was used for preserving and embalming as well as for the choicest food. It was used as a sacrifice to the gods. It was an important part of the folk ceremonies of all nations. In some countries the bee was regarded as sacred. In most countries the beehive was considered such an important part of the household, not so many years ago, that special ceremonies were held there on holidays. And should a tragedy or some great blessing befall the family, someone was dispatched immediately to notify the bees!

In 1747 the use of beet sugar for sweetening was introduced by Markgraf. With humanity's usual broad assumption that anything new is necessarily better, we took to using sugar rather than honey for baking and cooking. The full story of the results in terms of health will probably not be known until that happy day when refined white sugar is outlawed in every nation of the world. Then perhaps many of our modern diseases may disappear.

In 1942 according to T. Swann Harding, writing in the *American Journal of Pharmacology* for May, 1942, the average annual American consumption of white refined sugar was from 100 to 104 pounds per person. That is, the average American eats about one pound of sugar every three days! Our average consumption of honey is about 1½ pounds per person per year. Yet in 1941 the 4½ million hives in this country produced 206 million pounds of honey. An average bee colony may produce as much as 400 pounds of honey a year for its own use, the surplus of 50 pounds or so being what the beekeeper has for sale or for personal use.

If you want some fascinating reading, get yourself a book on bees and read the incredible story of the lives of these little creatures whose society is organized perfectly and ruthlessly for work and production, with no time for loafing or pleasure. Bees process the nectar and pollen of flowers to make honey. This complex and not-fully-understood procedure involves gathering the nectar and pollen on sunny days, packing it into the bee's pollen basket and honey stomach, then transferring it to the symmetrical wax cells of the hive. Somewhere along the line the flower nectar is changed by enzymes into the sweet, fragrant, nourishing honey that we know, which never spoils, molds or ferments.

How Honey is Produced and Processed

We are told that bees visit about 10,000 different kinds of flowers, acting of course as pollinators to these flowers in the process of gathering the pollen (protein) and nectar (carbohydrate) for their food. One pound of honey requires about 37,000 trips of the honeybees and one bee colony may travel 17 million miles back and forth in one year to provide honey for the population of the hive. In addition, of course, each colony collects 40 to 100 pounds of pollen each year.

We don't often get honey in combs these days. Most honey has been removed from the tiny geometric cells of the comb in which the bees placed it. To extract the honey, the tops of these cells are sliced off and the open comb is placed in a centrifuge which whirls the honey out in liquid form. This is called "extracted" honey. When the comb is crushed and the honey strained from it, this is called "strained" honey. Morris B. Jacobs in *Food and Food Products,* the monumental book on the production of all different kinds of foods, tells us that commercially-bought honey may be adulterated with cane sugar or corn syrup. So check carefully on the source of your honey.

We have heard marvelous stories of its curative powers. Down through the ages, it has been used as a medicine. Pythagoras advocated a honey diet, declaring that honey brings health and long life. Charles Butler in his *History of the Bees,* written in 1623, says, "Hooni cleareth all the obstructions of the body, looseneth the belly, purgeth the foulness of the body and provoketh urine. It cutteth up and casteth out phlegmatic matter and thereby sharpens the stomach of them which by reason have little appetite. It purgeth those things which hurt the clearness of the eyes and nourisheth very much; it storeth up and preserveth natural heat and prolongeth old age." It has been used to treat inflammation, kidney diseases, disorders of the respiratory and digestive tract, bad complexions, liver trouble, infectious diseases, poor circulation, and as an ointment for wounds.

Vitamin Content of Honey

What is the food value of honey that has led people for so many thousands of years to believe in it as food and medicine? In modern times the first answer to such a question must be given in terms of vitamins. White sugar contains no vitamins. Does honey? Indeed it does. H. A. Schuette of the Department of Chemistry of the University of Wisconsin, is one of the outstanding investigators of vitamins in honey. In an article in the *Journal of Nutrition* for September, 1943, he, George Kitzes and C. A. Elvehjem describe the determination of B vitamins in honey. Each of the samples varied in its vitamin B content, according to the locality from which it came and the kind of flower the honey was made from.

Here are the results of all honeys examined:

Riboflavin	from 7 to 60	micrograms per 100 grams
Pantothenic acid	from 9 to 110	micrograms per 100 grams
Niacin	from 72 to 590	micrograms per 100 grams
Thiamin	from 1.4 to 12	micrograms per 100 grams
Pyridoxine	from 0 to 27.7	micrograms per 100 grams

A few honeys were tested also for their biotin and folic acid content and traces of these were found.

These researchers turned up some other interesting aspects of vitamins in honey. They found that some of the B vitamins might be destroyed in storage over a period of years. They found that the vitamin content of pollen is much higher than that of honey, suggesting that perhaps the vitamins in honey are contained in the small pollen grains found in it. They also remind us that clarifying honey reduces the vitamin contents up to 35 to 50 per cent of the original values. Clarifying is a process which removes the slight cloudiness that may be present, resulting in crystal-clear, brilliant honey, but less nourishing than unclarified honey.

The vitamin C content of honey varies, too, with the kind of honey and the locality from which it comes. Some researchers have found as much as 311.2 milligrams and as little as 0 milligrams of vitamin C in 100 grams of honey. An orange weighing 100 grams contains from 25 to 50 milligrams of vitamin C. Naturally one cannot eat 100 grams of honey as casually as one might eat an orange because of its concentrated sweetness.

Minerals and Amino Acids in Honey

Honey contains minerals, too. Here, interestingly enough, the mineral content depends largely on the color of the honey, those dark honeys, like buckwheat, being richer in minerals than the lighter ones. H. A. Schuette and D. J. Huenink in *Food Research,* Volume 2, 1937, tell us that honey contains silica, phosphorus, calcium and magnesium as follows:

	Milligrams per kilogram			
	Silica	*Phosphorus*	*Calcium*	*Magnesium*
Light honeys	14 to 36	23 to 50	23 to 68	11 to 56
Dark honeys	13 to 72	27 to 58	5 to 226	7 to 126

In this survey 35 honeys were selected from nine different states and about 14 different blossoms. These writers point out that other investigators have found even larger concentrations of calcium and phosphorus.

In *Food Research* for July-August, 1939, Dr. Schuette and Warren W. Woessner report on sodium and potassium components of honey. Here too the minerals exist in much larger quantity in the darker honeys.

	Milligrams per kilogram	
	Sodium	*Potassium*
Light honeys	average of 18	average of 205
Dark honeys	average of 76	average of 1676

Working again with different colors of honey from a widely selected group, Dr. Schuette and C. L. Baldwin, Jr., reported in *Food Research* for May-June, 1944, that amino acids (forms of protein necessary for life) are also present in honey as "minor components." Once again the darker honeys are richer in amino acids than the light honeys. It is an interesting aspect of our study of foods to note that nature likes color and lavishes her richest abundance of health-giving nourishment on foods in which color is most intense. Keep this in mind when you're shopping for food. Take the bright orange sweet potato in preference to the pale yellow one. Buy the head of cabbage with the greenest leaves. Use the outer, dark green leaves of endive rather than the bleached white ones in the center. Pick the reddest watermelon and the pinkest cantaloupe. And, if you're buying honey for its mineral content, choose the dark honeys, even though you may not at first care for their stronger flavor.

Honey and Anemia

We uncovered several other interesting facts about honey in its relation to health. For instance, in an experiment with laboratory rats reported in the *Proceedings of the Society of Experimental Biology and Medicine* for May, 1943, M. H. Haydak, L. S. Palmer and M. C. Tanquary of the University of Minnesota discovered that dark honey added to a milk diet will increase the hemoglobin count and hence prevent or cure nutritional anemia in rats, whereas light honey added to milk caused the hemoglobin count to fall, meaning that the rats became even more anemic. Rats fed milk and sucrose also became anemic. So it sounds as though the famous milk and honey diet might be effective provided only that the honey is dark honey. Incidentally the iron content of honey ranges from 2.4 milligrams per kilogram in light honeys to 17.5 milligrams in dark honeys. And the copper content of honey ranges from .29 milligrams in light honeys to 1.4 milligrams in dark honeys.

In performing these experiments the researchers found that honey also contains an anti-hemorrhaging factor, suggesting the presence of vitamin K. Using vitamin-K-deficient chicks, they tested alfalfa hay and honey and found that they could indeed increase the chicks' store of vitamin K by the addition of alfalfa and honey to their diets.

Honey and Calcium Retention

Perhaps most valuable of all, from the point of view of human beings, is an experiment in feeding honey to infants as the carbohydrate part of their "formulas." Over the first six months of their lives fourteen healthy babies received formulas consisting of evaporated or half-skim milk, breast milk or dried protein milk for the protein part of the diet. The carbohydrate part consisted of corn syrup or honey. Vitamin D in cod liver oil was added at varying levels. E. M. Knott, Ph.D., C. F. Shuckers, M.D. and F. W. Schultz, M.D. of Chicago, reporting on this experiment in the *Journal of Pediatrics* for October, 1941, tell us that allowing for all other possible variations in the diets, honey came out well ahead of corn syrup as a preserver of calcium for the infants, which is, of course, good news for honey-lovers.

The infants were tested each day for calcium retention. Naturally the amount of vitamin D used that day affected the retention of calcium, for it is well known that vitamin D is essential for proper retention and use of calcium by the body. But it was found that wherever infants were fed under comparable conditions to make the comparison of these two types of carbohydrates completely valid, the average retention of calcium *was always higher if honey had been included in the formula rather than corn syrup*. The authors conclude that "honey is indeed a type of carbohydrate which is well suited to the infant's needs and therefore probably deserves a wider use in infant dietaries."

In general meats, eggs, cereals and nuts are acid in their reaction in the body's metabolism. Vegetables, fruits and milk are alkaline. Starches, sugars and fats are neutral. We should strive to maintain a balance in the kinds of food we eat, for most of us tend to lean too heavily on the acid-producing foods and don't eat enough fruits and vegetables to keep the proper alkaline balance in our blood. So it is cheering to know that honey, like fruits, has an alkaline reaction in the body. Even though it is sweet, it contains, like fruits, certain organic acids which react in the body's chemistry by producing alkalinity. So if you are hesitating over whether sugar or honey should go on the youngsters' breakfast cereal or on the fruit salad for tonight's dessert, don't hesitate for another minute. Sugar—white refined sugar, contains no vitamins, no minerals and no other healthful food elements. It makes enormous demands on your body's store of the elusive B vitamins, for it requires B vitamins for its digestion and they just aren't present in sugar. In addition, sugar is neutral in the acid-alkaline balance. But honey contains all the B vitamins necessary for its proper use by the body, contains minerals and amino acids and, in addition, will have an alkaline effect on the body.

Is Honey a Cure For Arthritis?

Now we come to two letters we received one day which were actually the cause of this investigation of honey. We heard from Mrs. Ida Crowther of Cass City, Michigan, and F. H. Young of Long Beach, California. Mrs. Crowther owns an apiary—that is, she raises bees. She told us that she had been suffering from a quite severe case of arthritis for months and had tried every known combination of foods in an effort to cure it. She noticed that the pain disappeared when she was helping her husband extract honey—and of course eating some honey while she worked—and appeared again when she was not working around the honey. Then one day she read in the *Bee Journal* an article on honey and arthritis, written by D. C. Jarvis, M.D., who said that honey had been used many times as a cure for arthritis. She at once began to take five tablespoons of honey per day. Within two weeks the swelling in her knee was gone. "And now a year later," says Mrs. Crowther, "I have never quit taking the honey and I can sit on the floor now with both my knees lying flat. . . . I would advise all who suffer from arthritis to turn to honey and use plenty of protein and whole milk, plenty of wheat germ and enough of brewers' yeast and a generous green salad, with an occasional fruit salad, all with lemon juice dressing and a little honey added for taste." Incidentally, Mrs. Crowther is on a reducing diet and has had no trouble in losing many pounds, even with her high-calorie honey every day.

Mr. Young's letter, in the same mail, told us just the opposite. He had noticed the beginnings of arthritis about five years ago, and changing his diet around, found that by omitting his usual honey on his morning cereal and toast, he could cause the pain of the arthritis to disappear. A friend had the same experience. Mr. Young wrote us suggesting that we do a study on honey and see what we could find. Would any of our readers like to make an experiment?

The article from the *Bee World* to which Mrs. Crowther referred talks about the ratio of calcium to phosphorus in the blood stream. We know that this ratio is important and that too much calcium or too much phosphorus will throw it off balance. Dr. Jarvis states that inflammation in the body is caused by a high phosphorus level, with not enough calcium to balance it. Cereals, beans and other seed-foods are high in phosphorus and many of us have far too much of this kind of food in our meals to the exclusion of calcium-containing foods. In fact it is accepted among nutritionists that most of us lack calcium.

Dr. Jarvis says that when the phosphorus level is high, the intense pain of arthritis is present. Honey raises the calcium level and lowers the phosphorus level. He says that one tablespoon of honey taken to relieve the pain will lower the phosphorus level of the blood for as long as 24 hours, after which it will return again to its original level, unless of course you take more honey. This, then is the explanation for Mrs. Crowther's almost miraculous cure.

Conclusions on Honey

Several questions remain in our minds. How does it happen that other foods high in calcium do not have this same effect? Why won't milk produce relief from swelling, or eggs, or any of the vegetables that are high in calcium? Or could it be possible that Mrs. Crowther's honey was superior—honey from her own hives which she knew contained no adulterant? Perhaps Mr. Young's honey contained sucrose artificially added, perhaps it contained residues of insecticides.

We don't have the answer to the whole problem of honey in its relation to arthritis. But, as you know, for some reason, bees have consistently been associated with arthritis cures. Bee venom, containing formic acid, is used in many parts of the world as a rheumatism cure. Honey contains an infinitesimally small amount of this acid. We'd suggest that, if you suffer from arthritis, you try the suggestion of honey with meals. But make certain you are getting pure honey, as free as possible from insecticides and make certain too that it has not been heated, clarified, or treated in any other way.

One word more on insecticides. We found in our research that residues of insecticides are found in honeys—very small residues, it is true, but enough to appear in laboratory tests. Lead and arsenic were found in the honeys tested. Nowadays, of course, many other insecticides are used which may be even more harmful than lead and arsenic. So we caution you, if possible, get your honey from a source where there is no possibility of contamination with insecticides.

As you know we cast a disapproving eye on sweets of all kinds, except those natural sugars found in fruits and vegetables. The research we have done does not convince us that you should deliberately add honey to your diet, unless you are experimenting for a relief from arthritis. Honey is a carbohydrate food and most of us get too much carbohydrate food in proportion to our protein. But, if you or your family feel definitely that you must have some sweetening, on fruit salads or cereals, for example, by all means use honey instead of sugar. Use it for freezing fruits. Use it in any recipe that calls for white sugar. We can guarantee that the unhealthy after-effects of sugar-eating will not stalk your footsteps. And, who knows, perhaps the ancients were right. Perhaps honey really does contain as yet undiscovered potentialities for health. At any rate, if it is produced and marketed with careful attention, it is a completely natural food. The bees thrive on it—and bees are mighty smart, hard-working insects!

Hormones and Cancer

Possible danger in feeds now given to meat animals.

This article is reprinted, by permission, from *The New York Times* for January 29, 1956, where it appeared in the column *Science in Review* by Waldemar Kaempffert.

We think it is highly significant that one of the researchers who testified showed that hormones given in very small quantities over a long period of time *may be more effective in inducing cancer than larger doses given intermittently*.

At last week's symposium on medicated feeds, organized by the United States Department of Health, Education and Welfare, and the Food and Drug Administration, Drs. Granville F. Knight, W. Coda Martin (American Academy of Medicine), Rigoberto Iglesias (Santiago, Chile) and William E. Smith (New York) sounded a warning against feeding animals with diethylstilbestrol, a female sex hormone. The hormone is known to induce cancer under some conditions. It is fed to food animals to stimulate growth and bring about an increase in weight.

More than 30,000,000 chickens and half the beef cattle of the country are now given diethylstilbestrol. What will be the effect of poultry and beef thus treated on a populace that consumes them as food? There is no evidence that hormone-fed chickens and cattle have actually induced human cancer, but Drs. Knight, Martin, Iglesias and Smith contend that the possibility cannot be dismissed.

Administration of female sex hormones to mice, rats and guinea pigs has induced polyps, fibroids and tumors. If no estrogen can be detected in the tissues of an animal that has been stimulated to put on more flesh it is not to be concluded that there is no danger of generating cancer.

Experiments conducted by Dr. Iglesias over twenty years show that continuing administration of minute doses of estrogen is more effective in inciting cancer than intermittent injections of larger doses. "The introduction of estrogens into the food supply presents the problem of exposure of human beings from birth onward," is the conclusion reached. The reason is that we eat meat from childhood to old age. The longer we live the more likely is cancer to be incited, this because cancer is primarily an affliction of middle and old age.

Hunger

"In the ideal state the living organism is directed by hunger to secure food in amounts sufficient to replenish the bodily materials that have been destroyed by oxidation or have been excreted. This primitive mechanism does not give rise to sensations which are primarily pleasurable. It is, so to speak, more businesslike than that. With the passage of time hunger has come to be so closely associated with other feelings called appetite that the mind of man no longer distinguishes clearly between the two. Appetite, strictly speaking, is a sensation produced by happy memories. The desire for food may be the expression of real hunger, but it is more generally a response to habit or the anticipation of pleasure." So say Norman Jolliffe, M.D., E. F. Tisdall, M.D., and Paul R. Cannon, M.D., in their monumental book, *Clinical Nutrition* (published by Paul B. Hoeber, Inc.).

There seems to be a lot of general agreement among the experts as to what hunger is not. But they cannot seem to agree on exactly what hunger is. We know it is not the same thing as appetite. As one writer puts it, hunger is felt in the stomach, appetite in the mouth. Hunger is unpleasant; appetite is pleasant; hunger can be satisfied only with food in quantity; appetite is more interested in the quality of food.

Hunger has been defined as an unpleasant feeling of emptiness pressure, discomfort or pain in the stomach region. It may also bring about weakness, headache and other unpleasant symptoms. In our well-fed country we are told that we rarely experience real hunger, unless we have avoided meals, have been exposed to extreme cold or have been engaged in hard muscular activity. We know, too, that hunger contractions appear to be the actual instruments of our hunger— that is, we feel hunger when the walls of the stomach are contracting. These contractions were first discovered by a most ingenious and not especially inviting experiment in which the subject swallowed a balloon which was then blown up inside his stomach. As his hunger increased the contractions were forceful enough to press air out of the balloon and this compressed air was measured as each contraction took place.

The only gap in our knowledge is: Nobody knows what causes the stomach to contract. There must be some chemical substance, some nerve, some muscle, some hormone or enzyme that is the watchman. When the stomach has been empty long enough, this watchman must somehow signal the stomach muscles to contract, resulting in a feeling of discomfort which the nerves carry to the brain and the brain interprets thus, "Boy, I'm hungry, must get something to eat." It seems there has to be a "hunger center" located somewhere in the brain, but this has not as yet been discovered.

Interestingly enough starving people, while they suffer from many distressing symptoms, do not experience hunger after the second day or so without food. This is quite different from the experiences of people going without water, for the sensation of thirst becomes stronger and more unendurable with every passing day.

An experiment was once performed on a group of normal subjects to find out something about hunger. They were all served with the same meals at the same table and were allowed to eat all that they wanted. For a time the meals were abundant in bulky foods—mostly vegetables. All the subjects lost weight, for they ate only the same quantity they were accustomed to eating and ate only until they felt "full." Then the diet was changed to a more concentrated one. Cream and butter were substituted for milk, and sugar (a highly concentrated food) was added. All the subjects immediately gained weight, not only because the food was more concentrated, but also because they enjoyed the taste of it so much that they ate more than they normally did. What a fine lesson this experiment is for would-be reducers!

The emotions have an effect on hunger as well as on appetite. Severe emotional stress causes some people to eat more, for they use food as a solace for their distress. Fear, anxiety, grief or worry can produce total lack of appetite which, if not checked, may finally result in starving to death from *anorexia nervosa*—as the doctors would say—in other words, from lack of appetite. *Hyperorexia* is the medical term for a pathological state of intense hunger soon after eating. This state of affairs may be the result of a badly deranged metabolism (such as might happen in cases of goiter) neurosis or some disease that causes a very rapid evacuation of the contents of the stomach, so that stomach contractions begin almost immediately. There are also a large number of infections which stop entirely or greatly depress the stomach's contractions—ranging all the way from the common cold to severe infectious diseases.

Someone suffering from hunger pangs or contractions to whom food is not available can stop the contractions, we are told, by chewing, swallowing, smoking, by putting alcohol or water into his stomach, by literally tightening his belt or applying cold compresses to his stomach.

One of the surest ways of losing appetite is to eat a diet that is deficient in the B vitamins, especially thiamin. It is believed that this may be partly responsible for the curious lack of appetite in children at certain stages of development. At any rate, one sure thing is that no complaint of lack of appetite no matter how genteel its proud possessor can long withstand the effects of a couple of tablespoons of brewer's yeast daily—or some other food rich in the B vitamins. It seems that vitamin A also has a great deal to do with appetite and its lack may result in "pickiness" where food is concerned.

One final point—if you suffer day after day from strong hunger pangs a considerable time before meals are served, this may be an indication that your blood sugar is low, for this condition may produce a pathological hunger. Meals high in protein and low in starches and sugars are the answer and between-meal snacks of cheese, nuts, meat, milk or fruit. Stay away from sweets and starches if you would keep your blood sugar normal!

Immunity

The subject of immunity is one of the most complex, least understood and most hotly debated subjects in all of physiology. The main theory concerning it was formulated some years ago by Paul Ehrlich, after the invention of the microscope had demonstrated the existence of bacteria. In general the theory goes like this: Bacteria cause infectious diseases by entering the body and attacking healthy tissue. Antibodies destroy these harmful bacteria. Antibodies are created in the liver and circulate through the blood and cells.

However, a sudden attack by a lot of bacteria may not leave the individual time to manufacture sufficient antibodies or he may not be in condition to do so. So why not inject him with dead bacteria or bacteria so weakened that they cannot cause a serious disease, but will force him to produce antibodies. Then an epidemic comes along and his antibodies will be all primed and ready and he won't get the disease. In very simplified form, this is the basis for our present-day "shots" and vaccinations.

Right away a lot of questions occur to any health-minded person. First—What about babies who have not been exposed to infectious diseases? How do they go about making antibodies against them? Supposedly babies can't do this and this is one reason why infectious diseases used to take such a toll of sickly babies. Nowadays infants are given shots—from the age of 3 months to 12 months they may get as many as five or more injections of vaccines against various diseases.

On the other hand, it has been clearly demonstrated that mother's milk contains an immunity factor against disease. In epidemics of often fatal diseases it has been found that as many as 75 per cent of the breast-fed babies recover while less than 30 per cent of the bottle-fed ones recover. In an epidemic of polio that once swept a settlement of Eskimos fatalities were high except among children who were still nursing. None of these children got the disease. Colostrum, the milk given during the first five days after birth is three or four times more powerful against disease than the mother's later milk.

Other powerful components in the body's defenses against disease are vitamin C and protein. The antibodies are made of protein and experiments have shown that people and animals lacking certain of the amino acids or kinds of protein are not nearly so immune to diseases as those who get plenty of complete protein in their foods. One writer tells us that even one week on a high protein diet will create a hundred times more antibodies than before. Although we do not know just how it works, vitamin C definitely has something to do with creating immunity. People and animals who get an abundance of vitamin C are less likely to "catch" infections than those who are consistently short on this vitamin.

Recently scientists at Western Reserve University, Cleveland, announced the discovery of a substance in blood which, it is believed, is the actual substance that destroys harmful bacteria in the body. They named it "properdin" from the Latin word meaning "to destroy." This substance has to work with other materials in the body. The researchers found that the rat has the highest amount of properdin in its blood, the guinea pig has the lowest. Rats are known to be very resistant to infection, guinea pigs "take" almost any disease that comes along. So perhaps scientists are on the trail of something very significant in investigating properdin.

But here again we are fearful that properdin will be used as vaccines are used. Instead of finding out why some of us have more properdin than others, and what we can do to increase our supply, scientists will probably go injecting properdin indiscriminately, with no regard to the other substances that must accompany it. And who knows what may result?

In view of our national preoccupation with "shots" it is surprising how many physicians have expressed grave doubts about the wisdom of vaccinations and other injections. Among laymen, of course, there is a large and vociferous minority who are violently opposed to vaccination. And there is an increasing body of medical evidence showing that vaccinations may be directly or indirectly responsible for the high incidence of such diseases as polio, cancer, encephalitis, hepatitis and so forth.

Another aspect of immunity that seems to us the most promising field of all for further investigation is the recent report by Eugene H. Payne, M.D. of the many places in South America which are "islands of immunity." Heart disease, cancer, malaria, hookworm, tooth decay, mental illness are unknown in one or another of these localities. Why? We do not know. But we do know that it is *not* because the residents have been vaccinated against the disease. And we feel very definitely that the finest contribution any philanthropist or foundation could make would be to investigate fully these islands of immunity and discover the secret which could possibly lead to greatly improved health for all of us.

Infections and Good Nutrition

How did any physician first come to the conclusion that lack of proper nutrition has anything to do with infectious disease? Was it when he visited a child in the slums, saw the completely inadequate diet this child ate, observed the dull hair and eyes, the bad skin, the rickety bones, the poor teeth, the listless attitude, and said to himself "There's a likely candidate for tuberculosis?"

Perhaps we originally get our association of good nutrition with resistance to infections from stories about the great plagues and famines that have ravaged one country after another. We know that no century —even the 19th—has been without its famine. As far back as 503-443 B.C. in India there are records of famines followed by plagues. It seems logical therefore that famines bring about plagues, but some investigators have questioned whether the diseases are brought about only by lack of proper food. During a famine, they tell us, there is a let-down in living conditions. Sanitation gets worse. The rats, who are hungry too, move in closer to the human population so that they can more easily share whatever food there is. Rats carry lice which carry typhus germs. Perhaps the reason for plagues following famines is not necessarily lack of proper food. But somehow we still incline to the opinion that food which does not properly nourish us leaves the door wide open for many different kinds of infections.

Modern nutritionists recognize the very definite relationship between nutrition and resistance to infections. By "infections" we mean all those ailments that are caused by a "bug" of one kind or another. We even know which elements of diet appear to be most effective in protecting us against infections.

Vitamin A and Infections

W. L. Aycock, M.D. and G. E. Lutman, M.D., review experimentation covering infection versus vitamin deficiency, in an article in the *American Journal of Medical Science,* Volume 208, 1944. They take up first vitamin A and ask whether it is really an anti-infective vitamin. Xerophthalmia is the disease produced by severe vitamin A deficiency. It is practically unknown in this country because even the poorest diets in this country somehow manage to contain enough vitamin A to prevent this disease. However in India and China patients suffering from xerophthalmia also suffer from numerous infections. Pneumonia, bronchitis, infections of the middle ear and so forth are common. All investigators have found that lack of vitamin A brings about an unhealthy condition of the skin and the mucus membrane such as the lining of the throat and nose. With little or no vitamin A in the diet, this mucus lining becomes hard and dry. The fluid that would normally wash off germs and carry them away is not present.

So it seems logical that such dried out tissues, lacking in their protective fluid, might much more readily become infected by the germs that surround us all the time. In an article in the *British Medical Journal,* Volume 2, 1928, H. N. Green and E. Mellanby describe experiments with young rats who were fed a diet rich in all known nutriments except vitamin A. They invariably died of infections—an abscess at the base of the tongue, pneumonia, and infections of the genito-urinary tract, the middle ear, and so forth. In most cases ample amounts of vitamin A added to their diets relieved their symptoms.

In an experiment by A. L. Daniels, M. E. Armstrong, and M. K. Hutton, reported in the *Journal of the American Medical Association* Volume 81, 1923, rats kept on a diet inadequate in vitamin A were killed at intervals and examined. All of the experimental rats had infections somewhere—in the ear, throat, at the base of the tongue or in the nose. The control rats whose diet contained enough vitamin A showed none of these symptoms. Many, many other experiments have been performed, some of them indicating that vitamin A deficiency does not affect susceptibility to infection, most of them indicating that it does.

Vitamin A in Human Nutrition

In case of human beings, it becomes more difficult to assess results. You can always say, well, the vitamin A content of this person's blood is low and he is suffering from an infection. But perhaps the lack of vitamin A is the *result* of the infection rather than the *cause*.

Experimenting with human subjects, E. L. Gardner and F. W. Gardner in the *American Journal of Children's Diseases,* Volume 47, 1934, describe giving vitamin A in the form of halibut liver oil to 50 school children, with another 25 acting as controls. These 25 children who did not take the vitamin A had a history of being highly resistant to colds already. However it was found that the 50 children taking vitamin A showed a decrease in incidence and severity of colds compared to the 25 who did not. In addition, the vitamin-taking children also increased in weight and in general health.

In some other experiments the decrease in colds is phenomenal. In one experiment 185 workers in industry took a tablespoonful of cod liver oil every day, with 128 other workers acting as controls. In the vitamin-taking group no colds developed in 55.1 per cent. Only 32.8 per cent of the non-takers developed no colds. The cod-liver oil group reduced their hours of time lost from work 51.9 per cent as compared to 40.6 per cent in the controls.

So far as colds are concerned, another observation appears to be equally important. F. Hoelzel, writing in the *Proceedings of the Society of Experimental Biology and Medicine,* Volume 25, 1928, tells us from his personal experience he has found that during fasting or marked undernutrition (note that we did not say malnutrition) colds did not develop. But they appeared after periods when not enough protein had been eaten. And, by restricting the carbohydrate level of the diet and maintaining an adequate protein level, colds could be prevented. This appears to be one excellent explanation for the rash of colds that break out after holidays when all of us, especially children, have been stuffing ourselves with holiday goodies at the expense of the protein, protective foods we need.

The American Medical Association Council on Pharmacy and Chemistry defined its attitude to vitamin A as the anti-infective vitamin in 1935 thus: "By virtue of its (cod liver oil's) vitamin A content, it promotes growth and as indicated by experimental studies, may be an aid toward the establishment of resistance of the body to infection in general, though it has not been shown to be specific in the prevention of colds, influenza and other such infections." L. J. Harris, in his book *Vitamins in Theory and Practice* (Macmillan, 1935) has this to say: "If you take insufficient vitamin A, you are certainly liable to develop special kinds of localized infections. It is wise therefore to take care that your diet is adequate and well-balanced. But this has nothing to do with ordinary infectious diseases as commonly met with; and in any case most people in this country do appear to get ample vitamin A, so that in such circumstances it seems futile to try and treat ordinary infectious diseases and septicemias with vitamin A medication."

Prevalence of Vitamin Deficiencies

Now right at this point we part company with the reasoning of the researchers such as Dr. Harris. In the first place on what do we base the statement that not many Americans suffer from vitamin A deficiency —the fact that practically none of us have xerophthalmia? This particular eye disease of course occurs only in the last extremities of vitamin A deficiency. But does it not seem that we are all probably suffering from a lesser vitamin A deficiency?

The minimum daily requirement of vitamin A is 5000 International Units. By this is meant that 5000 units will prevent symptoms of deficiency such as xerophthalmia. It is generally understood, however, that far, far more than this is necessary for good health. If you eat liver several times a week you are probably getting enough vitamin A, for an average serving contains about 11,000 units. Three-fourths of a cup of carrots contain 12,000 units, a medium sweet potato 7700, half a cantaloupe 5100. Green leafy vegetables contain an average of about 560 units per serving, a pat of butter represents 330 units, an egg 570 units.

A housewife who is very conscious of diet needs and works hard to balance the family meals probably sees to it that her family will get enough vitamin A, for she will serve carrots, sweet potatoes, liver, eggs and so forth frequently. But what about the other housewives who may not buy a bunch of carrots in a month, use margarine instead of butter, find eggs too expensive and tell us their families don't like liver? Talk to your neighbors and you'll find a shockingly high number of them in this category. Now where are these folks going to get their vitamin A? It is simply impossible to assume that they are not suffering from a slight vitamin A deficiency.

In addition, what of all the elements in daily life that use up our store of vitamin A? Mineral oil destroys vitamin A and other fat soluble vitamins as well, and the taking of mineral oil as a laxative is widespread. Peroxides used in bleaching flour and other foods are destructive of vitamin A, and those of us who eat processed foods are getting peroxides all the time. Several drugs are potent enemies of vitamin A. Pasteurization destroys about 19 per cent of the vitamin A in milk. All of the vitamins have their enemies, and these enemies surround us in our daily life.

McCollum, dean of nutritionists, writing in his books under such titles as *Common Sense and Nutrition* and *What is the Right Diet?* continually stresses *the necessity for the right food*—rather than depending on supplementary vitamins. With this, of course, we are in complete agreement. The ideal condition—and one in which we believe there would be precious little if any difficulty with infections—would be a life in which we eat organically grown vegetables and fruits fresh from the garden, eat many of them raw to conserve all the vitamins and enzymes, eat animal foods that are fresh and untreated with any preservatives or other chemicals that may react unfavorably in our body's chemistry, destroying the activity of vitamins. But how many of us can live like that?

Even those of us who have our own farms and gardens—if we live in the north—must depend on some other source for vegetables and fruits in the winter. Most of us must buy meat, cheese, milk and so forth from the big food companies which process everything. And, considering the almost universal use of all kinds of poisons—not only in insecticides and fertilizers, but in chemical preservatives, processing methods, coloring matter and even the containers in which our food is packed—how can we depend on this dead devitalized kind of food to give us ample vitamins? It seems to us absolutely necessary that all of us take supplementary vitamins and minerals—but here again, we continually stress the fact that these should come from natural food products—they dare not be synthetic.

B Vitamins and Infections

What about the B vitamins in prevention of infections? Two articles from the *Proceedings of the Society of Experimental Biology and Medicine* (volume 67, 1948 and volume 62, 1946) describe experiments on animals made deficient in pyridoxine, thiamin and biotin—all B vitamins. In all cases, the rats who were deficient in the vitamins were able to produce fewer antibiotics in their blood, for fighting off germs.

In an article from *Medicine,* volume 13, 1934, Elizabeth Chant Robertson of the University of Toronto devotes almost a hundred pages of discussion to experiments which have been done on vitamins protecting against infections. In her summary on vitamin B she says "a great variety of experimental infections have been shown to be more frequently fatal or more easily induced in animals lacking vitamin B than in normal animals. Very few reports have been published which have not shown this reduced resistance."

Vitamin C and Infections

Discussing vitamin C in relation to infections, Rhinehart, Connor and Mettier in *International Clinician,* volume 2, 1937 and *The Journal of Experimental Medicine,* volume 59, 1934, tell us they found that guinea pigs suffering from scurvy (vitamin C deficiency disease) who were infected with a streptococcus infection, developed a condition similar to rheumatic fever and rheumatoid arthritis in human beings. They suggested that a "sub-clinical" degree of scurvy may make up the rheumatic tendency which, with an added factor of infection, causes the development of rheumatic fever. This means that infections develop more readily in persons who lack vitamin C—not to the extent of producing scurvy, but just to the extent that most of us lack it—a "subclinical" deficiency.

It has also been found that diphtheria susceptibility is commoner in guinea pigs who lack vitamin C. Children with scurvy are more susceptible to diphtheria. Lawrynowicz, in the *Journal de Physiologie et de Pathologie Générale,* volume 29, 1931, suggests that scurvy may so reduce the resistance that a diphtheria carrier may become the victim of bacteria which it previously carried without any ill effects. Three investigators showed that added amounts of vitamin C assist animals on normal diets in their reactions against tuberculosis.

An experiment in a tuberculosis sanitarium was carried on during the months of March, April and May, when deaths most often occurred there. Patients were grouped in pairs, as closely alike as possible in age, sex, etc. One patient was given an orange each day, while his control was given a pastry. It appeared that addition of vitamin C (even in such small amounts) assisted in healing the tuberculosis symptoms. Testing patients who suffered from intestinal tuberculosis, a cod liver oil concentrate was given and no improvement was noted. But as soon as orange juice was added, immediate improvement began. In a second test, brewer's yeast (vitamin B) was given and again no improvement was shown until vitamin C was given too.

S. W. Clausen, writing in the *Physiological Review,* volume 14, 1934, throws light on the subject from the point of view of natural products supplying the vitamin content. In testing guinea pigs, several researchers have found that an abundance of fresh green fodder (containing, of course, natural vitamin C) has protected against infections. In a study of 400 animals one scientist (Wamoscher, *Zeitschrift fur Hygiene und Infektionskrankheiten* CVII—1937) showed that sub-acute scurvy predisposes to spontaneous pneumonia. Cure sometimes followed the administration of vitamin C in orange juice. L. T. Webster and I. W. Pritchett in the *Journal of Experimental Medicine,* volume 40, 1924, describe putting one group of mice on a complete, nutritious diet, as recommended by McCollum, the famous nutritionist. The other group ate bread and pasteurized milk, oatmeal, buckwheat and dog biscuits. The first group was more resistant to typhoid fever, mercury bichloride poisoning and botulinus poisoning.

McConkey and Smith (*Journal of Experimental Medicine,* volume LVIII, 1933) showed that animals on a diet lacking natural vitamin C developed ulcers of the intestines if they were infected with tuberculosis germs. If they received an adequate amount of tomato juice they almost without exception remained free of the infection. Dr. Clausen points out the significant fact that very few studies have been done on animals only partially deficient. Yet he says "partial deficiency in man is far more likely to occur than total deficiency." He says too that multiple deficiencies have not been adequately studied and reminds us that probably multiple deficiencies are frequent and important in human beings.

Experiments With Multiple Deficiencies

Finally let us examine an article in the *Journal of Laboratory and Clinical Medicine,* volume 30, 1945, in which L. J. Berry, J. Davis and T. D. Spies discuss the influence of the B vitamins on the resistance of rats to infection. We were glad to find the name of Dr. Spies listed as an author of this article, for we have come to expect from him most unusual and very practical experiments which add greatly to our knowledge of how human beings manage to get along. He did not disappoint us in this article. These researchers tell us that "single vitamin deficiency studies are important in elucidating the metabolic function of the vitamins, but single deficiencies seldom occur naturally." That is, in terms of human nutrition, a person who suffers from a lack of one B vitamin is certain to lack the others too, for they occur mostly in the same foods.

And they react with one another in the body. Someone who lacks vitamin B will probably lack the other water soluble vitamin C as well. If a person does not get enough vitamin A in his food, he almost certainly will not get enough of the other fat soluble vitamins—D and E, for they occur in many of the same foods.

In their experiment these nutritionists decided to place one group of rats on the diet commonly eaten by many of the patients who visit their clinic in Birmingham, Alabama. They divided the rats into ten groups—two of which received only the basic diet as eaten by families in the neighborhood. Two other groups received this basic diet plus casein (a protein). Two other groups received the basic diet plus casein and minerals. Two other groups ate the basic diet plus casein, and B vitamins. The final two groups received the basic diet plus casein, minerals and B vitamins.

The basic diet consisted of cornmeal, white flour, pork fat and cane sugar. Yes. this was the diet the researchers had discovered their clinic patients were eating every day. The animals were permitted to remain on the diets for two months before they were checked. The pictures taken at that time indicate more clearly than any words what condition the rats were in by then. Those on the basic diet were small, scrawny, weak. Their coats were rough and ugly. As the various elements were added to diets, the appearance of the rats improved. The final picture shows a handsome, sleek, healthy-looking rat who was of course eating the minerals, vitamins and proteins as well as the basic diet.

Laboratory tests showed that the leucocytes (disease-fighting blood corpuscles) decreased steadily in the rats on the deficient diets. As the diets became progressively better, the number of leucocytes increased and the total number of leucocytes was normal only in the rats on the best diets. "These studies support the working hypothesis that resistance to bacterial invasion may be depressed by inadequate nutrition," say these investigators. "Their importance is enhanced by the fact that the animals were eating the same diet that gives rise to the mixed deficiencies seen in patients in the clinic. . . . Therefore in mixed deficiencies, the importance of restoring the organism to a balanced nutritional regime becomes apparent if that organism is to be able to defend itself against the onslaughts of bacterial invasion."

How To Guard Against Infections

What should we conclude in summing up all the facts we have reviewed? That taking vitamin A in fish liver oil perles will guarantee you against colds this winter? Not entirely, if other factors in your diet are still inadequate. Do we mean to indicate that rose hip tablets and lots of fresh fruits and vegetables rich in vitamin C will guard you against colds and other pesky infections? Well, certainly, vitamin C is enormously important in the fight against infections, but only if other elements in your diet are adequate as well. Vitamin D is important, vitamin B is important and, as the last experiment showed, minerals are important, too.

So perhaps the investigation done by early scientists showed only that individual vitamins do have some potency against infection. But they can be completely effective only when all the other factors of a good diet are in proper balance as well. We hope this doesn't sound too impossible of attainment. Actually it's not difficult to arrive at a really and truly balanced diet that includes all of the important vitamins and minerals. Basically it boils down to this:

1. Your diet should contain nothing that does not contribute to nutrition. With this one statement we eliminate white sugar and white flour and all products made from them. We cannot stress too sharply the harm that these two villains (refined sugar and flour) commit. They have no food value, except calories. They take up valuable space on your menu and in your digestive tract and, especially in the case of children, they are so filling and appetite-satisfying that children who eat sweets and baked goods simply don't have room or appetite for nutritious foods. Perhaps even more important, these two "foods" have been stripped of all vitamins. But your body needs B vitamins to digest them, so it steals from your store of the tremendously important B vitamins, resulting in a certain deficiency.

2. Your diet should contain lots of the protective foods: meat (the organ meats such as liver at least once a week) cheese, eggs, milk (for children), fresh green leafy vegetables (raw), plenty of yellow vegetables and other vegetables, raw whenever possible, raw fruits in abundance.

3. Because of the "devitaminizing" that occurs before even the freshest food reaches your table, and because of all the substances that rob you of vitamins every day, you should take food supplements—not synthetic vitamins, please! Fish liver oil contains vitamins A and D, brewers' yeast and desiccated liver contain all the B vitamins, rose hips contain vitamin C, and wheat germ oil contains vitamin E. Bone meal is a source of abundant minerals—all you need.

Take them all, every day. Watch your diet, take your food supplements and say goodby to infections!

Infections and Vitamin C

We know that vitamin C is powerful against poisons of various kinds that are likely to attack the human frame. The poison of nicotine, for instance, uses up vitamin C, when one is smoking. This means, probably, that the vitamin C neutralizes the poison and is itself used up in the process. In general this is the way vitamin C works against poisons. It combines chemically with the poisons, researchers believe, to make a substance that is not poisonous and this substance is harmlessly oxidized. Of course you lose a lot of vitamin C that way.

Does vitamin C perform the same function against harmful bacteria that would otherwise cause infection? Many scientists believe that it does and their experience certainly bears out their contention. As long ago as February, 1951, F. R. Klenner, M.D. of Reidsville, North Carolina made a speech before the Tri-State Medical Association of the Carolinas and Virginia in which he described his own experiences giving vitamin C for a wide variety of infectious diseases with such dramatic success that you would think his speech on the subject would have shaken the medical profession to its foundation.

Dr. Klenner used vitamin C in treating virus pneumonia, measles, a pulmonary virus infection, virus encephalitis-meningitis, polio, influenza and other infectious diseases. In his address, Dr. Klenner describes many cases of his own patients treated with vitamin C alone. Two children with measles (or rather with premeasles symptoms) were completely cured within several days and no measle rash occurred. Virus pneumonia complicated by encephalitis affected a 28-year-old woman and a 19-months-old baby. In the first case the woman was clinically well of her pneumonia within 72 hours. The baby, who had been partially paralyzed, was able to drink fruit juice two hours after the first injection of vitamin C. Several other cases of respiratory illnesses responded almost miraculously to injection of vitamin C.

Vitamin C for Polio

Most important, however, Dr. Klenner feels, is the response in cases of polio. He says "Many physicians refuse to employ vitamin C in the amounts suggested, simply because it is counter to their fixed ideas of what is reasonable; but it is not against their reason to try some new product being advertised by an alert drug firm. It is difficult for me to reconcile these two attitudes. On the other hand, many physicians who have been willing to try vitamin C against the virus of poliomyelitis have obtained the same striking results as we reported."

His story of a diabetic boy is particularly revealing. This 7-year-old lad had been diabetic since the age of four. Any infection produced alarming changes in his blood sugar balance. He contracted measles and was forced to take six times the regular amount of insulin. Injections of vitamin C, right at the height of the disease, improved his condition at once and gradually brought his insulin requirement back to normal.

Dr. Klenner's idea of the way vitamin C works in cases of virus infection is that the vitamin joins with the toxin and/or virus to form a new compound which is then destroyed by oxidation—that is, combining with oxygen. Therefore, anyone suffering from an infection is bound to be short on vitamin C, for the vitamin is used up faster than it can be replaced by food. It has been found, says Dr. Klenner, that patients with infectious diseases do indeed have very low amounts of vitamin C in their blood.

Cold weather may mean you need more vitamin C! Yes, it's true, at any rate for guinea pigs who are the only creatures, aside from apes and human beings who cannot manufacture their own vitamin C inside their bodies. Jolliffe, Tisdall and Cannon in their monumental book *Clinical Nutrition* (Paul B. Hoeber, Inc., 1950) tell us that rats exposed to cold weather, develop more vitamin C, inside their bodies, to protect them from this stress of cold. Those rats who, for some reason, cannot produce the required amount of vitamin C, may begin to show a decrease of vitamin C in their tissues which may indicate that the cold actually uses up their store of vitamin C. Guinea pigs, who, like man, cannot make their own vitamin C, must depend on an increased intake in their food if they are to be able to survive cold weather. The lower the temperature the more vitamin C is required.

An amount of vitamin C that is perfectly adequate for a guinea pig at room temperature is reported to be completely inadequate at a temperature of freezing or 32 degrees Fahrenheit. The small animals can adapt themselves to cold and manage to live healthfully only if their supply of vitamin C is increased. In studying the guinea pigs it was found that this vitamin C supply was in the tissues of the bodies, especially the adrenal glands, of those which managed to survive. And when their supply of vitamin C was discontinued, those who had taken a large supply of the vitamin previously were found to survive longer than those who had not.

In our file on colds we found a letter from the *British Medical Journal* for April 21, 1951, written by John M. Fletcher and Isabel C. Fletcher, expressing surprise that more material does not appear in medical journals on the potency of vitamin C in protecting against cold germs. These two physicians state that in their own practice they have found vitamin C an excellent preventive of colds. Perhaps, they say, the general disregard of the vitamin as a cold preventive results from the difficulty among the experts in reaching agreement as to what actually is the daily requirement of vitamin C. With adults, they say, the disease of scurvy will occur when the adult is getting less than 10 milligrams of vitamin C daily. But, they continue, this represents far less than "saturation level." By this they mean that to soak all the tissues of the body in vitamin C a much larger amount than 10 milligrams a day is necessary. In cases of fever or hard physical exertion, the body uses up vitamin C much faster than usual. So it is not ever possible to set one figure as the absolute daily requirement for all people under all circumstances.

We agree wholeheartedly with the Fletchers only, as usual, we would carry their argument a little farther. Aside from fever and exertion, modern adults are subjected to countless other hazards that deplete their vitamin C—sleeping pills, for instance, tobacco-smoking, exposure to lead, benzene and other industrial poisons. And since no one has ever suffered from too much natural vitamin C, why in the world should we limit ourselves to a daily minimum when, apparently, the more we take the better we will feel in every way? We know from laboratory experiments that animals suffering from infections have a very small amount of vitamin C in their bloodstreams. We know, too, that animals deliberately kept on diets low in vitamin C develop more infections than those who are getting enough. These two facts alone are sufficient indication that vitamin C in large quantities is necessary in the fight against any infection—including, of course, cold infections.

Preventing Infections With Vitamin C

The Fletchers go on to tell of a number of experiments in Holland, Germany and Australia in which colds were prevented by the administration of vitamin C. In the German experiment there was a marked fall in the amount of illness over a period of eight months among factory workers given 100 to 300 milligrams of vitamin C a day, a benefit not found when they were given 20 or 50 milligrams.

In the *British Medical Journal* volume II, page 617, 1942, Doctors A. J. Glazebrook and S. J. Thompson report an experiment in an institution in England caring for boys. At this institution the handling of food—that is, the way it was stored, prepared, served and so forth—had resulted in a vitamin C intake of 15 milligrams per boy per day—just barely enough to prevent symptoms of scurvy. Some of the boys were given vitamin C for six months. The other boys went on eating their regular diet. During the brief period of six months there was no appreciable difference in the incidence of colds in the two groups, *but* the boys who had the vitamin spent only an average of two and one-half days in the infirmary whereas those who had received no vitamin C spent an average of five days being sick. So the additional vitamin C, even for this brief period, apparently strengthened the children's resistance to germs so much that they were able to throw off the effects in half the time it took the untreated children.

From the *Journal of the American Medical Association,* volume 120, 1942, page 1268 comes information about an experiment in which college students were given 200 milligrams of vitamin C daily and the colds they had were compared with those of another group of students not taking vitamin C. The vitamin-takers averaged 1.9 colds per year to 2.2 for the non-takers. Markwell, writing in the *Medical Journal of Australia,* volume 2, page 777, 1947 reported that the sooner vitamin C is given after the onset of a cold, the better. He successfully gave 750 milligrams at the start, then gave 500 milligrams or more, three or four hours later. Three other investigators, writing in the *Journal of Nutrition,* volume 23, page 309, 1942, had found that the higher level of vitamin C in the blood lasts only about three or four hours, even when a very large dose is given. So the doses must be given at frequent intervals, according to them, to keep the blood and tissues saturated with vitamin C.

H. W. Holmes, M.D. writing in *Science,* volume 96, page 497, 1942, describes his own experiences in relieving hay fever, food allergies and asthma with vitamin C. He gave it in large doses—200 to 500 milligrams every day for a week. Does this perhaps demonstrate that the usual daily requirement we casually accept as correct for adults (about 75 milligrams per day) may be far too low?

W. J. McCormick, M.D., of Canada uses vitamin C in enormous doses for curing disease. He tells us in an article in *The Archives of Pediatrics* for April, 1952, that vitamin C is important for the healing of wounds, the prevention of hemorrhaging and the building of a barrier against germ invasion. It contributes to the building up of disease fighters or antibodies in the bloodstream; it neutralizes toxins in the blood—that is, it helps to build a natural immunity to infectious diseases and poisons. In the rapidity with which it stops the course of some diseases it compares favorably with the sulfa drugs, says Dr. McCormick, and it does not have any after-effects that may be unpleasant or dangerous. Dr. McCormick uses injections of vitamin C to completely saturate tissues. Any excess is carried away by the kidneys. Dr. McCormick has used vitamin C successfully in treating tuberculosis, scarlet fever, pelvic infection, septicemia and so forth.

Since we are not physicians we cannot take vitamin C by injection to cure infectious disorders. Our doctors could, however, and possibly would undertake this kind of therapy if we were to tell them how the vitamin has been used successfully against infections. We ourselves can see to it that we get more than enough vitamin C every day in food and in food supplements. Dr. Klenner and the other physicians mentioned above used synthetic vitamin C. It can be given easily in massive doses that way, whereas it is a little more troublesome to take a considerable number of rose hip tablets to get the same amount of vitamin C. However, don't forget for a moment that other things come with the vitamin C in rose hips—rutin and hesperidin for instance. If synthetic vitamin C in large doses will give the results described above—it seems likely that even better results might come about from the use of natural vitamin C in a high enough concentration.

Insecticides—Systemic Sprays

By J. I. Rodale
Editor of *Prevention*

(A clipping from the *Washington Daily News* for September 2, 1955 states: "The Food and Drug Administration today approved a new type bug killer which a plant absorbs through its roots, making all of it poison to hungry bugs. The chemical is a trialkyl trio-phosphate with a trade name of Systox. It originated in researches in organic phosphates in Germany some 20 years ago. It's expected to prove a boon to truck gardeners, orchardists and other commercial growers, who'll get first chance to buy it.

"It won't be available to home gardeners, at least for use on food crops, until officials are satisfied it can be handled safely in the home. It also kills bugs on ornamental plants like roses and chrysanthemums.

"In concentrated form, the chemical is a deadly poison, related to a number of the chemicals internationally considered in the weapons class by chemical warfare specialists . . . The new killer won't wash off because it's absorbed into the plant itself. Sprayed on the leaves or poured in a weak solution around the plant roots, it quickly becomes a part of the plant. . . . F.D.A. officials are insisting that the quantities used and the methods of application be such that only the faintest traces can remain in any finished food product. 'We're setting our tolerances deliberately low,' one official said.")

Three years ago Editor Rodale wrote an editorial on systemic insecticides which becomes even more timely today than when it was written, for today we are finally faced with systemic insecticides in food. The new chemical, which poisons the whole plant, has been released for use on apples, broccoli, brussels sprouts, cabbage, cauliflower, muskmelons, oranges, pears, potatoes, strawberries, and walnuts. Other crops may be added to the list. We reprint herewith Editor Rodale's earlier comments:

Something sinister is occurring in American agricultural practice, far worse, in my opinion, than the imagination of anything agronomical science has conceived thus far, and which should be a cause for great alarm. It concerns a new method of preventing insect infestation in plants by means of poisonous insecticides and involves such a dangerous mode of action that I wonder if, adopting it, financially hungry industry isn't going a bit too far, or are the men who guide these concerns sick in the conscience? Is it possible also that the ignorance of these men in matters of diet plus the fact that they are consuming devitalized and poisoned food as a result of the products sold by their very own companies, is causing their mental powers to decline so that they cannot clearly see the effect of what they are doing? An English scientific organization has recently made a study in their country and America and has found that the mental ability of people has been declining two per cent per generation. Is this fact related to the quality of food produced by modern industrialized agriculture and the food processors?

About seventy-five years ago the poison spraying of apple trees was practically an unknown procedure in orcharding. Some insects came to plague the apples, but nature provided enemy insects that kept the trouble-makers in check. But, as is always the case in nature, it was not a 100 per cent effective arrangement and some fruit damage occurred. The public was used to seeing and even eating an apple here and there that exhibited an insect bite or two. However, a trend was developing in American life which demanded perfection of appearance. It was part of the movement that gave America automobiles with beautiful chromium fittings. The public began to demand white eggs, thinking they were "purer," and willingly paid a premium for them. Apples had to be large and perfect, without an insect bite, or other disfiguring blemish. The citrus interests began to add color to oranges and the dairy people put the cancer-causing butter-yellow into butter (now banned). Industry scandalously pandered to the consumer's taste for beauty and added eye-appeal to all items of food regardless of how it damaged their nutritional values. This tendency encouraged the chemical interests to play a big part in the beautification of food products.

Upsetting Nature's Applecart

As the years went on the problems in the orchards became more perplexing. The chemist mastered one insect, and another appeared from nowhere. In one season Chemical X destroyed insect Y but the next year insect Y developed a tolerance to poison X. This led to the perfection of more and more powerful chemical compounds and the need for increasing the number of applications to about fifteen or sixteen a season, disturbing the balance of nature to such an extent that even the bees that were needed for the orchardist to pollinate the apple blossoms disappeared, so that the farmer had to hire additional people to hand-pollinate his trees. And when this insecticidal bludgeoning with poison sprays got beyond the physical capacity of the farmer to handle, he took to the air and in 1951 the farmers of the U. S. used 6,500 airplanes to shower upon the earth these expensive chemical poisons.

The entomologists—those people who spend their lives trying to prove that man is superior to the insect—are having a tough time. They are frantically attempting to breed varieties of fruits and vegetables that are more resistant to disease and insects. They are working feverishly to discover magic formulas that will stop the insect dead in its tracks. But for a long time they have had a dangerous idea in the back of their heads. Why not feed some kind of poison to the plant instead of to the insect, so that every cell and bit of tissue becomes saturated with it. Thus when an insect feeds upon the plant it will be done for. This would be science with a vengeance. They thought of it so long that they actually did it.

Early in 1952 such a product, called *Systox,* was launched with powerful hullabaloo in the ballroom of New York's Waldorf Astoria hotel, by the Pittsburgh Coke and Chemical Co. This product, made from coal, has the chemical name of *octamethyl pyrophosphoramide.* This pesticide is either put on the soil around the roots or is sprayed on to the plant itself. In either case it forces itself into every cell of the entire plant. One can judge the potency of such a chemical which has the power of forcing itself so thoroughly and saturating every part of a plant.

Several years ago this idea was discussed in agricultural literature and it was announced that soon such a product would be placed on the market. When I was called as a witness, a few years ago, in a hearing in Washington conducted by the Pure Food and Drug Administration for the purpose of determining permissible residues of poison sprays on foods, I expressed alarm at the possibility that such a practice would be encouraged on food crops, that the public would be eating foods every cell of which was tainted by these systemic chemicals. Up jumped a representative of one of the insecticide companies and stated that it was not the intention that this product be used on food crops. It was only thought of for ornamental plants. But in my mind I harbored misgivings. It was a dangerous trend. I was sure that it was bound eventually to be used on edible crops. And that is exactly what is happening.

A Promise Not Likely to be Upset

Professor R. W. Leiby, entomologist of Cornell University, in the June, 1952, *Country Gentleman,* speaks of experiments with Systox on potatoes and apples, and states, "Much more experimentation must be made with the systemic insecticides before they will be approved for use on fruits, vegetables, or crops fed to livestock." But, in the demonstration at the Waldorf-Astoria, mentioned above, Systox was applied into a garden plot of widely assorted plants, including green beans and tomatoes. I feel certain that, unless some powerful consumers' group files an injunction against a few hundred farmers who begin to use systemic poisons on food crops, in a short time every mouthful of food eaten by the public will carry a quota of poison distributed in every cell of it.

The U. S. Department of Agriculture, at the time Systox was announced, advised that the systemic types of insect poisons were definitely not for use on edible crops, although it did state that some day these might be recommended for such crops. If that day ever comes it will be the most formidable blow ever struck against the public interest and the health of our citizenry. It will be the biggest step yet taken towards race suicide through the sterilization of the reproductive functions of man by the irritating effect of these harmful systemic chemicals upon them.

The experts say that systemic insecticides do not remain long inside a plant and that if you wait a few weeks after fruit and vegetables have been treated, they will be safe to eat. But in the same breath they state that the systemic insecticides last three to four times longer than ordinary poisons. I have seen so many of these sales talk statements prove to be false that I do not trust this one. I do not think that all of this poison will be excreted by the plant, and if it does, what effect will it produce on the plant's tissues while it is tarrying in its midst? And who is going to fence in all the orchards and farms to keep innocent wayfarers from this deadly produce *before* the poison is excreted?

The company that makes Systox states that its investigations have shown that bees tapping the nectar of plants treated with this systemic poison were not affected by it. Perhaps they were not affected outwardly or immediately, but careful study might indicate that they are less healthy. They might become lethargic and produce less honey. And did the Pittsburgh Coke and Chemical Company check on the quality of the honey produced by these bees? Does it contain a residue of these poisons?

Farm Chemicals magazine in its June, 1952 issue says that Systox is approximately as toxic to mammals as Parathion, and brother, Parathion is extremely toxic, having in only a few years time killed many orchardists who were applying it to their trees.

Will It Really Save Money?

A newspaper states that Systox will save the nation's farmers millions of dollars worth of crops a year, but I might add it might cause the people who eat Systox-treated foods, tens of millions in medical and hospital costs. Business is in the form of a monetary equation and we must not fail to study that formula in its every aspect, paying attention to both sides. The agricultural press widely acclaims this new product mouthing the prepared statements of the manufacturer to the effect that the product is not dangerous to human beings in the quantity present in harvested crop. But if it is added to all the food preservatives, all the germ killers, the benzoates of soda, the chlorine and alum in water, the sodium nitrite in frankfurters, the chemicals in bread and in every item of food on the daily menu, what then would be the total cumulative effect? The Pittsburgh Coke and Chemical Company, I am sure, has not made such a test.

This is a situation that calls for immediate action. The public must speak out boldly and at once. It must write to congressmen, senators, newspapers, agricultural colleges and the Pure Food and Drug Administration, asking that an unqualified ban be placed on this type of insecticide, even for ornamental plants, because there are too many uneducated farmers and truck gardeners who will be tempted, in bootleg fashion, to use it on food crops if they can purchase it for ornamental use. I say again that our readers must take immediate action to protect the public. It must be brought up for discussion in public forums and at parent-teacher meetings. The public has an inalienable right to eat unpoisoned food, and industry must learn to make profits without infringing upon that right.

Are We Going To Stand For This?

I am horror stricken as I observe the activities of these conscienceless chemical companies—truly organizations without souls, coldly proceeding with their devious money-multiplying devices, regardless of the effect it has upon people's health. I am shocked and never have I been so shocked before. Chemical fertilizers are bad, but the chemical fertilizer companies do not ask you to eat the fertilizers. But Systox and now Pestox and a hundred other competitors are chafing at the bit in order to force their share of this new poison down the public's gullet.

I cannot emphasize this warning sufficiently—we are in the greatest danger we have ever been. It is worse than military war. The public must become aroused and act at once to prevent this disaster from overtaking us.

Of late we have been leading the world in finance and to a certain extent in science. Many countries look to us for inspiration in regard to innovations in technology and culture. If we begin to use these systemic poisons many nations will undoubtedly blindly follow in our footsteps. Are we ready to accept the responsibility for the possible ruinous effects of such false leadership? We must be careful what we do, not only for our own sake, but for the sake of the effect it has on the rest of the world. We must cast out this idea before it takes strong root!

Insecticides Included in Household Polishes

A U. S. Patent has been taken out for a new liquid polish, invented by a gentleman from Iowa. According to *Chemical Week* for September 25, 1954, the formula consists of petroleum oil, whiting and liquid with about 5 per cent chlordane added to give it insecticidal qualities. *Chemical Week* adds the remark that the Department of Agriculture's views on such a product are not known.

So far as we know, there is no existing law to prevent this wax from being sold. Perhaps it is on your grocer's shelves at this moment. Why are we concerned? Chlordane, which composes five per cent of this polish, is one of the deadliest substances known to man. Can anybody come up with any reason at all why it should be included in a polish? It's spine-tingling to think of unknowing mothers putting such a polish on the floor or furniture where their kids are playing.

Chlordane is favored for use in insecticide vaporizers, too. Several states ban the use of these gadgets altogether. Delaware is the latest, whose Board of Health has become concerned and is planning to forbid the sale of vaporizers. These vaporize the insecticide electrically, you know, spreading substance around in a fine mist which settles on everything in the room. Your grocer and favorite restaurant probably use such vaporizers. Check with them. If they do, protest. Then write to your state board of health suggesting that they forbid the sale of vaporizers as other states have done.

Insecticides and The Law

"Last year more than two billion pounds of insecticide were manufactured in the United States. Some 30,000 registered formulas, containing some 100 pesticidal chemicals, have become virtual necessities to American agriculture. These are poisons, yet small quantities of them inevitably get into food." With these words Ralph G. Martin introduces his excellent article "How Much Poison Are We Eating?" in the April 1955 issue of *Harper's Magazine*.

He tells us that a new law will make it necessary for the producer of a new insecticide to ask the Food and Drug Administration to "set a tolerance" for his product. This means the FDA must decide how much residue of this insecticide may be left on fruits and vegetables in interstate commerce, and the manufacturer must abide by their decision. We suppose this also means that, if the FDA should decide that the substance is so poisonous that no residue dare remain on foods, the insecticide would be withdrawn.

The interesting thing is that we have never had any law of this kind before. Up to now, any manufacturer might put an insecticide on the market with no proof at all of its possible safety for human consumption. The government had to prove that the insecticide was harmful by showing in court cases that individuals had been harmed (perhaps fatally) by the substance, or that animal experiments demonstrated considerable toxicity. As you can see, such procedures were extremely expensive in time and money and, of course, no one knows how much damage had been done before the poisonous product was withdrawn.

One example is given by Mr. Martin. At the testimony before the Delaney Congressional Committee from whose hearings the bill evolved, Dr. W. C. Hueper of the National Cancer Institute revealed that the discovery that a certain insecticide was cancer-causing was made quite accidentally. So its use was forbidden. But had this accident not happened, the insecticide in question might now be used on food without anyone being any the wiser. How many cases of cancer might it have caused?

Against the pressure of the agricultural forces for more and better and hence more poisonous insecticides are pitted the efforts of many food companies who are trying to keep insecticides out of their products. Beechnut alone spent 100,000 dollars a year trying to buy foods free from insecticides for their baby foods. Other big food companies such as A and P, Quaker Oats and so forth, maintain large laboratories. A recent article in *Fortune* magazine described the new two million dollar duPont laboratory—the largest industrial center for toxicological research in the nation.

Said *Fortune*: "There is, unfortunately, no simple yes-and-no answer to a toxicological question since there is no such thing as a completely safe or non-toxic material. Thus ordinary water, a chemical in its own right, will ruin the kidneys if too much is drunk day after day. For many individuals, the 'natural' chemicals in a strawberry shortcake are enough to make it an allergic poison. The task of industrial toxicology is to find, quickly and harmlessly, the tolerable extent to which any new material should be introduced into mankind's complicated environment."

The Long Term Effects Are Important

Mr. Martin in *Harper's* goes on to tell us that "the reason for all this anxiety is not the microscopic bit of insecticide residue on any one apple you eat. It is fear of the unknown cumulative effect, the long-range build-up inside your body of the vast variety of toxic materials that may crop up in every meal. In his testimony, Dr. Francis E. Ray, director of the Cancer Research Laboratory of the University of Florida, explained why in his field this problem is particularly difficult to solve. 'Long continued application of small doses,' he said, 'is more effective in producing tumors than are large doses frequently applied. . . . Cancer of the internal organs may pass unnoticed until it has progressed to the fatal stage. In human cancer therefore it might be very difficult to prove that a tumorous growth was initiated by the long-continued ingestion of small amounts of chemicals in food'."

How can you judge what the poisonous effect of any chemical will be over a period of years? How much of it is retained by the body? Does it change into any other substance inside the body that may be even more dangerous? Can we assume that tests with experimental animals will give the same results as tests with human beings?

And, in this respect, how is it possible to know in a laboratory experiment how much poison any one individual may be getting from his environment—all of it cumulative. Laboratory animals are raised in safe air-conditioned cages, with a carefully prepared diet and distilled water, protected against any possible poison. Then they are given only one chemical as a test. But the unfortunate human inhabitant of the twentieth century has met with a score of poisons (and may have begun to store them in his body) before he is even born! Every hour of the day and night from then on he is constantly bombarded with one poisonous substance after another. Who is going to test his ability to withstand *all these poisons at the same time* especially if they are all accumulating inside his body?

About DDT Mr. Martin says: "Here is an insecticide that has been almost wholly integrated into our way of life, as familiar as orange juice. Last year we used at least a hundred million pounds of it and sprayed it on everything from hotel beds to whole cities. We eat DDT all the time, all of us. An investigation reported at a recent meeting of the American Public Health Association revealed that no meal had been found on which some trace of DDT did not appear, and that the daily menu for the average American contained 181 micrograms of it. . . .

"What particularly concerns the doctors is the tendency of DDT to store up in the fatty tissues of all animals, humans included. Dr. Francis Pottenger, Jr., secretary for the Los Angeles County Medical Commission for the Study of Environmental Contaminants, made a random sample in his community, 'If people after four or five years,' he reported, 'who have no reason to suspect that they have DDT in their bodies are found to have from zero to thirty-three parts per million of DDT in their fat, what is going to happen after we have been using DDT from ten to fifteen years'?"

The Staying Power of the New Insecticides

"With chlordane—as with other poisons in common use, like toxaphene, aldrin, dieldrin and heptachlor—the residues are powerfully difficult to remove; you cannot wash them off most foods even with a hot detergent bath. Worse still are the poisons that have staying power in the soil. Even if they are banned for use on edible food, crop rotation may bring them out in foods grown years later on the same ground."

It was found, for instance, that benzenehexachloride (BHC) caused cancer-like growths in test animals. The Department of Agriculture urged all growers not to use it on edible foods. Mark you—this is all the government could do—"urge." It could not *forbid* the use of BHC. But as long as three years later the BHC in the soil maintained up to half of its original concentration. BHC is still used on cotton. If peanuts are planted in rotation between cotton crops, the BHC shows up in the peanuts, causing an off-flavor and of course adding a little bit of deadly poison to be stored in the tissues of the people who eat the peanuts.

Systemic insecticides are so horrible that the mind wavers in an attempt to contemplate them with equanimity. "A systemic poison is absorbed into the plant itself, not merely sprayed on the outside, so that insects sucking the sap from the foliage get it into their own systems and are killed . . . Only two and a half parts per million of the poison kills an insect who feeds on the leaf so grown. . . . Under the new law, approval for thousands of new systemics will be sought," says Mr. Martin.

Sir Edward Mellanby, the world-renowned nutritionist, speaking before a medical school in London in 1951, said "Phenyl mercury compounds are used as fungicides on fruit and vegetable crops. It has been pointed out that as little as 2½ parts of chlordane per million in the diet produces pathological (disease) changes in the liver in rats, that 3 parts of the selenium compounds per million in the diet will produce cirrhosis of the liver and, if continued, cancer of the liver in animals; and that in the case of phenyl mercury compounds as little as .5 parts of mercury per million in the liver in the form of phenylmercuric acetate leads to measurable storage in the kidney with damage to that organ in animals."

What Chemicalization is Doing to Our Food

Mr. Martin continues: "Nonetheless there is a growing group of agricultural experts who feel that too heavy a use of insecticides may lead us into a downward spiral toward disaster. Many of them belong to what is generally known as the Organic Farming school, which holds that healthy plants in naturally fertilized soil can resist insects and disease without the aid of chemicals. There is often much mystical philosophy in this view; its claims cannot all be supported; and for large-scale farming the composting method would be prohibitively expensive. (*Editor's note:* We suggest you ask some of the large-scale organic farmers about that, Mr. Martin!) But despite the violence of the discussion Organic Farmers have aroused, there may be much to be learned from the questions they raise . . .

"For example, Dr. William Albrecht, the nationally-known nutrition expert of the University of Missouri, points out that you can kill insects and get more pounds of corn per acre, but the total amount of protein taken from that acre remains the same. And author-farmer Louis Bromfield, with much-publicized success, has operated farms in France, Ohio and Texas without using insecticides at all. Other 'organicists' have warned that insecticides could backfire (as they may already have done) by creating super-insects, bred from those that are immune, and thus increasing the ultimate pest population."

In spite of the seriousness of the situation, in spite of the fact that the chemical and insecticide manufacturers themselves know what a tough problem they have on their hands, you will find people all over the country rising to announce in loud tones that there is little if any danger and that more and more poisons must be made and spread around on our soil and food, as fast as we can manufacture them. An editorial in the Shreveport (Louisiana) *Journal* for February 15, 1955 praises the chemical industry, saying (believe it or not!) "Chemical fertilizers are putting back into our soils increasing amounts of the plant food removed by crops and erosion. Chemical pesticides are now dramatically reducing the losses caused by pests. . . . Chemicals likewise enhance food values . . . retard molding . . . keep foods soft and moist . . . give better texture." The editorial ends with a strong denunciation of any law which would "require prior government approval of every new ingredient going into food" for it would "hamper new research and drastically limit the nation's hopes for progressing toward its goal of greater abundance."

For this editorial writer we have only one suggestion—that he offer to be the human guinea pig for the new insecticides. The rest of us will wait for half a lifetime or so and see how he makes out.

What Can We Do About Poisons in Food?

What can readers do in the face of this kind of thinking? First of all, protect yourself and your family if you possibly can. Have your own garden and grow as much of your food as possible, organically. If this is impractical, buy as much organically grown food as you can afford. Make certain your diet is rich in the B vitamins, calcium and vitamin C—three things that will help to protect you against the doses of poison you get every day.

We do not know of any definite set of experiments proving that vitamin C protects against the evil effects of DDT. But we do know that it is necessary in the fight against any poison. That is one of its main functions in the body—detoxification. So one of your best guards against the possible devastating effects of DDT over a long period of time is plenty of vitamin C in your diet. Fresh raw fruits and vegetables are the best source—and, of course, rose hips and other completely natural food supplements.

Finally, we agree with Mr. Martin when he says that the new law for testing toxicity *first* before allowing insecticides on food "will be effective only if public pressure makes it effective. So far, the chemical companies and the food processors have been much more conscious of the need for the law than the average consumer, for the press gave the hearings almost no coverage. . . . The hope of the new law is severe enforcement. . . . And it is the hope most of all that public awareness will maintain constant pressure to keep the new law strict and strong, so that never again will the American people be 160 million guinea pigs."

Letters to your congressman, your senator, the Food and Drug Administration, your newspaper, your favorite magazines (especially the women's magazines which should be deeply concerned with the wholesomeness of our food) should help to put on pressure. Write to the people from whom you buy your produce. Tell them you would rather have a wormhole now and then, you would rather have beans and peas not quite so full-podded, if you could only be certain they did not contain deadly insecticides. Finally, remember that a federal law protects only food that crosses state lines. Local produce may be loaded with poisons unless you have an equally effective state law forbidding it. Talk to your state representative about it.

Insomnia

By J. I. RODALE
Editor of *Prevention*

I have been interested in the mechanism of sleep for over twenty years, but it was about a year ago that I suddenly became aware of a certain fact which has completely revised my attitude toward insomnia. For the last twenty years I thought I was suffering from this condition, but one day I received a shock. I had always thought that it took me hours to fall asleep but my wife told me that ten minutes after my head hit the pillow she heard me snoring. I began to see that I must study anew into my problem of lack of sleeping ability. A week after this there was an auto smash-up outside our house, in the middle of the night, that made a terrific noise. It awakened the whole family, but I slept through it all, oblivious to everything. I gave myself away in the morning when I pleaded ignorance to the whole thing.

"And you an insomniac!" taunted my spouse.

This required some study. I recalled the story of the old lady who had told her doctor that she never slept a wink all night. She insisted that she did not get any sleep at all. Since the old lady did not have any diseases that would cause a total lack of sleep the doctor told her that that was impossible.

"In fact," he said, "to prove to you that you *do* sleep I'll tell you what I'll do. I will get a nurse to stay with you one whole night. Each hour, on the hour, she will come into your bedroom, and wake you from sleep."

And that is exactly what was done. Every hour, on the hour, the old lady was awakened from deep slumber. I began to feel there was something that old lady and I had in common. What was it? We were both sure that we didn't sleep well, although she was a bigger liar than I was. Then one day I found the answer. I figured that we must be awake only in short periods, and we sleep only in short periods. *But we don't know the exact moment when we fall asleep!* We know when we are awake but we don't know when we're asleep. We have no feeling of being asleep.

Try and think back! Can you remember any one point during a night of recent sleep when you can say, this was the exact split second when I fell into sleep? No! No one in the world at any time has ever done that. It is a physiological impossibility. Try it tonight and prove it for yourself. But this is not the whole story of my observation. We also usually do not know the exact moment when we awaken, unless it is done by an alarm clock or someone nudging us. There may be a rare exception to this, but I think that by and large we do not know the exact split second during the night when we wake from our little doses of sleep. So, since we do not know when we fall asleep, nor when we awaken, and since there are so many of these short periods of being awake, we imagine we have been awake all the time. We then think we are insomniacs, and make matters worse by fighting sleep with the negative effects of such incorrect thoughts.

I have read dozens of books on sleep. There must be hundreds of them, but not one has ever come within a mile of expressing the particular aspect of the sleep mechanism to which I have drawn attention. They go into complicated scientific descriptions of what sleep is. Here is a typical example: "Dr. X reviewed the physiological aspects of sleep, stating that sleep was a conditioned reflex depending on fatigue of a waking centre rather than on stimulation of a sleep centre; he remarked that control of waking had not been assigned to the reticular substance of the brain stem." So what! And then the doctors tell you to count sheep. I will show you later how ridiculous and wrong that idea is!

In discussing my theory with Marshall Ackerman, our Advertising Manager, he drew my attention to the fact that James Whitcomb Riley had written a poem showing that he was aware of the fact that no one knows exactly the moment when they fall asleep. Here it is:

NO BOY KNOWS

By James Whitcomb Riley

There are many things that boys may know—
Why this and that are thus and so,—
Who made the world in the dark and lit
The great sun up to lighten it:
Boys know new things every day—
When they study, or when they play,—
When they idle, or sow and reap—
But no boy knows when he goes to sleep.

Boys who listen—or should, at least,—
May know that the round old earth rolls East;—
And know that the ice and the snow and the rain—
Ever repeating their parts again—
Are all just water the sunbeams first
Sip from the earth in their endless thirst,
And pour again till the low streams leap.—
But no boy knows when he goes to sleep.

A boy may know what a long, glad while
It has been to him since the dawn's first smile,
When forth he fared in the realm divine
Of brook-laced woodland and spun-sunshine;—
He may know each call of his truant mates,
And the paths they went,—and the pasture gates
Of the 'cross-lots home through the dusk so deep—
But no boy knows when he goes to sleep.

O I have followed me, o'er and o'er,
From the fragrant drowse on the parlor-floor
To the pleading voice of the mother when
I even doubted I heard it then—
To the sense of a kiss, and a moonlit room,
And dewy odors of locust-bloom—
A sweet white cot—and a cricket's cheep.—
But no boy knows when he goes to sleep.

Amazing, isn't it? But I am also amazed at the fact that Riley talked about sleep on the parlor-floor. You may recall the new mattress that I was instrumental in developing which took the floor and put it on top of the bed. Say, this boy Riley was good!

Now let us go a step further. What causes us to sleep in short periods? What is behind these alternating periods of waking and sleeping, when we go from the conscious to the unconscious and back? If a person slept in one position for too long a time, the blood would stagnate to that spot due to the pressure of the bed exerted against it. But through our elaborate nervous system, signals are sent commanding the sleeper to correct the condition, and he usually moves. There are certain paralyzed cases and others in various conditions in hospitals who cannot move, and they develop what are called bed-sores, unless the nurse changes their position every once in a while. Today there are mechanical moving beds available in which the point of contact between patient and bed changes gradually by automatic means.

In order to describe more fully what takes place during sleep with regard to changing our positions, I am going to quote from my 32-page booklet called *Sleep and Rheumatism:*

"According to popular belief a good sleeper sleeps like a log. Down through the years doctors and laymen alike have shared the notion that when healthy persons are undisturbed in slumber they lie practically motionless throughout the long hours of the night. Modern scientific investigation, however, has made clear beyond a shadow of a doubt that this belief is without a shred of foundation in fact. The time-honored phrase, 'sleeping like a log,' is an entirely incorrect description of healthy sleep. H. M. Johnson, Ph.D., head of the Simmons Investigation of Sleep, a branch of the Mellon Institute, says the only person he and his investigators ever found who slept like a log, was an insane patient in a hospital in Pittsburgh. Says Dr. Johnson, 'This patient actually lay still for seven hours on one night, but it was after extremely heavy medication. The facts are clear that it is abnormal to "sleep like a log." Healthy sleep is characterized by comparatively frequent changes of body positions.'

"The average person in good health experiences a 'crescendo' type of sleep in which there are involuntary body movements that increase as the sleep goes on, reports Dr. Donald A. Laird, professor of psychology at Colgate University, in a recent issue of *The Medical Record.*

"Contrary to popular belief, the average healthy sleeper changes his body position from twenty to sixty-five times in the course of an eight hour sleep and under unusual conditions even more times. Dr. Johnson, in collaboration with Dr. T. H. Swan and G. E. Weigand, writing recently in the *Journal of the American Medical Association,* reports that in a healthy sleeper the average time between movements is about two and a half minutes. About half of all the positions a sleeper takes are held for under five minutes; about a fifth of the positions for from five to ten minutes; about a tenth for from ten to fifteen minutes. Less often than once a night does he lie still for as long as an hour at any one time. Of course there are large variations among individuals, and the same individual also varies considerably from night to night. These observations completely upset the notion that healthy sleep is taken in a few positions, each of which is held for a long time.

"The studies Dr. Johnson and his assistants have made of movements in sleeping persons are not based on theory or guesswork but upon scientifically accurate observation. A motion picture camera was arranged so that it would automatically take a picture of a sleeper when he first touched the bed. A second picture would be automatically taken one minute after he ceased to stir, and a third when he stirred again, and so on. By means of this ingenious contrivance as much information was obtained in 7 or 8 feet of film as might be secured on several miles of film if the camera had been operated continuously. The face of a clock hanging beside the bed was photographed with the sleeping individual, thus enabling the scientist to determine to the second how long each sleeper maintained a posture that he kept as long as a minute. The scientists were not interested in the briefer movements."

Please note that in the foregoing quotation mention is made that in a healthy sleeper the average time between movements is about 2½ minutes, that about half of all the positions a sleeper takes are held for under 5 minutes; about a fifth of the positions for about 5 to 10 minutes; about a tenth for from 10 to 15 minutes, and that less often than once a night does he lie still for as long as an hour at any one time. Here you see the basis for my theory. A person sleeps for 2½ minutes, then when he has to move, it awakens him. He stays awake for a little while and then is off again into slumber, but doesn't know it. Now, if he is a sheep counter, when he awakens at these turning points, he says to himself, "Dawgone it, I can't sleep. I'm a hopeless insomniac," and he begins to count sheep. So, instead of remaining awake at this point for, let us say, a couple of minutes, he probably doesn't finish with his sheep for 10 minutes. I can express it perhaps a little better with some drawings.

Here is my conception of the sleep experience of one type of sleeper.

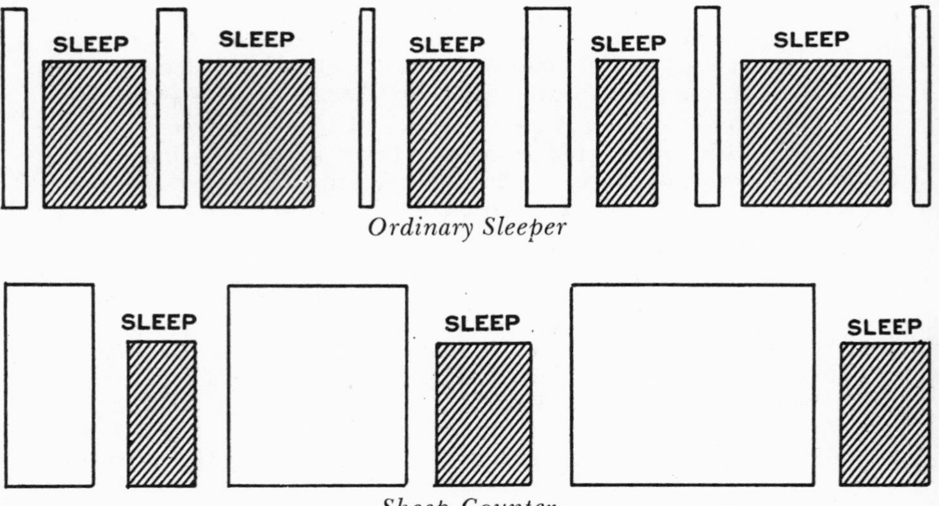

Ordinary Sleeper

Sheep Counter

The higher blocks represent the periods of wakefulness, the lower ones periods of sleep. Note the longer periods of wakefulness of the sheep counter who spends too much time in the pasture. If he forgot all about his flock of sheep, and were to concentrate on the fact that in a moment he would be in the soothing arms of Morpheus, he would get there much sooner.

Why do we think we are not sleeping? For after all, we're up, then we sleep. Then we're up. Even though we don't know exactly the point of falling asleep. The question arises why do we think we didn't sleep?

It seems to me the answer lies on the closeness between the tall points on the diagram, which represent waking. When the periods of waking are close together and the sleep period is short, even in the subconscious mind there is not time for the sleep period to etch itself on the consciousness. The closeness of the two waking periods erases completely the effect of the short sleep period.

Having found out what I now know, overnight I have become an entirely different kind of sleeper. No longer do I class myself as an insomnia sufferer. But I am willing to confess that I know my limitations. I am not the best sleeper in the world. But an insomniac definitely not!

When I go to bed I now have the confident feeling that in about ten to twenty minutes I may begin to catch those little periods of snoozes of perhaps only a minute of duration or so, but they will be the beginning of a process that will get me deeper and deeper into progressively more intense conditions of lethargy. That is the point I wish to make. The sleeper should look forward to the fact that he will at some time or other (sooner if he will help along) reach a state of lethargy or semisleeplessness. If you know about it, it is like hypnosis. A belief in the science and logic of what I am explaining will create a relaxed condition that will put you into a state of deeper lethargy. It is the power of mind over matter.

At this point may I say that there are some persons who have no sleep problems, God bless them. They turn a lot during the night, but they are in such a state of deep lethargy that they are not aware of being awake. Such type of sleepers can slap a mosquito while sound asleep without waking up. This type sometimes claims that he does not change his position during sleep, but even Rip Van Winkle regularly stirred in his long slumber, I am sure.

In laboratory sleep tests it was found that the deep lethargic type of sleepers could not remember hearing peals of thunder, yet they were seen changing their position at such times. In other cases investigators have actually talked to sleepers and received an answer. Yet on the following morning the sleeper could not recall that there had been a conversation.

It is a case of the extent of lethargy that you get into. There are probably three types of sleepers, with gradations, in between. *One* is the deep lethargic type; *two* the medium lethargic; and *three* (in my case) the light lethargic. But even if you are in class three you are getting much more sleep than you think you are.

Here could be the chart of a deep lethargic type of sleeper:

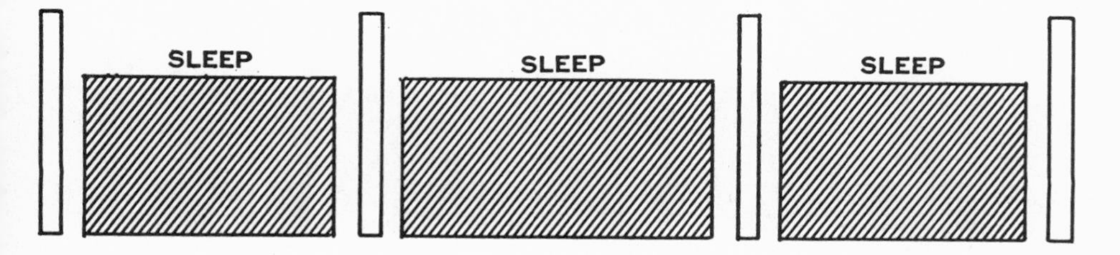

This type falls into a deep sleep very soon after he has made his turn.

The greatest mistake you can make in the periods of wakefulness is to begin to worry about the fact that you are awake. Your eyes may be open, but you may be in a state of lethargy in which nine-tenths of the body and its faculties are asleep. At this point, do everything you can to continue in that lethargic state. Above all, don't count sheep! Don't start to think of ideas! Don't give your mind any problems! Just keep thinking that in a few moments you will be asleep again and remember the thought that you will never know the exact second when that happens. If you don't disturb your periods of wakeful lethargy, the periods of sleep will be longer. Your body will gradually create an improved sleep pattern.

Perhaps you can recall getting up during the night and staggering about. That is because you are in a state of sleep lethargy. You are half asleep on your feet, and it will take a little time to get out of it. Lying in bed, during the night, you are in a much deeper state of lethargy which is giving valuable rest to your mind and body. Knowing this, and not trying to awaken yourself out of this semisleepless state, will aid in giving you a better night's rest. Incidentally I think it is undoubtedly true that the deep lethargic type I mentioned above is most groggy and staggers most when he gets up during the night. The medium lethargic type staggers not quite so much. And the light lethargic, such as I am, is wide enough awake so that he is hardly groggy at all.

Here is another interesting angle on the subject of insomnia. If you find yourself in a sleeper on a pullman car or at a hotel, you may tend to exaggerate the situation, when you awake at the time of making these switches of position. You will imagine that you are awake because of the lurching and rumbling of the train, or because you are not used to the bed. I have often heard people say that they never sleep a wink on a pullman sleeper. Yet they do sleep, although possibly not as soundly. But if they had the right mental attitude, their sleep on trains and in strange beds would be much better. I find in my own case that I am now able to sleep fairly well on a moving train. Yet I used to think that I hardly slept at all.

Only a few days ago I had an excellent example of this type of false insomnia. I had decided to set my alarm clock a half-hour earlier than my usual waking time, which is five in the morning. When the alarm sounded at 4:30 I did not feel like getting up, so I set the alarm for five o'clock, figuring that I would catch an extra half-hour of sleep. But it seems that I lay there wide awake for the whole half hour.

Actually, however, I am sure that I slept a good part of the time, for the alarm went off again in what seemed to be only five minutes of lying-in-bed-time. I must have been asleep for short periods, but I was not aware of it. In this case, especially, the memory of the first alarm was etched into my consciousness as well as subconsciousness. It stood out as a beacon tower of remembrance. Each time I awoke from a short period of sleep (without knowing it, of course) I still vividly remembered the last ringing of the alarm. If I had been really awake for the entire period, it would have felt like thirty minutes, not like five minutes.

Of course there are genuine cases of insomnia. A duodenal ulcer or a loaded colon will cause sleeplessness. In cardiac disease there can be genuine insomnia. When there is continuous unrelieved pain, sleep is difficult. We know that it is harder to sleep in very hot weather, or if it is too cold and you are not well taken care of with blankets. There are cases where a fairly good sleeper will suddenly be handed a puzzler of a situation, a real worrying problem. Then there is very little that can be done. But under ordinary circumstances and in the absence of disease or pain, everyone should get an adequate amount of sleep.

There is another situation where sleep is interfered with. Let us say you have to make a very early morning train and are afraid you will oversleep. Even the soundest sleeper will think of the train all during the night at the "change of position" points, with the result that he becomes more awake each time. The poor sleeper in such a situation may be awake for hours at a time. The answer is to set your alarm clock, or take the train the night before.

In a book called *How to Sleep,* by James Bender, (Coward-McCann, 1949) the methods of famous people for preventing insomnia are given. Bob Hope depends on a clear conscience, correct diet and rubdown at bed-time. When Milton Caaniff gets into bed he reads extremely complicated textbooks. Dr. Wilfred Funk thinks of the way the Chinese used to torture their victims to keep them awake. When Paul Gallico finds himself awake during the night he tries to work out an idea for a story. John A. Hartford tries to divert his mind with various things, and so on and on ad infinitum. But as you now have seen, these are not the best ways to court sleep. They actually accomplish the opposite of what one should strive for. When one finds oneself awake during the night one should know that it is but to be a short-lived, fleeting halt in the sleeping process. One will soon be asleep again. So don't fight it. Work with it! Relax! Let yourself go!

Remember that you are in bed and are resting. Your body will benefit even though you are not fully asleep. You are partly asleep. You are in a state of lethargy in which the processes of the body are reduced to the lowest ebb. Repairs are going on. So don't fight! And help matters along from a psychological point of view. Keep thinking that at any moment you will fall off to sleep.

But you will not know exactly when that moment is.

The French Blanket

I had an interesting "experience" a few weeks ago that will throw a little more light on the mechanism of sleep, and perhaps aid us in our conceptions of insomnia. This is one subject regarding which literature is not lacking. Hundreds of books have been written about it—a confused mass of conflicting ideas—but there is no reduction in the amount of insomnia that plagues the world. Or should I have said, there is no reduction in the amount of insomnia that people think they are suffering from, for much of it is either imaginary or not as bad as people think it is. I say *much of it*—a good part of it, I am sure.

Regarding my new "experience," at times I have mentioned a new method of studying French, Spanish and German that we have developed at the Rodale Press which is now on the market. Up to now we have been doing our own printing, but recently sold our entire printing plant because our business had developed to such an extent that the printing part of it had been getting too much for us.

We had already set a terrific amount of type for this foreign language system, and this posed several problems. Some of it had been proofread, some had not. Some of it was still in the long galleys and had not been made up into pages. We had sold our type. Now we had to find a shop which had fonts of type similar to ours so that they could make corrections in the unproofread portions. There were several other problems, too, and before I knew it, they assumed such importance that I was taking them to bed with me every night.

I recall the particular night on which I had my "experience." It was a night of nervous sleep at best. I kept turning and turning. In my mind, vaguely, there floated reams and reams of proofs, but the French proofs seemed to stand out from the rest. Why, I do not know. There were periods of sleep, I am sure, but when I awoke there were the French proofs again. Soon I began to imagine my blanket as one large French translation. It was not a French proof exactly, but in my mind the blanket was a translation.

I knew I was not dreaming, for I could faintly see and feel the blanket itself, and could see the dim light diffused at the windows. And the blanket was a French translation to me, in every sense. I absolutely did not consider it a blanket. My mind however, was somewhat in the distance. I could say that I was about a half or a quarter asleep, and my consciousness was not fully co-ordinated with the quilt. For several hours I wrestled with that blanket, thinking it was a French translation. I know that I wasn't in dreamland. That I am positive of. I was in a state of semi-consciousness, let us say—not quite in the land of fantasies, but next door to it.

Suddenly I shook my head and made an effort to think. Then I became aware that I was fully awake and that the blanket was a blanket and not a French translation. I smiled to myself, and spent the next hour mulling over what had happened. Then it dawned upon me that this was a beautiful illustration of the fact that man goes through several stages of consciousness in falling asleep, until he gets to the final stage where he is fully asleep. In my own case, because of my problem, I got hooked up in this first stage of semi-consciousness and went no further. And I don't need any psychiatrist to tell me that the blanket as a French translation represented no symbol of any kind, nor was of any interpretive value, except to express the fact that what was strongly in my mind before I fell into this state of torpor, shall I say, came out while I was in that state. We know of what strange stuffs dreams are made, now we must learn that in the semi-conscious state of awakeness or sleep, the stuffs are somewhat less fantastic. The simple fact of a blanket's being considered as a French translation cannot hold a candle to the fanciful and grotesque goings on in dreams.

Another example of being in such a semi-awake state has happened very often and has been mentioned in some of the writings on sleep. A person is awakened and is asked a question. He replies sometimes vaguely, sometimes more rationally. Yet the next morning, when he is told about it, he cannot recall the incident at all. The reason for this could be that when one is suddenly awakened, one is in the last stage of semi-consciousness, equivalent to the state one is in just prior to the moment of falling fully asleep, and therefore can recall very little of what takes place. In my blanket translation episode I evidently was in the first stage of semi-consciousness, and therefore more aware of what was going on, although had I not had a meeting with myself, immediately, right then and there, and thus impressed the whole thing indelibly in my mind, I could have considered it more as a dream, or probably not even remembered it the next morning at all.

We can learn one important thing from all this—that the person who has trouble falling asleep goes through six or seven stages in which he becomes progressively less and less aware of reality until he falls into the final stage, which is sleep itself. The stages are not clearly defined because the sleeper is only partly conscious. And it is even possible that the person who falls asleep as soon as his head hits the pillow may go through the same six or seven stages, but he does it very quickly.

Here is another experience I had many years ago which will throw a little more light on the principle I am trying to write about. About twelve years ago I had a special little device made which I placed at my bedside for taking notes during the night. Many a time I would get an idea during the night, and by morning it would have been completely lost. The device consisted of a little light, a pad of paper, and a pencil dangling on a chain, all mounted on a tiny wooden "counter." But it failed, and is gathering dust somewhere in our attic. Why? Well, I would get the idea in a condition of semi-awakeness. I would put on the light, all right, but when it came to take hold of the pencil and write, I found that I didn't have strength enough to grip it sufficiently to write with it. This illustrates that in such a state, not only is the mind not hitting on all cylinders, but the other parts of the body are also half asleep. This gives me an idea. I must experiment with a dictating machine at my bedside.

Another example illustrating the stages before sleep is that when a person gets out of bed during the night to go to the bathroom, he may stagger quite a bit in getting there. He is not fully awake yet. In fact, that is the case with some people when they awake in the morning. They find it hard to get out of bed. Their limbs are not yet awake. Thus we see that in falling asleep there are several progressive stages of deeper and deeper lethargy, while in awaking there are just as many progressive stages of lesser and lesser lethargy.

Another example is that of a baby a few months old. When it is born, it is like a person who has just been awakened from sleep. Its hands can barely grip an object. As the months go by it goes from stage to stage until it is gradually able to navigate on its own steam. I got this idea from playing with my own grandson, David Rodale, who was then about four months old. When he was a month or so old, and I would give him my fingers to grab hold of, he would not grab them. Later, at four months, he grabbed hold of the index finger of each hand, but if I pulled he let go. In another few months, in a similar situation, he held on strong enough to be pulled up.

Now, what should all this teach us? What can we learn from it? We should know that when we think we are awake during the night, we may be partly asleep. So, at such a time do not aggravate the situation by saying to yourself that you are not sleeping. Do everything possible to be as relaxed as you can. Keep thinking that in a few moments you will be completely in the arms of Morpheus. And then you will be, that much sooner.

Iodine

You do not need nearly so much iodine as you need of calcium and iron—actually you need only about one-one-hundredth as much iodine as iron. This is fortunate, for iodine occurs in extremely small amounts in food and water. It can be stored in the thyroid for a considerable length of time, so there is little danger of an over-dose—in food, that is. Of course, as we all know, tincture of iodine, prepared as an antiseptic, is poison.

About three-fifths of the body's supply of iodine is stored in the thyroid gland. But it is used also in the lymph, the cerebrospinal fluid, perspiration, chyle (a fluid used in digestion), in fluids which collect in the body when abnormal swelling is present, in fluids of the membrane that surrounds the lungs, and breast milk. Milk contains iodine in order to provide the newly born child with a supply, which must last for some time after birth.

From earliest days people have known about the relationship between lack of iodine and goiter formation. We are told that an ancient Hindu collection of incantations dating from 2000 B.C. gives the proper spells that should be said for curing goiter. Far back in history people must have suffered from this disease. During the Napoleonic wars it was discovered that iodine was the element involved in the whole complex business. This is how it happened: a chemist was processing seaweed for use in the war emergency and found that his copper kettles were corroding. When he tested the material to see what was causing the corrosion, he found that it was iodine. Now seaweed, sponges and other sea products have been used for centuries to cure goiter, and with this discovery scientists first began to realize that it is the iodine in the seaweed that is powerful against goiter.

For almost a century further investigation was made of iodine which was meanwhile being used for the treatment of goiter, although no one knew why nor how it acted. Then in 1896 Baumann isolated iodine from the thyroid gland and showed that it is necessary to the work of this gland for producing thyroxine. Later thyroxine was synthesized—that is, chemists broke down the hormone until they discovered what chemical substances were in it. Then they put these substances together to make a synthetic hormone. This hormone is 65 per cent iodine, showing how extremely important iodine is to the functioning of the thyroid.

Iodine and Goiter

The story of the geographic distribution of goiter is fascinating. Goiter occurs naturally in localities where there is not enough iodine in the soil and water. Goiter incidence is highest in the Alps, the Pyrenees, the Himalayas, the Thames Valley in England, certain districts in New Zealand and our own Great Lakes and Pacific Northwest regions.

During the last war in Yunnan Province in China workers on the Burma Road were cut off from their usual supply of salt, due to blockades. They began to use a salt containing less iodine, and within six months there was enlarged thyroid in 80 per cent of the workers. Regional differences in food habits have shown up the necessity for iodine in the diet. In Japan where there is little iodine in food and water, there is no goiter. In Formosa where there is also little iodine, goiter is widespread. The answer to this seeming contradiction is that the Japanese eat large quantities of seafood and seaweed, both rich in iodine. The Formosans do not.

In countries such as Switzerland where iodine is scarce in soil and water, goiter and cretinism have become national health problems which the Swiss have largely solved by using iodized salt. Cretinism occurs in children of parents who lack iodine and hence have goiters. Cretinism results in dwarfed children, with varying degrees of mental retardation, apathetic, with defective speech, clumsy gait, rough skin, sparse hair, brittle nails and a tendency toward constipation, poor teeth, pallor and anemia. Cretinism can be prevented by seeing that mothers have plenty of iodine in their diets before their children are born. It's just that simple. You can see from the symptoms listed above how extremely important iodine is in the diet, for lack of it in a mother influences all these different things in her child—personality, speech, mentality, skin, hair, nails, teeth, digestion and so forth.

Just as there appear to be other causes for goiter so there are other diseases that are believed to be due to iodine deficiency, for iodine is used in other glands, tissues and fluids aside from the thyroid. In animals, a deficiency of iodine results in serious breeding difficulties. Offspring may be stillborn and there may be difficulty with lactation. The administration of iodine brings health and vigor to mothers and children alike.

Goiter From Other Causes

Sir Robert McCarrison, a famous British physician devoted his life to the study of the causes of goiter. He travelled to far corners of the world looking for clues as to the cause of this disease.

He visited the country of Hunza described in Editor Rodale's book *The Healthy Hunzas*. He found that in nations in the territory surrounding the Hunzas goiters were common. The terrain, the amount of iodine in soil and water, the climate of these nations were similar to those of Hunza. Yet among the Hunza people, goiter is unknown. Sir Robert studied the water supply of Hunza and found that it was carefully guarded against pollution. Aside from the fact that the Hunzas themselves are meticulously clean in their way of life, they know that water for drinking must be pure. They keep their drinking water in roofed tanks or closed cisterns inaccessible to animals and well protected from any kind of contamination.

In nine villages about sixty miles from Hunza, says Sir Robert, "the water comes from a single source and is conveyed to the different villages in open kuls or channels . . . it will be observed that there are two main channels on the banks of which the villages are situated one below the other. Each village in this way receive the drainage of the village or villages above it, till at the last village, Kashrote, the drinking water has been polluted by the six villages above.

"The water in these open channels not only supplies the inhabitants with drinking water but it irrigates their extensive crops, serves as an open sewer, is used for the cleansing of their bodies, household utensils and wearing apparel. The drainings from cultivated and manured fields flow into it. It can readily be imagined, therefore, that considerable organic impurities find their way down to the lower villages."

Sir Robert then gives the goiter statistics for each village and says "From this table it is seen that the percentage of infected houses, of infected individuals in these houses and of the total population suffering from goiter, goes on increasing from the highest to the lowest village in the water-channels."

It seems that the pollution in the water uses up or nullifies the iodine in the body so that, unless large amounts of extra iodine are taken, polluted water will surely lead to goiter. It would be best, therefore, to check carefully on your water supply, especially if you live in the country, for government statistics show that the majority of old, shallow wells still in use are definitely polluted.

Sources of Iodine

Drinking water contains iodine, although in the northern part of our country it is present in very small amounts. In southern United States iodine is more plentiful in water. Vegetables and fruits grown in any one locality tend to reflect the amount of iodine available in the soil of that region, so there may be great differences in food content of iodine depending on where the food was produced. Here are some figures of iodine content of various foods raised in goitrous and nongoitrous regions:

	Goitrous	*Non-goitrous*
Milk	265-322	572
Potatoes	85	226
Carrots	2	170-507
Wheat	1-6	4-9
Oats	10	23-175

Most foods, we are told, contain so variable a supply of iodine that they are not reliable as a source of this element—except of course, seafood. Anything that comes out of the sea—plant or animal life—has absorbed so much iodine from the sea water that it is a rich source. Mushrooms and Irish moss are rich in iodine if they are growing in a soil where iodine is plentiful. Watercress absorbs iodine from the water in which it grows. Fish roe is rich in iodine. The liquors from canned fish, such as salmon, contain a lot of iodine. The iodine in plants is higher in winter than in summer. Onions and asparagus absorb more iodine than cabbages do and cabbages more than legumes. Legumes absorb more iodine than cereals and cereals in general contain more iodine than fruits do. Experiments have shown that the body absorbs and uses most readily the iodine present in fish liver oils, then the iodine from plants, and lastly the iodine from the meat of fish.

How Much Iodine Do You Need?

There is disagreement about the amount of iodine one needs every day. No set minimum daily requirement has been established. But it is approximately from .04 to .10 milligrams. Of course if you live in an area where goiter is common and eat the food grown locally, you will need to watch your diet more closely than if you live in a goiter-free area. No ill results have ever resulted from too much iodine as it naturally occurs in food or water. However iodine prepared as a drug or medicine must be very carefully prescribed, for an overdose can be extremely serious.

For those of our readers who live in goitrous regions or who, because they are eating very little salt, may feel they are not getting enough iodine, we suggest fish liver oil (which you should be taking anyway, for its vitamin A and D content) or kelp tablets, made from seaweed which contain other valuable minerals too.

Here are some foods relatively rich in iodine:

Food	*Parts Per Billion*
Abalone	1053
Asparagus	180-1080
Beans, dried	994-1315
Bluefish	260-1870
Catfish	420-1940
Chard, Swiss	992
Clams, hard	1370-6200
Codfish	1000-5350
Cod liver oil	3370-7670
Conch	290-1140
Crabmeat	148-3150
Eel	800
Flounder	290-1180
Haddock	290-9070
Halibut	250-830
Herring	214-1000
Lobster	322-11000
Mackerel	400-1410
Oysters	1160-6000
Perch	420-1420
Salmon	210-2010
Shrimp	375-1100
Spinach	32-1079
Turnip tops	340-2296

NOTE: We have listed shellfish here although we do not recommend eating them, on account of the danger that they may come from polluted waters.

Iodine—More Facts About Iodine

We know that iodine in the diet is of utmost importance for many reasons. Lack of iodine in food predisposes to goiter, a disorder of the thyroid gland. But when we say "a disorder of the thyroid" we should not think only of a swelling in the neck, even though this may be one outward manifestation of an unhealthy thyroid gland. The thyroid gland controls either directly or indirectly many functions of the body and when it is out of order, all these functions are thrown out of gear.

Cretinism is one result of thyroid disorders existing through a generation or two (cretinism is a most unpleasant and deformed condition, with accompanying idiocy or feeble-mindedness which used to be fairly common in regions where iodine was scarce in food and drink). The thyroid apparently has a lot to do with regulating sex functions; animals who lack iodine have difficulty in childbirth and lactation. The thyroid gland regulates body metabolism—that is, it is responsible for the rate at which you burn your food. If your metabolic rate is too rapid, you tend to be active, nervous, irritable, jumpy. If it is too slow, you may be sluggish, glassy-eyed, chubby and lazy. So just making sure there is plenty of iodine in the diet can make a tremendous difference in one's personality.

The thyroid gland has a lot to do with the body's regulation of heat. If you suffer from cold hands and feet; if you must wear excessively heavy clothing in winter and can't change to summer clothes until long after everyone else has, perhaps you lack iodine to keep your thyroid gland healthy. If you gain weight too easily and have difficulty reducing, perhaps lack of iodine is your trouble. We have much information indicating that disorders of the thyroid gland, resulting in too much or too little thyroid activity, may cause acne. We know, too, that the body's demand for iodine is especially heavy during adolescence, when the body is growing rapidly. Doesn't it seem likely that acne, which is widespread among our adolescents, may be caused partly by lack of iodine? Beginning goiters often are first noticed during this troublesome period. Perhaps the acne is merely another symptom of thyroid disorder.

Mentality, speech, the condition of hair, nails, skin and teeth—all these are dependent on a well-functioning thyroid gland and this in turn is dependent on the amount of iodine you get in your daily food.

We have found some other evidence of the importance of iodine—this time in relation to heart and blood vessel health. An article in *Science News Letter* for September 22, 1951, tells us that lack of iodine in the diet plays an important part in the production of hardening of the arteries, according to a prominent physician from the University of Iceland, reporting at the Second International Gerontological Congress. A normally functioning thyroid gland is of utmost importance for preventing or delaying artery hardening, he said.

Signs of this link between the thyroid, iodine and artery hardening come from comparisons he made between Icelanders and people living in sections of Austria where goiter is common because the people do not get enough iodine. Icelanders have less hardening of the arteries, especially of the aorta (the largest) than the people living in the goiter region. In fact, he said, as a result of 2,000 autopsies, he had found that it is not rare at all to find old people in Iceland with smooth aortas whereas in Austria there is almost marked calcification or hardening—often in people as young as fifty.

In addition, Dr. Dungal said, the thyroid gland usually weighs less in Icelanders, and they have a normal amount of iodine in their thyroids. We know that a thyroid which is functioning badly has a tendency to swell and become overweight, so the fact that the Icelanders' thyroid glands are small indicates a splendid condition of health. People who live in the goiter regions of Austria, on the other hand, have enlarged thyroids. This surely does not leave much room for doubt as to the effect of iodine deficiency on blood vessel health. We have no idea how the iodine may work in the body to bring about this effect in blood vessels. But it seems certain that it does.

A most unusual suggestion for the use of iodine in medical therapy comes from M. Kovnat, M.D. of Staten Island in *The Medical Record* for March 5, 1941. Dr. Kovnat uses iodine in the treatment of the common cold! When he first studied the possibility of using iodine in this way, he injected it. But he soon found that the injections must take place when the cold has just begun and they must be given at least twice a day for the first three days. It was, of course, well nigh impossible for patients to come to his office that often, so he decided to give the iodine by mouth.

He prescribed Lugol's solution, which is the drug form of iodine most often used in medicine. But here, too, the patient had to get the prescription filled at his drugstore and valuable time was lost. The iodine was not effective unless it was given at the very first sign of the cold. So Dr. Kovnat advised his patients to take tincture of iodine (five to eight minims) every three or four hours for the first three or four days of the cold. Eight minims is about one half a cubic centimeter—a very small amount indeed.

He tells us that almost at once the patient notices relief from the dryness of the mucous membranes and the other cold symptoms. The relief lasts for about an hour. Instead of progressing into the usual later stages of congestion and discharge, the cold gradually diminishes and finally fades away completely. To insure success, he says, several conditions must be observed. First, one must use the iodine at the earliest possible sign of the infection and before the second stage (runny nose) has established itself. Adequate dosage must be maintained for several days.

Dr. Kovnat had been using this technique on his own patients for four years when he wrote the article. He thinks it was successful in aborting the cold in the majority of cases. He suggests that other physicians try out this method and report their results. We could not find any indication in our medical indexes that other physicians had.

How You Can Make Use of This Finding

We would not under any circumstances advise readers to take tincture of iodine, no matter how violent a cold seemed to be coming on. First of all, vitamin C is the best cold preventive, we believe. And we are sure that taking massive doses of vitamin C when the first cold symptom appears will nip any cold in the bud. So there seems to be no reason for resorting to a strong drug preparation such as tincture of iodine. But it seems to us that Dr. Kovnat's story indicates that iodine, if taken regularly in sufficient quantity in the diet, will help to prevent colds. Perhaps one cause of colds may be some disorder brought about by too little iodine in the body. Since iodine is so important for so many other functions perhaps its regulatory powers go even so far as to preventing colds.

Another indication of the importance of iodine to basal metabolism comes to us in an article in the *Western Journal of Surgery, Obstetrics and Gynecology* for July, 1947. Three researchers from the University of

Oregon Medical School reported in this article that the basal metabolism rate in pregnancy was found to be higher than average. Giving iodine to pregnant women kept the metabolic rate within normal bounds. If it was high, the iodine lowered it; if it was low, the iodine raised it.

The same three scientists also reported in the *Proceedings of the Society for Experimental Biology and Medicine,* volume 45, 1940, that the mothers who got the iodine felt better during their pregnancies, were able to nurse their babies with little difficulty, and returned to a normal pre-pregnancy state much sooner than those who had not received iodine. Apparently much more iodine is required by the body during pregnancy than at other times.

Women who do not receive iodine supplements when they are pregnant often suffer from obesity and/or menstrual disorders of various types after the birth of their babies. This may be caused by exhaustion of the glands. Occasionally, they tell us, the work done by the thyroid gland during pregnancy and labor is so severe that the mother may suffer from a toxic hyperthyroid condition. Pregnancy, then, seems to be another of those human "stress" situations (like adolescence) where extra food supplements are essential.

For the rest of us, the lesson is apparent, too. Iodine regulates the body's use of food. If you are desperately trying to lose weight or gain weight or keep your weight constant throughout some particular strain to which you are subjected, look to iodine for help! Get it in a natural food supplement such as kelp, along with all the other minerals with which it occurs in foods.

Iron

Three or four hundred years ago you might have seen a warrior soaking his sword in water or wine, or scraping rust from an old weapon so that he might drink the liquid concoctions resulting. Old-timers believed that the strength of the iron went into their bodies when they drank iron water. Their belief was rooted in folklore, but the idea of drinking water in which a sword has been soaked is sound scientifically. The old warriors were preventing anemia which is caused by a lack of hemoglobin in the bloodstream. Iron makes abundant hemoglobin.

We stay alive because we breathe in oxygen all day long. The oxygen travels to every cell of the body in the red blood corpuscles. This entire respiratory system would fail and we would die from lack of oxygen were it not for iron. Iron is the most important ingredient of hemoglobin—the red pigment of the blood that carries the oxygen. This is why symptoms of anemia, or lack of iron, may involve shortness of breath or heart palpitations. Fatigue is another symptom of iron deficiency, for not enough oxygen is getting to the cells to prevent fatigue. Depression and lassitude are symptoms of iron deficiency, because oxygen is lacking in the brain cells, due to decrease in the hemoglobin.

If their mothers are healthy, children are born with a large supply of iron stored in their bodies, since it must carry them over during the period when they are living on milk. Milk contains very little iron. Children whose milk diet continues until they are several years old almost invariably become anemic, although we might point out that breast-fed babies are much less likely to suffer from lack of iron. Modern pediatricians advise feeding children a wide variety of food as soon as it can be managed—meat, liver, eggs, whole grain cereals and green vegetables contain iron which babies need desperately as soon as their original store of iron has been used up. Phytic acid in whole grain cereals has been shown to prevent the absorption of some iron, just as it prevents the absorption of some calcium. So, in case your children have a great fondness for large amounts of whole grain cereals and milk, you'd better make certain they don't overdo this part of their meals and that they get meats and green vegetables as well.

As people grow older, men appear to need considerably less iron in their meals than women do. For, unless he has some disease which causes continual loss of blood, a man does not lose blood. Very little iron is excreted in feces or urine, so the average male does not have to worry much about anemia. But girls and women lose blood every month in the menstrual flow and this hemoglobin must be replaced by iron in the diet, or anemia will result.

The Red Cross has done an analysis of low hemoglobin levels among recent blood donors. They found that of 73,783 women, they had to reject 12.6 per cent as donors, because their hemoglobin levels were too low. Of 165,408 men, they rejected only one per cent. Projecting these figures, it has been estimated that of a probable total of 47 million women between the ages of 18 and 59, perhaps six to ten million may have low hemoglobin levels—that is, they may have anemia or a tendency toward anemia.

Iron—Its Use and Absorption By the Body

While children are growing rapidly they need a large supply of iron. A diet that contains fruit juice, milk, vitamin A and vitamin D will not protect against anemia, remember, for none of these is high in iron. So unless a child has a good supply of iron in his food he may exhibit alarming symptoms which simply indicate lack of iron. He may have pallor, lack of appetite, restlessness, fatigue. He may eat dirt and stones, in his instinctive search for food containing iron.

The normal adult has about 4000 milligrams of iron in his body, over half of which is in the hemoglobin or the red coloring matter of the blood. The rest is stored in the liver, spleen and bone marrow. The average adult takes in about 15 milligrams of iron per day in his food. Iron is part of every body cell. Since little or none of it is excreted, the body's level of iron is adjusted by the way it is absorbed and the amount of iron that is absorbed.

In the blood stream of a normal adult seven million red blood cells die every second and must be renewed. The life of a red blood cell is from 40 to 120 days. As an indication of how precious iron is to human needs, we find that the body uses over and over again the iron that has appeared in red blood cells. As fast as these cells disintegrate their iron goes into the making of new red blood cells, so that not an atom of iron will be wasted.

Although we have considerable knowledge of the absorption of iron, still there is apparently a great deal that we do not know as to why and how iron is absorbed. We know that it must be in an acid medium to be absorbed. This means there must be hydrochloric acid in the stomach or iron will not be absorbed. As we grow older we tend to have less and less hydrochloric acid, so a slight anemia is rather common among elderly folks. In fact, about 25 per cent of people in their seventies suffer from achlorhydria, or lack of hydrochloric acid in the stomach.

However there must also be certain "reducing agents" in the digestive tract to reduce the iron chemically into the form which the body can use. Certain proteins and ascorbic acid, or vitamin C, are reducing agents for iron. In other words, if you want the best possible absorption of iron better make certain that you are eating plenty of vitamin C-rich foods. Something else important—iron occurs in two different chemical states—ferrous and ferric, depending on the chemical kind of iron that is present in any given substance. Ferrous iron compounds are easily absorbed. Ferric iron compounds must be changed to ferrous iron before they are used.

The body knows quite well, we are told, the difference between ferrous and ferric iron. Ferrous iron is allowed to traverse cell walls and otherwise move around in the body. Ferric iron is the form that is bound to one place and held firmly there by protein carriers. If the stored iron is to be moved to some other part of the body, it must first be changed to ferrous iron. Iron occurs in food chiefly in the form of ferric hydroxide or ferric phosphate. So the iron in food must be broken down by hydrochloric acid and vitamin C into ferrous iron. However even when ferrous iron compounds are given by the doctor, they may not be absorbed, for there are other obstacles in the way sometimes.

Importance of Good Diet For Iron Absorption

If digestive processes are out of whack so that food is hurried through the intestine, the iron will be badly absorbed and, no matter how much is taken, it will do little good. The regular taking of laxatives can thus result in anemia, for as the food is flushed out by the laxative it does not pause long enough in the intestine for the iron (or, for that matter, other valuable food elements) to be absorbed. Conditions such as diarrhea, dysentery, celiac disease and sprue also bring about little if any absorption of iron.

A great deal of the iron we eat is never used, even if we are in good health, However in an emergency the body knows to take up and use more iron. So in a case of acute loss of blood, up to 80 per cent of the iron in foods can be retained. McLester in his book *Nutrition and Diet in Health and Disease* (Saunders, 1949), tells us that minute amounts of copper are also essential for the best absorption of iron. Calcium is needed, also vitamin A.

So you see why we keep insisting on the absolute necessity for an all-'round adequate diet. Perhaps if your trouble is anemia, the reason might be any of the following: You do not eat enough foods containing iron. You do not eat enough foods containing vitamin A or vitamin C.

You do not eat enough foods containing copper. Your general diet is not guaranteeing an ample supply of hydrochloric acid in your stomach. Your diet does not contain enough calcium, or part of the calcium and iron too is being stolen by phytic acid, if you eat large quantities of cereals. You are not eating properly to avoid constipation and the laxatives you take are destroying iron. All of these angles should be taken into account if your doctor tells you you are anemic. And, once again, our recommendations boil down to several basic ones: eat fresh fruits and vegetables, meats, poultry, fish and nuts if you would be healthy. Notice at the end of this article how high in iron are the green leafy vegetables. Eat a big hearty salad every single day!

One interesting angle we have turned up concerns iron and vitamin E. It seems that the action of vitamin E is made ineffective when medicines containing iron are taken at the same time. This suggests that possibly food that is very rich in iron may not react favorably with vitamin E. If you are taking vitamin E for a heart condition, we'd suggest that you go easy on foods rich in iron and of course do not take any medicines containing iron. In case you are anemic and must take iron in some form, speak to your doctor about the possibility of taking the iron at some widely separated interval from the time when you take your vitamin E so that they cannot possibly mix in your digestive tract.

The How and Why of Anemia

Just what are the symptoms of anemia or iron deficiency? And what might bring about such a condition in a person who has been healthy heretofore? In general, people who are anemic are listless, easily tired, pale, have difficulty concentrating, have no appetite and may suffer from unreasonable fears and weeping spells. A sore mouth with cracks around the lips may indicate an iron deficiency or it may indicate a lack of both iron and one of the B vitamins—riboflavin. One authority tells us that a decline of 10 per cent in hemoglobin is not anything to worry about. But a decline of 50 per cent is serious enough to warrant a stay in the hospital.

What are some of the circumstances that may bring about anemia? As we have mentioned, anemia is prevalent among those children whose diets contain milk exclusively or too large a proportion of milk, so that they cannot eat enough of other kinds of food. Pregnant women may become anemic if they are not getting enough iron, especially if they have many children in a short period of time. The babies simply use up too much of their mother's iron.

In cases of hemorrhaging, anemia soon results and it is interesting to note that constant slight bleeding from some hidden disorder is apt to cause anemia sooner than an obvious large loss of blood such as one might have in an accident. So, in cases of anemia, one should always check carefully to make certain than no internal bleeding is going on. Diseases such as purpura, scurvy and hemophilia result in loss of enough blood to cause anemia. Peptic ulcers may bring on anemia. Any form of malignant disease in the digestive tract will probably produce enough bleeding to result in anemia.

Infections are a common cause of anemia. A tooth infection or some chronic (and perhaps unrecognized) infection of the genito-urinary tract can bring on anemia, for in cases of infection less iron is used to make red blood corpuscles and more is used for storage. In these cases, the anemia will not clear up until the infection is taken care of. So the infection should be treated and cured, first. Any other condition of the body that interferes with bone marrow or bone marrow ability to make red blood corpuscles can cause anemia.

Remember, too, that iron deficiency is only one kind of anemia. In pernicious anemia, taking enormous quantities of iron will do no good, for pernicious anemia is a deficiency of the bone marrow. It can be cured with vitamin B12, but iron has no effect on it at all.

Iron in Food

It has been estimated that the average well-balanced diet in the United States contains 10 to 12 milligrams of iron daily, out of which about one-half to one and one-half milligrams are absorbed. In the light of this statement it is surprising to remember that about six to ten million American women are anemic! Obviously they are either not getting enough iron in their food or for some reason the iron is not being properly absorbed. Here are the foods that contain the largest amounts of iron. Make certain that your family gets enough of all of these every week.

Food	*Milligrams of Iron*
Apricots, dried	4.9 in about 3 apricots
Almonds	4.4 in about 80 almonds
Beans, dried	10.3 in ½ cup
Beans, snap	1.1 in ½ cup
Beef, lean	3.0 in 2 slices
Beefsteak, medium fat	2.0 in 1 piece
Beet greens	3.2 in ½ cup
Dates	5.07 in about 20 dates
Honey	3.20 in 5 tablespoons
Heart, beef	6.2 in 2 slices
Eggs	3.1 in 2 eggs
Egg yolk	8.7 in 6 yolks
Kale	2.2 in 1 cup
Kidney	7.10 in ½ cup
Lamb	2.6 in 2 slices
Lentils	8.60 in 1 cup
Liver, beef	12.1 in 1 piece
Liver, calf	21.70 in 1 piece
Mushrooms, dried	16.10 in 7 mushrooms
Molasses, cane	6.7 in 5 tablespoons
Oatmeal	5.2 in ½ cup cooked oatmeal
Oysters	7.1 in 4 medium oysters
Peas, dried	6.0 in ½ cup
Peas, split	6.0 in ½ cup
Peaches, dried	6.9 in 1 medium peach
Parsley	19.21 in 100 parsley sprigs
Pecans	2.4 in about 80 pecans
Peanuts	1.9 in about 80 peanuts
Prunes	3.9 in about 12 prunes

Food	Milligrams of Iron
Raisins	3.3 in about 1 cup of raisins
Rice, brown	5.5 in ½ cup
Soybeans	8.0 in ½ cup
Spinach	3.0 in ½ cup
Swiss chard	4.0 in ½ cup
Turnip greens	2.4 in ½ cup
Walnuts	2.1 in about 80 walnuts
Wheat, whole	5.7 in 100 grams
Wheat, bran	12.70 in 100 grams
Wheat, germ	10.00 in 100 grams
Yams	7.40 in 1 small yam

Kelp

In the Chinese *Book of Poetry* written in the time of Confucius (between 800 and 600 B. C.) there is a poem about a housewife cooking seaweed. During this period in Chinese history seaweed was considered a delicacy, worthy of being offered to the gods as a sacrificial food. Several kinds of seaweed were used in ancient China. And seaweed still forms an important part of the diet in eastern countries.

In Japan, we are told, seaweed is used to a far greater extent than in any other country and provides about 25 per cent of the daily diet! The brown seaweeds are incorporated into flour and are used in almost every household as noodles, toasted and served with rice or in soup. Two other kinds of seaweed are used for sweetening and flavoring. Relishes, beverages and cakes are made from them.

In western countries seaweeds have never been generally accepted as part of daily meals, although in Ireland, Iceland, Denmark, Wales, Scotland and the Faroe Islands, seaweeds have been eaten extensively. The national dish of South Wales is laverbread, which contains seaweed. The Irish eat dulse, a seaweed that is called "sea lettuce" because it is tender, crisp and tasty like the land variety. W. A. P. Black, writing in the *Proceedings of the Nutrition Society* of England, volume 12, page 32, 1953, says that a certain seaweed, porphyra, is eaten in Scotland, grilled on toast. He tells us it looks like spinach and tastes like oysters.

Dr. Black also tells us that there may be present in the intestinal tracts of the Japanese people a specialized bacterial flora, giving the seaweeds a greater nutritional value. The bacterial flora are the beneficial bacteria which live in the intestines and manufacture certain vitamins there, as well as helping in the digestion of food. Dr. Black says that in digestibility tests with cattle it has been found that when seaweed is first introduced into the diet it is completely undigested and appears unaltered in the feces. After a few days, however, no seaweed as such is found in the feces. So it seems that the bacteria in the intestines have an important part in the digestion of seaweed. In Japan it appears that children develop the proper intestinal bacteria since they are fed seaweed products from infancy on.

Back in 1920, according to *Popular Mechanics,* for July, 1952, a man named Philip Park who was touring England was startled to see cattle passing over rich, lush grass so that they could feed on kelp or seaweed. He investigated the food content of this seaweed and went into business to produce it for animal food and human consumption as well. At his non-profit research organization, experiments are carried on to find out even more about this remarkable plant.

Kelp is harvested by special boats equipped with a great hook which pulls the plant up out of the sea. Special cutters then mow off the tops of the kelp plants which are carried back to the boat on a conveyor belt arrangement. At the processing plant, the kelp is chopped fine, dried, sterilized and shredded. There is no boiling or draining off of water. Everything in the way of minerals remains that was in the original plant. We are told that kelp plants are so vigorous in growth that plants cut to a depth of four feet will reach the surface of the sea again within forty-eight to sixty hours.

We are well acquainted, all of us, with the fact that plants growing on the land form, or should form, a large part of the diet of the healthy individual. What of the plants that grow in the sea? Is there any indication that they may be good for us too?

Something About Seaweeds

Sea plants go under the collective name of "algae." There are three kinds, depending on color—the green, the brown and the red. In some ways they are like land plants but in other ways many of them have little in common with what we are accustomed to thinking of as plants. They have no roots. They cling to stones, wharves or pilings with "holdfasts." They do not have stalks and branches in the same sense that land plants do. In many seaweeds there are no special parts of the plant either for support (like the stems of land flowers or the trunks of land trees) or for conducting nourishment from one part of the plant to another. Many seaweeds have structures that look like leaves, but they are not leaves in the same sense that we use for leaves of land plants. They do not manufacture food for the rest of the plant to eat. In seaweeds almost every part of the plant can make its own food. Seaweeds have nothing that looks like flowers, fruit or seeds.

They grow tall, some of the largest kelps stretching up for a hundred feet or more from the floor of the ocean. Because of their simple structure and the fossils in which they have been found, paleontologists (scientists who decide about the age of earthly things) have said that algae probably represent the first form of life that appeared on our planet. The seaweeds you find today have developed considerably since those first primitive times, of course, but even so, they still retain many of the primitive characteristics of early life. They are not nearly so complicated as the land plants which came much later in history.

The brown seaweeds are the ones we are going to talk about, for they are the commonest and the ones used most widely for food. Many of them are thick and leathery. Kelp comes in this category. Just as people in far corners of the world have eaten seeds, bones, insects and other foods that seem peculiar to us, just so have many peoples of the world eaten seaweed. And now it seems likely that kelp will become an important part of American diets.

What do seaweeds contain that might make them valuable as food? First of all, of course, just like other plants, they contain carbohydrates—that is, starches and sugars. The sugar of seaweed is called mannitol. It is not very sweet, has a mild laxative effect in large doses and does not increase the sugar content of the blood. This would be an important factor to diabetics if the seaweed-sugar should ever be used to a wide extent. Fats and proteins also exist in seaweed, the proteins about as useful to human bodies as the protein of land plants—that is, not as useful as protein that comes from animal sources, such as meat and eggs. Seaweed is not a very fatty plant but it does contain at least one of the unsaturated fatty acids necessary to human health.

In the way of vitamins, there seems to be some vitamin A and a certain amount of the B vitamins. Dr. Black of the British Nutrition Society tells us that the vitamin C content of seaweed is comparable with that of many vegetables and fruits. With some Eskimo nations seaweed was at one time used as their chief source of vitamin C. One test showed a vitamin C content of 5 to 140 milligrams of vitamin C per one hundred grams of wet seaweed. Oranges contain about 50 milligrams per hundred grams.

However, our main interest in seaweed or kelp as food is not in its protein, carbohydrates or vitamins—although it is good to know the status of any new food in these categories. What interests us mainly about kelp is its mineral content. It seems reasonable, does it not, to expect sea foods to be rich in minerals? Aside from the fact that sea water as such is a veritable treasure trove of minerals, land minerals are constantly washing into the sea, enriching it still further. Every river in the world carrying silt and soil that has washed away or eroded from the land runs eventually to the sea, giving up its minerals into the salty depths.

Plants that grow on land take up minerals from the soil. By testing the amount of minerals in any given plant we can get a good idea of how many minerals were in the soil in which it grew, for vegetables and fruits from mineral-rich land will also be rich in these so-important food elements. The same is true of sea plants. So we can expect seaweed or kelp to be a good source of minerals. How good it is surprised even us. Dr. Black tells us that the ash of seaweed may be from ten per cent to as high as 50 per cent. This means that if you burn seaweed you may have half the volume of the seaweed left as minerals! Compare this to some other foods. Carrots leave an ash of 1 per cent as minerals. Apples have a mineral ash of .3 per cent, almonds 3.0 per cent, beets 1.1 per cent.

Dr. Black says further, "It can be said that seaweed contains all the elements that have so far been shown to play an important part in the physiological processes of man. In a balanced diet, therefore, they would appear to be an excellent mineral supplement." We know that, of the minerals which are needed in relatively large amounts like calcium, iron, phosphorus, potassium and so forth, the average fruit or vegetable contains an amount approximate to the amounts listed on the tables and charts in nutrition books.

But, as important as these minerals are, perhaps even more important are the trace minerals—iodine, copper, manganese, boron, zinc and so forth. These minerals appear in minute quantities in food. Our bodies need only microscopically small amounts of them. Yet if that tiny amount is not there, the consequences may be fatal. Our land is becoming trace-mineral-poor. Floods and poor farming practices are causing our soil to be washed away. And with it go the trace minerals. Applying commercial fertilizer to the soil does not improve the situation, for this does not, cannot, contain the trace minerals. Only by organic farming—that is, returning to the soil everything that has been taken from it—can we be certain that our food contains all of the precious trace minerals necessary for health. What happens to the trace minerals that wash away from our farmlands? They wash into the ocean and are taken up into seaweeds. So the worse-off we become so far as trace minerals in foods are concerned, the more do we need a substance like kelp as a food supplement. Those of us who farm organically probably need it less than those of us who must buy all our food from a store.

Iodine in Kelp

From the point of view of nutrition the most important single trace mineral in kelp or seaweed is iodine. Why do we say this? How can one be more important than the others? It isn't that iodine is more important, exactly. It's simply that there are whole sections of the world where iodine *is completely lacking* in the soil. No food grown there contains any iodine at all. Many parts of the middle inland section of our country are deficient in iodine so far as soil is concerned. These localities are called "The Goiter Belt." We know that iodine is an absolute essential for the body, for it is the main ingredient of the product of one of our most important glands—the thyroid gland. Goiters are just one of the possible unhealthful results of too little iodine in the diet. There are many others.

For a long time public health authorities have promoted the use of iodized salt to prevent goiter. This is plain table salt to which potassium iodide has been added by chemists. Our objection to this is our objection to all medicated foods. Table salt (sodium chloride) is a drug—a pure substance denuded of everything that accompanies sodium chloride in nature. To this we add another drug—potassium iodide. Such a product still has no relation to nature, so far as we are concerned. Besides we believe that most of us get far too much salt. So we recommend not using table salt either in cooking or at the table. Where then can someone who lives in the "goiter belt" get the iodine that is so essential for his well-being? Why not from kelp?

In Borden's *Review of Nutrition Research* for July-August 1955 we are told that to get 100 micrograms of iodine (estimated as the normal daily requirement for human beings) one would have to eat

10 pounds of fresh vegetables and fruits, or
8 pounds of cereal, grains and nuts, or
6 pounds of meat, freshwater fish, fowl, or
2 pounds of eggs, or
.3 pounds of marine fish, or
.2 pounds of shellfish

They go on to state: "The problem of obtaining sufficient iodine from food of non-marine origin may be seen from values shown in this table. Iodine-rich seaweed is an abundant source on a limited scale for some peoples. Kelp contains about 200,000 micrograms per kilogram (about 2 pounds) and the dried kelp meal nearly ten times as much, or .1 per cent to .2 per cent of iodine. Used as a condiment this would provide ten times as much iodine as American iodized salt."

Kelp, then, it seems to us is the perfect answer for a mineral supplement for health-conscious folks. It is practically the only reliable food source of iodine, aside from seafood. It is rich in potassium and magnesium. It contains, in addition, all of the trace minerals that have been shown to be important for human nutrition and many more whose purposes we have not yet discovered.

It does contain sodium chloride, true. So does almost everything else that you eat. It contains more sodium chloride than vegetables and meats because it comes from the salty sea. But its content of sodium chloride is not high compared to table salt which is of course one hundred per cent sodium chloride. We do not believe that the salt in kelp is harmful, because it occurs along with the other minerals as a natural part of the food. We do believe that the other minerals, especially the iodine in kelp, make it one of our most valuable food supplements.

Here is an analysis of an average sample of kelp, neither especially high nor low in minerals: In some cases we have compared the mineral content of kelp with that of some other food especially rich in this same mineral: You will note in every instance how much higher is the mineral content of the kelp.

	Kelp	*Other Food*	
Iodine	.18%	Clams	1900 parts per billion
Calcium	1.05%	Milk	.001%
Phosphorus	.339%	Wheat Germ	.01%
Iron	.37%	Eggs	.0005%
Copper	.0008%	Eggs	.0000023%
Potassium	11.15%	Almonds	7%
Magnesium	.740%		
Sodium	3.98%		
Chlorine	13.07%		
Manganese	.0015%		
Sulphur	1.%		

Trace minerals in kelp, not listed above are: barium, boron, chromium, lithium, nickel, silicon, silver, strontium, titanium, vanadium and zinc.

Kidney Stones

A century or so ago kidney stones were an important cause of illness especially among young people. Today kidney stones are far less prevalent in this country and the emphasis has shifted from youth to age. Today kidney stones are a disorder of older people. But in some parts of the world this condition exists among most of the population. Such a background cannot help but lead one to believe that the development of kidney stones shows a background of poor nutrition.

No one knows exactly how or why the stones are formed, but it is generally, if grudgingly, agreed among the experts that diet plays a part. It is known for instance that stones formed chiefly of calcium oxalate may be related to a high content of oxalic acid in the diet. In Bridges' *Dietetics for the Clinician,* (Lea and Febiger, 1949), the editor Harry J. Johnson, M.D., F.A.C.P., says, "It is a matter of common observation that calcium oxalate sediments will appear in the urine of nearly every patient in a ward after ingesting oxalate-rich food as spinach and rhubarb." Now most of us don't eat enough spinach and rhubarb to cause this kind of trouble. But there are other foods rich in oxalic acid that we do eat in quantity, perhaps every day. Chocolate, for instance, and cocoa both contain lots of oxalic acid. Plenty of children (and adults too) have a cup of cocoa for breakfast, chocolate milk for lunch and dinner and possibly a couple of chocolate bars or chocolate cupcakes between meals. So it is well to keep in mind this possible cause of stones. Oxalic acid foods are undesirable as well because they cause the body to lose calcium.

Dr. Johnson goes on to say that vitamin deficiencies probably contribute to the formation of stones. The effect of vitamin A on the cells lining various passages in the body such as the urinary passage is well known and an adequate amount of the vitamin must be ingested in order to keep the urinary mucous membrane in good condition. Urinary stone occurs frequently following peptic ulcer therapy and the dietary restrictions involved.

Rose's *Foundations of Nutrition,* a classical nutrition textbook (The Macmillan Company, 1944) says that when animals are kept for some time on diets low but not entirely lacking in vitamin A, kidney and bladder stones are frequently found. They have not been found in animals on other types of deficient diets. According to McCarrison there are certain areas of India which are known as "stone areas" because of the prevalence of kidney stones among the people. It is a poor man's disease occurring among those whose chief dietary staple is cereal of some sort, but is most frequent where vegetation is relatively scanty, where grazing for cattle is poor, and where wheat is the chief food crop. McCarrison has produced stones in rats in 90 days from weaning time on diets low in vitamin A and consisting chiefly of wheat.

W. J. McCormick, M.D., of Toronto, whose matchless work on vitamin therapy we have reviewed many times in *Prevention,* has something further to contribute in the way of dietary prevention of stones—whether they form in kidneys, bladder, gall bladder or elsewhere. Dr. McCormick points out in an article in *The Journal of the Canadian Dental Association* for August, 1946, that vitamin A was the only vitamin known during some of these early investigations. Hence researchers who had removed all the vitamin A from the diet of their laboratory animals might think they had the answer, when as a matter of fact, they had also removed other necessary vitamins at the same time. He says that McCarrison found that if vitamin C were also removed from the diet, kidney stones were more likely to be produced. He reminds us that the diet of the Tibetans, the people of West China, India, Labrador and Newfoundland is almost completely lacking in vitamin C, and among these people kidney stones are common. The Easterners live on rice, barley flour, butter and tea with few or no vegetables and fruits. In Labrador and Newfoundland white flour, fish, game, lard, oatmeal, tea and sugar make up the bulk of the diet and here again fresh fruits and vegetables are all but unknown.

Retarding Calcium Deposits With Vitamin C

Dr. McCormick tells us further that the teeth of people living on these diets are covered with tartar. Even very young children have heavy tartar deposits on the teeth. This might happen, he says, because lack of vitamin C leads to a breakdown of the body tissues, including those of the mouth. The mucous lining scales off and, mixing with remnants of food, creates the unsightly and unhealthy deposit that clings so tenaciously to the teeth, resulting in pyorrhea and inflammation of the mouth tissues which have already been seriously weakened by lack of vitamin C.

Is it not possible, he asks, that the urinary tract goes through the same process when there is not enough vitamin C in the diet—the mucous lining scales off and forms the nucleus of the stones? And if this is true of kidney stones, might it not also hold true for gall bladder stones, and stones in the appendix, pancreas, prostate gland, mammary glands, uterus, ovaries and even the calcium deposit that brings about hardening of the arteries and arthritis.

Observing his own patients, Dr. McCormick found that cloudy urine containing phosphates (which constitute some kinds of kidney stones) and pieces of sloughed off mucous from the walls of the urinary canal went hand-in-hand with vitamin C deficiency. Giving large doses of vitamin C (much larger than one would get even in a daily diet relatively high in vitamin C) he could clear the urine within a matter of hours. During this treatment his patients reported to him that the tartar deposits were clearing from their teeth and dentures. Nurses in hospitals reported that patients whose urine had formerly caused calcium deposits on the urinary utensils now found that the utensils remained free from deposits. He interjects at this point a reminder that these particular patients were also getting a diet and dietary supplements high in the complex of B vitamins but his investigations seemed to show that it was the vitamin C that was responsible for the change in the appearance of the urine.

If Dr. McCormick is correct in his theory that ample vitamin C in the diet prevents the formation of stones and tooth tartar, how should we interpret the fact that Americans as a whole have less trouble of this kind than formerly, and the age accent has shifted from youth to middle age? It's very simple, says Dr. McCormick. American mothers these days have had it drummed into their heads that their children must have vitamin C. Summer and winter, infants and youngsters must drink their orange or tomato juice, and eat other fresh raw fruits. But how many of their fathers and mothers get a sufficient amount of vitamin C? We add that adults today are subjected to hundreds of substances that rob them of vitamin C. Smoking one cigarette, as Dr. McCormick himself has demonstrated in his laboratory, uses up 25 milligrams of vitamin C from the bloodstream. Drugs, insecticides, minor infections, sleeping pills, and scores of present-day industrial products (such as lead, paint and benzene) are enemies of vitamin C. So, while we protect our children from scurvy by giving them fresh fruits and vegetables, we forget that adults need vitamin C in even larger amounts than children. Might this not explain very satisfactorily why the incidence of kidney stones has shifted from children to adults?

Correcting Mild Vitamin C Deficiency May Be the Answer

McCormick quotes J. W. Joly in his book, *Stones and Calculus Disease of the Urinary Organs* (C. V. Mosby Co., 1929): "I believe the hypothesis that stone is a deficiency disease is the most plausible and probable that has yet been advanced. It explains not only all the principal features of the conditions today, but also the changes in incidence during the past years. I believe that vitamin starvation acts primarily on the renal epithelium (the lining of the kidneys) and through it on the colloidal mechanism of the urine; also that once this mechanism is deranged, stone formation must follow as a direct result of the laws of physical chemistry."

Since the time of the early Roman scientist Pliny, physicians have been searching for the cause of kidney stones, looking generally for some medicine that could be taken orally that would dissolve the stones. Pliny's remedy was the ashes of snail shells. One of the main causes for surgery during the past century, stone formation has been so common a disorder that there are in medical dictionaries some 80 words beginning with "lith" which is the prefix referring to stone formation.

Yet how simple the answer may be! And not just for kidney stones, but, as Dr. McCormick suggests, for every kind of unhealthful calcification process that takes place in the body! At first glance it may not seem easy to get enough vitamin C. The vitamin is extremely perishable. It disappears from food in the presence of heat and water. Fruits and vegetables that lie for a long time on the grocer's shelves lose vitamin C with every passing hour. Exposure to air, when you are chopping or slicing foods, destroys vitamin C. It is wasted when cooking water is thrown away. You must get a supply of it every day—your body cannot store it.

Yet, if you should decide that from now on you are going to get enough vitamin C, it isn't really an impossible task. Fresh raw fruits and vegetables are the answer—and the sooner you can eat them after they are picked, the more vitamin C you will have. Citrus fruits are rich in vitamin C. We do not advise eating too many citrus fruits. Eating whole oranges and grapefruit is much better for you than drinking juice, for the vitamins are concentrated in the tissues of the fruit. But cantaloupe is rich in vitamin C. Broccoli, mustard greens, kale, green peppers, turnip greens, watercress, parsley, strawberries, Brussels sprouts and cabbage are good sources.

Pyorrhea and deposits of tartar on teeth are so common in this country as to be almost universal. No one has ever been able to find that you can get too much natural vitamin C. So why not get rid of that ugly scum on your teeth right away and prevent the possibility of pyorrhea and stones forming later on, by being sure you get many times more than the accepted daily minimum requirement of vitamin C which is about 75 to 100 milligrams. Even if you eat ample amounts of the vitamin C–rich fruits and vegetables, take a natural vitamin C food supplement made from rose hips or green peppers . . . just to be sure. You'll find it's well worth it.

Laxatives

One reason why people take laxatives is that they fear their health may suffer from an accumulation in the lower bowel. Autointoxication is the word that was formerly used to describe this condition. The implication was that poisons from the accumulated feces would work their way through the wall of the bowel and spread throughout the body. More recent investigations indicate that nothing like this occurs.

Dr. Abrahams in *The Practitioner* for March, 1953, tells us that convincing people of the non-existence of autointoxication is difficult. He says that a contemplation of the material voided will usually make the constipated person believe that he has been absorbing this material through his bowels. "And no amount of argument will persuade the constipated that there is no absorption through the intestinal wall from solid contents unless the mucosa is seriously diseased . . . It is true that bacterial action upon amino acids in the large intestine produces powerful poisons, but this is a normal process and the body is provided with the means to render them innocuous."

Why then does one feel tired, headachy and so forth if he is constipated? Apparently the mere pressure of the feces upon the walls of the intestine and the nerves in that region produces the symptoms. Experimenters have produced the same symptoms in volunteers by packing the lower bowel with cotton. In another experiment five normal men voluntarily refrained from bowel movement for four days or so. They felt entirely normal within an hour after securing a bowel movement by enema. Surely if dangerous poisons were being absorbed during these four days it would have taken longer than an hour to be rid of them.

But it is perfectly true that constipation produces unpleasant, perhaps even painful, consequences. Why then should you not take a laxative to get relief? As we have explained in another article, one laxative is almost bound to lead to another. And once the habit has become established, the muscles of the intestine (like the muscles of an arm in a sling), become lax and unhealthful. Far from promoting intestinal health, the laxative eventually makes it almost impossible to secure a normal bowel movement without using a laxative.

How the Different Laxatives Work

There are a number of different kinds of laxatives. The irritants do their work by irritating the wall of the bowel. These are castor oil, cascara and phenolphthalein. If you are using a laxative, look on the label to see if it contains any of these. Then decide whether you want to continue to irritate and inflame this very delicate part of you. In cases of spastic constipation where there may be a cramp in the colon, the irritating laxatives may make such a condition much worse.

The second category of laxative, the salines, includes such things as epsom salts, citrate magnesia and so forth. These work by attracting water from the body store into the colon or large intestine. This tends to liquefy the fecal mass so that it may more easily be pushed toward the rectum.

Mineral oil represents the third category of laxative—the lubricants. Readers should by now know well all the serious disadvantages of using mineral oil. One researcher, Dr. Abrahams in *The Practitioner* for March, 1953, lists them thus: nausea, regurgitation, rumbling in the bowels, intestinal discomfort, itching anus and seepage from the anus. He says further that there are more serious disadvantages. There may be interference with the normal process of defecation. Leakage results in the rectum being continuously partially full, its volume not exercising sufficient pressure to initiate the defecation reflex but enough to cause irritation. There is evidence of interference with digestion. The system is depleted of the fat-soluble vitamins. Giving mineral oil to pregnant women and to those undergoing surgical operations may be regarded as particularly unsuitable; for in addition to malnutrition there is the danger of hemorrhage from lack of vitamin K.

It seems, too, that in the case of elderly people confined to bed, there have been reports of mineral oil getting into the lungs. In addition, the possibility that mineral oil may cause cancer should be mentioned, although at present the evidence seems to indicate that it is not cancer-causing.

Finally, there are the laxatives that are bulk-producers. These seem to be the least harmful of all, although there are medical reports of some strange accidents in the use of these. Trouble arises when individuals take these preparations without taking enough water along with them. There are several reports in the recent medical magazines of people who had to be taken to the hospital to have the mass of bulky stuff removed bit by bit from esophagus or throat. Any lack of water farther along in the digestive tract could well lead to impaction and serious trouble.

An article by Leonard Engel in *The Nation* for June 30, 1951 charges that irresponsible laxative advertising may be responsible for an "uncounted number" of deaths from cancer of the colon, which kills about 50,000 Americans a year. Says Mr. Engel, the ads encourage you to take laxatives for "middle-age irregularity." Now any radical change in bowel habits before or after middle age may be an indication of something seriously wrong—yes, even cancer. Apparently many people take to laxatives rather than having a physical examination which might indicate what is wrong.

He goes on to tell us that saline laxatives (Epsom salts and so forth) have an alkaline reaction in the stomach and may eventually neutralize all the stomach acid which is so necessary for good digestion. Psyllium seeds are tough and sharp and can tear the lining of the stomach or intestine. Lemon juice in water taken on arising in the morning has been widely advertised by citrus fruit packers. No one has ever been able to discover any laxative action of lemon juice and, of course, its acid can be highly erosive to the teeth. A glass of any kind of liquid first thing in the morning appears to be good food, for it seems to stimulate the bowels.

An article by Charles Bruce Morton, II in the *Virginia Medical Monthly,* May, 1951, describes the case of 90 patients (most of them over 40 but under 60) each of whom had such a small anus that the usual medical examination was almost impossible. All of them gave a history of taking laxatives or enemas or both over a long time, even many years. The occasional laxative had led to frequent laxatives and finally these patients arrived at the sorry state of taking a laxative every day or oftener, sometimes supplementing this with enemas. "Many patients stated they had not passed a formed stool or had a spontaneous defecation for many years," says Dr. Morton.

After dilating the anus under anesthesia, Dr. Morton laid down a prescription for these patients which resulted, he says, in regular normal bowel movements in the majority of patients. This regime was:

1. No laxatives of any kind and no enemas.
2. Some vegetable bulk at both noon and evening meals.
3. Some fruit or fruit juice at each meal.
4. Some fluid, a cup to a glass full, each hour during the day.

Lecithin

Our interest in lecithin at this particular moment in history springs almost entirely from our interest in another fatty substance—cholesterol. Because of cholesterol we have come, during the past ten years, to think of any fat in the diet as being dangerous, even possibly to the point of being actually poisonous to us.

As a result, diets are being prescribed right and left in which fat has been reduced to a minimum. A recent issue of a women's magazine carried a reducing diet which had obviously been worked out with great care to include all the vitamins and minerals for which official daily minimum requirements have been set. We checked it closely and found indeed that vitamins A, B_1 and B_2, vitamin C, calcium and iron were all plentiful in this diet. But most of the other B vitamins, vitamin E and the essential unsaturated fatty acids, sometimes called vitamin F, were practically non-existent in the menus for the simple reason that the diet was low in fat. No salad dressings were used, foods were prepared without vegetable oils, and whole grain cereals (one of our best sources of vitamin-rich fats) were not recommended.

Why this furor over fats? The reason is simple. Not so long ago it was discovered that cholesterol, a fatty substance, that occurs only in animal fats, is largely responsible for hardening of the arteries. Investigating the thick chunks of matter that clog hardened arteries, researchers found that it consisted mostly of cholesterol. So right away everybody became panicky about cholesterol. The popular magazines carried frightening articles about it. Fat-free diets became the rage. Fat—any and all kinds of fat—became anathema.

We have published in past *Preventions* some hair-raising stories about cholesterol. The *American Heart Journal,* volume 39, 1950, tells the results of a survey of the cholesterol content of the coronary arteries and blood of a group of patients who died of coronary thrombosis (a blood clot in the coronary artery). It was about four times the average of that of normal patients. Since an over-abundance of cholesterol was found in patients who died of coronary thrombosis it seems reasonable to believe that for some reason the bodies of these individuals are not able to handle fatty substances properly.

Another article in *Archives of Pathology*, volume 47, 1949, states that cholesterol is constantly present in the disordered blood vessels of a patient with hardening of the arteries. And it seems to be true, too, that the amount of cholesterol in the blood vessels increases with age.

Suppose we delete all food that contains cholesterol. Will we then be free from any menace? No, we won't, because cholesterol is produced in the body at a much faster rate than we could eat it. Apparently it is necessary for many body functions among them the formation of vitamin D, the sex hormones and the adrenal hormones and the bile salts, so important for the proper digestion of all kinds of fats.

It has been shown that, by eating a high-fat diet, approximately 800 milligrams of cholesterol are obtained daily. But the perfectly normal human liver produces 3000 milligrams of cholesterol or more per day, all by itself! So even though you cut out any and all foods containing cholesterol your body will still continue to manufacture it—and probably will also continue to misuse it so that you will still get deposits of cholesterol where they are not wanted—in the walls of blood vessels and in gall stones.

You see, once you cut out all fatty foods you also cut out all foods that contain lecithin, which is the substance that apparently can control cholesterol, keep it going its helpful way and prevent it from depositing where it is not wanted.

Adelle Davis, in her book *Let's Eat Right to Keep Fit* (Harcourt Brace and Co., New York, N. Y.) has this to say about lecithin. "Another cousin of the fat family, lecithin, is supplied by all natural oils and by the fat of egg yolk, liver and brains. Lecithin is an excellent source of the two B vitamins, choline and inositol; if health is to be maintained, the more fat eaten, the larger must be the intake of these two vitamins. This substance can be made in the intestinal wall provided choline, inositol and essential fatty acids are supplied. Lecithin appears to be a homogenizing agent capable of breaking fat and probably cholesterol into tiny particles which can pass readily into the tissues. There is evidence that the major causes of death, coronary occlusion and coronary thrombosis are associated with deficiencies of linoleic acids (essential unsaturated fatty acids) and the two B vitamins, choline and inositol and perhaps with a lack of lecithin itself. Huge particles of cholesterol get stuck in the walls of the arteries; they might be homogenized into tiny particles if sufficient nutrients were available for the normal production of lecithin. When oils are refined or hydrogenated, lecithin is discarded."

Lecithin is pronounced *less-i-thin* with the accent on the first syllable. The word comes from the Greek *Likithos,* meaning the yolk of an egg, for lecithin is abundant in egg-yolk. This is one reason why we have only recently begun to hear about lecithin—egg-yolk was too expensive a source of it to be very plentiful for experimentation. Quite recently another less expensive source has been found—soybeans.

Doesn't it seem significant that lecithin should appear in such quantities in egg-yolk which is also so rich in cholesterol? Doesn't it seem like a most beneficial provision of Mother Nature (who knows nothing about refining foods) to provide two substances that the body needs together in one food so that you could not possibly get harmful amounts of cholesterol without also getting enough lecithin to keep the cholesterol in a proper fluid state?

According to Adelle Davis a study at the Almeda County Hospital involved patients who were given fat from egg yolks *equivalent to 36 eggs* daily, and in no case did the blood cholesterol level rise above normal. The egg yolk, you see, contained also the B vitamins, the lecithin, and the other natural substances necessary for the proper use of the cholesterol by the body.

So we come back again to the only possible conclusion—we ourselves have created the threat that cholesterol poses—by our arrogant meddling with natural foods. Hardening of the arteries, heart disorders, gall stones —these are the results of our meddling.

Cholesterol appears in foods of animal origin—fat meats, butter, oils from fish, eggs and so forth. So far our brilliant food chemists have not found any way to meddle with these fats. We cook them and if we raise the temperature to an excessive high degree, the fats are bound to be harmful to us. Deep fat frying and browning butter are two cooking processes that should be forbidden by law. But aside from this, fats of animal origin have not been tampered with to any great extent.

What about fats of vegetable and cereal origin, so rich in lecithin, the B vitamins and the essential fatty acids sometimes called vitamin F? We have done everything possible to destroy completely these vitally important fats and not just destroy them but render what remains of the food positively harmful to human cells.

First we remove all the health-giving fats when we refine grains. The germ of the cereal contains the lecithin, the B vitamins, the essential fatty acids and vitamin E. So we throw this exceedingly important part of the grain away (because it spoils easily!) and eat only the starchy remnant, practically vitamin-free, which bakes into white, pasty bread with just about the same nutritive value as laundry starch. Your baker will tell you how they have "enriched" this pasty mass by adding some synthetic vitamin B_1 and iron. Ask him how much of the fatty part of the cereal grain has been replaced! This part is used instead for stock feed. Animals thrive on it.

And what of other natural sources of lecithin and all its accompanying vitamins? Seeds are rich sources. What seeds does the average American ever eat that have not been tampered with? Nuts are the only ones we can think of at the moment and even these he seems unable to eat unless they have been roasted almost to nothingness. Primitive peoples eat seeds of all kinds—melon seeds, sunflower seeds, cereal seeds, corn kernels, acorns, millet, whole rice and so forth. We smart Americans take the perfectly good seeds and other healthful foods Mother Nature gives and press out the oil. So far so good. If we stopped there (cold-pressed olive oil for instance), all would be well. Such oils are rich in lecithin, vitamin E, the unsaturated fatty acids and the B vitamins. And research seems to prove that in lands where cold-pressed oils are the basic fatty foods, hardening of the arteries, heart disease, gall-stones and other diseases involving cholesterol deposits are not common.

But our food technologists have developed ways of "improving" our vegetable oils. And you can be certain when that word "improve" comes in the front door, Mother Nature goes out the back. We "improve" oils by hydrogenating them. What does this give us? Hydrogenated shortenings—those lifeless (and, we are firmly convinced, deadly) solid white shortenings you buy in a can and use for making pastry, frying, cake-baking, deep-fat frying and so forth. They don't spoil; they're so economical; they're so much more convenient than messy liquid shortenings. You have all the arguments for them on your television commercials.

But unfortunately for you and me, all the lecithin, the B vitamins, vitamin E and the essential fatty acids have been destroyed in the process of hydrogenation. How is your body going to handle fats such as these without the natural substances that accompany fats in nature? It's an obvious impossibility. And all of the other food substances that depend on fats for their proper absorption—calcium, phosphorus, vitamin A and so forth—all these are going to be used improperly, too.

Consider for a moment all the conscientious mothers who "bake" for their families. To worthless white flour, completely denuded of all its nutritional value, they add white sugar (a drug with no food value but calories). Then, adding insult to injury, they cream into their cake hydrogenated shortening. The women's magazines supported by advertising for these very products, devote themselves to dreaming up new horrors in the way of cake-making, to persuade the completely unaware housewife and mother that she is not "doing her duty" to her family if she doesn't whip up one of these monstrous pieces of nutritional rubbish this very day.

Is it any wonder we as a nation shudder at the word "cholesterol" and bring children into the world afflicted with heart disease? What can we do to avoid cholesterol deposits? Stop eating eggs, fish and meat? No, of course not. Stop eating any fat that has been tampered with by food technologists. Read labels looking for the word "hydrogenated" and don't buy any product so labelled. Incidentally margarine is of course hydrogenated vegetable oils. And any packaged foods you buy like crackers are probably made with hydrogenated shortenings. Get completely natural oils from plant sources. If you can, buy and use cold-pressed oils. Olive oil is often available from Italian importers in large cities. Cold-pressed oils are available in many health food stores. Sunflower seed oil is available from *Prevention* advertisers.

And what's the matter with getting most of our quota of healthful untampered-with vegetable oil from sunflower seeds anyway? They're delicious to eat, a wonderful between-meals snack because they "stick to your ribs," being high in protein. And they contain the finest oil you can imagine, untouched by any human hand but yours.

Lettuce

If you've ever walked down a garden path on a fresh spring day between rows of green ruffled lettuce, you can never afterwards eat "store" lettuce with any satisfaction. Lettuce, perhaps more than any other vegetable, suffers from being picked, handled, transported and stored before it is eaten. Crispiness is the most important quality of lettuce. If it isn't crisp there doesn't seem to be any point at all to eating it.

Commercially grown lettuce can be stored (if it is in excellent condition) for three weeks or longer at a temperature of 32 degrees. It freezes at eight-tenths of a degree lower than that, so the storage temperature must be carefully watched. Usually what you buy at the store has been packed in ice for the trip from the farm. Even so, it's a pretty sorry looking head of lettuce as you select it and put it in your shopping bag. For five minutes away from the garden is enough to start the wilting process in lettuce. Some brands hold up longer than others, true. But it should always be your aim to eat lettuce as newly picked as possible for of course wilting means loss of vitamins and minerals.

So even if you can't have a garden, at least make some room somewhere to plant lettuce and the other greens you will need for salad during the spring, summer and fall. Then don't pick them until it's time to make the salad and put it on the table. If you must buy lettuce and other greens at the store, wash them as rapidly as possible and put them in a covered container in the refrigerator. Never, never soak them. True, it does "crisp" them, but it also drains off all the vitamins and minerals into the soaking water.

Many readers have inquired about insecticides used on lettuce and other greens. Of course the commercially grown greens have been doused with insecticides and perhaps preservatives as well to keep them from wilting. Furthermore, it is next to impossible to remove these bug killers, for they lurk in every little wrinkle and crevice in every leaf. In many cases the oily insecticides are not affected in the least by water. Another excellent reason for growing your own salad greens. You should wash carefully any lettuce you get at the store and wipe it with a dry towel as well. It's up to you to decide whether the benefit you will get from the greens will outweigh the possible harmful effects of whatever insecticides are on them. Personally we believe it does. But growing your own lettuce is the best answer of all. Of course taking your vitamin supplements regularly will help to protect you against harm from insecticides.

One final word on lettuce in the diet. We don't suppose anyone lives on lettuce. But is might be dangerous to do so especially during the hottest of the summer months. Lettuce grown on soil fertilized with nitrates contains nitrates which the hot sunlight may change into nitrites, a substance which, in sufficient concentration, can be dangerous. It unites with the red pigment in the blood that is supposed to carry oxygen. So don't eat leafy vegetables exclusively during the summer months. Eat plenty of the others as well.

Lettuce is not excessively rich in all of the important nutriments. But it does contain a goodly allotment of the B vitamins and vitamin A, and of course it makes the best possible base for salads of all kinds. Its protein content is low—only 1.2 per cent. But, considering the fact that its water content is 94.8 per cent, the protein in the remaining solids is quite high. The carbohydrate in lettuce is only 2.9 per cent—good news for dieters. One hundred grams contain 22 milligrams of calcium which is a little less available to the body than the calcium of milk, 25 milligrams of phosphorus and .5 milligrams of iron. Loose leaf lettuce is generally thought to be more nutritious than head lettuce because it is generally greener and also has access to much more sunlight. Green leaves are, of course, richer in all the vitamins and minerals than pale white ones.

The vitamin content of 100 grams of lettuce (about four large leaves) is:

Vitamin A	540 International Units
Vitamin B	
Thiamin	.06 Milligrams
Riboflavin	.07 Milligrams
Niacin	.2 Milligrams
Vitamin C	8 Milligrams

Lima Beans

Lima beans are a fine year-'round food, high in protein, vitamins and minerals, inexpensive, and highly satisfactory to most peoples' palate. In these days when the cost of meat, eggs and cheese is so high, it is well to remember that legumes, such as beans, are a splendid meat substitute. They do not contain all the various amino acids that make up "complete" protein—no vegetable foods do. But they are sufficiently rich in four of these amino acids to qualify as very high grade protein.

Lima beans came to us from South America. The fact that they are shelled out of their pods before they are eaten is a good recommendation for them in these days of ever-present insecticides on food. The actual lima bean kernel probably contains very little of whatever insecticide has been dusted or sprayed on the pods. Served fresh from the garden, not overcooked, there are few vegetables that equal them for flavor. Dried, they retain most of their vitamin and mineral content, with the exception of vitamin C. But they must be prepared correctly if they are to retain all these valuable food elements right up to the dinner table.

Until recently it was good cooking practice to soak dried beans overnight, throw away the water in which they soaked (and the B vitamins along with the water) then parboil the beans in fresh water to which baking soda was added for some obscure reason. The soda removed what was left of the vitamins, the parboiling removed the minerals, and the beans were served almost devoid of any food value, except that they filled you up. Nowadays we know that dried beans should be cooked in the water in which they are soaked. No soda should be used in preparing them and they should be cooked at very low heat so that their protein will not toughen. Adelle Davis in her excellent cook book *Let's Cook It Right* (Harcourt, Brace & Company, 383 Madison Ave., N. Y.) suggests not soaking the beans at all, but dropping them very slowly into boiling water, so that the water continues to boil. This will soften them, so that they can be cooked. Soaking them, then freezing them before cooking will subtract from the time necessary for the cooking process. There are endless tasty ways lima beans can be served—baked, boiled with meat, made into loaves and so forth.

Here are the vitamins and minerals found in one-half cup of lima beans, fresh and dried. Eat more of them!

	Fresh Lima Beans		*Dried Lima Beans*	
Calcium	63	mg.	72	mg.
Phosphorus	158	mg.	386	mg.
Iron	2.20	mg.	7	mg.
Magnesium			1.07	mg.
Copper			.86	mg.
Vitamin A	900	Int. U.	0-100	Int. U.
Vitamin B				
Thiamin	225	mcg.	300	mcg.
Riboflavin	250	mcg.	250	mcg.
Niacin	1	mg.	2.1	mg.
Pantothenic acid	95	mcg.		
Pyridoxine			550	mcg.
Biotin			9.8	mcg.
Vitamin C	42	mg.	2	mg.

Liver—Desiccated

Since the days of earliest history man has been looking for a wonder food—a food that would completely satisfy his needs, keep him young and strong and protect him from disease. We doubt if such a food exists, for we require a wide variety of foods to keep us healthy. But we believe that the closest thing to a wonder food that is available is probably liver, rich in the B vitamins, vitamins A, C, and D, iron, calcium, phosphorus, copper and the extremely important amino acids, which are elements in protein.

Liver has been known as excellent food for many years, but it seems that scientific research has not as yet nearly exhausted the possible findings as to the virtues of this food. We are going to review here some information received and add some new material we have uncovered on the subject.

Liver Protects Against Poisons

It is well known among physiologists that the liver is the detoxifying organ of the body. It destroys poisons we take in. For instance, according to an article in *The Journal of Nutrition* for March 10, 1954, whole liver in the diet or even fractions of liver have been found to be very powerful against the effects of massive doses of strychnine, sulfanilimide, promin, atabrine, dinitrophenol, diethylstilbestrol, alpha-estradiol, cortisone acetate and so forth. All of these long names refer to one or another industrial substance or medical drug to which we may be exposed. The liver is constantly on guard to protect us against these products.

According to the article in *The Journal* there is apparently a protective factor in that part of liver that is insoluble in water. In fact, it seems to be at least two factors which are not part of any of the known nutrients, whose requirements may be increased under conditions of stress, such as poisoning of some kind.

In the experiment described in the *Journal of Nutrition,* the author, Benjamin H. Ershoff of the University of Southern California tested desiccated liver, milk protein and all of the known B vitamins to see which would protect his laboratory animals from the effects of large doses of thiouracil, a drug that interferes with the workings of the thyroid gland. Now, as we know, it may be necessary to take this drug under certain conditions of illness. But physicians who prescribe it understand well that an overdose can have serious effects on the thyroid glands. So they prescribe it with great care. Dr. Ershoff, however, deliberately gave his rats large overdoses to see whether or not he could then protect them against this overdose by feeding them special things.

He found that there was indeed something in certain batches of desiccated liver that protected the rats against the ill effects of the drug. This substance was not present in casein (the milk protein) or in kelp or in any or all of the known B vitamins. Apparently the substance in the liver is thyroid hormone and it occurs in connection with iodine in the liver. Apparently there is a considerable amount of it in some batches of liver, and little or none in others.

Now of course, none of us is taking harmful doses of this particular drug. But, we know well that liver protects against other poisons to which we are subjected—insecticides, for instance. Testifying before the Committee to Investigate Chemicals in Foods, Bernard Krohn, M.D. of Long Beach, California, described many cases of poisoning from insecticides, which he was treating with injections of liver extract and also large amounts of liver given by mouth. Said he "Treatment of the disease is largely a matter of repairing damaged tissues. High protein and high vitamin diet, especially the B complex of vitamins, is useful. Injections of crude liver extract speed the process."

Recent articles on insecticides indicate that all of us are exposed to them almost continuously and that it is well nigh impossible to escape from some exposure to DDT, chlordane, lindane and the other new insecticides no matter how careful we individually are to avoid them in our homes. Now, if liver is part of the treatment for insecticide poisoning, there is every reason to believe that including plenty of liver in your diet will protect you against the poisoning.

The Liver and the Endocrine Glands

A further testimony to the power of liver in the diet is given in *The Lancet* for February 16, 1952. According to this editorial, the human liver is closely connected with the proper functioning of the endocrine glands. We all know how extremely important these glands are to our welfare. It appears that the liver regulates the functioning of the glands. Two vitamins, riboflavin and thiamin, and one amino acid or form of protein have been named as the absolute essentials for the proper functioning of the sex hormones, for instance. In other words, these food substances are necessary to keep the liver healthy and the liver must be healthy for the sex hormones to do their work.

In a series of 450 cases studied by Morton S. Biskind, M.D. (New York) and reported in *Vitamins and Hormones,* volume 4, page 147, disturbance of sex hormones had resulted in an excess of the female sex hormone—estrogen. In the women patients this brought about various menstrual disorders, painful breasts and acne; in the men, excessive development of the breast, softening of the testes, loss of hair in the armpits and so forth. In both sexes there was infertility. Dr. Biskind treated the patients with desiccated whole liver which resulted in completely healing all their symptoms of vitamin deficiency as well as the sex hormone disturbances.

In another series of cases described in *Archives of Internal Medicine,* volume 88, page 762, R. S. Long and E. E. Simmons tell of similar symptoms in persons who apparently had perfectly healthy livers and were not lacking in any of the vitamins. However, in these cases, too, the disorders of sex hormone functioning were cured by a diet high in protein, low in fat, richly supplemented with the B vitamins and crude liver extract. In the two cases where there was liver disease the effect of the diet was "truly impressive," say these authors.

Suppose you don't like liver for some reason or other and can't eat it. Is there anything you can take instead that will give you the same good results? Apparently not, for literature is full of comparisons of liver with other foods, showing the great superiority of liver and also showing that there are apparently many as yet unidentified substances in liver which are not known vitamins or minerals but which have astonishing characteristics. For instance an article in the *Journal of Nutrition* for January, 1949, shows that there is something in liver which is essential for the growth of laboratory animals. This element is not present in brewer's yeast or wheat germ (for the animals fed these two substances did not respond) and it is not in any of the known vitamins. Could it be vitamin B_{12}, the newly discovered miracle vitamin used to cure pernicious anemia? Apparently not, for in the June 28, 1952 issue of the *British Medical Journal* appears the account of feeding desiccated liver to a group of children and comparing their growth to that of an evenly matched group of children who did not get the liver. The author, John Mudkin, M.D. of the University of London, tells us that the liver factor which produced this result is not vitamin B_{12}, since vitamin B_{12} given alone does not have this effect. The children who got the liver showed 20 to 40 per cent gain in growth than those who did not.

Liver Combats Fatigue

Now we want to review two other experiments. The first concerns fatigue and liver. B. H. Ershoff, M.D. writing in the *Proceedings of the Society of Experimental Biology and Medicine,* July, 1951, tells of testing for an anti-fatigue diet in his laboratory He used three groups of rats on three different diets which he fed for 12 weeks. The first group ate a usual laboratory diet to which were added nine synthetic and two natural vitamins. By this we mean that the synthetic ones were made in a laboratory of the various chemical substances of which the vitamins are made. The natural ones were extracted from foods—brewer's yeast, wheat germ, or something like that.

The second group of rats had this same diet, added vitamins and all, with, in addition, a batch of B vitamins added—all the known B vitamins. The third group ate the original diet with 10 per cent desiccated liver added instead of vitamins. Desiccated liver is liver dried at low heat (to conserve vitamins) and powdered.

Now for the test. Each rat was placed in a drum of water from which he could not climb out. He had to keep swimming or drown. So, as you can see, this was a real test of endurance and anti-fatigue. The first group of rats swam for an average of 13.3 minutes before they gave up and indicated that they had no strength left. The second group swam for an average of 13.4 minutes and gave up. The third group—those which had the desiccated liver in their chow—broke all records. Three of them swam for 63, 83 and 87 minutes. The other rats in the group were all swimming vigorously at the end of two hours when the test was ended. Now, notice please, we did not say that Dr. Ershoff gave these super-rats a shot of something, nor did we say that they took liver for a day and then could perform this feat of endurance. We said that Dr. Ershoff fed them liver for a period of 12 weeks, which corresponds to a number of years in human beings, and *then* they were able to swim almost ten times longer than the ordinary rats, or the ones which had been taking synthetic B vitamins.

Liver Protects Against Cancer

Experiment number two concerns cancer. It took place at the Sloan-Kettering Institute for Cancer Research over many years. It was written up in the *Journal of Nutrition* for July 10, 1951. Kanematsu Suguira who conducted the experiments tells us that he tried out various food substances to prevent cancer in laboratory animals. As you know, there are certain coal-tar substances which are sure cancer-producers. One of these is butter-yellow, which at one time was used in food, but which is today prohibited. Mixed with rice, it will produce cancer when it is fed to laboratory rats in given quantity.

A group of rats was put on a diet of butter yellow and rice. Another group was given the same diet plus 10 percent desiccated liver. After a suitable period of time the rats were examined for cancer. All fifty of the animals in the group receiving no liver had cancerous livers within 150 days. The rats to whose diet desiccated liver was added were completely protected from the cancer. But when the amount of liver was cut to 2 per cent rather than 10 per cent the protection was less. It was also found that the liver supplement did not make for permanent protection. After it was stopped, cancer later developed in most of the animals. So it would seem that liver should be a permanent part of a good diet.

So liver actually seems to be the "wonder-food" or as near it as we will ever come. Does this mean you should attempt to live entirely on liver? No, although we have heard of people who were at death's door who cured themselves by eating liver three times a day—every single meal—for the rest of their lives. Didn't seem to mind it, either!

Growth, regulation of hormones, protection from poisons, protection from cancer and an assurance of strength and endurance—these are the health reasons we have uncovered so far which indicate that liver is an absolute necessity for anyone who would be healthy these days. You and your family should eat liver as often as possible—and surely at least once a week. If you don't like it, you will be amazed at how soon you can come to like it especially if you experiment with different ways of fixing it until you discover which one pleases you most.

Somewhere along the line of American cookery there arose a tradition of soaking liver. Someone wrote us the other day inquiring how long she should soak liver before cooking it—"to draw out the poisons"! *Of course no fresh food should ever be soaked.* But soaking liver is probably the worst crime against good health that you can commit. For most of the vitamins in liver are water-soluble. Many of the unknown factors (such as the anti-fatigue factor) may be water-soluble. This means that they dissolve in water. By soaking liver, you dissolve away—down the drain—all the precious food elements which make liver valuable! Cook liver the very day you get it from the store. Whisk it out of the refrigerator and on to the stove. Cook it at slow heat, for as little time as possible, to preserve vitamins. If you have it sliced thin, it will take less time to cook through.

Statistics in nutrition books indicate that there is a widespread vitamin B deficiency in this country, due to the processing all of our foods go through before they reach us. For this reason we advise all readers to take vitamin B as a natural food supplement every day. Brewer's yeast and liver are the two substances richest in all the B vitamins. Desiccated liver is more expensive than brewer's yeast because of the infinite care needed to dry it so that none of the vitamins will be lost. But it does contain food factors not found in yeast, as we have shown above. By all means, take desiccated liver as a food supplement, especially if, for one reason or another, you cannot eat liver at meals at least once a week.

Longevity

By W. CODA MARTIN, M.D., New York City, N. Y.

We are proud to present this article, reprinted from *The International Record of Medicine and General Practice Clinics,* September, 1953, covering the subject of nutrition in Geriatrics (the study of old age). Readers may remember Dr. Martin as the physician who made headlines all over the country recently with his sensational exposure of the fact that he had found DDT in the tissues of patients who had not been knowingly exposed to it.

It is in geriatrics that physicians are mostly brought face to face with medicine's greatest unsolved problem, that of the degenerative diseases in elderly patients. While infectious diseases may be said to have been basically conquered and while as a result the average life expectancy has been raised to 65 years, two painful facts remain: (A) To judge by such figures as those of rejections for military service in World War II (50 per cent unfit for armed services), the average health of the population is becoming worse rather than better. (B) The incidence of degenerative diseases is increasing by leaps and bounds.

Are we prolonging men's lives only to leave them at the mercy of cancer, arteriosclerosis, liver disease, arthritis, and heart disease? Can these and similar diseases be averted by preventive treatment, or even relieved after they have developed?

While the average physician today regards diet as a secondary factor in the treatment and prevention of these degenerative diseases, the author believes that a study of the findings of biochemists will show that a large share of this type of disease is the end result of prolonged malnutrition and can be averted by early adoption of an adequate diet.

Is our present diet so defective that the wealthiest and most bountifully fed people in the world are actually starving in the midst of plenty? The United States Plant, Soil, and Nutrition Laboratory at Cornell has pointed out that some of the principal truck-and-fruit-growing regions of our eastern seaboard are so deficient in essential minerals that the actual nutritive content of the "protective" foods which they supply to our great cities may be questionable.

In 1840, one ounce of genuine whole bread made of stone-ground wheat contained 20 units of vitamin B-1. In 1950, one ounce of white bread contained only five units of B-1 before the addition of synthetic thiamin. The Food and Nutrition Board of the National Research Council considers an intake of 1.5 to 2 mg. (445-660 IU) of B-1 per day as necessary for maintenance of good health.

The refinement of white bread has removed not only vitamin B-1 but other known and unknown dietary factors such as proteins, other parts of the B-complex, vitamin E and essential minerals. There has been added to what is called "enriched" bread only synthetic B-1, riboflavin, niacin, and iron. This is replacing only a part of the whole and cannot be expected to give the complete nutritional protection as the natural whole grain bread. Other grain food and cereals including polished rice are subjected to similar drastic processing.

Doctors Williams and Spies, who studied diets in various parts of the United States, state in their book, *Vitamin B-1,* published in 1938, that there is much sameness in diets all over the country. This sameness is largely in the enormous consumption of nonvitamin, nonmineral foods composed of white flour and white sugar. The average diet furnishes a vitamin B-1 intake of from 200-300 IU, which is just enough to prevent beriberi and pellagra. To have the optimum benefit from vitamin B-1, a person of 150 pounds weight should have a daily intake of 750-1000 IU.

The presence of mouth, teeth, and gum diseases in school children and adults needs no confirmation by laboratory test of the fact that nutritional deficiency is universal in civilized countries. It is also obvious that this condition does not improve with age. Doctor Alice Bernheim has shown that the average person's usual diet, being composed of refined foods, does not contain the needed amount of calcium. This deficiency is universal in all civilized countries. The figures from the *Food and Drug Journal,* which keeps an accurate record of the export and import of food products into New York City, showed that the food intake of the population measured only 25 per cent for the vitamin—and mineral-containing protective foods as against 75 per cent of devitaminized foods composed of white flour and white sugar.

If such depleted diets continue over a period of years the body will develop tissue changes that will inevitably lead to degenerative diseases.

What good nutrition can accomplish is shown in a report by Dr. Robert McCarrison. In 1918, speaking of the Hunza people in India, he writes: "My own personal experience provides an example of a race unsurpassed in perfection of physique and in freedom from diseases in general. Amongst these people the span of life is extraordinarily long; and such services as I was able to render them during the seven years I spent in their midst were confined chiefly to the treatment of accidental lesions, the removal of senile cataract, plastic operations for granular eyelids, or the treatment of maladies wholly unconnected with food supply. These people are long-lived, vigorous in youth and age, capable of great endurance and enjoy a remarkable freedom from disease in general. . . . During the period of my association with these people, I never saw a case of asthenic dyspepsia, or gastric or duodenal ulcer, appendicitis, mucous colitis, or of cancer."

Later, McCarrison made experiments in which rats were given the type of diet eaten by the Hunza people. This consisted of chapattis, or flat bread, made of whole meal flour lightly smeared with butter, sprouted pulses or legumes, fresh, raw carrots and fresh, raw cabbage *ad libitum* (as much as wanted), unpasteurized whole milk and soured milk, a small ration of meat with bones once a week, and an abundance of water. This food was grown on special soil prepared with organic fertilizers. No chemical fertilizers, insecticides or pesticide sprays have ever been used on the soil.

In this experiment 1,189 rats were watched from birth to the twenty-seventh month, an age in the rat which corresponds to that of about 55 years in man. His report states: "During the past two and a quarter years there has been no case of illness in this 'universe' of albino rats, no deaths from natural causes in the adult stock, and but for a few accidental deaths, no infantile mortality. Both clinically and at post mortem examination this stock has been shown to be remarkably free from disease."

McCarrison then took the customary inadequate diet of the poorer peoples of Bengal and Madras, consisting of polished rice, pulses or legumes, vegetables, condiments, and a little milk. He fed 2,243 rats on this diet and they developed all the diseases suffered by these people. They got diseases of every organ of the body, eyes, nose, ears, lungs, heart, stomach, intestines, kidneys, bladder, reproductive organs, blood, special glands, and nerves.

Later, McCarrison gave a set of rats the diet of the poorer classes in England, consisting of white bread, margarine, sweetened tea, boiled vegetables, white sugar, tinned meats and jams. He reports: "On this diet, not only did the rats grow badly but they developed what one might call rat-neurasthenia. They were nervous and apt to bite their attendants, they lived unhappily together and by the sixteenth day, they began to kill each other and eat the weaker ones amongst them." Because of this cannibalism in the rats, the experiment was discontinued.

This report shows the effect of various diets on experimental animals and humans. It reveals that foods grown on properly prepared soil, so that they contain adequate vitamins and minerals as well as complete proteins, will prevent degenerative diseases. The question then arises whether we can do anything to correct the pathological disease changes once they have developed. Recent experimental and clinical work shows that it is possible to control and retard some of these conditions and to prolong the life of the patient. This is true of liver dysfunction and its associated arteriosclerosis, hypercholesterolemia (excess of cholesterol in blood), and coronary disease. These conditions and many allied diseases of the human organism are recognized as being due to dietary deficiency, especially of the lipotropic factors (those that deal with fat), B-complex, and an excess intake of fat.

Morrison reviewed evidence that arteriosclerosis is a metabolic error and not the inevitable accompaniment of advancing age, and that it may be preventable. He maintained that arteriosclerosis develops through a triad based on (a) high cholesterol-high fat diet; (b) malfunction of the liver, involving disturbances in lipid (fatty substances) and lipoprotein metabolism, and (c) deficiencies and imbalances in endocrine function implicating the thyroid and sex hormones. He advised a program of low fat, low cholesterol diet and lipotropic therapy, choline, inositol combination and where indicated, estrogen and androgen hormones for coronary artery disease. Under this treatment mortality was reduced to one-third, angina pains decreased or disappeared, and patients returned to work or normal activities with a feeling of well-being, optimism, and better morale.

Doctor Boris Sokoloff states that not long ago it was believed that longevity of an animal or man is determined chiefly by heredity, but now scientists are placing greater emphasis on nutrition as a paramount factor in the prolongation of life in man and animal alike. The results of McCarrison's experiments showing that diet influenced the life span of man and rats have been dramatically confirmed recently by C. McCay and M. Crowell of Cornell University. They were able to double the normal span of life in rats by keeping them from birth on a low calory diet rich in vitamins. In other words diets high in protective foods and low in refined foods, depleted of their nutrient factors, improve the health and prolong the life span.

Henry C. Sherman believes that "old age can be deferred and man's life span lengthened." He further states: "The indicated improvement of the adult life expectation from 70 to 77 years is apparently well within the scientific probabilities for those who use the newer knowledge of nutrition in their daily food habits, beginning early enough in life. It is not merely a longer lease of life that is offered, but a life cycle both longer and lived on a higher plane of positive health, efficiency, and happiness throughout." Sherman stated many times that the larger the percentage of total calories in the form of protective foods, the smaller was the percentage of failure in the preservation of the characteristics of youth.

It is then apparent that when we learn to eat day after day, month after month, year after year, all the essential nutrients, a higher degree of health will result and there will be a marked decrease in the degenerative diseases, and a prolonged, healthy life span will follow. Progress of the science of nutrition and growing knowledge of vitamins, minerals, and enzymes places the physician in possession of facts that enable him to prevent and control the ever-increasing danger of degenerative diseases in geriatric patients.

Food intake should be based on what materials the body needs for its health and efficient function rather than on present-day perverted taste habits. The diet should be low in carbohydrate, low in fat, high in proteins, and high in foods that contain natural vitamins and minerals, such as whole grain products in the form of bread and cereal, fruit and fresh vegetables, and the intake of refined foods and sugars must be restricted or eliminated. Albrecht states: "We are constantly in danger of deficiencies of proteins and minerals relative to carbohydrates and fats." This he believes results in lowered powers of growth and lowered capacity for reproduction. He also states: "Life is not passed from one fat globule to another, nor from one starch grain to another, but only from one protein molecule to another protein molecule. Proteins are the foods that rebuild the body, carry life and guarantee reproduction."

There is need for a better understanding of how to choose a diet which will contain the factors essential to good health.

1. Delete from the diet any food which has the basic chemistry altered by the removal of those elements essential to human nutrition.

2. Do not depend on "enriched" or fortified foods. These foods replace only a small fraction of the vitamins and minerals removed in the process of refining.

3. The diet should be high in protective food. These include fresh fruits, vegetables, and dairy products, whole grain bread, and cereals. A large portion of the fruits and vegetables should be eaten in the fresh raw state to assure an adequate intake of the important heat labile enzymes.

4. Daily intake of lean fresh meat, fish, fowl and eggs.

5. Daily intake of milk and dairy products. Whole unpasteurized milk is preferable.

6. Adequate intake of fresh fruits.

7. For adequate intake of important B-complex factors, the diets of geriatric patients should be supplemented with a good natural source of these elements, such as (1) desiccated whole liver. This substance contains not only all the known and identified fractions of the B-complex but a number of unidentified substances that are at least as important to nutrition as those already known. It also contains the antifatigue factor which is so important in elderly people. (2) Brewer's yeast, which is probably the cheapest source of the natural B-complex and is also high in complete proteins. (3) Wheat germ is another excellent source of the whole natural B-complex and also rich in vitamin E.

8. The foregoing diet should supply sufficient vitamins A and D, but if there is a doubt supplement it with a preparation of aqueous natural A and D for better absorption.

9. Organically-grown foods are advisable when available for consumption. Organic foods have 20-40 per cent greater vitamin and trace mineral content than those grown in depleted soils. They are also free from chemical insecticides and pesticides which accumulate in human fat and produce liver damage. For optimum health this type of food is essential. Organically-grown foods contain many unknown protective elements that have not yet been identified. Many feeding tests in humans and animals have proved this fact. If this type of food is not available, a vitamin and mineral supplement is recommended.

In conclusion the diet must be optimum in its protein, vitamin, mineral, enzyme content to assure optimum health, protect against degenerative diseases, and prolong the life span.

Magnesium

Magnesium is one of the mineral substances in food. There is a great deal of uncertainty as to its place in nutrition, but we do know that it is present in bones and muscles and that it is a necessary part of the diet. Actually it seems that about .05 per cent of the body's content is probably magnesium.

Magnesium appears to be widely distributed in foods, chiefly in vegetables. It is present in the green coloring matter, or chlorophyll. Of course magnesium, along with other minerals, is removed when grain is milled and refined, so none of the natural magnesium of the wheat germ remains in the flour from which white bread is made, or in refined and processed cereals. The amount of magnesium in milk is quite small and varies with the season and the time of lactation. So pre-school childrens' diets which consist largely of refined cereals and milk are of course almost completely lacking in magnesium.

There is a peculiar antagonism between magnesium and calcium in the body's chemistry. E. V. McCollum, who has done much research on magnesium, says in his book *The Newer Knowledge of Nutrition* (Macmillan, 1947) that too much magnesium in the diet interferes with the body's use of calcium, when there is not enough phosphorus present. We have stressed many times in these pages the importance of both calcium and phosphorus in nutrition, as well as the great importance of their relationship to one another. That is, they should be present in a certain proportion to one another. Now it seems that this proportion is even more important than we thought. Not only is it essential for the proper metabolism of calcium, but also that of magnesium.

Possibly many of us are not getting enough magnesium for the simple reason that we do not eat enough green vegetables. From the research that has been done it appears that magnesium is responsible for the health of the nerves and the muscles; it is necessary to maintain the normal structure of growing tissues; it participates in the formation of bone in children; it activates certain enzymes in the body—a process very important to digestion, especially the digestion of carbohydrates. It is also used, in chemical form, as a laxative and antacid. Magnesium citrate and magnesium sulfate are laxative in their action, while magnesium hydroxide (milk of magnesia) is an antacid.

Symptoms of Magnesium Deficiency

It is difficult to plan a diet that will not include some magnesium. But in order to discover the results of a magnesium deficiency, McCollum and his co-workers devised such a diet and fed it to laboratory animals. They found that the animals developed the following symptoms, which the control animals did not: dilation of blood vessels, nutritional failure, kidney damage, loss of hair, rough sticky coats, diarrhea and edema. They also found that the rats whose diets were short on magnesium suffered from great excitability and also a form of tetany, or convulsions.

The variety of grain or vegetable being raised has a lot to do with the magnesium content. Also the soil on which it is grown. For instance, in a test made in 1933 by Graves and Graves and published in the *Journal of Nutrition,* it was found that the two varieties of wheat *planted in the same soil* varied as follows in their calcium, phosphorus and magnesium content:

	Calcium	*Magnesium*	*Phosphorus*
Kota wheat	.08	.182	.308
Turkey wheat	.055	.159	.153

This brings us to a consideration of several papers presented in France in 1934 and reprinted in the *Bulletin* of the Academy of Medicine there. In these papers, M. L. Robinet discusses the French vital statistics in regard to suicides, cancer, tuberculosis, senility and their relation to magnesium in the soil. "In one of my first communications," says M. Robinet, "I said that the use of magnesium permitted one to support adversity with more serenity." Comparing suicide statistics with charts on soil composition, M. Robinet discovered that "the comparison of geological maps and statistics establishes therefore in a striking manner the influence of the magnesium content of the soil on the number of suicides. . . . It is evident that one doesn't commit suicide because the soil is poor in magnesium. But those who regularly absorb a good amount of magnesium salts have a more stable equilibrium, they support adversity with more calm and do not renounce everything to avoid some sorrow."

With the exception of three regions where the figures do not hold true, the statistics show clearly that in regions rich in magnesium suicides are nearly three times less frequent than in regions where the soil has little magnesium. This finding is interesting in view of the experiments in which animals were deprived of magnesium and suffered from super-excitability—to such an extent that they became hysterical at the sound of small noises or the sight of shadows.

In studying the incidence of tuberculosis in its relation to the magnesium in the soil M. Robinet did not come to the same conclusion. In fact the statistics showed that for lands rich in magnesium and those very poor, the only difference in tuberculosis incidence is about 15 per cent—which is insignificant. For suicide and cancer it is 60 per cent.

Studying deaths from senility M. Robinet tells us that he knows how unreliable such statistics can be and he makes allowance for probable errors. However it is still evident that deaths from senility are much more rare in regions poor in magnesium. His final conclusions are that the curves in the graphs concerning cancer and suicide overlap almost exactly. On the contrary the curves indicating tuberculosis and senility are exactly the opposite. Therefore, says M. Robinet, "Deaths from cancer and suicide are the more frequent, deaths due to senility are more rare when the soil is poor in magnesium. In other words, there are more cancers, more suicides and fewer old men in regions poor in magnesium."

We plan some day to do more research on the subject of magnesium in the soil. But meanwhile you can see how important to human welfare this mineral must be if eminent scientists can find such a relationship between diseases and soil deficient in magnesium. Also if we would be healthy it seems essential that our food should be grown in soils rich in magnesium as well as the other important minerals.

If you want to check and make certain you are eating foods that contain magnesium, here is a partial list. Remember we said above that green vegetables contain magnesium and that it is present in a wide variety of foods, but is not present in refined or processed foods.

Food	*Milligrams of Magnesium per 100 Grams*
Almonds	252
Barley, whole	171
Beans, dried limas	181
Beet greens	113
Brazil nuts	225
Cashew nuts	267
Corn	121
Endive	380
Flour, whole wheat	122
Hazelnuts	140
Honey	386
Kohlrabi	370
Oatmeal	145

Foods	Milligrams of Magnesium per 100 Grams
Peanuts	167
Peas, dried	149
Pecans	152
Rice, brown	119
Soy flour	223
Walnuts	134
Wheat germ	511
Wheat, whole	165

Meat

Historians and nutritionists have theorized that the American pioneers who settled our continent were able to endure the many hardships, the cold, the hard work, the loneliness, the fear, because their diet consisted almost entirely of meat. Today we know that they lacked, in wintertime especially, many of the food elements needed for good health—vitamin C, for example. But in general their meals were high in the complete protein of meat and it seems fairly obvious that this was one reason, at least, why they survived and triumphed. Of course, we must not forget, too, that none of their food was refined or processed, as we think of processing.

Why exactly is meat such a good food? Or is it, for modern man? Perhaps the outstanding reason for the superiority of meat as food is the fact that it is a complete protein, as are all other animal proteins except gelatin. By "complete protein" we mean that meat contains all the amino acids which we human beings cannot manufacture inside our bodies. These are called the "essential amino acids"—for it is essential that they be present in our food since our bodies do not synthetize them.

Some vegetables contain some of these amino acids; other vegetables contain others. Soybeans have been found to be the only non-animal source of complete proteins. If you are skilled enough in nutrition it is possible to arrange entirely vegetable meals to include all the essential amino acids—but this requires infinite knowledge, patience and attention to the planning of each meal. For you cannot make up at lunchtime the essential amino acids that were lacking at breakfast. You must eat them all at the same time to achieve best results, nutritionally speaking.

Our bodies are made of protein and to be healthy we must provide them with sufficient protein to keep cells and tissues in good repair. These are constantly breaking down and wearing out. If good complete protein is not available, how can they be repaired? Vegetarians believe that we are able to manufacture protein from vegetables and fruits, as horses and cows do. It is our belief that, since our digestive tracts are not made like those of the vegetarian animals, we need to get our protein from animal sources, rather than from vegetable sources exclusively.

Vitamins in Meat

The second valuable food element in meat is its vitamin content. All meats, but especially the organ meats, are high in B vitamins. The different kinds of meat vary in their B content, but, as you can see in the chart following, all rank extremely high. For a country like America where refined carbohydrates make up so much of the diet, meat thus becomes doubly important. For the B vitamins that have been removed from these starches (white flour and white sugar) during their processing must be supplied somewhere in the diet, for they are necessary for the proper digestion of the carbohydrates. There is a chemical laboratory in each body cell where certain substances must be put into the test tube before other necessary substances can be manufactured. The B vitamins and carbohydrates are linked. One cannot benefit the body without the other. And the B vitamins that have been removed from refined foods are present in meat in large quantity.

We sometimes hear of folks who have broken many of the rules of good health. They drink, they smoke, they eat starchy desserts and soda fountain food, and still they are healthy. Probably no one will ever solve this mystery. It may have to do with the glands, arteries and other physical equipment they were born with. It may be that they are just naturally able to resist much of the nutritional degeneration that should affect them. But we have a strong suspicion that, if you look closely into their diets, you will find they eat lots of meat, fruits and vegetables. And perhaps this alone protects them from the results of their other bad habits.

Meat For Infants and Young Children

Meat is now a recommended food for babies. We uncovered a very revealing article on meat diets for infants in which milk was not given at all. Mildred R. Ziegler, Ph.D. of the University of Minnesota writes in the *Journal of the American Dietetic Association* for July, 1953, of the successful results obtained. She tells us that many infants cannot drink milk for one reason or another. (We rather suspect it may be the quality of the milk these days.) These children must have lots of protein, of course, and meat seems to be the answer. She tells us that the American Indians used to feed their infants on meat—pounded dried meat mixed with pounded dried choke cherries and the fat skimmed from boiled bones of the buffalo.

Dr. Ziegler also tells us that animal proteins have a much higher digestibility than vegetable proteins—up to 98 or 100 per cent. Meat, which is very rich in iron (needed after the infant is a year or so old) and the B vitamins, is not rich in calcium. Milk is of course very rich in calcium. So in preparing the diet Dr. Ziegler had to add calcium and trace minerals to the meat. She used the ash from veal bones. This contained not only calcium and phosphorus in their proper physiological proportions, but also all the various trace elements whose possible importance to nutrition we do not know as yet. The meat was cooked and strained.

All the children on the enriched meat diet throve. Dr. Ziegler describes the cases of two children—one with an allergy to milk, the other with a disorder called *galactosemia* which is an inability to use properly the galactose—a sugar occurring in milk.

The two-and-a-half-month old boy who was allergic to milk had had diarrhea almost since birth. He was in an extremely serious condition, with a distended abdomen, bad color, feeble cry, and no gain in weight. He was put on the enriched meat formula and began to improve almost at once. At the end of five months he had gained normally and there was no diarrhea. He continued on the meat formula with added fruits and vegetables as he grew older.

The second infant had jaundice, indicating possibly that some liver disorder had brought on the *galactosemia*. "The child showed marked clinical improvement with an amazing change in her activity and in her disposition, after the mineral-enriched meat formula was substituted for the previous milk diet," says Dr. Ziegler.

In an earlier experiment, reported in *Pediatrics* for October, 1952, we learn that the only illnesses that occurred among the healthy children eating the meat and milk diet were respiratory and digestive disorders. Those on the meat diet had considerably fewer of these and they were much less severe. Drs. Jacobs and George who wrote the article estimate that the disease rate for the meat-fed children was about 40 per cent less than that of the milk-fed children. Dr. Ruth Leverton and associates, writing in the *Journal of Pediatrics* for June 1952 tell us of another group of children part of whom were fed milk, the others meat. The hemoglobin and red blood cell count were better in the infants who got the meat. She also says "The infants receiving a dietary supplement of meat had approximately one-half as many colds as the control subjects and the duration of the colds was reduced. All infants were reported to have slept better and appeared more satisfied when they received the meat supplement."

Today's Meat is Chemicalized

We must consider for a moment all the various things that happen to meat before it reaches our tables to make it unhealthful. Cattle and other meat animals are not always fed the most nutritious diet, just as gardens and farms are not always fertilized properly. However, in general it is well known among breeders that healthy animals are profitable. So there is much less than there used to be of selling diseased or half-starved animals for meat.

However, scientists have recently discovered that animals grow faster when they are fed antibiotics along with their meals. So many farmers use feeds spiked with antibiotics. For years poultry raisers have used a hormone preparation to fatten poultry. By injecting a pellet of stilbestrol into the neck of the chicken, they produced an artificial castration which made the chicken grow fat and big much earlier than previously. During the Congressional Hearings on Chemicals in Foods, there was a lot of discussion of stilbestrol and the possibility that it might be harmful to individuals eating the poultry. It was felt generally among the experts that carelessly injected pellets could easily be eaten by poultry buyers with resulting harm. In fact, there was one government cancer expert who believed there was serious harm, perhaps even the possibility of cancer, to be feared as a result of the use of stilbestrol.

Now we read that stilbestrol is being used to fatten cattle. The aim of course is to save the cattleman money, by causing the cattle to grow much more rapidly so that they can be taken to market much sooner, hence a lot of feed will be saved. But the question of course is—what will be the effect of the stilbestrol on the person who eats the meat? And how much nutrition does one get from meat produced to some extent by the action of stilbestrol?

We do not have the answer to any of these questions as yet. We can only assume that any and all unnatural tinkering with animals meant for food is not good. The only way to avoid chemicalized meat is to buy your meat from someone you know, preferably an organic farmer.

Talk to your butcher about the kind of meat he sells you. If you buy from a large super market find out where their meat comes from and write to the source. Inquire what treatments their animals are given—do they get antibiotics, do they get stilbestrol and so forth? Indicate that you do not want to buy meat from animals that have been treated with any of these substances. One letter will do little good, of course. You will probably get an answer assuring you that there is no harm in any of these things. But if many people write—if you and your friends and neighbors and relatives and health club members write, perhaps the meat producers of this country will wake up to the fact that doping their animals is not really economical.

We have merely scratched the surface of all the things that are done to meat, for of course other processes are involved before the meat reaches your grocery store. You may well ask if it is really healthful to eat meat, considering all these outrages. Don't forget that similar things have been done to plants, too. Vegetables and fruits are subjected to hormone treatments, poison sprays, artificial fertilizers, various methods of breeding and forcing that are just as unnatural as the processes the meat goes through. So do not make the mistake of turning from chemicalized meat in disgust and eating nothing but chemicalized vegetables and fruits. For the meat contains much that will keep your body strong against the unhealthful things in your diet—the proteins and B vitamins of meat are necessary to protect you against the possible harm you may suffer from any or all of our modern chemicalized food.

Glance at the table below, which shows the vitamin and mineral content of the various meats. Note that the organ meats contain far, far more nutriments than the muscle meats. Make certain that you serve an organ meat at least once a week—oftener if possible. Get accustomed to using the less popular ones—kidneys, brains, sweetbreads, heart. There are many appetizing ways in which these can be served. They are economical and nutritious.

B Vitamins in Poultry and Meat

Milligrams per 100 grams (In general 100 grams equals an average serving)

	Thiamin	Riboflavin	Niacin	Pyridoxine	Panto-thenic acid	Biotin
Chicken	.90 - .150	.070-.260	8.6	.100	.550	.005-.009
Goose	.150	Good	3	?	?	?
Turkey	.120- .150	.190-.240	7.9	?	?	?
Duck	.360	.230	3	?	?	?
Beef	.100- .220	.120-.270	4.5	.077	.490	.002
Lamb	.80 - .210	.230-.266	5.9	.081	.600	.002
Pork	.90 -1.040	.040-.240	.9-4.4	.086-.270	?	?
Veal	.170- .180	.140-.280	3.1-6.5	.056-.130	.110-.260	.001

Mineral Content of Organ Meats

Milligrams per 100 grams

	Calcium	Phosphorus	Iron	Copper
Brains	8	380	2.3	0
Heart	10	236	6.2	0
Kidney	14	262	15.0	.11
Liver, beef	8	373	12.1	2.15
Liver, calf	11	205	5.4	4.41
Sweetbreads	14	596	1.6	0
Tongue	31	229	3.0	0

Vitamin Content of Organ Meats

Milligrams per 100 grams

	A	Thiamin	Ribo-flavin	Niacin	Inositol	Pyri-doxine	Panto-thenic acid[2]
Brains	0	.25	.26	6.0	200	?	
Heart	0	.54	.90	6.8	260	.120	1.8-3.6
Kidney (I.U.)	750	.45	1.95	7.4	0	4.0	2.0
Liver (I.U.)	19,200-53,000	.27	2.80	16.1	55	.170-.730	37.0
Pancreas	0	.320	.590	.584	?	?	4.4-7.6
Sweetbreads	0	.150	.550	3.3			?
Tongue	0	.15	.23	4.0		1.25	10.6
Tripe	0	.006	.12	.003			

	Biotin	Folic acid	Choline	Vit. C	Vit. D
Brains	.0074	.052	?	14	0
Heart	.0049	.130	?	14	0
Kidney (I.U.)	.92				
Liver (I.U.)	.096-.112	3.25-3.80	.380	31	15-45
Pancreas					
Sweetbreads				20	
Tongue	.003				

Menopause and Vitamin E

"The menopause, or climacteric, is another period when a lot of women take a beating. The elaborate machinery of fertility grinds to a stop, often like a streamliner, but sometimes like a freight train with loose couplings and dragging brakes. The secretion of hormones by the ovaries slows and stops, and estrogen production is taken over by the adrenal cortex." So say H. J. Berglund, M.D., and H. L. Nichols, Jr., in their book, *It's Not All in Your Mind,* published by North Castle Books, Greenwich, Connecticut.

Sometime, generally during the fifth or sixth decades of life, women experience what is known as the menopause. The word means literally a pause or stopping of the menstrual flow. In describing some of the symptoms of the menopause, John Bell Williams, D.D.S., writing in *Oral Hygiene,* for July, 1952, has this to say: . . . "While the process is normal it carries with it abnormal disturbances. Likewise these disturbances may be mild or they may be severe and distressing. . . . The so-called 'hot-flash,' as everyone knows, is the common symptom of this distressing period. It consists of a sudden flash of heat which covers the face and neck like a blush and even pervades the entire body. . . . Other disturbances attributed to the nervous system are palpitation of the heart and a feeling of fullness in the head. Also, the victims of these curious torments are in a constant state of fear. . . . Indeed it is only to be expected that the cessation of a powerful glandular secretion would be attended by extraordinary symptoms, but there are other factors that make the period extremely difficult."

He goes on to speak of the psychological difficulties many women have in adjusting to the changes brought by the menopause—chiefly, the fact that they cannot have any more children. "Simultaneously," says Dr. Williams, "wrinkles, double chins and gray hairs appear; hips, waistlines and other parts of the anatomy lose their youthful contour." Dr. Williams is speaking of the various difficulties of the menopause, for the benefit of his fellow-dentists. For, as he says, very often a woman plagued by all these symptoms visits her dentist and is told that, in addition, she must lose her teeth. He pleads for understanding and gentleness on the part of the dentist for, says he, the woman's symptoms are real—not imaginary—and she needs as much understanding and help as possible.

What actually happens during menopause is that ovulation ceases—that is, the ovaries no longer release the egg for possible fertilization. This means that menstruation (which occurs automatically in relation to ovulation) also ceases. Depending on the individual, it may cease gradually or it may stop suddenly without any preliminary warning. We have not been able to uncover any statistics about how prevalent among women are the very distressing symptoms of menopause but it appears that many women have little or no difficulty. Others may suffer from menopause difficulties for ten years or longer. And the health, mental or physical, of some women may be permanently impaired.

There are a lot of aspects to the whole problem, not the least of which is the psychological one. We want to cover these various aspects in this series of articles. First let us talk about the actual physical treatments given for menopause symptoms. The commonest present-day treatment is to give estrogens—the female sex hormone. You can see the reason for this. At the time of the menopause, the woman's body ceases producing this female sex hormone. It seems reasonable to suppose that the menopausal symptoms occur because the body is deprived of this hormone. So doctors give the hormone, in pills or injections. There are serious disadvantages to this kind of medication which we will discuss in another part of this book. Meanwhile, let us talk about another form of therapy which is being used by more and more doctors, because there are no uncomfortable or dangerous aftereffects—vitamin E therapy.

Examples From Medical Articles

Here are some sample (and these are only samples out of quite a considerable fund of material) of writings in medical journals on the effectiveness of vitamin E for menopausal symptoms. Dr. N. R. Kavinoky, writing in the *Annals of Western Medicine and Surgery,* volume 4, pages 27-32, 1950, describes the treatment of 92 patients with vitamin E in doses ranging from 10 to 25 milligrams daily. Thirty-seven of the patients complaining of hot flashes were relieved. Sixteen of those who suffered from backaches were relieved. Thirty-four subjects had had very heavy menstrual flow; in 16 the flow diminished.

Using vitamin E in doses of 50 to 100 milligrams daily, Dr. Kavinoky reports that even better results were obtained in another group of 79 patients. The treatment was very effective in relieving high blood pressure and muscle pains. Even fatigue and nervousness were reported by more than half the patients to be reduced. From 50 to 82 per cent reported relief from restless sleep and insomnia. In almost 100 per cent of the cases there was relief from dizziness, heart palpitations and shortness of breath. It took as long as two or three months in some cases to produce results, but in others it took only two weeks.

Dr. Gomez Haedo, writing in *Revista espanola de obstetricia y ginecologia,* volume 8, pages 421-8, 1949, tells us that he studied the effects of vitamin E for a period of a year on 27 women. He says that objectionable pains, irregularity, irritability and so forth were completely controlled by the vitamin E therapy. He also mentions the fact that certain disorders of the thyroid glands in these patients were apparently cured by the action of the vitamin E on the thyroid and other glands.

Dr. H. H. Cummings in the *Journal of the Michigan State Medical Society,* volume 47, page 1373, 1948, reports that in two years of vitamin E therapy he found it to be effective and free from undesirable aftereffects. W. H. Perloff, writing in the *American Journal of Obstetrics and Gynecology,* volume 58, pages 684-94, 1949, reports on the treatment of 200 women with vitamin E in doses of 75 to 150 milligrams daily. He claims that this therapy completely relieved the undesirable symptoms of 26.1 per cent. Another 26 per cent were improved. He believes that higher doses might well relieve some of the patients who did not respond to 150 milligrams. Once again we have the report that the vitamin E treatment produced no unpleasant aftereffects.

Dr. E. V. Shute of Canada is a pioneer physician in the use of vitamin E therapy for reproductive disorders. He and his brother are at present treating heart conditions with vitamin E and are the two outstanding specialists in this field today. Dr. Shute reported in *The Summary,* volume 2, pages 34-7, 1950, that vitamin E in doses of 30 to 75 milligrams daily decreased the intensity and severity of hot flashes and relieved the characteristic headaches of menopause. The skin conditions that are also typical of menopause (itching anus or vulva) were relieved by large doses of 300 to 5000 milligrams of vitamin E. In these cases he states that it is necessary to continue the treatment for some time, for no improvement may be noted for two to four weeks after beginning the therapy. Also, nine out of ten cases of *kraurosis vulvae* (dryness of the vulva) and *leukoplakia vulvae* (a whitening) were cured and remained so as long as treatment with vitamin E continued.

Dr. Pauline Harris, writing in the *Journal of the American Osteopathic Association,* volume 50, pages 586-8, 1951, says that she believes there is justification for the use of vitamin E for the circulatory disorders of the menopause. But she also believes that the therapy is in the experimental stage and she asks for a great deal more investigation to justify fully the use of vitamin E.

C. J. Christy in *The American Journal of Obstetrics and Gynecology,* volume 50, pages 84-7, 1945, reports on 25 patients to whom he gave from 10 to 30 milligrams of vitamin E daily for from one to six weeks. He says that the entire group benefitted and showed either complete relief or very marked improvement. He states that, since vitamin E has no possible cancer-causing aftereffects, it may be used freely in menopausal patients.

Further Proof of Vitamin E Effectiveness

M. P. Z. de Camara reports in the *Medical Woman's Journal,* volume 54, pages 43, 45, 1947, that she gave 150 to 200 milligrams of vitamin E daily to patients who had severe and prolonged bleeding from the uterus. In all cases the bleeding was stopped within three to six days. Then she says "A good diet was prescribed" and there was no recurrence of the hemorrhaging. Dr. H. E. Ferguson in the *Virginia Medical Monthly,* volume 75, pages 447-8, 1948, reports on 66 menopausal patients, 60 of whom were completely relieved of their symptoms when they received 15 to 30 milligrams of vitamin E per day. No objectionable side effects were noticed.

H. C. McLaren gave an average of 500 milligrams per day to a series of 47 menopausal patients over 37 days. Thirty of these patients found relief, according to an article in the *British Medical Journal,* volume 2, pages 1378-82, 1949. Of seventeen cases that were followed up, five remained cured, twelve had further hot flashes which were quickly controlled by more vitamin E. B. B. Rubenstein writing in the *Proceedings of the Federation of the American Society for Experimental Biology,* volume 7, page 106, 1948, states that he gave 75 milligrams per day of vitamin E to 17 patients with severe vascular disorders resulting from menopause. In 14 of these, marked reduction of the symptoms occurred. Only six obtained complete relief. Henry A. Gozan of New York tells us in the *New York State Journal of Medicine,* for May 15, 1952, that he treated 35 menopausal patients with 300 milligrams of vitamin E daily. He says "There was improvement in every symptom in some cases, but *pruritus vulvae* (itching vulva) was the only symptom which was improved in all cases. It was also noted that those cases which responded well did so in two to four weeks." He concludes by stating that vitamin E improved menopausal condition symptoms in slightly more than 50 per cent of the cases and that it is especially valuable in cases where estrogens absolutely cannot be used.

Using Vitamin E For Menopause

Do we need to go on—or do you have some idea now of the really significant contribution to medicine that has been made by the discovery that vitamin E will possibly bring relief in these most stubborn and unpleasant cases of menopausal disorders? You will notice that some doctors had more success than others. This is true, we suspect, with almost any kind of medicine. Even the administration of such things as insulin (which is taken so much for granted these days) must be very carefully worked out by the attending physician. In fact, there are some doctors who prefer not to give insulin at all and refer their diabetic patients to specialists.

You will note, too, that no two doctors we have mentioned gave the same dosage. It seems surprising that one patient could find relief from taking as little as 10 milligrams of vitamin E per day and another might be cured only with a dose as high as 300 or 500 milligrams. But this, too, is to be expected. Just as no two people eat exactly the same diet, so no two people have exactly the same physiology or symptoms. Undoubtedly many other factors, such as environment, income, emotional characteristics, past health and so forth are involved in the final outcome of what benefit is derived from the taking of any medicine.

But vitamin E is not exactly a medicine. Given in large doses, or injected, it is being used in the same way a drug is used, you might say. But it is actually something that occurs in food! And it seems likely that a woman who is getting ample vitamin E in her daily food may progress through the menopause without any unpleasant symptoms at all. Does it not seem plausible that most of the difficulties of modern women at the time of "Change of Life" may spring from many different factors in our modern lives, not the least of which is the fact that vitamin E has just about disappeared from our food?

Some researchers state that it has not as yet been proved that human beings need vitamin E. But we know that animals need it and it is included in one form or another in practically all commercial animal food, all the way from dog and cat food to food for cattle.

We know that vitamin E is being used successfully to treat heart and vascular disorders. Medical literature also includes ample mention of it in relation to disorders of the muscles, the joints, the liver, the kidneys and glands. We know that it is effective in reducing abortions and premature births in human pregnancies.

What application can we make of all these medical facts in relation to good health and the prevention of menopausal disorders? First, certainly, is to make sure that we are getting as much vitamin E as possible in daily meals. Vitamin E is most abundant in the following foods:

(These figures are from an article by P. Harris, M. L. Quaife and W. J. Swanson in the *Journal of Nutrition,* volume 40, page 367, 1950):

Vitamin E (Alpha Tocopherol) Present in Foods

Milligrams	*Food*
.72	1 medium apple
.44	12 slices of bacon
.37	1 medium banana
.10	1 cup steamed navy beans
.47	1 serving beef steak
1.40	1 serving of beef liver
.45	1 cup carrots
.46	1 cup diced celery
.21	1 serving roast chicken
3.60	about 6 tablespoons cocoanut oil
.84	about 1 cup cornmeal
7.	about 6 tablespoons corn oil

Milligrams	*Food*
56.	about 6 tablespoons cottonseed oil
1.16	1 whole egg
.25	¼ medium grapefruit
.35	1 serving haddock
.62	2 rib lamb chops
.29	6 large lettuce leaves
1.94	¼ cup uncooked oatmeal
.21	1 large raw onion
.23	1 small orange
11.	about 6 tablespoons of peanut oil
.10	1 cup steamed peas
4.0	1 small sweet potato
.63	1 serving pork chops
1.20	¾ cup cooked rice (brown)
10.	1 small tomato
2.24	½ cup steamed turnip greens

Secondly, it seems to us that all of us should be taking vitamin E and/or wheat germ as food supplements. Wheat germ, rich in vitamin E, also contains many other food elements, some of them undiscovered as yet, which contribute greatly to health. It is nothing more or less than the oil pressed from the germ or living part of the wheat berry. It is present in freshly-ground, whole meal flour. So if you are making your own whole wheat bread you are getting a certain amount of wheat germ and vitamin E.

How Much To Take

The Shute Brothers, pioneers in vitamin E history, have this to say about how much vitamin E can or should be part of one's daily food supplementation:

"What we tell patients is that in the large doses we use for the treatment of heart disease, there can be danger under two circumstances (1) if there is hypertension (elevation of blood pressure) present and (2) if the patient has had rheumatic fever and has had heart damage as a result, particularly if he is close to or in heart failure. We tell patients that, if these two dangers are not present, they can safely take any dose whatever of vitamin E. Certainly there are no people who cannot take 50 milligrams of vitamin E a day safely. There are virtually no people who cannot take 100 milligrams safely, unless a third condition exists, namely an allergy. When the dose gets above that level, there is danger in using it in a blanket fashion. Fifty to 100 years ago the average person probably ate about 35 milligrams of vitamin E a day. Now with increasing deficiency, it may take a large dose to prevent trouble."

If you are approaching the age of menopause, we would suggest that you watch your diet carefully and check on the amount of vitamin E you get daily from meals. Then we suggest that you take vitamin E and/or wheat germ oil, as a food supplement. You will notice that one of the physicians we have mentioned in this article, Dr. de Camara, relates that she prescribed "a good diet" for her patients who were treated successfully with vitamin E. Undoubtedly a good all-'round diet, with plenty of the other vitamins and minerals, will be a great help in preventing symptoms of menopausal disorder, along with vitamin E. If you are already experiencing some of the uncomfortable and alarming symptoms of menopause, suggest to your doctor that he give you vitamin E, especially if you are taking estrogens and having distressing aftereffects. It has been shown beyond a doubt that vitamin E given for menopause does not produce any disagreeable or dangerous side-effects.

Menopause and Good Nutrition

In the preceding article we discussed the relation of vitamin E to menopause symptoms, and showed that many researchers have had excellent results in treating menopause symptoms with vitamin E. This is not surprising since it appears to us that most of us must be deficient in vitamin E, for it has practically disappeared from our food supply, with the refining of grains and the processing of grain and vegetable oils.

It seems that there are other vitamins whose lack may predispose to uncomfortable, unpleasant or downright dangerous menopausal symptoms. The first article we found indicated that vitamin D may be powerful against menopausal symptoms. Nathan Freedman, M.Sc., M.D., of Montreal, writing in the *American Journal of Obstetrics and Gynecology* for December, 1951, tells us of an experiment in which 27 women were given massive doses of vitamin D and tests were then made to determine the effect on their physiology and on their "subjective symptoms"—that is, those disorders that the patient must describe to the doctor, like headache. In the tests performed, these patients were tested for estrogen which is the female hormone that disappears gradually during the menopause. It is believed that the loss of the activity of this hormone may be responsible for many of the unpleasant symptoms of menopause—hot flashes, headaches, irritability, nervousness, loss of appetite, dizziness and so forth.

The women who were given vitamin D ranged in age from 39 to 68 years. They were given massive doses of the vitamin—far, far higher doses than any of us should take unless it is under the supervision of a physician, for vitamin D can be toxic in doses that are too high. Thirty-seven different tests were then done on these women of which 22 were positive for estrogen. The symptoms of which the patients were complaining were also improved in many cases. Hot flashes were relieved in 18 out of the 27 women. All who suffered from rheumatic pains found relief. Altogether the record shows the following cases of improvement or complete relief: excessive perspiration—3, dizziness—2, nervousness—2, headaches—1, weakness—3, drowsiness—2, and rheumatic pains—12. It is interesting to note, too, that the vaginal tissue of the patients was greatly improved, even in those cases where the women had had their ovaries removed. So it appears that vitamin D works on the tissues whether or not the reproductive system is functioning or has been partially removed.

Oral Health During Menopause

A provocative disclosure about the possible deficiency of another vitamin in menopause patients comes to us from the pages of *Oral Surgery* for October, 1951. Written by Dr. Maury Massler of the University of Illinois, this article describes, for the dental surgeons who read it, the onset of menopause and the typical disorders that may result. It then discusses the oral symptoms that were observed in 86 women who were passing through some stage of menopause. It is well to keep in mind the great importance of the tissues of the mouth and throat as indicators of vitamin deficiency. Some vitamin deficiency states are detected first or perhaps solely because of certain conditions in the mouth, lips, gums and throat.

Many of these patients had been referred to Dr. Massler because they complained of ill-fitting dentures or bridges. Although apparently their dentists had done an excellent job and mechanically the dentures were perfect, yet the women declared their mouths burned, they had abnormal taste sensations, their meals didn't taste like they used to, they had chronic canker sores, gingivitis (gum disease) or some other symptom which to them indicated that the denture, or possibly even the fillings in their teeth were faulty.

Eighty of the patients suffered from burning mouth, the burning sensation being concentrated either on the tongue, the mouth tissues or the gums. Sixty-two suffered from abnormal taste sensations. Seventy-seven had a rabid fear of cancer which doctors call *cancerophobia.* It is understandable, of course, that they would worry about mouth-cancer, considering the symptoms they had and the fact that cancer becomes more frequent after middle age. But burning sensations, inflammation of the tongue and the gums may indicate vitamin deficiency. So Dr. Massler treated the patients with vitamin B therapy. In some cases he administered hormones as well. In about one-third of the cases the patients responded quickly and dramatically to the vitamin therapy. Two-thirds responded slowly or not at all. A second group responded only when hormones and vitamins both were given.

Dr. Massler says that it is fairly obvious that the majority of post-menopausal women suffer from a distinct vitamin B complex deficiency. Biskind showed that an intimate relationship exists between the vitamin B complex and the hormones of the body. Dietary neglect and peculiar dietary habits during the menopause may lead directly to malnutrition. Vitamin B deficiency itself leads to fatigue, mental aberrations, deterioration of personality, decreased libido and premature aging.

He also tells us that in every case, previously rejected dentures became acceptable and burning sensations disappeared. And the patient experienced marked improvement in general health and well-being. There was a marked increase in vitality, cheerfulness and the disappearance of neurotic complaints.

Now if, as Dr. Massler says (and we believe him) the majority of post-menopausal women suffer from a vitamin B deficiency, why do you suppose it is not regulation practice to give vitamin B to menopausal patients automatically, just in case it may relieve symptoms? Especially since the vitamin B complex has been found to be closely related to the production of hormones by the body, you would think that prescribing vitamin B as a preventive measure would be first on the doctor's list of recommendations!

In the next article we shall discuss a further investigation of vitamin B deficiency in middle-aged women, which may bring about some of the menopause symptoms.

Menopause and Vitamin B

The final medical article that we studied on the subject of nutrition and menopause dealt with vitamin B. This article appears to us so important that we wanted to print it in its entirety except of course that much of it is written in highly technical language. J. E. Ayre of the Royal Victoria Hospital of Montreal, tells us in this article in the *American Journal of Obstetrics and Gynecology,* volume 54, 1947 that he believes he may have found a clue to the formation of all cancers. And his theory sounds reasonable to us.

It concerns one hundred patients, fifty of whom had cancer of the cervix and fifty of whom were normal individuals used as controls. Dr. Ayre discovered that there was an abnormally high concentration of estrogen (the female sex hormone) in the cervices of the women with cancer. The research he had done indicated that in laboratory animals the estrogen will concentrate and fix itself in inflamed tissues. This suggests, he says, that women who have experienced some degree of inflammation in the cervix may have high concentrations of estrogen there. He found indeed in 125 cases, 87 per cent showed higher concentrations of estrogen in the cervix than in the vagina. He also reveals the amazing fact that "probably all parous cervices (that is, the cervices of women who have had one or more children) and many nulliparous cervices (that is, those of women who have not had children) have been subjected to some degree of cervicitis at some time during sex life and some residual disease doubtless remains in the glands as a chronic cervicitis." In other words, practically all women have at one time or another suffered from inflammation of the cervix. If excessive estrogen has concentrated there, the predisposition to cancer may be great.

Now Dr. Ayre discusses three patients who came to him with severe menopause or menstrual disorders—one of them only 14 years old, the others 29 and 64. In every case he tested for thiamin deficiency and found them all deficient. Liver tests showed that their livers were not functioning properly. Checking back on the diets of the patients, he found, sure enough, that there was every reason for them to be deficient in thiamin, since their diets had included little of this important vitamin. And in one case, the consumption of large amounts of alcohol had robbed the body of what little thiamin was present in the food.

Vitamin B Deficiency Leads to Over-Production of Estrogen

He tells us further that Biskind and Biskind report that vitamin B deficiency interferes with estrone inactivation in the liver of female rats. While these animals were fed a normal diet, no "heat" developed. When the diet was changed to one totally deficient in vitamin B complex, it was observed that, within two weeks on this diet, irregular "heats" began to occur. This was interpreted as indicating that the estrone was not being completely inactivated, and after three weeks on this diet, the rats remained in a state of constant "heat."

What we seem to have here is another of those infinitely complicated nutritional matters which demonstrates just how little we really know about how our bodies function. The liver is involved in regulating the production of the female sex hormone. So long as the diet is adequate and the liver is functioning properly this mechanism flows smoothly enough and all is well. But when the diet is deficient in vitamin B (of which thiamin is an important part) the liver is unable to regulate the production of this hormone and too much of it circulates in the body. As Dr. Ayre has pointed out, it may be attracted to parts where there is or has been inflammation, and may collect there. It is generally accepted among researchers that an excess of the female sex hormone may produce cancer. So it appears that, indirectly, the lack of vitamin B may be the cause of the cancer.

Dr. Ayre says that it seems remarkable that deficiency would occur irrespective of the economic status of the patient. Gynecologists have long believed that dietetics were not directly concerned with the production of pelvic diseases and the need for vitamins in particular was generally over-stressed. It would seem logical that the average person with a normal appetite for the various staple foods would not develop a deficiency. A study of the way thiamin is used by the body reveals evidence to indicate that this substance would appear to be particularly vulnerable to intermittent or chronic depletion without gross deficiency in the diet as a whole. A daily intake of thiamin is necessary and the organism absorbs only enough for the immediate needs. The excess is destroyed or excreted. More is required when a high carbohydrate diet is taken or when alcohol is imbibed. A vicious cycle may develop as loss of appetite and constipation frequently develop in the presence of even a mild deficiency. Therefore, the more persistent the lack of appetite, the more chronic the deficiency becomes.

As readers know, we have presented much evidence showing that vitamin B deficiency is widespread in our country, even among people whose income and education would seem to guarantee that they would eat a good diet. Refining of foods and transporting foods over long distances, then storing them before they are available for our tables practically assures us that our meals will be deficient in the B vitamins. Add to this the alcohol, the tobacco smoke and the hundreds of other poisons that rob our bodies of B vitamins and you can easily understand why Dr. Ayre found that, of his 50 cancer patients, *86 per cent were deficient in thiamin*. Of his perfectly normal controls only 10 per cent showed thiamin deficiency.

We Need Not Have Vitamin B Deficiency

"It must be remembered," he says, "that the cases we have analyzed have not been starvation victims, but rather mild, probably chronic deficients." Then he says, "It has long been recognized that chronic irritation is a contributing factor leading to the development of many types of cancer. It is accepted knowledge that infection alone will not produce a malignant growth without the addition of other unknown factors. It would appear that both nutrition and estrogen have a role to play . . . May it not be that in all cancers there are two essential combinations of forces? First a general body metabolic disorder characterized by a nutritional deficiency, possibly liver changes and resultant hormonal changes. This metabolic disorder may exist with variable intensity and chronicity for years without producing cancer. Ultimately the second factor is added to the picture, namely the focalizing factor of any chronic damaging or irritating condition which provokes growth response. Whether due to infection or inflammation or damage, an aberrant type of growth response results, varying in character with variation in force, intensity and chronicity of the particular carcinogenic (cancer-causing) factors which influence that particular organ. It may be then that the blow to the breast, which the patient recalls, is of more than coincidental significance. While it may prove harmless in the presence of a normal nutritional and hormonal balance, in the presence of the abnormal metabolic status, the resultant healing growth-reaction may result in growth of a malignant character."

Finally it is noteworthy that after Dr. Ayre gave thiamin to these patients, there was a definite change for the better in liver function within 10 days. In the cancer cases, he says, regardless of how far advanced they might be, there was improvement in appearance and appetite, some of the patients gaining as much as 20 to 30 pounds in weight. He also reminds us that patients who have been receiving vitamin B therapy are much less likely to be injured by x-ray or radium treatment.

Let us add vitamin B (as in brewer's yeast or desiccated liver) to our diet in order to avoid the disorders of menopause and the fear of cancer that, understandably, begins to gnaw away at so many of us at this time of life. We do not know how many other physicians or dental researchers have reported vitamin B deficiency in their menopause patients. Undoubtedly a search through medical literature would reveal a great many more. There is no need for us to sit back and bewail the fact that many physicians do not prescribe vitamin B for their menopause patients. Vitamin B is a food element, not a drug. We should be getting enough of it every day in our daily meals. But it is perfectly apparent that we are not. Let us therefore remedy this situation at once by seeing to it that we get more and more of this tremendously important vitamin. There is no possibility of getting too much of vitamin B from a natural food source. Every day your body excretes what it does not use.

Vitamin B occurs most abundantly in liver, eggs, fresh, raw, leafy vegetables, milk, meats, legumes and whole grain cereals. It has been removed from refined cereals. The easiest and most economical way to make certain you are getting enough vitamin B is to take desiccated liver or brewer's yeast—in tablets or in the powdered form which can be sprinkled over food.

Menopause and Hormones

"The fortress of the human personality is under assault from the cradle to the grave; in childhood, feelings of relative insignificance; in adolescence, doubts of capacity to face impending responsibilities; in adulthood, all the slings and arrows of outrageous fortune in both the material and spiritual fields." So says S. G. Sandes of Sydney, Australia in an article published in the February 20, 1954 issue of the *Medical Journal of Australia.* He is speaking of the psychological difficulties that may accompany the menopause and he draws attention later on to the fact that menopause is actually a kind of reversal of adolescence. Just as we must try to understand and sympathize with the oftimes dismaying characteristics of adolescence, when reproductive life is beginning, so must we be understanding and sympathetic for the symptoms of menopause, when reproductive life is ending.

"The menopause is the signpost that foreshadows many a threat to the female ego," says Dr. Sandes. "To all it means the loss of reproductive power and thus the loss of woman's main biological purpose, and life without some purpose is nothing. To the spinster it marks the point of no return, and the final abandonment of her hopes of motherhood. To the mother it frequently coincides with a period when dependent children grow up and leave the home and no longer require maternal care. Husband or contemporaries and friends may die, and new friends are harder to make, whilst any economic difficulties become harder to combat. In addition, when emotional control is unstable, guilt feelings experienced earlier in life may be reactivated and add their depressive quota of attacks upon the ego."

In the medical literature about the psychological aspects of menopause, we find wide difference of opinion. Some physicians tend to believe that most symptoms are imaginary and are purely the result of the shock to feminine vanity. Others contend that the physical changes that take place in menopause have a great deal to do with causing the frame of mind. We are inclined to go along with this idea. The female sex hormone, estrogen, ceases to be produced when menopause begins. All hormones are powerful substances which have far-reaching effects on nerves, glands, and so forth. It seems quite reasonable that when the supply of sex hormone ceases, either suddenly or over a period of time, a wide variety of symptoms, both physical and psychological, would ensue.

According to some estimates, about 80 per cent of all women may have unpleasant symptoms at the time of menopause, but only about 10 per cent of these have severe symptoms. Judging from their own literature, physicians have a tendency to ascribe any and all symptoms in any woman past the age of 35 as being due to menopause. If she is 35 or so, they tell her it is an early menopause. If she is sixty or over, her symptoms are described as post-menopausal. Needless to say, the medical journals deplore this tendency and urge meticulous examinations to pin down the symptoms, be they menopause or something else.

The Use of Hormones for Menopause

In general, it is the practice these days to give hormones for menopause difficulties. The reasoning is that, since the symptoms arise because the natural female hormones are decreasing, giving hormones will prevent the symptoms, because they will take the place of the natural ones. Well and good. But the gradual decrease in the production of sex hormones is a perfectly natural process and the body must eventually adjust to it. If hormones are given by the doctor, will it not simply postpone the time when the body must adjust to doing without? And is it not possible that many women will not be able to stop taking hormones without causing all their symptoms to appear again?

J. M. Habel, Jr. writes in the *Virginia Medical Monthly* for October, 1948, that the excessive or prolonged use of hormones will often cause prolongation of readjustment. He tells us that most of the symptoms of menopause are thought to arise not from a lack of female hormones, but from a surplus of hormones put out by the pituitary gland because of the lack of sex hormones. So, he says, "the long-continued use of estrogenic substances only tends to retard the readjustment to the lack of estrogenic substances." He also tells us that he believes the long-continued use is more dangerous than large doses for a short period of time. He suggests giving vitamin B to any and all patients who are taking hormone preparations.

Speaking quite frankly to his fellow-physicians, Dr. Habel says further that only a small percentage of women going through the menopause will need any therapy. Too many doctors, especially during the years when they did not have time to examine patients carefully, have been prompted to label every ailment a woman has between the ages of 35 and 50 as due to the menopause. Their symptoms were due to "change of life," doctors say, and, as a great many listen to their friends explain their symptoms as due to menopause, they would accept the diagnosis. Then, the patient is given numerous injections of estrogenic substances and, in most cases, it is given by the nurse, the patient not seeing the doctor again for a long period of time. "Another factor which may cause this long-continued course of estrogen is financial," says Dr. Habel, "I have often heard physicians say that their office expenses were paid by injections of estrogenic hormones given by their nurses. If most of these patients had been adequately examined, they would have been found to have something entirely different from the menopause." Dr. Habel titles his article "Indiscriminate Use of Estrogens in the Menopause." And we begin to understand what he means by that.

The Dangers of Hormone Medication

There is considerable evidence that the administration of sex hormones can cause cancer in women who are predisposed to it. Dr. Habel refers to an earlier article by Ayre which showed definitely a relation between nutritional deficiency, too much estrogen and inflammation as possible causes of cancer. We discussed this information in our last article on menopause.

There is one aspect of the taking of hormones that is exceedingly important. Considering their potency, it becomes obvious that just about the most dangerous thing anyone could do is to try to treat herself with hormone preparations. Yet these powerful substances are available at drugstores. They are sold through the mail. Even though articles in current magazines warn of their dangers, how many women are at present dosing themselves with synthetic hormone preparations for real or imagined menopause symptoms?

In addition, since menopause is a perfectly natural result of becoming middle-aged, does it not seem foolish to keep administering sex hormones after the body has stopped making them? Wouldn't it seem just as logical in the case of a young girl who had trouble with menstruation, to give her some anti-hormone preparation which would keep her from developing into a woman? We suppose there are cases of such severe menopause symptoms that a course of hormone injections is necessary to preserve health. But, it seems to us that a woman in good health, eating an adequate diet, need have no dread of menopause, any more than the healthy adolescent needs to fear the onset of menstruation.

Of course the mental point of view involved in the two experiences is exactly opposite and perhaps that is the crux of the matter. The young girl is at the beginning of life, full of hope and youth and beauty. The middle-aged woman is at the end of a certain period of her life—perhaps the most pleasant and satisfying period. But surely there is no need to face what is ahead with panic or terror. The menopause, while it ends reproductive life, does not affect the woman's enjoyment of sex life.

While the menopause may mean the beginning of wrinkles, gray hair and "middle-aged spread" for some women, it need not, if one eats and lives properly. A diet rich in protein, vitamins and minerals and completely devoid of the starchy concoctions made of white refined flour and sugar will keep anyone looking young and slim, almost indefinitely.

Dr. Chapman whom we quoted earlier suggests the following in the way of diet: attention to the health of the reproductive tract which means plenty of vitamins C and D in the diet, reduction of overweight if it is present, a high protein diet which means of course a diet relatively low in carbohydrates and fats, as little salt as possible, for salt causes water to collect in the body tissues. We, of course, would add vitamin E and wheat germ oil, both so important for the health of the reproductive tract, bone meal for steadying and calming the nerves, the B vitamins in a natural food supplement such as brewer's yeast or desiccated liver, and vitamin A in fish liver oil because vitamin A has been found so effective in preventing the ravages of old age.

The final recommendation made in all the literature about menopause is "keep the patient busy." At a time when her children no longer need her constant attention, many a mother finds herself sitting at home with little to do or think about. So, understandably she worries about her own condition. On the other hand, many women find that this is the time of life when they can enjoy themselves most. Up to now they have been too busy to engage in all the many activities that have beckoned. But now, at last they have time for all the things they have always wanted to do—gardening, music, art, painting, craftwork, club work, flower arrangement, embroidery, travel—the world is full of hundreds of activities to investigate and new skills to learn. For the healthy woman this can be the pleasantest and most rewarding time of life.

Menstruation

"The bleeding phase of the menstrual cycle rarely appears unannounced. Signs and symptoms that herald its approach are experienced by many women. Anxiety states, depression, lower-abdominal pain, thirst, breast fullness and personality changes of a mildly anti-social nature announce the approaching condition," say two researchers writing in the *New England Journal of Medicine* for September 20, 1951. They go on to tell us that these symptoms are accepted philosophically by most women but a minority group of perhaps twenty-five per cent (which, incidentally, we think is a rather large minority group) require medication. Hippocrates believed that premenstrual symptoms were caused by "agitated blood" seeking to escape through the uterus. Police records of Paris show that there is a striking increase in criminal acts of women during their premenstrual period.

Other medical writers give different estimates of the number of women who suffer uncomfortable symptoms at the time of menstruation. Dr. S. Leon Israel writing in the *American Practitioner* for October, 1951, states that two-thirds of all normal women suffer to some degree from premenstrual symptoms. He lists them as fatigue, irritation, backache, fullness of the breasts, and a vague sensation of pelvic discomfort. It is difficult to assess the amount of discomfort, says Dr. Israel, because every individual's ability to bear pain is different and many personality factors are involved as well. Not the least of these is the aspect of anticipation. One fairly painful menstrual week will cause almost anyone to expect discomfort when the cycle swings around to the next period and this very anticipation may well increase the discomfort. Also, says Dr. Israel, disorders of menstruation usually occur in asthenic childless women who have a low threshold for pain.

The Physiology of Menstruation

What is menstruation and why should any distress be connected with it? In the woman's reproductive cycle, ovulation consists of the ripening or maturing of an egg in one of the two ovaries. This egg is detached from the ovary and proceeds down the tubes that connect to the uterus. If the egg is fertilized by a male sperm cell, it remains in the uterus and grows into an embryo child. Meanwhile, the lining of the uterus is preparing for a possible fertilized egg. It becomes thick and many other changes take place in it. If the egg is not fertilized, and no pregnancy is to take place, the lining of the uterus sloughs away and becomes the bloody discharge we know as menstruation.

Menstruation occurs on an average of every 28 days. This differs, of course, in individuals. Some completely healthy women menstruate every twenty-one days, some only four times a year. Thirteen is the average age at which menstruation begins. This too is variable. There are cases on record where the beginning of menstruation (the menarche) was delayed until the age of 17 or 18. When the cycle begins there may be considerable irregularity before it is established. This is nothing to worry about. Then, too, a great change in environment or kind of work may cause menstruation to stop temporarily. Girls going away to college, women moving to an entirely different climate should not become concerned if they experience considerable irregularity in menstruation.

What causes menstruation? We do not know. Says Dr. G. W. Theobald in *The Medical Press* for January 23, 1952, "We are only beginning to comprehend dimly the profound, complex and rapidly varying physicochemical changes which are associated with the menstrual cycle, which are evinced by such easily measurable factors as changes in temperature and in basal metabolism and blood sedimentation rate." We do know that hormones are chiefly responsible for the series of events that takes place—ovulation, menstruation or pregnancy, then ovulation once again. The sex hormones, progesterone and estrogen, are involved, the pituitary hormone and the thyroid hormone appear to have a great deal to do with the whole process, too. So it seems that all-round good health would be the best guarantee against menstrual distress.

The young girl, menstruating for the first time as she passes through adolescence is, in our culture, a law unto herself. Given to dreaming or stormy weeping, giggling or completely unreasonable fits of depression, she has been immortalized in literature as the eternally incomprehensible adolescent. But in other cultures this is not necessarily so. We are told that in Samoa the young girl passes through the most uneventful and serene period of her life during adolescence. There is none of the turmoil and stress that we associate with this age group. So perhaps some of the storminess of modern American adolescence is due to upbringing. We are also tempted to wonder how much our modern diet has to do with it.

Loss of Iron May Cause Anemia

What is the normal menstrual flow and what is its significance? It is difficult of course to get any exact idea of the amount of blood lost but it is generally assumed to be somewhere in the neighborhood of 50 to 100 grams. Dr. Theobald says, "It is truly surprising how much blood a woman can lose month after month over a period of years without becoming anemic, but sooner or later her powers of regenerating blood become exhausted and severe anemia may ensue with dramatic suddenness."

Some nutritionists believe that many women have an excessive flow of blood for many years without ever knowing it. Figures given out by the Red Cross at blood donor stations indicate that a big percentage of American women are too anemic to give blood safely. This is one of the reasons why women must pay very special attention to diet, whether or not they have children. The drain of losing blood (perhaps excessively) every month will certainly result in anemia unless the diet is very carefully chosen. Iron is the single most important mineral for preventing anemia.

Whole grain cereals are a rich source of iron. But it is removed in the refining process. Leafy green vegetables contain considerable iron. Liver is the richest source of all. Assimilation of iron is a whole story in itself for the body must have ample vitamins A and C and copper, for proper assimilation of iron. There must be plenty of hydrochloric acid in the stomach for absorption of iron—this means plenty of vitamin B in the diet. Diarrhea or taking laxatives can interfere seriously with the assimilation of iron.

Let's see if a good diet is related to menstrual disorders other than excessive loss of iron. Dr. Alexander Pou of Uruguary writing in the *American Journal of Obstetrics and Gynecology* for June 1951, tells of giving large doses of vitamin A to 24 patients, with very considerable improvement in their premenstrual symptoms. In 13 patients the results were very good, the most remarkable being the relief of breast tenderness. In four others, all symptoms were partially relieved and all breast tenderness was eliminated. Three more noticed considerable improvement but still had some distress. And the final four patients did not respond to the vitamin.

Restricting Fluids and Salt May Help

Dr. Bickers whom we quoted above has quite a different idea as to the main cause of premenstrual discomfort. It is caused by retention of fluids, he says, and he tells us that it is not unusual for women to gain as much as seven pounds during the premenstrual days. The hormone activity that goes on during this time appears to cause retention of water. We know, of course, that sodium in the diet also tends to cause water retention. So Dr. Bickers advises giving a drug which will cause sodium to be excreted from the body. Of course the more obvious procedure for us to follow is to stop eating salt which is the main source of sodium in our diets. Other researchers have found that a salt-poor diet during the days before menstruation does much to ease the bloating that frequently takes place.

In *Bridges' Dietetics for the Clinician* (Lea and Febiger) we read that lack of vitamin A has something to do with the storage of water in tissues, so getting enough vitamin A may help in preventing this source of distress in menstruation. We know that deficiency in vitamin A is widespread in this country. We also learn from *Bridges'* that there is a "diminished tolerance" for carbohydrates during menstruation. So the diet recommended here is high in protein and vitamins, fairly low in carbohydrates, low in fats and low in salt, with a limited amount of water. The suggestion is made to take 5,000 to 10,000 units of vitamin A daily in concentrated form, such as fish liver oils.

Calcium in Bone Meal is Important, Especially during Adolescence

Adelle Davis in her book *Let's Eat Right to Keep Fit* (Harcourt Brace and Co.) gives another sound reason why lack of vitamin A may contribute to unhealthy menstruation. Vitamin A is necessary for the health of the tissues. When not enough of it is present, dead cells may accumulate in the tissues of the reproductive system and cause profuse menstruation. She goes on to remind us that vitamin E too is an absolute essential for the health of the reproductive tract. In animals deficient in vitamin E the entire reproductive cycle may stop, only to start again normally when vitamin E is added to the diet.

Calcium is another food element involved somehow in all the various changes that take place during menstruation. The calcium level of the blood falls during the week prior to menstruation. This may very well be the reason, we believe, for irritability and nervousness, for calcium-lack always brings jittery nerves. When menstruation begins, the calcium level of the blood may fall still farther, resulting in "cramps"—the regular accompaniment of menstruation in countless women. During adolescence cramps are especially distressing and this may be because the growing body of the adolescent is already making heavy demands on her supply of calcium. Menstruation increases the demand and muscle cramps—the sure indication of calcium lack—result.

In this connection it is interesting to note a paragraph in *Bridges' Dietetics for the Clinician.* We are told that canker sores often accompany menstruation, just before and on the first days of flow. It seems that bone meal will do away with these pesky things within 48 hours. Says Dr. Johnson, who writes this article, take 15 grain tablets of bone phosphate twice daily. This is, of course, bone meal. He has also gotten excellent results using half dicalcium phosphate and half bone phosphate. We know of course that calcium makes up the largest part of bone. Could lack of calcium be the cause of all canker sores, we wonder? Would any readers like to experiment? Next time a canker sore appears, increase your daily ration of bone meal to approximately 30 grains and see whether you can do away with the canker sores.

Are there psychological reasons for menstrual distress? We believe there are, but we are inclined to believe they are less important than most doctors would have us believe. Fear of pregnancy can result in menstrual irregularity. Severe emotional strains can bring on menstrual pain and depression. Unhappy conditions at home, at work or at school make the situation worse. But, generally speaking, women who are well nourished can take these things in their stride. We noticed all through our research on menstruation that difficulties in this field are usually encountered in women who are "asthenic"—weak, sickly, nervous, without much endurance. Now people don't become asthenic because they want to. In at least nine cases out of ten, and maybe even that tenth one too, you can change asthenia into robust, bouncing good health with a good diet.

Consider the diet most of our adolescent girls eat today. They are fearful of putting on weight, but the attractions of the chocolate sundae and the bottle of coke are strong. So after they have indulged they cut down on other foods—healthful foods. Butter is fattening, they think. Their cereals and sandwiches are refined. The amount of fresh fruit and raw vegetables they eat is sometimes non-existent. Where can they get the calcium, the iron, the vitamins A, C and E that are necessary for regular painless menstruation? And their mothers, who have been eating this kind of diet for perhaps twenty or thirty years, can expect not only to have difficulty with menstruation, but with menopause, as well, when that time comes.

To summarize: Menstruation, like other normal body functions, seems to go along smoothly and naturally without undue distress in those women whose bodies are healthy. Here are the nutriments that seem to be specifically most involved in the mechanism of menstruation: Iron (available in liver and other organ meats, leafy vegetables, egg yolk). Vitamins A and C (available in fresh raw fruits and vegetables, fish, liver oil and rose hips), vitamin E (in whole grains, but lost in the refining), calcium (bone meal as a food supplement is your surest source). It boils down actually to a good diet—the kind of diet we are recommending all the time in these pages. And finally, for those who wish to avoid much of the distress of menstruation, why not begin to get along with much less salt? Reduce your salt intake gradually over a period of several months until you are finally adding no salt in cooking or at the table. Perhaps this will do away with much of the feeling of heaviness and discomfort.

Mental Health and Vitamins and Minerals

Mental illness! What dread the very words bring! Mental patients are at present so numerous that they fill more than half of our hospital beds. Not one of us can honestly say that mental illness has not struck close—someone in his immediate family or circle of friends. As readers know, we believe that today's impoverished diet has much to do with mental disease. Editor Rodale's book *Whither Mentality* (Rodale Press, $1.00) discusses evidence that we have uncovered showing the relationship between increasing mental disability and a diet that gets worse every year as we introduce more and more synthetics into food and, by our methods of farming, deplete the farmer's produce of more and more trace minerals.

Always on the lookout for more material on this subject, we were gratified to find the other day an article in the *Journal of Psychology* for October, 1954, describing the experiments done by two members of the faculty at the University of Southern California and the University of California. George Watson and Andrew L. Comrey stated the problem they hoped to throw some light on by saying that most people believe that mental illness is not subject to physical treatment. They think it must be treated by a psychotherapist. For, since it has to do with the mind and the personality, it seems that conversation and persuasion by trained therapists should be curative. On the other hand, say our two authors, we know perfectly well that mental illness can be produced by semi-starvation and we know that patients suffering from pellagra have serious mental derangement. Pellagra is a disease that comes from deficiency of the B vitamins.

None of the patients in this experiment was suffering from starvation. They all had what is known as "an adequate diet"—that is, the kind of diet many Americans eat all the time. So the experimenters were not trying to feed these folks *more* food, or to increase the amount of calories they were getting. Instead they wanted to improve the quality of the food —to put in large amounts of all the vitamins, minerals and amino acids that are known to be necessary for good health.

They used a food supplement that contained 54 of these food elements: vitamin A, vitamin D, the B vitamins, vitamin E, vitamin K, unsaturated fatty acids (vitamin F) lecithin, rutin, the trace minerals such as copper, zinc, fluorine (from bone meal, incidentally) yeast, liver, bone marrow and so forth. They included in the formula all the food elements that have been shown to be necessary to human nutrition along with the parts of food in which they appear, such as alfalfa, kelp, watercress and so forth.

They divided the patients into two groups. One group got the dietary supplement, the other group got a pill that looked the same but did not contain anything of food value. Of the eleven patients who got the *imitation* pills nine showed no improvement, one improved for two months and then suffered a relapse and one believed she felt better. It was expected incidentally that some of the patients would feel better by suggestion. Of course none of the patients knew who was getting the real pills and who was getting the fake ones.

Improvement in Mental Symptoms

Of the 32 patients who took the pills containing all the vitamins and minerals there was what the doctors call "marked clinical improvement" in 13. Fifteen other patients showed moderate improvement. In the personality test that was given, the patients getting the vitamins showed a gain of 22 points, while those who got no added vitamins showed an improvement of only 1 point.

What do we mean by "improvement"? Here are some case histories that will show you what we mean. One woman of 75 had been confined to her bed for two years, was severely depressed, suffered from uncontrollable weeping, hallucinations and extreme mental confusion. After only one month's treatment she was able to leave her bed for breakfast and took up gardening. Her mental confusion, depression and hallucinations all departed.

Another case is that of a boy of 18. He had had encephalitis and could not go to school. He could not get along with people, required care at home and was graded in the psychological test as being seriously ill mentally. After treatment with the vitamin-mineral preparation he was well enough to go to college and did well there. At present he bears little resemblance to the person he once was, according to observers.

A woman who had just been released from the hospital after unsuccessful treatment had a history of twenty-five years of mental illness. When she began to take the supplement she was dazed, incoherent, disorganized and suicidal. By the end of the second month she was alert, "careful of her appearance, and facing adjustments at an entirely different psychological level." She got a job and then the experimenters had difficulty in contacting her. When next they found her she was in much worse shape. She had practically stopped taking her nutrition supplements. She agreed that her condition was much worse and began to take them again, with great improvement within two months.

Another woman was started on the fake pills and showed no improvement. So she was put on the vitamin and mineral pills, without, of course, knowing that any change had been made. After eight weeks most of her worst symptoms had disappeared. She no longer "ached all over." Her vague aches and pains had disappeared and her irritability was gone.

Another subject was afraid to go to sleep or to be alone. She felt "as though she were walking through space alone." Within two months from the time she began to take the vitamin and mineral pills, her fears were mostly gone and she reported that she was getting better all the time.

What Does the Experiment Mean?

The researchers tell us that the conditions for their experiment were certainly not the best possible. Patients were not under close supervision as they would have been in a hospital. They undoubtedly skipped their pills often. "It is difficult to say what further improvements would take place over longer periods of therapy," say the researchers. Some of the patients appeared completely normal after only three months of treatment. Others were still taking the pills after six months and may continue to improve. It is possible that results might have been much better if the vitamins and minerals had been started earlier rather than after a long history of mental trouble. It seems that years of mental illness may bring about physical changes that cannot be reversed. Yet one of the patients in this study was seventy-five years old! This woman had been given up as hopeless by literally dozens of doctors. Her family had spent thousands of dollars on hospitals and doctor bills.

Drs. Comrey and Watson are careful to point out that this experiment is only "exploratory" in nature. They plead for further experiments along these lines. And they conclude that the evidence presented in this account "may justifiably be considered as partial confirmation of the hypothesis that some mental illness can be at least partially relieved by employing purely physical, as contrasted to psychological therapy."

The preparation used in this experiment was made up specially for the experiment. But there is no mystery at all as to its contents. It contains in general those food elements we are always recommending to readers—all of the known vitamins along with the foods in which they are most plentiful such as yeast, alfalfa, etc. All of the minerals known to be necessary for human health along with the foods in which they appear, such as bone meal, wheat germ and so forth. We checked the formula used by these doctors against the formulas of several *Prevention*-advertised all-in-one products and found them to be very similar. In addition, of course, the *Prevention*-advertised products are all made entirely from natural food—no synthetics. We assume that some at least of the doctors' formula was synthetic.

Can we guarantee that you can get results such as these doctors got by giving vitamin and mineral supplements to someone who is mentally ill? Of course not. But we do think this experiment shows clearly that years of not paying enough attention to diet can produce tragic results in mental illness and that good diet plus vitamin and mineral supplements may do much to prevent mental disorders.

Our country is spending millions and millions of dollars every year taking care of our mentally ill. We build grand new hospitals, and introduce all the latest developments in psychiatric therapy, electric shock treatment and so forth. It would cost but the smallest fraction of this enormous expenditure to provide vitamin and mineral supplements for all the patients in these hospitals. Why do we not make use of this inexpensive and simple kind of therapy? How long will it be until we recognize that nutrition is the single most important element in health—physical or mental?

Milk—The Case Against Milk

By

J. I. Rodale

Editor of *Prevention*

I don't drink milk, and am not ashamed to admit it. I have been away from milk-drinking now for over 5 years and as yet there have been no signs of any deficiences or repercussions of any kind. So far my body has taken no reprisals against me. At first there was a feeling of anxious uncertainty. Would lightning and thunder figuratively come and destroy me for such sacrilege? Not only has nothing of the kind happened, but I am going my merry way, thriving healthfully without milk, full of buoyant energy and with the confident feeling that (pardon the grammar) me and the cow, (that is, its liquid white portion) have parted ways forever.

Now, from whence comes my calcium if I do not get it from milk? I have news for you. I now get it from *bone meal!* If there had been no bone meal substitute, there could have been trouble unless in expert fashion the rest of the diet had been tailored to make up for that calcium deficit.

For many years I would come across an item here and another there in health magazines, and in an occasional health book, disputing the value of milk as an item of diet, and I put them down as the unscientific talk of rabid physical-culturists. There were many of them, and I wish I had preserved them all. But one day, about ten years ago, a man from Boston visited me and related the following story:

He had obtained a position with a mining company in an isolated section of Montana, and in a few months a very bad case of arthritis which had plagued him for over ten years mysteriously cleared up; but completely! However, when he went back to Boston a few years later, his condition returned in full virulence. At first he put it down as being caused by living again in "civilization," but finally he recalled the fact that in the section of Montana where he had worked there had been no source of milk. For two years he had lived without it.

He decided to eliminate milk again and see what happened. Miracle upon miracles! In a few months his arthritis vanished. Again he began to drink milk and again his malady returned. No wonder he began to shout from the housetops, what he had learned and had to come all the way to Emmaus to tell me, first hand, what he had observed.

This made me think again about all those items I had read in the health literature, attacking milk as an item of our diet. Now arthritis is no mere result of an allergy. It goes deeper than that. I became thoroughly convinced that there were thousands of other persons suffering from this disease merely because they were drinking milk, and I was quite sure that the medics to whom they went were approaching their problem purely through palliation with drugs.

I found confirmation of this idea in a booklet by C. Ward Crampton, M.D., formerly Associate Professor of Medicine of the New York Post-graduate Medical School and Hospital and Chairman of the Subcommittee on Geriatrics and Gerontology, Public Health Committee, Medical Society of the County of New York. Dr. Crampton says, "The daily need of calcium is about one gram or 15 grains. A quart of milk daily will supply this. It is the natural food of the young. Cream, however, may be bad for the 'gouty and arthritic.' This is not as yet fully established but some arthritics seems to do better without any milk. Calcium is not harmful in arthritis even though there are some calcium deposits in and around the joints."

My Wife's Story

I recalled the case of my own wife who hasn't drunk milk or eaten any cheese since she was weaned from her mother's breast. For some mysterious reason or other she developed a deep-rooted aversion to milk and its whole family of related products. Yet, today, at the age of 52, she is as hard as a rock. Where other women have already had an appendix removed and a hysterectomy performed, friend wife has a perfect record in keeping the surgeon's knife at a respectful distance. And how that woman hates milk and cheese! I have seen her in a restaurant returning a luscious-looking stuffed potato because her sharp nose detected that it had been surfaced with a microscopic amount of cheese. Which reminds me of her keen sense of smell—five times better developed than my own. Can its sharpness have something to do with her no-milk diet? I would not rule the possibility out, yet I cannot submit this as a scientific affirmation. Oh, I forgot! My wife seems to have gotten along without milk and without having had the benefit of bone meal, until about five years ago when we all began to take the latter. During all those former years she must have gotten her calcium from something else.

It is a strange thing, though, that although she got along so beautifully without milk, yet she tried to stuff it into our three children. Somehow or other she felt that it was wrong not to drink milk. She wanted to go along with the herd. On the other hand, for at least 15 years I had heard rumblings against milk and therefore was a considerable force in subduing this overpowering desire of hers to compel the children to drink milk. As a result, Nina, who is now over 18, merely takes a little milk with which to help her swallow her vitamin pills, and she has a practically perfect set of teeth.

Septic Sore Throat

In thinking back about milk I recalled a visit I once made many years ago to a farming school where a herd of cows was kept. This was a school, mind you, not a private farm or dairy. When I went into the place where the cows were being milked I immediately experienced a suffocating tightness. I will admit that the ventilation in the barn was poor. The next morning I had the most beautiful case of septic sore throat of my entire life. As you read the various articles about milk in this book you will come across some statements about septic sore throat being transmitted through milk, in spite of pasteurization.

A few years ago while I was taking a summer course in geology, the students took a field trip to nearby quarries, and we took our lunches along. One of the teachers, after he finished his sandwiches, began a mad search for a grocery store. Soon he returned with a whole quart of milk which he drank down with an avid fervor as if his life depended upon it. I am sure he felt that unless he drank at least two quarts of milk a day he was doomed to get cancer at the earliest possible moment.

I sized him up. I could see that his nose was a little on the stuffed side. When I questioned him I found that his nose gave him more torment than a human should ever endure—sinus, colds, catarrah and what have you. And when I told him that his overconsumption of milk could be at the bottom of his trouble he laughed so loud that he must have scared some rabbits a mile away.

Still—Hesitation!

Looking back at all these facts I still hesitated to take up my cudgels in print against milk. For years I thought and thought about it, debating whether or not we should tell our readers what we knew against milk drinking, but it seemed too revolutionary a thing to do. There had been built up such a sacred attitude towards milk that it had become more than a fetish. Down through the ages it had become a powerful symbol. It had grown into a magic belief, a refuge, a sort of sacred fountain from which one drank and imbibed eternal youth. How could we snatch away this source of comfort from our friends?

But my conscience could not remain quiet. When I saw people breaking every rule of health and then resorting to milk as if it would quench out all this error, I became aroused. When I realized how many persons are needlessly suffering through an overconsumption of milk, I came to a decision. I would do it regardless of consequences. I would cast the data I had upon the waters. If it comes as a shock to some, I hope that they will study the matter most thoroughly, possibly experimenting a little before they make up their mind.

I will say one thing most positively—if you think that milk, as it is produced under modern conditions, will be an appreciable factor in giving you health, I must tell you that you are not basing your belief on reality. Today's emasculated product is not fit for human consumption, not to mention the needs of the calf itself for whom the milk was intended. Poor thing! The modern calf is not growing up into a healthy cow.

The Use of Antibiotics

This is proven by the increasing use of the antibiotic drugs given to cows. No one can tell me that this doesn't affect the cow's meat and its milk in some detrimental way. I have before me several strange circulars issued by the Tarkio Molasses Feed Co. of Kansas City. In one of them dated March 22, 1955, and addressed to "Dear Cattle Feeder," the company says, regarding the stilbestrol drug that was approved a few months ago by the U. S. Food and Drug Administration, that it causes meat to go "soft" and not to age properly, and that their company did not intend to put any stilbestrol into its cattle feed. The other circular is a letter from the Williams Meat Co. of Kansas City, one of the outstanding meat provisioners of our country today, who furnishes the best of meat for many large fancy restaurants. Here is what Mr. Williams of that company said in a letter to the Tarkio Molasses Feed Co. on March 14, 1955: "As you know we specialize in prime quality meats, making Kansas City meats nationally famous. For some reason in recent months, the texture of the meat is exceptionally soft and not responding to proper aging. Are feeders experimenting too much with drugs?"

Much of this sort of wonder drug feeding is happening to cows and I wonder what it will do to the milk? At any rate, the whole thing is so unpredictable that one will never know at what moment Bossy will be given another "wonder" treatment, without waiting the necessary time in laboratory checking of dangers.

Propaganda

A great part of milk's popularity is due to the propaganda of the milk interests. They are powerfully organized. They send their tons of literature to the schools, the P. T. A.'s and to other places where it will do the most good. I recall an experience I had about seven or eight years ago which will throw some light on this activity. When we started the Soil and Health Foundation I had some correspondence with a professor in a dental college who wished to know whether I could run an experiment on our farm, feeding two groups of mice—one with food raised with chemical fertilizers, the other with foods raised by the organic method. Then he came to the farm for further discussions. He advised that the experiment would be financed by a big milk foundation, but when he said that milk had to be one item of food for each group of mice, and when I expressed a few negative thoughts about milk, he left, never to return. I received no more letters from him.

Much of our opinion regarding the healing quality of milk stems from this endless stream of propaganda—a torrent of advertising costing hundreds of millions of dollars. We are bombarded by it at every turn, through the newspapers, radio and television until milk has become crowned with a halo. But it is a halo purchased with dollars, and therefore I do not feel guilty when I tarnish it a little.

There is no question that milk has a delightful, satisfying taste, but so has strawberry short cake and ice cream. However, one cannot live by taste alone if one wishes to live a long, healthy life, although there is nothing wrong with the taste of apples, carrots, and roast beef.

How about those who do not drink coffee? If they also eliminate milk, they might complain of the loss of a hot or cold liquid with which to end the meal. But there are always the various kinds of mint and herb teas that one can come to enjoy highly. I occasionally drink an alfalfa mint tea and rose hip tea and find them satisfying from both a taste and a health standpoint.

My own diet consists of meat, eggs, vegetables (mostly raw, some cooked) and a lot of fruit. I do not eat anything that has gone through a factory, and to me, milk is a highly factoryized thing—not only in the aspect of pasteurization but also in the fact that a high production factory has been made out of the cow's udders. I eat no bread or cakes, and no soups, because I am on a reducing diet. But my diet is a very satisfying one especially since I have stopped drinking coffee. I used to drink considerable amounts of coffee because it apparently helped a heart condition. I have discovered, however, that I am better off without it. Vitamin E and desiccated liver are good substitutes. I take a great many different natural vitamins, plus bone meal.

I am on a low salt, no sugar diet, and because of this and my general diet, my blood pressure is like that of a new-born babe—120 over 65, Before I began all this I had a very high blood pressure.

Now a few words of advice. What you intend to do is entirely up to you. Read the articles that follow. Then make up your own mind. Some will cut milk out entirely. Others will merely reduce the amount they consume. But do not let nostalgia influence you, for nostalgia has filled too many a grave. You can point to some persons who are heavy milk drinkers and yet who are perfectly healthy, but it is possible that it is the way they are built. Perhaps they have wider arteries than the average person and a more tuned up set of glands. It is the way they were born, due to their heritage. Those are the people who smoke and drink and live to over 80. But you and I may not be in that class.

It is too bad about the cow! If there were only a way that we could start to unbreed her—to breed her backwards so to speak, to progressively reduce the size of her udders so that one day again she could become a scrub cow. Then, and only then, would I consider taking a drink of her milk. In such a day, perhaps ways could be found to keep her healthy and clean and by some other method, milder than pasteurization, to preserve her milk's nutritional qualities as well as kill its germs. Man has abused a good thing.

Milk, Further Arguments Against

I say to you who are really health-conscious, who want to live to 100 and over without the usual signs of crippling senility—don't drink milk, which means also, don't eat butter or cheese or any other dairy product. If you are satisfied to live to only 70 or 80, or even 85, and if you have been endowed since birth with a body structure that enables you to snap your fingers at the average health-producing procedures, and if you feel that you must drink milk, then drink it! But you will probably pay for it in some other way or another. You won't have that elastic step. You will dodder more. Your eyes may grow dimmer, your ears may lose their hearing edge.

After all, we are in search of something, and our search is not yet complete. We are looking for a program that will give us 100 active healthy years, and more. If we want that, then why take a chance? There is so much medical evidence against the drinking of milk, that where there is smoke there may be fire. Remember that half the world, the eastern half, does not drink milk. I was talking to a Chinese professor the other day and he confirmed this fact to me and more. He stated that the average Chinese student who comes to this country, and hears about the supposed health-giving qualities of milk, begins to drink it, and as a result, he gets gas on the stomach and many other digestive ills. But he does not get it from eating meat, fruits or vegetables!

A while ago I spoke of raw milk. Only the other day I was told of the case of the wife of an advertising executive who visited her uncle's farm where there was a herd of 200 purebred cows. They kept one cow for themselves under unusually sanitary conditions and did not pasteurize its milk. The lady in question, who drank some of this milk on this visit, contracted a severe case of undulant fever which took three years to cure. But the people who were drinking this milk all along had become inured to it. Somewhere, years back, they may have experienced some kind of trouble, unless they may have had some natural immunity.

I would like to speak about another phase of milk drinking—the heart disease question. In a recent study of this disease, the unusual amount of heart attacks in this country was attributed to the large amount of fat consumed in our diet, namely 40 per cent. The authors found that in Italy the consumption of fat is only 20 per cent of the total food consumed, and heart fatalities there are not one-third of what they are in this country. There can be no question that the total fat consumed is an important factor in bringing on heart attacks to vulnerable cases. This is brought out in hundreds of medical researches which I have gone over.

The usual practice is to tell the heart patient to cut down on eggs, but from what I have seen, as between eggs and dairy products, I would say to the average heart case, cut out all dairy products completely, but by all means eat eggs, for eggs are a seed from which a chick will come out. The egg contains terrific, living, nutritional elements. It is a complete package. There is sufficient food in it to feed the emerging chick for a few days and the poultryman does not have to do it. Anyone who passes up eggs is denying himself one of the finest foods that God made.

Of course both eggs and dairy products contain fat. And the body needs some fat, to be sure. We cannot eliminate all fat from our diets. Another angle to remember about cheese is that most cheeses are quite high in salt—also bad for the heart patient.

And the Government encourages the farmer to so feed his cows that more butterfat will be in the milk. That is the Government standard as to how the farmer should be paid for his milk. It is based on its butterfat content. Less would be better. Of course, the physician will advise his heart patient to drink skimmed milk. Yet in restaurants he will put regular milk—even cream—in his coffee.

Another thing that militates against milk, as far as I am concerned, is the fact that practically all milk today contains traces of penicillin, from shots given to the cow to prevent or cure disease. If we keep drinking such milk, the effect of this cumulative penicillin will be to kill all the body's protective bacteria, and already there is evidence that this will cause trouble when a real emergency arises. But now some research scientists are speaking of a new practice that they wish to see inaugurated with respect to milk—a practice which should be killed dead in its track by public outcry. It is based on researches conducted at the University of Minnesota, aided by the American Dairy Association of Chicago, which may set off such a dangerous trend in nutrition that anything that has gone before will pale into insignificance.

What is suggested now is that disease germs be injected into cows. They will then give milk containing large quantities of disease-fighting agents, or antibodies, which would protect people against certain diseases if they drink this milk. Already 10 years have been spent in these researches, all with animals, and the idea has worked, according to the research scientists.

However, two questionable thoughts arise in my mind. One—what will be the ultimate effect in the human body of twenty or thirty years ingestion of such antibodies? Will it completely inactivate the body's own mechanism to produce the protective antibodies? Disuse encourages petrification. The day may arise when something will happen to the cow. She may become unable to pass on the antibodies. What will happen then, if the body has become so coddled and weakened that it has "unlearned" its ability to fight for itself? Modern practices tend to continually weaken the ability of the individual to assert the resistive qualities of his body. He has been called a machine, and is being treated purely as a machine in this case. But it is far safer to improve our primitive qualities in regard to the physical operation of our bodies, rather than to reduce them.

Number two—The dangerous trend set off by the fluoridation of drinking waters (namely, the concept of preventing something by doing something to that which we take into our bodies every day) is given another shot-in-the-arm. There is no telling where this idea will end up. What will the Christian Scientists think of such milk? Nothing, I am sure. Such procedure is a threat to the liberty of the individual who has a right to decide for himself whether he wishes to be "medicated" in such unorthodox ways.

Another hidden defect in this milk treatment is (and the same is true of fluoridation to reduce tooth cavities in children) that it lulls us into a false sense of security, it prevents us from searching out the real causes of disease and rooting them out. If it were not for the prejudiced money-tainted commercialism of the large-scale food-producing factories, the public would today know the simple basic causes of cancer, polio, heart disease and the host of other ailments that are bringing prosperity into the doctors' offices. *Prevention* magazine and its readers already know their causes, but the problem is to get the general public to know them and to resist the fancy pseudo-scientific Salk vaccines, the water chemicalizations and the attempt to put a white coat on cows. That's what they are trying to do—to make doctors out of cows. This is really laughable, for if you knew the extent of disease that exists today in cows, you would see how badly *they* need the doctors themselves.

I, therefore, urge you to write to your congressmen, to your senators, both federal and state, and to other interested officials, write to the University of Minnesota and to the American Dairy Association of Chicago, telling them of the dangers involved and that it may cause many persons to stop drinking milk.

Milk looks innocent in its innocuous whiteness, in its wonderful taste, but still waters flow deep. There are 48 states and the dairy laws differ in each one. God alone knows what the dairyman already is doing to the cow and to the milk. There are far better, and more certain ways of getting the finest nutrition. And that's what you are entitled to—the finest.

Milk, Story of

Most Americans have been told since they were youngsters that milk is the perfect food, that everyone should drink milk every day—children a quart, adults at least a pint. In school health classes, in home economics courses, in diet and health columns in newspapers and magazines, in radio and television, we are urged to drink milk, to use more milk products if we would be healthy.

Because we believe readers get enough and more than enough of this information everywhere else, we are presenting in this book some less well-known facts about milk, with a question in our minds as to whether or not milk is a good food. As Editor Rodale puts it—"We want to tarnish the halo a little." Most of us think of milk as one of the oldest of foods, since it has obviously been in existence since the first baby was born to the first mammal. But how long have adults been drinking milk? Not long, relatively speaking, according to reseachers. Grains and flour date back to more than twenty thousand years in history, but man has probably been drinking milk for only about five or six thousand years. One good reason for this is undoubtedly the fact that the animals from whom man gets his milk were not domesticated until then.

One writer, Mark Graubard, hazards the opinion in his book *Man's Food: Its Rhyme or Reason* (published by The Macmillan Company, 1943) that cows were not domesticated for their milk—or their skins, meat or any other practical reason. Says he, man domesticated animals because he liked them and liked their company. Then too, he could not have thought of drinking the milk of the cow, for no animal in nature has milk to give away. In wild cattle certainly the mother's flow of milk stops as soon as her calf is weaned.

In our country cow's milk and goat's milk are accepted kinds of milk to drink. Would you want to drink the milk of a pig or a horse? Imagine then the feelings of the first man to drink cow's milk! There is no reason to believe, of course, that cow's milk was the first milk our ancestors drank. In many other parts of the world cow's milk is unknown. Reindeer milk and the milk of buffaloes, donkeys, camels and mares is drunk. Perhaps the ancestor of one of these animals was the first whose milk was taken for food by our human ancestors.

In very early times, historically speaking, milk was apparently used more for medicine and for religious rites. Egyptian records show milk (from the cow which was sacred in Egypt) being used in religious ceremonies. The Bible speaks of Abel bringing milk for his sacrifices. Greek writers mention flocks of cows kept for their milk which was used sacrificially.

The Ways in Which Milk is Processed

In modern times we have refrigeration so that we alone of all the people who have used milk as food could use fresh raw milk, for it would keep easily in our efficient refrigerators. But paradoxically we are the ones who have done most to process, preserve and change the basic nature of milk. Most milk these days is pasteurized. This is usually done by heating the milk to the temperature of 145 degrees Fahrenheit, for 30 minutes then cooling it rapidly to 45 or 50 degrees.

Ordinary milk if pasteurized and kept at a temperature of 34 degrees Fahrenheit will keep without any great change for about a month, according to Hutchinson's *Food and Principles of Dietetics.* This is one reason why milk is generally pasteurized. The most important reason is, of course, that pasteurization kills germs of some diseases that are undoubtedly milk-borne. It is well to keep in mind, however, that pasteurization does not mean boiling the milk or keeping it at high heat for very long. The temperature at which milk is pasteurized is about that of the water from your hot water faucet. True, it is enough heat to destroy much (about 20 per cent of the vitamin C and perhaps 10 per cent of the vitamin B_1 in milk. But in general we do not depend on milk to supply us with these two vitamins. So their loss in pasteurization is not overwhelming. However, it does represent one more deletion from food of valuable food elements, sacrificed to modern methods of production, transportation and distribution of foods. The farmer who milks his cows before dawn and drinks the milk for breakfast gets milk as nearly as possible as it should be drunk.

In addition to pasteurizing milk, we process it in other ways. In evaporated milk, the water content of the milk is reduced 60 to 65 per cent. In this process, 50 per cent of the vitamin B_1 is lost, 10 per cent of the vitamin B_2, and about 60 per cent of the vitamin C. The milk is then sealed in a container and processed by heat as are other canned foods, so that it will not spoil. Then, according to Morris B. Jacobs in *Food and Food Products,* "To ensure smoothness, disodium phosphate or sodium citrate or both, or calcium chloride may be added." Evaporated milk may also be fortified with vitamin D, a fact which will be indicated on the label.

Condensed milk (and the term is generally used only for sweetened milk) is the product that results from evaporating the water from milk to which sugar or dextrose have been added. The composition of condensed milk is: fat—8.5 per cent; protein—8.1 per cent; lactose and sugar—54.8 per cent and water 27 per cent. The sugar is added to prevent spoilage.

Other Milk Products

Cream is the fatty portion of milk which rises to the top if raw milk is left standing for any length of time. Light cream, table cream or coffee cream must contain at least 18 per cent and not more than 30 per cent butterfat. Light whipping cream must contain not less than 30 per cent and not more than 36 per cent fat. Over that, it is called heavy whipping cream.

Commercial sour cream is produced by inoculating the sweet cream with a bacterial culture. It is generally made from the cream surplus of the spring months which has been frozen, then thawed. After homogenization and pasteurization the cream is cooled and lactic acid bacteria are put in it. It is allowed to stand at room temperature until the proper acidity is reached. Refrigerating it stops the action of the bacteria. Whipping cream is generally most successful if the cream has a large fat content, is cold and has been "aged" somewhat, which increases its acidity. Of course the whipping must be done rapidly.

Yogurt, buttermilk and sour cream are examples of fermented milk products. In these cases, special bacteria are put into the milk or cream to sour it in a certain way. Buttermilk was formerly a product that remained when butter was churned. But these days buttermilk is made by souring milk with bacteria. Skim milk is milk from which enough of the fat has been removed to reduce the fat content below 3.25 per cent. Most skim milks actually have a fat content as low as .2 per cent. Dried milk products, also called powdered milk, are made by spray-drying fresh milk. Butter is made from the butterfat of milk. And cheese is made from the curd (or solid matter) which separates out when milk is coagulated.

The dairy industry is a mammoth even in America, the home of big business. Milk and cream alone, or as milk products, or in combination with other foods, comprise about one-sixth of the weight of food eaten by an average American family. About 40 per cent of the milk produced in this country is used as fluid milk and cream, while about half is used in making other dairy products. Milk products are also used for industrial purposes as in the manufacture of casein, casein paint, lactic acid and so forth. The dairy industry is the largest source of agricultural income. Its income was equivalent to one billion, seven hundred million dollars of farm income in 1939.

Milk From the Modern Cow

By J. I. Rodale*, Editor of *Prevention

The cow that went aboard Noah's Ark was a far different critter from what she is today. Noah's cow did not have heavy milk bags to carry around to plague her. Noah's and Father Abraham's cows had only small teats, like those of a horse. There was no dairy business in those days. Those that wanted milk kept their own sheep, goat or cow. But in the Eastern part of the world, milk even today is generally not drunk.

Now, why does a cow give milk? A cow gives milk for the same reason that a woman does—to provide food with which to nurse a new-born thing. As soon as a woman or a cow becomes pregnant, forces are set in motion in the body to build a milk supply. After a certain period goes by and the calf gets to the age where it can forage for itself, the cow's supply of milk dries up. You can see, therefore, that in order for the cow to give more milk, she must have another calf. Thus, keeping a cow in milk involves maternity.

Most people are of the opinion that the cow has a set of spigots to be turned on and off when one needs milk, and that's what most city folks believe. Now, in the old days a family that kept a cow sometimes appropriated some of the milk for their own use, but the wise, all-seeing Creator foresaw this propensity of man's for taking things, without asking, and he gave the cow a bountiful extra reserve of milk. But as the centuries rolled on, man saw an opportunity of making money from the cow's milk supply, and with that devilish cunning he shows wherever money is concerned, he found a way to force the cow to give more milk.

He observed that some cows give more milk than others, and by closer study, discovered that such cows had larger teats than others. He found also that this ability to give more milk ran in families. So he mated cows from such families to bulls from similarly endowed families and, that, still further, increased the capacity to give milk.

The result was that from generation to generation, cows gave more and more milk and their udders thus gradually became larger and larger. Now, by the time of George Washington, the cow's udders were at least 20 times the capacity of a cow in the days of King David. In Revolutionary War times you could already begin to call them milk bags, though they hung down only about five inches or so. But today, by further breeding the cow's milk bags have been enlarged to ten times the size they were when George Washington was president. Yes, sir! Today the milk bags of some cows are so huge that they pretty near drag the ground and you will find listed in Sears Roebuck's catalog girdles for cows to hold up their udders so that they won't drag or crack.

Man has made a factory—a milk machine out of the cow. Where, in Noah's time, a cow gave about 200 pounds of milk in a year, today there are cows that give 15,000 pounds or 75 times as much milk. And this overproduction is causing more disease in cows. A lot of cows are getting leukemia today and many other diseases which they never used to get.

Now, getting back to what we moderns call milk—it is very diluted because of the large quantity the cow has to give. Milk is a very delicate thing, inter-related to almost every gland and organ of the cow's body. It is a part of the function of the animal in creating life. All of the best elements in its body must be assembled to make it, so that the calf can have a good start.

Our scientists do not seem to be aware of what they are doing. They are shallow fragmentists. All they are after is to secure increased volume of an opaque white liquid, with a reasonable amount of butter-fat content, but are they worried over the fact that its vitamins and hormones are below a safe level? No! Why, there were more vitamins in a thimbleful of milk at the time of King David than in a whole beer mug of today.

When we force a cow to give 75 times the amount of milk that God intended her to it must be a kind of milk that is not up to snuff. That is point number one. Now we come to point number two. Artificial insemination.

The dairymen seem to delight in making the cow a completely artificial animal. Formerly a bull mated with a cow in order to give her a calf, but that is too much trouble for dairymen today, so they have this artificial insemination. The bull is masturbated, and the amount of semen ejaculated is used to inject into forty or fifty cows or even more. It is nothing but male prostitution. It is an irreligious, impious trick if I ever saw one. First they hang a hundred pound weight under the cow, then they deprive her of her gentleman friend! What next? They are piling artificiality upon artificiality. Poor bossy, with her big sad eyes waiting for the father of her children who never comes. One day she may realize that she has been let down, deceived, tricked, cheated out of the natural biological satisfaction which is her inherent right. Can the milk of such a cow be any good?

And the bull—what of him? There are going to be disastrous effects upon his character. Already bulls are refusing to work and are becoming obstreperous. Recently near Winchester, Indiana, a bull gored the auto of the county's artificial inseminator.

God does everything for a purpose. He makes fruit colorfully attractive and sweet so that the birds will seek it out and scatter the seed. Thus fruit trees spring forth all over creation. He has put glorious colors in the flowers so that the bee will be attracted to pollinate them and they will grow in profusion on the face of the earth. He has made the cow and the bull for each other but who is man to say "I will change what God hath intended?"

When God promised the Land of Canaan to the children of Israel, describing it to Moses as a land flowing with milk and honey, did he mean milk from cows artificially inseminated and with oversized milk bags? According to Leviticus the cow offered up for sacrifice in the temple was supposed to be absolutely pure and without a single blemish anywhere. Would a cow begotten in artificial insemination be an acceptable animal for the temple ritual? Would you consider her bloated milk-bag a blemish? Should a good Christian drink milk produced in such a profane, ungodly way?

Now, since the practice of artificial insemination began there is much more disease in cows. They are dropping dead from unknown causes, and there are all kinds of reproductive diseases—mastitis of the udders for one. A cow's life is 20 per cent shorter than it was 30 years ago.

But God has methods of his own. In artificially inseminated births more male calves are being born than ordinarily, and this tendency will keep on increasing even with human artificial insemination births—we call them test-tube babies—60 per cent more boys than girls.

Do you realize what this means? If the percentage of males in births keeps on increasing, and it will if these dairymen insist on continuing this suicidal insemination practice, God will see to it that eventually no females will be born at all. The species will die out.

You would think that scientists would be more careful. They should have tested artificial insemination for 50 years before letting it loose on the public. But science is running ahead of human wisdom and the public is not without blame, either. The public is lazy. It shirks its responsibilities. And that's not all about artificial practices and cows. Already there is a new and vicious thing that is being used. Instead of spraying insecticides in the barn and on the outside of the cow's skin, they are now injecting this chemical right into the cow's blood stream, so that if a fly or mosquito bites her anywhere, it will automatically get a dose of the chemical and die.

This chemical that is powerful enough to kill a fly at one bite will be present in every cell of the cow's body, and will get into the milk. How brave these scientists are at the public's expense. Cato the Elder was right when he said, "There is a wide difference between true courage and a mere contempt of life." Nor have I mentioned the formaldehyde preservative that some dairies put into milk. Formaldehyde is a chemical used to embalm people.

There are many other artificial practices that are perpetrated against the cow, but it is all part of the processes of chemicalization and artificialization which have been thrust upon us—people as well as cows. The scientists are in the woods and cannot see the cows. And as far as I am concerned, I am through with milk. I have been through with it for many years now and feel as fit as a fiddle. Of course, I see to it that my diet is well balanced—the bone meal taking care of what was in the milk far more effectively than the milk did.

Milk and Alkalis

Ever hear of something called the Milk-Alkali Syndrome? Doctors put that mouth-filling name to a disorder that is often associated with stomach ulcer. Taking it apart, the phrase means just a certain condition that is apparently caused by taking too much milk and something alkaline.

In ulcer cases there is generally too much hydrochloric acid in the stomach. This is one of the digestive juices—absolutely necessary for good digestion. It is of course strongly acid. Minerals and water soluble vitamins like vitamins B and C must be mixed with plenty of hydrochloric acid in the stomach or they will not be absorbed. You also need it to digest protein.

However, there can be too much of a good thing. Some doctors think stomach ulcers cause too much hydrochloric acid; others think that too much of the acid is responsible for the ulcers. No one knows for sure. But at any rate, we do know that having ulcers generally means as well having too much hydrochloric acid for your own good. So doctors frequently prescribe alkaline substances to counteract the hydrochloric acid.

Many ulcer diets have milk as their base, if not their sole item. You have probably known people who lived on milk and cream for at least several weeks while the doctor was treating their ulcers. And probably they were taking alkaline powders at the same time.

Then, too, many patients take alkalis without their doctor's advising it. In *The Southern Medical Journal* for February 1948 there is the story of a man—an ulcer patient—who took bicarbonate of soda at the rate of a third of a box a day! He did not drink milk, but he ate as much as a fourth to a half of a pound of cheese a day. What exactly took place in this man's digestive tract as he drank down the bicarbonate of soda followed by the cheese? (And remember, any other so-called "alkalizer" would have done just the same thing.)

The cheese is rich in calcium. But the alkalizer neutralizes the acid in the stomach so that the calcium cannot be utilized. Of course all the B vitamins in the cheese are wasted, too. In the book *Diseases of Metabolism,* edited by Garfield G. Duncan, M.D. (W. B. Saunders Company, 1952) we are told that calcium absorption is governed by three things: (1) Other substances in the diet. (2) Vitamin D and (3) The acidity of the intestine where the food must be digested. The acidity of the normal duodenum (the opening of the intestine) is from 2.3 to 7. That is very acid indeed. And the more acidity, the better the calcium is absorbed.

The higher the phosphorus content of the diet, the less calcium is absorbed. This is one reason why diets high in cereals tend to rob the body of calcium—for cereals contain lots of phosphorus. But so does milk. So what little calcium might be absorbed in these decidedly unacid surroundings is cancelled out by the high phosphorus content of the milk.

So our poor patient gradually gets into a state where all the fine and necessary calcium which should have dissolved and gone into his bloodstream where it could nourish nerves and cells, has not dissolved at all. It is collecting at various spots and what is actually happening to our patient is that he is gradually turning into limestone. He may get calcium deposits in his kidneys. Certainly all of the various minerals and vitamins whose functions are related to those of calcium in the body go out of balance. Magnesium, for instance, gets entirely out of control and much larger quantities of it than normal appear in the blood stream. Now all these various food elements are not just circulating around for lack of a better place to go, you know. Each of them has a number of jobs to perform in the body. And when one is thrown out of balance, it is bound to affect all the rest.

What Happens to Patients Living on Milk and Alkali?

In *Archives of Internal Medicine,* volume 95, page 460, 1955, there is a report on eight patients who had had ulcer symptoms for from many months to several decades. All but one consumed in excess of a quart of milk a day. Several took as much as three or four quarts. In addition each of them took alkaline powders frequently. One patient estimated that he took as much as two and a half pounds of "sippy powders" a week. It was not unusual for the patients to state that for weeks or months they had lived on milk and alkaline powders.

In another article in *Annals of Internal Medicine,* volume 42, page 324, 1955, several patients are discussed who have deposits of calcium in eye tissues, the tissues just underneath the skin, in the lungs and the walls of the arteries. Why do not the kidneys excrete the calcium harmlessly? It it not known why. Perhaps the kidneys have already been damaged. Usually as soon as the diet is stopped and all alkaline medicine is forbidden the kidneys return to normal and no permanent damage is done.

We have another suggestion as to why the part that calcium should be healthfully playing is so distorted under these abnormal circumstances. Vitamin C is destroyed in an alkaline medium. There is practically no vitamin C in a diet of milk to begin with, especially if the milk has been pasteurized or boiled. Whatever small amount happens to remain in the milk is promptly destroyed by the alkaline powders once it arrives in the stomach. We believe that vitamin C has a lot to do with the proper disposition of calcium in the body. We think that lack of vitamin C can cause kidney stones and deposits of calcium in the arteries. So it seems reasonable to suppose that when the diet contains not a bit of vitamin C, the calcium supply is going to get completely out of control in a very short time.

As you have gathered by now we do not approve of milk and alkali diets for ulcer patients. It seems that the medical profession is rapidly coming to that conclusion too. *Time* magazine for March 21, 1955, reported Dr. Edward Kessler as saying that "ulcer victims who swill milk and assorted alkalies can do themselves more harm than good." He had seen three patients, he said, who were petrifying themselves by clogging their kidneys with excess calcium. The danger from the treatment increases with the duration and degree of the self-medication, especially sodium bicarbonate which is, of course, baking soda.

The news that physicians are concerned about what may develop on the usual ulcer diet is encouraging. But we must not forget all those ulcer victims who prescribe for themselves and will continue to take medicines that "alkalinize" them, along with enormous amounts of milk.

There is a large amount of research indicating that we human beings cannot have too much calcium in our diets, provided that other elements in the diet are in balance. In other words, you can take as much calcium as you can get, provided that everything is in order to use the calcium properly. You should have the right amount of phosphorus in the diet, enough vitamin D and enough fat, too, for proper use of the calcium. Then vitamin C is also extremely important. The milk-bicarbonate diet contains very little vitamin D, plenty of phosphorus and fat. But, after the alkali has counteracted the natural stomach acid, can either the phosphorus or the fat be used by the body? The diet contains no vitamin C. We have read in medical journals of ulcer victims who eventually showed signs of scurvy (the disease of extreme vitamin C deficiency) after they had been on such a diet.

Taking bicarbonate of soda or any other "alkalinizer" is extremely hazardous to health. You are bound to get into serious difficulty, for nothing will be properly digested or absorbed into the body. You need to keep a certain "alkaline balance," true. By this we mean that you should eat not only foods which cause an acid reaction in the body, such as meats. Plenty of fruits and vegetables will adjust your alkaline balance.

Milk and the Dangers It Holds

By Emanuel M. Josephson, M.D. of New York City

This article is reprinted (with permission of the author) from the book, *Your Life is Their Toy*, published by Chedney Press, 127 East 69th Street, New York City. The book was published in 1940 and undoubtedly the situation in regard to the cleanliness of milk has improved considerably since then.

Milk is Nature's food for the new-born. Its high dilution and its weakness adapt it to the delicate and undeveloped digestive system of the young infant. For adults, it is both uneconomical and inefficient as a food because of its dilution, and is not an essential element of diet. Loss of weight on milk reduction diets attests to the inadequacy of milk as a diet for adults.

Indeed, milk is not even an adequate food for infants. Infants fed on milk alone almost invariably develop rickets, scurvy and tetany. For though milk has a good calcium content, it contains little or no vitamin C even when absolutely fresh; and without the vitamin the lime (calcium) is not assimilated by the intestines. Because of this and other deficiencies of milk, infants are given orange and tomato juice, cod liver oil, vegetables and other foods at the age of one or two months, or as soon as they can tolerate them. This procedure has done much to make our children healthier and stronger. It is apparent from the brief period of lactation of mothers that Nature did not intend milk as a diet beyond infancy.

Man is the only mammal that habitually consumes milk after the stage of infancy during which the mother lactates. In Japan male children are nursed at the breast during childhood and sometimes to the age of nine years. The physique of the Japanese fails to reflect any advantage in prolonged nursing and milk feeding.

Milk is not Essential in Diet after Infancy

Much that has been said and written about milk is untrue. (Dr. Josephson goes on to say that the famous nutritionist, Dr. E. V. McCollum has pointed out that the inhabitants of Southern Asia have no herds and do not drink milk.) They subsist on rice, soybeans, sweet potatoes, bamboo sprouts and other vegetables. They contrast sharply and favorably with milk-drinking folks and, according to the doctor, for their development, physique and endurance they are exceptional, their capacity for work is extraordinary, they escape skeletal defects in childhood, and have the finest teeth of any race in the world—with no milk.

Dr. Rabinowitz, Director of the Metabolism Department of the Montreal General Hospital, points out that milk is totally absent from the adult diets of many virile nations, and cannot be regarded as a necessary item in the adult diet. He also points out that milk is not a good diet even for children. He wrote in *The New England Medical Journal* of September 13, 1934:

"Now milk is not a natural beverage of the human being, or of any other mammal, after the period of infancy . . . Some children, after drinking the milk and orange juice which are their required (by the fashion in pediatrics) quota for breakfast, have little appetite or room left for the bacon, bread, cereal, egg and fruit which should be the chief staples of their meals."

Chemical Dangers of Milk for Adults

Man may pay a severe penalty for the drinking of milk. Milk contains a high content of the chemical cholesterol. Many research workers, including Dr. Timothy Leary, have traced the origin of hardening of the arteries (arteriosclerosis) and one of the most deadly diseases of the heart (coronary sclerosis) to an excess of cholesterol. He points out that man is the only animal who dies early in life from coronary sclerosis and who almost universally acquires arteriosclerosis in later life; and he is the only animal who continues to drink milk throughout life.

Because of its cholesterol and hormone content, milk may also play a role in the causation of cancer. Statistical studies indicate that cancer occurs with higher frequency among peoples who are steady and habitual milk drinkers. Cholesterol is closely related chemically to substances which are known to be the most potent chemicals for causing development of cancer.

Disease and Death May Lurk in the Milk Bottle

Those qualities which make milk an ideal food for infants also make it an ideal food for germs of all varieties—both the harmless and those which cause dangerous disease and death.

Milk is potentially the most dangerous of all foods. This does not imply that in every glass of milk there lurks danger or death. But it does mean that one cannot be sure that these risks are not present. *Milk is probably the food most frequently responsible for disease and death.* So many are the risks and possibilities of danger in milk that some of our leading medical authorities who are courageous and independent of the control of medical organization, of milk companies, and of "educational foundations," absolutely prohibit the use of any form of loose or pasteurized milk for their infant patients.

Pasteurization is not Absolute Protection

Contrary to propaganda and popular belief, pasteurization does not make milk sterile or serve to effectively protect against these dangerous infections. On the contrary, pasteurization may sometimes increase the danger. Boiling, however, does sterilize milk and make even polluted milk safe.

The false popular belief that pasteurization makes milk absolutely safe has been fostered by intensive, high-priced propaganda participated in by both the milk distributing companies and by some States, such as New York State. This propaganda is a deliberate fraud upon the people in which both the medical and social service rackets play important roles.

The textbooks generally state that pasteurization reduces the bacteria in milk by about 99 per cent. This much is true under ideal conditions of pasteurization, which often do not prevail in commercial practice. But the statement is a half truth which conceals the fact that the one per cent of germs which survive even ideal pasteurization rapidly multiply. Within several hours after pasteurization the number of bacteria present in the milk may be larger than the number prior to pasteurization.

Pasteurization May Make Milk More Dangerous

Numerous studies and investigations have proved the deficiencies of pasteurization. The works of Rogers and Frazier, and of Prucha reveal that certain types of the dangerous streptococci and other groups of bacteria may actually flourish at the temperatures of pasteurization. Ayers and Johnson of the U. S. Department of Agriculture stated in their official publication, *A Study of Bacteria Which Survive Pasteurization* as follows:

"Four distinct groups of bacteria, the acid-forming, the inert, the alkali-forming and the peptonizing, survive pasteurization . . .

" . . . Streptococci from milk and cream were much more resistant than those from other sources."

The diseases borne by milk are many. These may be divided into two groups—human diseases originating in diseases of the cow that are conveyed by milk, and disease due to contamination of milk.

Among the diseases of the cow conveyed to the human by milk are the following:

Colds, Septic Sore Throat, Rheumatic Fever and Heart Disease

Septic sore throat is caused by streptococci on the cow's udders, which may or may not give rise to disease of the cow or they may be introduced into milk by contamination. The disease which these streptococci cause in the human is generally virulent, and dangerous to health and life. It may cause rheumatism, heart disease, St. Vitus dance, kidney disease, and even death through the blood stream infection, so-called "blood poisoning." Periodic epidemics of septic sore throat recur as often as three or four times a year among milk drinkers.

There is little room for doubt that the streptococci of milk are the most frequent cause of rheumatic fever the most deadly disease of childhood. It ranks first as the cause of death in girls and third in boys. Characteristically, little mention is made of this fact by our corrupted public health officials or intimidated "authorities" in the current exploitation of rheumatic fever. Instead they tell the public: "Drink more milk."

Danger to health and life could be avoided if the public were notified of the epidemic and warned to boil milk. But seldom, or never, do public health authorities who are dominated by milk interests notify the public of the prevalence of these epidemics. They seek to avoid damage to the milk business, even though it be at a sacrifice of health and life.

Many mothers ask their physicians, "Why do my children have frequent colds, although they are well fed and get plenty of milk?" The answer is not infrequently that milk, laden with virulent streptococci, is the cause of the colds.

Streptococci-laden milk is probably the most frequent cause of heart disease which kills and maims children. Public health organizations pretend to fight juvenile heart disease. But due to subsidy by milk companies and allied foundations, this danger of milk is not mentioned to the public.

Almost regularly, each year, whole towns must be quarantined because of epidemics of septic sore throat. These epidemics are seldom announced in the press except when they affect only small rural communities. Such epidemics also occur in the larger cities; but information regarding them is suppressed because of the resultant financial loss to the milk interests.

Thus during the winter of 1937, there occurred in Owego, N. Y. an epidemic of septic sore throat which was so severe and widespread as to lead to a quarantine of the whole town. This was announced in the press dispatches. During the epidemic, the milk from the same herds as caused the disease was shipped to New York City. The epidemic which was caused in New York City by this highly infected milk was labelled "influenza" by health authorities.

Tuberculosis Due to Milk

Tuberculosis is as widely prevalent in cattle as it is in humans, and the bovine form of tuberculosis is readily transmitted to humans by milk. Students of the subject have estimated that over six per cent of the deaths from tuberculosis in this country are due to bovine tuberculosis, even though that form of tuberculosis is less deadly than the human form.

In 1930 the Massachusetts Department of Health reported that one-fifth of the population of Massachusetts, a million persons, each day consumed milk derived from cows that might have been tubercular. In London a study of milk samples before pasteurization revealed that 83 per cent showed virulent tubercle bacilli; and three per cent showed it after pasteurization.

Calmette of the Pasteur Institute devised a method of immunizing calves against virulent tuberculosis. It consists of the injection of a weakened strain of tubercle bacilli into the calves shortly after birth. This gives them a mild form of the disease which protects against the more virulent form. It protects the cows. But it is not absolutely proved that cows thus infected may not transmit the disease to humans. Tuberculin testing is not entirely adequate for the elimination of the danger of transmission of tuberculosis. Lax inspection of cattle by health authorities considerably enhances the menace.

Undulant Fever—A disease of Milk

Bang bacillus infection, or brucellosis, is a disease which causes abortion in cattle. It is highly contagious among cattle, and may ruin whole herds. It is widely prevalent among the herds of this country. It is even present in certified herds. Five per cent of milk samples from certified herds of Detroit showed the bacilli.

The disease is conveyed to humans by milk; and there have been quite a few cases of the disease recognized in the human, although it is difficult to diagnose and frequently goes unrecognized. It is characterized by recurrent attacks of low fever, shooting pains, sweats and weakness which may continue for months or for years. In the chronic form it causes weakness, loss of weight, lassitude, occasional fever and other vague symptoms. There is no method of treatment which assures any degree of success, and the disease must be left to run its course. The disease also causes abortion in the human.

Undulant fever is spreading rapidly in this country. At times and in some communities it has attained epidemic proportions. For a long time the matter was hushed even in the medical press, so that even many doctors were not aware of the existence of the disease or its nature. But its spread is forcing it on public attention. A recent survey among the school children of Detroit showed that one-third of those examined were affected with unsuspected chronic undulant fever.

Deadly Milk Trembles

Epidemics of ulcers of the stomach and intestinal tract in children from one to six months of age were traced by Dr. H. F. Helmholz and Dr. E. W. Saunders to germs which cause inflammation of the udders of cows and which survive pasteurization. These germs were found also to cause ulcers in animals to which they were fed.

A new infectious disease borne by milk known as Haverhill Fever has recently come to light. It starts with chills and fever. Soon a rash develops and joint pains which jump from one point to another.

A mysterious and deadly disease which is known by the name of "milk sickness" or "trembles" seems to be peculiarly American. It occurs generally in Virginia, Ohio, Indiana, Kentucky, Tennessee, the Carolinas, Georgia, New Mexico, and Arizona. Dairy products and meat from cattle fed on white snakeroot, which they may eat in dry spring weather, convey the disease. It comes on acutely with sudden loss of appetite, nausea and weakness of the muscles in the arms and legs. After two or three days severe abdominal pains develop. The victims become dull and apathetic and may lapse into unconsciousness or coma. Historical interest attaches to the disease because it was the cause of death of Nancy Hanks, the mother of Abraham Lincoln.

Diseases Due to Milk Contamination

Diseases which may be borne by milk contaminated in the process of handling are numerous. Such contamination is in some measure unavoidable. Few persons who could see the amount of filth removed from milk at the point of collections, by a process of centrifuging, would care to drink milk. Manure, hay, hair, scabs, occasionally even drowned mice, and a large assortment of foreign bodies are thus removed from the milk. There cannot be removed in this manner the bacteria conveyed by those substances and by the dirty milk cans. These bacteria breed prolifically in the milk.

Disease of milk handlers may contaminate milk and be transmitted by it. Typhoid fever, scarlet fever, measles, the human form of tuberculosis and many other dangerous and deadly diseases can be thus conveyed by milk to the human.

Dysentery and Milk

Recent widespread epidemics of dysentery and gastro-intestinal disorders have been traced to milk; and there the matter was dropped by health officials. Thus G. M. Fyfe reported a milk-borne epidemic of dysentery affecting one hundred and fifty people in 1927. Since then, numerous epidemics have recurred, many of them directly traced to pasteurized milk.

Milk, both raw and pasteurized, plays a large role in causing diseases of the digestive organs. Thus Dr. Horace W. Soper writes.

"About four years ago I became convinced that raw as well as pasteurized milk contained pathogenic bacteria and advised boiling milk and cream. In time, I employed the evaporated milks particularly in cases of gastric and duodenal ulcer, ulcerative colitis, catarrhal colitis, etc. The results were so satisfactory that I prescribed the canned evaporated milks exclusively in my diet-lists for such conditions. Ulcers healed more quickly and recurrences were less frequent. Ulcerative colitis patients responded especially well and relapses which formerly were so common are now rarely encountered. Many cases of catarrhal colitis are quickly corrected by this simple change in dietary habits."

Processed Milk is Safe and Better

Unprocessed milk, even though pasteurized, is so fraught with potential dangers to life and health that were it not nature's diet for infants, its use would probably be eliminated for the protection of public health.

Competent authorities have arrived at the conclusion that since milk is potentially the most dangerous of foods, it should be used only after sterilization and packaging in sealed containers, in condensed, evaporated or dried forms. They alone offer protection against the array of disease conveyed by milk.

Former Commissioner of Health of New York State, Dr. Hermann M. Biggs, predicted more than thirty years ago that eventually milk would be sold in concentrated sterilized form. Only milk that is actually sterilized, he stated, is safe for human use; and the sale of only such milk should be permitted. The objection that the vitamin content of milk may be affected by these methods of preparation is not very valid; for the destruction of vitamins scarcely equals that of universally adopted adulteration of milk for urban consumption.

There are other advantages to processed forms of milk. They have a higher concentration of solids and a higher food value than milk. They are generally prepared from fresh milk, and are less likely to be adulterated. And they are also more economical in some respects although the distributors maintain the retail price at the same level as an equivalent amount of bottled milk.

Approximately 85 per cent of the contents of milk is water. The sale and distribution of the water in the milk entail a huge waste. Advances in science and technology now make it possible to sterilize and concentrate milk, or even to reduce it to a powder before shipment. If racketeering is ever eliminated from the milk industry these preparations should make possible a safe and inexpensive milk for use when required, also safe cheeses and other dairy products.

Milk, Its Food Elements and Their Effect on Adults

"There is probably only one subject upon which all dietitians agree, viz., the value of milk—generally speaking, cow's milk—in human nutrition. Milk is a food developed in nature for the feeding of the immature mammal. The only doubts which can arise about its use by man are: (1) Is it wise to divert the food intended for the young of other mammals to man, and (2) should adults take a food intended for the immature? The answer to these two questions, from the dawn of history to the modern experimental era is undoubtedly 'yes'." So say two famous writers on nutrition V. H. Mottram of the University of London and George Graham, M.D. of St. Bartholomew's Hospital, London, in the book *Hutchinson's Food and the Principles of Dietetics* published by Edward Arnold and Co., London.

There is no doubt that milk contains a formidable array of nutritious elements. It would have to, for it is the sole food of the infant mammal for some time—a time when growth and development are taking place at a rapid rate. Good nutrition is necessary for any living thing to grow and develop.

Let us consider first the vitamins in milk. A quart of milk from cows on green pasture contains about 3,500 International Units of vitamin A. This compares favorably with 4,500 units in a half cup of cooked carrots—a food we think of perhaps first in relation to vitamin A. Summer milk may contain twice as much vitamin A as winter milk. And—a noteworthy fact—human milk is richer in vitamin A than cow's milk. So the baby that is fed from a bottle does not get as much vitamin A as he needs unless he is given a supplement.

Vitamins in Milk

Milk is also rich in the B vitamins. A quart may contain 600 milligrams of thiamin and 2.1 milligrams of riboflavin. Twice as much thiamin as beef liver and about a fourth as much as you will get in a half cup of wheat germ.

Riboflavin is the vitamin that gives milk its characteristic yellow color. And this is the vitamin in which you are almost bound to be deficient unless you are paying very special attention to your diet. You should have 2 milligrams of riboflavin a day as the very minimum that will protect you from disease. Kidney and liver contain considerable riboflavin. You could get it from three cups of cooked soybeans, about 15 eggs, 2 cups of cooked beet greens or kale. And that's about all, with the exception of brewer's yeast and wheat germ, both of which are rich in riboflavin. Brewer's yeast, richer in all the B vitamins than any other food, contains relatively enormous amounts of riboflavin. Some yeasts are grown especially with riboflavin in mind, so that they are even richer in this vitamin than the average yeast. Remember, when we recommend brewer's yeast, this is not the kind of yeast you buy at the grocery store with which to raise bread. It is rather a food yeast, specially dried and prepared to conserve all the B vitamins.

Niacin, another B vitamin, occurs in milk. Pyridoxine, pantothenic acid and biotin are also very plentiful in milk. Milk should not be depended upon for its vitamin C content. Physicians discovered this fact long ago when pasteurized milk was first used to feed babies. Much of the vitamin C in the original milk (and there is only a fair amount to begin with) is destroyed in the pasteurization process.

Milk contains little vitamin D. And why should cow's milk contain any vitamin D at all? Nature has provided for the calf to be born out of doors and it receives sunlight from the moment of its birth. This can of course be changed into vitamin D in the skin. But the human baby needs vitamin D. So these days most milk is treated to assure a standard amount of this vitamin. It can be achieved (expensively) by feeding irradiated yeast to the cow or (less expensively) by exposing the milk to ultraviolet light or putting a synthetic vitamin D concentrate in it. Four hundred International Units per quart is the standard.

In some localities, other vitamins and minerals are added to milk. This is called "fortifying" the milk. Some dairymen add vitamin A, thiamin, riboflavin, niacin, vitamin C and calcium. Needless to say we consider this adding of synthetic vitamins a tampering with food that should be made unlawful.

Here is what we consider a very significant statement from Jacobs in his monumental *Food and Food Products* (3 volumes) published by Interscience Publishers, Inc. N. Y.: Not all of the known growth factors of milk have been isolated. That is, although we have a fairly good idea of the vitamins, minerals and enzymes in milk, we do not know whether these are the factors that bring about the growth of the young mammal or whether there are many more yet-to-be-discovered elements which may be responsible. We think it is well to keep this in mind in considering milk as food for an adult—what possible harm might these unknown growth factors do him? Adults do not grow. Their growing time is over. What function, then, do the growth factors in milk perform in the adult?

Minerals in Milk

Minerals are plentiful in milk. These are necessary to build the bones, teeth, nerves and so on of the young animal. Calcium is the outstanding and most important of these. According to *Clinical Nutrition* by Jolliffe, Tisdal and Cannon (Paul Hoeber, Inc.) about 75 per cent of our calcium, nationally, is obtained from milk. Why should this be? There are many countries in the world today where milk is unknown. How do these folks get their calcium? Can it be that our methods of fertilizing and refining foods have so depleted our other foods of the calcium they should have that we *must* rely on milk? Could we, in our country today, get enough calcium without drinking milk?

It's all very well for some writers to say (and one dentist we quote in this book says it) "get your calcium where the cow gets hers—from green leafy plants." But the adult needs about one gram (1000 milligrams) of calcium daily.

How much of the green leafy vegetables should one eat to obtain this every day? Well, you would have to eat about four cups of raw cabbage, five cups of chard leaves or collards, cooked, five cups of cooked soybeans, 30 eggs or 10 fresh oranges. We have named foods high in calcium. We also want to remind you that we are not made like cows. We do not have the same kind of digestive tract and there is doubt as to how much of the calcium found in vegetables we assimilate. But seriously, does it seem to you that any of us, adult or child, can depend on our usual food sources for one gram of calcium per day—which is the very lowest minimum that can possibly keep us free from disease, and it is generally agreed among nutritionists that we need much more for good health!

Long ago convinced that you cannot indeed get enough calcium from other foods in this day and age and not at all convinced that adults should get it from milk, we advocate the use of bone meal—high in calcium and other minerals, a completely natural food.

In many of the countries where milk is unknown, bones are the main source of calcium. They are eaten whole in small fish; they are chewed along with meat, or they are ground into powder and used as food. There is no waste fluid involved in bones as food—they are mineral through and through. In other articles in this book, we discuss bone meal more thoroughly. For those readers who want even more information, we recommend our booklet *Bone Meal for Human Consumption,* available from Rodale Press Inc., Emmaus, Pa.

There is one further aspect of the calcium content of cow's milk that should concern us. We can assume without much doubt that human milk is perfectly designed for human babies. Then we run squarely up against the question of the suitability for children of cow's milk which contains much more calcium than human milk. A chart showing the calcium content of the different kinds of milk and the time required to double the weight in each of the animals involved reveals that the human child doubles his weight in 180 days and the calf in 47 days. Does it seem wise to give the child cow's milk? Is it the large amount of calcium in the cow's milk that causes the calf to double its weight in 47 days, or is it the "mysterious growth factors" which we have not as yet investigated?

There is also much more phosphorus in cow's milk than in human milk—something else that should concern us as we contemplate the almost universal use of cow's milk for American infants.

One other significant difference between human milk and cow's milk. Human milk contains three times as much iron as cow's milk and three times as much lecithin (a fatty substance found along with several of the B vitamins). This seems to indicate that the human baby needs three times as much of these substances as the calf needs, in proportion to body weight. Where does the average child get the extra iron he needs if he is on an exclusive or almost exclusive milk diet? Where does he get the extra lecithin?

Milk is also low in copper, another mineral needed (along with iron) to prevent anemia. Phosphorus, sodium, potassium, magnesium, chlorine, sulfur, zinc, manganese, aluminum and iodine appear in milk in varying amounts.

Enzymes in Milk

Enzymes are those elusive substances that occur in everything associated with life. Milk has its share—amylase, catalase, peroxidase, lipase, phosphatase. Each of these has a specific job to do in some chemical change that will take place during digestion. Phosphatase, for instance, is necessary for phosphorus to be handled properly by the body. This brings us to an interesting fact about milk pasteurization. The enzymes are destroyed or inactivated during pasteurization, for they are very susceptible to heat. In fact, the inactivation of phosphatase is the standard test as to whether milk has been pasteurized. They test the milk for this enzyme. If it is not there, then they know that the milk has been pasteurized.

Now keeping in mind that the enzyme was placed in milk to perform some function in digestion what do you suppose happens to that function when pasteurized milk is drunk? Of course cooking destroys all enzymes, so all of us present our bodies with a trying problem when we eat any cooked food. This is one reason why we must make certain that we get a goodly portion of our food raw—because of the enzymes. And don't forget, when you are adding up your raw food total for the day—pasteurized milk is *cooked food*.

Proteins and Carbohydrates in Milk

About 4.5 per cent of milk is protein. Carbohydrates account for about 6 per cent and fat about 7.8 per cent. This varies, of course, with the different breeds of cows and their feed

The sugar in milk is lactose which occurs in no other food. It digests less readily than other sugars so it does not cause overweight. It is broken down into two other sugars inside the body—glucose and galactose. Galactose is important for building the complex and delicate nervous system in the human child. Perhaps that is the reason why human milk contains far more sugar than cow's milk—6 per cent compared to 4.9 per cent. Could this be another reason why feeding the baby a formula made of cow's milk is not nearly so healthful as breast-feeding? Additional sugar must be added to the cow's milk and it goes without saying that no sugar is going to be as effective in this formula as the sugar in the human mother's milk. It wouldn't be so important what kind of sugar we use if its purpose was just to supply calories. But this sugar is going to be used for building a nervous system!

Is milk a good food for adults? We have presented above considerable evidence both pro and con. The nutritionists, by and large, are convinced that it is. But every once in a while in the midst of their glowing tributes to the wholesomeness of milk we run across statements like the following. On page 376 of the ninth edition of *Hutchinson's Food and Dietetics,* which we mentioned earlier, the author is describing some of the infectious diseases and epidemics traced to milk. He ends by saying "These are but a small sample culled mainly from one medical journal during six months. It is no wonder that (the) many medical men look upon milk as a highly dangerous food." At this point in our research we gaped and blinked and muttered, "Come again?" These are the same authors who told us at the beginning of this article that all nutritionists are agreed on the value of milk in human nutrition. After pages of fulsome praise of milk as the well nigh perfect food, a statement that many medical men consider it dangerous leaves us wondering indeed.

Milk and Antibiotics

The Food and Drug Administration in Washington has forbidden until recently the use of antibiotics as preservatives in food, because "the consumption of food so treated may cause sensitization of the consumer to such antibiotics and may result in the emergence of strains of pathogenic microorganisms resistant to these drugs." Within the past few years we have seen the use of antibiotics as food preservatives. There is a lively debate as to the possible harm that may result, even though the F.D.A. insists that all the antibiotic disappears in cooking. We are already getting too much antibiotics in food. Listen to this:

"A new form of aureomycin . . . (an antibiotic) that can be given orally to small animals and to calves is now being marketed . . . said to be especially effective in treatment of scours and pneumonia." This article appeared in *Chemical Week* for February 27, 1954

In the *Drug Trade News* for December 7, 1953, came the warning "Antibiotics No Panaceas, Animal Men Warned. A caution on over-dependence on antibiotics by cattle, sheep and poultry raisers was sounded at a meeting of the Agricultural Research Institute here recently by George H. Hart, dean of the University of California veterinary school."

Dr. Hart emphasized that he was not advising farmers to give up the use of antibiotics entirely, either in animal feeds or as drugs, but he warned against placing sole dependence on them. We gather from this that antibiotics are administered to farm animals just about as indiscriminately as they are given to human beings. Dr. Hart seemed to think that lack of attention to nutrition and sanitation may result in trouble.

The Lancet (a British medical journal) reported in August 22, 1953, that the American use of antibiotics in animal food had finally resulted in England adopting regulations that permit the use of penicillin and aureomycin in food for quick fattening of pigs and poultry. Mind you, this is not just drugs for sick animals. Antibiotics are now being incorporated into *food* for animals. They get a small amout of antibiotic every day. According to *Nutrition Abstracts and Reviews* for volume 23, 1953, no one knows just how soon the intestinal bacteria of the animals will develop resistance to the antibiotics, nor is it known whether the farmer actually saves money on the deal because of the cost of the antibiotics, but "it is reasonable to expect a small margin of profit."

Sensitivity to Penicillin is Increasing

Our file on antibiotics is crammed full and running over with clippings on the dangers of widespread use of antibiotics. The November 9, 1953 issue of *Time* magazine carried the story of a meeting of the world's top authorities on antibiotics where Dr. Harry F. Dowling sounded the keynote by saying "as each antibiotic is introduced, we hear first of miraculous cures, second of deleterious reactions and third of the appearance of resistant strains (of bacteria)." There was plenty of talk about the increasing numbers of serious or fatal reactions to antibiotics. Dr. Ethan Allen Brown of Boston called today's use of antibiotics "appalling." He said that it is misleading to speak only of patients who appear to have died instantaneously from reaction to antibiotics. There are more deaths which never make the headlines. Still more numerous are the reactions short of death. And finally, most frequent of all are the allergic reactions which are never reported anywhere because the patient did not die. He continued, "What the medical reports fail to stress is how many had wished themselves dead. Of these exquisitely sensitive-to-penicillin patients, I am one."

From the *Pittsburgh Press* for June 6, 1954, comes the news that antibiotics are now being used on plants—to combat hitherto incurable plant blights which have been destroying millions of dollars worth of crops. Terramycin and streptomycin are being used to cure "fireblight" in apple trees, for instance.

We found another yellowed clipping from the Kansas City *Star* for February 22, 1951, revealing that Dr. Alton Ochsner (whose recent book on smoking and lung cancer is making history) stated at a meeting that the incidence of blood clotting had doubled in the past five years, the chief reason for which was the use of the antibiotics which tend to increase the clotting tendency. "Because of penicillin and other infection-fighting drugs, the medical profession will have to find new methods to save lives from blood clots," said he.

Penicillin dog tags were proposed in all seriousness by the chief of an allergy clinic in New York in a statement released by the American

Foundation for Allergic Diseases on December 22, 1953. Said Dr. Horace Baldwin two out of every hundred patients now suffer penicillin reactions ranging from hives to high fever and severe joint pains that may last several months. Among the million or so Americans who suffer from asthma and the six million allergics the rate is considerably higher and shock and death may result from exposure to antibiotics. He suggested that dog tags be worn by persons known to be penicillin-sensitive.

Does your Milk Contain Penicillin?

This is but a smattering of the material on penicillin and the other antibiotics that we have in our files. Then we have a quote from *Food* for July, 1952, written by the director of the Express Dairy Company, London. Says he: "The general use of penicillin for combatting mastitis (in cows) from about 1945 onwards has resulted in considerable trouble in the cheese industry, due to the antagonistic effect of the residual penicillin in the milk used for starter cultures. Instances have been known where farms and factories have been forced to discontinue cheese-making. The same effect may occur with yogurt manufacture. Ordinary pasteurization has little effect on any penicillin-milk and even autoclaving (heating at high temperature and pressure) will not remove it."

We have not been able to find any investigation that has been done on the possible residues of cleaning fluids in milk. Of course all the equipment involved in processing milk—from the milking machine right on down to the bottling machine—must be cleaned often and thoroughly. Since milk is a fluid in which bacteria can grow and flourish, the materials used for cleaning must be strong and antiseptic indeed. We suppose that each local dairy has its own cleaning methods. How much of the cleaning fluids remain in the milk? We have no way of knowing, but we think you should take this into account when you are adding up the pluses and the minuses where milk is concerned.

Milk From Goats

Everyone has his favorite food and everyone should be allowed to cheer for whatever special food it is that he enjoys, that makes him feel good or that has apparently helped him to recover from an illness. Goat's milk is that favorite food to lots of health-conscious folks in this country. We have received many letters asking, nay, demanding that we publish full information about goat's milk, since it is the wonder food, according to these correspondents.

We have done careful research and we report below the facts about goat's milk as we found them. We're sorry that they don't seem to add up to the extravagant claims made for goat's milk among the champions of this food. From what we could discover, goat's milk is just about the same as cow's milk except for a few differences which we will discuss.

First of all, so far as vitamin and mineral content is concerned, here are the figures on the two kinds of milk, both in the fluid, whole state:

	Cow's Milk	*Goat's Milk*
Calcium	118 mg.	129 mg.
Phosphorus	93 mg.	106 mg.
Iron	.1 mg.	.1 mg.
Sodium	50 mg.	34 mg.
Potassium	144 mg.	180 mg.
Vitamin A	160 Int. Units	160 Int. Units
Vitamin B		
Thiamin	.04 mg.	.04 mg.
Riboflavin	.17 mg	.11 mg.
Niacin	.1 mg.	.3 mg.
Vitamin C	1 mg.	1 mg.

These figures indicate that the vitamin and mineral content of the two milks is very similar. A little more calcium, phosphorus and potassium in the goat's milk seems to be the only difference worth mentioning. So sweeping statements about the vast superiority of goat's milk over cow's milk so far as nutrition is concerned seem to be unjustified.

Goat's Milk is Naturally Homogenized

There is one characteristic of goat's milk that does recommend it especially for babies and invalids. The globules of fat in goat's milk are considerably smaller than those of cow's milk. This makes for easier digestion. The curd of the milk is softer. So it seems quite possible that infants who could not digest cow's milk due to the size of the fat globules might take goat's milk with a lot less trouble. However, when cow's milk is homogenized, the fat globules are broken up until they are as small as those of goat's milk. So drinking the latter should have just about the same effect as drinking homogenized cow's milk, so far as digestibility is concerned.

It seems quite possible that before milk was homogenized, goat's milk was the only answer for infants who could not digest the larger globules of the cow's milk. And perhaps from this circumstance came the reputation of goat's milk as the wonder food. Any mother whose baby has kept her awake night after night vomiting, crying and apparently starving would surely hail as a wonder food any food that the baby could digest, and keep down. No one can blame those mothers for declaring that goat's milk saved their babies' lives. It did, obviously. But it seems probable that today's homogenized cow's milk might work just as well, doesn't it?

A. K. Besley, Ph.D. of the U. S. Department of Agriculture, Beltzville Station, did a very careful study of the nutritive value of the two kinds of milk which he reported in the *American Journal of Public Health* for February, 1940. Rats and goat kids were used for the experiment. One group received goat's milk and the other cow's milk. Dr. Besley tells us that there was little difference in results. Gains in weight took place in proportion to the total energy contained in the milk, regardless of which kind it was. This was true of both raw and boiled milk. All of the experimental animals eventually developed anemia, for both kinds of milk are deficient in anti-anemia factors. Another experiment involved four babies fed goat's milk and three fed cow's milk. Once again, there was no difference in the health of the babies. These were of course normal healthy babies to start with. They had not shown any allergic tendencies or any inability to digest cow's milk.

Dr. Besley tells us further that the bacteria count in the goat's milk they used (from the Beltzville herd) was extremely low so a goat milk producer should have little trouble meeting the standards for the production of milk.

Goat's Milk and Anemia

The *Journal of Biological Chemistry,* volume 77, page 797, 1928, mentions the fact that a different kind of anemia may be produced by goat's milk. As we know, a diet consisting entirely of milk will produce anemia for there is very little iron in any kind of milk. But, according to E. B. Hart and his fellow workers, iron and copper will not cure the anemia brought on by a diet of nothing but goat's milk. It seems that goat's milk lacks sufficient vitamin B_{12}. An investigation in 1951 indicated that it contains about .15 micrograms of the vitamin whereas cow's milk contains 3 to 4 micrograms per liter. Lack of folic acid (another B vitamin) may also be responsible.

An article in *Deutsche Medizinische Wochenschrift* for October 26, 1951, describes several cases of anemia caused by goat's milk. This is related to pernicious anemia. It involves the inability of the blood to renew itself. In these cases, vitamin B_{12} and folic acid together brought about a cure. However, say the authors, a diet of goat's milk alone can also produce iron-deficiency anemia, just as an exclusive diet of cow's milk can. Nutritional damage occurs more readily with goat's milk, they say. They also tell us that the goats whose milk caused the anemia had been kept in the stable and did not receive any fresh fodder. So the folic acid that is in fresh green leaves did not show up in their milk.

Does Goat's Milk Cure Infantile Eczema?

In another article in *Prevention* on milk we tell the story of some cases of allergies to cow's milk that were cured by drinking goat's milk. Or perhaps we should say they were cured by omitting cow's milk from the diet. If the child was not allergic to goat's milk, the eczema or whatever other form the allergy took would disappear. Stories like these apparently led some people to the conclusion that goat's milk would cure eczema.

A letter to the editor of the *British Medical Journal* for March 29, 1952, tells of a number of babies at a British hospital who suffered from eczema. Taking away the cow's milk from their diet and giving them goat's milk instead cured the eczema. And any attempt to return to cow's milk brought the eczema back again. This letter drew two answers in the May 3, 1952, issue of the *Journal.* One doctor reminds us that there are many crossed reactions between cow and goat lactalbumin. This is the substance in milk that supposedly is the allergic substance. In one series of cases, he says, of 44 infants with eczema who could not take cow's milk, 25 of them could not take goat's milk either!

The other answer tells of a two-month-old baby who could not drink any of the cow's milk available in England. The physician found out that the baby was allergic to fish and the cows were fed a fish-containing meal supplied by the government. He obtained a source of goat milk and extracted a promise from the owners of the goat that they would not feed it on government-supplied meal. The baby's allergy disappeared.

Goat's milk surely seems to be superior as human food in one respect. That is, the goat mother's milk was designed for a baby who weighs about eight pounds at birth, as a human infant does. Cow's milk is meant for a calf which weighs some 45 pounds at birth. One other aspect of the goat's milk reputation for healthfulness may be that, in this country, goats are raised chiefly by folks who know about the rules of good health. They are quite likely to be people who understand the reasons for organic farming, who know how important "live" food is compared with "dead" food, who would raise goats as healthy and strong as any animal could be. Perhaps milk from such animals has many advantages over cow's milk bought from a dairy where all the milk purchased that day is mixed together and the degree of health of every cow involved has something to do with the final product. So mass production may be responsible for much of our feeling against cow's milk as compared with goat's milk.

Milk, Insecticides In

Dairy animals exposed to DDT pass it along in their milk. According to Morton S. Biskind, M. D. writing in the *American Journal of Digestive Diseases* for November, 1953, the body fat is called a "biological magnifier" of DDT by Food and Drug investigators. When as little as one-tenth of a part per million is included in the diet, the body fat may reach concentrations up to 150 times as much. DDT can be found in all body tissues, in proportion to their fat content.

Dr. Biskind then tells us of the investigation of Dendy in Texas, who bought meat and milk from July through December. Every sample of these two staples contained DDT—the milk varying from less than .5 parts per million to 13.8 parts per million. As a result of this and other investigations, the Food and Drug Administration issued an order permitting no tolerance for DDT in milk or other dairy products. This means that, for milk shipped across state borders, no DDT is permitted in the milk. However, most of us drink milk produced and sold locally, over which the Food and Drug Administration has no control. The feed eaten by the milk cows may be contaminated with DDT, the barn may be sprayed with it, the cow herself may be sprayed. Unless there is a local law setting a fine for the occurrence of any DDT in milk, there is nothing to protect us from the virulence of gradual accumulation of this poison, for DDT accumulates in the tissues and we may not know for years what damage it has done.

Milk, Getting Enough Vitamins Without It

If you are planning to give up milk entirely, it will be well to check over your diet and make sure you are getting from other foods those vitamins that are in milk. The minerals of course you can get from bone meal. Here is a brief review of the vitamins in milk and the foods in which they are most plentiful.

Vitamin A is a fat soluble vitamin, which means that it can be stored in your body and you do not need to have it every day. But you must be certain you are getting enough of it, for lack of it can cause: night blindness, sensitivity to glare, difficulty reading in dim light, inability to store fat. It is absolutely essential for skin health, for fighting colds and other infections, for preventing kidney stones and for promoting growth and dental health in children. It is most plentiful in green and yellow foods, for it comes from a substance called carotene which is yellow. These foods are rich in vitamin A: carrots, collards, dandelion greens, endive, beef liver, mustard greens, sweet potatoes, turnip greens, watercress, egg yolk, and of course fish liver oil which is by far the richest source. We advise taking fish liver oil as a food supplement every day.

The B vitamins should always be taken together as they appear in food—don't ever let yourself be trapped into taking a pill that contains only one or several of the B vitamins— they are made synthetically when they appear this way and you may do yourself immeasurable harm by throwing your supply of the other B vitamins out of balance, for they all work together and your body must have all of them in the proper balance, which is the way they appear in food. The B vitamins are water soluble— this means that you excrete every day whatever you have not used that day. So they must constantly be replaced; they are not stored in the body. Our national shortage of B vitamins was brought about largely by refining foods. They have been carefully removed from all our cereals, breads and flour. True, a few synthetic B vitamins have then been added, but these cannot possibly make up for what has been removed.

The Importance of B vitamins

Milk is rich in several of the B vitamins, so if you do not drink milk you must watch closely to make certain that you get plenty of them in other food. In general the B vitamins are necessary for the following reasons: thiamin protects the health of the digestive tract and the nervous system, is good for the muscles of the stomach and intestines, prevents constipation, prevents beri beri. Lack of riboflavin may result in skin and mouth disorders, scaly patches and cracks at the corner of the mouth, burning feet, burning and dryness of the eyes, dislike for bright lights. Niacin prevents pellagra, diarrhea, depression, dermatitis, tender gums, insomnia, loss of appetite, neurasthenia, anxiety, dizziness, fatigue, backache and nervousness. Pantothenic acid is important for skin health and a youthful appearance, relieves some kinds of neuritis and alcoholic neuroses, may help to keep hair from graying. Lack of pyridoxine causes (in animal experiments) skin disorders, bad muscle tone, heart symptoms, anemia, insomnia, nervousness, irritability.

In animals choline, another B vitamin, help to prevent: high blood pressure, cancer, fatty liver, anemia, liver trouble, hardening of the arteries, goiter. Inositol helps prevent hardening of the arteries and protects the muscles, including the heart muscle. Vitamin B_{12} is the cure for pernicious anemia. It has also been used in the treatment of: multiple sclerosis, alcoholism, diabetes, arthritis, osteoporosis. Biotin, another B vitamin, is necessary to prevent: fatigue, muscular pains, loss of appetite, dryness of skin, nervousness. Para-amino-benzoic acid is necessary for the proper use of the other B vitamins by the body. It may also be involved in preventing gray hair.

The foods in which the B vitamins are most abundant are: dried legumes, liver, kidney, heart and other organ meats, egg yolk, wheat bran, wheat germ, soybeans, leafy vegetables, rice bran and rice germ, peanuts, and of course brewer's yeast and desiccated liver—two food supplements which we believe should be in everyone'e diet.

Milk is not important as a source of vitamin C. This vitamin you get from fresh raw fruits and vegetables. It is extremely important from all aspects of health. Get plenty of it. Rose hips and other vitamin C supplements made from natural foods are the richest sources in food supplements.

Vitamin D does not exist in very large quantities in foods. In general, children, who need vitamin D more than adults, get it from the sunshine, for it is formed in the skin by the action of sunlight on some substance in the skin. Its richest food source is fish liver oil. Vitamin E is extremely important for the health of all the body muscles, including the heart. It is also important for the health of the reproductive system. Vegetable and cereal oils are the richest sources. Vitamin K helps the blood to clot properly. It is most plentiful in green leafy vegetables. Vitamin P occurs along with vitamin C in fresh raw foods. It is important to prevent hemorrhaging.

Milk—Harmfulness of Artificial Insemination

By J. I. Rodale
Editor of *Prevention*

An article in the Spring, 1955, issue of *Arkansas Farm Research*, a journal published by the Arkansas Agricultural Experiment Station, begins: "The practice of artificial breeding has disclosed the occurance of sterility in dairy cattle, and resultant economic loss." (These agriculturists are atrocious spellers. *Occurrence* should have two *r*'s and an *e* instead of the *a*.) But God bless 'em for publishing this admission of the troubles ahead for artificially inseminated or test-tube cows.

A study was conducted from 1949 to 1951 in conjunction with the Arkansas Artificial Breeders' Association, and covered cows in 22 counties, mostly in northwest Arkansas. During that time it was found that in the artificially inseminated cows, out of a possible 100 per cent conception or birth rate, only about 66 per cent "took." This is far far below the normal conception rate and involves huge economic losses. In all, in this study, there were 31,045 attempts at conception by means of test-tubes instead of in the way that nature intended.

Many of the cows failed to conceive after three or more artificial attempts and too many of them showed signs of disease—pus in the vaginal mucus. What was most disturbing was that a lot of the cows did not have a "heat" period for from 2 to 4 months, and young heifers lacked the heat period at breeding age. We must bear in mind that agriculture is only at the beginning stages of this artificial insemination crime against the cow. What will happen in another 20 to 30 years?

Why doesn't agricultural science back out before it is too late? But no! It would be a disastrous loss of face. The usual procedure in science when an artificial practice produces reverberations, is to find something even more artificial to hold things in line, until finally the result is a fearful, synthetic Frankenstein which can run amok at any moment.

But let us return to the Arkansas Experimental Station article. What do they do to these sick, artificially inseminated cows? Do they tell them to go home and see a bull? Why, no, bless your heart. They dose them up with antibiotics. That's what they do.

The animals suffering from functional sterility were given penicillin G sodium, and later on penicillin and di-hydro-streptomycin sulphate. But this is hardly the place to give the complete list of stuff they shot into these poor, unfortunate defenseless cows. However, I *did* notice stilbestrol in the list, a drug which is known to *produce* sterility. In the meantime, what happens to the milk of cows who have been heavily dosed with medicaments and who, later, conceive and give milk? My opinion is to boycott milk until this lewd, shameless, dangerous practice is desisted from. I and thousands of others have been getting along beautifully without milk. One half the population of the world does not drink milk. So if you decide not to drink it anymore, don't worry about it. You won't die. There is always bone meal for your calcium.

Minerals

For thousands of years we have been eating trace minerals without ever being aware of them, without knowing that they are in the soil, in our food and in our bodies. Within very recent times equipment has been perfected for detecting and measuring trace minerals. And for the first time there is tremendous scientific interest in the whole subject. In many universities and colleges across the land careful studies are being made of the importance of each of the trace minerals, where it is found, what part it plays in the life of plants or animals, how it may be related to health and disease, with what other food elements it works, and how it can be used to promote health for soil, plants and living things.

And high time it is that such studies should be undertaken. For among many top-ranking scientists there is absolute conviction that one of the main causes of today's degenerative diseases is the lack of trace elements or minerals in the soil and in the food. This decrease or complete lack of certain trace minerals has not come about suddenly. And in some cases it is not the result of man's carelessness. For instance, there are parts of the world where sheep cannot be successfully raised. The lambs will, for no apparent reason, develop diseases of the nervous system. The reason turned out quite recently to be the fact that there is not enough copper in the soil and the lambs are suffering from a copper deficiency.

Now who would ever imagine such a thing as this! Copper is a bright, shiny, reddish metal that makes very pretty living room accessories. And copper is used to make pipes which some people have installed in their homes for water pipes, with a resulting greenish tinge to the water indicating that the folks in that house are probably getting a most unhealthful dose of copper along with their water. Now how could lack of such a metal have anything to do with the nervous disease of lambs? But it does. And copper is extremely important for human health. It helps the body to use iron. It's perfectly possible for you to develop iron-deficiency anemia if you aren't getting enough copper in your food, even though you are getting enough iron.

Cobalt is a trace mineral that nobody heard anything about until the past few years. Then, through the lengthy, patient work of a group of scientists, it was discovered that cobalt is necessary in cattle food or the cattle will develop anemia. But the dictionary defines cobalt as "a tough, lustrous, silver-white, somewhat magnetic metal related to and occurring with, iron and nickel." What could such a metal have to do with anemia? As more and more scientists and nutritionists delved deeper into the problem, it finally developed that cobalt is one of the important elements in vitamin B_{12}—the miracle vitamin which prevents and cures anemia. Is it the cobalt alone that does the trick? No, the other parts of the vitamin must be present too.

You Need Only a Small Amount of Each Trace Mineral

Perhaps the first and most important thing to understand about the trace minerals is that they are necessary in infinitely small quantities. That is one reason we have been so long in studying them. Calcium and phosphorus occur in food and in our bodies in relatively large amounts. A bone or a tooth looks as if it were made of calcium or lime and it is to a large extent. When you boil a bone, adding a little vinegar to the water, you finally come out with a bone that is honeycombed with small holes—the holes where the calcium was. The calcium has passed into the soup you are making. So it's fairly easy to understand that calcium is essential—we can see it with our own eyes.

But the trace minerals that go to make up that bone are just as important as the calcium, even though they leave no visible holes when you take them away. For without these trace minerals the calcium could not have combined with the phosphorus and you would not have a bone at all.

A couple of years ago two doctors at Cornell Medical College announced that they had given strontium to patients whose bones were too porous. And the strontium aided greatly in healing the bones. The patients were relieved of pain and went back to work. Strontium? Who ever heard of strontium as something desirable to eat? This is just an instance of the discoveries that are being made every day, now that, at last, we have begun to investigate the trace minerals.

Some of the trace minerals like iodine, for instance, occur in such extremely small quantities in food and water that we cannot measure them in terms of "parts per million," but can only speak of "parts per thousand million." Of course you could not see this small an amount of iodine in a teaspoon of bone meal let's say. You could not even imagine how infinitely small such an amount would be. But it is there and the fact that it is there probably has a great deal to do with your good health, if you are taking bone meal. For you need iodine only in infinitely small quantities. But you must have it for good health.

Another important thing to remember about trace minerals is that they are all beneficial to you when they are present in the right amounts in relation to all the other trace minerals and the vitamins. All of them are important, even though the amount needed may vary greatly in every case. Together with carbohydrates, proteins, fats and vitamins they make up everything necessary for the health of plants and animals. How they do this is still largely a mystery.

In the case of some of the trace minerals like iodine and iron we have a pretty good idea of what they do in the body. Iodine helps to manufacture thyroxine, the substance necessary for the thyroid gland. Iron helps in the manufacture of hemoglobin, the red substance in the blood that carries oxygen to the cells. In the case of many of the trace minerals we know that they combine with other minerals and with vitamins to form enzyme systems which carry on most of the physiological work that goes on inside our bodies. Without the trace minerals, these enzyme systems simply won't function normally. So it seems that the trace minerals are very important indeed so far as health is concerned.

But never forget that trace minerals in too large a quantity are dangerous. We all know how unhealthful it is to drink even a couple of tablespoons of iodine. Yet iodine in "trace" amounts is an absolute necessity for health. In just the same way, getting even a tiny bit too much of the other trace minerals is dangerous. Nature has very carefully doled them out in infinitely small amounts. Meddling, by way of using larger amounts, is likely to result in trouble.

Trace Minerals In the Treatment and Prevention of Disease

Doctor William A. Albrecht of the University of Missouri has been using trace minerals in treating cows for Bang's Disease. He had already determined that the sick cows had deficiencies of some of the trace minerals. Dr. Ira Allison of Springfield, Missouri has been working with

Albrecht and has treated human patients for brucellosis (milk fever). An article in the *Chicago Daily News* for March 13, 1950 tells us that of 1800 brucellosis patients a high percentage have been cured on a high protein, low sugar diet with trace minerals added. In some cases the cure took only 12 weeks. In almost every case, Dr. Allison said, there was indication of very bad habits of nutrition long before the disease appeared, seeming to indicate that the lack of these essential nutriments was responsible for the appearance of the disease.

Dr. Henry Trautmann of Madison, Wisconsin said in the same article, "Chemical farming overstimulates the soils to produce bountiful crops. Strange to say, however, disease continues apace. So it is evident that there are some vital elements lacking in the soil and the food it produces naturally lacks the same vital elements.

"Little is known of the effect of the various chemical fertilizers on the plant protein molecule. Since the protein molecule is the basis of life, its change of structure might well be the basis of ill health.

"The problems of malignancies may, sooner or later, be found in such chemical changes. It certainly is true that man's interference with nature processes has much to do with poor health."

Some time ago we received a copy of a beautiful Finnish magazine which contained the story of a little country town in Finland where a group of people were curing cancer with the ashes of the bark of a certain kind of birch tree that grew there. Now certainly there is nothing about ashes that has any curative property, except that when the bark is burned whatever minerals exist in it remain in the ashes, in concentrated form, for of course all the burnable part of the wood is gone. We had the article translated and made many efforts to get in touch with the folks whose names were given in the article, but without success. If any readers have further information about this, we'd appreciate their letting us know.

Is Multiple Sclerosis Related to Lack of Trace Minerals in Soil?

James A. Shield, M. D. of the Medical College of Virginia, writing in the *Southern Medical Bulletin* for January, 1947, says "In the occurrence of multiple sclerosis in Germany, England, Northern Europe in general and the United States where large amounts of inorganic incomplete chemical fertilizers are used by farmers, in contrast to the absence of multiple sclerosis in China, Japan and India where natural fertilizers or manures are used, nature presents us with a challenging fact.

"Farm practices which influence the total quality of the crop and, in turn, the quality of man's food, are the concern of this paper. Thus the soil, as a source of man's food, especially the trace elements, becomes the physician's problem. The doctor must demand that the agriculturist produce a food that will meet the multiple protoplasmic needs for optimal growth, development and function. Prescribing a good diet is not enough. There is a very wide variation in the composition of fruits, vegetables, grains and meats, milk and eggs when produced on different soils, in different sections of the country, on different farms, or even on different fields of the same farm. The Peckham Pioneer Health Service Centre in England discovered that feeding families in the Centre with ordinary, so-called balanced food diet bought from a shop was not enough. They were forced to grow the food themselves and to use not new methods but the ancient method of returning waste to the soil. Man's interference with the perfect balance between the natural processes of growth and decay may be largely responsible for the predicament of our malnutrition, in spite of adequate diet by the present standards."

We are one hundred per cent in agreement with Dr. Shield's theory. We believe that not only multiple sclerosis, but many other degenerative diseases, like arthritis, muscular dystrophy, cancer, heart trouble, polio and so forth may be due, in part at least, to a lack of trace minerals and a lack of balance of trace minerals in the food we eat.

Where Can You Get Your Essential Trace Minerals?

Look at the list of trace minerals in various foods on another page. You will notice that such foods as white bread, noodles, white rice, sugar, soft drinks, hot dogs, ice cream and so forth are not listed. They contain no trace minerals, for all the minerals have been refined out of such foods. So obviously people who live on this kind of food cannot be healthy for they lack any trace minerals at all.

But what about the health conscious folks who are careful not to eat refined and processed foods, who eat lots of fresh fruits and vegetables, no cereals but whole cereals, meats, eggs and the other foods that *do* contain trace minerals? Well and good, if the food they are eating comes from a farmer, or even a field of one farm where the trace minerals exist in the soil in a well balanced harmony. But what if, buying commercially grown food in their part of the country, they get the tomatoes with only one part per million of iron rather than those with 1938 parts per million? What if they have been eating, over the years, the cabbage that contains no cobalt, rather than cabbage that contains the infinitely small amount of .15 parts per million that may mean the difference between health and disease?

Do you see now why we urge readers to eat organically grown food, even if it means digging up the lawn or traveling out into the country to garden over weekends? We'd like to be able to tell you very definitely just why you need a certain amount of manganese, copper, potassium, magnesium, and so forth in your food. We'd like to be able to tell you how much of each of these you need. We'd like to be able to tell you just how much of each of them exists in every piece of food you prepare in your kitchen. But for the answers to the first two questions we must wait probably for years until the answers have been found in the laboratories. For an answer to the last question, we would have to place a battery of scientists and a laboratory of equipment in your kitchen to work night and day.

What is the answer, then? Must you do without these vitally important trace minerals? Must you take a chance on contracting a disease that results from a deficiency? No. The thing for you to do is first of all, get organically grown food if possible. If you can't possibly have your own garden, try to persuade a friend to garden organically. Buy as much food as you can from advertisers who farm organically.

In addition, eat only foods that *may* contain trace minerals. Soft drinks don't. White bread doesn't. White sugar and all the nuisance foods that spring from it are devoid of trace minerals. Eat vegetables, fruits, meats, eggs, fish, nuts, poultry. And finally take minerals with your food supplements. Bone meal contains trace minerals. Kelp contains trace minerals. In fact, if you live in a "goiter area," kelp tablets and ocean fish are essentials in your diet program. The sea contains many minerals which are absorbed by the seaweed, kelp.

It isn't hard to take bone meal or kelp. And it isn't expensive. It will cost you less than your weekly chocolate sundae which we urge you to relinquish anyway. You can buy these two mineral-rich foods in tablet or powder form. If you're squeamish about taste or if you have little time to fuss with foods, buy the tablets and swallow them down. If you don't mind going out of your way to do little extras in the kitchen, get used to including the powdered form (much less expensive) in all kinds of foods. Beat it into health drinks. Bake it in your whole grain bread. Sprinkle it over cereal or fruits. No matter how you may decide to take them, do get your trace minerals. There is nothing else in food that can substitute for them.

To demonstrate the difference in minerals and trace minerals available in food, we reproduce here a chart showing the highest and lowest quantity found in five vegetables tested at Rutgers University. This material was originally part of the Firman E. Bear Report:

	Percentage of Dry Weight		Millequivalents per 100 grams dry weight				Trace Elements parts per million dry matter				
	Total Mineral Matter	Phosphorus	Calcium	Magnesium	Potassium	Sodium	Boron	Manganese	Iron	Copper	Cobalt
SNAP BEANS											
Highest	10.45	0.36	40.5	60.00	99.7	8.6	73	60	227	69	0.26
Lowest	4.04	0.22	15.5	14.8	29.1	0.0	10	2	10	3	0.00
CABBAGE											
Highest	10.38	0.38	60.0	43.6	148.3	20.4	42	13	94	48	0.15
Lowest	6.12	0.18	17.5	15.6	53.7	0.8	7	2	20	0.4	0.00
LETTUCE											
Highest	24.48	0.43	71.0	49.3	176.5	12.2	37	169	516	60	0.19
Lowest	7.01	0.22	16.0	13.1	53.7	0.0	6	1	9	3	0.00
TOMATOES											
Highest	14.20	0.35	23.0	59.2	148.3	6.5	36	68	1938	53	0.63
Lowest	6.07	0.16	4.5	4.5	58.8	0.0	5	1	1	0	0.00
SPINACH											
Highest	28.56	0.52	96.0	203.9	257.0	69.5	88	117	1584	32	0.25
Lowest	12.38	0.27	47.5	46.9	84.6	0.8	12	1	19	0.5	0.20

Moles

It is believed that all human beings, except albinos, have at least one mole. Some people have hundreds of them, varying in size all the way from microscopic pin points to enormous discolorations covering a large part of the body. A mole is a growth or a tumor, which differs from other growths in that its cells collect melanin, the pigment that colors skin and hair. This gives the mole its characteristic color. Some moles are not raised from the skin while others look warty, and others appear to grow on a stalk almost like a mushroom. In general people have two distinct opinions about moles. Many people with moles go through life fearful lest the moles become malignant, and worrying constantly whether or not they should have them removed. Others ignore the moles entirely and may very well ignore a mole which is actually becoming malignant and should be removed.

By far the largest proportion of all moles are harmless and should give one no cause for alarm. The kind of mole that is flush with the skin, the brown mole, the one from which hairs grow—none of these is likely to become cancerous. But the black mole, especially the blue-black, green-black or slate-colored one, is a likely candidate for cancer, and should be removed. A mole on the sole of the foot can be quite dangerous too and should be removed. Then, of course, any mole that occurs at a place where there is constant friction or irritation (under the armpit, on the shaving area of the face, etc.) should be removed, for the irritation is likely to produce malignancy in the mole. Aside from these circumstances, there is no need to worry about any mole, unless it presents a cosmetic problem.

On the other hand, if you have any doubts about your mole fitting into one of the above categories, or if it suddenly begins to grow, you would do well to see your doctor at once and have the mole removed. For malignancy in a mole can result in the most deadly and rapid kind of cancer. Removal of a mole is easily done by surgery under local anesthetic or burning off with an electric needle. These operations should be undertaken, of course, before the mole has a chance to become cancerous, for after the cancer has begun to grow, desperate surgical measures may be needed, even to amputating an arm or leg.

So our advice on moles resolves itself to this: if you have a mole that falls into the classifications mentioned as dangerous, it might be best to have it removed at once before you have any trouble with it. For other kinds of moles, forget about them. In many countries they are considered a mark of great beauty.

Mouth

While it is healthy, probably no part of your body functions so efficiently and apparently so effortlessly as your mouth. You're not conscious of it, are you? The chomping teeth, the saliva that slips down every time you swallow, the tongue that helps you to swallow, chew and talk,—you accept these blessings without comment until the time comes when something goes wrong in your mouth. Perhaps nothing can be more annoying than a fever blister or a sore spot on the tip of your tongue. If you have the misfortune to suffer a really serious mouth infection, your troubles will be multiplied by the fact that you simply can't eat with a sore mouth. And, before you get well, you are likely to develop a full-fledged state of deficiency.

All by yourself, with the help of a mirror, you can discover a number of things about the health of your mouth that will tell you important things about your general health. Look first at the color. The tissues should be a healthy pink. If they are pale or whitish you may have some form of anemia and you should certainly have your doctor check to see.

Look at your gums next. Are they solid, firm, clinging closely around the stems of your teeth? That's how healthy gums look. Or are they boggy and swollen? Do they bleed easily? Do they fit closely around your teeth, especially right at the base? Are any of your teeth loose—can you move them back and forth with your finger? All of these symptoms indicate a sad lack of nutritional fitness. Vitamins A, B and C are all involved in the health of these tissues. Vitamin C is especially important, for scurvy—the disease resulting from vitamin C deficiency—produces many of these symptoms.

Now, look at your tongue. Is it pink and rough, with no deep indentations and no tooth marks on the sides? That is how a healthy tongue should appear. If it is scarlet red, beefy red or magenta in color, this is an indication of nutritional deficiency. If it is or has been swollen, you will see the indentation marks of teeth on it. This too indicates deficiency of the B vitamins.

The roughness of a healthy tongue is made up of the little nodules that occur there naturally. If your tongue is smooth and shiny, those nodules have disappeared or atrophied. This generally results from a deficiency of all the B complex vitamins, with special emphasis on riboflavin, niacin, vitamin B_{12} and folic acid. When there are deep indentations in the tongue, it is called "geographic tongue" by nutritionists, because it looks like a relief map of a mountainous land. This too is the result of deficiency in the B vitamins.

Do you have little red sore spots around the edges of your tongue or at the tip? Niacin deficiency can cause this. And, even though niacin is one of the B vitamins, don't make the mistake of getting niacin at your drug store and taking it by itself. All of the B vitamins work together and to make sure you have no deficiency in any of them, you must take all of them, as they occur in food, such as brewer's yeast. Canker sores in and around the mouth may result from too little vitamin B. If the condition becomes serious, trench mouth or Vincent's disease may result. This is a most unpleasant and painful ailment in which the entire inside of the mouth is covered with ulcers. It has been cured with niacin and the other B vitamins.

Your lips are indicative of good health, too. *Cheilosis* and *angular stomatitis* are two very common signs of vitamin deficiency. These are cracks at the corners of the mouth, which may remain open and sore for a long time. Perhaps they are not even painful, but when you open your mouth slightly, they are clearly visible at each corner. These are generally indicative of vitamin B deficiency.

But they may also indicate malocclusion. In these latter cases, the teeth do not meet as they should when the mouth is closed and the overlapping at the corners of the mouth invites the growth of fungus. Or it may be that badly-fitting dentures have caused the cracks. Or dentures that fit well are removed at night, leaving a fold at the corner of the mouth where saliva and bacteria can accumulate. Any of these may be the cause of cracks at the corner of the mouth.

The lips may appear to be chapped if there is serious vitamin deficiency. Flecks of skin scale off like sunburn peeling. At the same time there may be an increase in the number of vertical lines in the lips—those little wrinkles all of us have to some extent. The wrinkles may extend out beyond the area of the lips. And eventually the lips may gradually become smaller and smaller. You have often seen old folks whose nutrition is especially bad who appear to have no upper lip at all.

A nutritionist looks first at your mouth to make a diagnosis about the excellence of your nutrition. If you have one or several of the symptoms listed above, he knows that you are short on vitamin B, vitamin C and probably vitamin A as well. These are symptoms of deficiencies of these two vitamins. How do you prevent the symptoms and preserve a healthy mouth? Eat a good diet, high in protein, fresh raw fruits and vegetables. Skip the refined carbohydrates—products made from white flour and white sugar. Take food supplements—especially brewer's yeast for vitamin B and rose hips for vitamin C.

Multiple Sclerosis

Some time ago one of the women's magazines published an article on multiple sclerosis, written by a wife whose husband had, a short time ago, been supposedly dying of the disease. He was blind, paralyzed and so weak he could barely talk. Hospitals, operations, convulsions followed one another for years, and finally the doctors told his wife that he was suffering from multiple sclerosis and they gave him only a few years to live. Through a series of incidents, his case came to the attention of a doctor who told him he thought he didn't have multiple sclerosis at all; he thought he had hyperinsulinism. He began treatments for hyperinsulinism and within an amazingly short time the young husband was back at work, apparently cured.

This article indicated that the young man was put on a diet by the doctor who cured him, but it gave little or no idea of what the diet consisted. We thought we recognized both the doctor and the diet and, sure enough, in *The New York State Journal of Medicine* for June 1, 1954, we came across an article by E. M. Abrahamson, M. D. of New York City which seemed to give us the answer to our search. One of the cases given as illustrations in this article sounds like the case written about in the women's magazine, even to the initials of the patient

We have talked a great deal about Dr. Abrahamson in these pages, and we consider this article to be one of the most important he has ever written. He discusses 126 patients he saw over an 18-month period and states that in every case the multiple sclerosis patient was suffering from hyperinsulinism and also from lack of calcium. With injections of calcium and a diet to cure the hyperinsulinism, Dr. Abrahamson worked miracles.

What are all these long words—hyperinsulinism and multiple sclerosis? Multiple sclerosis is a disease involving the nervous system. It apparently brings about a hardening or degeneration of the nervous tissue, resulting in paralysis, blindness, dizzy spells, inability to walk properly and finally death in a wheelchair. Its cause, according to the medical books, is unknown. It may seem to be cured and then recur. Hyperinsulinism is another word for low blood sugar. It is the opposite of diabetes. The hyperinsulinism patient is releasing too much insulin for his body to handle, rather than too little, as is the case with the diabetic. Can such a disorder be related to multiple sclerosis? Dr. Abrahamson believes that it is.

How Low Blood Sugar May Bring About Serious Symptoms

He gives case histories of six patients, all of whom had been diagnosed as having multiple sclerosis. He tells us that in all the rest of the 126 cases the symptoms of hyperinsulinism were present. A doctor tests for hyperinsulinism, or low blood sugar, by giving what is called the glucose tolerance test, a rather elaborate test requiring six hours during which the blood sugar is tested hourly until the final check is made. However, one's own knowledge of oneself and one's food habits may give a very good clue as to the state of one's own blood sugar. Hunger, fatigue, headache, a few hours or less after eating strongly indicate low blood sugar, especially if the symptoms are relieved after you eat.

The process that takes place is simply this: taking food raises your blood sugar level. In persons whose apparatus is functioning well, the blood sugar drops a little after meals, then levels off to a plateau and stays this way until the next meal, when it is again slightly raised. This is one reason you feel good after a meal; you are less tired, less grumpy.

The person whose blood-sugar-regulating apparatus is not normal has a different experience. His blood sugar rises, too, right after a meal, but then it plunges far below where it should be. Result? Headache, fatigue, dizziness, grumpiness and/or hunger. He feels so restless and "all-gone" that he takes a piece of candy or cake. His blood sugar shoots up again and for a brief while he feels fine. Then it plunges and his symptoms return until his next meal. The ideal situation is to have your blood sugar level off to keep you happy and content with just a little hunger developing immediately before your next meal.

Why Do We Have Low Blood Sugar?

How does it happen that our grandfathers never heard of such a disorder? Dr. Abrahamson does not mince words as to the reason. He says "Two things have come into the human dietary in comparatively recent times—concentrated sweets and caffeine. Both of these cause an unnaturally rapid rise in blood sugar which may in time have a bad effect on the organs that regulate the blood sugar—the Islands of Langerhans. These organs may become so sensitized that they may begin to over-respond to normal stimuli which will result in quite wide fluctuations in blood sugar. The Islands of Langerhans are the organs that regulate the mechanisms for blood sugar control. Dr. Abrahamson tells us that many of the 126 patients described in this article reported that they consumed enormous amounts of candy or caffeine-containing beverages or both for many years. Then, too, it seemed that most of them had been through a period of great emotional stress which might also contribute to disordering the blood sugar apparatus. In addition they were short on calcium—a positive essential for healthy nerves.

The diet which Dr. Abrahamson prescribes for his low blood sugar patients is the Seale-Harris diet he made famous in his excellent book *Body, Mind and Sugar* (Published by Henry Holt and Co., New York). It is high in protein and fat, low in sugar and starch. For, strangely enough, it is an excess of sugar and starch in the diet that brings about low blood sugar. Eating protein and fat tends to cause the blood sugar to level off as it should.

The women's magazine we mentioned earlier did not describe the diet which worked such a miracle on their multiple sclerosis patient. For obvious reasons. The pages of their magazine are filled with ads and articles about the very items of food that are forbidden in the diet. We cannot blame the magazine. If people continue to buy and serve sugary, starchy delights, if they let their children live on sundaes, cokes, pie à la mode, candy and so forth, magazines will continue to carry ads for these very profitable items. But we find that Dr. Abrahamson's diet is very closely related to the kind of diet we are always recommending. Once again, the title of Dr. Abrahamson's book is *Body, Mind and Sugar,* the publishers are Henry Holt and Co., 257 Fourth St., New York City, and the price is $2.95. If your local library does not have the book on its shelves you can order it from your bookstore.

If someone in your family or circle of friends has multiple sclerosis, we would suggest that you make a note of where Dr. Abrahamson's article appeared—the *New York State Journal of Medicine,* June 1, 1954. Ask your doctor to send for a copy. Ask him to give the patient the test for low blood sugar. If it develops that the blood sugar is low, urge the doctor to recommend the diet Dr. Abrahamson recommends.

Preventing Low Blood Sugar

If you are interested in preventing low blood sugar with many of the disorders that may attend it—all the way from headaches to multiple sclerosis, why not follow the diet yourself? Put your whole family on it and take delight in the new health and vitality everyone will notice. We do not hesitate to recommend it as the best all-round diet we have ever come across, with only a few minor changes we would make in it.

If your blood sugar is not in any danger of getting too low, you need not of course eliminate honey, potatoes, rice, grapes, raisins, plums, figs, dates and cherries for your diet, all of which are excellent foods, except for their high content of natural sugar and starch which is what the low blood sugar patient must avoid. Of course you understand that you should be taking your food supplements along with the diet—especially bone meal for calcium. Here is our version of the diet. Get the whole family accustomed to eating this way:

On arising: fruit or vegetable juice.

Breakfast: fruit or vegetable juice; one helping of protein food such as eggs, cheese, nuts, etc. Only one slice of whole grain bread or toast with butter.

Two hours after breakfast: Vegetable or fruit juice or fruit.

Lunch: Meat, fish, poultry or eggs; salad of fresh raw vegetables and greens, cooked vegetables, if desired; only one slice of whole grain bread or toast with butter; dessert (see below which desserts are allowed); beverage.

Three hours after lunch: high protein snack—seeds, nuts, etc.

One hour before dinner: fruit or vegetable juice or fruit.

Dinner: Soup, if desired (not thickened with flour); vegetables, salad, meat, fish or poultry, only one slice of whole grain bread if desired, dessert; beverage.

Two or three hours after dinner: Protein snack.

Every two hours until bedtime: fruit or fruit juice, nuts or other high protein food.

Allowable vegetables: all except potatoes.

Allowable juice: Any unsweetened fruit or vegetable juice, except grape juice or prune juice.

Allowable fruit: all except grapes, raisins, prunes, figs, dates, cherries.

Allowable beverages: weak tea (teabag, not brewed), Postum, Sanka.

Allowable desserts: Fruit; D-Zerta or other unsweetened gelatine; junket (made from tablets, not the mix).

Avoid absolutely: sugar, honey, rice, candy, cake, pie, pastries, custards, puddings, ice cream, caffeine (ordinary coffee, strong brewed tea, cola beverages), spaghetti, macaroni, noodles, alcoholic drinks, and of course such starchy products as pretzels, doughnuts, crackers, and so forth.

Lettuce, mushrooms and nuts may be taken as freely as desired. Use salt sparingly—do not add it to food in cooking or at the table.

Muscles

One group of muscles works tirelessly for you all day and all night without your ever being conscious of them. Another group responds instantly whenever you decide to make a movement. A third group keeps your heart beating. Altogether you have about 400 muscles in your body, arranged in a marvelous design whereby one muscle contracts while its opposite is relaxing. This is why you can move easily and gracefully without ever consciously commanding your muscles to move.

The visceral muscles are those which line the digestive tract, blood vessels and so forth, and work continuously expanding and contracting to keep your blood flowing and your digestive processes in motion. Inside your chest are respiratory muscles, some of them designed to enlarge the chest (the inspiratory muscles) and others whose purpose is to decrease the size of the chest. Between them and the diaphragm, which is the chief breathing muscle, they take care of the whole process of breathing.

Skeletal muscles are made from fibers and liquid and are attached at each end to bone. These are the muscles responsible for your movements and many, many of them are involved each time you lift your hand, take a step, turn your head. There is a constant blood supply to all muscles, for each cell in every fiber comes into contact with a blood capillary. Almost every muscle cell contains a nerve ending, too, which brings the message from the brain when any muscle is to be contracted or relaxed. No one knows exactly what causes muscles to contract, although many theories have been advanced. One theory involves lactic acid, which is a waste product that results when muscles are fatigued. Muscles hard at work require more blood than resting muscles, and more oxygen. That is one reason why you tire more quickly when you are working in a stuffy room, rather than outside in the fresh air.

Muscles are made from proteins. That is, the muscle proteins are like the cylinders, pistons and valves in a motor. No change takes place in them while the muscles are working, but they are completely necessary if the work is to be done. In them the carbohydrate fuel is burned. Just like parts of a motor, muscles are worn by wear and tear and proteins must be forthcoming for the repair job. Proteins are not stored in the body, so there must be a daily supply if one's muscles are to be healthy. Extreme muscular activity raises the necessary quota of protein, so our grandfathers were wiser than they knew when they ate steaks and chops for breakfast, before a hard day in the fields. A protein deficiency results in flabby, weak muscles, no matter what your age. In persons who have been starved, practically no muscle is left, for the protein of which they are composed has been used by the body to stay alive.

When you consider the foods necessary for healthy muscles, it seems to include just about every category. Calcium and phosphorus are essential, especially in growing children, for the growing bones compete with muscles for the available supply of these two minerals. You have often seen teenagers who have suddenly become quite tall and at the same time have become stoop-shouldered, with very bad posture. This is because there is simply not enough calcium and phosphorus in their diets to supply both bones and muscles. A lack of calcium results in irritable muscles. In some kinds of rickets, calcium is so scarce in the diet that the child has "convulsions." His muscles are protesting their calcium-starvation. "Growing pains" are another indication of too little calcium for growing muscles. Calcium also regulates the action of the heart muscle.

Sodium, potassium and magnesium are important, too, for muscle elasticity. The necessity for all these various minerals is made abundantly clear in experiments in which hearts, removed from their bodies, are kept beating in a fluid that approximates body fluid in its mineral content. Vitamin A is important for good muscle tone and growth. The B vitamins, inositol, biotin and pyridoxine are essential for healthy muscles. The heart muscle is especially rich in inositol. Recently a great deal of work has been done investigating the relation of vitamin E to muscle function. Lack of vitamin E causes paralysis in animals. So might lack of vitamin E be partly responsible for such diseases as polio and muscular dystrophy? The investigation of vitamin E and muscular dystrophy seems to indicate that perhaps this disease is contracted because the patient is unable to assimilate or use vitamin E.

We cannot tell you, for no one knows, exactly why your muscles become stiff when you do unaccustomed hard work. We do know that you'll have less stiffness, better posture, less susceptibility to rheumatism and other muscular diseases if you make sure your diet contains ample mineral (as in bone meal) vitamin A (fish liver oils), vitamin B (brewer's yeast and desiccated liver) and E (wheat germ oil).

Muscular Dystrophy, Treatment For

Word from California leads us to believe that muscular dystrophy may soon be a thing of the past. Before we review these recent findings of Dr. VanMeter of the University of California School of Medicine, let us remind you of the meaning of the word dystrophy. It means, according to medical dictionaries, "imperfect or faulty nutrition." So it seems that we have known all along that muscular dystrophy results from malnutrition, that is, not enough or the wrong kind of food for the muscles.

So it is not surprising to find that Dr. VanMeter in the October, 1953, issue of *California Medicine* announces that he has used amino acids and selected vitamins in 10 patients over a period ranging from two months to a year, with noticeable improvement in the patients. No drugs are involved—no expensive treatments. Dr. VanMeter's reasoning went like this: he figured that there might be, in dystrophy patients, a failure of the digestive system to split protein foods into amino acids. Normally proteins (which are composed of amino acids) are broken down into these various amino acids by the digestive system. Then they are recombined by the various body enzymes, into new body-building tissues, like muscle tissue. If anything goes wrong in this process, the proteins cannot be utilized to build tissue.

Dr. VanMeter prepares amino acids by having them predigested so that the body does not have this job to perform. Certain doses of vitamins are also given in conjunction with the treatment, since vitamins form a part of the chemical structure in which enzymes can work in the body. The results obtained in patients included increase in size of wasted muscles, restoration of normal respiratory action, and relief of depression. Says *Science News Letter,* reporting on the article, one woman, a complete invalid, was able to resume all her household chores, after treatment.

We do not know what causes muscular dystrophy but all research has pointed to the fact that it is nutritional in origin. In 1861 it was first described as a disease separate from other forms of paralysis. Boys are affected more often than girls. The disease quite often afflicts members of the same family. Then too, it has been found that the mother often gives a record of very poor diet before the birth of the child who later develops muscular dystrophy. The child may be born after several recurrent abortions, for instance, which appear to indicate serious lack in the diet of many important factors, including vitamin E.

In general the disease may come on in the form of great muscular weakness in the legs and back, so that the patient has trouble walking. Gradually the paralysis spreads until he is unable to move at all. Respiratory muscles may be affected to such an extent that the patient is unable to cough, so if he contracts even a slight cold, he may suffocate since he cannot cough to remove mucous from his throat or chest. Weakness of legs, lateness in beginning to walk, slowness in running, frequent falls, lordosis (sway back) and prominent stomach—these are easily recognized symptoms of muscular dystrophy in children. In some cases, the disease attacks the arm, shoulder and face muscles before the legs, resulting in a strange expression on the face and possibly inability to close the eyes.

Muscular Dystrophy and Vitamin E

Franklin Bicknell, D.M., M.R.C.P. and Frederick Prescott, M.Sc., Ph.D., F.R.I.C., M.R.C.P., writing in the book *Vitamins in Medicine* (Grune and Stratton, 1953), tell us that past research indicates muscular dystrophy may be caused by inability of the muscles to use vitamin E. They can produce muscular dystrophy in an animal at any time by simply removing all traces of vitamin E from its diet. However, giving vitamin E or wheat germ oil (in which vitamin E is most plentiful) does not necessarily bring about a complete and certain cure in human beings. So, believe Drs. Bicknell and Prescott, muscular dystrophy patients cannot use the vitamin E in their food, so their muscles become wasted. We know that vitamin E is essential for the health of muscles and there have been some experimenters who have wrought near miracles using the vitamin. S. Stone in the American publication *Archives of Pediatrics,* volume 49, 1949, tells us of 25 children treated with fresh wheat germ oil every day, all of whom improved and one of whom recovered completely. Dr. Stone added the B vitamins and vitamin C to the wheat germ oil, incidentally. Other investigators have failed entirely to bring about any improvement with vitamin E or wheat germ oil.

Drs. Bicknell and Prescott tell us that children who have improved on the wheat germ oil treatment are in general children who have been given excellent, fresh diets including whole wheat and home made bread. In general, children whose diets remain unchanged except for the wheat germ do not show improvement. Yet, on the other hand, one patient was placed on an excellent fresh diet and then was given a whole set of variations in the form of food supplements for a period of two years and he failed to show any improvement.

However, it seems to us that, taking into account all these earlier investigations on vitamin E and the ideas of Dr. VanMeter, we will soon surely arrive at a decisive conclusion as to how muscular dystrophy can be cured. We believe we know how to prevent it. Cure will mean new life for those Americans, especially young people, who are at present confined to wheel chairs and beds, helpless, with wasting muscles. And, since we define the disease as "imperfect or faulty nutrition," there can surely be no excuse for ever treating it with a drug. We know that the diet must be good in every sense of the word to prevent muscular dystrophy, especially in those who may be predisposed to it.

Dr. VanMeter believes the answer lies in the body not being able to use proteins correctly. Earlier researchers have believed the cause of the disease is not being able to use vitamin E properly. Perhaps the two are related. Perhaps diseases that result in destruction of vitamin E (such as sprue, celiac disease and other diseases involving diarrhea) may also bring about inability to use proteins properly. Perhaps vitamin E is necessary for proper usage of protein by the body. At any rate, whether or not both these two factors turn out to be involved in producing this tragic disease, we can be sure that medical science is at last on the right track in ferreting out the cause of muscular dystrophy.

Human and Chemical Enemies of Vitamin E

Meanwhile what can we do to make certain we do not ourselves get M.D., or pass it along in inheritance to our children? Vitamin E is important—of this there can be no doubt. Vitamin E appears in many foods—chiefly in vegetable and cereal oils, and leafy greens. It is seriously affected by rancid fats in the diet. It is completely destroyed in the digestive tract by mineral oil.

Please remember, too, that the richest source of vitamin E and all the accompanying B vitamins was bread, up until the beginning of this century when we began to mill wheat to make white flour. Vitamin E and the B vitamins are contained in the wheat germ—that tiny, living part of the wheat which is responsible for the sprouting of the grain. Modern millers remove this wheat germ because (they say) customers want white bread and also because the wheat germ spoils, molds or becomes rancid very rapidly. So wheat flour that contains the germ cannot be stored for long periods of time—it is almost as perishable as milk. In our great modern economy where wheat may be raised and milled many miles from where it is to be baked into bread, the wheat germ must be removed for the sake of convenience to the bakers, regardless of what it may do to our health. If you eat lots of bread and if you would be healthy, buy real stone-ground, whole wheat flour and make your own bread. Or buy a small home-mill and grind your own flour from the wheat. *Prevention* advertisers sell organically-grown wheat and stone-ground flour.

In *Bridges' Dietetics for the Clinician* (Lea and Febiger, 1949), we find that vitamin E is also destroyed by ozone, chlorine, permanganate and ferric chloride. We wonder how the chlorine in urban water supplies all over the country may be affecting the vitamin E in the bodies of Americans who drink this water. Could chlorinated water be a possible contributing cause of muscular dystrophy, as well as heart disease? For we know that vitamin E is essential for the health of the heart and other muscles of the human body. Ferric chloride is one of the medicines containing iron that is given to anemia patients. Could it be that children who have been treated for anemia suffer from a shortage of vitamin E resulting in muscular dystrophy or heart trouble? Could it be that mothers who have been treated with ferric chloride do not provide their new-born children with enough vitamin E so that they soon develop these deficiency diseases? Perhaps the widespread use of mineral oil as a laxative is responsible for many muscle diseases. It is also true that defatted wheat germ does not contain vitamin E—the vitamin is in the fat or oil. So perhaps even those health-conscious folks who endeavor to protect themselves from a vitamin E shortage may not be accomplishing this, if the wheat germ they use has been defatted.

Considering how many enemies of vitamin E we may encounter in our everyday living, does it not seem worth while to supplement your diet with wheat germ oil or natural vitamin E, or both? As we have pointed out many times in the past, vitamin E is being used at present by many physicians for treatment of heart and blood vessel diseases. Surely a diet rich in this vitamin, along with wheat germ oil and/or natural vitamin E is the best safeguard against muscular dystrophy, heart disease or any other disorder of the muscles.

These are the foods that are richest in vitamin E: Dry navy beans, beef liver, butter, coconut oil, yellow cornmeal, corn oil, cottonseed oil, whole eggs, oatmeal, peanut oil, green peas, sweet potatoes, brown rice, soybean oil, turnip greens, wheat germ oil. Are you and your family getting enough of them every day?

Muscular Dystrophy, A Case History

Some time ago, writing about vitamin E used in the prevention and cure of various diseases, we mentioned the fact that it has been used to treat cases of muscular dystrophy. Quoting from Dr. Walter Eddy in *Vitaminology* (published by the Williams and Wilkins Company, Baltimore, Maryland) we said: "In 1940 Stone reported treatment with wheat germ oil of five patients with muscular dystrophy; one with muscular atrophy following anterior poliomyelitis; one with muscle atrophy after an attack of multiple neuritis." He found, Dr. Eddy tells us, that definite improvement was obtained in all cases with muscular dystrophy, the improvement being shown in gain in muscle strength, the disappearance of fatigue and muscle pain on slight exertion, change in muscle texture and displacement of the diseased muscles by normally contracting muscles. *He tells us further that the addition of the vitamin B complex to vitamin E appeared to increase the value of the vitamin E.*

Then we said, "Now this statement alone might very well answer our question about conflicting results in the use of vitamin E for human nutrition. One doctor giving vitamin E to patients might pay no attention to their diet, might make no effort to see that they are also getting all the other vitamins so necessary for good nutrition. This doctor might not get any results from giving vitamin E. But another physician, aware of the great importance of one vitamin in relation to another, might check carefully to see that his patient is getting all the vitamins in abundance. And in this case the addition of vitamin E to the diet might work wonders!"

For some time after we wrote this article we searched medical literature for some mention of a physician who had indeed used vitamin E in conjunction with an outstanding good diet, for muscular dystrophy. We did not find any. However, just the other day we received a letter from William Coda Martin, M.D., of New York City enclosing an article of his that appeared in the *International Record of Medicine and General Practice Clinics,* for February, 1954. Dr. Martin indicated that we might use this article if we wished to.

Imagine our delight when we saw the title of the article: "A Case of Muscular Dystrophy Responding to Therapy," and when we saw that the therapy was nothing more or less than a good diet well fortified with food supplements rich in vitamins and minerals. Dr. Martin believes that muscular dystrophy is the result of a disorder in metabolism which has been present since birth and hence indicates that the diet of the mother may have been seriously unbalanced. He reminds us that experiments with laboratory animals show that lack of oxygen in the unborn child can result in malformations in the child. Experiments have also shown that maternal diets which do not contain enough vitamin D, calcium, phosphorus, riboflavin, folic acid or pantothenic acid may produce deformities or disorders in the functioning of various organs. Experiments show that lack of vitamin A in the mother's diet can produce deformities of the heart, the eyes, the genital organs and the urinary tract.

Says Dr. Martin: "The importance of the mother's diet in the human being, in relation to well-being during and after pregnancy, occupies a prominent place among nutritional studies today. There is an increasing body of evidence that a relationship exists between the nutrition and the development and survival of the baby. Data seem to indicate that the weight of the liver of the fetus (the unborn child) bears a close relationship to the dietary intake of the human mother during the last month of pregnancy. This is especially true when there is a deficient protein intake." He quotes Elvehjem and Pottenger who showed that muscular dystrophy is one symptom of puppies whose mothers were fed on fortified pasteurized milk or evaporated milk.

He says further that in muscular dystrophy there is a fatty infiltration of the muscles. He believes that this condition arises from the liver of the child not working as it should because of the harm it suffered while still unborn, from its mother's diet. In the early stages of the disease, this liver disorder can be corrected and all the later tragic consequences of muscular dystrophy can be avoided. "It is well known," he says, "that dietary deficiencies are always multiple and therefore, the treatment must be based on adequate nutrition supplemented by multiple micronutrient factors." In other words, you cannot take a pill, or two or three pills a day and expect to prevent or cure muscular dystrophy any more than any other disease. You must completely revise your diet to include only those foods and food supplements which contain an abundance of all the vitamins, minerals and enzymes *and you must exclude from your diet those things which do not.*

Diet Therapy Must Be Complete, Intensive and Persistent

"To correct a multiple vitamin deficiency, the therapy must be complete, intensive and persistent," he states, and right here, we suspect, is where so many of us fail, especially when we are dealing with our children. If Junior is used to receiving a piece of cake or candy as a reward for eating his vegetables, surely, we say to ourselves, just this one little thing can't hurt. But we forget that glass of soda pop Junior has at bedtime and the white bread and jelly he eats when he comes home from school. Since refined cereals are the only kind he likes, surely there can't be much harm in just one bowl of "crunchies" for breakfast. And so it goes. *"Complete, intensive and persistent,"* says Dr. Martin and that is exactly what he means.

The case he describes is so dramatic that it certainly proves what can be done by diet alone—not just in preventing disease but in curing it. The patient was a baby girl who at 17 months could not stand without support. She had had pneumonia twice. X-rays showed that her bones were normal, but that her muscles were heavily overlaid with thick strips of fat. She was discussed at a pediatrics conference at Babies Hospital, New York, on January 4, 1952, "at which time it was decided that the picture was one of muscular dystrophy for which no therapy is known." So she was discharged. Her mother brought her to Dr. Martin on January 10, 1952. She was given a diet and diet supplements, and the record from then on is amazing. By January 25th she could stand with support; by April she could stand alone; by September her walking had improved, she was mentally alert and her speech had improved. By November she could walk and run but was still a little unsteady on her feet. By the end of January, 1953, she was very active; could run, play and dance; her speech had improved, her growth, weight and mental development were normal.

Now just think how different the story would have been, had the mother accepted the verdict of the pediatricians . . . "no therapy is known." Or if she had consulted Dr. Martin and instead of following the diet he gave her, had decided that what you eat doesn't really make that much difference and so had become lax and indifferent about the diet. That baby would today be another statistic to be quoted over the radio in appeals for the muscular dystrophy fund. That baby would have spent the rest of her life in hopeless invalidism. But her mother was apparently determined that the diet therapy would be *complete, intensive* and *persistent.* And you can see what results it brought.

The Diet That Was Used

The diet is simplicity itself. We assume the family lived in New York and managed to follow all the regulations of the diet using what foods could be purchased in that city. The diet follows:

1. Low cholesterol, low fat diet, free of refined sugars and carbohydrates. (The first provision is not to be recommended for normal children whose bodies can handle fat successfully, but the "free of refined sugars and carbohydrates" is surely an excellent recommendation for all.)

2. Only whole grain bread and cereal. (No bakery bread; no ready-to-eat cereal, in spite of all the inducements of the prizes every box top will bring.)

3. Certified raw milk (rather than pasteurized or evaporated milk).

4. Fresh raw fruits and vegetables daily—extra supplements of vegetable and fruit juices. (We suspect that most mothers these days try their best to get their children to eat lots of raw fruits and vegetables, but, we might as well face it, a child who has filled up on candy, ice cream and pop simply cannot be interested in a raw vegetable. And note that this child ate *not only fresh fruits and vegetables every day, but fruit and vegetable juices in addition, every day.*)

5. Raw fresh calves' liver (juice or rare broiled liver) daily. (It seems logical to expect that eating liver, especially raw liver, would work wonders for someone with a liver disorder. But liver is a wonderfully healthful food for all of us and how many children are brought up without ever having tasted it! Serve it at least once a week.)

6. Lean meat, fish or fowl. (To supply the protein. If your children get enough first-class protein they will not be so hungry for the forbidden sweets.)

7. Nutritional supplements: Vitamin E (natural tocopherols). Desiccated liver. (What, in addition to liver every day at meals? Yes, indeed.)

Multiple vitamins: (This we suppose would include the B vitamins, vitamins C, A and D.)

Lipotropic substances: Crude Liver and B_{12} intramuscularly daily. Thyroid.

These last three substances are the only medical preparations used—the only part of the treatment that you could not provide yourself in your own home. Surely the miracle of this baby's return to health is ample evidence of the healthfulness of such a diet for all of us. Prospective mothers especially should be certain that they eat plenty of the good foods mentioned above, avoiding completely the forbidden ones, if they would look forward to the birth of a baby perfectly formed and free from any threat of muscular dystrophy.

Mushrooms

Mushrooms are among the foods richest in iodine. This started us out on a search for other facts about these strange little objects. We uncovered some astonishing information, even though none of it has anything to do with iodine.

Did you know, for instance, that mushrooms are very rich in folic acid, the yellow vitamin which, along with vitamin B_{12}, is the most potent weapon ever discovered against pernicious anemia? The speed with which infinitely small doses of this vitamin rejuvenate patients of this dread disease has amazed doctors ever since the vitamin was first discovered. Brewer's yeast, raw wheat germ, soybeans, kidney and liver are other rich sources.

Mushrooms are fairly good sources of other B vitamins as well—¾ of a cup containing about as much thiamin as a bran muffin, as much riboflavin as an orange, and as much niacin as a serving of halibut. Also, surprising enough, we are told that mushrooms grown in the light are rich in vitamin D which does not occur in any other foods from non-animal sources. Vitamin D in mushrooms! This seems especially odd, since we automatically associate mushrooms with dark cellars, whereas vitamin D is the vitamin one manufactures from sunlight!

Mushrooms, as everybody knows, are not plants, as vegetables and grains are. They are fungi—a group of plants that includes also rusts, molds and mildews. They do not reproduce by seeds, but by spores. The spore is the fine black dust that is thrown off when a mature plant is laid on a white surface. The spore gives rise to the "spawn"—stringy white material which penetrates dried manure or similar substances and eventually develops into a mushroom. Mushrooms are grown in beds heavily fertilized with manure. We wonder whether or not this may have something to do with the abundance of the B vitamins, folic acid in the mushroom. We know that the vitamin is produced in the intestinal tract of the healthy animal. Could it be that the mushroom, growing on dung, takes up some of this precious substance that has been eliminated by the animal?

The other astonishing thing about mushrooms is the fact that they are so nutritious and yet grow without chlorophyll, the green life's blood of all other plants that we eat. The mushroom family apparently does not need chlorophyll.

One of the earliest introductions we as children have to mushrooms is the warning that we may by mistake get a poisonous one. And it is just as well, unless you are an expert in recognizing mushrooms, not to eat any you may find growing in the woods or fields. It is indeed true that there are deadly kinds of mushrooms. The poisonous material in this type of mushroom is a narcotic which induces nausea, drowsiness, stupor and pains in the joints. Mushroom growers sometime find that spores from other (and perhaps poisonous) mushrooms have invaded their planting beds and must be disposed of.

However, in general, one can feel quite safe in eating mushrooms sold in today's markets, for they are grown carefully.

Here is the vitamin and mineral content of 100 grams of mushrooms which is about ¾ cup:

Vitamin B

Thiamin	160 micrograms
Riboflavin	500 micrograms
Niacin	6 milligrams
Pyridoxine	45 micrograms
Pantothenic acid	1700 micrograms
Biotin	16 micrograms
Folic acid	considerable (no exact figure available)

Vitamin C	1-8 milligrams
Vitamin D	21 international units, if grown in dark
	63 international units, if grown in light
Calcium	14 milligrams
Phosphorus	98 milligrams
Iron	3.14 milligrams
Copper	1.79 milligrams
Manganese	.08 milligrams

Nicotine

Our campaign against smoking was reinforced by finding recently an article in the *British Medical Journal,* March 29, 1952, in which Ronald Bodley Scott, M.A., D.M., F.R.C.P., reviews the whole history of tobacco and gives us a glimpse into the various effects it may have on the different organs and systems of the body. Dr. Scott tells us that tobacco is "the only drug to which addiction is universally considered respectable."

A hundred years ago smoking was not the generally accepted social habit that it is today. As late as 1848 there were prohibitions against smoking in the streets of Berlin. Earlier, various legal measures were passed to discourage the use of tobacco. In old Russia smokers' noses were amputated. In the Swiss canton of Berne, the offense ranked only one degree less odious than adultery. But nowadays, Dr. Scott reminds us, the English government revenue from sales of tobacco provides some six hundred million pounds. "The moralist will find matter for reflection in the thought that over one-quarter of the country's income is now derived from the addiction of its inhabitants to tobacco and alcohol," he says. Undoubtedly the situation in this country is pretty much the same.

Dr. Scott tells us that there are some fairly far-fetched notions abroad about the reason for tobacco addiction—that it constitutes the remains of ancient fire worship; it pleasantly stimulates the nerve endings; it satisfies the need to hold something in the mouth as a reminder of childish pleasure in taking food. Then of course there is the plain unadorned fact that smoking consists of an addiction to the drug, tobacco.

Estimates differ as to the amount of nicotine entering the body during smoking. Early reports seemed to show that as much as 3.6 milligrams of nicotine were absorbed during smoking. More recently it seems that about one milligram may be absorbed during the smoking of one cigarette. Using a holder decreases the amount of nicotine absorbed. After the smoking of 20 cigarettes in seven hours, the quantity of nicotine in the blood reaches an average of .14 milligrams per liter and traces of nicotine can be found in the blood ten hours after the last cigarette has been smoked. In addition to nicotine, tobacco smoke also contains hydrocyanic acid, ammonia, carbon monoxide, pyridines, aldehydes and tars. In this country it contains as well residues of all the toxic insecticides that have been sprayed on it during growth. A correspondent wrote us recently that he lives close to a tobacco plantation and has seen the workers there wearing gloves to protect their hands from these poisons. Yet these same poisons are still on the leaves when we smoke them!

Smoking and the Heart

Smoking has a very definite effect on the heart. It causes a rise in blood pressure, an increase in the pulse frequency and certain changes in the pattern of an electrocardiogram. There are also changes in the circulation. The arteries narrow and the skin temperature falls when we smoke. Cigarette smoking leads to constriction of the small blood vessels, says Dr. Scott, possibly because smoking brings about a release of adrenalin into the bloodstream. "It will be obvious," he says, "that symptoms due to pre-existing cardiovascular disease may be aggravated by these (actions of tobacco)." We have printed in *Prevention* the opinion of Dr. W. J. McCormick of Canada, based on statistics taken in Canada, that smoking and drinking are responsible for large numbers of coronary thrombosis deaths.

Effects on Respiratory Tract and Digestive System

The irritant effect of tobacco on the respiratory tract has been estimated by experiments in which six standard "puffs" of smoke have produced swelling and irritation in the eye of a laboratory animal. We are all familiar with the "smoker's cough" which will certainly lead to chronic pharyngitis and will keep chronic bronchitis active in those who are predisposed to it. We know too that smoking reduces vital capacity—that is, chest expansion—so it is quite true that cigarettes are "bad for the wind." We have published much information on the relation of smoking to lung cancer. Dr. Scott points out that lung cancer has risen alarmingly in all countries except Iceland. In London it provides 27 per cent of all deaths from malignancy. In Iceland only 2.9 per cent. "It is of interest," he adds, "that the cigarette consumption in Iceland has been negligible until the last few years. . . . The moral we should draw is obscure. Perhaps we should caution all young men and women not to smoke more than 20 cigarettes a day. The popular reaction is illustrated by the subscriber to *Reader's Digest* who was so upset by an article on smoking and cancer that he decided to give up reading magazines.

Tobacco has a very definite effect on the digestive tract, aside from lip cancer which is commonly found among pipe and cigar (but not cigarette) smokers. Smoking one cigarette will diminish hunger contractions and gastric mobility. It decreases as well the volume and acidity of the digestive juices of the stomach. This may be the reason why an increase in appetite is noticed by those who stop smoking. Although we cannot definitely ascribe stomach ulcers to tobacco, says Dr. Scott, yet smoking definitely has been shown to produce dyspepsia closely resembling ulcer, which disappears when smoking is stopped. He recommends that those who suffer from gastric complaints of any sort stop smoking to see whether or not it relieves any of their symptoms.

The Nervous and Genito-Urinary System

So far as the nervous system is concerned, there seems no doubt but that nicotine affects it unfavorably. There have been reports, says Dr. Scott, of patients who have recovered from serious nervous symptoms after giving up smoking, of a boy who fell victim to a manic-depressive psychosis from smoking 20 cigars a day, "there are records of fleeting cerebral attacks, neuralgic pains, headaches, fits . . ."

One disorder definitely caused by tobacco is tobacco amblyopia which is a disturbance of vision commonly occurring in men between the ages of 35 and 55. This begins as a "blind spot" which spreads gradually to the center of vision. It is also interesting to note that malnutrition seems to make the symptoms much worse. And when vitamin B was given to one series of patients, their visual symptoms decreased even though they went right on smoking. The suggestion has been made that the toxic substances in the tobacco are removed by a healthy liver, so that the ordinary smoker does not have amblyopia. But when the liver does not function so well, because of malnutrition—which would of course involve deficiency of vitamin B—then the toxic substances remain to make trouble for the eyes.

Tobacco has apparently little effect on the genito-urinary system. In normal people it is inclined to have an anti-diuretic effect—that is, it decreases urine flow. Some researchers have claimed that smoking leads to infertility and abortion although other investigators have found high fertility among some special groups of pipe-smoking women. We do know that nicotine is secreted in human milk in proportion to the number of cigarettes smoked.

Dr. Scott reminds us that a physician's advice in regard to smoking is likely to be colored by how many cigarettes he himself smokes. "It is a matter which concerns us as doctors," he says, "for patients are constantly asking our advice about smoking. Most of us are prepared to give it without deep reflection, for the view the doctor takes is dictated rather by the number of cigarettes he smokes himself than a profound knowledge of the pharmacology of tobacco (its effect on the body)."

There is a relation between smoking and vitamins C and B—both are used up more rapidly in the body metabolism of the smoker. There is also a relation between smoking and low blood sugar. Like sweets and caffeine, nicotine brings about a momentary rise in blood sugar, but in half an hour or so causes it to drop far below normal, so that the smoker must quickly light another cigarette to bring his blood sugar up again. So, if you are a smoker, we'd recommend getting plenty of vitamins B and C, to make up for what tobacco steals from you. And in addition, put yourself on a high-protein diet with no sweets, starches or caffeine, for a few weeks, and see if you don't manage to overcome some of your craving for tobacco.

Nose

"To Jack and Jill Public, the nose is a buffoon among the organs of the human body, painfully wanting in drama, mystery and glamor. Long before Cyrano de Bergerac, it served as a subject for jesting; in reality the nose has been a target for invective and injury from early times." So says Noah D. Fabricant, M.D., in his book *Headaches,* published by Farrar Strauss and Company, 1949.

He goes on to defend this abused organ by telling us that it is the most efficient and compact air-conditioning unit in existence. The air we inhale is strained through the coarse hairs that line the nose passages. Dust and dirt are trapped. Finer particles of dust and some bacteria are caught in the secretions of the nose's mucous membrane and carried along to the throat. This job is performed by millions of tiny hairs called cilia that wave back and forth constantly—250 times per minute, sweeping all kinds of impurities before them. Cilia are organisms that need a constant supply of calcium if they are to be healthy. One good reason why taking bone meal may help to prevent colds.

Air is also moistened by the mucous membrane which secretes for this purpose about one quart of fluid each day. As the air passes through the nose, it is warmed to body temperature so that it can be immediately used by the lungs. The mucous membrane lining of the nose, which carries out all these functions is so important that its fluid is being constantly replaced. Approximately every twenty minutes the mucous is renewed. The nose also secretes a substance called lysozyme which is powerful against some germs. So the nose has the job of filtering, humidifying and warming all the air we breathe—about 500 cubic feet per day. This is one of the main reasons why mouth breathing is so unhealthful, for all these functions of the nose are by-passed when we breathe through our mouths.

The nose consists of two nostrils, divided by a wall called the septum. Its bones are attached to the skull bones. Its lower part is held in place by cartilage. The floor of the nose cavity is the roof of the mouth. At the back of the nose there is an opening into the throat. There are also five openings from the various head sinuses into the nose. And the tear glands open into the nose, too, which is the reason why every tearful heroine of every play or movie must always borrow the hero's handkerchief to mop up, when she is weeping.

The lower part of the nose is for breathing. The upper part contains the delicate sensory cells that are in constant touch with the olfactory nerve, allowing us to smell.

The two most familiar disorders of the nose carry the scientific names of *rhinitis* and *epistaxis* (colds and nosebleed to you). As you know, no one has discovered as yet just what causes colds, but we all know that the first symptom is probably dryness and irritation in the nose. This means that the protective mucous has dried out and the cold germs have a comfortable home in which to grow and flourish, unmolested by any of the body's policemen. We know too that vitamin A and vitamin C are most important to the health of these membranes that secrete mucous. So it is our belief that people who get more of these two vitamins than they need will probably not suffer from colds. If you should have a cold, it is best not to blow your nose violently and not to hold one nostril shut while you blow through the other, for you may, by so doing, cause an infection in the sinuses or in the ear passages. One last reminder about colds. Omitting grain products from the diet may tend to decrease colds. We do not know why this is so, but carefully controlled experiments have shown that it is true.

Nose bleed can arise from a number of different causes but, of course, before your nose can bleed there must be a rupture of one or more of the many blood vessels that supply blood to the nose membranes. Another good reason for making certain your diet contains enough vitamin C which keeps these blood vessel walls healthy. Vitamin K is important to prevent bleeding, too. Most serious nose bleeds occur in older persons and we might add that most older folks are notoriously lacking in vitamin C. And in many cases reported in medical magazines, nose bleeds have been stopped with massive doses of vitamin C.

In her book, *Let's Have Healthy Children* (published by Harcourt, Brace and Company, 1951) Adelle Davis tells the story of a little boy who was allergic to horse dander which always gave him a bleeding nose. His parents were in the horse business and he had to accompany them on many trips to stables. Large doses of vitamin C given every hour while he was in the stables brought about the complete prevention of the nose bleeds!

Two more cautions about preventing trouble with your nose. Avoid oily "nose drops" like poison. One famous physician has estimated that 85 to 90 per cent of all chronic nose ailments have been brought on by the patients themselves who tilt back their eager heads and spill oily medicine into their patient nostrils day after day whether or not they "feel a cold coming on." In children such a practice can lead to pneumonia and death, for some of the oily substance slides down the windpipe into the lungs from which it cannot be excreted. Then, too, beware of clipping or plucking the hairs that grow in your nose. They are there for a very important reason, as we have shown. In one case in our files a patient died from a nose infection after his barber had clipped out annoying hairs. With clean scissors, you may safely cut off the hairs that extend outside your nose, thus marring your beauty. But leave the ones inside strictly alone!

Nutrition—Soil Deficiency and Health

A new book on the work of Sir Robert McCarrison has recently been published in England—a "must" for the library of anyone vitally interested in nutrition and the organic method of farming. The chapter headings are indicative of the wealth of splendid material to be found in the book: *Researches on Fever, Researches on Goitre and Cretinism,*

Researches on Deficiency Diseases, Researches on Beri-Beri, Researches on "Stone," Researches on Human Diet in Relation to Health and Disease.

Sir Robert McCarrison is one of the greatest nutritionists of our time. He carried on his studies in India, discovering hitherto unsuspected aspects of the problems of food and nutrition in their relation to disease. Perhaps his most famous experiment is the one in which he fed laboratory rats a diet common in England—white bread, margarine, tea, sugar, jam, preserved meats and overcooked vegetables, and produced in the rats the diseases also common to modern Britishers. Another group of rats was meanwhile kept free from these diseases by feeding them a diet that contained all the necessary food elements in the proper proportion.

The chapter on "stone" in this newest book is particularly significant. Kidney stone is very prevalent in India. In 1926-28 there were more than 34,000 persons who came to Indian hospitals complaining of kidney stone. And undoubtedly there were many more who did not come to the hospitals. There are geographical areas in India where stone is more common than in other areas. But no connection could ever be traced to pin the causes of "stone" on geological, climatic or racial influences, nor on the fact that some areas where stone is prevalent are in the hills and others are in the plains.

However, Sir Robert noticed that in the areas where stone was common the principal cereal crop was wheat, corn or millet, while the other areas grew rice. He began a series of experiments using the various cereals to produce stone in laboratory animals. He found that stone is produced by a diet high in these cereals, in the following order: whole-wheat flour, oatmeal, North Indian millet, white flour, rice, South Indian millet. It seemed from the experiments, that the stone was produced probably from an excess of calcium or a deficiency of phosphorus in relation to calcium. Also a lack of vitamin A was evident.

Adding a very small amount of whole milk each day to the diet of every rat prevented the formation of stone. Butter and cod liver oil (both animal fats) had the same effect. But vegetable fats did not. It is not to be assumed from this, says Sir Robert, that milk alone is a protection against kidney stone or any other disease. No single food is a perfect food. Even whole wheat must be taken with other foods. Sir Robert clarifies this further as follows: "The truth is that no single food material is in itself a 'complete food'—even milk is not; if it be not faulty in one regard it is faulty in another. The best are those whose faults are least; and in the latter category both whole-wheat flour and oatmeal are to be included. Milk, as an exclusive food will cause anemia in rats; onions, anemia in dogs; cabbage, goitre in rabbits and oatmeal or *atta* will cause stone in rats; yet what better food can there be for mankind than a judicious mixture of all four?

"I claim for this experiment (on rats) that it proves conclusively that one-sided diets which are disproportionately rich in cereals and poor in animal fats, milk and fresh vegetables are capable of inducing in albino rats a large proportion of the diseases included in our calendar of human ailments I may add that of all the faulty diets I have used, that composed of white bread, margarine, tea, sugar, jam, preserved meat and scanty, over-cooked vegetables—a diet in common use by many people in this country—proved to be one of the worst, and most likely to be associated in rats with many of the morbid (disease) states I have mentioned, especially diseases of the lungs and of the gastro-intestinal tract.

"I lay stress on the food materials themselves (raw milk, butter, cod liver oil, carrots and fresh green vegetables used in nutritional experiments on animals) rather than on any particular ingredient of them, or any particular quality possessed by them, believing, as I do, that in nature's laboratory all elements and complexes needed for normal nutrition are combined in a way which we cannot wholly achieve, and that the health-giving properties of food are largely dependent on this combination. For my own part, I have been able to devise no synthetic diet which can equal in these properties a mixture of natural food materials such as that on which I feed my stock rats and on which some of the finest physical specimens of mankind are reared."

Nutrition Related to Method of Agriculture

The kind of soil that food is grown on is important, too, in assessing its nutritive value. The next time you are challenged to produce proof that the organic method produces food that is superior so far as nutrition goes, you can quote the following statements of Sir Robert McCarrison's—"Considerations of this kind led me, in the course of the inquiry on which I am engaged, to attempt, in a way as wide as my limited circumstances permitted, a study of the soil conditions which influence the nutritive value of the commoner food grains of India. Millions of people in this country rely from generation to generation on a single cereal as the main staple of their dietary. It seemed necessary, therefore, to be aware not only of those soil conditions which influence the yield of grains but of those which influence their nutritive quality. . . . The soil conditions which it was thought would be likely to influence the nutritive quality of food grains were (a) the chemical composition of the soil itself, (b) the manurial treatment to which it is subjected, and (c) irrigation as compared with normal rainfall. . . . The results already arrived at are of interest. It has been found in regard to millet—a common food grain in south India—that soil on which it is repeatedly grown, but which has received no manure for many years, yields a grain the nutritive value of which is so low that it may actually be harmful to the users of it; suggesting the acquirement by the grain of toxic qualities. It has been shown, moreover, that the nutritive and vitamin values of the millet grown on soil treated with cattle or farm-yard manure are markedly superior to those of millet grown on the same soil when treated with a complete chemical manure. In regard to wheat, it has been found that when it is grown on soil treated with farm-yard manure, its nutritive value is approximately 17 per cent higher than when grown on soil treated with complete chemical manure. The deficiencies of the wheat grown under the latter conditions are due in the main to an inferior content of vitamin A, that substance which is so essential in maintaining the resistance of man and his domestic animals to infectious diseases."

A Sad Cycle of Inefficiency

And, on the same subject: "Human and animal inefficiency is reflected in the soil; in its imperfect cultivation; in inadequate manuring; and in crops scanty as to quantity and deficient as to quality. Too few animals are kept by the cultivator (in India) as the scanty vegetation cannot support them; and so there is returned to the land too little of that organic matter, in the form of barn-yard manure, on which the continued fertility of the soil is so dependent. It has been shown in regard to plants, as in regard to animals, that they cannot thrive, nor their seed attain to the fullest 'reproductive quality' unless they be provided, in addition to the mineral constituents of their food, with certain organic substances known as 'auximones' These substances, which are akin to vitamins, are as essential to the normal metabolism of plants as vitamins are to the normal metabolism of man and animals. They not only enable the plant to build up from the simple ingredients derived from the soil those organic complexes required as food by men and animals, but they enable it to elaborate vitamins without which these organic complexes cannot be properly utilized by the animal organism. . . . So it is that such disabilities of mankind as are due to faulty nutrition are sometimes traceable to the soil itself, which has become exhausted and unproductive of the best kind of food through improper attention and cultivation. Malnutrition, thus, pursues its harmful course in an ever-widening vicious circle; the cultivator is too often ill-nourished and ravaged by disease which is commonly the result of his ill-nourishment; his beasts are alike ill-nourished, while both toil wearily in a heartless effort to extract from the ill-nourished earth enough to keep them from starvation. The solution of the problem of malnutrition, is thus, to a great extent, one of improvement in methods of agriculture."

Sir Robert's book is not all as easy reading as these portions we have quoted. His observations on his experiments and the diseases he studied in India are couched for the most part in scientific terms. If you have a medical dictionary handy you can become one of the best-informed individuals in your neighborhood by reading the book, *The Work of Sir Robert McCarrison.* We'd suggest that it would make an excellent gift for your family doctor, or some young medical student you know who will probably get nothing but a smattering of nutrition study in his medical courses. You can order the book from your local bookshop. It is published by Faber and Faber, Ltd., London, England.

Nuts

One pound of nuts is equal in calories to 2.3 pounds of bread, 3.7 pounds of steak, 12.3 pounds of potatoes or 15 pounds of oranges. One pound of oily nuts supplies all the calories needed for the day plus 40 per cent of the protein, 60 per cent of the phosphorus, 30 per cent of the calcium and iron and four times the daily requirement of fat.

What do you think of a food that has this kind of nutritive value, grows wild and free for the picking, needs little care while it is growing, is harvested by picking it up from the ground, needs no processing and no cooking, and keeps well with no refrigeration or preservatives? Doesn't this sound like the absolutely ideal food that we have been waiting for all these years? Well, its been here and waiting for us all these years. Why have we been so slow in recognizing nuts as one of our best and most practical foods?

Speaking generally, nuts are defined as hard-shelled seeds enclosing a single edible oily kernel. If you want to be technical about it, you will find that nuts are classified biologically as one-seeded fruits, such as beechnut, chestnut and so forth. But we have come to think of a lot of different products as nuts, including such varied edibles as cashews, peanuts, coconuts and so forth. Most of these are high in protein and fat and low in carbohydrate. Some nuts contain as much as 60 per cent fat. Some kinds of pecans contain as much as 76 per cent fat.

This high fat content would seem to indicate that nuts are an excellent food for those who are trying to gain weight. They are a source of natural fat, delicious to pick up as a snack between meals. They are high in protein as well as fat, which means that they do a good job of helping to regulate blood sugar, which is so important to good health. Pound for pound they contain more calories than most foods.

In general, nuts are high in minerals and have peculiar affinities for certain kinds of minerals. The hickory tree, for instance, accumulates aluminum from the soil. The ash of hickory leaves is high in this trace mineral. Hickory trees also accumulate the rare earths—*scandium, yttrium, lanthanum, dys prosium, holium, erbium* and so forth—names we lay folks seldom hear.

The Brazil nut contains much barium, another trace mineral. In fact, some Brazil nuts have been found to cause distress if they are eaten in quantity because of the large content of barium. There is a deficiency of zinc in the pecan, English walnut and almond and a deficiency of boron in the English walnut. The European beechnut contains a toxic substance in its seed coat. The shell of the cashew contains liquids and oils which are toxic and irritating to the skin, much like poison ivy.

However, we need not concern ourselevs with these analyses, for of course, we do not ever eat those parts of the nuts which contain toxic material. And, since none of us lives exclusively on nuts, we need not worry about getting too much or too little of one of the minerals or trace minerals. Our other foods will balance this. Tannins, which most of us associate with nuts, are found only in the shells, wood and bark of the trees.

Vitamins and Minerals in Nuts

Most nuts contain a good supply of vitamin A and thiamin, one of the B vitamins. Some of them contain vitamin E. Immature English walnuts have been found to contain large amounts of vitamin C, which disappears as the nuts ripen. The walnut hulls are an excellent source of vitamin C, containing as high as 1550-3036 milligrams of this vitamin for every hundred grams. Of course we can't eat the walnut hulls. In some parts of the world, we understand, efforts are being made to extract the vitamin C from the walnut hulls. The red skin of the peanut contains considerable thiamin, incidentally, so don't throw it away when you eat peanuts.

Nuts are not complete proteins, even though their protein content is high. We mean by this that they do not contain all of the amino acids, or kinds of protein essential for human health. Only foods of animal origin contain all these amino acids—they do not occur in any one vegetable food except soybeans But, even so, nuts are a most important food if you want to increase your protein intake, and most of us should.

The foods of animal origin that are high in protein such as meat and eggs have an acid reaction in the body whereas most nuts have an alkaline reaction. Filberts, peanuts and walnuts are acid. All others are alkaline in their effect in the body. They are a highly concentrated food.

Nuts have the reputation of being hard to digest. But they were often eaten at the end of a heavy meal by an individual who had stuffed himself on all kinds of indigestible desserts and the nuts took the blame for his over-indulgence Nuts must be chewed carefully. Otherwise they will not be properly digested, for the digestive juices cannot break down the tough kernels.

Rich in protein, they do not present any problem of decay or spoilage such as occurs with meat and other animal products. True, nuts eventually become rancid but there is no question of refrigeration and threat of poisoning from spoilage. Nuts are free from uric acid and other substances produced in the body by eating meat. Do keep in mind, however, that they cannot be used as a complete substitute for meat unless you are highly skilled in balancing menus, for their protein is not complete. And they do not supply the same bulk that meat and other foods supply, which is important for propulsion in the digestive tract.

How Nuts Are Processed

Nuts, like other natural products, should be eaten in as nearly the natural state as possible. But we civilized twentieth century folks must always prove our superiority by processing nuts until we finally almost destroy their food value. The cashew nut is shelled in India from whence it comes. First it is heated in liquid to make the shells brittle and to extract the oily substance inside. The shell of the English walnut is sometimes loosened by exposure to ethylene gas. Almonds are bleached by dipping in chloride of lime. Pecans are sometimes bleached, sometimes dyed.

Blanching the nuts—that is, removing the inner skin, is accomplished by soaking in hot water. But pecans and English walnuts are dipped in hot lye, followed by an acid rinse. Another process is to pass the kernels through a heated solution of glycerin and sodium carbonate, then to remove the skins with a stream of water and dip in a citric acid solution.

Cooking the nuts in oil causes considerable loss of vitamin contents. We are told that in an experiment macadamia nuts were cooked in oil at 135 degrees centigrade for only 12 to 15 minutes and lost 16 per cent of their thiamin. Modern commercial methods of processing nuts bring about destruction of perhaps 70 to 80 per cent of the thiamin.

So what can you do to secure nuts whose food value has not been ruined before you get them? First of all, pass by the fancy, toasty-smelling nut and candy shops as if they weren't there. Never buy nuts that have been shelled or roasted. Buy them in the shells and shell them yourself. And then, whatever you do, don't roast all the goodness out of them before you eat them! If you have ever tasted an almond right out of the shell, you will agree with us that there is absolutely no excuse for roasting them. We do not know where you can get nuts that have not been bleached or dyed, except from organic growers who do not use chemicals of any kind. But the dye or the bleach is only on the outside of the nut which of course you do not eat.

Where and How We Get our Nuts

The Southern European and Mediterranean countries are the world's largest producers of nuts. Brazil nuts are grown in Brazil and Bolivia. Cashews come from India and Mozambique. United States is the largest producer of English (sometimes called Persian) walnuts and almost the sole producer of pecans. Although the total value of edible nuts produced in 1949 was seventy million dollars, the people of this country used only about one and a half pounds of nuts per person that same year. So you see we do not begin to appreciate the value of nuts as food. In spite of the fact that they are generally presented to us commercially in candies, pastries, and so forth, we still eat only about a pound and a half per person per year, whereas we consume annually well over a hundred pounds of sugar per person. And sugar has no food value whatsoever except calories.

The peanut, which is of course not a nut at all but a plant whose nuts ripen in the ground, has recently come into its own as a food of surpassingly high quality from the standpoint of nutrition. Peanut flour contains over four times the amount of protein, eight times the fat and nine times the minerals that are in wheat flour. It can be used with great success in recipes. Adelle Davis in her excellent cook book *Let's Cook it Right* (Harcourt Brace and Company, New York) says she has never had a failure using peanut flour in baking recipes. For those who have difficulty of any kind with cereals and flours made from cereals, peanut flour would seem to be the perfect answer.

Acorn flour is used extensively in Europe and among the Indians of our Southwest. We are told that, in all probability, over the centuries, more human beings have eaten acorns than have eaten wheat. In Spain and Italy as much as 20 per cent of the food of the poor folks may be acorns. Some of them are edible as they grow. Others can only be eaten by first removing the tannins.

Nuts in their shells keep well. Shelled they become rancid in three or four months, especially in the summer. They can be kept at refrigerator temperatures for a year. With the exception of black walnuts and hickory nuts, those which are available to us in this country are not so hard to shell, so there seems to be no reason for not keeping them right in the shell until you use them. They are an excellent and unusual dessert.

For those housewives who feel lost somehow now that they no longer serve cakes, pies, puddings or cookies for dessert, why not get yourself a big bowl of the family's favorite nuts, a couple of nut-crackers and picks and bring them to the table after each meal along with fresh fruit as the best and most healthful kind of dessert! We often forget about nuts if we keep them in a bag in the kitchen cupboard. So try to keep a bowl of them handy for everyone to dip into for snacks—on a table in the dining room or living room.

Here is the composition of a number of kinds of nuts. Note, please, that some of them are relatively high in starch content while others contain little starch. Some are as high in protein content as meat. Others contain less protein. Remember, too, that, although the protein of nuts is excellent protein, it does not contain all of the essential amino acids that are present in foods of animal origin.

	Percentage of Carbohydrate	Protein	Fat	Calories per pound
Acorn	57.10	6.65	5	1909
Almond	4.3	20.5	16	3030
Beechnut	13.2	21.9	57.4	2846
Brazil nut	4.1	13.8	61.5	3013
Butternut	3.5	27.9	61.2	3165
Cashew	29.4	21.6	39	2866
Chestnut	36.6	2.3	2.7	1806
Coconut	27.9	5.7	50.6	2760
Filbert	9.3	14.9	65.6	3288
Hickory nuts	11.4	15.4	67.4	3342
Lychee	78	2.9	.80	1539
Macadamia nuts	8.2	8.6	73.0	3507
Peanuts	8.6	28.1	49	2645
Pecans	3.9	9.4	73	3539
Pine nuts	6.9	33.9	49.4	3174
Pistachio	16.3	22.3	54.0	2996
Walnut, black	10.20	27.6	56.3	3180
Walnut, English	5.0	12.5	51.5	3326

The percentage of the mineral content of nuts is given in the following chart:

	Phosphorus	Potassium	Calcium	Magnesium	Sodium	Chlorine	Iron	Sulfur	Zinc	Manganese	Copper
Almond	.475	.759	.254	.252	.026	.020	.0044	.150	.0019	.0008	.0015
Brazil	.602	.601	.124	.225	.020	.081	.0028	.198	....	....	.0014
Butternut	....	....	....	....	....	....	.0068	....	....	....	.0012
Cashew	.480	....	.048	....	....	....	....	....	....	....	....
Chestnut	.093	.560	.034	.051	.065	.006	.0070	.068	.0004	.0031	.0078
Coconut	.191	.693	.043	.077	.053	.225	.0036	.076	.0010	....	....
Hazelnut	.354	.618	.287	.140	.019	.067	.0041	.198	.0010	....	.0012
Hickory nut	.370	....	....	.160	....	....	.0029	....	....	....	.0014
Macadamia	.240	....	.053	....	....	....	.0020	....	....	....	....
Peanut	.392	.614	.080	.167	.039	.041	.0019	.226	.0016	.0020	.0009
Pecan	.335	.332	.089	.152	....	.050	.0026	.113	....	.0043	.0010
Pistachio	....	....	....	....	....	....	.0079	....	....	.0007	.0012
Walnut, black	.091	.675	.071	.098	....	....	.0060	....	....	.0033	.0032
Walnut, English	.308	.332	.089	.134	.023	.036	.0021	.146	.0020	.0018	.0011

Although they are not as rich in vitamins as some other foods, nuts provide some of the vitamins that exist in all natural food products that have not been refined. The B vitamins are scarce in modern American diets, for we have removed them from refined foods during the processing. So nuts, even in the small quantities in which we eat them, compared to other foods, are an excellent source of the B vitamins. Here is the vitamin content of some of the common nuts:

	Vitamin A	Vitamin B_1 Thiamin	Vitamin B_2 Riboflavin	Vitamin B Niacin
Almonds (3/4 cup)	0	.25 mg.	.67 mg.	4.6 mg.
Brazil nuts (3/4 cup)	trace	.86	....	....
Cashews (3/4 cup)	....	.63	.19	2.1
Chestnuts (40)	0	.108	.24	1.0
Coconut (2 cups)	....	.30 .60	1.0	....
Peanuts (3/4 cup)	0	.30	.13	16.2
Peanut butter (6 tbs.)	....	.12	.13	16.2
Pecans (1 cup)	50 I.U.	.72	.11	.9
Walnuts, Eng. (1 cup)	30 I.U.	.48	.13	1.2

In addition peanuts are rich in pyridoxine, pantothenic acid and biotin, three other important members of the vitamin B family.

The almond includes both bitter and sweet among its relatives. The sweet almond is the one we eat. Both are closely related to the peach tree. As a matter of fact the almond nut itself is almost identical with the peach stone. The bitter almond contains hydrocyanic acid, a toxic substance. Beechnuts too, as they are grown in Europe contain a substance that can be harmful in quantity. But the American beechnut has no such ingredient.

We usually eat chestnuts cooked almost like a vegetable, but they are delicious raw, once you get used to them that way. In many parts of the world chestnuts are ground into flour which is used as cereal flour is here.

Peanut butter is made of peanuts that have been roasted and halved. Then their skins are removed and they are ground. Usually oils are added to keep them in a smooth, buttery condition. If you have access to it, we'd suggest buying raw peanut butter or grinding your own from raw peanuts. The famous scientist, Carver, produced 202 different products from peanuts—not all of them food products, of course.

Non-food products are made from other nuts, too. A floor covering is made from nutshell flour mixed with pigment, resin. Loud speakers for radios are made from walnut shell flour. For some peculiar reason this substance seems to filter out vibrations more effectively than any other!

Oatmeal

In a section of rural Wales there is a legend of a famous giant who attributed his strength to eating oatcakes and buttermilk. In the same county, we are told, there were also two blacksmiths who used to walk 18 miles from Bala to Dolgelley carrying their heavy tools with them, shoe about twenty-five horses each and then walk back home the same day. As you surely do not need to be told, oats are staple fare in this part of the world, even today.

They are the second leading cereal of this country, corn being the first. The annual per capita consumption of oatmeal in the United States is today about four pounds. More oats are used in the breakfast cereal business than any other cereal. The part that we eat is called the groat and it is obtained by removing the tough hulls of the oat grains.

Interestingly enough, when oats are milled, the germ and bran remain in the portion used for human food. So actually oatmeal is a whole grain cereal, like brown rice, containing far more of the nutritional value of the original grain than white flour contains, or white rice. In the milling process the fibrous hull is first removed. Then, in making the slow-cooking kind of rolled oats, the whole groats are steamed, which partially cooks them. The quick-cooking oats are chopped with rotary cutters into varying sizes. Afterwards they also are steamed. Then both kinds are rolled to make the "rolled oats" we have for breakfast.

A number of years ago Sir Edward Mellanby, a famous British nutritionist brought down on himself the wrath of the Scottish people by publishing the results of experiments showing that there is a substance in cereals, especially in oatmeal, which robs the body of calcium. The substance is phytate or phytic acid. Mellanby proved in his experiments with puppies that a diet high in oatmeal (or other cereals to varying degrees) would produce rickets. The Scots were enraged that anyone dared to say such things about their national dish, oatmeal, or porridge as they call it. Their newspapers published satiric cartoons in which they made fun of Sir Edward. However, at the time rickets (a disease of calcium and phosphorus deficiency) was widespread in certain parts of Scotland where oatmeal was the staple food.

Many other nutritionists have since challenged Sir Edward's findings, but so far as we know, no one has managed to disprove them. So we must accept the fact that cereals, even cereals whose calcium content is high, such as oatmeal, do have an unhealthful effect on the calcium stores of the body, under certain circumstances. It seems that these circumstances are important, too. Plenty of calcium and vitamin D in the diet appear to counteract the effect of the phytate in the cereals. This, says Sir Edward, is the reason old-timers always ate plenty of milk with their oatmeal, for milk is rich in calcium. The fisherfolk who did not have milk ate fish livers which gave them vitamin D. And in the presence of plenty of calcium and vitamin D, perhaps the anticalcium effects of oatmeal would do little harm.

However, it is well to keep in mind when you are planning meals that cereal—any kind of cereal—prepared either as breakfast food or bread, should not have too large a place in your plans. Cereals are cheap, filling, easy to prepare and convenient to eat so we all tend to use more of them than we should, especially in children's diets they tend to replace the healthful fresh fruits and vegetables. So, even though oatmeal contains valuable food elements as we show below, remember that you are losing some calcium from your diet when you serve it. So make up for the calcium in some other way. Use milk rather than water for cooking the cereal. You can add powdered milk to the liquid milk. You can add powdered bone meal to oatmeal or to almost any kind of bread you are making. All these will add calcium to the meal you are making.

Three-fourths cup of cooked oatmeal (and we are speaking here of rolled oats, either the quick or long-cooking kind—we are not speaking of processed cold cereals made of oats) contain approximately the following vitamins and minerals:

Vitamin B:		
Thiamin	.55	milligrams
Riboflavin	.14	milligrams
Niacin	1.1	milligrams
Pantothenic acid	250.	micrograms
Choline	150.	milligrams
Vitamin E	2.10	milligrams
Calcium	54	milligrams
Phosphorus	365	milligrams
Iron	5.2.	milligrams
Copper	.50	milligrams

Organic Gardening and Health

By WILFRID N. SISK, M.D., M.P.H.
In charge of Industrial Medicine, the Upjohn Co.

An address delivered before the Lansing meeting of the Michigan Federated Organic Clubs

I would like to consider with you for a few moments the purpose of the Michigan Federation of Organic Clubs We are a group of people from all walks of life who have come together to study the *organic method* of *farming* and *gardening*. Now many of us are interested in different phases of the work. Some of us like flowers, others vegetables, others canning and freezing and others cattle raising. And there are even some of us who would just as soon let someone else do the growing of the various foods so long as we are able to buy the organically-produced products. It seems to me, however, that there is one central purpose which binds us all together and that purpose I believe might well be expressed in one short sentence: We desire to stimulate the production in the U. S. of the best food that it is possible to produce.

I'm sure no one would quarrel with our objective of producing the best food possible for America. In fact there are a great many other organizations, some of them much larger than ours, which share the same objective. The difference lies in the fact that we believe that the best way to accomplish our purpose is by the use of what we call the *Organic Method.*

Here again I believe a definition is in order. The *Organic Method* is not a static thing, but rather is changing from time to time as we learn more and more about the needs of plants and animals. Also, there are many shades of opinion within our movement so that not all of us agree on every single detail of what should be done. The binding part of our creed is found in the belief that we must *come as close to nature's own methods as is possible under modern conditions* and we further believe that much organic matter must be returned to the soil—just as nature invariably does. Our British colleagues believe that no fertilizer other than that coming from organic matter is needed. I must point out, however, that even they use ground limestone and ground bone. We in America, while admitting the soundness of the British attitude, are a little more impatient and find that we can get more rapid results by using ground rocks of various sorts along with our organic matter. In this way we are still cooperating with nature.

Here I would like to correct a mistake in many people's minds concerning our use of fertilizer. It is often said that we do not use *commercial* fertilizer. Another statement which is in error is that we do not use chemical fertilizers. We make both statements among ourselves and know what we are talking about, but outsiders misunderstand and feel that we are fighting *them* instead of fighting *for* them and their very welfare. There is no reason to be careful about the feelings of a crook who is purposely misleading the public. But we do not want to antagonize the person who is honestly doing the best he knows how but simply is not as well informed as we.

So what do we actually mean. We mean that we do not use soluble fertilizers. The ground rock, the ground bone, the prepared compost, yes, even the ground limestone that the British use and yes, the ground corn cobs some of us use are prepared by commercial interests and sold on the market, so we do use *commercial fertilizer.* And this ground limestone, ground rock and ground bone is certainly a chemical. And the organic materials we use are certainly among the most complex and perfect chemical substances on the face of the earth so we do use *chemical fertilizers.*

What then is the distinguishing characteristic of the substances which we use? The substances we use are not made artificially soluble and are not artificially concentrated. Most of the fertilizers to which we object have been treated with a strong acid such as sulfuric acid. Thus we seek to avoid *soluble fertilizers.* Many, many misunderstandings and arguments are caused by a careless use of words, sometimes just one word. Let us all make it a point to make it clear that we welcome the fertilizer manufacturer. It is only necessary to look at any organic publication to see their advertisements. We simply want quality fertilizer. We do not want the soluble fertilizers.

We think of life as a mysterious thing of great complexity, and indeed the processes we call life are the most complex processes on the face of the earth. Even though science has made more progress in the past 50 years in unraveling life's secrets than has been accomplished in all the thousands of years of man's previous existence, we have still only scratched the surface of knowledge about life.

Why then do we believe that organically-raised foods can help us maintain a better life? The answer to that question is in several parts. The first part is the observation concerning the origin of modern man. We must recognize that we are the product of man's struggle with nature for the past several thousand years. Among other characteristics of the human body is its need for the foods to which it has become accustomed. We must recognize that the needs of the body have been built up over several thousand years and cannot be changed in one generation without some harm resulting. Perhaps in another ten generations the human body can develop tolerance for large amounts of lead arsenate, but for the time being we must keep our intake of this and similar substances to a low level. Up until a little more than 100 years ago there was no such thing as a soluble fertilizer, so that all the food was raised in a manner very similar to what we now call the organic method. Comparatively little in the way of insect sprays were used before 1900. Therefore, if we look back to conditions as they were a hundred years ago, we should be able to see whether we are doing as well today as people did with more naturally grown food.

Unfortunately, so many factors have changed in the past 100 years that an exact comparison is not possible, but there are some very suggestive indications that in many respects our great-grandparents were living a more vigorous life than we. One indication is the life expectancy tables. It has become customary in the newspapers and magazines to compare the life expectancy at birth (or in other words, at age 0), of some previous period with the life expectancy at age 0 today. I think this is largely because of the fact that we want to pat ourselves on the back and these figures are best calculated to do the patting. For example, the white males born in 1850 had an average life expectancy of some 38.3 years, while white males born in 1950 had an average life expectancy of 65.9 years. This is a gratifying improvement and I would certainly not want to see us go back to the infectious disease and poor medical care of a hundred years ago which resulted in the death of so many thousands of babies.

Actually, those figures mean nothing in the world except the fact that we have saved the lives of many babies who used to die within the first ten years of life from poor medical care and because of the fact that no one knew what to do about infectious disease. The Government and the life insurance companies, however, do not stop with age 0 in figuring out their life expectancy tables, but there seems to be a feeling that the American public wants their facts sugar-coated, so that life expectancy tables for older ages are seldom published except in technical journals. So many wonderful things have been developed in the past 100 years that we certainly have enough things to brag about and we certainly can afford to look at the whole truth even if it is a bit sobering.

While all of us are interested in the fate of a new-born baby, it is only human to be more interested in the fate of people our own age. The life table for age 10, for example, only shows a moderate improvement between 1850 and 1950 and the improvement decreases as we go up the age scale. For men who manage to live to be 40 years of age, the life expectancy has increased exactly three years in the period between 1850 and 1950. This much improvement could be expected from the discovery of penicillin alone. In 1850 men who lived to be 40 years of age could expect on the average to live to be 68 years of age, while men 40 years of age in 1950 could expect to live to 71 years. At age 50 there has been an improvement in life expectancy of exactly one year. At age 60, 70, and 80 there has actually been a few tenths of a year decrease in life expectancy.

When we recognize the fact that medical attention and general care of all people has improved tremendously in the past hundred years, we certainly have a right to expect more improvement in longevity after age 40 than has been the case. In fact, to stay alive 100 years ago required a much more vigorous person than it does today. Life expectancy for the older ages hit its lowest point between 1900 and 1920.

These figures alone would not convince one that anything is wrong with present day American health, but they are a straw in the wind and there are other things indicating that we are not doing as well as we might. For example, there were 16,500,000 people admitted to hospitals in 1949. The average number of people in the hospital in any one day was 1,200,000, of whom more than half were in mental hospitals. According to Lawrence J. Link, over 10,000,000 persons are suffering from chronic illness and disabling conditions in the United States and the number of handicapped individuals exceeded 18,000,500, making a total of more than 28,000,000 handicapped or ill persons. Of course when we reduce infectious diseases we automatically keep alive some people who are otherwise ill or handicapped, but in my opinion at least, this factor cannot begin to account for the tremendous increase in mental diseases, diabetes, stomach ulcers, arthritis, allergy, cancer, and the other degenerative diseases.

As an example of what I mean, there was a recent report in the *Journal of the American Medical Association* concerning men killed in battle in Korea. Autopsies were performed on 30 such men and their hearts were very carefully examined. In 77 per cent of the hearts there was found some disease of the coronary arteries. The average age of these men was 22 years and there was only one man as old as 48 years. This is indeed a young group to be showing already disease of the coronary artery. The native Koreans by contrast to the Americans very rarely have heart attack, which of course results from disease of the coronary artery. Dr. Paul White of Boston, one of the leading cardiologists in the country who has spent his whole life in the study of heart disease, recently reported on the difference between the heart disease patients of 1925 and those of 1950. His figures do not give an exact percentage which can be applied to the population as a whole, but they show a decrease in heart diseases caused by infections and a sizable increase in the proportion of coronary artery disease.

Let us take the picture of cancer as another example. Cancer is increasing out of proportion to the increasing age of our population and it is reaching back farther and farther into the younger age groups. In the case of diabetes, survey indicates that approximately two per cent of the population is suffering from this disease. In the case of arthritis, approximately 7,000,000 Americans are affected. In the case of allergy there is some disagreement as to the exact extent of that disease, but a conservative estimate would be approximately 10 per cent of the population.

These figures still, of course, do not prove beyond a shadow of a doubt that food is the chief factor causing so much illness and disability. Dr. Weston Price, however, did a monumental piece of work in seeking out peoples of the world using what we might call an old-fashioned diet, and compared them with members of the same nationalities who were living on what he called the modernized diet. He visited small groups of people of all races and in all climates. He visited the Eskimos of northern Alaska, the Indians of northern Canada, a group of British people on some isolated islands northwest of the British Isles, some Swiss people in the high valleys of the Alps, some Negroes of Central Africa, the isolated natives of Australia, New Zealand, and the South Pacific islands, and he finished his study by examining the skulls of several thousand Italians who lived before Christ, and several thousand Indians of Peru who lived before Columbus. Being a dentist, Dr. Price paid first attention to the teeth, and in everyone of these 14 instances he found uniform and virtually perfect teeth so long as the individuals stayed on their traditional diet. When families from these same groups moved to places where they bought most of their food from the store, there was rapid degeneration of the teeth. Resistance to tuberculosis was much lessened, for example, when these people changed to the modernized diet.

One of the precepts of the organic teaching is that we should use a minimum of poison sprays. I am not sure that we will ever get completely rid of insect sprays, at least on commercial farms, but our spraying practices could certainly stand some intensive study. For example, the Bright Leaf tobacco which is the chief ingredient in cigarettes is bothered by a certain little worm-like parasite. In order to get rid of this parasite lead arsenate is the spray most frequently used. Now arsenic is known to be closely associated with the production of cancer. Cancer of the lungs and throat in both Great Britain and the United States has increased exactly in proportion to the increase in cigarette smoking. It even showed a greater increase later in women than in men. Would the arsenic-containing cigarettes cause this increase?

It is not only a matter of the growing of our food, but the processing. In food processing many chemicals are being added to our foods with what I consider to be inadequate testing of those chemicals. I'll cite two examples. For some 50 years or more a bleaching process was used in producing white and frequently whole wheat flour. Veterinaries for many years have warned against feeding dogs white bread. But it was only about four years ago that the running fits and the death which occurred in dogs fed white bread was definitely pinned down to this bleach. The Government has since insisted that the millers use some other bleaching method. For 75 years we have used coumarin as an artificial flavor instead of pure vanilla. Only within the past few months was coumarin examined carefully enough to show that it produced severe liver disease in rats. Only within very recent times has the Food and Drug Administration taken it off the market.

There is much more data which might be presented which would indicate that in spite of all of our technical improvements of the past 50 years, we could be doing much better than we are. But what I have given will indicate some of the things we should do. The first thing indicated is the improvement in the growing and processing of our foods.

We can all cooperate in the growing of our crops by as natural methods as possible and by using as little insect spray as possible and we can help ourselves by using these quality foods with as little processing as possible. We must recognize, however, the growing population not only of the United States but of the world, and must realize that the hand methods of a hundred years ago are not going to feed the populations of the future. We must encourage experimentation which gives bigger yields, while at the same time insisting that the quality be kept up. While there has been much sound and fury concerning the tremendous differences between the organic method and that advocated by the agriculture colleges, actually the two methods are constantly coming closer and closer together. For example, Dr. Albrecht and his staff at Missouri State College are doing excellent work, and his conclusions follow very closely the normal agriculture which we recommend. Even Dr. Wynd here at Michigan State College recently published an article entitled "Feed the Soil," which is so close to the recommendations which we make that in fact the article was re-published in *Mother Earth,* the publication of the British Organic Farmers.

In studying the diets of people having some type of degenerative disease, the dietary defect which is most frequent is an insufficient amount of protein-containing foods. I do not mean to imply that fruits and vegetables are not valuable foods, but the foods more frequently used in too small a quantity are meats, eggs, and dairy products. We have two problems here in Michigan. One is the problem of climate. This mid-western climate is the most stimulating climate on the face of the earth. It causes us to be energetic but at the same time the very climate puts stress upon our bodies, wearing us out before our time. The second problem is that of relatively little physical exercise. The people of a hundred years ago could eat and burn up virtually double the amount of food which we consume. However, this smaller amount of food must contain the same amount of minerals, vitamins, protein, and other nutritive elements that our bodies need. If we are going to keep up our vigor and keep down our "figger" we must use foods high in nutritive values. This means that we must use a relatively large amount of protein-containing foods.

In the past few minutes I have summarized extremely briefly some of the medical information which leads many to believe that Americans are not living as well nor as long as we might. While these figures show that we have done a remarkable job in the preservation of infants and small children and in the control of infectious disease, they also show that we are paying a price after we reach the age of 40. The life expectancy, for example, among people 40 years of age or over has not shown as much improvement in the past 100 years as I feel we have the right to expect. The 28,000,000 people either handicapped or ill do not leave much room for complacency. The increase in coronary heart disease, in diabetes, in cancer, and other degenerative diseases is out of proportion to the known aging of our population. We have laboratories all over the country in which people of great training and technical skill are studying all of these degenerative diseases and I do not wish to minimize the importance of this scientific investigation. These investigations are of extreme importance and it is only by the use of knowledge so gained that the world is going to be able to support the probable population of 25 or 50 years from now. We are worried by an agricultural surplus at the moment and falling agricultural prices, but if the present population trend continues, the United States will have 200,000,000 people or more by 1975. We will either need to tremendously improve our agricultural production or import food. I don't believe we will be worrying about parity prices.

I am sure that there are some farmers who will say "this business of producing high quality foods with organic matter is all very well, but I have to make a living and have to keep up my yield with soluble fertilizers. After all, I can feed these soluble minerals to the plant without worrying much about the soil." This is the oversimplified explanation of soil fertility, which unfortunately has been popularized between certain members of the fertilizer industry. This oversimplified statement is only true under very special circumstances and I am sure that it is the source of much of the argument which has arisen between the larger fertilizer producers and those of us in the organic field. Let me make an exact quotation from Dr. Wynd as his article is quoted in *Mother Earth.*

> . . . "Soil is alive, truly, actually, and literally alive. Soil is not soil until it is alive, and no amount of chemical plant food mixed with dead, finely ground rock particles would produce the equivalent of a productive soil. If soil were a lifeless thing, we would never concern ourselves with erosion, or leaching, or with any phase of soil conservation, as long, of course, as the physical texture of the mass permitted seeds to be planted and roots to explore. 'Plant food' would solve all the farmers' problems, and he could boast, as he frequently and foolishly does, that the soil on his farm is 20 feet deep. If he had eyes that could see the soil in all of its microscopic and sub-microscopic details, he would see that the living portion is only a few inches deep, and he would shudder when he saw muddy rivulets carrying it away . . ."

I would not pretend that Dr. Wynd in his complete article admits to being an organic farmer, but I believe you can see what I mean when I say that organic methods and the more traditional methods are coming closer and closer together.

I would like to point out one other phase of farming in which organic matter shows its great usefulness. At the Friends of the Land meeting a little over a year ago, one of the men from Missouri State College classified the various different clays for their ability to hold plant nutrients and to hold water. In that list he had only one substance other than clay, and that was humus, which as you know is the material resulting from the proper decomposition of organic matter. In nutrient-holding capacity and water-holding capacity, humus stood head and shoulders above the best quality of clay. In fact, in most of these respects, humus was about four times as good as the best possible clay.

In conclusion, let me say that if the growing population of the United States is to be fed and fed well, we must have scientific research and improvement in our methods of farming, gardening, and food processing. We must not fear the truth, but only be sure that it is the whole truth. All of the knowledge to date, whether from the organic organization or from the agricultural colleges, stresses the need for organic matter in the soil and I have no fear that in the foreseeable future any new development will overthrow this basic idea concerning the needs of our soil.

Organic Gardening—Properties of Organic Food

By W. C. Martin, M.D.

Dr. Martin is well known for his recent startling discoveries about the presence of D.D.T. in human tissues. This article was written especially for *Prevention.*

Nutrition should be studied as a whole, although special study of its individual parts is necessary for a more complete knowledge, it is not necessary to wait until the scientist investigates the multiple factors of the chemistry of food in order to utilize nutrition in medicine.

Unfortunately there is very little information acceptable to science as to the value of total organic nutrition; there is, however, much evidence available that shows the vital influence that organic foods have on health and resistance to disease.

The "magic bullet" theory of medical therapy is applicable to infectious disease where a specific organism can be isolated as the causative agent, but in degenerative disease there is no specific etiologic factor (cause). Degenerative disease is due to "metabolic error" the basis of which is usually nutritional deficiencies and imbalance, and is therefore multiple in nature. Dr. King has called these metabolic errors "Nutritional Time Bombs" which may explode into a disease entity at any time during the life span. This occurs usually following a period of physical or emotional stress. The treatment of such conditions must therefore, be based on a multiple nutritional approach.

The human body is a living organism and not a manmade mechanical robot. The body cannot long survive on inorganic and synthetic foods but must have living organic food elements. The chemist has not yet been able to instill into his laboratory products the life forces of nature that are essential for the survival of the human organism—neither can these essential factors be removed from the food or destroyed by processing without damage to health.

This life force can be obtained only from a dynamic living organic soil. Foods from such soil, free of chemicals and refinements have the power to prevent degenerative diseases and increase the body resistance to infectious disease. If organic foods are of better quality and nutritional value, what constitutes these extra factors?

One of the most important factors in quality food is the protein content. Protein is the food constituent that makes the body grow. It helps combat invading organisms by producing active antibodies for protection and immunity in biochemical ways yet unknown. Numerous studies have shown that, unless all the essential amino acids are available at the same time, normal protein synthesis cannot take place in the body.

In fact, it has been found that simultaneous feeding of all the amino acids, non-essential as well as the essential is more effective than feeding the essential amino acids alone.

What part does organic farming play in the protein synthesis in the plant? There is much evidence to show that deficient soils upset the process of building proteins in the plant; whereas in organic soil the proteins are properly synthesized. The proteins are not only increased in amount but contain a more complete supply of amino acids, especially tryptophane and lycine. Analysis reveals that wheat is producing less protein and more starch each year. A recent report shows that our hybrid corn grown on regular soil contains only about 6-7 per cent protein while corn grown organically contains from 11-12 per cent protein. It is believed that the low grade protein is imperfectly formed and thus will reflect in the health of animals and humans.

Research is now being done on water extracts of organic matter in the soil. This extract is being tested on plants for its growth hormone factors. Tests have also shown that pigs grow more rapidly if allowed to root in pastures or if they are fed sod soil. Only recently has the "dung factor" from cow manure been discovered, which is now considered an excellent factor in poultry foods. This factor is associated with the "animal protein factor" (APIL.) or the "antianemia factor." This is now believed to be the cobalt containing vitamin B-12. All this gives a clue that organic soil contains an additional amount of essential unidentified micro-nutrients needed for better plant and animal nutrition. This is then transmitted to the human when this source of food is used for nourishment.

Trace Minerals In the Soil

There are 60 trace elements that are known to be essential for plant nutrition and approximately 24 of these are known to be necessary for human health. Dr. Wm. Albrecht has shown that many plant and animal diseases are caused by a deficiency of these trace minerals in the soil. In a test he varied six essential minerals in the soil. Whenever calcium, magnesium, sulfur, phosphorus or nitrogen was varied the plants varied in the concentration of the amino acids that made up the proteins. The variation was at times as high as 80 per cent—this reveals the difference in the quality of proteins in foods on soils deficient in trace elements. This will reflect on the health of the animals and humans living on this food.

Dr. Albrecht has also cited evidence to show the importance of trace minerals in the soil and plants in the prevention of Brucellosis or Bang's disease in cattle. Dr. Allison was able to repeat these findings in chemical tests in humans. A large percentage of the soil in the U. S. is deficient in some of these trace minerals, a condition which reflects on our health today.

Maximum of organic matter in the soil has been shown to increase the vitamin content of plants—Sir Albert Howard found that grain produced with organic material contained more vitamins than when grown with regular commercial fertilizer. This was true particularly of the important B complex vitamins. Dr. Pfeiffer found by analytical test that carotene, vitamin A and vitamin C content of organic food was increased from 20-80 per cent.

Do we have any evidence that organic soil contains any protective factors against disease? It is known that the organic matter of the soil is the habitat of teeming millions of organic life in the form of fungi, bacteria and macro- and microscopic animal life. Dr. Selman A. Waksman, one of the discoverers of streptomycin, says that it has been found that many disease-producing bacteria do not survive long in the soil. They are destroyed through the action of other organisms. He also gives many examples of antagonism between plant pathogens and other soil organisms such as the Dutch Elm disease, potato scab, turnip rot, etc.

There are also present in organic soil certain ultramicroscopic substances, parasitic upon bacteria. These are called bacteriaphage. Many of the soil fungi have been isolated and cultivated and their antibiotic properties used in medicine to cure diseases. Many plant experiments have shown the value of soil fungi as a protection against disease. Sir Albert Howard stated in *An Agricultural Testament* the presence of mycorrhiza (root-fungus) in the roots of the plants is associated with health, its absence is associated with diminishing resistance to disease.

Is it not possible to assume that small amounts of these antibiotic substances are absorbed by the plants and will retain their protective properties when consumed by the humans?

Earthworms and the Soil

Another important organism in the soil that has not been studied for the beneficial effects on health is the earthworm. It has been estimated by E. J. Russell that the addition of manure to the soil will increase the worm population from 13,000 to 3,000,000 to 5,000,000 per acre.

Dr. E. E. Pfeiffer stated that he has found that the earthworm digestive enzymes will destroy T. B. bacilli. He feels that this possible protective factor needs further investigation, to see if these earthworm enzymes will have the same bactericidal effect on other pathological bacteria. These findings suggest the many possible complicated integrations by which nature maintains a balance in the life cycle.

How does this then affect the argument for and against organic farming? The natural food of fungi and earthworms is the organic matter in the soil. As this is depleted the food supply for these organisms is reduced and their number is reduced. Also the commercial fertilizer as used today is a strong irritant and, when applied to the soil will destroy a large proportion of these organisms. This is also true of the chemical sprays used as insecticides today. The sprays are absorbed into the soil and poison the fungi, bacteria, worms and other microorganisms. When this happens then the plants become unhealthy. A recent report reveals that when one application of D.D.T. is made to the soil, 80-90 per cent will remain for 8 years and still affect the growth of certain plants. The insecticides not only interfere with the growth of the plants but the residue on the plants is cumulative in the human tissues. The author has shown by biopsy that

D.D.T. is present in human fat. Twenty-three out of twenty-five human tissues analyzed showed D.D.T., and 28 per cent of the cases had 5 P.P.M. or more which has been shown to be toxic in animal tests. These chemicals produce liver and nerve damage. Organic farming eliminates this health hazard and must be considered as a protective factor.

Organic Foods and Health

Is there chemical evidence that organic foods will improve the health and increase the resistance to infections? There are many such examples in animals and some in humans. Unfortunately these tests have not had scientific controls and therefore must be accepted only on their apparent value. One of the early animal tests was by Sir Albert Howard in India. He showed that his cattle fed on organically-grown foods developed resistance to virus infections such as hoof-and-mouth disease. He allowed his oxen to rub noses with infected cattle and they did not contract the disease.

Another example which covers an overall picture of increased health and vitality is the report from a breeding stable in Kentucky. This stable for decades had produced champion race horses, then in 1930, things changed; fewer horses won races and mares began to drop still-born or deformed colts. By 1941, the owner was advised to sell the horses and start with new ones. This he refused to do. Instead he started a program of soil restoration and an increase in organic matter. Within two years, a marked improvement was apparent, and by 1946 the stable stood third among the winners of the country, and the trouble with still-born colts had disappeared.

Dr. Weston Price in his book, *Nutrition and Physical Degeneration,* cites groups of people all over the world that have nearly perfect health, who live on organically-grown unrefined foods. The best known of this group are the Hunza people in Northern India. Dr. McCarrison stated after a seven-year study of these people, that they were "unexcelled in health and physical fitness."

To compare this with the physical fitness of the people of the U. S. where 47 per cent of the young men of draft age are rejected because of physical or mental defects should make us take a new look at our nutritional status.

There are many other unknown and unidentified accessory food factors that are necessary for good nutrition. Also, these numerous nutritional factors must be in harmonious balance for optimum health. This can only be obtained by encouraging natural ecology of the soil. (The science of vegetable and animal economy and activity.)

Optimum health implies maximum reserve capacity for each and every structure and function of the body. This ideal health should be our ultimate goal. It is the duty of the doctor to apply this new nutritional knowledge but the burden of production of quality foods is on the American farmer.

Organic Gardening—A Book Review

***Organic Gardening; How to Grow Healthy Vegetables, Fruits and Flowers Using Nature's Own Methods*, by J. I. Rodale, published by Hanover House, Garden City, New York reviewed by William Albrecht, Ph.D., Chairman of Department of Soils, University of Missouri**

This is another book by an author and editor who has been calling attention for years to the organic matter as an important, but sadly neglected, part in gardening and farming. It indicates the author's increasing study of this more dynamic segment of the soil body, and his attempts to bring together both the practice, or empiricism, and the science, or causes and effects, for production of nutrition and health in the plants we grow. He draws from experiences and many publications, especially those on soils.

This publication explains what organic gardening is in principle and in practice. It is the attempt to use the soil but also to maintain it in a highly fertile state by applying nature's activities in soil construction to offset man's activities in soil destruction. For this, the adding of organic matter to the soil as a mulch, as crop residues worked into the soil, or as composted materials partially changed from organic matter toward humus are all emphasized and discussed as foremost. Distinctions are clearly made between "organic matter for the soil" and "humus within the soil." The former materials vary widely in their nitrogen contents as the tables show. But once they are composted, used as a mulch, or worked into the soil they approach a more nearly constant figure of five per cent, common for the less dynamic humus within the soil. The author points out that the varied concentrations of nitrogen in organic matter are significant in terms of their ratio, to the concentrations of carbon. This ratio determines the rate of decay, the disturbance of that process to crop growth via microbes as competitors with the crops for nitrogen and for other fertility elements. The ratio relates itself to all these dynamics of nitrogen and carbon "on the move" in making the soil organic matter valuable. The oxidative release of the carbon, as carbonic acid, gives nature's most abundant and most universal acid. It is the force for rock breakdown. By this and other acids the limestone, the less readily soluble other minerals, and rocks like rock phosphate, granite dust, basalt powder and others are naturally chemically treated by this acid to make their fertility contents available for plant nutrition.

All of this is presented by the author as more "natural" than is the treatment of the soils with chemical fertilizers. Fertilizing with the commercial salts is a kind of "dousing the soil" at the time of seeding. The organic method is a seasonal timing of the increasing rate of fertility delivery by decay in correlation with the crop's needs for its increasing growth rate. The organic method is a natural "automatic" aspect in contrast to the chemist's over-enthusiastic efforts, mainly at the crop's outset.

The author puts into simple, more common language what is so often presented in terms too technical for most folks. It is his challenge for more science to be put under the practice affecting the organic phase of the soil, which is a small but all important part not yet put under most searching light by research workers. He has been struggling to learn the lesson of the organic matter in the soil which comes hard, like organic chemistry for college students in which too many refuse to enroll because of the difficulties in the clearer comprehension of the facts.

Emphasis is well put in the need for balance of all the factors in plant nutrition, but especially for all those of fertility, both organic and inorganic. The imbalances as they are reflected by growth of much plant lead but less fruit, many destructive fungus diseases or few of them, serious insect attacks or their absence, excessive nitrate in the plant to approach poisoning by the forage, and many other symptoms shown by plants under deficiencies and excesses of any factors, are called to the reader's attention. Lists of diseases, insects, methods of making composts at different rates of decay and quality of the product, let this book serve much as a handbook as well as a plea for better understanding of how valuable more organic matter built into most soils may be.

Mr. Rodale emphasizes organic matter for natural values not yet understood and therefore neither approved nor accepted. He speaks of a march of artificial practices which are becoming more artificial each year. They could not have come into existence without having been preceded step by step, technique by technique, with untested theories and methods which have become more standard and acceptable with more passage of time, but whose real value is absolutely questionable. When antibiotics are organic and of soil origin, we are slowly turning our ear to those who speak up in defense of the organic matter which may well be considered the "constitution" of the soil, or the ability of the soil to remain a living body in spite of, rather than because of, all the chemical treatments the soil doctors are prescribing for it. A new significance in the conservation of the soil in terms of its organic matter will stand out in the minds of all who read this book, regardless of whether one is in the "organic camp," or in the "chemical clique," or among those who compromise between these. Reading it will give new emphasis and effort to making our soils more productive.

Osteopathy

An article about the benefits of osteopathy in a medical journal? Impossible, you will say. Yet the March 19, 1955, issue of the *British Medical Journal* (corresponding to our *Journal of the American Medical Association*) carries an article by J. F. Bourdillon, B. M., F.R.C.S., Consultant Orthopedic Surgeon, North Gloucestershire Clinical Area, on this very subject. There are no apologies, excuses, or explanations from the editors of the magazine. It appears from this that they may take to printing other articles like this in the future.

The article begins by announcing that back disorders very often require manipulative treatment, and members of the medical profession "have actually recommended osteopathy to their patients." Dr. Bourdillon then goes on to relate the incident that started him on the trail of his investigations.

He was working with a surgeon who manipulated spines while the patient was under anesthesia. He had, in addition, a patient who was away from home and so could not go to her regular doctor. She was suffering from low back pain and sciatica. She showed Dr. Bourdillon how her own doctor treated her back and he did the same, bringing the patient relief.

Another patient had had a fractured vertebra. In the four years since the accident she had suffered from intermittent pain in the back of the leg. She had already been treated in a plastic jacket for four months. Physiotherapy and wearing an orthopedic corset seemed to achieve nothing. So Dr. Bourdillon manipulated her back, while she was anesthetized. Her relief lasted a week. Then he repeated the treatment a number of times at weekly intervals. Realizing that he could not continue to anesthetize this patient week after week, he began to give the treatment without anesthesia. The patient was eventually completely relieved.

Well, said Dr. Bourdillon to himself, there's something to this spine-manipulation after all. He began to use the treatment on other patients, with surprising results. One patient in particular had a pain on the inner side of the knee and could not stretch his leg out straight. The more treatments the doctor gave, the better his results, but he was still concerned about some cases that did not seem to improve. He followed up some of the patients. *They told him they were later cured by osteopaths.*

Now right here is the point at which, we are afraid, most medical men would turn their backs on the whole idea. And our story would then be over. But Dr. Bourdillon says, "I decided that I must learn more about osteopathy in spite of my early indoctrination against it, and by chance I met a qualified doctor now practicing osteopathy in London. I spent a week seeing his patients with him, and very quickly realized that there was a lot that I could learn from him." What glorious words! Here at last is an orthodox medical man who admits that he can learn much from one of the other healing professions! This is the kind of humility and liberal-mindedness we cherish in medical men. This kind of thinking throughout all medical circles could soon end much of the heartache and suffering that at present is not being relieved by the medical profession.

The Osteopath was Thorough and Skilled

Dr. Bourdillon was surprised, he says, by the way his osteopath examined a back. He tested every joint for movement and tenderness. He also showed Dr. Bourdillon that the sacroiliac joint (at the bottom of the spine) is mobile, not stiff. And when it is stiff this may indicate that something is wrong. He also showed him a method for testing its mobility. Then the osteopath went on to demonstrate his methods to the wondering and appreciative M. D. He showed him exactly how each joint is to be manipulated. He demonstrated the treatment for patients with recent acute back pain.

Dr. Bourdillon goes on for a couple of pages of fine print, revealing to his medical colleagues some of the things he has learned about examination and treatment of the spine with osteopathic methods. We find comments like this, "Personally I use the technique (one of many the osteopath has showed him) although I cannot explain its effects, because I find its helps some patients very much." Later on he says, "As, however, every joint in the back is examined, the likelihood of missing infective or neoplastic (possibly tumor-forming) processes is much less than with the orthodox type of examination." And "I am satisfied, however, that my results are much better than they were by orthodox methods alone."

He continues to list the various conditions for which he has used osteopathic manipulation, including migraine headache, "tennis elbow," frozen shoulder and various kinds of difficulty with sacroiliac joints. He concludes by saying that his peculiar interest in back disorders may spring from the fact that he himself has had chronic back pain. So he knows just how painful it can be and how essential it is that we find a remedy for it.

We think this is one of the most extraordinary articles we have ever read in a medical magazine. In this country the American Medical Association at its convention in June, 1955, disapproved a proposal that would have merged osteopaths into the medical association. This was defeated, says the *Times* of June 10, 1955, "in the express belief that the 'osteopathic concept' shows evidence of 'cultist' healing. The attempt to unite osteopathy and medicine was defeated by a vote of 101 to 81 by representatives of all the state medical societies. (This is not what one would call an overwhelming vote incidentally. In fact, had only eleven men voted differently, the motion would have passed.)

The Situation is Different in This Country

However, it goes without saying that American medical journals never mention osteopathy, except in terms of "cultism." One cannot imagine such a thing as a lead article in the *Journal of the American Medical Association* recommending, as this article indirectly does, that medical doctors should study chiropractic methods. Why is it, do you suppose, that in the case of England and osteopathy and in the case of Germany and chiropractic (as we report elsewhere in this book), such encouraging events can take place, while in this country our medical society steadfastly turns its head in the other direction?

Time Magazine for March 26, 1951, reported that in that year the U. S. Public Health Service made teaching grants of $25,000 and $20,000 to two osteopathic colleges. The A.M.A. "made no objection," says *Time.* "In osteopathy's long, slow climb toward respectability, every nod has helped. The nation's six accredited schools of osteopathy require four years of professional training as medical colleges do, and two years of college-level pre-training for a doctor's degree. . . . In all but eight states, their graduates may now prescribe drugs and perform surgery." *Time* goes on to tell us that the A.M.A. still holds it unethical for an M.D. to refer his patients to an osteopath (unless the osteopath also happens to be an M.D.).

Do osteopaths want to be absorbed into the general practice of medicine? Not according to Assistant Executive Secretary, Eldon McKenna of the American Osteopathic Association who told *Time* that they would never be absorbed, "at least never so long as medical men refuse to accept the osteopathic cause and cure of disease. M.D.'s treat symptoms. D.O.'s treat structural integrity and they will never forget the concept they were taught."

If you want to know more about osteopathy, there is a fine little magazine called *Osteopathic Magazine.* You can find out about it from the American Osteopathic Association, 221 East Ohio St., Chicago, Ill.

Peaches

So far as we can tell, peaches originated in China about the tenth century, B. C. They were known in Persia by the fourth century B. C., then were introduced into Europe and America. Today they hang, luscious and golden and juicy, on trees all over our country, even in the northern sections. Peaches contain three of the fruit acids—malic, tartaric and citric. But, as do other fruits, they have an alkaline reaction in the digestive system of the body. The sugar in peaches increases as they ripen, is least in the early varieties.

Peaches can be stored successfully at 32 degrees Fahrenheit, but they soften rapidly at temperatures higher than this and do not keep well even at optimum temperature for longer than two to four weeks. Commercially grown peaches are ripened by being exposed to gas, and are sometimes stored in this way to preserve them longer. Peaches that are bagged when they are just blossoms do not spoil as rapidly as those which grow in full sunlight. Bagged Elberta peaches develop higher vitamin A content than those not bagged.

Since they are difficult to store, peaches are preserved in many different ways. Canned peaches are a favorite American dessert. Peach jam and butter is popular. Freezing peaches is the best solution for those who have freezers. Peaches are dried commercially by the use of sulfur dioxide. They are exposed to these fumes for five or six hours, so that the color will remain and the vitamin A and C will be preserved. Then the peaches are exposed to the sun's rays for two to nine days. Before they are packaged, they are put through a brushing machine that removes the fuzzy part of the skin. Then they are sulfured a second time.

Dried peaches are concentrated food. One pound of dried peaches can be made from six or seven pounds of fresh ones. So the vitamin and mineral content of dried peaches is also greater than that of fresh ones. We prefer not to eat fruit that has been sulfured for it seems to us that the concentration of inorganic sulfur remaining in the fruit is most harmful. Fresh peaches contain about 5.7 milligrams of sulfur per hundred grams of fruit. *Dried peaches contain as high as 240 milligrams of sulfur.*

The skin of a peach contains more vitamins than any other part of it. But we must caution against eating the skins, unless you are sure your fruit is grown organically. Many different kinds of insecticides are sprayed on peaches for there are many pests that attack this soft and tender fruit. Since the skin is fuzzy, it is almost impossible to wash off the spray and we don't doubt that some of it penetrates into the meat of the peach as well. Just beneath the skin is the next highest concentration of vitamins, and the flesh around the stone has the least. As hard peaches ripen, their vitamin C content increases. It differs according to variety and also according to growing conditions within the different varieties.

Peaches are valuable chiefly for their content of vitamin A and vitamin C. Yellow peaches contain more vitamin A than white ones. Here is the approximate vitamin content of one average-sized peach:

Vitamin A:

White Peaches—5-100 International Units
Yellow Peaches—880-2000 International Units

Vitamin B:

Thiamin—20-40 Micrograms
Riboflavin—50-60 Micrograms

Vitamin B:

Niacin—.9 Milligrams
Pantothenic Acid—35-45 Milligrams
Inositol—96 Milligrams

Vitamin C:—8-10 Milligrams
(An orange contains about 25)

Here is the mineral content of one average-sized peach:

Calcium	10 Milligrams
Phosphorus	21 Milligrams
Iron	.36 Milligrams
Copper	.01 Milligrams
Manganese	.11 Milligrams
Chlorine	4 Milligrams

Peanuts

Junior is showing good judgment when he insists on peanut butter sandwiches rather than jelly or jam. As a matter of fact, if he must eat sandwiches, peanut butter is better as a filling than anything else except meat. Two tablespoons of peanut butter contain more protein than an egg.

In addition peanuts contain large amounts of the B vitamins and vitamin E. They are rich in minerals. Peanut flour is a very excellent supplement for wheat flour. It contains four times as much protein as wheat flour, eight times as much fat and nine times as many minerals. In recipes using wheat flour you may substitute peanut flour for 15 to 20 per cent of the wheat flour without making any special change in the recipe.

As yet we have hardly begun to appreciate the value of peanuts as food. You know, of course, that they are not actually nuts, in that they do not grow as the fruit of trees, as other nuts do. Peanuts are legumes, like soy beans and peas. They grow on a peanut plant. As the plant matures, the ends of the branches bury themselves in the ground and the peanuts are formed underground. When the plant withers it's time to dig the peanuts. They're easy to grow. If you have a garden, by all means plant a few rows. Only be sure to buy peanuts meant for seed—roasted peanuts won't sprout. Peanuts will keep, in their shells, in a covered container at about 35 degrees Fahrenheit for two years, losing only little of their food value.

As everybody knows, peanuts are delicious, eaten either straight from the shell or toasted in butter. (Go easy on the salt!) Peanut flour, peanut butter and peanut oil are as nutritious as the peanuts themselves. We have read somewhere that raw peanuts are far better for you than roasted ones. Personally we don't like the taste of raw peanuts, but if you find that you do, by all means eat them raw! In the figures below, we are talking about roasted peanuts:

Vitamin B content	*per 100 grams*
Thiamin	300-400 micrograms
Riboflavin	160-500 micrograms
Niacin	16.2 milligrams
Folic acid	280 micrograms
Biotin	39 micrograms
Choline	145 milligrams
Inositol	180 milligrams
Pantothenic acid	2500 micrograms (more than any other food except liver)
Pyridoxine	300 micrograms
Vitamin E content	26-36 milligrams
Calcium	71 milligrams
Phosphorus	399 milligrams
Iron	2.31 milligrams
Copper	.96 milligrams
Chlorine	56 milligrams
Potassium	700 milligrams
Sodium	120 milligrams
Sulfur	226 milligrams
Zinc	2 milligrams

Peanuts are also rich in the essential amino acids—those eight forms of protein that contribute so much to human health. About 100 grams of peanuts are about 100 peanuts.

Peas

June peas! Fresh from the vines, sweet and crisp and tender! What city-dweller could possibly know the delights of eating a dish of June peas right from the vines in his own garden! We're sure that farmers and gardeners will agree with us that the first peas of the season are a real event.

In addition to their delectable taste, peas are excellent food. They are, of course, seeds, so they are well equipped with all the nourishment the new plants will need to grow and carry on the next generation. They are a plant with a long history, well known to the Greeks and Romans, the ancient Egyptians and Ethiopians. In fact, we are told that evidence of the pea as human food has been found in that area of Switzerland inhabited by the Lake Dwellers during the bronze age.

The kind of pea most generally eaten in this country is the seed, wrinkled or smooth, of the *pisum sativum*. Then, too, there are sugar peas whose pods are eaten right along with the seeds. Peas suffer extensively so far as nutrient value is concerned with every hour they remain on the shelf after picking. Not only do vitamins disappear from them as they grow old, but their sugar is decreased and their starch content increased. As a matter of fact we are told that the sugar content of the pea is greatest when the pea is too immature to be eaten.

Peas are an excellent food for freezing. It has been shown in carefully controlled experiments that if they are frozen raw and kept at below zero temperature, they deteriorate within a very short time. This is, we suppose, because of the enzymes they contain. So they should be blanched briefly before freezing. Of course eat them fresh if you can get them that way. But if you are deciding between frozen or canned peas, the decision should be easy. First of all, you should not eat any canned foods—but least of all canned peas which certainly bear little resemblance, either in taste or nutritive value, to fresh or frozen ones.

When you are cooking fresh peas, cook them just until they are tender (a very short time) and use all the water in which they cooked—as little as possible. If you're cooking frozen ones, by all means leave them frozen until you pop them into the utensil. They lose vitamins if they are allowed to thaw.

Undoubtedly the best way to eat peas is raw. Here is what Editor Rodale said on this subject several years ago in an article on raw food: "One of my first experiences with raw vegetables was with peas. It is ridiculous to cook them. They are so easy to take raw and any child will agree that in cooking, something is lost. When you eat them raw you get everything. Don't overlook the fact that peas are seeds. They are living things and will grow if placed in the soil. When you cook them that living quality is destroyed. Its germination power is annihilated. You are then eating a dead food."

Nightshade, a poisonous weed, often grows near or in the rows of peas at the big canning plants. The seed of the nightshade gets in with the shelled peas and up until recently there was no practical way to remove it. Then somebody invented detergents—yes, the kind we use for washing dishes—and a mix of detergents solved the pea-packers' problems. The peas, soaking in the detergent, sink to the bottom of the sorting racks. The nightshade seeds don't absorb the detergent. They float and can be skimmed off. How much detergent you eat in the can of peas you buy at the store is anybody's guess. We suggest strongly you make your own garden and grow your own peas if you possibly can. However, if you must eat commercially grown peas, it is comforting to know that, when you remove the pod you also remove much of the insecticide residue, so peas and shelled beans are thus probably safer from this point of view.

Peas are fairly rich in protein—a characteristic of all the legumes. But, they are deficient in two or three of the essential amino acids, so they cannot be counted on to supply whole protein, such as one gets from animal foods like meat and eggs. Here is the vitamin and mineral content of about a cup of peas:

- Vitamin A—680 International Units
- Vitamin B
  - Thiamin—340 to 400 micrograms
  - Riboflavin—160-200 micrograms
  - Niacin—2.1 to 2.7 milligrams
  - Pyridoxine—79-190 micrograms
  - Pantothenic acid—380-1040 micrograms
  - Biotin—3.5 micrograms
- Vitamin C—26 milligrams
- Calcium—14-22 milligrams
- Phosphorus—17-122 milligrams
- Iron—.46-1.9 milligram
- Copper—.10 milligrams
- Sulfur—50 milligrams
- Bromine—.21 milligrams
- Iodine—9 parts per billion
- Sodium—1 milligram
- Potassium—370 milligrams
- Carbohydrate—7.5 to 17.7 per cent
- Protein—4.2 to 6.7 per cent
- Fat—.2 to .4 per cent
- Calories—40 to 90

Penicillin

With every passing month the medical magazines add one or two more pieces of evidence to the case against the antibiotics. In recent days we have come upon a great deal of information on harmful reactions to penicillin among hospital personnel who are not taking the antibiotic themselves, but have been so exposed to it while they were giving it to patients that they are now extremely sensitive to it. Of course the rest of us do not come in contact with the antibiotics every day. But what proof do we have that a dose of penicillin from time to time—for a cold, for a cut finger, or for almost anything else—may not in time make us sensitive, too?

In addition we have been warned over and over again by anxious medical men that we are now developing a much more powerful and stubborn kind of germ that can withstand the antibiotics. After a few more years of dosing with these medicines, we are likely to find that they are no longer effective against anything. What will we invent then to destroy these virulent germs? Another stronger poison? And what will happen when the germs become resistant to *that* poison, too? No, it seems to us that a far wiser course is to develop instead bodies strong enough to withstand germs without any help from antibiotics. And certainly the most foolish course we can take is to rush for the penicillin at the slightest pretext, such as a common cold!

Allergic Reactions To Penicillin

Reporting in the *Armed Forces Medical Journal* for October, 1950, R. L. Gilman, M.D., calls attention to the fact that the severity of reactions to penicillin, currently being administered as a last-minute cure-all in the treatment of even noninfectious complaints, is greatly increasing. Whereas previous sensitizations produced by the wonder-drug had resulted principally in skin eruptions such as itching, wheals, nettle rash and hives, the list of newly observed post-injection effects now includes prostration, symptoms of arthritis, shock, chills and fever. All require protracted periods of readjustment for recovery which may be marked by still further irritations. Dr. Gilman calls for a renewed and careful study of the use of the powerful antibiotic and states flatly that he considers its administration prior to any and every surgical operation to be unsound. He also demands that it not be employed in the case of maladies that have no infectious origin.

An army medical man warned the medical profession and the general public of the current misuse of the antibiotic drugs, says the *New York Times* of November 2, 1951, reporting on a meeting of New York surgeons. Colonel Edwin J. Pulaski of the Walter Reed Hospital disclosed that one hospital recently reported that 40 per cent of its pharmacy bill was for antibiotics!

Colonel Pulaski goes on to say that resistant strains of disease organisms are appearing which have acquired immunity to the antibiotic drugs, such as penicillin and aureomycin. Continued misuse of the drugs will increase the number of resistant strains. Actually, he tells us, all the wonder drugs do is halt the growth of germs which the body's natural defense mechanisms then destroy. The usefulness of the drugs depends therefore on the condition of the patient, his state of nutrition and his general stamina. "If the natural defense is at a low stage, the antibiotics are not apt to help much," he says. He also declares that antibiotics in powder or ointment form are probably of little benefit and the combined use of several antibiotics together appears to be of little value.

Peppers

What do we demand of foods that we prefer to eat raw? They must be crisp or crunchy, have a distinctive flavor, be easily chewed and not too inconvenient in the way of skin or seeds. No vegetable fills all these demands so well as the bell pepper—a food many of us neglect simply because we have never learned to appreciate its value.

Peppers are not actually vegetables. Botanically they fit in the category of berries, because they have numerous seeds. They grow, as any gardener knows, on tidy plants with luscious shiny, dark green foliage. They can be eaten any time after they have attained any size at all, but actually they are not ripe until they are red. Peppers are picked green for marketing, so those of us who shop for vegetables seldom see a red one.

The chief claim to fame of the pepper is its phenomenally high vitamin C content. The vitamin C increases in the fruit as it ripens, so that in a pepper which is half red and half green, the red side will contain more vitamin C than the green side. One ripe bell pepper may contain as much as 300 milligrams of vitamin C. An average-size orange contains about fifty.

We hardly need to add that the vitamin C begins to dwindle almost as soon as the pepper is picked from its bush, so it is best to buy peppers as freshly picked as possible. At its best, a pepper is crisp and firm, thick-fleshed with a good color. The limp, wilted, shriveled pepper has lost most of its food value and probably all of its vitamin C. Of course, your peppers should go in a closed container in the refrigerator as soon as you bring them into the house. They lose vitamin C when they are cut or shredded, so serve them soon after they are prepared.

Vitamin P was first extracted from paprika, peppers and citrus fruits, so we know that this valuable vitamin accompanies the vitamin C in our tasty bell peppers. When vitamin C was first discovered, peppers were used extensively as a source of it. Many natural vitamin C preparations are today made from peppers rather than rose hips or other vitamin C-rich foods.

You can cook peppers if you must, and of course there are many cooked dishes which owe their tastiness to peppers. But serve them raw as often as possible. They make a fine addition to any vegetable salad, they add a lot to cole slaw and they are most nutritious and attractive stuffed with cheese or meat filling. Of course don't forget to add them to the plate when you are slicing "finger salads," for their lovely color contrasts beautifully with raw carrots, radishes and celery.

Pimentos, and hot peppers are related to bell peppers. All of them, and paprika too, give you an abundance of vitamin C and other vitamins. Here are the vitamins and minerals you will find in an average-sized green pepper, which weighs about 100 grams:

Vitamin A	700-3000	International units
Vitamin B		
Thiamin	30-70	milligrams
Riboflavin	40-100	milligrams
Niacin	.4	milligrams

Vitamin C	120-180 milligrams
Calcium	12 milligrams
Phosphorus	28 milligrams
Iron	.4 milligrams
Protein	1 gram

Peppers fall in the category of the 5 per cent carbohydrate vegetables and one medium sized pepper contains only 25 calories!

Phosphorus

Phosphorus is present in all foods except refined sugars and fats. It is present in all body cells. Calcium and phosphorus stand first and second respectively in the quantity of mineral elements present in the body. Phosphorus is perhaps the most important single element for a healthy soil and is the one most likely to be deficient in soils. The phosphorus of the earth's soil is unevenly distributed so that some localities may contain ample amounts while others have a deficiency. Phosphorus in nature may exist as a soluble substance which can easily be taken up by plants as food, or as rocks whose phosphorus is more slowly dissolved in order to become available to plant life. For this reason phosphorus is used in most fertilizers and the maintenance of enough soil phosphorus becomes one of the most pressing of agricultural problems.

The use of phosphorus in the body is closely interrelated to the use of calcium, so that when we are speaking of one we must constantly refer to the other. The amount of phosphorus needed by the body is not so important as the relationship between the calcium and phosphorus. In other words, a certain constant balance between the two minerals should be maintained at all times for perfect health. This ratio is two and one-half to one—there should be two and one-half times as much calcium as phosphorus.

Functions of Phosphorus

The body of an adult contains from one to one and a half pounds of phosphorus. Whereas most calcium in the body is contained in bones and teeth, only about 70 to 80 per cent of the body's phosphorus is in bones and teeth. The rest is distributed in muscles and nerves. We do not know as yet all the functions of phosphorus in the body, but here are some that we do know:

It exists in bones and teeth along with calcium and other minerals. It is present in fluids and soft tissues—that is, blood and cells contain phosphorus. It is necessary for the assimilation of fat by the body, for it combines with the fat to form a substance that can be digested. It also combines with proteins so that the protein can be absorbed by the body. You cannot digest niacin or riboflavin (two B vitamins) unless phosphorus is present. Aside from all these functions, phosphorus is also used for many other chain reactions and interrelationships in the body.

Perhaps the most important functions of phosphorus from the point of view of present-day Americans are those relating to carbohydrates and certain of the B vitamins. Our American diet is high in refined carbohydrates—white flour and white sugar. As we know, the B vitamins must be present if these carbohydrates are to be handled easily by the body's digestive processes. Now we find that we must also supply our body with plenty of phosphorus if carbohydrates are to be used successfully. The same is true of fats and proteins, both of which combine with phosphorus in the complicated chemical mechanism of digestion.

And yet, we must keep in mind that the calcium-phosphorus balance dare not be disturbed. White sugar is one of the most powerful "disturbers" of this balance. Melvin E. Page, D.D.S., of Florida who has done extensive laboratory work on the calcium-phosphorus balance tells us a story in his book, *Degeneration and Regeneration* (published by the Biochemical Research Foundation, 2810 First Street North, St. Petersburg, Florida), showing the disastrous results of even a little sugar in a modern diet. After several of his patients had not progressed as they should, he found they had been taking candy without letting him know. So he set up some experiments on patients for whom he had done a number of blood tests—for calcium and phosphorus balance. "Immediately after taking a blood sample each was given all the candy she wanted and other blood tests were taken at intervals. There was no change in two hours, but in two and a half hours the phosphorus level dropped five-tenths of a milligram. This was after eating nine pieces of chocolate candy—one-fourth of a pound. This was enough to make a difference of nine points in the usable product of calcium and phosphorus," says Dr. Page.

Dr. Page believes that diseases such as arthritis, pyorrhea, tooth decay and so forth, are brought about by disorders of the calcium-phosphorus balance. So you can see that it is mighty important for us to keep this balance regulated. And if such a seemingly slight matter as nine pieces of candy can make such a difference, what are most of us doing to the calcium-phosphorus balance of our bodies every day, especially so long as we continue to eat white sugar and flour products which we know definitely will throw that balance off!

Phosphorus is especially important for growing youngsters, for it must be present in sufficient quantity to make healthy bones, teeth and muscles. During the teenage years while the body is growing very rapidly, there is competition for the available supply of phosphorus. If the bones take up all of it, the result may be sagging weak muscles. If the muscles succeed in getting their share, the bones may be weakened. And, most important of all, if the calcium and phosphorus ratio is not maintained, both these vitally important minerals may be drained out of the body without being used. In other words, if there is too little calcium in the diet or too much phosphorus, both calcium and phosphorus supplies will suffer. If some condition in the body results in calcium not being retained, phosphorus will not be retained either, so our health will suffer a double set-back. During pregnancy, calcium is withdrawn from the bones and at the same time (so closely related are these two elements) just about the same amount of phosphorus is withdrawn, too.

Phosphorus is an important constituent of the brain. The brain consists of 80 to 85 per cent water. The solid matter is made up of phosphorized fats. These increase in proportion as the nervous system grows older and the brain becomes more learned. Recent researches have also shown that phosphorus may be important in cancer prevention, for investigators have discovered that phosphorus is more easily lost from cancer cells than from normal cells.

Assimilation of Phosphorus

Even though you get enough phosphorus in your food, there is a chance that you may have a deficiency, for certain conditions are necessary in your body for you to assimilate phosphorus. In general, these are the same conditions necessary for proper calcium assimilation. In cases of diarrhea, for instance, all the mineral elements may be lost to the body—calcium and phosphorus among them. Phosphorus must be in an acid medium to be properly absorbed, so there must be the correct amount of hydrochloric acid in the stomach during digestion. Vitamin D must be present, for phosphorus, like calcium, is absorbed only in the presence of vitamin D. For this reason, either a lack of calcium, phosphorus or vitamin D can bring about rickets, for all three are necessary to prevent this disease. High fat diets or digestive conditions which prevent the absorption of fat increase the absorption of phosphorus in the intestine, but such a condition is not healthful, because it also decreases the amount of calcium absorbed and throws off the calcium-phosphorus balance.

Phosphorus Deficiency and Daily Needs

It is difficult for laboratory workers to devise a diet that contains no phosphorus. But several workers have accomplished this and have found that phosphorus deficiency results in serious difficulties and eventually in death. The animals eating such a diet showed all the symptoms of calcium deficiency, too. They grew slowly, had difficulty in walking, were sensitive to the touch, had difficulty in breathing (because the rib bones were too soft to expand and contract) and showed signs of rickets. The phosphorus which goes to the brain, liver, heart and muscles is retained longer than that in the bones when there is a diet deficiency.

Finally, how much phosphorus do we need daily and how can we be certain we get it? In general, nutritionists agree that any good wholesome diet will contain enough phosphorus without any special attention. Since phosphorus appears in all foods and is especially rich in cereals, it is difficult to imagine a diet in this country that would not contain enough phosphorus. But—and it is a big "but," the one food element in which Americans are most likely to be deficient is calcium. And lack of calcium is bound to affect the calcium-phosphorus balance, so that, no matter how much phosphorus-rich food one eats, there will not be enough phosphorus for body use, so long as there is a shortage of calcium. It has been estimated that we should have daily 1.32 grams of phosphorus for every 70 kilograms (or roughly 140 pounds) of weight. Children need about 1 gram of phosphorus daily.

Phosphorus in Foods

Before you look at the table below which gives the approximate amount of phosphorus in various foods, let us remind you that all we have said above about the important relationship of calcium and phosphorus underlines the necessity for taking bone meal. It is course impossible for any of us to regulate our diets so carefully that we can measure every day the amount of calcium and the amount of phosphorus we are getting in our food. So by far the easiest and best way to make certain that you are getting the right proportion of calcium and phosphorus is to take bone meal. In these ground-up bones of healthy young cattle, the proportion of calcium to phosphorus is correct—otherwise the animals would not have been healthy. So by taking bone meal you too can be assured that you are getting enough calcium and phosphorus, every day. In addition you will be getting those other minerals that make up bones which are also important for good health.

Here are some foods rich in phosphorus:

Food	*Milligrams of Phosphorus*
Almonds	475 in 80 almonds
Beans, dry	463 in ½ cup
Beans, kidney, dried	475 in ½ cup
Beans, lima, dry	380 in ½ cup
Beans, lima, green	158 in ½ cup
Beef	167-208 in 2 slices
Beef, dried chipped	376 in 8 slices
Brain	380 in 2 pieces
Bran, wheat	1215 in 5 cups
Brazil nuts	592 in 15 nuts
Bread, whole wheat	270 in 5 slices
Cashew nuts	480 in 70 nuts
Cheese, hard	610 in 5 one inch cubes
Cheese, cottage	263 in 5 tablespoons
Cheese, Swiss	812 in 4 slices
Chicken	218 in 3 slices
Corn, sweet	120 in ½ cup
Eggs, whole fresh	210 in 2 eggs
Fish	218 in 1 piece
Heart, fresh	236 in 2 slices
Liver, fresh	373 in 1 slice
Milk, fresh, whole	93 in ½ cup
Milk, powdered	712 in 12 tablespoons
Oatmeal	365 in ¾ cup cooked
Peanuts	393 in 80 peanuts
Peanut butter	393 in 5 tablespoons
Peas, split	397 in 1½ cups cooked
Peas, green	122 in 1 cup
Pecans	324 in 80 pecans
Rice, brown	303 in ¾ cup steamed

Food	*Milligrams of Phosphorus*
Salmon, canned	286 in ½ cup
Soybeans, whole mature	586 in ½ cup
Sweetbreads	596 in ¾ cup
Tuna fish, canned	290 in ½ cup
Turkey	320 in 2 slices
Veal	200 in 2 slices
Wheat germ	1050 in 12 tablespoons

A milligram is one-thousandth of a gram, so you can see that a daily serving of meat, cheese and beans would give you your daily quota of phosphorus. But remember, the meat and the beans are short on calcium, so you would need to eat lots of calcium-rich foods too, so that the calcium-phosphorus balance would not be disturbed. Taking bone meal is a simple way to regulate this balance.

Pineapple

Did you ever wonder why so many old bedsteads, chairs and desks carry a stylized pineapple as their major decoration? In colonial America this beautiful fruit was carved, painted and embossed on furniture because it was thought of as a symbol of hospitality. So a carved pineapple on the bedstead indicated to the guest that he was welcome. And of course its graceful form and handsome tuft of leaves made the pineapple an ideal subject for carving, just as it is a beautiful centerpiece for a table decoration.

But quite apart from its beauty, a pineapple is good food. Possibly its greatest appeal to northerners is that it is available in winter and early spring when the vitamin C content of our food reaches its lowest ebb. True, it is picked when it is green so that it can be transported to our markets from its faraway tropic home. And picking green means with the pineapple, as with other fruits, that vitamins are lost. We are told that there is a very great difference in the vitamin C content of pineapples depending on the variety, the way they are grown and the condition in which they are picked.

Investigators have found in one study of pineapples that some contain as much as 165 milligrams of vitamin C compared to only 24 milligrams in other varieties.

Fresh pineapple contains a protein-digesting enzyme. Enzymes are substances formed in our saliva, stomach and intestines for digesting various food. We are all familiar with the enzyme from the papaya which is sold commercially as a meat tenderizer. The enzyme in pineapple will perform the same job. That is, sprinkling some fresh pineapple juice on your tough steak a little before you cook it will tenderize the steak. Or eating fresh pineapple as the first course of a meal will assure you of good digestion for the meat course.

As readers know, we do not advise eating canned foods. There seems to be little or no reason for eating canned pineapple when it is so widely available in the fresh state. However, the way pineapples are canned in Hawaii seems to guarantee that as much food value as possible remains with the fruit, for they are picked when they are ripe and every effort is made to have them in the cans within 36 hours. But of course the very process of canning is bound to destroy water-soluble vitamins—the B and C vitamins that we need so desperately. Canned pineapple shows up with about 10 milligrams of vitamin C to 38 of the fresh pineapple.

One reason why we recommend pineapple so highly is that its thick skin protects the fruit from poisonous insecticides that seep through the thin skins of other fruits. You can't eat the skin of a pineapple; it's too spiny and too tough. You lose vitamins when you peel it, but you can be fairly sure that you are not going to be eating a mixture of pineapple, lead, arsenic, chlordane and DDT, after you have the skin off!

In choosing a pineapple this is what you should look for. It should have a fresh, clean appearance, a dark orange, yellow color and a delicious fragrance. Usually the heavier it is, the better the quality of the fruit, provided that the pineapple is fully mature. The "eyes" should be flat, almost hollow.

Why not put pineapple on the menu for dessert or appetizer at least one day a week? And, for goodness sake, don't spoil it by burying it in sugar or sugar syrup. A normally ripened pineapple is 12.11 per cent sugar already—good, healthful fruit sugar that doesn't need any more sweetening from a sugar bowl.

Here is the approximate vitamin and mineral content of about ⅔-cup of fresh pineapple:

Vitamin A	150	International Units
Vitamin B	.1	milligrams
Thiamin	.1	milligrams
Riboflavin	.02	milligrams
Niacin	.2	milligrams
Some pantothenic acid		
Vitamin C	38	milligrams
Calcium	8	milligrams
Phosphorus	26	milligrams
Iron	.32	milligrams
Copper	.07	milligrams
Magnesium	1.07	milligrams

Poison Ivy

A reader sends us this suggestion for preventing Ivy Poisoning or curing it if you have already been poisoned.

If you are allergic to Poison Ivy and like to fish or picnic in the summertime, life can be miserable. But Ivy Poisoning can be cured—even prevented. The Indian medicine men knew how, and many present-day country people can tell you how. It is simple—and it works 100 per cent.

Just go to some cool, shady spot, probably along a creek anywhere from Maine to Florida and pick some Jewel Weed, often called Touch-me-not, (Scientifically known as *Impatiens*). Mash up the juicy stems and leaves in your hand and rub on the red, irritated or blistered part of your skin. Immediately the itching will stop and within 24 hours, the rash is gone and the skin is healed.

If you have been exposed to Poison Ivy but haven't started to blister, hurry and get some Jewel Weed juice on and you won't blister or even turn red. Even if you get Ivy Poisoning every time you go near it, you can now go fishing, hiking, picnicking with no fear—just pick some Jewel Weed plants and rub them on your exposed skin and you can walk right through Poison Ivy without its affecting you.

Try it some time on yourself or your kids and spread the word to your friends and neighbors.

If you are so extremely allergic to Poison Ivy that you get it in the middle of winter from old dead plants (as the writer did), go to a florist or greenhouse and buy some Flowering *Impatiens* and use it the same as Jewel Weed.

One warning: Material must be used freshly picked.

Polio and Iodine

By

J. F. Edwards, M.D.

Reprinted from the June 1954
Manitoba Medical Review

According to British Law, an individual is innocent until proven guilty. Applying the same legal dictum to Poliomyelitis its cause was adjudged, between 1905 and 1911, to be contagious and infectious; this, in the absence of a knowledge of its cause of spread, its only proven crime being that it could become epidemic. It was declared to be viral in origin.

This implication by the Public Health Laws of many of the Provinces of Canada and of the States of the Union made Poliomyelitis legally an infectious, contagious disease, and thereby opened the door for research, considering the disease as such; and closed the door to research along lines other than that which has been publicized and financed by endowment in the past forty years. This situation finds the Medical Profession in this year of our Lord 1954 in a position to declare "We have no treatment for Poliomyelitis." Truly nursing care has improved, dating from the initiation of the Kenny Method of therapy, but methods of treatment or prevention of the disease are conspicuous by their absence.

Viewing the disease from a clinical standpoint, in Manitoba's epidemics of 1952 and 1953 one notes that:

1. Few of our cases had a history of contact with an earlier case.
2. Few of our cases transmitted the disease to family contacts.
3. Few of Medical Personnel in attendance upon Polio patients acquired the disease or transmitted it to their families.
4. A state of fatigue frequently preceded the attack, yet many Medical Personnel working with these patients to a point of their exhaustion did not fall victim to the disease.
5. The disease is seasonal and may be geographical.

Animal experimentation has truly shown the disease to be transmissible, but no single means of transmission in the human animal has been proven.

The fact that polio is a seasonal disease occurring in late spring and summer, places it in a class apart from practically all other infectious diseases, which are most prevalent in those seasons when humans are confined within doors and congregate in groups. And the fact that epidemics fall off with the advent of cool fall days and nights, leaves one to consider if the then existing protection is not linked with body function; probably with stimulation of thyroid function.

An overall geographic picture of epidemics would place Winnipeg as the Canadian polio capital and St. Louis the American capital. A similar map drawn for encephalitis in horses would correspond favorably with the polio map.

Viewing the problem of spread from the geographic angle one is not a little surprised to see it compares favorably with our goitre area. Could iodine deficiency link in with polio's so-called infection?

Assuming this to be a fact and after confirming the assumption in animal virus diseases, in 1952 I treated three bulbar polio patients with intravenous sodium iodid. In these three, control of the disease was found to be most rapid and convalescence surprisingly brief. I was, at this time, convinced that the iodides acted as a virucide (a substance that destroys viruses) but the virucide theory was hardly tenable as the quantities used (grs. 7½) were hardly ample and the dosage was never given more than twice, and then three days apart. Further consideration and discussion brought forth from one of my confreres the suggestion that by the intravenous injection of iodides I was stimulating a defense mechanism, the iodides acting as a catalyst.

The 1953 epidemic was entered with this theory in mind. Numbers, and the varying severity of the disease, forbade intravenous therapy so I administered iodides orally depending on clinical examination for diagnosis, I having concluded in 1952 that spinal puncture only added insult to injury, with nothing gained.

The season advanced: gamma globulin stocks became exhausted; and my patients clamored for protection. Carrying the defense mechanism theory a step farther; "if I could control why could I not protect?" Of those seeking protection I formed an experimental group, giving one to three minims, according to age, of S. S. Pot. Iodide in milk daily for ten days (equivalent to 1.7 to 5 grains KI).

The season finally ended. I had seen some sixty cases. Two were sent to the King George Municipal Hospital because of the possibility of respiratory difficulties and lack of nursing care. The remainder were treated at home. Only one on home care developed paralysis, a paralysis that did not advance after oral iodide administration. None of two hundred contacts on prophylactic therapy developed polio. There were no deaths.

Can this theory fit our endemic cases and our Eskimo group? I believe it may. These people may be so low in iodine requirements as to have little or no defense against the invader if such there be.

The use of iodides in the control of known virus diseases affecting the central nervous system by no means is new. (In the following paragraphs the numbers refer to the articles listed in the bibliography at the end of this article.)

1. Manson, of England (1825) advocated its use in palsies, many of which cases must have been polio.

2. Coplan (1850) reports benefits in palsy, derived from potassium iodide in dosages as small as grs. 1 in twenty-four hours.

3. Brown-Sequard (1861) recommended potassium iodide as the only known remedy that could be used without danger in various forms of paraplegia.

4. Sinkler (1875) reported the treatment of an asthmatic with potassium iodide. The patient, who also had polio, improved with the therapy.

5. Elliott (1885) employed and recommended potassium iodide in combination with other medications in polio. Similar therapy was employed by Erb, Charcot and Hammond.

6. Webber (1885) recommended its use in polio.

7. Ridley (1925) employed Tincture of Iodine in the treatment of beriberi, a paralytic disease genetically related, according to 8. Braddon, to poliomyelitis. Beriberi was at one time declared like pellagra to be a virus disease.

9. Sir Thomas Horder (1927) reported the use of Colloidal Iodine intravenously in the treatment of poliomyelitis. He recommended its early use.

10. Breuil and Dartiguenave (1937) after trial with chemo-therapy failed in polio, reported improvement on iodine therapy.

11. Maberly (1939) reported complete recovery of four cases of polio on iodine therapy.

12. Mazzitelli (1939) gave a teaspoon of iodine-tannic acid syrup twice a day for several days to children in families with cases of poliomyelitis or in contact with them. None of these children who had preventive therapy developed poliomyelitis in that epidemic or in future ones. (Syrup Iodo-Tannicus contains 1.0% iodine.)

13. Scobey (1946) suggested the use of iodine in the prevention and treatment of polio and 14. in 1948 pointed out that iodine combined with ascorbic acid and calcium produced improvement in some cases in twenty-four hours.

The present writer in 1944 discussed with Dr. Fahrni of Winnipeg the possibilities of using intravenous sodium iodide in polio. Dr. Fahrni was then using sodium iodide, grs. 15, in 10 cc. distilled water (Parke-Davis) intravenously in thyroid crisis. Dr. Fahrni assured me that if given slowly it could at least do no harm. Not until 1952 did the opportunity arise to use it, with the previously recorded results.

15. In 1948 I reported to the Canadian Medical Association Journal a report of a number of experiments with iodine on humans and animals.

Iodine Therapy in Herpes Zoster

16. Head and Campbell (1900) described herpes zoster (shingles) as "Acute Posterior Horn Poliomyelitis." In this disease the anterior horn cells have not infrequently been involved and paralytic manifestations and atrophy have been observed. Epidemics of herpes zoster have been reported. These epidemics have sometimes paralleled polio epidemics.

17. Ruggles (1931) and 18. Beers (1939) reported early and dramatic relief of herpes zoster with intravenous sodium iodide.

19. Beckman (1953) approves the use of sodium iodide, Gms. 2 in 30 cc. of water intravenously at two day intervals for four or five treatments in herpes zoster.

Iodine in the Treatment of Encephalitis and Central Nervous System Diseases of Animals and Fowl

20. Lewitis (1935) states that iodides have been used with surprising results in cases of inflammation involving the spinal cord and brain.

21. Brinton, a poultry man (1931) reported that leg weakness in his flock following the feeding of excess wheat was cured with iodized buttermilk. Later he prevented the leg weakness and also coccidiosis with said buttermilk.

22. Grey (1940) used a 10 per cent solution of potassium iodide in distilled water in the treatment of fowl paralysis (lymphomatosis). After the first injection the birds became brighter, after the second muscular tone was restored and the birds rapidly progressed to normal.

23. Radeleff (1946) employed intravenous sodium iodide in the treatment of equine encephalitis. In his group so treated the mortality rate was less than ten per cent with no "dummies." Dummies are animals that survive, but have permanent brain damage. In his control group the mortality rate was 40 to 50 per cent. He reports rapid recovery and short convalescence in his iodide treated group.

McLoughry, a Manitoban veterinarian, during the epidemic of encephalitis in the later thirties and early forties paralleled Radeleff's findings. He employed potassium iodide. His success prompted my experiment reported in 1948 in the prophylaxis of equine encephalitis.

It is worthy of note that a number of workers including 24. von Economo (1931) employed iodine in the treatment of human encephalitis with favorable results.

Last summer Dr. Archie Kiteley of Nipawin, Sask., drew my attention to the fact that his area had no cases of human encephalitis during or since the epidemic years. This he argues may be due to the fact that in the early days, while we farmers were battling our stock breeding problems, he and his confrere, Dr. Max Scott, recognizing the deficiency of iodides, prescribed sodium iodide in practically every prescription they wrote. Is it possible epidemics of polio were suppressed by this very means?

25. In an editorial in the *Journal of the American Veterinary Association* the reports on the treatment and prophylaxis of equine encephalitis by Radeleff and myself are reviewed. In that editorial it is pointed out that 26. Holtman (1946) has made known his belief that there may be a relationship between the level of thyroid secretion and susceptibility to human poliomyelitis and encephalitis, due to the fact that these diseases occur in warm weather when natural secretions of the thyroid are the lowest.

Within our midst we may shortly have definite information to prove or disprove Holtman's belief. Dr. Brereton, Sr. is finding some startling data on thyroid function in children. And Dr. Elliott is conducting a survey in those areas of Manitoba which the Dept. of Health supplies with iodides to prevent goitre, to determine the incidence of polio in those children on iodides.

Comment

A summary is here presented of the uses of iodine in treating poliomyelitis and other central nervous system fevers in man, animals and birds. Its use in polio is viewed with definite doubt by a large portion of the medical profession and this with reason, for so many theories of therapy have failed, even our hopeful gamma globulin being questioned, not without reason.

My personal opinion is that iodine restores to normal a function probably thyroid in origin, which produces a chain reaction of defence and the patient is made to develop his own gamma globulin or its counterpart. I do not ask you to accept my theory without reserve until I have delivered further proof. I am planning should Manitoba have a polio epidemic in 1954, to place an experimental group of 10,000 on prophylactic therapy. May I ask your sympathetic observation and your extension of the experiment if you see fit.

I am in my own mind convinced that iodine constitutes a prophylactic means against polio; that its use in the treatment of polio tends to restore muscle tone early and reduces convalescence to a minimum. Its use as a prophylactic could be extended to large areas by using the present system employed by Provincial Health in goitre areas. This would bring the third halogen, iodine, into the field of preventive medicine with chlorine and fluorine.

Appreciations

27. To Dr. R. R. Scobey, 1411 South Salina St., Syracuse, N. Y. I extend my appreciation. I have used his article in the *Archives of Pediatrics,* 68, 1951, as my guide in tracing the Medical uses of Iodides in human therapy. I have indulged possibly in plagiarism in my quotations from his article. My only regret is that he does not quote his own cases. He may have been in a position not dissimilar to my own from 1944 to 1952 when I had no cases.

To Dr. Isa, of the Veterinary Department of the University of Manitoba, I am indebted for research of veterinary medical literature.

To Dr. Ormerod of the Manitoba School of Medicine, I am indebted for discussion and constructive criticism. He is responsible for the formulation of the protective mechanism theory.

To my best of all wives I am indebted for her patience in reviewing my records and assisting in my experiments. Her observations were most valuable.

To my patients who submitted to experimental therapy, I am indeed indebted.

References

1. Manson, Alexander: Medical Researches of the Effects of Iodine in Bronchocele, Paralysis, Chorea, Scrofula, Fistula Lachrymalis, Deafness, Dysphagia, White Swelling and Distortion of the Spine. London, 1825.
2. Coplan, James: On the Cause, Nature and Treatment of Palsy and Apoplexy, Lea and Blanchard, Phila. 1850.
3. Brown-Séquard, C. E.: Lectures on the Diagnosis and Treatment of the Principal Forms of Paralysis of the Lower Extremities. J. P. Lippincott & Co. 1861.
4. Sinkler, W.: *Am. J. Med.* Sc. 69. 348-365, April, 1875.
5. Elliott, G.: *Am. J. Med.* Sc. 89. 138-146, January, 1885.
6. Webber, S. G.: A Treatise on Nervous Diseases—Their Symptoms and Treatment. p. 200, 1885.
7. Ridley, H. W.: *J. Trop. M. & Hyg.,* 28: 102-103, March 2, 1925.
8. Braddon, W. L.: The Causes and Prevention of Beriberi, 1907.
9. Horder, Sir Thomas: *Lancet,* 1: 340-341, Feb. 12, 1927.
10. Breuil & Dartiguenave: *Bull. Soc. Med. Chir. de L'Indochine,* 15: 803, August-September, 1937.
11. Maberly, J.: The Health of the Nation and Deficiency Diseases, 1938.
12. Mazzitelli, M.: *Studium,* 29: 73, April 1, 1939.
13. Scobey, R. R.: *Arch. Pediat.* 63: 322-354, July, 1946.
14. Scobey, R. R.: *Arch. Pediat.,* 65: 131-166, March, 1948.
15. Edward, J. F.: *Can. M. A. J.,* 58: 210, February, 1948.
16. Head, H. and Campbell, A. W.: *Brain,* 23: 23, 1900.
17. Ruggles, E. W.: *Arch. Dermat & Syph.,* 23: 472-476, March, 1931.
18. Beers, N. T.: *J.A.M.A.,* 112: 2553, June 17, 1939.
19. Beckman, H.: Pharmacology in Clinical Practice, p. 257, 1953.
20. Lewitus, Victor: *Vet. Med.,* 31: 29-33, January, 1936.
21. Brinton, W. R.: Quoted by Chidester, F. E.; Ashworth, A. M.; Ashworth, G. A. and Wiles, I. A.; *International Clin.,* 3: 63-72, September, 1934.
22. Gray, E.: *Vet. J.,* 96: 28-34, 1940.
23. Radeleff, R. D.: *J. Am. Vet. M. A.,* 109: 129-132, August, 1946.
24. von Economo.: Encephalitis Lythargica, London, 1931.
25. Editorial, *Vet. Med.,* 37: 6, January, 1942.
26. Holtman, F.: *Science,* 104: 50-51, July, 1946.
27. Scobey, R. R.: *Arch. Pediat.,* 68: 309-321.

Polio—Review of Preventive Measures

We have much evidence in our files incriminating poisonous insecticide residues on fruits and vegetables as possible causes of polio. We know that the function of many of these insecticides involves paralysis of the insect. What makes us so sure they will not act in exactly the same way on human beings, even though we get them in small amounts? By the end of summer, when polio epidemics reach their height, how much of the various poisons has been ingested by people who eat their fruits and vegetables without washing or paring them? Buy organically-grown, insecticide-free produce, if you possibly can. If not, wash thoroughly and *peel* produce before you eat.

Ralph E. Scobey, M.D., of Syracuse who has devoted many years of his life to a study of the causes of polio, recently sent us this letter:

"Dear Mr. Rodale:

"I have just come across the following items regarding the causes of polio which will be of interest to you because it corresponds with our ideas.

"This is a translation of an article occurring in *Tidskrift for Halsa,* October, 1953 (Swedish).

"In the Danish Weekly Bulletin for Physicians, No. 32, Dr. A. Maag, staff physician in Copenhagen, takes a definite stand against the current concept of the spread of poliomyelitis. He states that there is no virus connected with the transmission. It is merely a matter of dead molecules, in other words, just dead chemical matter, and it enters the cell protoplasm through plain chemical affinity. He then points to the great epidemic of poliomyelitis in Denmark last year. Altogether 4,000 persons were engaged in one way or another, taking care of all the patients, and not one was infected by the disease. Dr. Maag states that all isolation, quarantine, closing of churches and schools is unnecessary and futile. Instead, he indicts the spraying of fruits and vegetables with chemicals as the actual cause of polio. As such spraying is steadily on the increase so are also these epidemics.

"In another newspaper, *Nationaltidenie,* also Danish, another municipal physician, Dr. R. Kjer-Petersen, comes out openly and announces that artificial fertilizer and the chemical spraying of fruits is the basic cause of infantile paralysis. He even asked the general public to go on a 'fruit-eating strike' until the growers would stop the spraying.

"I am very glad to note that our ideas are being upheld by these men in Europe because the virus theory has been so deeply embedded in the minds of the American people by the Foundation that outside influences may be very helpful. You will recall that the Australian and British physicians forced the recognition in this country of a relationship between inoculations and polio.

Sincerely,
RALPH R. SCOBEY"

Dr. Scobey has developed a sound theory on the possible relation of cyanide poisoning to polio. Cyanide is an ingredient of many insecticides. It is also a substance found in contaminated waters from which shellfish may be taken. It seems logical to assume that water draining from areas heavily treated with cyanide insecticides as well as water from industrial areas where cyanide is used might certainly contaminate shellfish taken from such waters. We recommend avoiding shellfish especially during the summer months.

Deficiencies in Vitamins and Minerals

W. M. Brumby, M. D., suggests that polio resembles in every detail a disease of cattle called loin disease which seems to be the result of deficiency in calcium, phosphorus and the other precious minerals we need for good health. In the bovine disease, cows carrying calves are particularly susceptible, just as pregnant women are susceptible to polio. The newborn calf and the newborn baby are not stricken, supposedly because they have enough minerals, at the expense of their mothers. Calcium deficiency is perhaps the most general diet deficiency in our present-day America. And the child who lives on soft drinks and ice cream during the summer months, rather than milk, meat, fruits and vegetables, is courting certain calcium deficiency and hence, perhaps polio susceptibility.

W. J. McCormick, M.D., of Toronto, Canada, cures polio patients with massive doses of the B vitamins. In every case he finds that the polio patient has been eating a diet containing an abundance of white-flour products and practically nothing in the way of vitamin-B-rich foods—liver, fresh fruits and vegetables. Hot weather causes us to use up B vitamins more rapidly, so we are more likely to be short of B vitamins in the summer time (polio time) than at any other time. In the summer time our children consume vast quantities of soft drinks which further rob their bodies of vitamin B, for this vitamin is absolutely necessary for digesting anything containing sugar.

Low Blood Sugar and Polio

A day spent in the company of a soft drink dispenser can do more harm than possibly anything else, especially in the summer time, when children are over-exerting themselves with strenuous games. For soft drinks, along with other food containing concentrated sugar lower the blood sugar to a dangerous level. Benjamin P. Sandler, M.D., in his book *Diet Prevents Polio* (available from the Lee Foundation for Nutritional Research, 2023 West Wisconsin Avenue, Milwaukee, Wisconsin) tells us of a polio epidemic in North Carolina which was stopped in its tracks when diet recommendations were broadcast through the press and radio and residents were terrified enough to follow them. "For the week ending July 31," he tells us, "there were 304 more cases than in the corresponding week in 1946. Then a sudden change occurred. For the next six weeks 1948 fell behind 1946 by 1,581 cases." From then on the number of cases fell rapidly. And the manufacturers of soft drinks and ice cream alone probably lost millions of dollars in that one area.

Dr. Sandler recommends the following as a diet that will keep blood sugar at normal high levels: eliminate all foods that contain sugar: soft drinks, ice cream, cakes, pastries, candy and so forth. Cut down on starchy foods, such as those made from white flour, and starchy vegetables. Eat plenty of non-starchy vegetables. Perhaps most important of all, eat plenty of protein foods: meat, fish, poultry, eggs.

As most of us know, surgical operations that are absolutely necessary should be done before, or postponed until after, the polio season. Medical journals are full of evidence of the increased susceptibility to polio after tonsillectomies and inoculations. The polio appears at that part of the body which suffered what doctors call the "insult." A tonsillectomy may produce bulbar polio. An injection may bring polio paralysis to the limb injected.

We have one final suggestion for avoiding any possibility of contracting polio this summer—get lots of vitamin C. Fred R. Klenner, M.D., of Reidsville, North Carolina, has successfully used massive doses of vitamin C in treating polio and other virus diseases. This appears to indicate that vitamin C in large amounts is very powerful against the disease. Might it not also indicate that an abundance of vitamin C in the diet would protect one against the ravages of the virus? Fresh raw fruits and vegetables (especially green, leafy ones) contain lots of vitamin C. Rose hip preparations are the richest natural food source. We need more vitamin C in the summer time, for we lose this water-soluble vitamin in perspiration.

To sum up: don't become over-fatigued, don't get too much sun, peel fruits and vegetables if you cannot get organically-grown ones, avoid shellfish, get plenty of the water-soluble vitamins, B and C, and plenty of the important minerals. One of the best ways of accomplishing this is to put the whole family on the Sandler diet which also guards against low blood sugar.

Polio and Civilized Living

Wrote an Associated Press reporter on September 11, 1954, "Polio was pictured Friday as the great leveler, attacking the highest and sparing the lowest of the world's civilizations. Its incidence rises with the standard of living. It seems to thrive where other diseases fail. Where infant mortality is highest, it is lowest. It probably will continue to advance along with civilization, until some dramatic new vaccine brings it to a halt.

"This phase of one of the world's problem diseases was presented Friday to the final session of the Third International Poliomyelitis Congress."

At the same congress Dr. Rivers, director of the Rockefeller Institute for Medical Research in New York, said it is now well known among medical researchers that in primitive countries and in communities where the economic and social levels are low, antibodies against polio appear sooner than they do among the "privileged" children of the higher civilizations and communities. Said Dr. A. M. M. Payne of the World Health Organization, "Until the infant mortality rate falls to about 100 per 1000 live births, the incidence of poliomyelitis is generally below 2 per 100,000. As the infant mortality rate falls from about 50 to 20 there appears to be a tendency for the incidence of polio to increase alarmingly."

In our file on polio, we have some of the most astounding theories you can imagine—for instance an observation that the paralytic aspects of polio may be much worse after the child has been transported in an ambulance to the hospital. We have theories on whether polio is hereditary, whether it attacks only certain racial groups and other equally nonsensical observations. And now we have the theory that, so long as children are living under the worst possible conditions of bad sanitation and squalor, they will somehow manufacture antibodies to combat polio when they are quite young and so will never get the disease when they are exposed to it later on. If there is indeed anything to this theory, then we see even less need for the programs of spraying with DDT which are carried out regularly in many parts of our country as a precaution against polio. We have never heard of any polio epidemic being stopped by spraying with DDT and we have heard of localities where the polio incidence rose after the DDT spraying.

But, to return to Dr. Rivers and Dr. Payne. You see where this line of thinking leads us—if we're just dirty enough and disregard even the basic laws of sanitation, our children will be safe from any threat of polio. Isn't that exactly what they imply in statements such as they made?

Polio is a "Civilized" Disease

Disregarding the theory about antibodies being formed in the blood only of children who live in filth, let's consider for a moment the well-known facts (for they are well known now) that children and adults in primitive countries simply don't get polio. And the more civilization they have, the more polio they have. The lower their infant mortality, as a result of wonder drugs and all the marvels of civilized medicine, the higher their rate of polio.

For instance, a letter from a Turkish correspondent in the *Journal of the American Medical Association* for August 6, 1950 assures us that polio is practically unknown in Turkey. Monthly reports submitted to the Ministry of Health and Social Assistance indicate that there are 2 or 3 cases of polio a year in the whole country. There is no evidence that an epidemic has ever occurred there. Medical students never observe the disease in its acute stage and seldom see a patient with recent paralysis. We are told that in the summer of 1947 the child of a prominent physician, returning from a summer resort in Istanbul was the first patient admitted to the Ankara General Hospital with polio. Remember those conditions—the boy had been away to a summer resort on a vacation.

In *Science News Letter* for October 4, 1947, we read of a group of university scientists visiting the orient to take blood specimens in an effort to discover why American troops in Japan, India and North Africa suffered from an increased incidence of polio, while the native populations had no polio at all.

Dr. A. B. Sabin, writing in the *Journal of the American Medical Association* for June 28, 1947, discusses the same puzzling aspect of polio. Why, asks Dr. Sabin, in the same year when polio epidemics are raging in cities like New York, Chicago, Los Angeles and Denver, do Chinese cities occupying the same latitude report only rare, rare cases of the disease?

Dr. Sabin tells how polio occurred among American troops in China, Japan and in the Philippines in spite of the fact that there were no outbreaks of polio at the time among the native children and adults. In 1945 there were 246 cases of polio with 52 deaths among American troops in the Philippines. There have never been any outbreaks of polio among the native Philippines. For many years medical magazines have been commenting and marveling on the scarcity of reports of polio among the races living in North China.

What About Civilization Contributes to Polio?

Isn't it discouraging how our experts will examine every aspect of the problem except the obvious one that is staring them in the face? They study the climate of Chicago compared to the climate of Shanghai. They study the blood of the children of China and compare it with that of American children. They note with care the number of flies in homes in Shanghai and on the South Side of Chicago. These and countless other angles have been investigated. Why have they never studied the food eaten by the people of these countries and compared it with the food eaten by Americans and Europeans, whether they are at home or abroad?

It's pretty obvious that American troops in all the fighting theatres of the last war ate in general the same foods they eat at home—including white bread, refined cereals, white sugar, soft drinks, ice cream, candy, canned vegetables and all the degerminated, devitalized, refined foods that "civilized" people eat. And the American troops went right ahead consuming their annual 103 pounds of sugar per person. Consumption of sugar in China is 3.2 pounds per person, annually. Why is it that no writers except the "faddists" have pointed out this fact?

What kind of food did the Turkish physician's son have at the summer resort that was different from the food he ate at home? Does it seem far-fetched to believe that, because he was a physician's son, his family could afford to buy him refined and processed food such as the other Turkish children could not afford to eat? What would a survey reveal about the food habits of this boy and those of the other Turkish children who apparently are not susceptible to polio?

We do not believe that the per capita consumption of 103 pounds of sugar annually is solely responsible for the high incidence of polio among Americans abroad and the low incidence of polio among the native peoples in the same countries. But when the Third International Poliomyelitis Congress announces to the world that the higher the scale of civilization, the higher the rate of polio, we believe that the time has come to investigate the part played in such a circumstance by "civilized" food as opposed to the more or less natural foods eaten by people who have not as yet attained our level of civilization.

We suggest that one of the best guarantees against polio this summer is to keep yourself and your family as nearly as possible on a diet which is not "civilized"—that is, avoid the foods that have been put through the mill of civilized processing. Avoid foods made from white sugar and white flour, canned foods, prepared "mixes," ice cream, bakery products, cold cereals or any cereals that are not completely whole grain. Stick to the natural foods—fresh fruits and vegetables, as many raw as possible, for cooking is actually a form of processing, remember. Eat fresh meats, nuts, eggs, fresh or frozen fish. Even though you live in a civilized country, you do not need to suffer the penalties for that, if you will take just a little trouble to avoid the foods that civilization has turned into health-menaces.

Pollution—Air

In New York City one spring day in 1952 a couple of thousand women walking in the vicinity of Penn Station suddenly found that their stockings had runs—runs which did not result from any snags or tears. Apparently something had simply eaten through the nylon and decomposed it. One summer morning in California a farmer and his wife were picking their spinach crop, went home for lunch and returned to find the spinach bleached to a sickly white and the stalks dried and curling. One horrible week in the winter of 1948 the little steel town of Donora, Pennsylvania, counted in the hundreds its victims of a strange respiratory ailment that brought disease and death to many while the town lay gasping beneath a heavy blanket of smog.

London, England, reported 9,000 deaths more than the average for that time of year during the five weeks ending January 3, 1953—five weeks during which London was smothered in a dense fog. A November 4, 1953, United Press dispatch reports "The polluted air breathed by city dwellers and not cigarette smoking probably is the 'principal' cause of the alarming increase in lung cancer in the past few decades, a cancer research scientist told the annual meeting of the American Cancer Society."

What have these stories in common? They are all concerned—yes, even the nylon stockings—with air pollution, which is fast becoming one of the major headaches of industry and private citizens alike. Do you have any idea of what you are breathing on any given day, if you live in a town or city? Every day you breathe into your lungs 30 pounds of air. In any community where there is any industrial concentration at all, you may expect to find in the air any or all of the following (according to *Scientific American,* May, 1952) : soot, fly ash, water vapor, carbon dioxide, carbon monoxide, sulfur dioxide, oxides of nitrogen, hydrocarbons, oxygenated hydrocarbons and organic acids. According to the *American Journal of Public Health* for May, 1952, there may be as many as 50 substances in solution in polluted air. The air over Los Angeles contains one part per million sulfur dioxide, 20 p.p.m. of carbon monoxide, .38 p.p.m. oxides of nitrogen, .32 p.p.m. of ozone, .4 p.p.m. of aldehydes, 1.2 p.p.m. of hydrocarbons and so forth. In other cities where the industries are different the air contaminants are different. Meanwhile, we know that some of these substances in concentrations the least little bit too high will prove dangerous or perhaps fatal. Formaldehyde irritates the eyes at a concentration of 1 p.p.m. in the air. Carbon monoxide is unsafe in a concentration of more than 100 p.p.m. Chlorine is dangerous at concentrations above 1 p.p.m. and fluorine above 3 p.p.m. Hydrogen fluoride in concentrations as low as 1 part in 200 million will damage some plants after an exposure of only a few hours.

The problem of air pollution is not a new one. *Industrial Hygiene and Occupational Medicine* for September, 1953, in speaking of England tells us "As long ago as 1257 Eleanor, Henry III's queen, was forced to leave Nottingham because of the coal smoke. Soon after this, the first smoke-abatement law was passed by Edward I (1273) who prohibited the use of coal as being prejudicial to human health. In 1306 the first smoke-abatement group was 'formed' by the lords spiritual and temporal and others attending Parliament who were annoyed at the increasing smoke; as a result a Royal Proclamation was promulgated prohibiting artificers from using coal in their furnaces. The following year one offender was condemned and executed for this offense."

There can no longer be any question, then, as to the possible harmfulness of air pollution. We know it is unhealthful. If we needed further confirmation, the tragedy at Donora and the fantastic rise in death rates in London would be ample proof of the deadly character of the air we breathe in any industrialized part of the world. The nylon stockings incident was caused by particles of sulfuric acid in the air created by moisture which attacked and combined chemically with the particles of grime that were falling Sulfuric acid eats through nylon and air pollution probably is responsible for some 5000 nylon runs per day in New York City, according to DuPont. What do you suppose that corrosive sulfuric acid does to the inside of your lungs when you breathe it?

In his book *Cancer, Can It Be Prevented,* Editor Rodale goes into detail on the subject of the Green theory of cancer. Mr. Green was a researcher in England who made remarkable studies of the incidence of cancer in relation to coal smoke. He discovered, for instance, that cancer deaths were higher in sections of the country where houses were situated in gullies or on the tops of hills, so that winter winds, circulating around the houses, brought some of the coal smoke back into the rooms. In comparatively flat countryside where the wind carried the coal smoke directly away from the chimneys, there was far less cancer. He found too that chimneys should extend above rooftops and over surrounding buildings or trees, so that the smoke would be carried away effectively. In cities where tall buildings mix with dwellings, the smoke is bound to be forced down by winds around the high buildings, with resulting pollution of the air inside the house.

He also discovered that in sections of the British Isles where peat is burned instead of coal there is less cancer, except in certain localities where the peat contains large amounts of sulphur. In France and Germany he found that cancer was far more frequent in the northern parts of the country and less frequent in the south where much less coal was burned. Then, too, he studied the occupational occurrence of cancer and found, without exception, that cancer deaths were more prevalent in occupations where sulfur or some of its compounds were handled daily. Of course the highest incidence of cancer was at that time (1917) found in chimney sweeps, who are in daily contact with coal soot from chimneys.

Pollution in Various Cities

Perhaps you think your locality is free from air pollution. Let us give you some figures on pollution in different towns and cities: In Louisville, Kentucky, approximately 470 tons of dust particles are scattered into the air every day. In South Charlestown, W. Va., factories used to discharge about 14 tons of sulfuric acid mist into the air every day. In the Detroit-Windsor area some 430,000 tons of sulfur dioxide contaminate the air each year. Each day in the Los Angeles area 125,000 tons of contaminated air emanate from the motor traffic alone, in addition to the contamination pouring from factories. In Grafton, W. Va., the annual pollution amounts to 1867 tons per square mile; in Baltimore it is 1800 tons, in Pittsburgh 1031 tons.

What do we mean by air pollution? We mean tiny, microscopic particles of matter that hang suspended in the air and, most of them, land somewhere eventually—on our clothes, faces, furniture, newly painted homes and newly washed curtains. The smallest of these particles of course are inhaled into our lungs. According to *Science News Letter* for August 1, 1953, fog in which visibility is limited to 100 feet contains about 200 particles per cubic inch. A "peasoup" fog may contain as many as 2000 particles suspended in every cubic inch of air. We are accustomed to thinking of air pollution as smoke. But today smoke from coal burning furnaces is only one of many pollutants. And as the chemical industry grows, new contaminants are added every day.

Masks and More Permanent Solutions to the Problem

As we go to press the newspapers are full of pictures of pretty British girls wearing masks designed to protect them against the London smog. Wearing a mask day and night may not be a very comfortable prospect, but if you can't move to the country, and if your local air pollution is pretty grim, perhaps it might not be a bad idea for you too. The mask consists apparently of gauze which covers the nose and mouth and is tied behind the head.

But masks are of course only a temporary and unsatisfactory solution. Everyone agrees that air pollution will not be licked until individual citizens get up on their high horses and demand an end to it. *Woman's Home Companion* (back issues available at your library) gives a suggested program for those of us who want to do something about air pollution right now. In general this is the program:

1. Get a survey made of your local situation even if it means calling in an outside expert. 2. Sponsor and vote for an anti-pollution ordinance with teeth in it. 3. Study sites where schools and other public buildings are to be erected before plans are drawn up, to make certain they are located in reasonably safe areas. 4. Keep your fight out of politics by getting all political parties to back it. 5. Check on the contribution you yourself may be making to air pollution. Is your heating equipment in perfect order and is it smokeless? Do you burn garbage and trash in your back yard? (It goes without saying that no *Prevention* reader would ever burn garbage—he makes compost out of it.) Is your car in good repair or does it blast the countryside with carbon monoxide gas every time you drive it? Do you report smoke and pollution instances whenever they occur, so that your local authorities have this information? In one city the League of Women Voters took over the job of notifying the authorities when chimneys were more than ordinarily troublesome.

In case you are interested in where your city may stand in the air pollution scheme, a survey by the Air Pollution Control Association made this report on the following cities:

Conditions were *poor* in Birmingham, Alabama; Boston and Suffolk County, Mass.; Canton, Ohio; Dayton, Ohio; Des Moines, Iowa; Erie, Pa.; Evansville, Ind.; Madison, Wisconsin; Miami, Florida; Montreal, Quebec; Ottawa, Ontario; Philadelphia, Penna.; Rochester, New York; Stamford, Connecticut; Trenton, N. J.; Vancouver, British Columbia. Conditions were *fair* in Akron, Ohio; Asheville, N. C.; Baltimore, Md.; Charlotte, N. C.; Chattanooga, Tenn.; Chicago, Ill.; Cumberland, Md.; Denver, Colo.; Detroit, Mich.; East Chicago, Ind.; Hamilton, Ontario; Houston, Texas; Indianapolis, Ind.; Kingsport, Tenn.; Knoxville, Tenn.; Los Angeles, Calif.; Nashville, Tenn.; New York, N. Y.; Niagara Falls, N. Y.; Peoria, Ill.; Roanoke, Va.; Syracuse, N. Y.; Tacoma, Wash.; University City, Mo.; Windsor, Ontario; Winston-Salem, N. C.; Wyandotte, Mich. Conditions were rated as *good* in Allegheny County, Pa.; Atlanta, Ga.; Buffalo, N. Y.; Cincinnati, Ohio; Cleveland, Ohio; Columbus, Ohio; Green Bay, Wisconsin; Kansas City, Mo.; Louisville, Ky.; Milwaukee, Wis.; Minneapolis, Minn.; Omaha, Neb.; Pittsburgh, Pa.; Providence, R. I.; Richmond, Va.; St. Louis, Mo.; and Toledo, Ohio.

In case the thought of the cost of air pollution control has you worrying, another expert assures us that we can control air pollution all over the country for an average cost of ten cents per person per year if we all cooperate and work at it! But don't wait for your community to become a second Donora before doing something about air pollution. Every day you breathe this pollution is doing you physical harm!

Pollution—Water

Here are some recent news stories about water. (1) *The Canadian Journal of Public Health* for April, 1951, reviews a survey made by a joint United States-Canadian commission to study pollution of boundary waters. The report shows that a daily discharge of more than two billion gallons of waste material is poured into water being used for drinking by four million persons.

(2) A clipping from a Seattle paper shows sewer pipes jutting out on a bathing beach and recites the grim story of a man who got paratyphoid fever from eating raw oysters he had gathered within 100 feet of a sewer opening.

(3) An article in *Time,* July 6, 1953, tells of 1490 Singer Manufacturing employees at South Bend, Indiana, threatened with amoebiasis, and four who died, as a result of drinking water from an old well whose cracked pipes were letting in sewage.

(4) The Detroit *Times* for September 15, 1953, displays a picture of millions of dead carp jamming a stream up to five feet deep leading into the Kalamazoo River. "River Pollution Killed These Fish" says the headline.

(5) The Oregon *Journal* for November 8, 1952, relates a tragedy that took place when some poisonous substance was dumped by an industrial firm—10,000 salmon headed up the Green River to spawn were killed. Investigators were trying to find out what firm was guilty.

Every week brings us new clippings, for water pollution is very much in the news at present. One reason for this is of course the fact that each day water pollution gets worse instead of better. In addition the recent extensive droughts have forced us to realize anew that life simply can't go on without water—clean, pure water. A new Public Affairs Pamphlet on water pollution, *Washing Our Water* by Helen Beal Woodward, (22 E. 38th St., New York 16, N. Y.) says: "The unprecedented growth of industry, together with our expanding cities, has burdened many of our rivers beyond their capacity to flush away waste. The seriousness of this, as it affects the health and general welfare of people and industry alike is the subject of the pamphlet. . . . Pollution from human sewage and industrial waste increases in two ways as citizen and industry grow. Less water is available to carry waste away, because of increased water demands and at the same time the water flushed back into the common supply carries a heavier burden of waste. *Modern chemical industries have made the problem even more imperative, as ordinary methods of water treatment do not always affect the complex new chemicals."* (Italics are ours.)

Now should we become concerned over the news above? Well, how do you feel about drinking water so poisonous that fish die in it by the millions? It seems to us there are two kinds of water poisoning we should discuss here—(1) the pollution that occurs in drinking water, either from natural sources or from industrial wastes, and (2) the chemicals that are added to water to remove the impurities.

Water Polluted By Human and Industrial Wastes

How dangerous can polluted water be? In the case of the Singer employees, they were drinking water from a well drilled 52 years ago when the plant was built. No one suspected drinking water as the cause of the four deaths until amoebae were found in stool samples. "A quick check of 138 Singer workers showed about half with amoebiasis." At present all workers who show evidence of amoebic infestation are being treated by the company at a cost of $77,000. How much less expensive in money and lives it would have been to check the old well and drill a new one.

The Journal of the American Medical Association for May 5, 1951, tells us that during 1949 there was an increase of 951 reported cases of waterborne diseases over the previous year. Total figures for the years 1938-1949 are 130,524 cases of disease, 94 deaths. We wonder whether these figures include such incidents as that which occurred at Rochester, New York, several years ago when untreated water from the Genesee River was mistakenly pumped into the city water supply and in a short time there were 35,000 cases of gastroenteritis a waterborne disease which inflames the stomach and intestines.

A clipping from *Time,* September 16, 1949, discloses that infectious hepatitis (inflammation of the liver) was the main nuisance of World War II. Disabling 30,000 G.I.'s in the Mediterranean Theatre alone, it is caused by polluted drinking water. This was discovered in a summer camp for youngsters where 350 campers came down with the disease, and its cause was eventually traced to a camp well into which cesspools drained.

Much has been written about pure water for country-dwellers and much literature is available from the government and in public libraries on how and where to drill wells, how to make certain that cesspools or privies will not contaminate the well, how to have the water tested for purity. Yet in spite of all this available information we are told that a large percentage of wells on farms are unsafe. "Dug" wells are the worst offenders since surface water can drain into them easily. But the water from drilled wells should be tested for safeness too, for it may be contaminated.

City dwellers are at the mercy of their water departments. Public Health Service Publication, No. 67 *Clean Water for the Western Great Lakes Region* tells us that in this area there are 610 municipal sources of pollution with sewerage systems serving 6,930,000 people. Only 168 of the industrial sources of pollution have adequate treatment facilities—that is, only 168 of the manufacturing plants treat their waste products so that they do not contaminate the water. This is the situation in just one section of the country. A long list of such pamphlets is available from the Superintendent of Documents in Washington. Write for some information on your own locality.

What is being done about pollution? Up to now it seems that very little has been done, but now the problem has become so serious that steps are being taken in some parts of the country. For instance, the *New York Times,* for October 14, 1951, describes the arrangement made by ten New Jersey cities to drain off and process all sewage in a jointly owned disposal plant. Seven of these cities had been under order from the state board of health to end pollution ever since 1934. The disposal plant cost 13 million dollars which is being paid off at the rate of $135 per million gallons by each community.

State laws on pollution are tightening up, according to *Chemical Week* for July 4, 1953, so tnere is continual pressure on industry to solve their pollution problems and constant urging by federal officials that plants that have solutions for their disposal problems should publicize them widely so that others can follow suit.

On the other hand we find in many localities an attitude of indifference, or we hear people saying "Why should we not throw our sewage into the river when all the other towns upriver do, so that the water is already filthy by the time it reaches us?" In cases where a water source crosses state boundary lines, the federal government can step in and, working with local authorities, can see to it that wastes from one state do not pollute the water of residents of another state.

Ways of Disposing of Sewage and Industrial Wastes

Here are some samples of ways in which industrial firms have solved their waste disposal headaches. (From an article by Sidney Katz in *Magazine Digest* for Octover, 1947.) Citrus canners who used to have mountainous wastes now use 80 per cent of the peel, seeds and so forth to make animal food. One large corporation making vaccines, liver extracts, and so forth now presses its animal wastes into blocks which are then sold as protein feed for livestock. A chemical company manufacturing 400 products separates each waste product carefully and treats it individually with a special process before discharging it into the water supply.

An interesting case is presented in *Water Works Engineering* for December, 1948. The engineers of the town of Ridgefield, Connecticut, were having trouble with algae (small water plants) growing on the walls of their reservoir, the pond which supplied water. From 1906 on they had treated the water with copper sulfate (about 125 to 130 pounds per season). The situation grew worse and worse until by 1933 the water was very discolored. Larger and larger doses of copper sulfate were used which finally resulted in killing the fish in the reservoir. More fish were ordered from a hatchery and within a few months all discoloration of the water disappeared. As more fish were added the water became clearer and there was no further trouble with the algae. And no more copper sulfate was needed. The engineer writing the article, Francis W. Collins, had no explanation for this natural solution to a problem that arose from a purely natural source. But it certainly suggests that natural means are far superior to chemical ones whenever possible.

A number of cities are transforming sewage into compost which they then sell to farmers (organiculturists, to be sure!) This is killing two birds with one stone, for wastes are returned to enrich the land and water pollution becomes a thing of the past. *Chemical Week* for July 18, 1953, notes that 80 industrialists met the previous week to discuss waste disposal regulations for the Ohio River basin. Hearings on pollution of North Carolina streams were held on July 28. Michigan and Ontario officials were reported to be on the brink of investigating pollution of the St. Clair River with phenol (carbolic acid) wastes which menace the Detroit water supply.

The Woodward pamphlet *Washing Our Water* which we mentioned above tells us of a steel company which decided to stop dumping furnace flue dust into the Ohio and spent $516,000 on a treatment plant. In its first year the plant recovered enough ore to yield $581,000 profit. At Florence, Alabama, through vigorous citizen action, a $90,000 sewage disposal plant was built even though the residents then had to accept a 50 per cent rise in the cost of water.

And so it goes. Water pollution is a live, burning issue all over the country and it's likely that any movement to investigate the pollution of your local water and do something about it will find many supporters. In some places the whole matter of pollution has been brought into the light of day during a fight over water fluoridation. And indeed, this is a skillful and unanswerable argument. "Let's put our money first to the job of getting pure healthful water to drink, before we start adding medicines to it" is the cry of these civic-minded anti-fluoridationists.

What About Chemicals in Water?

It may be that your community solves—or tries to solve—its water pollution headaches by pouring more chemicals into the water. For instance, here is a sample of how water in swimming pools is treated. The 27 pools in New York City are "purified" each year by the addition of the following chemicals (according to *Chemical Week* July 4, 1953): Chlorine, 59,000 pounds; Anhydrous Ammonia, 5,000 pounds; Sodium hypochlorite, 12,000 gallons; Ammonium sulfate, 80,000 pounds; Soda ash powder, 140,000 pounds; Soda ash cake, 20,000 pounds; Copper sulfate, 8,500 pounds; ammonium alum, 20,000 pounds. Yes, folks, this is the chemical brew in which New York children swim. It's a wonder there is any room left in the swimming pools for water, isn't it?

We don't know how many of these same chemicals are in drinking water in New York City. We have the word of a reader that Columbus, Ohio, adds these chemicals to its drinking water each year: 500 tons of aluminum ore; 8,000 tons of lime; 3,000 tons of soda ash; 1200 tons of sulphuric acid; 500 tons of coke and 8 tons of liquid chlorine. Now seems to be as good a time as any for all of us to get busy and do a survey on the water we are drinking. Why not find out, for your own information, just what chemicals are added to the water in your home town?

Some time ago we quoted a question that appeared in the *Journal of the American Medical Association* for July 28, 1951, asking what research has been done on the effects of chlorinated water drunk over a period of years. The answer was that no official research has ever been done to determine the possible harm to human beings of drinking chlorinated water. And most of the urban water supplies are chlorinated! But now we see that chlorine is one of the least of the villains we have to contend with. Apparently city drinking water contains as well untold amounts of copper sulfate, aluminum, sulphuric acid, and who knows what else! A clipping from Canton, Ohio, December 4, 1951, indicates that a chemical was added to the water in that city for removing iron which, we suppose, was causing the housewives trouble staining their washing and making rusty rings on their bathtubs. The treatment was sodium hexametaphosphate—170 pounds daily. Now if anybody has ever done any research on the effects of chlorinated water, whose use is almost universal, what research has been done, do you suppose, on chemicals like this sodium hexametaphosphate and its effects on infants, sick people and pregnant women who drink the water?

We don't believe the fault lies with the waterworks officials who impress us as overworked and extremely conscientious public servants, more dismayed than anyone else at the pass to which we have come. It is up to us, Mr. and Mrs. Average Citizen, to take up the cudgels and announce once and for all that we simply will not put up with water pollution, nor with thousands of tons of chemicals of unknown toxicity being dumped into the drinking water to counteract the pollution.

A Program For Pure Drinking Water

Where do you begin a program of this kind? We would suggest first of all that you write to the Superintendent of Documents in Washington, D. C., and ask for all the information available on water pollution particularly in your part of the country. An excellent pamphlet *Clean Water is Everybody's Business* is available as a starter for 20 cents. On the last page of this pamphlet you will find suggestions for how to investigate the condition of your own drinking water and what to do about it. Also send for the Public Affairs Pamphlet *Washing Our Water,* 25 cents. Write or call on your city health department and gather information. Your poor, beleaguered water officials have probably been trying for a long time to get public support for a program of pure water. Give them all the help you can. After you have gathered information and know the point of view of your local officials, begin to write letters to the editor of the local paper. You might even ask the editor to assign a reporter to do a series of feature stories on the local water situation. In this way you can enlighten other citizens and enlist their support.

Meanwhile, are you going to go on drinking this filthy, polluted chemicalized liquid that comes out of your water faucet? Are you going to go on giving it to your children to drink? We know, from scientific investigation, of the diseases that can result from polluted water—typhoid, amoebic dysentery, hepatitis, goiter, polio, gastroenteritis, and many more.

So far as we know, no one has proved as yet, with a scientifically controlled experiment that countless diseases of modern times may not be the result of the chemicals in the water we drink. Yet many cases are on record in medical journals of allergies, asthma, hives and other conditions brought on by chlorinated water. So why should we not assume that chemicalized water is unhealthful until it has been proved otherwise?

If you live on a farm, by all means have your well or spring water tested. Your local county agent can tell you how to have this done. If the water shows any trace of pollution, stop drinking it. And don't wait until next month or next year to drill a new well.

If you live in a city, buy bottled spring water for drinking and cooking. This is not expensive and will pay for itself many times over in your own additional peace of mind. If there is no source of bottled spring water available, canvass every country dweller known to you or any of your friends and see whether you can obtain water from his well or spring, making certain of course that you have this water tested for purity. Your city waterworks will test the water for you.

All of us want good health for ourselves and our families. We spend a great deal of time and money buying and preparing the best and most nourishing foods. But what does it avail us to have our own organic garden so that we won't be consuming, for instance, copper sulphate insecticides, if we then drink water loaded with copper sulphate? What good does it do us to avoid the chlorinated hydrocarbon insecticides, if we then fill our poor bodies with heavily chlorinated water? Under ideal conditions of life, exposed to no poisonous substances, we might be able to resist both the pollution and the chemicals in our water supply. But, exposed as we are every day to countless poisons, the least we can do for the sake of our health is to drink pure unpolluted and unchemicalized water.

Posture

Stand on a street corner and watch the people pass. The vast majority of them have attractive faces, nice clothes, pleasant smiles. What then is it that gives this parade of human beings such a sorry woebegone look? Their posture! You may find one person in a hundred—man, woman or child—who holds his body correctly and walks as if he were glad he's alive. And that one in a hundred will probably turn out to be a model or a dancer or a gym instructor. The people whose livelihood necessitates a good figure and good posture have no choice. But how about the rest of us? How does it happen that we can go along, year after year, slumping, sagging, slouching as if we were made from rags instead of flesh and bones?

All of us know, or should know, what good posture is. If you don't, stand in front of a full length mirror, look at yourself in profile and imagine a plumb line dropped from the lobe of your ear to your foot. Half of you should be on each side of that line. Or have someone take a snapshot of you full length in profile, standing as you normally do. Then take a ruler and draw a line on the print. How does your posture look compared with the immutable straightness of that line?

What happens when your posture is not good? If one part of your body slackens and slumps, other parts must, too, for otherwise, you could not keep your balance. The abdominal muscles are the part that is most likely to sag, especially in women who have had children. When these muscles sag, they pull on the small of the back so that a certain amount of swayback becomes almost inevitable.

It is part of the function of the abdominal muscles and those of the lower back to keep the pelvic bones held in the proper position. When these muscles sag, the pelvis tilts forward. Organs that should be held in perfect position for functioning are thrown out of place. How can the stomach or intestines function properly when, because of bad posture, they are thrown together in a heap, rather than keeping to their separate, well-balanced locations?

If the abdominal muscles are slack and the lower back muscles reflect this slackness, then the shoulder and chest muscles are affected, too. The upper part of the back protrudes to balance the lower part which has caved in. So shoulders drop, chests flatten, chins jut out and round lumps of flesh begin to accumulate between the shoulder blades. Sound familiar?

How do we permit ourselves to get into such terrible shape? How does it happen that primitive peoples everywhere still untouched by "civilization" walk proud and tall and even in middle and old age do not ever develop the paunches, stoop-shoulders and protruding buttocks that characterize just about everybody in our country? Food is important to good posture, of course. Lots of protein and calcium are absolute essentials for strong muscles. Boys and girls in their teens, using up what calcium and protein they get in their foods to add inches to their height, are likely to become round-shouldered. No amount of scolding will make them improve their posture—their muscles are probably not strong enough to hold their tall frames upright. Eating refined carbohydrates is responsible to a large extent for our bad posture. It puts on fat which makes a bigger load for our muscles and it contributes nothing to the strength or health of those muscles. B vitamins are important for muscle health and refined carbohydrates rob your body of B vitamins, too.

Another reason for our bad posture is, of course, the way we live. We are sedentary; we never walk when we can ride; we watch the dancing instead of participating ourselves; we walk on hard floors and hard sidewalks; we wear badly fitting and improper shoes. Primitive people walk barefoot. They carry loads, so they must learn to balance their bodies perfectly or the loads will spill. Shoes, sidewalks, floors, high heels—these attributes of civilization, are unknown to the gracefully, perfectly poised men and women of primitive nations.

Once you have corrected your diet (and we hope all readers will) is there anything else you can do about poor posture? Yes, of course, there is. Almost any good book on the subject from your local library will give you exercises that you can do for five or ten minutes a day or longer. As soon as we said the word "exercise" you probably lost interest. For it seems that the prospect of actually going through a set of exercises every day of your life is simply too much for most people to face. So, what about some exercises you can do while you are working, while you are reading the paper, traveling on the bus, riding in an elevator, washing the dishes?

The main object, remember, is to strengthen those abdominal muscles so that they will do their job of supporting the lower part of the body. The way to exercise them is to pull them in tautly and tightly. This may be impossible at first, if you have let them sag for years, but constant practice will help. Here's how to exercise those muscles. If you are standing—no matter what else you are doing—flex your knees slightly, tuck your lower back in as far as you can get it and pull in on your abdominal muscles. You will find that you automatically straighten your shoulders and lift your chest—can't help yourself.

A dozen times a day, back up against the wall of the room, place your feet about six inches out from the wall, bend your knees just a little, then press your back against the wall, tight as you can, all the way down. You will probably find that, right in the middle of your back there is a hollow place between you and the wall. Press back, trying your best to flatten that, too, against the wall. While you are doing this exercise, your abdominal muscles will be strengthened, and gradually—ever so gradually—your posture will improve.

You can do the same thing sitting in a chair. Sit straight, feet flat on the floor. Press your spine against the back of the chair trying to flatten it completely so that there is no space between you and the chair back. You can practice this exercise while you are working, watching TV, riding in the car, bus, or trolley.

The kind of mattress you use has a lot to do with posture, too. Soft beds are not beneficial. Your mattress should be firm, or, better yet, you should sleep with a bed board. One final word on posture. A friend of ours who is taking chiropractic treatments showed us x-ray pictures of his spine before and after a series of treatments. The very definite curvature in the "before" picture had been almost completely corrected in the "after" picture. It is well to remember that these members of the healing profession, chiropractors and osteopaths, specialize in adjusting posture, if you want to express it that way. They know better than anyone else what good posture is and they are better equipped to handle posture problems than anyone else.

Posture—General Principles of

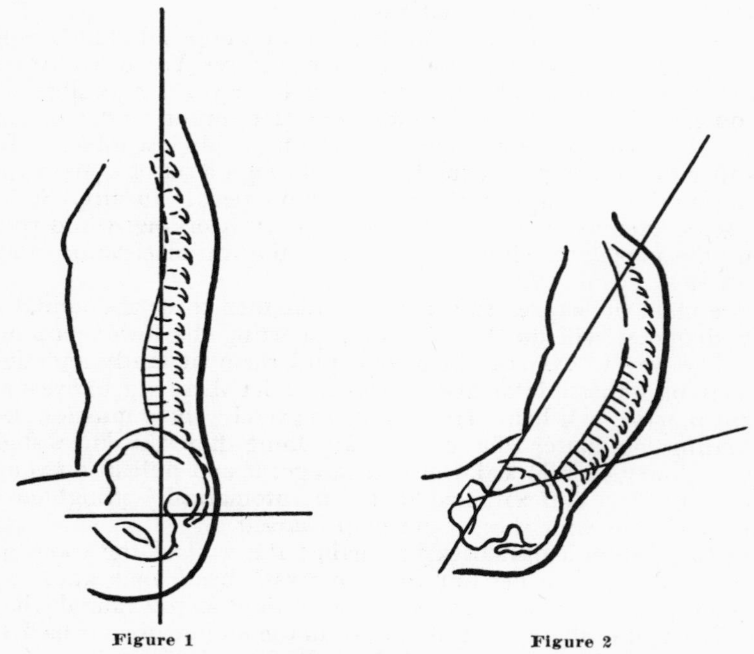

Figure 1 Figure 2

Here you can see what poor posture does to your spine.

Said Plato, "The most beautiful motion is that which accomplishes the greatest result with the least amount of effort." Leonardo da Vinci, one of the greatest anatomists that ever lived, believed that the center of gravity of the body was the most important single factor in good posture and graceful movement. Said he, "A man, in going upstairs, involuntarily throws so much weight forward and on the side of the upper foot as to be a counterpoise to the lower leg, so that the labor of his lower leg is limited to raising itself." He also pointed out that a man always throws the greatest amount of weight in the direction in which he is moving. So he is, in one sense, always pursuing his center of gravity. The faster he runs, the farther forward he leans, so that he throws more and more weight before him and then must catch up with it to keep from falling forward.

Later anatomists and physiotherapists decided that Leonardo was wrong—that movement in men was decided not by their center of gravity, but by the interplay of one muscle with another. If you want to step to the right, they said, the muscles of your right leg pull you in that direction, then the muscles of the left leg are activated to take the second step. Recently, however, we are beginning to return to Leonardo's theories concerning the importance of the center of gravity to movement and to posture.

Your center of gravity is, of course, the very center of your body if you were to draw imaginary lines horizontally and vertically through the middle of your silhouette. Your body is composed of certain masses grouped around your spinal column. So long as you keep these masses in alinement, so that your center of gravity remains actually *in the center of you,* you will have good posture. You will be able to move gracefully and efficiently and you will not be bothered with all the many disorders that can result from bad posture. But as soon as you let one section of your anatomy get out of line, you must automatically adjust other sections so that you can remain upright. This means that another part of you must go out of line to balance that part already out of alinement.

For example, consider for a moment the wearing of high heels. According to David H. Tribe, of the University of Queensland, writing in the *Medical Journal of Australia* for February 6, 1954, women who wear high heels spend the walking and standing part of their existence on an incline of about 30 degrees. To understand this, get yourself a board, prop it up at an angle of 30 degrees and stand on it barefoot. You will see at once that your whole body is thrown forward and you have to make certain adjustments in order to stay erect. You lock your knees, rather than keeping them slightly flexed or bent which is the proper and healthful way to stand. Your hips are thrown back, and at once you develop a sway back—an ugly hollow in your lower back. To compensate for this exaggerated curve in your spine, your stomach protrudes and your chest flattens and sinks.

During the moment you stood on that board you did yourself no harm, for your bones and muscles slipped back to normal as soon as you stepped off the board. But women who wear high heels force their bodies to assume this unnatural position all the time they are standing or walking. The harm that may be done can of course never be estimated, for who will ever be able to discover what drastic changes are brought about in internal organs when the bony cage that supports them is tilted at such an angle for four, six or eight hours a day?

How Do You Walk?

Take the matter of walking. During the past century it was considered polite to turn the toes out. As one anatomist of the 18th century, Peter Camper, put it, "The toes of gentlemen should always be turned out, those of peasants and particularly of boatmen, are always turned in." In the days when gentlemen wore knee breeches it was mandatory to show off a well-turned calf. This could be done only in profile, so "toeing out" became fashionable. And it is only quite recently that we have seen the fallacy of such distortion and begun to teach our children in gym classes that the feet should be parallel when one walks. But the damage done to millions of older feet by "toeing out" has already been demonstrated on our older generation.

We used to believe that the toe should touch the ground first in walking—a thoroughly illogical idea, according to Dr. Tribe—for why, he asks, should we try to proceed with the weight bearing area advancing from front to back, when we wish to go forward! The mass of the body, which is to be supported, should of course be placed first on the heel, which is equipped to bear it, then should be gradually transferred to the toes as the forward step is taken. Is this the way you walk? Sometime when you are walking in light snow or sand, check your footprints to see whether you toe out and whether your weight is borne first on your heel when you take a step. You may be surprised at what the footprints reveal. The best way to correct "toeing out" is to set yourself with great deliberation and care to walking "pigeon-toed" for a while. You can easily do this while you are walking around the house or in the country where no one can see you. When you are going about your work, do your best to plant your feet parallel to one another, pointing directly in front of you.

Do You Slouch When You Sit?

How you walk is but one indication of the state of your posture. How do you sit? Dr. Tribe gives an interesting diagram showing how the various bones are arranged when you are sitting correctly (Figure 1) and when you are slumped (Figure 2). Notice how the center of gravity is thrown completely out of line when you slump, and all the bony structure must adjust itself to this condition. See how the whole pelvic basin is tilted backward. Obviously such a position affects more than bones.

Dr. Tribe tells us that slumping in a chair eliminates the normal curves of the back, forces the intestines down on the bladder and genital organs. The ribs are in a state of collapse so that breathing is hindered. The kidneys and liver are no longer supported by the curve of the spine and you may stretch too far the tissues that hold them in place resulting in a "floating" kidney or liver. Not breathing correctly may result in too little oxygen, tenseness, fatigue and so forth. Reading in this slouched position may cause you to hold the book too close to your eyes, bringing strain to the muscles that regulate the way your eyes focus.

The kind of chair you sit in is important for good posture, too. It should permit you to sit erect, without strain and the bone on which you sit should have more cause to slide back in the chair rather than forward.

The back of the chair should not come below the hips as this may interfere with the lower curve of the back. You should be able to sit comfortably with both feet on the floor. And that is the way you should sit.

Dr. Tribe tells us that an investigation carried out by The National Health and Medical Research Council revealed that of 421 children examined 66.5 per cent had postural deficiencies and 46.3 per cent needed expert attention. We suppose that children in this country are not a bit better equipped so far as posture is concerned. "Yet the vast majority of people continue to sport postural defects unabashed and undismayed," says Dr. Tribe. "They suffer from the anatomical and physiological defects I have mentioned previously. Their vitality is poor, their appearance worse." Among the conditions they may be inviting are: flat feet, knock knees, bowlegs, sway-back, lateral curvature of the spine, protruding shoulder blades, humpback and osteoarthritis. He also tells us that a recent study has indicated that posture is related to personality. People with good posture have more self-reliance and self-respect than their slouching friends.

Dr. Green's Posture Measurements

We recently received a newspaper clipping about Dr. C. S. Green, a Chiropractor, of Rexburg, Idaho. Dr. Green has developed a method of measuring posture whereby he can tell how far the present posture deviates from normal and can spot a case of poor posture that is likely to cause trouble later on. He has tested 488 high school students at several Idaho cities and finds that only 4.5 per cent of them stand correctly. Dr. Green has published a booklet about his method—*A Simple Way of Measuring Human Posture.* He would like to get the cooperation of educators and doctors for carrying out the measurings of some 500,000 children so that an accurate cross-section might be obtained.

Dr. Green's measuring system is concerned with angles and squares and seems to us to be a bit hard to follow. But readers who have a mathematical bent would no doubt find it fascinating. They could do a lot of good by using this method to measure the posture of children in the family, neighborhood or school. In fact, it might be an excellent project for a Parent-Teacher organization and would be of great benefit for the physical education department in planning exercises and games for the children. Those children whose posture is shown by measurement to be very bad could then have corrective exercises. As Dr. Green has pointed out in letters to us, exercise would take on a much greater significance when the children themselves could see the measurements of their own posture and then see the change in the measurements as they progressed through exercise to better posture.

You can secure a copy of Dr. Green's booklet by writing him at Box 112, Rexburg, Idaho. We are sure he will be glad to answer questions and give whatever help he can, if you are interested in starting a community project for improving posture. You should, of course, keep in touch with him so that whatever measurements you take can be added to his cross-section total.

Potassium

This mineral is important for our good health, both because of the functions it performs in the body and because of the delicate balance that is found between potassium and sodium in the body tissues. Potassium is necessary for normal growth, for muscle function, and to preserve the proper alkalinity of the body fluids It is especially in demand when tissue is being formed—in children and young folks. During the oxidation or burning of carbohydrates and fats to make energy, a number of enzymes are involved—all of which depend on potassium for their stability. Potassium is necessary for the proper working of the digestive tract. A serious deficiency in animals leads to such severe constipation that the animals may die of it. In fact a lack of potassium is frequently found in people who are sick with some disease of the digestive tract.

We are told that the rate at which the nerve cells take up oxygen is increased when there is more potassium present. There are in all more than eight separate body enzymes that can function only when potassium is present in sufficient quantity.

Since potassium is concentrated mostly in the tissue cells of the body (whereas sodium is in the fluids) we would expect that it would be especially important for the health of the muscles. This is true. In fact a clipping from *Science News Letter* for July 10, 1954 tells us that a leakage of potassium from cells may be one cause for muscular dystrophy. A group of doctors at the University of California believe that a defect in the cell formation may permit the potassium to leak away, thus creating such a low level in the muscle cell that it is impossible for the muscle to function. We are also told that potassium is essential in order for the body to use protein properly. If enough potassium is not around, nitrogen will be lost, which means that protein is not being assimilated.

One reason why we find the study of potassium so fascinating and so puzzling, too, is that it is so closely tied up with sodium. As Adelle Davis puts it in her book *Let's Eat Right to Keep Fit* (Harcourt Brace and Co., 383 Madison Ave., New York, N. Y.) "Just outside the cell wall is sodium, which may have originally come from meat or table salt. In some way not understood, sodium carries on a lifelong duel with potassium, largely inside the cell. This mysterious duel is apparently fought over the water supply. When the sodium appears to be winning, the cell contains more water, but potassium is withdrawn and excreted in the urine; when potassium wins much sodium and water are lost. The referee for the duel appears to be a messenger from the outside of the adrenal glands."

This is actually what goes on in and around cells: when we engage in muscular activity of any kind (which of course we do every waking moment) cells lose their potassium and acquire sodium. In other words, the wall of the cell allows sodium to come in and the potassium leaks out. When the body is resting, the sodium is forced out of the cell and the potassium comes in again. But this requires considerable effort on the part of the body mechanism.

When the body is depleted of potassium, the sodium content of the heart and other muscles increases. So, in case you have a deficiency in potassium and you get a lot of sodium (table salt) in your food you are going to be in serious shape, for the lack of potassium automatically means that you had too much sodium to start with. This is the one note that runs through all the medical literature about potassium—as soon as there is a deficiency, sodium moves in and takes over.

One physician, Dr. Ian W. MacPhee in *The Medical Press* for December 30, 1953, expresses it this way: "For my part, I always picture sodium as masculine—bold, uncomplicated, obeying simple laws and making his presence felt, whereas potassium is a lady, devious and difficult to understand, now advancing, now withdrawing and obeying only her own whims, a veritable Gioconda."

The Complex Functions of Potassium

Under what conditions is one likely to encounter a deficiency in potassium? Chronic illness, malnutrition, extensive surgery, vomiting or diarrheal conditions, or as one M.D. puts it "as a result of lengthy abuse of purgatives!" (How many readers are guilty in this respect?) What doctors call a "hypermotile intestine" can result in loss of potassium. That is, the intestine which pushes food through too rapidly will be wasteful of potassium, as well as other minerals and vitamins, too. There is just not enough time for them to be absorbed in the brief time they spend in the intestine.

In addition to these conditions you lose potassium when you are taking hormone products—cortisone, DCA, aldosterone and so forth. Sodium is retained and potassium is excreted when you are taking these drugs. For some reason or other licorice extract also causes the body to lose potassium. In diabetic patients, when blood sugar rises in the urine, potassium is lost. Ulcerative colitis patients may have too little potassium. It has been found that the level of potassium in the blood is very low in leukemia and polio patients. No one knows why.

What happens in diabetes, in regard to potassium and sodium, is most interesting and proves beyond a shadow of a doubt that both minerals are very important to the functioning of the glands—for of course these are badly out of order in diabetes. In a normal person whose diet does not contain enough potassium, an excessive amount of sodium causes the blood pressure to rise. Substitute potassium for sodium and the blood pressure goes down. In the patient with *severe* diabetes giving excessive sodium causes the blood pressure to go up and the sugar in the blood to go down! As an experiment, 40 grams of sodium were given to a diabetic patient. There was an immediate rise in his blood pressure and fluid began to accumulate. The potassium content of his blood fell sharply. As soon as potassium was given, the blood pressure fell and the fluid was excreted.

Giving potassium to patients with *mild* diabetes causes a fall in blood pressure and in blood sugar, too. As the amount of potassium in the blood increases, just at this same rate the blood sugar falls. There can be no doubt that potassium is very closely related to the function of glands that are disordered in diabetes. In a diabetic coma fruit juice and broth are given, partly because they contain so much potassium. And the potassium apparently helps to bring the patient out of the coma.

How Does Our Salt Intake Affect Our Potassium?

We think that a lot more research in laboratories in the coming years will add, greatly to our knowledge of the workings of potassium in the body. Meanwhile, our chief concern is simply that most present-day Americans are getting more and more sodium in their meals all the time. As our commercially-grown and chemically processed food becomes steadily more tasteless, more and more salt is poured on to give the food some flavor! What is this doing to the potassium balance of our bodies? Could this excessive amount of salt in our diets be responsible for the widespread incidence of overweight which is our greatest health problem in America today, as well as many other diseases which may be related to not enough potassium?

Dr. Max Gerson, M. D. of New York City, cures cancer with diet—a diet rich in potassium, containing little or no sodium and containing in addition carefully measured potassium salts given as medicine which help to drive the sodium out of the tissues and hence restore health to cancer patients. Dr. Harry Hoxsey, at whose clinic in Texas cancer patients are being cured, uses an herb medicine, one of whose ingredients is potassium iodide.

The average book on nutrition dismisses the subject of potassium in the diet by saying that all of us get plenty of it, so we need not concern ourselves about it. We wonder. Considering how much sodium most of us get, and considering that potassium is richest in fruits and vegetables (not especially popular foods) doesn't it seem likely that many of us may be walking around with definite potassium shortage which may be responsible for fatigue, irritability, constipation, lack of appetite?

According to one authority, a grown man should get .58 grams of sodium and 1.28 grams of potassium a day, so that the ratio between the two should be roughly 2 to 1. Keep those figures in mind—a two to one relationship between the two. We should have *twice as much* potassium as sodium if we would be healthy!

One authority tells us that a survey of American diets showed that the average daily intake of potassium is from 1.43 to 6.54 grams a day. Another researcher tells us that the average intake of potassium is about 2.4 grams per day. Nobody knows for certain what the average is, it seems. And of course there may be many individuals who are getting far less than the average. To be completely fair, let's say that the average American gets three grams of potassium a day. This means that he should get only 1.5 grams of sodium, if the balance between the two is to be properly maintained.

Yet the lowest estimate we could find for sodium in the average American diet is four grams. Jolliffe, Tisdall and Cannon, in their classic book *Clinical Nutrition* (published by Paul Hoeber Books) tells us that the average American gets from 8 to 15 grams of sodium per day, from all sources! The individual who gets 15 grams of sodium per day is getting exactly ten times what he ought to have, provided he is actually getting 3 grams of potassium per day. If he is getting less potassium, then he is in even worse shape! Take the lowest estimate of sodium consumption—

4 grams. Such an individual is getting more than twice the amount of sodium he should have, in proportion to his potassium intake!

How is it possible, with these facts and figures before them, that medical men and nutrition experts can say "don't worry about your potassium intake—any old diet will have enough potassium in it—and don't cut down on your table salt—your body needs sodium!" The figures prove exactly the opposite—that we are all getting far, far too little potassium for the amount of sodium we take.

Well, you may say, sodium is easily excreted by the kidneys. It is given off in perspiration, too. So you needn't worry about getting too much, the body will take care of it all right. But why subject our bodies to all this extra work? And why take the chance of overburdening our organs of excretion? In addition, we have caught a glimpse of all the complex mechanism that goes into action to maintain the balance between sodium and potassium—glands, hormones, blood pressure, blood sugar are involved. And in each individual cell the battle between sodium and potassium goes on every second. Why should we deliberately give our bodies all this extra work to do by paying no attention at all to maintaining the proper balance of sodium and potassium in our diets?

Where do we get potassium? Here is a table showing the approximate sodium and potassium content of a number of foods. The value of this chart to you is for you to check to assure yourself that you are getting plenty of potassium every day to balance the sodium you get. We assume that you have already—or will soon—decide to stop using sodium chloride (salt) either in cooking or at the table.

Food	*Sodium Content Milligrams per 100 grams*	*Potassium Content Milligrams per 100 grams*
Nuts		
Almonds	2	690
Brazil nuts	.8	650
Filberts	.8	560
Peanuts (unsalted)	.8	740
Walnuts	2.0	450
Fruits		
Apples	.1	68
Apricots	.5	440
Bananas	.1	400
Cherries	1.0	280
Lemons	.6	130
Oranges	.2	170
Peaches	.1	180
Plums	.1	140
Strawberries	.7	180
Cereals		
Barley	3.0	160
Corn	.4	290
Oats	2.0	340
Rice	.8	100
Wheat	2.0	430

Food	Sodium Content Milligrams per 100 grams	Potassium Content Milligrams per 100 grams
Legumes		
Beans in pod	.8	300
Lima beans, fresh	1.0	700
Navy beans, dry	.9	1300
Fresh peas	.9	380
Green leafy vegetables		
Broccoli	16	400
Cabbage	5	230
Cauliflower	24	400
Lettuce	12	140
Spinach	190	790
Celery	110	300
Root vegetables		
Beets	110	350
Carrots	31	410
Potatoes	.6	410
Turnips	5	260
Eggs, whole	140	130
Milk	51	140
Butter, unsalted	5	4
Meat and fish		
Beef	53	380
Chicken	110	250
Codfish	60	360
Liver, calf	110	380
Lamb	110	340
Turkey	92	310

Potatoes

The other day a friend of ours was talking to us about the harmfulness of white bread. She agreed she'd better omit it from her diet from now on. "And potatoes, too, of course," she continued. We stopped her right there. "Why potatoes?" we asked. "Well, everybody knows that white bread and potatoes are just about the worst things you can eat, aren't they?" she asked. For some reason health literature of the past twenty-five years or so has, without meaning to, given the general public a completely erroneous notion about the food value of potatoes. How else can we explain the prevalent idea that potatoes are almost worthless as food?

Potatoes are about 20 per cent carbohydrate, that's true. Carbohydrate foods should not be used to excess, if it means cutting down on protein foods. But potatoes are about two per cent protein. In addition they contain so many minerals and vitamins that they are quite capable of sustaining life over a period of time, even if no other food at all is available.

A potato is defined as "a swelling at the end of an underground stem." We generally speak of them as tubers. While most kinds are brown, there are some pink-skinned varieties, one of which was cultivated and eaten centuries ago by the Incas who lived in Chile and Peru. Today, we are sorry to say, there are potato growers bent on making this fine food unfit to eat. We have in our file a label from a potato sack in Florida which indicates that the potatoes have been "protected" with a color wax which dyes them pink. A clipping from *Science News Letter,* October 7, 1950, tells us that 2, 4-D, the highly toxic weed-killer, is being used to "intensify red skin color and increase vitamin C content of Red McClure and Bliss Triumph potatoes." The weed-killer is sprayed on the vines while the potatoes are still in the ground. Of course the fact that the color of the potatoes changes indicates that the spray penetrates right through the plant and into the delicious spud which we then buy to feed our families. "Growers have been warned to be especially careful in use of plant-killing 2, 4-D" the article goes on. The poison is sprayed on the potatoes to make them more attractive to housewives! We have no idea why a poison spray should increase the vitamin C content of potatoes unless, as seems quite possible, the potato is forced to manufacture more vitamin C to protect itself against the poison. Thanks, we'll take our potatoes with a little less vitamin C, and we don't honestly think a poisonous red dye makes them the least bit more attractive! A number of deadly insecticides are used on potato plants, so we advise that you scrub thoroughly any commercially bought potatoes you eat.

Bread and cereal products produce an acid reaction in the body. Potatoes, along with other vegetables, are an alkaline-reacting food. As a matter of fact, they are one of the most alkaline of foods. Their vitamin and mineral content are as follows:

Content in One Medium Boiled Potato

Vitamin A	20 milligrams
Vitamin B_1	.11 milligrams
Vitamin B_2	.04 milligrams
Other B Vitamins:	
Niacin	.1 milligrams
Pyridoxine	320 micrograms
Pantothenic Acid	400 to 650 micrograms
Inositol	29 milligrams
Folic acid	140 micrograms
Choline	20-105 milligrams
Vitamin C	24 milligrams
Vitamin E	.06 milligrams
Calcium	5-11 milligrams
Phosphorus	33-56 milligrams
Iron	.46 to .70 milligrams
Copper	.15 milligrams

Cobalt	2-3 micrograms
Fluorine	20 micrograms
Potassium	410 milligrams
Sulfur	24.3 milligrams

The essential amino acids (forms of protein) are present in potatoes. The quality of the protein in potatoes has been the subject of lively debate. By this we mean, is the potato protein such that it will sustain life? In one experiment a researcher lived for six years with potatoes as his only protein and abandoned the diet only because he feared the spray residues were accumulating in his body and might poison him. An article in *Science News Letter* for September 3, 1949, tells us that scientists have discovered some substance in potatoes that may aid the body in using protein. In other words, eating potatoes, as well as meat, cheese and eggs, may help your body to make the best possible use of the meat, cheese and eggs.

Many people like raw potatoes and there seems to be nothing wrong with eating them raw if you like them and if they agree with you. Some people find that raw potato starch is almost indigestible. A Rodale employee who suffered from eczema reported to us that she cleared up a stubborn case by eating raw potatoes. We have no medical authority that indicates what in the potatoes might be responsible for this, but it certainly is worth giving a try, if you suffer from eczema. If you buy potatoes in quantity, they are best stored at a temperature of about 40 degrees in a dry, well-ventilated cellar. They lose some of their vitamin C in storage.

We're sure you've been told many times that potatoes cooked in their skins retain far more vitamins than peeled potatoes. To preserve the largest possible amount of vitamins and minerals, boil potatoes in their jackets. Pressure cooking and baking destroys only a little of these food elements. Paring the potatoes, then boiling them, results in 47 per cent loss of vitamin C. Mashing such potatoes then destroys another 10 per cent. And if, for some special recipe you must pare, slice, grate or cube potatoes, chill them in the refrigerator first, so that some vitamin C will be preserved. And never, never under any circumstances soak them in water, for all the B vitamins as well as vitamin C dissolve immediately in the soaking water.

If you find, toward the end of winter, that your potatoes have sprouted, cut deeply around the sprouts before using the potatoes. A substance called solanine accumulates in potato sprouts which in large amounts can be quite harmful. If you're reducing, you might be wise to avoid too many potatoes, but chances are it's mostly the butter, cream sauce or gravy you put on the potatoes that puts those extra pounds on you.

Pregnancy

Years ago grandmothers, mothers, doctors and midwives used to terrify prospective mothers with dire predictions about what would happen to their offspring if they did or did not do certain things. The pregnant woman who was frightened by a mouse was told that her child's body would carry on it somewhere the mark of this experience. If a child was born with a flaming red birthmark, the mother was reminded of a fire she had seen at some time during her pregnancy. This must have caused the birthmark! If she wanted her child to be musical the expectant mother was told to sing while she was carrying it. A literary child would certainly result if the prospective mother spent her time reading Browning and Tennyson.

Today we know that many of these notions are just notions. But, on the other hand, today's scientists are continually being surprised at how right the old-timers were about some things relating to the embryo child carried within its mother. (Embryo is the term used for the unborn child up to the fourth month of pregnancy.) Until very recently we had little information about the life of that embryo and no explanation for many of the unfortunate children that were born with one or another irregularity in their physical or mental make-up.

However we have now discovered a number of most significant things about the relationship of the mother to her unborn infant. We know for instance that there are illnesses of the mother which may severely injure the child. Rubella, or German measles, is one of these. In *The Archives of Pediatrics* for December, 1953, Edward E. Brown, M.D., F.A.A.P., discusses mongolism in its relation to maternal illness before birth.

Mongolism is a condition in which the child possesses the mentality of an idiot, along with certain definite physical traits such as a broad face, with a flat, stubby nose and eyes set obliquely (hence Mongolism, for the appearance of the eyes resembles those of the Mongol group of people). The mouth of the Mongol child hangs open, the skin is fat and soft, the muscles flabby.

Dr. Brown quotes other authorities for the statements that, in one series of eight mongol idiots, the history of four revealed bad health in the mother before birth. Another authority who studied 379 cases of mongolism reported ill health in 179, or 47.2 per cent of the mothers. Bleeding during pregnancy, the continuation of menstruation during pregnancy and severe vomiting were common symptoms. "With increasing frequency mongolism is being noted after virus and streptococcal diseases attacking the mother usually in early pregnancy," says Dr. Brown, "virus diseases include rubella, measles, mumps and influenza. Among the presumably streptococcal diseases are mastoiditis, pleurisy, otitis media (inflammation of the middle ear), sinusitis and nephritis."

Dr. Brown reports on eleven cases of mongols and "missed mongols" in which ten of the eleven revealed some history of maternal illness during the (most critical) early months of pregnancy. Inquiring into the history of eleven normal babies, he found nothing more serious than nausea as a pregnancy complication.

Of the mothers whose children were mongols—or deficient in such a way as to be almost mongols—he found that several had suffered from severe constant colds, influenza, nephritis, asthma, rheumatic pains or violent vomiting throughout pregnancy. His conclusions are: "Viral and bacterial diseases during the first three months of pregnancy may be a more common cause of mongolism than has been recognized previously.

Further studies of the health of mothers during the first trimester (three months) of pregnancy are needed to verify this suspected relationship."

Heart Deformities in the Embryo

Another study in *The Lancet,* December 12, 1953, discusses congenital heart defects that are associated with illness of the mother during pregnancy. Seventy-eight children who had congenital cataract were studied. It was found that 44 of these children had heart disease. In all cases the mothers had contracted German measles early in pregnancy. In another series of cases there were 21 children with heart irregularities among 61 born to mothers who had had German measles. It is believed, says the editorial in *The Lancet,* that heart defects in children result from arrested development of the heart of the embryo during the early months of pregnancy.

Now we come to the work of Josef Warkany of the University of Cincinnati which shows by means of scientifically controlled experiments in a laboratory what happens to embryo animals whose mothers are deprived of certain nutritional substances. In a report in *The American Journal of Anatomy,* July, 1949, Dr. Warkany and Dr. James G. Wilson of the University of Rochester describe their experiments with rats. They found definite irregularities in the heart and the aorta of rats born from mothers on deficient diets. The aorta is the large blood vessel that carries blood from the heart to all parts of the body. Dr. Warkany and Dr. Wilson fed female rats diets that were deficient in vitamin A prior to and during their pregnancy. The rats born from these mothers showed heart deformities in 75 per cent of the cases. In addition there were serious irregularities in eyes and organs of the genital and urinary tracts. After describing the form these various irregularities took, the doctors tell us that it appears they were caused on or after the twelfth day of pregnancy.

In another article in *The Journal of Nutrition,* June, 1944, Dr. Warkany and Elizabeth Schraffenberger describe experiments in which they produced different kinds of malformation in rats by omitting riboflavin (one of the B vitamins) from the rats' diets. They quote other authorities who worked with other animals and produced, for instance, pigs in which some limbs were completely missing (the diet was deficient in vitamin A), calves who were congenitally blind, pigs with harelips, cleft palates, accessory ears and misplaced kidneys due to a mother's diet before birth that was deficient in vitamin A. In Dr. Warkany's experiment under discussion, the deformities were prevented by the simple addition of riboflavin to the diet.

In an address before the Academy of Pediatrics, reprinted in *Pediatrics,* May, 1951, Dr. Warkany summarizes the knowledge we have up to now regarding malformation in human children which may result from malnutrition of the mother. He says, "Adverse factors acting in prenatal life contribute appreciably to the mortality of infants and many children go through life deformed or crippled because of unfavorable intrauterine (prenatal) conditions." He tells us that congenital (existing at birth) deformities are at the root of many chronic and some incurable diseases of childhood.

Many diseases of the urinary tract, for instance, are now recognized as proceeding from prenatal influences. That is, influences that were effective before birth. Intestinal disorders that were formerly just called "vomiting" or "malnutrition" are now known to spring from this same source. Heart disorders and disorders of the glands may result from maternal malnutrition. Nervous diseases and mental deficiency may be traced to the same cause. He tells us also that some congenital deficiencies may be traced to heredity, to be sure, for these appear regularly in families. However, he says "One can disturb the normal development of the embryo by depriving the pregnant female of certain essential nutritional elements. General starvation of the mother results in sterility, abortions or stillbirths. . . . However, under certain special experimental conditions, *when the pregnant animal is kept in a border-line state of depletion of a specific nutritional element, the embryo may be damaged without being killed.*"

Nutrition of Expectant Mothers in This Country

We have italicized this statement of Dr. Warkany's because we believe this "borderline state of depletion" is what we are dealing with in many of today's mothers. Dr. Warkany says that he does not believe that dietary deficiency of mothers in this country is a factor in producing congenital irregularities in children. However he believes that in countries where food is scarce and knowledge of nutrition is lacking conditions such as their laboratory animals endured may be prevalent.

In a book called *Ecology of Health,* edited by E. H. L. Corwin, Ph.D., from the proceedings of the New York Academy of Medicine, Institute on Public Health, 1947, published by the Commonwealth Fund, 1949, we find a chapter on maternal health and nutrition. This chapter describes three experiments in maternal nutrition conducted at the University of Toronto, the Philadelphia Lying-in Hospital and Harvard University School of Public Health. "That the dietary habits of the mother are related not only to her condition during pregnancy, labor and convalescence, but also to the condition of her baby has been demonstrated by these studies," says the account.

In the experiment ninety women were left on their usual diets which were apparently quite inadequate. Ninety other women were given special dietary supplements in the form of eggs, milk, canned tomatoes, cheese, oranges, vitamin D and wheat germ. Reviewing the various complaints of the women of both groups, we find that of those on the inadequate diet (by which we mean their usual diet at home, which was not improved). Anemia—24, as against 14 in the group with the supplemented diet; toxemia 24 as against 15; hemorrhage 13 as against 9 in the second group; pyelitis (inflammation of the pelvis of the kidney) 5 against 3, numerous other complaints—24 against 14 in the supplemented group. During childbirth the figures are equally revealing with 5 premature births in the first group compared to 2 in the second group, 4 miscarriages compared with one, 3 stillbirths compared with 1 in the supplemented group. The rate of deaths after birth was 15 per cent higher for infants whose mothers were in the first group.

In addition it was found that the children from the group whose diets had been supplemented were taller and weighed more. But Dr. Warkany has said that he does not believe the American diet is deficient enough to cause irregularities in unborn children. Yet a study at the New York Lying-in Hospital reported in *Ecology of Health* shows that while non-pregnant patients have a level of about 1 milligram of vitamin C in their blood, the level in the blood of pregnant women at the time of childbirth is about .3 milligrams or about one-third of a milligram. "Since a level of .5 milligrams of vitamin C in the blood is . . . indicative of a deficiency, many so-called normal pregnant patients are in reality subnormal with respect to vitamin C." In the New York hospital it has been found that patients who suffer from threatened abortions show no vitamin C at all in their blood! At the Philadelphia Lying-in Hospital it has been found that pregnant women with depression, fatigue, lassitude recover quickly when they are given vitamins of the B complex. So, either their diets were deficient in these vitamins, or they were not absorbing what vitamin B there was in their diets.

These facts, from the New York Academy of Medicine Institute on Public Health strengthen our point of view which is that many pregnant women in this country are suffering from slight vitamin deficiencies, or at any rate, their condition and that of their children could be greatly improved by supplementing their diets.

Other Observations About the Life of the Embryo

Finally, to get back to the theories of doctors and midwives of past centuries, we want to review an article that appeared in the *Ladies Home Journal* for February, 1954. Written by Ashley Montagu, Chairman of the Department of Anthropology at Rutgers, and Gertrude Schweitzer, this article is titled "There is Prenatal Influence." Dr. Montagu tells us that modern science has shown that the old-timers were not so far wrong, after all. We have found, for instance, that some profound emotional shock occurring to the mother during pregnancy can result in a nervous, perhaps neurotic child. We have found that the child in the womb can be trained to respond to external stimuli.

In this interesting experiment, a doorbell with the gong removed was used. The unborn child of a woman eight months pregnant did not respond when the doorbell was vibrated close to the mother's abdomen. When the gong was replaced, the baby jumped inside the womb. After repeating the experiment many times, it was found that the baby began to respond by jumping when the bell was vibrated, even when the gong (or sound) was not present.

We have also found that the pregnant woman's craving for certain kinds of food may result in definite damage to the child. Two cases are cited. In one the mother craved nuts and ate about a pound a day during her pregnancy. The baby was born normally and not until he was four years old did he develop any signs of allergy. Then he became allergic to—of course, nuts. A second mother ate a lot of wheat products when she was pregnant—a loaf of bread a day, cakes, pies, crackers and so forth. When the baby was seven months old and began to eat cereals for the first time, she developed a violent allergy to all wheat products. The explanation of this phenomenon appears to be that proteins, such as are contained in wheat and nuts, can pass through the placenta to the unborn baby. We know that adults may produce an allergy in themselves by overeating one food. In these cases, the allergy was produced in the children by the mothers' overeating.

Dr. Montagu covers the question of nutrition and, reviewing Dr. Warkany's work which we discussed earlier, he reminds us that maternal nutrition is of the utmost importance to the welfare of the baby. Then, because he is not a nutritionist, he does not go into all the ramifications of this problem. He mentions smoking. It seems to be definitely established scientifically that even one cigarette smoked by the mother may produce a change in the heartbeat of the unborn child. Dr. Montagu thinks it is quite within the realm of possibility that smoking by modern mothers may be responsible for part of today's big increase in heart disease cases.

The child's height we have always believed is decided by the genes—those tiny substances that carry hereditary traits from one generation to the next. But Dr. Montagu tells us that the genes carry only the height "potential" of the new individual. Taking into account the height of both the mother and father we might say that Junior could be six feet tall—no taller. But whether or not he actually reaches the height of six feet is determined by his mother's nutrition and economic status, as well as whether the birth is normal. It is also dependent on the kind and amount of love the baby receives. Says Dr. Montagu, "There are cases on record of children whose growth was arrested during periods when, for one reason or another, they were deprived of affection, and who began to grow again at a normal rate when they once more came under the influence of love."

Dr. Montagu believes there is nothing for prospective mothers to worry about in his findings. If the mother loves her baby from the moment of its conception and if the mother herself is loved, then the baby will be happy and well, or at any rate can grow into a happy and well individual. We go along with this theory up to a certain point. But what about all those mothers in the New York survey who, we assume, loved their babies, but simply did not know what foods they should have eaten during pregnancy? What about the patients nearing childbirth whose blood showed a complete lack of vitamin C, that most vital food element? No amount of love is going to provide the vitamin C unless the mother knows that the vitamin C is necessary. What about all the women who contracted virus diseases bringing heart disorders or mongolism to their babies? It seems to us that the prevention of virus diseases involves having a strong, healthy, resistant body. And the most important factor in perfect health is a good diet, well supplemented to prevent any possible deficiencies. After that, the love comes naturally, for people just naturally love healthy individuals, and healthy babies are the most beloved of all.

Primitive Diet—A Physician's Journey

Every once in a while an article appears in a medical magazine which is so enlightening and so astounding that we wonder why a meeting is not called immediately to discuss the facts revealed and to take steps through preventive medicine to use the information for promoting good health. Such an article is "African Journey" by L. S. P. Davidson, Professor of Medicine at the University of Edinburgh, Scotland, which appeared in the March 20, 1954, issue of *The Lancet.*

Dr. Davidson begins, "Last year, on my journey from Cape Town to Cairo, which took about three and a half months and covered twenty to thirty thousand miles, I visited medical schools and hospitals in South Africa, Rhodesia, East Africa and the Sudan and I was able to study the medical services in each of these lands. Naturally I also heard much about the background against which these services work."

He goes on to describe the economic and political problems of Africa which are troublesome indeed in comparison with those of Europe and this country. In describing hospitals in Africa, Dr. Davidson says, "The European hospitals are comparable to the average provincial hospitals in Great Britain, but they are, of course, antiquated compared with many of the newer hospitals in America, Sweden or Switzerland. The African hospitals all over Africa are usually overcrowded and with certain notable exceptions less well constructed than the European hospitals. They are also less well equipped with apparatus and laboratory facilities, and with nursing and technical staff." Discussing the medical facilities of the different sections of Africa, Dr. Davidson presents us with facts such as these—there are three medical schools in South Africa, no universities or medical schools in Northern or Southern Rhodesia and "the total revenue of East Africa is stated to be between 30 and 40 million pounds per annum, of which about a tenth is allocated to provide medical services. This amount is totally inadequate to provide Western medicine for even a minority of the 18 million Africans living in these territories, should they desire medical advice and treatment from European doctors."

In speaking of African witch doctors, Dr. Davidson says, "A medical specialist in Rhodesia who had made a special study of witch doctors and had taken an excellent colored film showing how they carried out their professional duties, assured me that by and large they were a respectable and responsible body of men and, as is not generally realized, women. On the whole, they carry out their work conscientiously. It is believed that 80 to 90 per cent of all Africans are treated by witch doctors at the present time. Their art and practice can be passed down from one generation to another of a particular family or it can be acquired through a system of apprenticeship.

"African patients who have obvious cause for an illness such as an injury to an external part of the body are able to understand the reason for their sickness and hence can usually be successfuly treated by the local application of fomentations and a bottle of medicine. When their illness is due to internal causes which are not visible, such as headache or pleurisy, the African patient usually ascribes it to being bewitched by some enemy. The only way of being relieved of the evil spirit which has entered his body is to have it removed by a witch doctor. Unless the patient can be convinced that the evil spirit has been removed, he not infrequently lies down and dies. European doctors who understand this African belief told me that they had on occasion called in witch doctors to help cure psychological disorders in Africans which had failed to respond to European methods of treatment, and that the witch doctor sometimes succeeded where the European doctor had failed."

So much for the medical background for the many millions of Africans living on the Dark Continent. Considering their poverty, lack of education, lack of sanitation, lack of all knowledge of nutrition and the primitive conditions under which many of them exist, it seems probable that the Africans would be oppressed with all manner of diseases, doesn't it? Listen to what Dr. Davidson has to say: "If it could be established that certain diseases were relatively rare in Africans compared with Europeans or Asians living in the same district, this would open new lines of research into their aetiology (causes) because the basic cause in this difference in incidence must be conditioned either by racial and constitutional factors or by environmental factors such as diet, housing, associated infections. Accordingly I sent a memorandum to all the medical centers from Cape Town to Cairo which I was going to visit, and at the end of my lecturing and ward rounds in each centre we held a clinicopathological conference at which physicians and pathologists gave their views on the comparative incidence of diseases in Africans and Europeans."

What Diseases Are Prevalent in Africa?

Do Africans suffer from disease? They do. The most common, according to Dr. Davidson, are: Disease of the liver, nutritional diseases, tropical diseases, respiratory diseases and venereal diseases. These are much more common in Africans than in Europeans. In our country venereal disease is well controlled with drugs which, we assume, are not widely available to the Africans. We have read medical articles showing that the widespread liver diseases of Africa may be due to a diet that does not contain enough protein. Many of them live entirely on grains or fruits and vegetables. Tropical diseases could, we suppose, be stamped out with proper sanitation. Respiratory diseases may, again, be the result of diet. But where are the blood vessel diseases, the heart diseases, the coronary thrombosis, the stomach and intestinal diseases, the rheumatism, the diabetes, the anemia?

On the subject of gastro-intestinal disorders, Dr. Davidson tells us that "Peptic ulceration of the stomach is relatively uncommon in Africans, but its two most serious complications—hemorrhage and perforation—are so rare that many physicians and surgeons who had spent years in Africa told me that they had never met them." Cancers of the stomach and intestines, appendicitis, gall bladder disease and gall stones are likewise practically unknown.

Angina, coronary thrombosis, cerebral thrombosis, diseases of the blood vessels and high blood pressure are also not common among Africans. Says Dr. Davidson, "So rare is classical coronary thrombosis in Africans that I did not see a case in any hospital I visited." Hardening of the arteries is much less common and less severe among Africans. Rheumatic fever occurs in Africa, but much less commonly among Africans than among Europeans. Rheumatoid arthritis is so rare in Africans that Dr. Davidson did not see a single case in any hospital. Osteo-arthritis is also uncommon and less severe among Africans. Goiter and diabetes are far less frequent among Africans.

The complicated anemias which afflict Europeans and Americans are very rare and iron-deficiency anemia when it does exist, is usually caused by some other disease such as hookworm or malaria, rather than from deficiency of iron in food.

Why Are Africans Immune?

Can it be that Africans have some mysterious immunity to the "diseases of civilization" such as heart and vascular trouble, appendicitis, rheumatism, stomach ulcers? No, for Dr. Davidson says, "I have been told by doctors who have practiced in America and by Europeans and Indian doctors who have practiced in India that diseases which are rare in Africans now living in Africa are also rare in African and Indian peasants living under poor conditions in America and India, but that when Africans and Indians become successful and adopt European customs, eat the same kind of food and are submitted to the emotional strains of modern civilization, the incidence of the vascular, gastro-intestinal and endocrine diseases among them shows a remarkable increase. If these observations are true they suggest that environmental factors rather than racial factors are largely concerned in the aetiology (cause) of these diseases.

"Environmental factors such as bad housing, nutritional deficiency or infection do not appear to play an essential part in the causation of those diseases which are rarer in Africans than in Europeans, since Africans are worse housed, worse fed, and suffer from infectious diseases, especially tropical diseases and helminthic (worm) infestations much more often than Europeans living in the same district.

"Two other causes may be responsible for the high incidence of certain diseases in Europeans—namely (a) the excessive consumption of calories or the excessive intake of some particular food such as fat or protein; or (b) an excessive or uncontrolled production of emotional stimuli due to the competition and stress of modern life."

He concludes by asking for "intensive research" for discovering the reasons for the rarity of some diseases in Africans as compared with Europeans. How wonderful it would be if we might know that such research would be soon underway! And how does it happen that of all the enormous sums donated to cancer, rheumatism and heart research not a penny of it is spent in finding out more about why these plagues of civilized countries do not afflict primitive Africans?

Is it not logical to inquire into what kind of food the Africans eat and how that food is grown? A recent survey in the middle west disclosed the fact that the protein content of the grains being raised in that section of the country has decreased 10 per cent in the past ten years. Worn out soil, "hopped up" with chemical fertilizers, simply cannot provide the proper protein content in food grown on it. Perhaps the primitive Africans, growing their crops as their ancestors did and certainly without any access to modern commercial fertilizers, have food far richer in protein and mineral content than ours. Might this not have a great deal to do with their resistance to our modern diseases?

We do not hold with the theory of the "noble savage," nor do we believe that there is anything particularly healthful in living "primitively" as such. But we do believe—and every sentence of Dr. Davidson's article strengthens our belief—that modern degenerative diseases of the heart, the digestive tract, the muscles, the glands are caused directly and completely by eating food that has been refined and denatured until it is no longer food. Primitive Africans cannot obtain such food. White sugar and white flour, and the host of other artificial, synthetic flavored and doctored foods, are unknown to them. When they become wealthy and "civilized" and take on our habits of eating, then they at once become susceptible to our diseases!

How long must we wait for our researchers to take up Dr. Davidson's challenge and investigate the reasons (which are not very difficult to find) for the remarkable freedom from degenerative diseases among the peoples of the world who do not eat food that has been tampered with according to the latest technological findings of the food scientists!

Prostate—Preventing Disorders of the Prostate

The prostate gland is removable. Because prostate trouble can be cured by an operation, little definitive research has apparently been done on what causes such trouble and what, aside from an operation, can be done to help.

If the prostate gland were not situated as it is, the enlargement that occurs so frequently in later years might go completely unnoticed. But for some mysterious reason this gland is located around the mouth of the bladder. So when it swells it cuts off the tube leading from the bladder and, since urine cannot flow freely as before, complications arise rapidly.

The prostate gland is an auxiliary sex gland, concerned with manufacturing the fluid in which the sperm cells float. Hence the removal of the gland results in sterility, even though generally it does not otherwise affect the sexual powers of the individual. In some cases it may. Until quite recently removal of the prostrate gland was a dangerous operation with a high mortality. In recent years less than 2 per cent of patients die of prostate gland operations. The time in hospital has been cut to a minimum and, in general, members of the medical profession urge removal of the gland when it is causing difficulty.

Since disorders of the prostate occur mostly in the years past middle-age, it might seem likely that surgery mortality would be high because of the advanced age of the average patient. We have the word of John A. Taylor, M.D. of New York in the *Journal of the American Medical Association* for October 27, 1951, that prostatectomy (removal of the prostate gland) is not especially hazardous even for patients in their nineties. Since 1945, 41 operations have been done at St. Luke's Hospital on patients over eighty, and Dr. Taylor has performed 27 operations on his private patients over eighty. In one case the patient was 96 years old. Most of the patients had other diseases as well, the most common of these being hardening of the arteries and heart disease. There was a total mortality of 3.1 per cent among these elderly patients which seems to indicate that the operation, as performed today, carries little risk.

The decision to have an operation is generally the result of a lot of misery, for an enlarged prostate gland is both dangerous and painful. At first the only symptom may be a feeling of congestion and discomfort. Then there may be difficulty in starting the stream when urinating. There may be a feeling of fullness in the bladder, necessitating frequent trips to the bathroom, even though the amount of urine voided may be small. The residual urine—that remaining in the bladder—causes trouble. First there may be dribbling of urine. Then, as urination becomes more and more difficult, the contents of the bladder may accumulate to such an extent that they flood back into the kidneys, causing the very serious and immediate danger of uremic poisoning.

It is assumed that our patient will have consulted a doctor long before this last stage is reached. Actually, however, he will soon discover that, aside from an operation, there is little or nothing the doctor can do for him to bring permanent relief. A catheter inserted into the bladder will drain off the accumulated urine, but shortly it will accumulate again. Massage of the prostate gland is often helpful in reducing its size. This must be done frequently. Hot baths may relieve congestion. Some physicians suggest hot sitz baths—that is, baths in which just the lower part of the trunk is immersed, while the chest and legs are not.

Is Nutrition Important?

What possible role does good nutrition play in preventing disorders of the prostate gland? The fat soluble vitamins seem to be most concerned with the health of this gland, just as they are with the well being of cells and tissues throughout the lining of the digestive and reproductive tracts. We know that a lack of vitamin A has a very definite reaction on these tissues. One of the earliest symptoms of vitamin A deficiency is a sloughing away of cells on the lining of the digestive, respiratory and reproductive tracts. Just as the tissues of nose and mouth may clearly indicate a vitamin A deficiency, so the delicate and sensitive tissues of the reproductive tract reflect any deficiency.

We know, too, that vitamin E plays an important part in the health of the reproductive tract. Many experiments with animals have shown that a deficiency in vitamin E will create all kinds of problems in sexual life, for both the male and the female. In animal experiments these difficulties can be speedily corrected by giving vitamin E. This is one reason why good animal feeds always contain ample vitamin E.

Wheat germ oil, too, is noted for its effectiveness in preventing disorders of the sexual organs. It is given to both males and females in animal experiments and has proved itself of great value. It is believed that the natural hormones that occur in wheat germ oil are responsible for its powerful effect. It is made from the reproductive part of the wheat, of course, and carries with it all the substances that safeguard the reproductive processes of the grain.

Another fat soluble vitamin, vitamin F (the unsaturated fatty acids) has been named by two researchers as curative of enlarged prostate gland. James Pirie Hart and William LeGrande Cooper, M.D. of Los Angeles, California, conducted an experiment involving nineteen patients to whom they gave unsaturated fatty acids. No other treatment was given. Writing about this experience in a pamphlet published by the Lee Foundation for Nutritional Research, 2023 W. Wisconsin Ave., Milwaukee, Wisconsin, these investigators give their results as follows:

1. All cases showed a lessening of residual urine—that is, urine remaining trapped in the bladder. In 12 of the 19 cases there was no residual urine at the end of the treatment.
2. For 13 of the 19 patients, the treatments ended their getting up at night to urinate.
3. There was a decrease in fatigue and leg pains and an increase in sexual libido in all patients.
4. Cystitis or bladder inflammation cleared up as the residual urine disappeared.
5. Dribbling was eliminated in 18 of the 19 cases.
6. The force of the urinary stream was increased.
7. In all cases the size of the prostate gland was rapidly reduced.

We could find no confirmation of this experiment in other medical literature. In other words, no other physician seems to have gotten interested in the subject and decided he would experiment, too. This happens often in the scientific world.

Prostate Infection and Health

But there are other physicians who are experimenting with diet in relation to prostate gland disorders. We want to review in detail an article which appeared in the *American Journal of Digestive Diseases* for December, 1951. It is a preliminary report on a nutritional method *for preventing surgery* in cases of prostate enlargement. Benjamin F.

Sieve, M.D. of Boston, who wrote it, has done considerable work along nutritional lines and has contributed many articles to scientific magazines.

Dr. Sieve's theory in general is that vitamins and hormones (the substances produced by the body's glands) work together to create health. Infection, emotional upsets and mechanical interference with food intake prevent a proper nutritional state. In studying 200 cases, Dr. Sieve found that infection was one of the main causes of nutritional decline in 60 per cent of the cases. Among men the most prevalent source of infection was the prostate gland. Along with the infection went nutritional deficiency and disorders of the glands and hormones. All three had to be cleared up in order to get the patient back into a healthy state.

Dr. Sieve made a careful study of 100 patients who suffered from prostate trouble. The age range was from 15 to 75 years, with the majority in the 43-63 age group. In 70 per cent of these the stage at which it would have been necessary to operate was prevented and no operation was necessary. Dr. Sieve's treatment, by his own admission, is purely preventive. He does not guarantee anything in the way of cures for patients with advanced cases. Instead he suggests that treatment should be started in the thirties, especially in those men who have a history of recurring infections. The younger the patient, the easier it is to correct his nutritional state, hence the infection and hence the condition of the prostate.

The first patient he describes was 20 years old and suffered from headaches, lack of appetite and pain in his legs. He also had acne, brittle, ridged fingernails and other indications that all was not well, nutritionally speaking. Dr. Sieve prescribed a full and well-balanced diet, along with vitamin supplements containing vitamins A, C, D and E and the vitamin B complex. In addition, he was given another preparation containing vitamin B.

And, in case there might be difficulty assimilating these vitamins, vitamin injections were given once a week. The patient was also given by mouth and by injection various hormone substances that his condition indicated he needed. In addition a course of prostatic massage was given. Four years later the young man was quite well. He was still taking the vitamin preparations and Dr. Sieve says he hopes the youth realized their importance enough to go on taking them the rest of his life. He also stated that he could predict that this patient would never suffer from prostate enlargement, barring acute infection.

The second case was 35 years old, a man who complained of fatigue and extreme sluggishness as well as distress in his digestive tract resulting in gas, vomiting and abdominal pain. There were many other symptoms indicating wrong diet for a period of years. And the prostate was "boggy." In addition to the vitamins A, B, C, D and E in large amounts, this patient was given a capsule containing the fat soluble chlorophyll substance from alfalfa, buckwheat and soybean (did this possibly contain the precious vitamin F?). Furthermore, he was given vitamin injections and gland medication. He had prostate massage once a week. And his prescribed diet was well balanced.

Twelve months later he showed great improvement in many directions. He had not noticed any stomach distress for more than eight months. He had lost 12½ pounds of excess weight. He had not been absent from work for a single day in seven months. The prostate gland was much smaller and no possibly dangerous nodules were to be found in it. For five years he continued to improve. Dr. Sieve comments that "a good . . . clue to the type of case in which prolonged infection can be anticipated is for example the individual who gives a history of having had severe acne at puberty."

He reminds us further that these cases of nutritional deficiency he is describing are not "full blown, classic textbook cases," . . . but the findings all add up to "subclinical nutritional deficiency." That means, just enough deficiency to bring about countless ills, such as acne, prostate enlargement, fatigue, headaches and so forth, but not enough deficiency to result in scurvy or pellagra or one of the other vitamin deficiency diseases. This is the condition we talk about so much in *Prevention*—this dragging, listless, tired state of health that most of us have, which could, with proper nutrition, be changed to vital, glowing health.

Vitamins and Hormones for Prostate Enlargement

The third patient Dr. Sieve treated was 55 and had been warned by a number of specialists that an operation on his prostate was absolutely necessary. His complaints were dribbling and frequent urination at night. He had also suffered from an attack of coronary thrombosis. As Dr. Sieve examined him he noted many symptoms of vitamin deficiency (in nails, tongue, skin, etc.).

His prescription was similar to those mentioned before—large doses and injections of all the vitamins and treatment for glands. The prostate was massaged once a week. Five months later the patient looked and sounded like a new man—free from headaches, no pain in his heart, slept better and had lost all symptoms of the prostate difficulty. At this time he was also given the tablet made from soybeans, alfalfa and buckwheat . . . At eight months even greater improvement was shown and, says Dr. Sieve, the patient looked twenty years younger.

The fourth patient was 71. He had been advised when he was 53 that he should have the treatment described above if he wanted to avoid surgery. However, he was just plain ornery and refused to take any preventive treatment whatsoever. In addition to his prostate trouble, this patient ended up with a plethora of other complaints—constipation of 30 years duration, bloating, gas, belching, headaches, cough, dizziness, swelling of the ankles, palpitation of the heart and so on and so on. He was suspicious and apprehensive of everything that was suggested to him. But he was finally convinced to change his diet and to take diet supplements, which included incidentally 150 milligrams of vitamin E taken twice daily. He also had massage of the prostate but refused to go for the massage as often as he was asked to go.

So the prostate symptoms did not clear up and this patient at last ended in the hospital (after eighteen years of a miserable existence) for a prostatectomy. During the course of convalescence there were complications and it took upwards of 19 months for him to regain his strength. Says Dr. Sieve, "Had this patient not been so fearful, and started treatment as recommended eighteen years before, he could, in our opinion, have gone along with a normal prostate gland . . . A healthier, happier and undoubtedly younger appearing patient would have resulted."

We have given these four examples from Dr. Sieve's experience to indicate as clearly as we can the tremendous importance of correcting your diet early—don't wait until you are ill and run down. If a proper diet can prevent trouble with your prostate, isn't it sensible to undertake just such a diet now, rather than waiting until something goes wrong and you get panicky fearing you may have to have surgery?

You will notice that Dr. Sieve did not give his patients just one or two vitamins—they got them all, and in large quantity. And in addition to a good, well-balanced diet. By a good, well-balanced diet we mean a diet high in protein (meat, fish, eggs) with little or no food made from white sugar and white flour products, a diet that includes plenty of fresh fruits and vegetables and nothing that is refined, processed, degerminated or chemicalized. In addition, get your extra vitamins as Dr. Sieve's patients did: fish liver oils for vitamins A and D, brewer's yeast or desiccated liver for the B vitamins, rose hips for vitamin C and, perhaps most important of all, wheat germ oil, vitamin E and the unsaturated fatty acids, otherwise known as vitamin F. If you buy them at your local health food store, insist on completely natural products—not synthetic.

Protein

A contractor builds houses out of many different materials, but if he is a man who deals mostly in brick houses, we might say that the most important single material necessary for his houses is bricks. If the design of each of his houses is different, the arrangement of the bricks will be different. Some houses will have brick chimneys, others brick porches, in still other houses the bricks will be arranged in designs to form railings or terraces. Some houses have brick floors, brick fireplaces or brick walls in the garden. There is a wide variety of color and kinds of bricks for the contractor to choose from.

If you buy the house and do not like the design, you can take apart the bricks and put them together again to form an entirely different house, out of the same bricks. If you were to number each brick in the house and then rebuild the house, putting each brick in a different place, you would be able to continue for thousands of years, combining and recombining the different bricks and never getting quite the same house as the original one, for each time you would make some slight change in the arrangement of the bricks.

As your house grows older some bricks would have to be replaced, and after a certain length of time you would probably have replaced all of the original bricks at one time or another. Now regardless of what plumbing, insulation, roofing, wallpaper you use in the house the bricks are still the most important part for you must have them or there simply will be no house.

Just like a house, the human body is made up of building blocks or bricks, if you want to call them that. These bricks are the amino acids which go to make up the protein of which the human house is made. Although they can be arranged and rearranged in thousands and thousands of different combinations, they are still protein and they are still the essential part of your human house. Without them life could not go on. No living thing survives without protein. When it comes to building a fire to keep your house warm you use materials that are largely carbohydrate. But the house itself must be made largely of protein.

What exactly does this mean in terms of body physiology. Your blood is protein, your tissues, organs, skin, hair, nails are protein. Your bones are made of protein which supports all the various minerals that give them strength. The fluids your body secretes are protein—hormones, and enzymes. Your nerves and brain are made of protein. Obviously when you were an infant, then later through childhood and adolescence, you needed large amounts of protein, for then you were building the house and every day you needed more and more bricks for the bricklayers to use. But as a house grows older, bricks crumble and must be replaced. Human protein—marvelous substance that it is—does not have the hardness and durability of bricks. It is subject to terrific stress and strain, and some of it wears out a little each day. So there is no reason to believe that, as you grow older, you require less protein. Quite the opposite is true.

Now taking a look at your human body it is difficult to believe that fingernails are made of the same substance as blood or nerves. They don't look the same. Well, neither does a brick chimney look like a brick floor, but both are made of bricks. The difference in your body lies in the various combinations in which the amino acids, or bricks, are put together. And if you can have many different designs of houses, all made of brick, just think for a moment of all the different kinds of protein you can have by re-arranging the various amino acids. Of course you can't actually imagine such a number, for it is bound to be astronomical.

What Is Protein?

In 1839 a chemist first isolated a substance containing nitrogen, which he announced was the basis of life. He named it protein, meaning "primary substance." It was not until 1906 that other chemists first demonstrated an essential amino acid—a building block of the substance protein. The carbohydrates that we eat are made of carbon, hydrogen and oxygen. Proteins are made of carbon, hydrogen, oxygen and nitrogen. It is this nitrogen apparently that makes all the difference between proteins and carbohydrates—building blocks and fuel. After the first amino acid was discovered a great deal of research was devoted to this branch of biological chemistry and many more amino acids have been discovered. We do not have any idea of how many there may be. We have so far discovered about 21 in protein food products.

The study of protein is extremely complex, as you can imagine, for it deals with all the different combinations of these amino acids, which may be put together by nature in different quantities and different arrangements to make up any given kind of food product. Then, of course, in most foods the protein amino acids are combined with fat and carbohydrate, as well. When we speak of protein, we are not talking about something like vitamins which exists in infinitesimally small quantities and which are necessary just to cause certain processes to take place inside the body. *You can see protein.* The white of an egg is almost pure protein, composed of a series of different amino acids. So the *bulk* of protein food you eat is quite important—for this is the substance from which the body makes or replaces actual body structure.

After you have eaten protein, the digestive juices of the stomach and intestines go to work on it and break it down into its amino acids. This is because the actual cells of a human body are put together differently from the white of an egg, for instance. So the digestive juices, the enzymes and the body hormones are all involved in putting these amino acids together once again in a different combination so that they can form part of the body. One re-constituted protein substance will go to make-up red blood cells. Another will be rushed to the fingernails which are constantly growing so that they need new protein constantly. Another will be sent to the brain where a lot of thinking has worn out a number of cells. Still another protein will be transferred to a gland where it helps to form a gland secretion or hormone. And so forth. You can easily see why we must have protein every day, and must have it in quantity.

The Quality of Protein is Important

But it appears, from later research work, that the most important thing about protein is not quantity, but quality. What do we mean by "high quality" protein? We mean protein containing all the essential amino acids in the proper proportion. If one of them is missing, the protein will not sustain life in laboratory animals. If one of the essential amino acids is present in too small a quantity, this protein will not maintain health. It is as if you were building your brick wall and trying to use a brick that is smaller than the other bricks. In a wall, you might fill up the gaping space with mortar, but there is no mortar that will replace protein in body structure. So your wall, with several bricks too small, will sag and be out of line.

Practically, in selecting food, how does this amino acid set-up work out? You should try to eat as much "complete" or "high quality" protein as you need. Foods containing an incomplete quantity or proportion of one or another of the essential amino acids will not sustain health. Complete proteins appear in foods from animal sources—meat, fish, milk, cheese and eggs are complete proteins. In the vegetable kingdom these are the protein foods that most nearly approach completeness: nuts, soybeans, wheat germ. You can see that a completely vegetarian diet presents hazards. In order to maintain good health a vegetarian must know the amino acid content of all the vegetables and fruits. If he is going to eat a vegetable that is short or completely lacking in one of the essential amino acids, he must eat something that contains this amino acid, even though it may be short on another. So a constant vigilance is necessary and a great deal of knowledge about the quality of the protein in the various vegetables and fruits.

The names of the essential amino acids are complicated and not especially meaningful to those of us who are not chemists. But it is well to be familiar with them, for you often run across them in articles dealing with food or health and if you do not know what they are you may become confused and think they are vitamins or enzymes or something else. The essential amino acids are those that have been found to be absolutely necessary in the diet of human beings. Nothing can substitute for them. They are: Arginine, histidine, isoleucine, leucine, lysine, methionine, phenylalanine, threonine, tryptophan, valine. The amino acids that at present are listed as unessential are: alanine, aspartic acid, cirrulline, systine, glutamic acid, glycine, hydroxyproline, hydroxyglutamic acid, norleucine, proline, serine and tyrosine.

As researchers progress in their study of the proteins, it is quite possible that they may discover that one or more of the unessential amino acids also have important functions in the body and should be considered essential. However, it seems that we may be able to manufacture within our bodies some of these unessential ones. We cannot manufacture the essential ones, so they must be supplied in food. However, just as in the case of the vitamins, the amino acids work together and, if you are getting a lot of the unessential ones it seems that this makes up somewhat for a slight deficiency in the essential ones. But keep in mind that you can get amino acids—essential or unessential—only from protein. They do not exist in carbohydrate foods. White sugar is the one outstanding example of a so-called food that is pure carbohydrate, without any protein whatsoever. This is one of the main reasons why white sugar is worthless as food. Your body cannot use it to build or replace any cells. And the more sugar you eat, the less you can eat of the protein foods that have so much value for your good health. Vegetables and fruits contain in general far more carbohydrate than protein.

You can make a quick check on all the foods you eat, so far as protein content is concerned, by sending to the Superintendent of Documents in Washington, D. C., for a copy of the Agricultural Handbook, Number 8 which lists all the common foods, along with their protein, carbohydrate and fat content.

What Results From Protein Deficiency?

The list of diseases resulting from protein deficiency is almost endless. Jut stop and think for a moment of all the things that would go wrong with the house you tried to build of bricks if there were few or no bricks available. The hemoglobin of blood is 95 per cent protein. Lack of protein will produce anemia. The antibodies your blood manufactures to fight germs are made of protein. Lack of protein leaves one an easy prey to all kinds of infections. Proteins protect the liver against poisonous chemicals to which we are all exposed all the time. Protein regulates the amount of water in body tissues. The unhealthy swelling or dropsy that accompanies so many diseases (especially of the heart or kidneys) may be simply an indication of too little high quality protein in the food: And speaking of kidney disease, researchers used to think that people with kidney disease should not eat protein. The kidneys were already excreting a great deal of nitrogen (one of the main constituents of protein). Therefore, reasoned these physicians, the nitrogen is irritating the kidneys, so we will eliminate nitrogen (protein) from the diet. But patients died, for of course all the diseased tissues of their bodies needed the nitrogen desperately to rebuild themselves. Nowadays kidney disease patients are placed on a high protein diet. And the protein replaces the nitrogen lost through the kidneys.

If you have a wound, cut or burn, protein is lost in the fluid and blood that escape. Furthermore to remake healthy tissue over the site of the injury the body must have protein, for this is what the cells are made of. So ample protein in the diet helps hasten the healing process. Muscles are made of protein. Lack of protein breaks down these muscles faster than they can be replaced, resulting in fatigue and lack of stamina. The poor posture of adolescents may often be the result of lack of protein. For flabby muscles simply cannot hold the body erect. The health of your skin, hair and nails depends on protein supply—they are made of protein and cannot grow or replace dead tissues unless they are supplied with the necessary substance, protein. Constipation may be the result of flabby muscles in the stomach and intestines that cannot contract and expand as they should to move the food along our digestive tracts. Protein in the diet will firm and strengthen these muscles. Finally, we know that vitamins and mineral will not be used in the body unless the proper hormones and enzymes are there to combine with them. Hormones and enzymes are made of protein. So all the vitamin and mineral preparations in the world will not make you healthy unless you also provide protein so that these substances can be used.

The subject of absorption of proteins is an important topic in itself. People who suffer from diarrheal conditions do not absorb protein properly, so whatever protein they eat may be partly wasted. Bacteria in the intestines can make the amino acids of protein unabsorbable. Protein must be digested in an acid medium, so if hydrochloric acid is lacking in the stomach, protein food will be wasted. Then, too, those folks who follow every meal with a dose of bicarbonate of soda, or one of the other so-called "alkalizers" will produce a condition in the stomach where the protein simply will not be digested. It has been found that the proteins of some foods are more thoroughly digested than those of others. Ninety-seven per cent of the meat you eat is completely digested (in a healthy person), only 85 per cent of the protein of cereal is digested, only 83 per cent of vegetable protein, 78 per cent of legume protein and only 85 per cent of the protein that appears in fruits.

How To Get High Quality Protein

How are you going to know how much protein you need every day and which proteins contain the essential amino acids? And, perhaps just as important, how are you going to pay your grocery bill once you start living on t-bone steak? First of all, there is no necessity for living on t-bone steak, pleasant though the prospect sounds. In general all meats contain the same amounts of the essential amino acids. Liver, heart, kidneys and brain actually are a little higher in amino acid content.

And hamburger may be even more acceptable to the youngsters and oldsters in your family because it is easier to chew. Whole wheat bread contains far more protein than white bread and is no more expensive. Can you substitute beans or soybeans for meat? Sometimes, but remember no vegetable food is as rich in all the essential amino acids as food of animal origin, so don't depend on beans day after day for protein. Can you substite macaroni or spaghetti for meat? No, you cannot, despite all the attractive recipes offered in the women's magazines during Lent. Cereal foods (especially refined ones) are largely carbohydrate foods and cannot be used as building blocks for a healthy body. Fish is cheap and an excellent source of high quality protein.

What about gelatin as a source of protein? Often we hear recommendations for taking one or two packets of gelatin every day for a good supply of protein. It's cheap, certainly, but we must report that gelatin is the one animal protein that is not complete. In other words, it does not contain all of the essential amino acids. It will not sustain life in laboratory animals when it is used as the sole source of protein. Now of course, if you were living under extraordinary circumstances where you could not obtain any protein except gelatin, it would be best to eat the gelatin, because it will sustain life longer than a diet completely lacking in protein. And of course if you are hesitating between a dessert made of white sugar, corn starch or corn syrup, and another dessert made of gelatin, you should choose the gelatin dessert for it does have protein value and the others do not. But don't depend on gelatin, cheap as it is, for protein, for it simply cannot fill the bill.

How Much and What Kind of Protein?

How much protein do you need? As you know our pioneer ancestors lived chiefly on high quality protein in the days when they hunted game, before they had gardens or farms. Many people believe this is the reason they were able to endure such hardship and perform such prodigious feats of work. Arctic explorers have lived healthfully for as long as two years on meat, lean and fat. Nothing else. No carbohydrates at all. So there is no chance of your getting too much protein. There is every chance of your getting too little. Recent surveys have indicated that as many as 60 to 80 per cent of Americans get far too little protein in their diets. The official recommendation of the National Research Council is 40-100 grams of protein every day for children, depending on age and 60-70 grams of protein for adults. It is generally agreed among nutritionists that these allowances are far too low and actually may only be enough to keep one from suffering some kind of deficiency disease.

When you are planning menus, your Agricultural Handbook, No. 8 will indicate in grams the amount of protein in any given food. For instance, five tablespoons of dried skim milk give you 34 grams of protein. Four ounces (one-fourth pound) of lean beef give you 22 grams of protein. One cube of cheese 2 by 1 by 1 inches, gives you 12 grams of protein. And so forth.

One final word about amino acids. Scientists have learned how to synthetize them. We say it with regret. Our information comes from an article in the *Herald-Tribune* for December 27, 1952, in which it was announced: "Four cheap factory-made chemicals can double the protein value of the world's food supply, a chemist said here today." The synthetic amino acids, made from coal tar, are to be added to foods like wheat, corn and so forth to double their protein value. However the scientific journals are full of warnings about the possible harmful effects of tampering with proteins. Says *Borden's Review of Nutritional Research,* "Recent investigations, however, indicate that indiscriminate supplementation with amino acids may precipitate a dietary imbalance having dangerous consequences." The articles goes on to tell of an experiment where, by adding synthetic amino acids, the proper balance of the protein was thrown completely out of line and the experimental rats developed a serious nervous condition very shortly. Protein is the fabric from which living tissue is made. Isn't it obvious to even the most unenlightened of us that you cannot make something out of coal tar and substitute it for living tissue? Be on your guard against any food to which synthetic amino acids have been added. Shun it as you would shun synthetic vitamins.

However do not confuse synthetic amino acids with natural amino acid preparations made from food. Food supplements exceptionally rich in all the essential amino acids have been made from food substances such as meat, yeast and so forth. These are no more artificial than are dried milk or powdered eggs. And the amino acids are so concentrated in them as to provide a wealth of these valuable food elements in the proper proportions as they occur in nature. If you are in doubt about the source of any amino acid preparation or any individual amino acid, such as methionine, that your doctor may have prescribed for you, check on whether the amino acids came from a food source or whether they are synthetic. The synthetics are not for you.

Prunes

Plums (from which prunes are made) were grown originally in the region of the Caucasus and the Caspian Sea. Later they were brought to central Europe and the Balkans And today they are grown mainly in California. The French prune, with a small pit, is the most sought-after one for drying. Prunes drop from the trees of their own weight when they are ripe, are gathered carefully and dipped in a milk alkaline solution to boil, so that tiny cracks will be formed in the skin. From these the moisture escapes evenly while they are dried. Some prunes are sun-dried, but most of them today are dried in dehydrators in 18 to 24 hours, at an even temperature. Be sure not to buy prunes that have been dried with sulfur.

The prunes are packed according to size. Just before being packed, they are dipped into boiling water to sterilize them. Statements on the labels indicate the size of the prunes inside the packages. Small prunes pack 85 to the pound, medium 67 to the pound, large 53 and extra large 43 or less to the pound. So a label reading 30/40 means that there are 30 to 40 prunes in the package.

Prunes have long been noted for their laxative qualities. There seems to be nothing about prunes to produce this effect except for their cellulose content which is very high. It is well known that foods high in cellulose tend to regulate the bowels. And it is also true that most modern foods are low in cellulose, because of the refining and processing they undergo. So perhaps prunes deserve their wide fame as a laxative.

One further reminder about prunes. When you are considering the acid-alkaline content of your diet, keep in mind that prunes (like plums and cranberries) produce an acid reaction in the body, rather than the alkaline reaction resulting from all other fruits. So if you are trying to arrange for a more alkaline diet, prunes are not for you. But if you eat lots of fruits and vegetables, so that you have plenty of alkaline material to work with, prunes will be highly beneficial, for they will contribute to the acid balance.

They should be cooked quickly. And there is no need to soak them these days, for the treatment they are given when they are packed guarantees that they will cook in a very short time without soaking. If you allow them to stand for a time in the cooking liquid before serving them, they are softer and plumper and generally tastier, for they have absorbed some of the cooking water. Of course you should always eat this cooking water along with the prunes, for it contains much food value.

Prune juice is made by cooking the prunes in water, just as you would at home, then pressing the whole business through a strainer. The pulp may be left in the juice, or strained out. We imagine that juice which contains the pulp would probably be richer in vitamins and minerals.

Prunes are richer in some of the B vitamins than any other fruit. They contain large amounts of vitamin A and minerals, especially iron. And they contain a trace—the merest trace—of vitamin C.

Here is the vitamin and mineral content of 100 grams of prunes which would be about 12 medium-sized ones:

Vitamin A	1890 International units
Vitamin B	
Thiamin	.10 milligrams
Riboflavin	.16 milligrams
Niacin	1.7 milligrams
Pantothenic Acid	60 micrograms
Vitamin P	300-400 units
Vitamin C	3 milligrams
Calcium	54 milligrams
Phosphorus	85 milligrams
Iron	3.9 milligrams
Copper	.41 milligrams
Manganese	.18 milligrams

Pulse

By J. I. Rodale

A few months ago I completed the manuscript of a 64 page book called *This Pace is not Killing Us.* It is based on a series of articles by the same title that appeared in *Prevention,* but with much additional data. The main contention of the book is that not only are we *not* traveling at a faster pace, but that it is not the pace that kills. In fact, I showed that the reverse was true. Most heart cases die because of a killing inactivity. Their hearts cannot take such indolence.

When the book was completed I realized that I was the worst offender in regard to what I had written. I was the most typical example of the sendentary businessman that I had been so loudly censuring. Being over 50, and a heart case, I can now see from what I have learned about the evils of inactivity, that unless I change my way of life I am in for consequences. Only ten months ago I was turned down for life insurance. When I walk upgrade there comes a feeling of pressure in the chest region. It is difficult to pin down the exact nature of my condition. The doctors seem to be vague about it. One of them called it coronary sclerosis.

So there I was, the author of a book proclaiming that lack of movement is a cause of heart disease while I kept sitting in cushioned comfort. This will never do, I said. After all, even in the irresponsibilities and impracticalities of authorship there is a limit! To regain my self-esteem I would have to take a dose of my own medicine.

So I began to walk—ten minutes the first few days, then fifteen and in about a week I was doing a full hour every morning, covering about two or three miles—briskly. One day, as I heard my heart pounding, I decided to stop and take my pulse. To my surprise I found it to be 112. At rest it was usually between 76 and 80. Walking, therefore, had upped it about 35 beats a minute.

Thinking that danger might be concealed somewhere in this fact, I decided from this point on to keep a record of my pulse during these walks. I did it scientifically, that is, I took it eleven times each day during the hour, at exact predetermined spots, so that the comparative daily record would mean something. Each day I added up the eleven figures and divided by eleven. Here are the average daily pulse results for the seven weeks of record keeping:

Date	Pulse	Date	Pulse	Date	Pulse
July 12	95.6	July 29	87.0	Aug. 15	86.0
July 13	101.0	July 30	89.8	Aug. 16	86.3
July 14	97.5	July 31	92.3	Aug. 17	84.8
July 15	98.5	Aug. 1	95.5	Aug. 18	91.4
July 16	94.1	Aug. 2	95.1	Aug. 19	90.7
July 17	94.8	Aug. 3	....	Aug. 20	96.7
July 18	96.1	Aug. 4	95.2	Aug. 21	90.0
July 19	96.7	Aug. 5	94.5	Aug. 22	85.4
July 20	97.7	Aug. 6	93.1	Aug. 23	83.6
July 21	96.1	Aug. 7	90.9	Aug. 24	85.1
July 22	96.3	Aug. 8	87.4	Aug. 25	....
July 23	93.3	Aug. 9	....	Aug. 26	83.4
July 24	93.6	Aug. 10	87.3	Aug. 27	84.7
July 25	94.4	Aug. 11	86.7	Aug. 28	82.7
July 26	....	Aug. 12	87.5	Aug. 29	81.3
July 27	93.8	Aug. 13	....	Aug. 30	80.7
July 28	94.4	Aug. 14	86.6		

For those who do not like to analyze figures, I have made a chart. Note the remarkable reduction in the last few readings. To me this is nothing short of miraculous. After only six weeks, I can walk an hour with my pulse about ten beats per minute less than its high at the beginning of this period. I am also certain that as more time elapses, there will be much more improvement. I will be able to subject my heart to this hour of exercise with a much lower rise in its pulse action.

I can also say that after the second week I began to finish off the walk with a wonderful feeling of euphoria, with no pounding of the

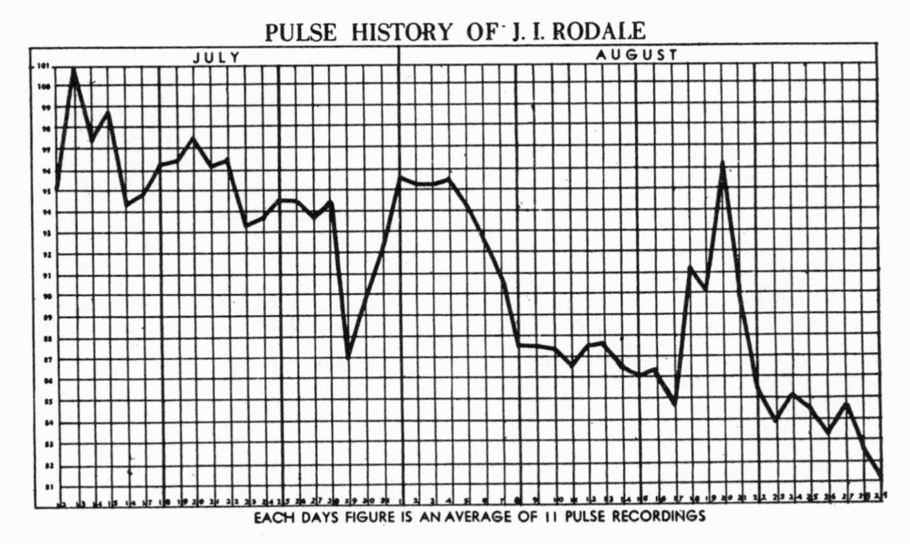

PULSE HISTORY OF J. I. RODALE

EACH DAYS FIGURE IS AN AVERAGE OF 11 PULSE RECORDINGS

heart. I would feel thoroughly relaxed with no suffering of fatigue or exhaustion.

A word about the method of taking my pulse. When I stop, I wait about twenty seconds, and then count the beats of my heart as I note the ticking off of 30 seconds by the watch. I then take the count of the next 30 seconds and that is the one I record. This, of course is then multiplied by two. It is best to plan a walking course which has a few up-grades in it. I stop for a rest of about a half minute to a minute half way between each pulse recording stop, thus making about 20 stops in all. However, if I experience any pressure symptoms I will stop for a moment wherever necessary. Remember, I am still a heart case.

The most unusual thing of all is that in the last six days my chest pressure symptoms have all but disappeared. For the first five weeks or so I continued to experience these symptoms—more on some days, and less on others, but I felt them only in the first 15 minutes of walking, as this part of the walk contains several up-grades. After this first quarter of an hour I could make the other hills with rarely a pressure pain. Evidently by this time the body had become thoroughly oxygenated, and the physical exercise had caused the blood to flow more vigorously through the coronary arteries.

But, in the last six days there have been practically no pressure symptoms even during the first 15 minutes, and you can imagine how I feel about it. It will be sensational if this keeps up. If I never again experience the pressure pains on movement of any kind, it would be stupendous! And, of course, it would add to my life. Is it possible that I will be absolutely cured? I cannot believe it, but will continue with this experiment. As long as I am physically able, and the elements permit, I will walk my brisk hour and more every day.

It is interesting to study the chart and to note the successive waves, each one going lower than its predecessor. With regard to the sudden leap upwards of August 18, 19, 20, I have a theory. In order to explain it, may I say that during all these walks I found no direct relationship between the experiencing of a chest pressure symptom and the pulse at that moment. I could have a low pulse when there was a chest pain, and a high pulse when there was none, or vice versa. Now, it was beginning with the morning of August 17, the start of the period of the banishment of heart pressure symptoms, that my pulse suddenly began to shoot upwards. For three days it kept leaping. This set me to wondering. What could be the reason for it? I have come up with a possible explanation, although I know that it is rank theory. But it is worth while talking about it.

As my walks progressed, from day to day, there occurred a reduction in the pulse, and a development gradually of a sense of well-being towards the end of each walk. This indicated possibly that the flabbiness of the heart was turning into muscle. But there was still something wrong either with the heart, or the arteries leading in and out of it, that gave me the pains during the first fifteen minutes of walking each day. Then these practically disappeared, and at the same time there was a sizable increase in the pulse. Does this indicate a second step in the rebuilding process? Have the heart muscles become so strong that they can do some function that they could not do before? Have they been able to close some kind of gap? Have they engaged in some additional physical building of something in the heart, an action which required the help of the whole heart to pump more blood for its accomplishment? Such a project would definitely raise the pulse.

Then the thing is done. The heart goes back to its previous pace. It goes down as precipitately as it went up. Is this fantastic reasoning? Perhaps. But it will have to do until someone works out a better reason. Perhaps it was not the heart alone. Is it possible that my lungs were strengthening themselves, being able to perform more efficiently so as to give more oxygen to the heart with less physical action of taking breaths? Is it possible that on August 17th something physical happened with regard to my lungs, something that knitted together, something in which the heart had to take part by furnishing more blood for the building?

It is interesting to be aware that when a man-made machine has to be fixed it must stop working and outside forces do the job. But the heart performs the job of reconstruction itself and at the same time it pumps blood to the rest of the organs of the body.

One more observation. Beginning a few days ago, I noticed that the pulse during the second half minute of its taking goes down more than it used to. Before this, the pulse in the second period would be almost as high as that of the first. It indicates a newly acquired ability of the heart to snap back to normal after exertion. Another thing. I note that I breathe better while working at my desk.

I also wish to say that I can recommend the taking of vitamin E, based on a four year detailed study of conservative medical researches regarding it. If you are interested, read *Alpha Tocopherol (Vitamin E) in Cardiovascular Disease,* by Drs. W. E. Shute and E. V. Shute, Ryerson Press, Toronto, Canada, $7.00. This is a scientifically documented book of 236 pages which proves conclusively that vitamin E is a specific for practically all heart cases. Like exercise it oxygenates the tissues, and I have taken this vitamin in big doses for over ten years. The trouble with the average heart case no doubt is a stagnation within the body, a lack of circulating oxygen, due to a sedentary life.

During my daily walk, I perspire profusely. Perspiration is one means the body employs to get rid of toxins, or poisons. Is it possible that such poisons, remaining in the body because of a sedentary daily regimen, make the heart work harder to rid the body of them through other means and channels?

Is it also possible that these toxins by remaining in the body and distorting the blood chemistry on a permanent, continuing basis, further interfere with various internal processes, which throw additional strain onto the heart, thus forcing it to pump more rapidly in an attempt to reduce the condition?

There must be a reason why my pulse is going down and I choose to think that a good sweat-out each day is part of it. By the sweat of thy brow shalt thou earn thy daily bread. Is this why farm workers are far less subject to heart disease than office-inhabiting men? Of course they exercise more, but I think it is the combination of the two. Exercise breaks down old cells, causing new ones to form. It gives rise to an increase in the blood-flow. Breathing is extended, and body functions stimulated. Muscles are kept in good repair, and their "tone" improved. There is a great improvement in the coordination of muscles and nerves. The circulation and elimination processes of the body are stimulated.

The late Dr. Raymond Pearl, of Johns Hopkins University, who studied the pulse records of thousands of individuals who died young, found that on the average their pulse rates were higher than normal. In the *Journal of the American Medical Association* of August 7, 1954, (Drs. Hammond & Horn) appears the following: "A Study Conducted by the Society of Actuaries revealed that, among persons with a high pulse rate, the number of deaths from cancer was about 60 per cent above the expected amount."

If you want to see an example of a heart shouting for help, examine my pulse readings for July 12, 13 and 14. A few weeks later I am able to do the same walk without the pulse once going over 100. It now looks as if it will be kept below 90 within a week or two. An hour a day of walking exercise must be a remarkable tonic to the body. I believe it is better than playing golf once or twice a week.

I was surprised, on August 1, 1954, to read in the Sunday *New York Times* magazine section that Roger Bannister, who recently broke the one-mile running record, was able to do so by a method he used of reducing his pulse. "By making his heart a more muscular pump, he was able to reduce his pulse beat from its original 72 in repose to below 50," says this magazine.

By making his heart a more muscular pump! That must be what I am doing to mine.

Incidentally, my doctor, who examines my heart action and blood pressure once and sometimes twice a week, is quite satisfied with what he observes. Action is definitely improved, and my heart murmur is all but eliminated. Blood pressure which, when I began was about 135/85, recently came down to 120/70, a figure which is well nigh perfect for any age, and which I never had before that I can remember.

Not every heart case will be permitted to do what I have done. The physician must be the judge. Mine may be the ideal form of heart disease for this method of treatment. But there are more serious cases, and I would urge extreme caution. There are leaking hearts and oversized hearts. There are hearts damaged in various ways, and some that have had thrombosis, or blood clots. These people must depend on their physicians for guidance. I will say, however, that many individuals who have been suffering from a variety of heart ills and who have been immobilized, should have been set moving and walking as soon as possible. I further believe that vitamin E can be a great insurance against a heart attack during these walks, but within the medical profession this is a subject of violent controversy. Why? I cannot understand.

What I have thus far done for my heart has two implications—one, I have built up the heart muscle: that is, improved the heart itself. Two, I have induced a condition in which the body can exercise with less effort, with less pumping on the part of the heart. Note also, in the extended tables, that the first reading which is the pulse at rest at home before starting on the daily walk, has gone down considerably. Eventually, this walking may greatly reduce my "at rest" pulse. The other day I ran after a bus and was able to do it with the greatest of ease. There was no aftermath of pounding, nor the feeling that I might get a heart attack.

One more thing about the pulse: What we eat affects it. Dr. Coca of Oradell, N. J. has worked out a whole science about it, and a few years ago, following his ideas and checking the effect of each food individually on my pulse, I discovered six that were causing my heart to pump more whenever they entered my stomach. By eliminating them I was able to get my pulse at repose from about 86 to 76. By combining both methods, that is, diet as well as exercise, phenomenal reductions in the pulse rate could be brought about.

A few days ago I made a startling observation. My first heart symptoms had appeared in 1937, but it was in 1949 that they became really temperamental and troublesome. It was then that I increased my vitamin E dosage astronomically in order to relieve the chest pressure symptoms. I now know the reason why. A friend and I used to go on hikes, sometimes for eight or nine miles. It was in 1949 that he moved to Philadelphia and from then on I fell into a most sedentary routine—no long walks; and my heart rebelled.

I was told recently of a man who for forty years was a track-walker for a railroad. For eight hours each day he walked the tracks to check for imperfections. A few years ago he retired and said, "Now I will rest." He then sat on his porch all day long. He was a healthy man, but within a year they laid him away to eternal rest. He had a heart attack. His heart could not stand the killing inactivity.

I look forward to these daily walking periods. It has become a time for thinking. One day when it rained and I could not walk I felt depressed about it all day, so that on a later day of inclement weather I went for my walk with an umbrella. It was a little difficult taking my pulse and holding the umbrella at the same time, but the actual readings were lower than for the previous day.

Food and the Pulse

About a year ago, I purchased a book called *Familial Nonreaginic Food-Allergy* written by Arthur F. Coca, M. D. which was published by Charles C. Thomas Co. of Springfield, Illinois It is an extremely technical piece of work and is not suggested for the average layman. It describes a method of reducing the pulse by eliminating foods to which a person is allergic. However, it does not do it by the usual needle-skin-scratch system. With the method outlined I was able to reduce my pulse from about 86 to about 76.

In following the system you choose a time about an hour and a half after you have eaten and eat a small portion of one food that you wish to test, taking your pulse immediately before the test. You then take your pulse a half hour later, and again a half hour after that, recording the figures in a ruled blank book, with the date, time etc., and leaving room for a list of the food eaten, and other comments. It will become a valuable record for later study. If the figures are kept on pieces of paper, it is easy for them to get lost.

It is best to take your pulse-reading at the wrist using the two fingers. Never use your thumb because it has its own pulse.

I found that the average food raised the pulse from three to five points per minute, although there were some that did not raise it at all, but that when a food caused the pulse to run up eight or nine points it was one of the allergy-causing ones. In my own case I had a high pulse, but no apparent allergies. Through years of study and analysis of my condition I was able to become so healthy that I no longer suffered from headaches or colds and my blood pressure had gone down more or less to near normal, but it still was worth while to reduce my pulse.

I discovered that figs, honeydew melon, whole wheat, and fried foods of any kind were the basic trouble-makers. It was absolutely fascinating running them down. For example, at first the indication showed that chicken raised my pulse unduly. But after I had accumulated sufficient records, showing in each case whether the chicken had been fried or broiled, I found that my pulse went up only when I ate fried chicken. I could eat broiled chicken without any trouble at all.

In the case of wheat, I made a rather thorough study. I found that whole wheat bread raised my pulse, but white bread did not. I could also eat wheat germ, which is present in whole wheat and not in white bread, without having the pulse go up. I therefore concluded that it was the bran that was difficult for my stomach to handle. This would indicate that, for me, the best kind of bread would be one with everything in it but the bran—a branless whole wheat bread. However, I found that I could eat raw wheat without raising the pulse.

French fried potatoes would send my pulse up, but not mashed or baked with the skins. It was the oil used in frying that I seemed to have a difficulty in handling. I could eat cantaloupe but not honeydew, and regarding figs, I used to eat them by the pound. No wonder my pulse had been around 85 and sometimes 95. (Note: A few weeks ago I checked my pulse again on figs and found that now I could eat them without raising it. It may indicate a gradual strengthening of the body.)

I found that coffee did not raise my pulse even a point, and was surprised. I am not a regular drinker of alcoholic beverages but, just to test, I drank some scotch and soda and beer, and was amazed to find that such drinks also kept the pulse down.

Regarding coffee, I discovered that the way we made it, in glass, it did not raise my pulse, but if boiled in an aluminum utensil it *did* raise it unduly. In this respect I would like to mention the fact that Dr. Coca, in the book which I have mentioned, cites the cases of six patients whose pulses were raised by eating foods cooked in aluminum pots. Coca says, "Vaughan in his *Practice of Allergy,* p. 831, mentions 'the cure of cases of long-standing refractory colitis following change from aluminum cooking utensils to enamel or glass vessels'."

Since there seems to be such a strong vegetarian movement and at times I have been tempted to try a vegetarian diet I made sure to observe carefully the effect of meats on my pulse. In no case were they unfavorable. In other words, in my stomach, meat is digested very easily. It is a known medical fact, incidentally, that meat does not have to be chewed much. It is the carbohydrates that need lots of work in the mouth. Bear in mind, however, that these idiosyncracies with regard to food vary with different persons. I may have an allergy to honeydew, for example, while you might eat it with impunity. So it is important that you check your own case thoroughly.

It is terrific in its implications when one considers what a reduction of the pulse actually means. In my own case the pulse was reduced by 15 points per minute. This means that every hour my pulse beat 60 x 15 or 900 times less. And in a full 24 hour day my heart had to expand and contract 900 x 24 less times or 21,600 less times a day. Merely by eliminating a few foods that I can easily get along without, my heart saves 43,200 movements in only one day. This is 21,600 expansions and 21,600 contractions. The heart actually moves between one and two inches each time in such expansion and contraction. Can you visualize this? Try and open and close your fist 21,600 times, moving it each time from one to two inches.

This means a saving of 15,768,000 movements a year for my little old heart. Is it any wonder that Dr. Raymond Pearl found that people who die young on the average have high pulses?

It certainly will pay everyone who reads this to check his or her pulse immediately, and if it is above 75 to try to discover what is raising it. In Coca's work he is able to bring patients' pulses down to as low as 65.

If you do decide to study your pulse, my suggestion is to note down the record of your pulse before and after each meal (½ hour and one hour after) for about one week so that you can have something to shoot at. After you have found the five or six offending foods that have been playing havoc with your pulse, you will note the effect of their elimination on the pulse recordings after full meals.

In my own case I had one extremely interesting experience which is worth telling. Several times, my pulse went up after a meal more than it should have according to what I ate, and after thinking about it I discovered that at those meals I had forgotten to take my vitamins. I then proceeded to check on it by alternately taking my vitamins and leaving them out after meals, and it worked every time. It would indicate that the vitamins I was taking were aiding my digestion. This also shows that it was best for me to take my vitamins at my meals. I checked the effect of each vitamin separately. Some worked and others did not. But bone meal worked every time in keeping the pulse down. It would be interesting to have readers experiment on this phase of pulse checking.

In his book Coca describes symptoms which disappeared by lowering the pulse, in conditions of migraine, fatigue, nervousness, indigestion, dizziness, constipation, neuralgia, canker sores, chronic rhinitis, heartburn, urticaria, epileptic seizures, overweight, psythic depression, asthma, and many others. It looks to me as if here we have a method that may revolutionize our entire conception of health and disease. Physicians should get a copy of Dr. Coca's work which is now in a new edition.

In Connection With the Heart

Shall we do away with labor-saving devices and the automobile? No! But let us keep moving as much as possible during our leisure hours. Let us form hiking groups for young and old.

Regarding vegetarians—many of them live long and I believe it is because they are generally health-conscious. A great many vegetarians are physical culturists, and know the value of exercise and walking. Witness the fantastic activities of Bernarr MacFadden who lived to be way above eighty.

I knew a vegetarian who lived to be 94. He would have lived to be 100 if he hadn't fallen out of a nut tree that he was pruning at the age of 92. He came to see me about five years ago and explained the value of his diet which was practically limited to fruits and nuts, but I believe it was his keeping on the move which was an important part of his formula for long living.

At the time of his visit to my farm he was 90 and spent most of his time prowling about the fields. He was more active than a barrel of monkeys, and if it had been pruning time, he would have "done" all our trees. I have to smile now when I recall him, but I was blind at the time, being an enemy to all forms of exercise. However, it is not too late.

Thus far I have stressed nutrition and physical movement. If we wish to live to be 90 or more I believe there should be added one more plank in the platform—something spiritual. Without it, not only would it be difficult to attain to a nonagenarian state, but you wouldn't want to. It would be boring. There must be a belief in the idealistic way, a tolerance toward your fellow man, a lightness of spirit, a strong belief in God and a sense of humor. Given nutrition, movement and spirit, there would be far less of disease and far more of life.

My final advice to all—keep moving, but stay out of trees after you are 90.

Pyorrhea

Would you be very much surprised to learn more teeth are lost because of pyorrhea than because of tooth decay? One authority (Don Mosher, D.D.S., in the *Military Surgeon* for April, 1942) tells us that more teeth are lost from the ravages of this disease than from all other sources combined. Pyorrhea has been known by physicians since the days of Hippocrates—(the Fifth Century B. C.). The Egyptians, the Greeks, the Romans and the early Chinese suffered from pyorrhea, judging from descriptions of the disease in their medical literature.

Dr. Mosher goes on to tell us that the beginning of pyorrhea can be detected five years before it becomes serious—by the use of X-ray. The disease resembles tuberculosis in that it progresses very slowly, giving no warning by pain or discomfort. Normal gum and mouth tissues are light pink, firm and in firm contact with teeth, all spaces between teeth being neatly filled in with gum tissue. Pyorrhea might be defined as chronic gingivitis or gum disease. In pyorrhea the gums are swollen and red, they bleed easily and are tender to the touch. As the disease progresses, the gum tissues detach themselves gradually from the teeth, the gums become thick, hard and leathery and eventually the bony foundation of the tooth roots is destroyed, the teeth become loose and must be extracted. Tooth decay is a disease of youth, claiming the majority of its victims among teen-agers. Pyorrhea is a disease of middle age and old age, which leads us to believe, of course, that it is a degenerative disease and hence that it *can* be prevented.

Very often pyorrhea is not accompanied by tooth decay. It can occur in mouths which have been carefully tended from the point of view of hygiene. Sorry, but we can't go along with the toothbrush and dentifrice ads that hold out hope for the "four out of five" that have "pink toothbrush." Apparently there are mechanical reasons for some cases of pyorrhea. Chewing always on one side of the mouth can bring it on. Malocclusion (and most of us suffer from some degree of malocclusion) can produce pyorrhea, because the stresses and strains of chewing can work havoc with teeth and gums alike when teeth are not arranged in the proper pattern to share these stresses. Excessive tartar can cause pyorrhea by accumulating along the gums and irritating them until pus pockets are formed. Yet we are acquainted with people who take meticulous care of their mouths, brushing their teeth carefully after each meal and these folks still have excessive tartar on their teeth. Hence they are likely candidates for pyorrhea. Periodontists have developed many treatments for dealing with gum disorders caused by malocclusion, such as filing off any teeth which may be out of line just enough to throw the rest of the teeth "out of occlusion."

There are other gum diseases, among them Vincent's Disease or Trench Mouth (so-called because during World War I it was common among soldiers). Trench mouth begins with a germ that may be passed from person to person on cutlery or dishes. It results in ulcers of the gums, mouth and throat, which are extremely painful and pus-laden. The business of curing it may take weeks or even months for, if the victim is to go on eating, it is impossible to keep the inside of his mouth sterile.

Readers will remember that in many articles on vitamin C we have described the deficiency disease of scurvy in which gums are affected and teeth loosen. It seems likely to suppose that scurvy may be related to pyorrhea, so far as the mouth symptoms are concerned. We hope to show that this is indeed the case.

In spite of all the wonders of modern medicine, tooth decay, which affects almost everyone in civilized countries is still a mystery. We do not know what causes it. Some scientists claim that it is caused by the acid formed when carbohydrates are eaten, some say it is the result of refining foods so that we do not have as much chewing to do as our ancestors had, some say it results from lack of calcium and other minerals, some persist in affirming that brushing teeth faithfully will arrest tooth decay. Pyorrhea presents us, we believe. with a much easier problem to solve and we are convinced we know how pyorrhea can be prevented. If you have pyorrhea already, your dentist is probably giving you treatments. You should by all means continue with these treatments. But this does not prevent you from undertaking a health program of your own which may make the dentist's treatments unnecessary! Look at the evidence we have assembled on preventing pyorrhea and judge for yourself.

Vitamin A Is Important

J. A. Sinclair, D.D.S., in an article in the *Journal of the American Dental Association* for October, 1939, tells us "Experiments conducted by May Mellanby showed that pyorrhea develops readily in dogs on diets deficient in Vitamin A, while on similar diets with this vitamin added the gums remain normal. 'The fact that nerves are affected by a vitamin A deficient diet' she writes, 'suggests that possibly diseases of the gums develop in the first place as the result of loss of neurotrophic control (that is, the control of the relationship between nerves and nutrition) and later lead to pyorrhea'." Dr. Sinclair reminds us that just getting enough vitamin A in the diet is not enough. We must be sure, too, that the vitamin is being absorbed and properly used. In cases of digestive and liver trouble, vitamin A may not be assimilated. In youngsters who are growing fast, more vitamin A is needed. In patients with severe infections, vitamin A is used up so rapidly by body tissues that there is never enough left for ordinary functions.

Paul E. Boyle, D.M.D., Otto Bessey, Ph.D., and Burt Wolbach, M.D., writing in the November, 1937, issue of the *Journal of the American Dental Association,* tell us that "experimental rickets and vitamin A deficiency in laboratory animals have been shown to affect the peridental (gum) structures," although they believe that these disorders are not similar to human gum disease. J. D. King, Ph.D., D.P.D., L.D.S., in the *Medical Journal of Malaya,* December, 1946, has this to say about vitamin A and pyorrhea: "As regards the use of vitamin A in the prevention and treatment of human peridental (gum) disease, little reliable information is available. On the basis of the animal investigation, however, we should be well advised to insist on a liberal supply of this food factor in the dietary of the expectant and lactating mother and of her offspring at least up to puberty, in order to insure that the gum epithelium and alveolar bone are properly formed."

Vitamin B and Pyorrhea

The relation of vitamin B to healthy gums is discussed at length by Dr. Sinclair who reminds us that Vincent's Disease occurs often among people afflicted with pellagra—a vitamin B deficiency disease. He describes cases in which the redness and soreness disappeared almost miraculously within a day after the pellagra patient was given niacin—the B vitamin most concerned in pellagra. He also tells us that a gangrenous condition of the gums was produced in monkeys on a diet deficient in vitamin B. And once again, he mentions that it is not enough just to get ample vitamin B in the diet—there are times when a great deal more is needed. Certain patients who preoperatively showed few or no signs of vitamin deficiency developed deficiency following operation. Fever increases the vitamin B need and in an individual whose vitamin intake has for any reason been impaired prior to operation, fever occurring postoperatively may result in a very rapid development of deficiency, particularly if the intake of food is inadequate during this time. Patients with achlorhydria (lack of hydrochloric acid in the stomach) show evidence of deficiency even when the dietary intake is adequate.

Dr. Sinclair tells us, too, that sensitivity of teeth and gums to thermal changes and to instruments seems to depend entirely on their supply of vitamin B. Time and again, he says, patients who could not drink hot or cold liquids and suffered anguish at the touch of a dental instrument were relieved of all these symptoms by a large dose of vitamin B. He has found that in every case of Vincent's Disease and pyorrhea, his patients who were treated with vitamin A, B and C responded well.

Dr. King has personally treated 500 patients with Vincent's Disease, using niacin (one of the B vitamins) which, he says, seems to restore some link in the chain of tissue respiration. He once gave himself Vincent's Disease so that he might observe it first-hand. And he came to the conclusion, he says, that "the condition is likely to occur only in persons whose general resistance is depressed by defective nutrition or other illness." . . . We were glad to find, too, that Dr. King agrees with us as to *how* one should take vitamin B. . . . "One important point of agreement appears to be that in many animals the sum of the known vitamin B_2 components in their synthetic state is by no means as effective as the whole complex in the form of less artificial products, such as yeast and liver preparations." If you are not getting enough vitamins in your daily meals, take natural food supplements in which these vitamins are concentrated—but don't take synthetic vitamins!

Relation of Vitamin C to Pyorrhea

It seems to us that any researcher seeking to prevent or cure pyorrhea would think first of vitamin C, because of the serious gum disease that accompanies scurvy. And so we find that a great deal of constructive work has been done along these lines. We know for instance that pyorrhea is almost universal in Newfoundland and is accompanied with heavy deposits of tooth tartar. The diet of Newfoundland is remarkably lacking in fresh fruits and vegetables which, of course, contain vitamin C. In the British West Indies, on the other hand, where vitamin C-rich fruits are eaten in great quantity the year 'round, there is little or no pyorrhea.

Dr. Sinclair reminds us that vitamin C deficiency destroys the body's ability to rebuild tissues and fibers such as the tissues of the gums. He tells us that he completely cured two patients of pyorrhea by giving them 150 milligrams of vitamin C daily for 30 days. Dr. Boyle tells us that among 66 patients examined at the Harvard Dental School, more than half had far less vitamin C than normal in their blood. And all of these patients had marked disease of the gums. "Ten of these patients in the low level range were given pure vitamin C by mouth and showed clinical improvement in the periodontal structures coincidental with increase in the blood ascorbic acid (vitamin C)."

In another *Dental Association Journal* article (October 1, 1944) J. S. Restarski, M.D.S., D.D.S., and M. Pijoan describe an experiment in which they induced scurvy in six volunteers. The diet was complete in every way except that it lacked vitamin C. Within five or six months, these subjects showed the classical signs of scurvy—hemorrhage, fatigue, etc.—but did not seem to have any gum disorders. From this Dr. Restarski and M. Pijoan conclude that, while gum diseases might have developed if they had been left on the diet longer, a lack of vitamin C cannot be taken as one of the causes of pyorrhea. Of course we differ in this conclusion. Let us relate one more experiment and then we'll tell you why we disagree.

C. D. Marshall Day, Ph.D., D.M.D. and K. L. Shourie, M.B., B.S., describe in the *Indian Journal of Medical Research* an experiment at an orphanage in India. All the children were on the regular orphanage diet—high in cereals and low in fruits and vegetables. Many of the children suffered from gingivitis and tooth tartar. Fifty of them were given 100 milligrams of vitamin C per day for 100 days in addition to the regular diet, while 50 others who acted as controls, ate the regular diet with no added vitamin C. The results were disappointing, say Drs. Day and Shourie. There was some slight improvement in the children taking the vitamin C, but not enough to make much difference.

What is your own conclusion? Do these two experiments prove that vitamin C is not important in preventing pyorrhea? To us they prove exactly the opposite—vitamin C is vitally concerned in the prevention of pyorrhea, *but*—pyorrhea is a disease of several deficiencies, not just vitamin C! The volunteers who gave themselves scurvy did not get pyorrhea because their diet contained ample vitamin B and A and other important factors. The Indian children were already eating a diet so low in vitamins A, B and C that the mere addition of one of these—vitamin C—could not stop the disease. On the other hand, Dr. Sinclair brought about astounding cures by giving his patients large doses of all three vitamins! And mark that fact well—Dr. Sinclair did not just tell his patients to eat a well-rounded diet and let it go at that. He took for granted that they were simply not getting enough of these three important vitamins in their diet and he gave them *large doses* of all three vitamins.

Minerals Are Involved Too

Other researchers have turned up valuable material concerning mineral deficiency and pyorrhea. First Lieutenant William A. Musgrave, D.D.S., writing in *The Military Surgeon* for February, 1941, tells us that the calcium-phosphorus balance is an important consideration in pyorrhea patients. Testing his patients for the amount of calcium and phosphorus in their blood, he found that by far the largest number of those with pyorrhea had a high phosphorus—low calcium ratio. That is, their diets contained far too much phosphorus in relation to the amount of calcium they obtained. Meat and cereals are high in phosphorus. Milk and green leafy vegetables contain calcium, so it is not surprising to find many American soldiers with their calcium-phosphorus balance upside down.

Dr. Musgrave found congested, bleeding gums, soft tissue pocket formation and excessive tartar deposits above and below the gums. "The high phosphorus pulls the calcium out of the body with loss of bone density" says he, "if the calcium leaves the body by way of the saliva, heavy salivary and serumal (serum) deposits are found on the teeth. If the calcium is lost by way of the urine, the saliva may be so low in calcium that erosion or gingival caries may result with very little tartar found." He advises diets with meat and eggs six times per week, whole grain cereals, very little candy or sweets, one raw salad per day, one or two non-starchy cooked vegetables per day, raw fruits for dessert, plenty of cheese and butter, and one or two glasses of raw fruit or vegetable juices per day.

Allison G. James, D.D.S., of Beverly Hills, writing in the *Annals of Western Medicine and Surgery,* September, 1947, states "With the understanding that nutrition is the process by which growth is promoted and health maintained, and that disease represents disturbed nutrition of the cells, part or organism affected, dental pathologic lesions receive a more logical consideration than is possible from the mechanistic point of view." Dr. James believes that the inclusion of refined foods and sugars in our diet is responsible not only for pyorrhea but also for tooth decay. Here are the conclusions he comes to: "1. Inclusion of a proportion of refined grain and sugar products in the diet beyond the tolerance of the patient appears as the chief causative factoı in dental caries and peridentosis (gum disorders). 2. Proportionately as the phosphorus intake increases beyond the one and one-half ratio to calcium, the vertical atrophy (disease) of peridentosis increases. 3. For prevention and control of dental disease, diets of 2000 calories may not safely be diluted by refined grains and sugar products."

In conclusion we want to quote from a most encouraging and sensible article by Anna P. Boudin, D.D.S., which appeared in the *Medical Woman's Journal* for April, 1943. It is especially gratifying to know that this article was written ten years ago when vitamin research had not progressed nearly to the point where it is today. Yet Dr. Boudin courageously lays the entire blame for tooth and gum disease right where it belongs—in faulty nutrition. She describes an experimental study in which four groups of monkeys were maintained on different diets. The first group ate a regulation laboratory diet, supplemented with *all the vitamins.* They showed no gum disease, even though the germs of gum disease were found in their mouths. Their good nutrition enabled them to withstand these germs. The second group had a diet deficient in vitamin C, with added supplements of vitamins A and D. They all developed diseases of the mouth and lost their teeth. The third group was given a diet deficient in vitamin C plus supplements of vitamins A and D and several of the B vitamins. They developed "slight to moderate" diseases and all showed a definite increase in the number of germs present. The fourth group was given a diet deficient in one of the B vitamins, but with plenty of vitamins A, C, D and other members of the B group. Fifty-four per cent of them developed gingivitis in addition to anemia, loss of appetite, weakness and diarrhea. Germs from the mouths of diseased animals were transferred to the mouths of the first group on the full diet with all the vitamin supplements. These well-nourished animals did not become diseased and the injected areas healed promptly.

Dr. Boudin says, "It has been found that a diet completely lacking in vitamin C produces extensive gingivitis (in guinea pigs, monkeys and man). However, vitamin C therapy alone failed to produce a cure. Generally, when the vitamin C intake is low, multiple deficiency may be present. Therefore, each patient suspected of vitamin C deficiency should be studied from all aspects."

It seems to us that any reasonable person, studying the evidence we have presented, can come to only one conclusion—pyorrhea is indeed a deficiency disease—not a disease involving deficiency of one food element but many. So, if you wish to prevent pyorrhea as you grow older—and remember it destroys more teeth than all other causes put together—do not decide to do it by taking one food supplement alone. That won't work. Vitamins A and D are contained in fish liver oil. All the B vitamins are in brewer's yeast and desiccated liver. Vitamin C is most abundant in rose hips and other natural vitamin C supplements. The proper ratio of calcium and phosphorus is found in bone meal, along with other important minerals. You can't get along without *all* of them. And by taking just one or just two of these supplements, you may be leaving out the very vitamin or mineral in which you are most deficient.

We repeat what we have said so many times in these pages: If you possibly can, get all your vitamins and minerals in your daily food. But because most of us eat some food that has been refined and denatured and hence is lacking in vitamins and minerals, we believe sincerely that most of us should take natural food supplements which will guarantee rich amounts of all the important food elements. Certainly, if you suspect that your gums are not as healthy as they might be—and remember pyorrhea progresses silently and without warning—be sure to supplement your meals with the food supplements we have mentioned above. Be one of the five out of five that can prevent pyorrhea, rather than one of the "four out of five" with "pink toothbrush."

Rice

Rice is an extremely important cereal from the point of view of humanity in general, for about one-half of the world's population considers rice as their basic food. In some countries it is eaten at every meal, almost to the exclusion of all other foods. So we must admit that rice has great value as a nourishing food, even though no nutritionist would advise eating it exclusively.

The best possible use that we, in western countries, can make of rice is to use it oftener than we do for the starchy part of a meal. If you're hesitating between rice or potatoes for dinner tonight, for instance, you should take into account what else your family has eaten during the course of the day. If cereal for breakfast and several slices of bread per meal are the rule in your household, then potatoes would be a better choice, for rice is a cereal and has the disadvantages as well as the advantages of other cereals. Like other cereals, it has an acid reaction in the body's metabolism, whereas potatoes, being a vegetable, have an alkaline reaction. On the other hand, if you're hesitating between noodles, macaroni or spaghetti versus rice, your choice should be rice. Products like noodles, macaroni and so on contain little real nourishment if they are made from white flour which all commercially-prepared products are. On the other hand, rice—brown rice, that is—contains all the original nutriments of the grain.

The chief crimes committed against rice in the name of civilization are those same ones we commit against wheat when we mill it. The original brown rice, as it comes from the rice plant, contains protein, starch, fat, minerals and vitamins, chiefly in its bran, endosperm and germ. As brown rice is milled to make white or polished rice these important nutriments are changed for the worse. Milling results in a loss of about 10 per cent of the protein, 85 per cent of the fat and 70 per cent of the minerals. What happens to the vitamins is even more drastic. Brown rice contains approximately 2.93 milligrams of thiamin, .67 milligrams of riboflavin and 49.2 milligrams of niacin for every hundred grams. These are the major B vitamins. White rice contains only .60 milligrams of thiamin, .26 milligrams of riboflavin and 18.5 milligrams of niacin.

The milling of rice was the accidental cause of an important discovery in vitamin research more than 50 years ago, when a disease called beriberi first became widespread in oriental countries. Investigations showed in 1884 that milling and polishing the rice caused the disease by removing the B vitamins mentioned above. Since rice is the staple food in these countries there was no possibility of making up this loss in other foods, and beriberi, a disease which often proves fatal, became common. Reverting to brown rice completely cured and prevented the disease. Since all this has been known for half a century, you might wonder why we still sell white rice in stores. There is no logical answer to this question. Processors tell us that people won't buy brown rice because they've become accustomed to white, and we consider this answer an insult to the intelligence of the average American woman who simply does not know which foods are nutritious, but would gladly buy them if she did know. In the orient and in this country as well, we have resorted to "enrichment" of rice—that is, we first remove most of the vitamins and minerals from the rice to make it white, then we replace only a part of the vitamins and minerals by a synthetic process which leaves the rice still looking white.

This is how this process is accomplished. After the white, gleaming, polished rice has come from the mill it is coated with a "premix" of zein (a protein substance obtained from corn) and alcohol. Then iron pyrophosphate is added (to replace the natural iron just removed from the rice). Then the rice is dipped into the mix again and a synthetic vitamin is added, and so forth. This "mix" has been so cleverly compounded that it is not affected by washing, cooking or storage. How it affects your stomach has probably not been studied. We don't know.

However, we do know that "enriched" rice does not contain the original substances put there by nature and we believe it is no improvement over white or polished rice.

You can obtain brown rice in most grocery stores these days. If your grocer does not have it, ask him to order it for you. Perhaps we can convince the food processors that we are more than eager to have nutritious food, regardless of color. Incidentally brown rice, after it is cooked, looks only a little darker than white rice. There is so little difference that your family or guests will never suspect that a wholly nutritious food is being served them in place of a dead, starchy mockery of food.

Wild rice is a rare delicacy. It is unrelated botanically to cultivated rice and grows in this country chiefly in Minnesota where it is harvested by the Indians of the Great Lakes region. Only about 350,000 to 500,000 pounds are for sale every year and the amount of labor involved in finding the rice and harvesting it make the price very high. If you can afford wild rice at about a dollar a pound you can be sure that you are getting the very finest and most nutritious food, for wild rice contains twice as much protein as white polished rice, four time as much phosphorus, eight times as much thiamin and twenty times as much riboflavin. And it has not been tampered with.

Here is the nutritional story on rice and of course we are speaking of brown rice. These are the minerals and vitamins contained in about ¾ cup of cooked brown rice:

Calcium	22 to 39	milligrams
Phosphorus	112 to 303	milligrams
Iron	1.6 to 5.5	milligrams
Copper	.36	milligrams
Magnesium	1.70	milligrams
B Vitamins:		
Thiamin	190	micrograms
Riboflavin	75	micrograms
Niacin	4.6	milligrams
Pantothenic acid	2200	micrograms (in the bran)

Rice Germ

The story of rice bran and rice polish is actually the story of how scientists first came to suspect the existence of the minute substances we now call vitamins. It was in 1883 that a Japanese naval officer, Baron Takaki, discovered something important about the disease that was the scourge of sailing men in the East—beriberi. The Baron declared that the disease was caused by the sailors' diets. He added other foods to their daily fare of polished rice and the disease was soon conquered.

Baron Takaki thought the answer was simply that the diet he prescribed contained more protein. It was up to other investigators to show that, although the protein was important and although polished rice was nearly entirely starch, still something else that existed in *unpolished* rice was necessary for human health.

A Dutch physician, Eijkman of Java, did some experimenting with pigeons. He could give the pigeons beriberi in a short time by feeding them polished rice. He could cure them by giving them unpolished rice. Three workers at the school of Tropical Medicine in Liverpool, England, found that laboratory animals got beriberi when they were fed exclusively on either polished rice or white bread. They recovered when they got whole grain bread or unpolished rice. So it appeared that there was some important substance in the unrefined grains that the refined ones did not contain.

Years later Casimir Funk named the substance a "vitamine"—a food element present in minute quantities which is absolutely necessary for human health. Today we know that the vitamin in rice polishings is thiamin, a B vitamin. It exists there along with the other vitamins of the B complex which are present in considerable amounts in unrefined grains of all kinds. Beriberi as such has been all but wiped out in civilized parts of the world where there is any knowledge of nutrition. But a slight deficiency in thiamin is still widespread, even in America, because most of our grain and cereal products are refined.

Why You Need More Thiamin if You Eat Refined Foods

As Mark Graubard says in his book *Man's Food, Its Rhyme or Reason* (Macmillan Company) "Nature apparently saw to it not to make life too easy for us. The amount of thiamin needed depends on the other items of our diet. Also, the higher the energy expenditure of the body the more thiamin is required. The more sugar or starch we consume, the more of that vitamin is needed. If we feed largely on protein or fat, for example, we need less thiamin to maintain our system in good shape. Thus, eating polished rice or white, unenriched bread or potatoes cooked in much water which is discarded, makes for quite a vicious circle. Not only is the thiamin thrown out or destroyed in the preparation but because these foods are all starches, the body requires more thiamin than normally."

Thiamin is needed for the body to digest starch. So as soon as you remove that vitamin from a starchy food (like grain) the food becomes a peril, for eating it can produce a dangerous deficiency in thiamin.

Rice is grown chiefly in the Orient and is staple food for more than half the world's population. After the rice is thrashed the "rough rice" consists of a kernel contained in a hull. When the hull is removed you find that the rice grain is made of a pericarp (the outer bran) and the seed, which includes the inner bran, the endosperm and the germ. In this state the rice is called "brown rice." When it is milled into polished rice the bran and germ are removed. Nothing but the pure starchy endosperm remains. This is white rice, or polished rice, such as you buy in the grocery store. This is the food that devastated eastern countries for many years before it was discovered that the milling and polishing of the rice had removed the necessary part of the cereal.

What Is Lost When Rice is Polished

When rice is converted to white rice about 10 per cent of the protein, 85 per cent of the fat and 70 per cent of the minerals are removed. Here is a chart showing how the B vitamins disappear during the refining process. It represents micrograms of the vitamin per gram:

	Thiamin	*Riboflavin*	*Niacin*
Rough rice	2.93	.67	49.2
Brown rice	3.02	.53	55.1
White rice	.60	.26	18.5
Pearling cone polishings	22.88	1.62	290.3
Brush polishings	20.95	1.34	368.0

The chart also makes perfectly clear just what happens to the B vitamins. As the rice is polished the bran and the germ are removed. These contain the vitamins, minerals and much of the protein. So it is easy to see that the fluffy white starchy grains we serve regularly at dinner contain none or practically none of the real food value of the rice. It has departed into the bran, germ and polishings.

It's very much the same story as what happens when wheat is refined. Here, too, by far the best part of the wheat is left in the wheat germ which was generally sold for cattle and stock food. That's what happens to the rice polishings, too. Except, of course, that some of those food faddists eventually came along and asked a very pertinent question. "Why," they asked "should we keep our cattle and pigs healthy by taking away the best part of the grain and feeding it to them, while our people get only the starch with none of the value left in it?" So they began to package wheat germ and rice germ and polishings and sell them as "health foods." Now actually, as you can see, they are not special "foods"—they are simply what originally was in the grain and then was removed. So they are really far more natural "foods" than white rice and white flour. And you can tell that to anybody who laughs at you as a food faddist for eating wheat germ or rice germ.

According to Marinus C. Kik of the Department of Agricultural Chemistry of the University of Arkansas, the nutritive value of wheat and corn germ has been well investigated. So, in an experiment reported in the November, 1954, issue of *Agricultural and Food Chemistry* he tested rice germ and compared it to the two other foods from the standpoint of nutrition. It rated high. For instance, its thiamin content is about twice as high as that of wheat or corn germ. It contains good protein, including ten of the amino acids which are essential for human beings to have in their food. We manufacture some of the amino acids (or blocks of protein) ourselves. The rest we must get from food. Rice germ has some of all of these.

Here is a table, according to Professor Kik, showing the vitamin and mineral content of rice germ:

B vitamins	
Thiamin	65 micrograms per gram
Riboflavin	5
Niacin	33
Pantothenic acid	30
Pyridoxine	16
Biotin	.58
PABA	1
Inositol	3725
Folic acid	4.3
Choline	3000
Calcium	.275%
Phosphorus	2.10
Iron	.013
Protein	14.93
Fat	11.52

What should all this mean to you in terms of your own daily meal planning? First of all, we hope you never serve your family white rice. Your grocery store probably sells brown rice. If not, they can surely order it for you. Your health food store probably sells rice germ or rice polishings.

Perhaps your family is already eating wheat germ. You might want to include rice germ or rice polishings along with the wheat germ, or alternate the two. We have demonstrated how vitally important it is for you and all the members of your family to get plenty of the B vitamins the rice products contain. If you are not taking brewer's yeast or desiccated liver, this is doubly important. Don't neglect them, especially if you eat any refined carbohydrates at all. By this we mean products made from white flour or anything that contains sugar, refined cereals (the kind you get at the grocery store) prepared or packaged "mixes" or any other processed food. The more of these you eat, the more B vitamins you need to be healthy.

Rose Hips

Most American books on nutrition ignore the rose hip as if it did not exist which seems to us a very short-sighted and wasteful point of view. What kind of a hue and cry would be raised if our nutrition books were to ignore the citrus industry as a source of vitamin C! The rafters would ring and the newspaper headlines would shout that the nutritionists had betrayed the people of America by not telling them of the wealth of vitamin C to be found in citrus fruits.

Yet the vitamin C in citrus fruits is inconsequential in comparison with the vitamin C in rose hips! And still the rose hips are allowed to rot and dry on the bushes year after year, eaten only by the birds and the woods animals, while our school children regularly show up in tests—deficient in vitamin C.

In England and all over Europe the value of rose hips for their vitamin C content is well-known. And we dare say that few rose hips go to waste there. According to *The Chemurgic Digest* for June 15, 1944, "even wild roses which thrive through the English countryside, have a vital war job. According to the *New York Times,* the British Information Services recently reported that these blooms, lately recognized as even richer natural sources of vitamin C than citrus fruits, were gathered extensively last year for nutritional purposes.

"The vitamin is extracted from the rose's flesh red fruit or seed case, which is ripe for picking late in the fall. In addition to vitamin C which protects against scurvy, the rose hips also contain some vitamin A and an unexpected amount of recently isolated vitamin P, it was stated.

"In 1943 a 500-ton harvest of rose hips was gathered commercially, according to the information service. This crop is reported to have equaled the vitamin C content of 250,000 oranges and was the source of 2,500,000 bottles of national rose hip syrup for children."

This shows you what a nation can do in an emergency when lack of fresh fruits cuts off the main supply of vitamin C in this island country. But why should we in America wait for an emergency? Why not make use—full use—now, today, of this wealth of vitamin-rich fruit that is free for the asking!

What Are Rose Hips and How Much Vitamin C Do They Contain?

Rose hips are the fruit of the rose bush, left after the flower has disappeared. Just like other fruits, the different kinds of roses produce a wide variety of hips. Some are small, some large. Rose hips grown in northern countries always contain more vitamin C than those grown farther south—as if nature were going out of her way to take special care of her creatures during cold weather. Your friends (unless they are from Europe) will probably laugh at your new enthusiasm for eating rose hips —but why not? Who decreed that we should eat apples, pears, and plums, but not rose hips? We have in our files notes from many countries in Europe where rose hip soup, jam, jelly and purée are used as freely as we use apple sauce and fruit salad.

The vitamin content of 100 grams rose hips is as follows:

Vitamin A	5 milligrams
Vitamin E	47 milligrams
Vitamin K	100 units
Vitamin C	500 to 6000 milligrams
Vitamin B_1	.10 milligrams
Vitamin B_2	.007 milligrams
Vitamin P	240 to 680 units

(The vitamin C content of one orange weighing 100 grams is about 50 milligrams.)

Rose hip preparations are difficult to prepare, for the elusive vitamin C is not easy to capture in powder forms. If you want to grow your own roses or if you have access to roses whose hips you can use, it is not advisable to try to dry them yourself. You lose so much vitamin C during the long process that drying the hips at home is very wasteful. The best idea is to make a puree of them which you can then use by the tablespoonful or can stir into fruit juices.

Here are two recipes for rose hip puree. The first comes from Adelle Davis' excellent cook book *Let's Cook it Right* (Published by Harcourt Brace and Company, 383 Madison Ave., New York, N. Y.). Says Miss Davis:

"Gather rose hips; chill. (This is to inactivate the enzymes which might otherwise cause a loss of vitamin C.) Remove blossom ends, stems and leaves; wash quickly. For each cup of rose hips bring to a boil 1½ cups of water. Add one cup of rose hips. Cover utensil and simmer 15 minutes. Let stand in a pottery utensil for 24 hours. Strain off the extract, bring to a rolling boil, add 2 tablespoons lemon juice for each pint, pour into jars and seal. (Remember, don't make the mistake of using copper or aluminum utensils when you are cooking rose hips.)"

The second recipe is much like this. It is from the *British Medical Journal* for May 29, 1954. (Of course we recommend omitting the sugar from this recipe.)

"Two pounds of hips are put through a coarse mincer, and at once placed in three pints of water which has been kept briskly boiling in readiness. The water is again brought to the boil, and the saucepan is then put aside to cook for 15 minutes. The water and hips are next poured into a jelly-bag made of flannel or linen, crushed, and allowed to drip until most of the fluid has come through. If the first drippings from the jelly-bag contain hairs from the insides of the hips they are put back into the bag. When the flow of fluid has ceased, the hips are returned to the saucepan and are stirred up with another 1½ pints of boiling water. After standing for 10 minutes, they are put back into the jelly-bag and more fluid is collected. The combined extracts are boiled down to a volume of 1½ pints and a final boiling of five minutes is given after the addition of ¼ pound of sugar. While still hot, the syrup is poured into small bottles, which must be hot and sterile. If they are sealed with corks, these should be boiled for a quarter of an hour just before use, and should be covered with melted paraffin wax.

"About two teaspoonfuls of the extract should supply the daily dose of vitamin C. The syrup should be stable if kept in full bottles in a cool darkened cupboard, but the vitamin deteriorates in a few weeks after the bottles have been opened and air admitted. Cooking utensils made of copper or uncovered iron should not be used for making the syrup, since these metals accelerate the destruction of vitamin C."

Where Can You Get Rose Hips to Grow?

Here is a list of roses high in vitamin C:

	Milligrams of Vitamin C per hundred grams of rose hips
Rosa Laxa	3000-4000
R. acicularis	1800-3500
R. cinnamomea	3000
R. rugosa	3000
R. Eddieii	2780
R. Moyesii	2383
R. arkansana	1300-2000
R. woodsii	1300-2000
R. nutkana	1200-1370
R. canina	711-1338

	Milligrams of Vitamin C per hundred grams of rose hips
R. mollis	1260
R. Sherardi	1260
R. nipponensis	1180
R. megalantha	694-1124
R. spaldingii	694-1124
R. cariifolia	1080
R. Afzeliana	1000
R. tomentosa	690
R. dumetorum	590
R. multiflora	250

Andrew Nursery, Faribault, Minnesota—Rosa rugosa.

Bobbink and Atkins, 588 Paterson Avenue, East Rutherford, N. J.—Rosa rugosa.

Farmer Seed and Nursery Co., Faribault, Minnesota—Rosa rugosa.

Henry Kohankie and Son, Painesville, Ohio—Rosa acicularis, rugosa, moyesii, eglanteris, canina, coriifolia, woodsii, multiflora.

Lester and Tillotsen Rose Gardens, Watsonville, California—Rosa rugosa magnifica, moyesii.

Manitoba Hardy Plant Nursery, Dropmore, Manitoba, Canada—Rosa laxa, acicularis, arkansana, cinnamomea, rugosa, canina.

F. W. Schumacher, 579 Center Street, Jamaica Plain, Massachusetts—Species roses.

Royal Jelly

For thousands of years honeybees have occupied a unique niche among all the living creatures that have come to live with man. Because of their intricate and fascinating community life, we human beings have always known that there was something special about bees—something not quite comprehensible to mere man. In all parts of the world in times past, and in many agricultural countries even today, the bees share in family celebrations. At Christmas and Easter, for weddings and funerals, special ceremonies must be performed near the beehives. If a disaster or a blessing befalls the family, the bees must be told, first of all.

It is not surprising that men have such reverence for these furious and conscientious little insects. Bees not only organize their community life along the strictest lines, not only do they work at unbelievable speeds and collect incredible amounts of food in the way of nectar and pollen, but they communicate with one another. They have their own system of mathematics, geometry and geography so well worked out that the bee who discovers a cache of honey can describe to the other members of the hive exactly where the honey is located, how much there is and what is the shortest and best route to take to get there. All these facts have been verified by scientists.

Recently another fabulous aspect of bee-life has been getting publicity—royal jelly, the food of the queen bee. We have been reading a lot about royal jelly, *Look* for October 19, 1954 carried a feature story on it. The New York Sunday *Mirror* for June 27, 1954, carried a syndicated feature story. *The News* from Sarasota, Florida for October 21, 1954, carried a front page story on a beekeeper there who shipped in 20 million bees, in the hope that he can produce royal jelly commercially. We have received clippings on royal jelly from state after state. And many letters from readers asking where they can buy this miracle food.

Apparently the answer is not at the corner store. For there is a peculiar problem involved in producing royal jelly which will invariably limit its usefulness so far as human consumption is concerned. Royal jelly is the food produced by the worker bees to feed the queen bee. A queen bee is both mother and ruler of an entire hive. During one season she may become the mother of as many as a quarter of a million bees. A queen bee has been known to lay more than 2000 eggs (more than her own weight) in a single day. Of the eggs she lays, the fertile ones may develop into either worker bees or queens. Their development depends entirely on their food. All the eggs are fed royal jelly for the first two or three days after hatching. But the egg destined to be a queen bee, and then the queen bee herself, receives royal jelly throughout her life. So it seems reasonable to assume that the food is solely responsible for the great difference between the queen bee and the workers, for no other circumstances of their growth are different, except for food.

Worker bees grow up in from 21 to 24 days. Queen bees mature in 16 days. Worker bees work furiously and live from two to six months. Queen bees, working just as hard at their egg laying, may live as long as eight years. What a powerful force of longevity and fertility must be contained in royal jelly!

But here is the catch to the whole thing. Worker bees feed royal jelly to create a queen only when they need a queen—that is when the old queen is dying or they have decided to get rid of her, or when, for some other mysterious reason of their own, they want a new queen. To produce royal jelly for experiments, scientists must first remove the reigning queen. The bees know at once that she is gone and they work desperately feeding royal jelly to several more larvae in order to produce a new queen. The experimenters again remove the royal jelly and the bees must frantically produce more.

As more and more royal jelly is removed it seems to us that the frenzy and frustration of the bee colony must become frightening. And which of us can predict what will be the final effect on the well-ordered life of the bee colony after this process has gone on for some time? Can we afford to endanger the whole structure of bee society and possibly do serious damage to the bees in order to procure for ourselves the marvelous royal jelly that has such potency so far as bees are concerned?

What Does Royal Jelly Contain?

Well, then, you might say, let us study the royal jelly, find out what it contains, and manufacture our own! Easier said than done. For royal jelly has so intrigued scientists of recent years that they have conducted extensive researches on it, without finding in it any substance that would explain its marvelous power. They have taken royal jelly apart until they know what all its ingredients are, they think. Then they put these ingredients together in the laboratory and what they get is not royal jelly at all! So apparently there are substances in the jelly with which we are not only unfamiliar, but whose presence we cannot even detect.

Melampy and Jones reported in the *Proceedings of the Society of Experimental Biology and Medicine,* volume 41, page 382, 1939, that they could detect no vitamin A in royal jelly. There was some vitamin B_1 (thiamin). Pearson and Burgin in the same magazine, volume 48, page 415, 1941, reported that royal jelly contains more pantothenic acid than any other known substance. Between 2½ and 6 times as much as yeast and liver. Pantothenic acid is another B vitamin.

Other investigators have reported little or no vitamin E in royal jelly, and no detectable amount of vitamin C. Thomas S. Gardner, writing in the *Journal of Gerontology* for January, 1948, tells of experiments involving fruit flies which were fed royal jelly. According to him, the pantothenic acid in royal jelly increased the life span of the flies. He goes on to say that no one knows as yet how much of the valuable B vitamin is needed by the average human being, but it has been estimated that we need about 11 to 15 milligrams a day. In the average American diet most of us obtain only about 5 milligrams a day. However, no one has done any research apparently to find out whether pantothenic acid, either in or out of royal jelly, will increase the life span of human beings.

We Welcome Scientific Material on Royal Jelly

And so the story goes. When we first began to collect clippings about royal jelly, we wrote to some ten or fifteen laboratories where, according to the clippings, research is in progress. None of them could give us any help. They referred us to the information we have given above, but without exception they told us that they know of no research involving human beings. We also wrote to all our advertisers who sell honey. More than anyone else, beekeepers are respectful when they speak of all the marvels of bee-life and community organization. And they are all sure that royal jelly must be a truly miraculous substance, for they see what happens in their beehives to those individual bees that feed on royal honey as compared with those which do not. But none of our beekeeper friends had heard of any research involving human beings. And most of them stated that royal jelly is not very tasty. It is a white milky paste with an acid flavor.

Rutin

One of the most recent subjects for investigation in cases of hypertension (high blood pressure) has been rutin—a substance found most plentifully in buckwheat. Rutin is a part of vitamin P. Apparently vitamin P, like the other vitamins has many parts called "flavones." All of them are more or less related and have many of the same properties so far as human health is concerned, but some parts appear to be more effective in the treatment of certain disorders.

High blood pressure brings with it certain dangers, not the least of which is hemorrhage—including cerebral hemorrhage which we speak of as a "stroke." In cases of stroke, the small blood vessels or capillaries rupture, due to the pressure upon them and the hemorrhaging of the blood from this ruptured vessel brings about the unconsciousness and other symptoms of stroke. Doctors sometimes refer to strokes as "cerebral accidents."

It would seem that more is involved in this rupturing of a blood vessel than just the pressure being put on it by the blood. Perhaps, researchers have reasoned, part of the fault may lie in the weakness of the actual walls of the blood vessels, or capillary fragility. Interest in rutin was aroused by the discovery that apparently it had a lot to do with maintaining the walls of the blood vessels so that they do not become fragile and hence are less likely to rupture and cause serious illness or death.

Immediately, a whole series of problems in research presented themselves. First of all, how can the fragility of the blood vessels be measured? It is relative to the blood pressure of course, and the higher the blood pressure goes, the more hardy the vessels must be not to rupture. In a patient suffering from stroke, one may assume that perhaps his blood vessels were indeed fragile, but how can one discover this *before* the accident takes place so that the patient can be treated for fragile blood vessels and so perhaps never have a stroke? The problem of measuring the fragility of blood vessels has never actually been solved satisfactorily and this is one reason for the doubt and confusion around the whole subject of rutin for high blood pressure patients.

Working with laboratory animals there are several methods of measuring fragility of capillaries and these have been used in experiments. H. K. Hellerstein, M.D. and his colleagues at several hospitals in Illinois and Ohio experimented by producing in animals blood pressure high enough to cause hemorrhaging from the blood vessels. To one group of animals they gave rutin ten days before inducing the high blood pressure. Another group received no rutin. As reported in *The American Heart Journal* for August, 1951, all of the animals died as a result of the high blood pressure but those which received rutin did not show any evidence of hemorrhaging as the other animals did.

Vitamin P For Hemorrhagic Disease and Cancer

It is well known that patients exposed to X-ray may hemorrhage, supposedly because the X-ray has affected the walls of the tiny blood vessels. John Q. Griffith, M.D., and James F. Cough, Ph.D., writing in the magazine *Blood,* for June, 1951, describe experiments in which they gave rutin to rats before they were exposed to X-ray. The rats which received the rutin did not hemorrhage, while those which did not receive rutin suffered the usual hemorrhagic disorders. Boris Sokoloff and his associates at the Florida Southern College in Lakeland, Florida, tested various vitamin P compounds on rats and found that the mortality from X-ray was reduced to 10 per cent in the group of rats receiving the vitamin P as against a mortality of 80 per cent in those rats which did not receive the vitamin. Say these authors, in commenting on their experiments in the *Journal of Clinical Investigation,* April, 1951, "capillary injury is by far the most frequent cause of clinical hemorrhagic disease," and this injury "may be due to infection, drugs, toxemia, allergy or nutritional disturbance." Increased capillary fragility appears to come, they say, from some defect in the intercellular cement—that is, the substance between the body cells which holds them together. They say, too, that vitamin P factors (rutin among them) appear to "affect the capillary system directly perhaps participating as a principal in the 'wear and tear' of a part or all of the capillary system, inhibiting its degeneration and taking part in its regeneration, specifically as far as the intercellular cement is concerned."

In another article in the *Archives of Pathology* for September, 1951, Dr. Sokoloff and his fellow-workers discuss the effect of vitamin P on experimental cancers. They note that many years ago researchers mentioned the possibility that the intercellular cement might be an important factor in the occurrence of cancer. In their experiment, they gave a vitamin P compound to animals with cancer and discovered that it had a moderate effect on the growths—that is, it decreased them. They also noted that the vitamin P had apparently no bad effects at all.

Bicknell and Prescott in their book, *Vitamins in Medicine* (Grune and Stratton, 1953) relate a number of experiments having to do with vitamin P in cases of high blood pressure. In one case rutin was given in a dose of 20 milligrams three times daily for periods up to four years. In seventy-five per cent of those tested, capillary fragility became normal. In the majority of cases the blood pressure was not reduced by the rutin. The authors are careful to point out that *rutin is not given to lower the blood pressure*. It is given to prevent accidents in which hemorrhages might occur in high blood pressure patients. In other words, it seems that rutin prevented the possibility of "stroke" in 75 per cent of these patients. It did not cure their high blood pressure.

Bicknell and Prescott give numerous other examples of vitamin P being used successfully in the treatment of cases involving hemorrhaging due to disease or due to drugs which the patient was taking for some disease. Hemorrhages due to drug poisoning, for instance, can be relieved by giving some vitamin P compounds.

Eye Disorders and Rutin

Rutin was also administered to a group of patients with glaucoma—the tragic eye disease in which the pressure inside the eyeball rises. Among 26 patients who received 20 milligrams of rutin three times a day, 17 noticed a fall in the pressure inside the eye, in four the results were not definite and five subjects noticed no change.

We found an extremely interesting article on the use of rutin in Ophthalmology by L. B. Somerville-Large in the *Transactions of the Ophthalmological Society of the United Kingdom*, volume 69, pages 615-617, 1949-1950. Dr. Somerville-Large states that "in the eye we have what appears to be the only opportunity the human body affords of actually observing lesions (disorders) associated with capillary dysfunction. We must, therefore, forgive our medical colleagues for their caution in recognizing the value of rutin." He goes on to tell us that the tiny blood vessels in the eye can be studied by the ophthalmologist. It is actually the only place in the body where blood vessels can be directly observed. These tiny capillaries in the eye are packed closely together and they have a wider "bore" than other capillaries in the body.

He says that the commonest conditions in which the capillaries seem to be out of order are diabetes, toxic and inflammatory conditions, high blood pressure and hardening of the arteries. Although hypertension (high blood pressure) of itself has no relation to capillary fragility, he says, six to ten per cent of those hypertensives who do have increased capillary fragility suffer from hemorrhages in the retina of the eye, and cerebral or brain hemorrhages. He gives doses of two sixty-milligram tablets of rutin three times a day making a total dosage of 360 milligrams daily. "I find," says he, "that the larger doses give a more rapid and more complete negative result to capillary fragility tests." Incidentally he always combines the rutin with 200 milligrams of vitamin C daily.

It is interesting to note that throughout the discussion of vitamin P and rutin in medical literature, it is suggested that vitamin P and vitamin C work closely together and better results are always obtained when they are given together. Note, too, that Dr. Somerville-Large gives quite a large dose of vitamin C—200 milligrams. At the present time the official recommendation for the minimum daily intake of vitamin C is only 70 milligrams and it is believed that most of us don't even get that much! Does it not seem reasonable that two or three times this amount of vitamin C every day might do a lot to prevent the capillary fragility which is responsible for so much distress today? Remember that vitamin C is also involved in keeping the intercellular membranes healthy.

In conclusion, Dr. Somerville-Large states that in his experience he has not yet "met a case in which the capillary fragility skin test has not been reduced with rutin to well within normal limits." In speaking of the length of time it is necessary to continue taking the rutin, he says, "To me at the present time it looks like a life sentence. Whenever rutin has been discontinued the capillary fragility has again increased. Also if the rutin is discontinued and the vitamin C alone persisted with, again the capillary fragility increases."

One last example of the use of rutin in treating capillary fragility. Bicknell and Prescott in *Vitamins in Medicine* tell of twelve children in a group of 100 allergic children who were treated with 100 to 150 milligrams of vitamin P daily for six months. At the end of this time their capillary resistance became normal.

How Much Vitamin P Are You Getting in Everyday Meals?

What application can we make of all these experiences to our daily life? First of all, if vitamin P (of which rutin is a part) is really a vitamin, how much of it do we perhaps need every day? The Federation of the American Societies for Experimental Biology have voted to discontinue the use of the term "vitamin" in relation to vitamin P. They declare that it has not been proved as yet that these substances (the flavones) are essential to good health and that their absence in diet will cause any disorder that can be cured by administering them. However, it is interesting to note that people in other countries, and this country as well, go right on calling the flavones "vitamin P." Bicknell and Prescott state that the daily requirement may be not less than 33 units daily "and possibly considerably more."

Just like vitamin C, vitamin P is destroyed by cooking in an open vessel. So, much of the vitamin P value of food is lost in cooking. Once again we are faced with the absolute necessity for eating plenty of fresh raw fruits and vegetables, for it is in these that vitamin P is found in the largest amounts, along with vitamin C. The rutin concentrate used by doctors in treating hypertensive patients is made from buckwheat. Rutin occurs chiefly in the leaves of buckwheat which may contain as much as seven or eight per cent of rutin. It is rapidly destroyed when the leaves are dried slowly, so they must be processed with the greatest care. After the leaves are completely dried, there seems to be no further loss of rutin.

If you are suffering from high blood pressure and your doctor advises taking rutin to avoid any possibility of a stroke, we would certainly go along with his advice, on the basis of the evidence we have collected. If you are perfectly healthy and interested in preserving the state of your blood vessels so that you will not suffer from these disorders later on, then by all means see that you get, every day, plenty of the foods in which vitamin P (hence rutin) occurs, along with vitamin C. Of course, we are always urging readers to get enough vitamin C, for we believe it to be one of the food elements most essential for good health. Now it appears that vitamin P, always associated with vitamin C in foods, may be of great value as well.

Here is a list of foods that are rich in vitamin P and we have given you their vitamin C content as well. We hope you notice that, just as rose hips are many, many times richer in vitamin C than any other food so too they are especially rich in vitamin P.

	Vitamin P Content in Units	*Vitamin C Content in Milligrams*
Apricots	75-100 in 8 apricots	4
Blackberry	60-100 in ¾ cup	3
Black currant	200-500 in 1 cup	150
Cabbage (summer)	100 in 1 cup, raw	50
Cherry, black	60-100 in 12 large cherries	12
Grape, black	500-1000 in 1 small bunch	3
Grape, white	500-1000 in 1 small bunch	4
Grapefruit	100 in ½ grapefruit	45
Lemon juice	450-750 in 8 tablespoons	25
Orange	300-500 in 1 medium orange	50
Parsley	130 in 1 cup	70
Plum	50-200 in 3 medium plums	5
Prune	300-400 in 8 medium prunes	4
Rose hips	240-680 in 100 grams	500 to 6000

Saccharin

We say a positive and unequivocal "no" to any and all sugar substitutes—that is, the various chemicals you can buy labeled saccharin, sucaryl, dulcin, sodium cyclamate and so forth. All these are many times sweeter than sugar. A small tablet of one of these chemicals dropped into your coffee or dissolved in your pudding gives you no calories, hence no energy, and absolutely nothing else, either, except a sweet taste.

They are all products made from coal tar. Applying to them our two rules for what we should and should not eat, we discover that these chemicals give us nothing that is needed nutritionally and do much that is harmful. So we cannot possibly recommend that you use them even for a short period of time to tide you over the uncomfortable few days when you are learning to get along without sugar.

We have done considerable research on saccharin which we will review here rather than going into an individual discussion on each of the sweeteners. New sweeteners are being discovered all the time, out of the busy test tubes of our chemists in a nation where the largest portion of the population suffers from overweight. These sweeteners are announced with great fanfare as they appear. We are told we can eat them with safety while we are reducing; we can give them to children and sick people; we can feed them to diabetics. What we have to say about saccharin applies with equal force to all these synthetic sweeteners. *Leave them alone if you would be healthy.*

Since its discovery about 70 years ago, saccharin has been the subject of endless investigation, because, apparently, most researchers have had serious doubts as to its harmlessness in the human body. In our large file on saccharin we cannot find a single article that does not caution that we should use saccharin "with care." Its use should not be abused, they say. Now all this means only one thing. If it were harmless we could eat all of it that we happen to want and suffer no ill consequences. In Europe country after country has forbidden its use in food and drink. In 1912 our Food and Drug Administration forbade its use in foods because, they said, it would constitute an adulteration. People might think they were getting sugar which, as we know, has a certain value in calories which saccharin does not.

Early in our medical history physicians advised the use of saccharin because it has no food value, which seems to us just as idiotic as if a coal dealer should advise us to fill up our winter furnace with steel because it will not burn! Why in the world should we take anything into our bodies *because* it has no food value? And what is our body supposed to do with something that scientists agree cannot possibly be called food?

Here is a quote from our earlier article on saccharin: "In the *British Medical Journal* of October 9, 1915, H. C. Ross, M.D., whose address given at the end of the article is 'Lister Institute' tells us that recent research there has shown that saccharin is a powerful auxetic, like several other constituents and derivatives of coal tar; and there is now strong evidence that it is these auxetics in tar and pitch that give rise to the predisposition to the cancer known as pitch and sweepers' cancer. The next reference we find to it appears in Dr. B. M. Gupta's article published twenty years later in the *Indian Medical Gazette* (September, 1935) : 'Although this statement (of Ross') does not seem to have been contradicted in any medical journal it appears from a private communication that the suggestion that saccharin may predispose to cancer is not accepted by the present authorities of the Lister Institute.' Who lost the evidence in a file somewhere? What became of the records of the experiment proving the association of saccharin and cancer? Is it possible that they have just been overlooked all these years?"

Effect of Saccharin on Plants and One-Celled Animals

We discovered several experiments revealing the deadly effect of saccharin on plants and one-celled animals. E. Verschaffelt, M.D., writing in the Dutch Medical Journal, *Pharmaceutisch Weekblad,* Volume LIX,

1915, describes an experiment in which he soaked dry seed peas in four different solutions: plain water, salt, sugar and saccharin. Two days later 94 per cent of the peas treated with water had sprouted; 87 per cent of the peas treated with sugar had sprouted; 44 per cent of those soaked in salt water germinated and none of the peas soaked in saccharin solution sprouted. Using a saccharin solution only half as strong as the salt solution, Dr. Verschaffelt once again found that the salt-treated peas germinated twice as fast as those soaked in saccharin. His conclusions are that saccharin is a protoplasmic poison. That is, regardless of how long the process may take, saccharin eventually poisons protoplasm, which is nothing more or less than the substance of which plants and animals are made.

Dr. W. A. Uglow, M.D., tested saccharin on one-celled animals and his experiments are reported in the German medical magazine, *Archiv fur Hygiene,* Volume XCII, 1924. Testing saccharin solutions and phenol (carbolic acid) solutions of varying strength, Dr. Uglow found that saccharin is 12 times as deadly to bacteria as carbolic acid which is another coal tar derivative and a deadly poison. In a further test he found that a solution of one part of saccharin to 500 parts of distilled water almost corresponds in its toxicity to a .05 solution of sulfuric acid—another violent poison.

In a solution of one part of saccharin to 400 parts of water Dr. Uglow placed some cyclops quadricornis (a microscopic one-celled animal). They died within 40 minutes. In a solution of one to 800 parts of water, they died within an hour and so on until he found that it took a solution of one part of saccharin to 8000 parts of water just 24 hours to kill all the cyclops. Incidentally one part of saccharin to 10,000 parts of water is approximately the solution we get when we slip a saccharin tablet into a cup of tea or coffee.

A one-celled animal is made up of one tiny cell of protoplasm—the same protoplasm that makes up all the many tiny cells of your body. Cancer research deals largely with what goes on in cells. Certain coal tar products are known to produce cancer through their effect on the cells of the body. Saccharin is a coal tar product. Saccharin means certain death to a one-celled animal. Do you need further proof of the harmfulness of saccharin and all other synthetic sweeteners?

Incidentally, although saccharin instead of sugar is illegal in food and drink so far as interstate commerce is concerned, there is nothing to prevent local food processors from using it in all their sweet products unless your state has a law which forbids it. Why not write to your state department of health and check?

Only one word more on saccharin. We can present testimony from healthy people who are getting along happily and serenely without ever using sugar or any other kind of sweetener except fruits and vegetables. We can show that saccharin is a poison. What possible excuse can there be to continue to prepare foods for diabetics (desperately sick people) using saccharin? Why do we continue to propagate the fable that Americans simply can't get along without a sweet taste in their mouths at every meal and most of the time between meals? In many parts of the world whole nations have never tasted sugar or sugar substitutes. In our own country thousands of people have not eaten sugar or sugar substitutes for years. Why must we continue to feed the poisonous sweet-tasting sugar substitutes to sick people?

Salt

How many diseases could be prevented if our bodies could cry out "Too much salt" as our taste senses can when food is too highly seasoned. With the evidence we have against salt and its effects, how much wiser we would be to break ourselves of the salt "habit"—for it is a habit like tobacco and liquor—than to wait for the sword to strike and then run for the cure.

Enough salt can be obtained from most foods in their natural form. R. Ackerly, M.D., in *Proceedings of the Royal Society of Medicine,* 1910, states that the body requires only from two to three grams of salt a day, and that "western nations eat, on an average, seven to ten times as much salt as is necessary, and frequently more." Dr. Egon V. Ullmann in his book *Diet, Infections and Colds* (Macmillan, 1933), shows how 5 grams of salt a day may be obtained from food without added table salt, and gives a list of everyday foods and their sodium chloride (salt) content. Dr. L. Duncan Bulkley, editor of the medical journal *Cancer,* believes that one-quarter of an ounce of added salt per week "is ample to supply the body with the actual needs in the replacing of chloride of sodium lost in modern methods of cooking and the preparation of food."

Why Is Excess Salt Bad?

(1) *Excess Salt Causes Hyperacidity.* The formation of hydrochloric acid in the stomach depends on the salt intake. The chlorine of the sodium chloride goes to make up part of this hydrochloric acid. So if too much salt is taken, too much of this acid will be produced (hyperacidity). Too much hydrochloric acid is generally accepted as one predisposing cause of stomach ulcers.

(2) *Excess Salt May Prevent Proper Use of Calcium in the Body.* Much of the sodium of the sodium chloride will be held in the tissues and will reduce the effect of calcium, which is so badly needed in the body. Where salt is reduced, calcium action will prevail and will counteract inflammations. These two points are made by Dr. Ullmann in his book mentioned previously.

(3) *Excess Salt Stimulates the Body and Nerve Cells.* We know how salt irritates an open wound, or salt water stings the eyes. In the same way it irritates delicate membranes throughout the body. Dr. Henry C. Sherman in his book *Chemistry of Food and Nutrition* (published by Macmillan, 1952), states that "through overstimulating the digestive tract, salt may interfere with the absorption and utilization of the food." He also states that an excess of salt may disturb the osmotic pressure of tissues, involving almost every portion of the body. Although some salt is needed to keep the tension of the body fluids at a normal level, we get enough in our foods in their natural content to serve the purpose.

(4) *Excess Salt Causes the Retention of Fluid.* Every gram of salt binds and holds 70 grams of water. The bad effects of this accumulated fluid may be seen as the cause of many diseases.

(5) *Table Salt Contains Chemicals.* Most of us are wary of ordering just any old chemical from the druggist's shelf without competent advice, but how many of us have looked into the effect of the chemicals that have been added to packaged table salt? One box of salt listed the following added items: .01 per cent potassium iodide, .05 per cent sodium bicarbonate, and .90 per cent tri-calcium phosphate. Sometimes hyposulphite of soda is added. Though the individual chemical added may not be harmful in itself, the combination of all of them may well be.

(6) *Chemicals Must Be Used To Combat Bad Effects of Salt in the Body.* There are research findings that may eventually prove the prescription of salt-free diets unnecessary. Work along this line was described in *Science News Letter* for September 16, 1950. In brief, the researchers found that certain chemicals called "ion exchange resins" can combat the accumulation of fluid and the inability of the body to get rid of too much sodium, such as is contained in common table salt. These resins, they found, can remove the salt from the body, and "in order to avoid robbing the body of potassium as the sodium is being removed, a combination of ammonium and potassium forms of the resin was adopted." However, as we have said before many times, why put something irritating into the body that needs something else to undo the harm? And who knows the effect of these added chemicals over a long period of time?

(7) *Salt Contains Bacteria.* "Refined salt from various sources was found to contain up to 8,300 bacteria and 400 mould (spores) . . . and toxic cultures were obtained in some cases. Brines of various sources and ages were badly contaminated," according to the *Analyst,* June, 1926. Commenting on this, Frederick L. Hoffman, M.D., a member of the American Association of Cancer Research, in his book, *Cancer and Diet* (Williams and Wilkins) stated: "If this should be substantiated, it might be a clue to the injurious effects of common salt in introducing irritating bacteria into the human body, directly operating as causative factors in tumor growth."

Diseases and Salt

Cancer. Because cancer is still baffling medical science, we have come to assume that its cause must be tremendously complex and mysterious. But there is evidence that the seemingly harmless substance, common table salt, is held in positive suspicion by medical authorities.

One of the earliest writers on Cancer, Dr. James Braithwaite, of Leeds, England, tells of the increase in diameter of a tumor from 2⅜ inches to 3¼ inches when one of his patients resumed daily use of salt, even in small quantities. He says that salt, being an inorganic chemical and not a food, is dangerous in oversupply. It harms the body tissue as it is a powerful stimulant to cell metabolism. This information is from his book, *Excess of Salt in the Diet and Three Other Factors, the Probable Causes of Cancer.*

Frederick T. Marwood, a layman, made the interesting observation that in Denmark, where the consumption of salted fish is the highest in Europe, the cancer rate is also the highest in Europe *(What Is the Root Cause of Cancer—Is It the Excessive Consumption of Common Salt, Salted Foods and Salt Compounds? 1910).*

In contrast, Dr. L. Duncan Bulkley tells us of the low incidence of cancer in Mexico and among the Indians, where the use of salt is relatively small. He describes how "chloride of sodium, or common salt, in any excess with the food may disturb the balance of mineral ingredients of the blood, replacing the tissue of the cells when worn out, instead of a potassium salt, thus starting them on their riotous malignant action, in response to local irritation, and ending in fully developed cancer." This statement appeared in the publication *Cancer,* July, 1927.

As salt has the property of holding fluid about it, a diet rich in water again favors cancer cell growth. The tissue of the tumor contains a larger amount of fluid proportionately than any tissue in the body according to Frederick L. Hoffmann, M.D., in *Cancer and Diet,* quoting Dr. Bernhard Fischer-Wasels, Director of the Pathological Institute of the University of Frankfort.

High Blood Pressure and Kidney Disease. Dr. Frederick Allen, who introduced the low-salt diet for this disease into this country in 1922 has had consistently good results from the restriction of salt. He also conducted animal experiments which proved that with the feeding of salt, blood pressure increased causing hypertension. This research is reported in the *Journal of the American Medical Association* for June 4, 1949.

"Twenty-one patients treated with low-salt diet were observed by Svith for one to five months. In all cases the blood pressure was reduced from 20 to 75 mm., usually in two to four weeks, "and the patients' other symptoms disappeared, too," according to an article in *Ugeskrift For Laeger,* Copenhagen, March 30, 1950.

Dropsy. Doctors now believe that the cause of dropsy is not too much water, but too much sodium, which prompts the body to hoard water in abnormal amounts, usually as a result of a heart or kidney ailment. Dr. Ferdinand Ripley Schemm's salt-free diet has won wide acceptance and his tireless work on the disease resulted in the establishment in 1947 of the Western Foundation for Clinical Research. Dr. Schemm believed that if the sodium taken in with food were cut down, the body itself could in dropsy cases regulate the sodium already in the body and give the kidneys enough water so that they could work properly and flush out the sodium salts through the urine. The "restriction of water is harmful and a cause of suffering," he said in cases of dropsy.

Heart Disease. Though a low salt diet is not infallible, there is definite evidence of its beneficial effects in many cases. Wheeler, Bridges and White in *The Journal of the American Medical Association* for January, 1947, describe the treatment of 50 cases of congested heart failure with a diet low in salt, containing about five-eighths of a gram of sodium per day. Patients were chosen for whom all other treatments had failed. Of the 50, only 35 followed the diet honestly, and out of this number 22 received definite benefit, while 13 did not.

Pregnancy. Seventy patients, put on a salt-free diet in the latter weeks of pregnancy, showed a definite reduction in the length of labor and, as far as could be measured, in the severity of the pains. It is believed that the decreased sodium and chloride (from salt) resulted in removal of water from the maternal tissues, bringing about a lessening in excitability of the nerve centers and a definite sedative effect, according to an article in *Hospital Topics,* 1940.

Deafness and Sinusitis. Here is a beautiful "believe-it-or-not," the more beautiful because it is backed up by scientific, medical knowledge. Dr. Frank Graham Murphy, of Mason City, Iowa, had as a patient a woman who had been deaf for years and according to the specialists was apparently incurable. Questioning her eating habits Dr. Murphy found she was a heavy consumer of salt, and advised that she drop it completely. After three weeks she returned—her hearing restored, as good as ever!

Dr. Murphy says that the ears and sinuses are affected when there is an excess of salt in the body tissues. When free perspiration does not help get rid of the excess, the kidneys force the salt into other organs or tissues. As salt collects water about it, a waterlogged condition may result in the ears and sinuses. Other fluid-retention foods, with a high number of calories, such as bread and sugar, when eaten in excess, may also play a role, he says in *Clinical Medicine* for August, 1944.

Obesity. A drastic reduction of salt is advised because of its water-holding properties. Fluid adds to the weight. Salt also excites thirst, making for a greater intake of water, and excites appetite by increasing the flow of saliva.

Headaches. Migraine and other headaches are attributed by Dr. Max Goldzieher to pressure caused by an increased flow of water to the tiny blood vessels in the head because of abnormal retention of salt in the tissues.

Other Diseases. Hives, epilepsy, insomnia, nervous tension states, and rheumatic swelling also respond to the restriction of salt intake, says the magazine *Good Health.*

Forbidden Food on the Salt-Free Diet

The following is a list of foods commonly forbidden by physicians to patients on a low-salt diet: Processed meats: salted, smoked, canned, spiced, and pickled foods, bacon, ham, sausages, bologna, frankfurters, liverwurst, salami; shell fish: clams, oysters, lobster, shrimp; processed fish; canned vegetables (unless specially packed without salt); beets, celery, endive, spinach, kale, sauerkraut; broths, meat soups; regular commercial bread and rolls, salted crackers, pretzels; peanuts; all salted cheeses, salted butter; commercial ice cream. Also forbidden are olives, raisins, catsup, mayonnaise, pickles, relish, salted meat gravy and salted meat sauce.

This list is for sick people who have to be extremely strict. An ordinary healthy person may use his judgment as to how far he wishes to go. Remember that in their raw state fruits, vegetables, meats and cereals naturally provide all the vital food salts we need for our well-being and preservation. If a person will go to a little pains to figure out an appetizing diet, the saltless features of it won't be hard to take.

Salt Substitutes

There are two kinds of salt substitutes, if substitute you must. First there are the non-chemical substitutes like Vege-Sal which is sold in health food stores. This contains some sodium chloride (which is what you are trying to avoid) soybean extract, sea salt and vegetable powders. This is far safer than the chemical salt substitutes such as Diasal, Gustamate,

Neocurtasal and so forth. But it is our opinion that no salt substitutes should be used. By omitting salt in cooking and not adding any at the table you will find, after a matter of several weeks, that you do not miss the taste of it. As a matter of fact, you will begin for the first time to appreciate the actual taste of many foods whose flavors you have up to now been drowning out with salt. Honestly, you'll soon begin to enjoy food more without salt! There are many primitive nations in the world whose people have never tasted salt and many other people, such as the Eskimos, who will not eat food that has been salted!

There are diseases such as Addison's disease where the body mechanism is so badly disordered that salt is necessary. If you are suffering from any of these diseases, of course, follow your doctor's direction about the amount of salt you need. Otherwise you are perfectly safe in cutting down on the salt you add to food in cooking and at the table, for you are already getting all the sodium you need in food.

Heat and Salt Tablets

Many people believe they should take salt tablets during the summer months. Taking salt tablets to prevent heat shock or prostration started with steel workers who stand before searing furnaces all their working day, losing a large amount of salt and water in perspiration. In our usual haste to take up anything new, many employers provided salt tablets even in cool offices where employees were not being especially active physically. Recently the tendency has been to swing away from taking salt tablets. The National Research Council, official authority on matters of nutrition and health, has concluded that the average American gets from 10 to 15 grams of salt a day which is easily enough to make up for loss in perspiration. In addition it has been found that one soon becomes accustomed to hot weather and one's perspiration becomes less salty. So it now appears that, for the average person, exerting himself in an average way, there is no need for extra salt during the summertime.

If you eat a purely vegetarian diet, you may feel the need of a little more salt than those of us who eat meats, butter and eggs, for the fruits and vegetables do not contain as much natural sodium as the animal products. Our final word on salt—and we believe the facts we have presented prove our case—throw away your salt shaker, gradually begin to use less and less salt in cooking and enjoy the increased health and good flavor of natural foods that will be your reward!

Salt and Colds

In his excellent book, *Diet in Sinus Infections and Colds,* (Macmillan Co., 1942), Egon V. Ullmann, M.D., advises among other things the use of a salt-poor diet for chronic cold sufferers. We have long recommended giving up the use of salt in cooking or at the table, regardless of whether or not one is suffering from any disease. Dr. Ullmann is very emphatic about not using salt if you would be free from colds.

Part of his explanation is this: The chemical content of table salt is sodium and chloride. The chloride serves no purpose in our bodies except that it may go to form hydrochloric acid in the stomach, a certain amount of which is necessary for digestion of proteins. An excess of salt in the diet can result in too much hydrochloric acid in the stomach which will surely produce stomach ulcers.

The sodium part of table salt is the part most of us have been warned against. It seems that, to a certain extent, sodium cancels out the excellent and necessary functions of calcium. "If large amounts of sodium chloride are taken," says Dr. Ullmann, "a good deal of it will be stored in the skin, mucous membrane and other tissues, and calcium will be liberated. Therefore each sodium molecule retained in the tissues will diminish the calcium effect. . . . On the other hand, with a reduction of sodium chloride in the diet the calcium action will prevail and lead up toward an anti-inflammatory effect. . . . To sum it up, it can be said that the secret of calcium action lies in the relation of calcium taken with food to the other minerals, especially sodium, magnesium and phosphorus. If any of those are taken in too large amounts the calcium effect may be impaired."

We want to point out here the importance of calcium in relation to cold susceptibility. Sir Robert McCarrison in *The Journal of the Royal Society of Arts* for September 4, 1936, shows how malnutrition can contribute to a condition in the nose that might create susceptibility to cold catching. He says:

"Let me draw your attention to the kind of change that is brought about in epithelium (skin or mucous membrane) by the lack of this vitamin (vitamin A). This membrane is covered by tall epithelial cells, each of which has a fringe of cilia. A function of these cells is to secrete mucous which not only traps bacteria but permits the cilia to perform their movements—this they can only do when the membrane they fringe is moist *and the moisture contains calcium* (italics ours). The function of the cilia is, by their rapid movements in waves, to propel bacteria or foreign particles, as of dust, towards the exterior of the body, whence, in normal circumstances, they are ejected. It has been estimated that the cilia move at the rate of about 600 times a minute. Now when the food is deficient in vitamin A the cilia slough off and the cells themselves lose their secretory character, becoming horny or keratinised, as it is called. Figure to yourself what this means: no longer is this trapping, this propelling of harmful particles, whether of dust or bacteria or both, possible in the areas so affected. For, unless the deficiency be very grave, it is only at certain places that these changes occur. Where they do occur the local defenses are broken down and bacteria are free to implant themselves in the soil thus made ready for them and to invade the tissues."

In the diet Dr. Ullmann outlines for chronic cold patients, he specifically recommends that no salt be added either in cooking the food or at the table. He suggests ways of making food tasty with herbs and seasonings other than salt. He also advises against the use of non-sodium salt substitutes. They are generally not liked by patients, he has found, they may leave an aftertaste, are hard to get used to and are expensive. He advises instead, and we agree completely, that the best way to learn to get along without salt is simply to stop using it. Within a few weeks you will be used to the taste of food without salt and will, in fact, for the first time in years begin to appreciate the real taste of food, for you will be tasting the food itself rather than the salt you used to douse it with.

Do We Need To Salt Our Food?

He covers in his chapter on salt all the old arguments offered against the practice of doing without it. People will tell you, "But animals have to have salt. Human beings cannot get along without salt. Throughout history salt has been a valuable commodity and wars have been fought for possession of it." Spices have also been a valuable commodity down through the ages—so valuable that the voyages of explorers like Columbus were undertaken to find new sources of spices or shorter ways of reaching the old sources. But surely no one would claim that man cannot live without spices! There are whole nations of people whose languages do not contain a word for salt. There are many parts of the world where salt has never been eaten and where just the taste of it sickens the people. Animals who do not get enough sodium chloride in their food frequent salt "licks" because they have a need for the sodium and the chloride. But we human beings get plenty of both in our daily food. The only reason why we add more salt is the same reason why we add sugar—we like the taste of it.

It is generally agreed among authorities that we do not need more than five grams of sodium chloride per day. Adding up the sodium chloride in the foods eaten by the average American for a week, Dr. Ullmann lists the sodium chloride content of meat, milk, eggs, rice, wheat, peas, cream, bread, potatoes, fruits and vegetables and finds that we get, from a diet like this, without salting the food, 5 grams of salt per day. "The trouble is," he says "that most of us consume about 15 grams or more per day, an amount which is in excess of what the body really requires. There is hardly a dish to which the cook does not add just 'a pinch of salt' and at the table salt is frequently added in amounts which remind one of the salt licks of the animals."

Here is a chart showing the amount of sodium chloride in a number of common foods. Study it and you will agree with us that you do not need any more salt than your food naturally contains:

Food	*Usual Portion and Weight*	*Milligrams of Sodium Chloride Per Ounce (A milligram is 1/1000 of a gram)*
Almonds	20=1 ounce	7.4
Apples	1=1⅓ ounce	2.8 to 4.2
Asparagus	6=2½ ounces	.5 to 4.5
Bananas	1=5 ounces	.02 to 12
Barley, pearl	3T=1 ounce	.7 to 16
Beans, butter	¾ cup=2½ ounces	17.4
Beans, green lima	½ cup=2½ ounces	.28 to 25.4
Beans, dried lima	½ cup=2½ ounces	47.7 to 80.5
Beef, lean	½ pound	15 to 24
Beets	⅔ cup=3⅓ ounces	15.1 to 31.4
Bluefish	½ pound	19.4
Cabbage, red	½ cup=⅚ ounces	1.4 to 10.8
Cantaloupe	¼=3⅓ ounces	3.4 to 13.7

Food	*Usual Portion and Weight*	*Milligrams of Sodium Chloride Per Ounce (A milligram is 1/1000 of a gram)*
Carrots, raw	½ cup=2⅔ ounces	8.8 to 27
Celery stalks	2=1⅓ ounces	28.8 to 38.9
Cheese, American Swiss	⅛ inch=1 ounce	120.0
Cheese, Cheddar	⅚ ounce	154.2
Chicken breast	½ pound	15.4 to 26.0
Chicken, leg	½ pound	15.4 to 31.4
Coconut, fresh	1 inch=⅓ ounce	4.7 to 11.4
Cream	1T=½ ounce	8.8 to 11.4
Dandelion greens	½ cup=1⅔ ounces	21.7 to 48
Duck leg	½ pound	27.4
Eggs	1 average=1⅔ ounces	31.7 to 40
Flounder, steamed	¼ pound	32.6
Goose, roasted	¼ pound	41.2
Haddock, steamed	¼ pound	34.4
Halibut, steamed	¼ pound	31.5
Kale	1¾ cup=6 ounces	14.2 to 31.4
Kidney, beef	5 ounces	60 to 69.5
Kohlrabi	½ cup=1⅔ ounces	14.2
Lamb, without fat	1 chop=3⅛ ounces	14 to 31.4
Lentils	¼ cup=2 ounces	16.2
Liver, beef	½ pound	6 to 24.8
Liver, calf	½ pound	24.8 to 31.4
Mackerel	½ pound	43.7
Milk, fresh whole	1 cup 8 ounces	13.4 to 14.5
Oatmeal	¼ cup=1 ounce	.5 to 20.5
Pork, without fat	½ pound	16.5 to 23.1
Radishes	6 med.=1⅔ ounces	2.3 to 23.7
Spinach, boiled	½ cup=3⅓ ounces	34.9
Trout, steamed	4 ounces	25
Turkey, breast	8 ounces	11.4 to 37.1
Turkey, leg	8 ounces	26.2 to 37.1
Turnips, white	¾ cup=4 ounces	10.5 to 29.7
Turnip greens	1 cup=3⅓ ounces	2.8 to 74.2

Salt—Iodized

Years ago when it first became apparent that lack of iodine in diet and water might render inhabitants of certain parts of the world susceptible to thyroid disorders, it was suggested that we solve this nutritional problem by adding iodine (as potassium iodide) to common table salt. In this way, it was argued, we could be sure that everyone got enough iodine to prevent any thyroid difficulties.

So in many sections of the world today iodized salt is available and in some countries its use is mandatory. However, a booklet entitled *Iodine in Drinking Waters, Vegetables, etc.* by G. S. Fraps and J. F.

Fudge published by the Agricultural and Mechanical College of Texas, tells us that potassium iodide added to the rations of various animals "rarely gave any beneficial results and sometimes gave detrimental ones." The surveys and experiments were done in areas where it was known that iodine was low in food and where goiter was prevalent. Nevertheless among sheep fed a daily ration of iodine, reproduction was abnormal; in the case of hogs, no beneficial results were found and there was some indication that the animals' use of calcium was disordered. Calves that had the iodine ate less hay and made considerably less gains in weight than those which did not. And so on. The conclusion of researchers Fraps and Fudge is "The use of iodized table salt for human consumption in Texas is not recommended, except under the supervision of a competent physician. The use of iodized mineral mixtures for livestock in Texas is not recommended."

In a book called *Trace Elements in Food,* (published by John Wiley & Sons, NYC), G. W. Monier-Williams, formerly of the Ministry of Health in England, has a great deal to say about the results of using iodized table salt. He says that it is pretty well agreed that the thyroid gland is of importance primarily in childhood and that treatment with iodine has not the same effects later on in life, except during pregnancy with the object of preventing goiter in the unborn child. Children tolerate iodine much better than adults, he says, and their iodine requirements are three times as great. It is alleged, he says, that adults constantly receiving small doses of iodine are likely to develop toxic symptoms.

One researcher in 1936 for instance found that there was a marked increase in cases of hyperthyroidism (overactivity of the thyroid gland) in adults after iodized salt was introduced, which could be ascribed only to the action of the iodine in the salt. She believes that sensitivity to iodine is apparently quite common among adults, especially in goitrous regions. Other authorities have argued that the dose of iodine from table salt is very small indeed—far less than that given in medical treatment and that any excess of iodine over that required to maintain the thyroid gland in good health is promptly excreted in the urine.

However, Monier-Williams reminds us that iodine belongs to the same chemical family as bromine (and fluorine, too, we might add). Bromides are excreted very slowly indeed from the body. "It may be that occasional massive doses of iodides cannot be considered in the same light as daily small doses continued for many years, and that the habitual use of iodized salt, while beneficial and even essential to children, is not altogether without risk to a certain small proportion of adults," he says. "Hyper-sensitiveness to iodine may be commoner in some districts than in others, but even if it affected only 2 per cent of the population this would seem to be sufficient reason for objecting to the compulsory iodization of all household, or even all table salt." We go along with Dr. Monier-Williams one hundred per cent in this opinion.

There are a number of other reasons why we object to iodized salt. One of them is that the potassium iodide is lost very rapidly from salt in cardboard containers. We are told that salt containing 5 parts per million of potassium iodide may lose as much as one-third of that within six weeks depending on the atmospheric conditions. So one never knows how much iodine may actually be in the box of salt he purchases. If he depends on the iodine to protect him from iodine deficiency, perhaps he will be cruelly deceived.

If, on the other hand, he is sensitive to iodine, the very small amount that may remain in that salt carton may be just enough to start trouble for him, taken day after day and year after year. Consider for a moment—if two per cent of our population suffer from iodine sensitivity—that is more people than suffer from most of our great chronic diseases, so of course it is important to consider the reactions of these two per cent before we arbitrarily decree that everyone everywhere should take iodized salt.

"Doctored" Foods and Iodine Sensitivity

Our principal reason for avoiding iodized salt stems from another reason, however. We do not like "doctored" foods. The potassium iodide placed in table salt was not placed there by nature. So it is not accompanied by all the other substances that go along with iodine in foods. And it is not in what we call "organic combination" with the other ingredients of salt. This makes it a drug, from our point of view.

We know that potassium iodide is used extensively in medicine. In fact, one of the principal ingredients of several very famous cancer treatments is potassium iodide. But this, mark you, is treatment, given under the strict supervision of doctors, to very, very sick people. This is surely no indication that we should all be taking potassium iodide every day of our lives along with food!

Iodine sensitivity is nothing to joke about. We have an article from the *Journal of the American Medical Association* for July 2, 1955, in which two Buffalo, New York, doctors discuss the case of a young patient who was suffering from a horrible dermatitis involving ulcers, eyelids swollen shut and so forth. He had been taking potassium iodide as an expectorant. It was believed that taking iodized table salt had sensitized the patient over a period of years so that when he got medicine that contained potassium iodide he reacted immediately with a serious allergic response. The authors go on to tell us that fatalities have resulted even from the application of iodine *to the skin of sensitive persons.*

Now, of course, this does not mean that we should all stop getting any iodine at all in our diets. We must have iodine—a certain very small amount of it—or we will perish. But doesn't it seem that nature is trying to warn us not to take iodine in the concentrated, non-organic form in which it appears in iodized salt? We have never heard of anyone reacting negatively to iodine in food—sea food or seaweed or mushrooms, because here the iodine is part of the food and combined with it in nature's proper way.

Of course it may have occurred to many readers to ask why we should mention iodized salt at all, since we do not think any of us should salt food, either in cooking or at the table. A highly pertinent comment to make. Of course those of us who have stopped using salt or have cut down drastically will not need to worry about iodized salt. Yet, from letters we know that these are the very people who worry most, for they write us in great concern "Since I am not taking salt I am not getting any iodine—how shall I make up the loss?" Of course our answer is "Go right on skipping the salt and get your iodine from some organic source—seafood, kelp or seaweed." In fact, it seems to us that powdered kelp would be the best possible salt substitute for those readers who are trying desperately to cut down on salt but haven't yet conquered that all-American gesture of reaching for the salt-shaker before eating anything. Fill the salt shaker with powdered kelp—far, far richer in iodine than iodized salt, and with a pleasant taste, too.

We Shouldn't Salt Our Food Anyway

We have a new story about salt restriction which we think is extremely important. It is generally widely known these days that doctors prescribe salt-poor diets for heart patients. Now we find in a lead article in the *Journal of the American Medical Association* for November 26, 1955, that salt restriction helps greatly in cases of cirrhosis of the liver, too. The treatment was given to 30 patients in Bellevue Hospital by Dr. Charles S. Davidson. All of them suffered also from *ascites,* which means an accumulation of fluid in the abdomen. Of the thirty patients, 28 were known alcoholics, but two clearly were not, although the cause of their disease was not known. Four of the patients were considered well nourished. In 16, undernutrition was moderate and 10 of the patients were definitely severely undernourished.

These patients were put on a good nourishing diet rich in vitamins and minerals and their salt intake was restricted to 200 milligrams per day—that is about one-fifth of a gram.

The results were uniformly excellent. All of the patients improved. It took longer in some cases than in others—as long as sixteen months in some cases until the patient was free from the terrible swelling that deformed him and of course distorted all his body functions immeasurably. At the same time, the nutritional status of all the patients improved, too, and the liver began to function much more normally. The doctors believe that the livers of the patients were actually regenerated. Improvement in a feeling of well-being, return of appetite and successful readjustment of many body functions went along with the salt-poor diet.

Many disorders may be related to the consumption of too much salt. We have told of deafness, sinusitis, miscarriages, headaches, insomnia, hives, kidney diseases, Menière's Syndrome, dropsy, pregnancy toxemia, epilepsy, migraine, high blood pressure and heart conditions relieved when a low-salt diet was taken.

There is no medical or physiological evidence that the human body needs more sodium chloride (table salt) than is contained naturally in foods. Our continual daily over-consumption of salt (the only food we eat which has neither an animal nor vegetable source) may well be the cause of many more troubles than we know. Don't depend on iodized table salt for your iodine. Get it from a natural source like kelp or salt water fish. And cut down on salting your food until you arrive at that happy stage where you will not miss the taste of salt at all and will, instead of tasting salt, be tasting the food you eat.

Seeds

By

J. I. Rodale

Editor of ***Prevention***

This is being written on the last day of 1955. About four or five months before this, there developed in my left eye a slight quiver, which did not seem to want to go away. That was bad for an editor of a health magazine. I let a few weeks pass, thinking that, like a ship that passes in the night, it would go away. I closed my eyes to it, but it persisted.

I thought back to my pamphlet *Sunflower Seed—The Miracle Food,* written about ten years ago, and re-read the following in it: "About a week later (that is, after beginning to eat sunflower seeds) a slight intermittent quiver in my left eye went away. I usually suffered from this only in the winter, when there was little opportunity for exercise or sunshine. As this is written two winters later I am glad to report that it has not returned, thanks to the fact that I still eat sunflower seeds practically every day."

Well, I seemed to have gotten careless, and had stopped eating sunflower seeds somewhere along the line. So I began eating them again. But I had none of our own organically-raised ones. The previous year's crop of them had been fed to the chickens. So I began to eat some hulled seeds that we had around the house and that had been purchased some months before. I ate them for several weeks, but nothing happened.

Along about October our new crop ripened and I began to eat our own seeds. Within three days my eye quiver vanished, but before I could start crowing, that is about two days after that, it returned in fairly full vigor.

"Hm," said I. "This is more serious than I thought. But I must track this thing down. There must be *some* cause." There always are causes and they can be found if one keeps one's mind at it. It is a matter of a little thinking plus a little of trial and error.

The next thing that I tried to incriminate was my pillow. Years ago I had a pain in the neck which evidently was caused solely by sleeping on a pillow. Crooking the head causes a bend in the jugular vein of the neck. The veins become wrinkled at the point of bend, and congestion of the blood circulation occurs there. There is not a free flow of blood to and from the head. Within a few days of learning to sleep flat, the pain completely cleared up—but completely. A few months ago I heard one of the girls in our circulation department complaining of a pain in the neck. I described my own experience to her and in a very short time she completely rid herself of it—solely by sleeping without a pillow.

Here again I had gotten careless, and a few years ago had resorted to the pillow again. Nothing happened by sleeping on a pillow this time; that is, the pain in the neck did not return. But now I began to suspect the pillow in connection with my eye quiver. If there was a congestion in the mechanism that feeds blood to the head, perhaps the eyes weren't getting enough blood. So I began to sleep without a pillow. A few weeks went by but the quiver remained—and I was exactly where I started.

I noticed, however, that when I took my glasses off, the quiver was less marked. I don't want to give you a wrong impression. The eye did not quiver constantly—it was an intermittent thing. But with the glasses off it was a little more intermittent. My glasses could have something to do with it, thought I. The next day saw me at the optometrist, my personal friend. "It could be one of two things," he said. "Either it is a calcium deficiency, or your left eye has either improved or gotten worse, that is, the lens for your left eye might need correction."

Vision Improved

Now I knew that it couldn't be a calcium deficiency, with all the bone meal I take, and the doctor knew it too, for he is a subscriber and believes in *Prevention*. I now felt sure that the vision of my left eye had improved. Why? Because on the several previous occasions that I had gone up for routine eye check-ups there had been slight improvements in my vision. The doctor began the test, and lo and behold, he found that the vision in my left eye had improved. Within three or four hours, after wearing the glasses with the new slightly weakened lens, my eye quiver disappeared. That was on October 24, 1955. Today, December 31, 1955, the cure has held with nary a quiver.

Here are the comparative measurements of my lenses:

Sept. 18, 1951				
	Right	3.50 SPH	1.75 Cyl. Axis	180
	Left	4.00 SPH	1.25 Cyl. Axis	12
Oct. 24, 1955				
	Right	3.00 SPH	1.50 Cyl. Axis	180
	Left	3.50 SPH	0.75 Cyl. Axis	7

It seems to be a progressively improving trend and I can attribute it mainly to my nutritional program. I believe the fact that I take no artificial sugar, that I am on a no-salt diet, that I eat no bread or dairy products, that I drink no carbonated beverages, that I take many vitamins and minerals, are all factors in the improvement of my eyesight. Vitamin A (Halibut liver oil perles) is specific for the eyes. Vitamin E, of which I take huge amounts, is also very important. It oxygenates the tissues everywhere in the body. It, therefore, helps the blood circulation to the eyes. The minerals in bone meal help in the mineralization of the blood, and make it a chemically better food for the eyes; etc., etc., etc.

May I pause a moment in regard to soft drinks and quote from our *Health Finder,* page 749: "We report on the point of view of Dr. Hunter H. Turner in an article in the *Pennsylvania Medical Journal* for May, 1944, on the subject of prevention of myopia or degenerative nearsightedness. Lamenting over the large numbers of Americans who are doomed to wear glasses, he suggests that incorrect diet undoubtedly plays an important role in producing myopia. Furthermore he believes that carbonic acid is the eye's worst enemy and he attributes the alarming increase in cases of myopia to the pernicious guzzling of carbonated beverages by young children today. As we showed in this earlier article, carbonated beverages exposed to air break down into their basic ingredients of water and carbon dioxide so that such drinks would be much less harmful if they were allowed to stand until they were 'flat.' But of course their most attractive characteristic is their 'fizz.' So they are taken into the stomach while they are still actively effervescing. . . . A large amount of the acid is assimilated by the body."

And yet medical journals regularly accept the advertisements of soft drink manufacturers. Here is one sponsored by The American Bottlers of Carbonated Beverages, which appeared in a medical journal recently. The heading is, "The 'catalyst' of everybody's love of carbonated soft drink is CO_2!" It says further that CO_2 "speeds up the digestive processes . . . ," but what does it do to the eyes? And who wants to speed up the digestive processes?

Now let's go back to my eyesight. I have not gone in for eye exercises because I did not wish to confuse the issue. I would like to know whether eyesight can be improved solely through nutrition. I feel certain that, had I added eye exercise to my program, the improvement would have been greater, but then I would never have been sure—was it my nutrition, or was it the eye exercises?

Another fact: Many persons believe that over-use of the eyes in close work will eventually ruin the eyesight. Cases in point are the famous authors Thurber, Tarkington and Milton. That may be so where the nutrition is poor, but given the proper nourishment based on the newer knowledge as we know it, the eyes will be able to stand a terrific amount of abuse. In my own case, I have been terrifically over-using my eyes in close work for the last five years, and yet my eyesight is actually improving, and what is of even more importance, my doctor tells me that examination reveals an unusually healthy organic condition of the whole eye organ; that is, there is not the slightest evidence of cataracts or other eye disease.

Sunflower Seeds in the Diet

Now let's go back to sunflower seeds. Although they did not cure my eye quiver, I observed a remarkable effect through eating them. About five years ago, a heavy book feel on my left foot, hitting the right half of the big toenail, and blacking that part of it. After about six months, as the blackness did not show any signs of going away, I went to an Allentown surgeon who treated it by cutting the right half of the nail right down to the base. I would come to see him each week, and as the nail grew back, he would continue to cut it back. But the blackness remained. After a few months of this unsuccessful treatment, I stopped going.

For four years I watched that nail and the right half of it continued to remain black. There was absolutely no pain to it, and I felt a feeling of security due to my excellent nutrition. I knew that my vitamin E was keeping the circulation active in my feet. One day, early in the morning, while I was indulging in my usual one-hour walk on the soft turf of the Allentown Fair Grounds, whom should I meet but my old surgeon friend, riding his horse! He stopped, and we exchanged a few words. I told him that my nail was still black and asked him if there was any danger in it. He said absolutely not. I was resigned to carry a black toenail to the grave.

But then I began to eat sunflower seeds in an attempt to stop my eye quiver. Within about ten days I noticed a lighter region in the newly grown nail, only about a sixteenth of an inch from its base. I kept watching it. Gradually the lighter section kept going higher and higher until, about a week ago, it reached to the top. The blackness is completely gone and the color is only slightly darker than that of a natural nail. What do you think of that? I can attribute it to nothing else than the effect of eating sunflower seeds, my own organically-grown ones. There must be something extremely potent about them. They are a seed from which a huge amount of plant tissue will grow. They contain a living element, a germ, which represents life and which you do not get when you eat such foods as lettuce or carrots. In the old Czarist days, Russian soldiers were given what was called an iron ration—sunflower seeds. I do not know whether this custom has carried over into modern times.

What About the Electric Potential of the Seed?

I like another thing about the sunflower seed. The sunflower plant usually turns with the sun as it grows, the head containing the seeds always being exposed to it. It thus becomes sun-drenched. A friend has an electric machine that tests the electric potential of plants. He has found that foods growing in the sun contain a higher electric potential than foods like the potato that grow in the ground. He also has found that apples growing on the outside of the tree, that get the sun, have much more electric potential than those growing in the interior of the tree where it is shady.

The ash of the sunflower seed shows a tremendous amount of phosphorus (35 per cent), calcium (7½ per cent) and a trace of fluorine. The sunflower seed has more vitamin B than wheat seed and it is very rich in vitamin A.

In my opinion the sunflower seed, unroasted and unsalted, is dynamite in its wonderful effect on the body. It is a specific for the eyes. May I quote from my sunflower seed booklet, written in 1945: "My eyes are not my strongest point. In the winter I would have trouble in walking on snow-blanketed roads. Before I became aware of the value of eating sunflower seeds I left the house on the farm one day for a walk but had to return after being out only a moment, as the excessive brightness of the snow interfered with my vision. In fact, it made the snow seem a pink color. After being on the sunflower diet for about a month I noticed I could walk in the snow without distress. A little while later my car broke down and I had to walk over a mile on a snowed-up highway in bright sunshine with no trouble at all for the first three-quarters of the way. On the last stretch the eyes smarted a little."

I will eat a handful of sunflower seeds every day for the rest of my life, and advise you to do likewise—about 50 of them a day should be enough. And if you have the tiniest bit of grass you ought to grow your own sunflower plants organically. The sunflower plant is the easiest thing to grow. If you don't have any compost, use a liberal amount of dried blood and bone meal, which are available at chain stores, nurseries and seed stores. Even with compost, add a liberal amount of dried blood and bone meal. If you can get some kind of seaweed fertilizer so much the better, or rotted manure. Write to *Organic Gardening,* Emmaus, Penna. for its list of publications on the organic method. Think of eating highly potent sunflower seeds which you can grow yourself! What a wonderful item to add to your diet!

A word of caution. The bone meal that you buy for use as a fertilizer is not for human consumption. It may contain disease organisms that are harmful to a weakened human body. Another word of caution—some people have trouble cracking sunflower seeds with their teeth, either through having false teeth or because it might result in chipping sensitive teeth or separating the two front teeth. I would suggest two things: Either soak the seeds in cold water with their shells on, or open them with a pair of pliers. Will someone develop a little hand tool that could open these seeds easily?

In conclusion, I have related three things in one package. The cure of the quiver, the improvement of my eyesight, and the getting rid of the black toenail. If I continue improving at this rate I will live a long time. It is my ambition to live to be 102 years and one day. Why the extra day? I was born in 1898. If I live to be 102 years and one day, I will have lived in three centuries.

"And God said, Behold, I have given you every herb bearing seed, which is upon the face of the earth, and every tree, in which is the fruit of a tree yielding seed; to you it shall be for meat."

This is Genesis, Chapter 1, Verse 29 . . . The seed is life itself. It contains the spark which is extremely vital to the functioning of our bodies. The perpetuation of the species is accomplished through the seed. The seed is the vehicle for storing life's reserves. The seed is the crucible wherein the alchemy of life works its magic. In this tiny place is contained the condensed germinating energy, the life-giving elements, including as yet undiscovered gleams. Science still knows very little of the vast and intricate interplay of life forces that lie within the seed.

Its living substance can be preserved for many years, and during the entire life of the seed, which in the case of certain legumes is more than fifty years, there is a continuous respiratory action, showing that it is a living organism. The seed of the Indian lotus plant buried for over 200 years in peat bogs has been known to germinate successfully. Melon seeds carefully stored, packed between paper, have germinated after thirty years. There must be very important life-giving elements that will resist the passage of such long periods of time and this should make a very healthful food for homo sapiens. All seeds are rich in vitamin B, and the sex and fertility factors. That is why the wheat germ is fed to women who do not seem to be able to bear children.

Everyone knows that vegetables are an essential to a properly balanced diet, but their maximum vitamin content is only found in really fresh produce. Compare a crisp lettuce straight from the garden with the limp faded thing it becomes two days later. Its "living" quality has gone, and with it, most of its food value. This cannot be said of seeds.

To get an idea of what nutrition is packed in the average seed we must bear in mind that nature has placed an extra store of concentrated feed in it to nourish the emerging plant for a few days. There is enough food in the seed to be used by the young plant to form a root, stem and several leaves without having to get food from the soil.

Seed foods are wonderful for city folk who are faced with the necessity of eating so much processed foods. They can protect themselves by making seed foods a liberal part of their diets. They are also a protection in winter when one is eating stored vegetables that have lost much of their potency.

Much data is available to prove that seeds are a food of high nutritional value. Let us take one instance: In the magazine *Science* in 1932, volume 75, page 294, Davidson and Chandbliss wrote an article called "Chemical Composition of Rice and its Relation to Soil Fertility in China and Japan." It is an astounding article of far-reaching significance to nutritionists. But it was read and promptly forgotten. Davidson and Chandbliss in experimental work discovered that "variations in the nutrient content of soils have less effect on the seed than on any other part of the plant." The best food elements in the soil will be saved for the seed so that the plant will be sure to reproduce itself. Nature wants to be sure of that. This would indicate that seeds have a higher nutritional value than the leafy parts of the plant

The Nutritional Content of Seeds

R. C. Collison, writing in the *Journal of Industrial and Engineering Chemistry* (August, 1912) proved the same thing. He showed that the proportion of organic to inorganic minerals in the seed is much higher than in the rest of the plant. This is necessary because the seed must have sufficient potency to carry on into the next generation. Therefore, where there is a given amount of organic minerals available, as much of it as can possibly be spared will go to the seed. Even in an infertile soil, whatever organic minerals the roots of a plant can forage out will be available first for the formation of seed.

Thomas H. Mather, writing in *Scientific Agriculture,* volume 10, 1929, about an experiment in which the effect of a chemical fertilizer, superphosphate, was measured on a crop of alfalfa, in comparison with a similar crop on which no fertilizer was used, discovered that all of the inorganic phosphorus of the fertilizer went to the stalk and leaves. In this experiment it was proven that the seed actually turned back the inorganic phosphorus. It would have none of it. Nature cannot build a strong race of alfalfa plants with minerals that are inorganic. If there is not a sufficient supply of organic minerals the plant will either produce seed which is defective, or it will not produce seed at all.

I wrote to Prof. Wm. A. Albrecht, Chairman of the Department of Soils, University of Missouri, about this question and he replied: "It is significant to remember that the chemical composition of seeds does not flocculate as widely as the chemical composition of vegetation. The seed is the means of survival of the species, hence this survival will not be possible unless a minimum of food materials are stored in the seed. We well know that when the fertility of the soil drops to a low level less seed is produced. Seemingly the amount of seed is the variable, while the quality of the seed is more nearly a constant. It is the fertility of the soil as a growth-providing substance that seems to determine the seed production rather than the air, water and sunshine that contribute the starches and the energy materials."

Schrumph-Pierron, in the *Bulletin of the Institute of Egypt* (Jan. 4, 1932) says, "Let us observe, however, that the mineralization of seeds is always more stable and less susceptible to wide digressions than that of the leaves or the roots."

This is an extremely important point to be carefully considered. Those of you who are worried about having to purchase food raised with chemical fertilizers, should see to it that a certain portion of your diet consists of seeds, because the seed is not anywhere nearly as much affected by the use of strong chemicals as the leaves or stalks, and thus contains significant amounts of organic elements.

Luther Burbank, the great plant wizard, realized the value of the seed as human food, but he merely mentioned it casually and then proceeded to forget all about it. In his book *Partner of Nature* (Appleton-Century, 1939) he stated, "Fruits ripen, not to make food for us, but to encase and protect the seeds inside—pips or pits or kernels. But we pay no attention to Nature's purpose and revel in the delicate flavors and delicious flesh of apples, pears, peaches, tomatoes, melons and all and throw aside carelessly the seeds that the plant went to so much trouble to build and in which it stored the life-giving germ and a reserve of starch to help it start in life again as a baby plant."

Dr. Henry C. Sherman, Columbia University's outstanding nutritional authority, has said that in studying the nutritional needs of man you cannot deal exclusively in terms of known chemical factors. You have to include "natural articles of food" he says, to "ensure adequate supplies of any possible factors which may not yet have been identified and listed in chemical terms. We must give emphasis to those foods which, as the 'natural wholes' to which our species is nutritionally adjusted by its evolutionary history, will furnish us, along with the known essentials, any unknown factors which may also be essential to our nutrition." Could Dr. Sherman have been referring to seeds? They certainly are "natural wholes."

Two other nutritional experts, Burr and Burr, have shown that a diet may be complete in all essentials, including minerals, vitamins, proteins, etc., but if it lacks the unsaturated fatty acids, which are obtained chiefly from seeds, nutritional deficiency will result. Of course, the average eater is bound to get *some* seeds in his diet such as peas, beans, nuts, wheat, corn, etc., but if he is conscious of their importance he will find ways to add more of them in his total food intake.

Seeds, Apple

By J. I. Rodale

Editor of *Prevention*

I have another little story to tell you. Many years ago I read in a medical journal that a physician was curing a certain disease with an extract made of apple seeds. At the time I was already eating sunflower seeds, and knew their health-giving properties, so I figured, why not add apple seeds to my diet. Since this doctor was curing diseases with them, I imagined that there might be something in apple seeds more potent even than in sunflower seeds. And there was!

I left instructions with the maid one morning to have ready at suppertime a whole teaspoonful of apple seeds, and that night I had them for dessert. It must have been the seeds of about 12 apples. The next day the whole left side of my face felt terrible, from my head down to my chin. I wouldn't call it a paralysis, but it was the closest thing to it that I ever experienced. And it could have come from nothing else than eating those apple seeds.

I re-read the item in the medical journal about the use of the extract of apple seeds. Ah, an *extract* made from the apple seed! It was not the whole apple seed! I decided to look into this matter, in the meantime eating no more apple seeds. I soon found an article in a German medical journal *Zeitschrift Fur Untersuchung Der Lebensmittel,* (*Journal of Food Study,* issue 70, 1935, pp. 255-258). That solved the mystery. In connection with the search for a war-scarce item—fats, German scientists studied apple and pear seeds as a source. They found that about 20 to 26 per cent of the seeds was oil. The article said, "We could use the fat fruit seeds either as fodder or, because of their pleasant taste, even in human nutrition, that is, as a substitute for almonds." I was beginning to wonder, when the author continued, "In this connection Mach observed that apple seeds could not be directly used for this purpose, because of their content of amygdalin, a crystalline principle existing in bitter almonds, etc. Relative to this, we tested apple seeds and actually found prussic acid and benzaldehyde in them . . . Amygdalin was not to be observed in pear seeds."

Prussic acid! That is another name for hydrocyanic acid, one of the most violent poisons known to man. It checks the oxidation process in living matter (protoplasm). Herman Göring, one of the big three Nazis, cheated the gallows with a little phial of this poison. A heavy dose will kill in two minutes, and antidotes are practically useless. In the case of one who has committed suicide with cyanide, there hovers the faint odor of bitter almonds.

So, the mystery was solved. I had taken a dose of the prussic acid almost sufficient to paralyze the left side of my face!

However, I was in no mood to start eating pear seeds, regardless of the opinion of my esteemed German professor. But I cannot stop you from eating them, especially if you are in pear-growing country where they might be obtained from canning plants or in other commercial places. If you try them, however, don't eat them by the spoonful. At any rate, the next time you eat a pear you might chew up and eat the pear seeds also. I have done this frequently with no negative consequences.

Note that the German article said that apple seed contained amygdalin, a crystalline principle existing in bitter almonds. In other words, almonds, another seed, contain some hydrocyanic acid. I recall, in the days when I would get headaches at the slightest provocation, I could easily get one after eating a goodly quantity of almonds. However, hydrocyanic acid is found only in bitter almonds which are not the kind we eat.

We see, therefore, that we cannot rush in and eat seeds indiscriminately. I recall a grocer once telling me of a customer, an old man, who would eat nothing unless it was a seed. He would not eat beets, lettuce, celery, carrots, etc. I think that his nutrition was somewhat off balance. We do need other kinds of foods for various reasons, but I do think that not enough emphasis has been placed on the fact that there is a certain amount of insurance in eating a fair amount of live raw seeds full of enzymes as well as their maximum quota of vitamins. The effect on the intestinal flora must be a very beneficial one.

Seeds as Human Food

By J. I. Rodale

Editor of *Prevention*

You have just read some of my experiences with sunflower seeds, a miracle food if there is one. Another seed that I would like to suggest is wheat—raw wheat seeds. These could very well be substituted in the raw form instead of bread, for in them you get everything, including the living germ. The defect of whole wheat bread is that baking destroys the living qualities of the germ. Bake a wheat seed and then plant it in the ground. Nothing will grow out of it. A few years ago I had a graphic illustration of the value of wheat used as an item of diet.

If you will refer to page 663 of our *Health Finder,* you will find described a method of screening out foods to which you are allergic by means of your pulse. A few years ago, by this method, I checked all the foods I was eating and found that I was allergic to wheat bran. But, strange to say, I was allergic only to baked wheat bran. Eating whole wheat bread raised my pulse unduly, but eating the wheat seed that contained the same bran, but in a raw state, did not. I could eat white bread without raising my pulse.

Of course, the pulse is not the only measure of whether a food is desirable. I would not eat white bread because of the chemicals it contains and for other reasons. If you wish to eat the raw wheat seed, take a handful into the mouth but keep them there for a few moments before you start to chew them. They will soon become thoroughly softened by ensalivation, and then will make a delightful chew. They must be thoroughly masticated and not swallowed till practically a liquid. You have to be careful not to buy wheat seed destined for the farmer's fields. Such seed has been treated with mercury poisons to kill out the rust and smut disease organisms. Buy organically produced wheat seed from advertisers in *Prevention or Organic Gardening And Farming.*

May I quote from *Food, Health, Vitamins,* by R. H. and V. G. Plimmer (Longmans, Green and Co., 1936): "Wellington's soldiers were famous for their fine figures and good looks, yet the food they ate would be scorned nowadays. They received one pound of wheat per day. They ate the whole grain as it was issued, or if time allowed they pounded it up and made a coarse bread."

A popular health writer has written, "A few people have gained notoriety by not cooking or baking starchy foods, thinking they thereby draw closer to nature and enjoy better health. The result of this practice, however, is that such people must suffer with gas collection in their stomach and intestines, and many develop a griping pain. Their uncooked food undergoes fermentation within their systems, causing intestinal toxemia. Another result is considerable loss of weight." I wonder.

My suggestion would be to start with a small amount daily of raw wheat seed and watch developments.

Raw wheat is better than baked wheat, for many reasons. When wheat is ground and stored, serious losses of vitamin set in as the air begins its destructive process of oxidation, or burning out. Where the outer coating of the seed is preserved until it is in the stomach, this cannot occur. The whole seed will preserve its living qualities for a long time. According to Drs. Sherman and Lanford in their book *Essentials of Nutrition* (p. 212), wheat seeds have been known to retain their vitamins after 100 years.

In the *Science News Letter* of March 24, 1955, there is an item that wheat "kept over 20 years, still makes good bread if properly stored, report scientists of the U. S. Department of Agriculture." In tests made it was found that wheat kept 14 to 22 years in a dry, unheated room still had a high content of vitamin B (thiamin).

Food Elements in Wheat Seeds

Let us compare the whole raw wheat seed as far as its wheat germ is concerned with wheat germ oil. Wheat germ oil is not as complete as the wheat germ in the seed. The latter contains the outer layer of the germ which is full of minerals. Of course, the reproductive capacity lies in the oil, but the minerals are valuable too from a dietary point of view. So to receive the full benefit, if you do not care to eat raw wheat seed, take wheat germ oil, plus raw wheat bran which can be purchased from advertisers in *Prevention* magazine.

One writer says, "The entire grain is a complete food and contains within itself the factors of equilibrium. During the process of digestion the starch and the protein part, yielding an acid reaction that becomes immediately neutralized by the mineral factors contained in the outer layer, which has an alkaline reaction."

The wheat seed contains a desirable type of non-soluble fluorine, which is in the mineral-carrying outer layer of the seed. May I quote from the October, 1944, issue of the *News Letter on Compost,* published in England: "The time seems to have come when we should reconsider the present practice of extracting the 'crease dirt,' that is, the minerals, including fluorine, from our flour; and whether fluorine derived from sunflower seeds is what benefits the teeth of the Russians who chew them. The minerals are absorbed from the soil, they pass up the vascular bundles to the seed, and in the case of wheat they enter the 'staff' or leash of vessels at the base of the groove or 'crease' and are there deposited. The miller's 'break rolls' break the staff, the minerals fall out. He sieves them from the flour, and calcium, phosphates, fluorine and all, he throws them away."

In 1951 I spent several weeks at the plant of the Madaus Company, a large drug firm in Cologne, Germany, studying their methods of making drugs. They combined their efforts entirely in making drugs from plants, a great part of which they grew in the fields surrounding the factory. I went there on their invitation because they found out about our movement against the use of chemical fertilizers in growing food crops. Over a period of 20 years they had discovered that organically grown plants were more potent in producing drugs that would cure than plants grown with chemical fertilizers.

My trip there was an enjoyable vacation, as I watched them making compost heaps, and learned many things about growing plants and drug-manufacturing methods. They were a health-conscious bunch. I recall one day, when we were discussing the nutritional value of raw foods, that one of their medical scientists said he would show me something. He lived in a house, German style, that was in the park-like factory grounds. He left and in a few moments returned with a dish of fermented rye seed. As he described it, you fill a plate with seeds, either wheat, rye or millet, or a combination of the three. You then pour a goodly quantity of fruit juices on it and permit it to ferment for a few days. The seed then becomes quite soft and juice-saturated and makes a delicious dish. He has three sets of plates going all the time so that one is ready every day.

May I suggest that health-conscious vegetable gardeners consider growing wheat, rye or millet for personal consumption. Millet is the healthiest of the three with rye second. Wheat and rye seeds are sown in the fall and mature sometime around July 1st to 5th. It is then still time to put in many vegetable crops.

The Hunzas of India, regarding whom I have written in my book *The Healthy Hunzas,* make a wheat product called *chapattis.* Like wheat cakes, this is made out of ground wheat, but is permitted to be heated on hot plates for only a matter of seconds. Thus the vitamins are conserved.

May I mention one more thing about wheat? According to an experiment that I saw performed with white rats, it was found that where bread could be constipating, raw wheat was not. It was done with white rats by Dr. Robert Mick of Laurel Springs, New Jersey. A careful record was kept of the rat droppings in the two groups. Since the droppings of the bread-fed group were less, they became fatter. Those who are on diets to reduce their weights should remember this. Cut out all bread and other cooked or baked grain foods. Eat raw wheat seeds instead.

In concluding on this subject we must bear in mind that the wheat seed has enzymes which are valuable when it comes to its digestion. Cooking kills every one of them. Enzymes die at a temperature of about 130 degrees Fahrenheit or over. Then the body must produce a new set of them to do the work of digestion.

So—I make sure to eat about 50 to 60 sunflower seeds and about three or four mouthfuls of raw wheat seed every day, seeds that are grown organically on our farm. You can also either grow them or buy them, organically produced.

THE NUTRITIVE CONTENT OF SOME SEED FOODS

Seed	Calories	Protein	Fat	Total Carbohyd.	Minerals: Calcium	Phosphorus	Iron	Sodium	Potassium	Vitamins: A	Thiamine	Riboflavin	Niacin	C	E	K	Average Portions Measure
		Grams	Grams	Grams	Mgs.	Mgs.	Mgs.	Mgs.	Mgs.	I.U.	Mgs.	Mgs.	Mgs.	Mgs.	Mgs.	Mgs.	
Grains:																	
Barley, pearled	711	17	2	161	33	386	4.1	6.12	326	0	2.4	1.6	6.3	0	6.5-10.8	....	1 cup
Buckwheat Flour	341	6.3	1.1	77.9	10.8	86	.98	....	......	0	.08	.04	.4	0	......	....	1 cup
Cornmeal, whole	459	18.4	4.3	94.5	7.6	226	2.3	....	......	588	.4	.10	2.4	0	3-12	....	1 cup
Millet	332	6.2	1.4	78.2	329	254	5.3	....	......	.....	.33	.10	1.3	....	......	....	1 cup
Oatmeal, cooked	150	5.5	2.9	26.1	21.4	160	1.7	.7	131	0	2.4	.05	.5	0	4.8	....	1 cup
Rice, brown	748	15.6	3.5	161.6	81	630	4.2	18.7	312	0	.67	.10	9.7	0	4.9	....	1 cup
Rice, converted	677	14.2	.6	148	44.8	254	1.5	7.5	318	0	.37	.07	7.1	0	.74	....	1 cup
Rice, wild	593	23	1.1	123	30.9	552	....	11.4	358	0	.73	1.03	10.1	0	.76	....	1 cup
Rye flour, dark	254	13	2	54.5	43.2	429	3.6	.8	108	0	.49	.18	2.2	0	1.8-2.8	....	1 cup
Sesame seed	610	19.3	51.1	18.1	1,125	614	9.5	....	......	.....	.93	.22	4.5	0	......	....	100 grams
Sorghum	332	11.0	3.3	73.0	28	287	4.4	....	......	.....	.38	.15	3.9	....	......	....	1 cup
Wheat flour	400	11.5	1.1	83.7	17.6	9.6	3.2	1.1	95	0	.48	2.9	3.9	0	2.2-3.5	2.4	1 cup
Wheat germ	246	17	6.8	33.7	57.1	745	5.5	1.4	530	0	1.39	.54	3.12	0	......	2.5	1 cup
Vegetables:																	
Chickpeas, dry	359	20.8	4.7	60.9	162	344	8.4	....	......	90	.49	.18	1.6	Trace	......	....	1 cup
Corn, sweet, raw	92	3.7	1.2	20.5	9	120	.5	.3-.4	240-370	390	.15	.12	1.7	12	......	.01	1 ear
Corn, sweet, cooked	119	3.8	.98	28.2	7	73	.84	....	......	546	.15	.14	1.9	11.2	......	....	1 ear
Cowpeas	44	3.4	.3	9.2	53	65	1.1	2	560	1,520	.16	.10	1.1	34	......	....	1 cup
Lentils, dry, split	204	14.4	.72	36.2	20	175	4.4	1.8	720	342	.34	.14	1.3	3	......	....	¼ cup
Lima beans, raw	96	5.6	.6	17.6	47	118	1.7	.75	510	210	.16	.08	1.05	24	......	....	½ cup
Lima beans, cooked	76	4	.32	14.6	23	62	1.4	....	......	232	.11	.07	.88	12	......	....	½ cup
Mung beans, sprouts	23	2.9	.2	4.1	29	59	.8	....	......	10	.07	.09	.5	15	......	....	1 cup
Mung beans, dry	339	24.4	1.4	59.7	91	320	6.3	....	......	40	.68	.21	2.0	3	......	....	1 cup
Peas, green, raw	74	5	.3	13.3	16.5	92	1.4	.75	278	510	.26	.12	2	20	1.6	.52	½ cup
Peas, green, cooked	42	2.9	.24	7.3	13.2	73	1.1	....	......	432	.15	.84	1.3	9	3.6	Fair	1 cup
Peas, dry, split	344	24.5	1.0	61.7	33	268	5.1	42	880	370	.77	.28	3.1	2	......	....	½ cup
Popcorn	54	1.8	.7	3.1	1.5	39	.38	3	33.6	70	.057	.017	.31	0	......	....	1 cup, popped
Pumpkin seed	541	30.9	43.1	17.9	33	1,290	12.7	....	......	80	.25	.13	2.0	....	......	....	1 cup
Red Kidney Beans, cooked	230	14.5	1	42	122	316	4.8	....	......	0	1.3	.13	2	0	3.1	....	1 cup
Soybean, dry	695	73	38	73	477	1,230	16.8	8.4	3,990	231	2.25	.63	4.8	Trace	......	39	1 cup
Soybean sprouts, raw	50	6.6	1.5	5.7	51	72	1.07	....	......	192	.25	.21	.85	14	......	....	1 cup

Seeds and Mental Power

By J. I. Rodale
Editor of *Prevention*

Is there such a thing as a brain food? It used to be thought that fish was such a food. Nutritionists in discussing it refer to the phosphorus contained in fish as being a brain stimulant. But this idea has been more or less debunked. Let us, however, consider seeds as a food for the brain. Seeds will also satisfy the requirements for phosphorus. In fact, they contain ten or twenty times more phosphorus than fish. Seeds are truly a brain food.

It is a known fact that animals that are fed raw grain seeds can perform much more work than those grazing pasture grass exclusively. This, of course, is work, not brain power, but let us look a little further.

I will quote G. A. Sutherland, M.D. in his *A System of Diet and Dietetics,* 1925: "Thus among the rodents, the stupid rabbit, unable to climb and with little prehensile power, has to be content with a bulky diet of comparatively innutritious herbs, while the more intelligent squirrel, a nimble climber and possessed of considerable prehensile power, is able to procure highly nutritious seeds and a considerable amount of animal food as well. The intelligence and nimbleness of rats, again, enable them to procure highly concentrated and palatable foods, and to place under contribution even those that man has stored for his own use."

Again, later on, this author states: "The frugivora, which include animals like the squirrel, the rat, and the monkey, consume vegetable food in its more concentrated forms, such as seeds and nuts. Being generally more intelligent than the herbivora, and gifted also with the inconsiderable prehensile powers, they are able to pick and choose their food more cleverly; and hence securing it in much more concentrated forms, they are provided with a much less bulky digestive system than the herbivora."

In the early primitive days of civilization, while man ate plants and fruit, a goodly part of his diet was in the form of seed which was consumed without any cooking, tampering or processing. In this regard Dr. James Empringham in his book *Intestinal Gardening for the Prolongation of Youth,* gives a remarkable instance of how food can sharpen the faculties of the human body. He says: "In the Pyrenean mountains, that separate France from Spain, there is the most interesting cave the writer has ever explored. At some remote time, masses of rock fell down, completely covering up the entrance to this natural, subterranean chamber, so that this marvelous museum of prehistoric art remained buried, according to geologists, for at least fifty thousand years, until rediscovered by accident some years ago.

"That the cavern had been the resort of human beings in former ages is evident from the crude drawings that still decorate the interior. These sketches consist, for the most part, of outlines of animals, long extinct, which hitherto were known to science solely by the fossilized remains found in the Earth's rocky strata. The roof of this cave is embellished with representations of the midnight sky. But among familiar constellations, such as the Great Bear, there appear stars that can be seen by no person now living, except with the aid of a telescope.

"Now, inasmuch as the savages of that distant age had no knowledge of glass, and possessed no instrument for assisting the eye, these pictures seem to prove that the people of that far off time, had much stronger vision than men of today.

"Strange as it may seem, there is much evidence to prove that, not eye-sight only, but all of the senses of modern man—hearing, feeling, tasting and smelling—are less acute than the faculties possessed by our remote ancestors."

Seeds Down Through the Centuries

In Biblical times a great deal of seed food was part of the daily dietary. Dill and cumin seeds were considered so important that tithes were paid with them. In his book *Jewish Magic and Superstition,* Rabbi Trachtenberg says that Baladur (Anacardia) was a memory-strengthener. He advises further for strengthening of the memory, "Eat hazlenuts for nine days, beginning with 6 and adding 6 more each day; eat pepper seeds for nine days, beginning with one seed and doubling the dose until it reaches 256 seeds on the ninth day, and each time before you consume them, recite Deut. 33:8-11 and Psalm 119:9-16; grind cloves, long peppers, dates, ginger, galanga-root, and muscot nuts in equal quantities, beat them with olive oil into a paste, and eat a little every morning before breakfast."

The Romans, at the end of their gluttonous feasts, ate spice cakes flavored with aniseed. Seed cakes charged with a large variety of seeds, were a standby of the Middle Ages. Vernon Quinn in *Seeds—Their Place in Life and Legend* describes an Englishman of Pepys' time commending seeds as "marvelously good for a melancholicke person, excellent fine for such as be of a cholericke nature even to free the sleep from monstrous nocturnal visions."

There seems to be some evidence of a dependence in olden days on eating seed to either strengthen the mind, to free it of conditions brought about by dissipation, or to cheer it up generally. Our common sense should tell us that the mind is nourished by the food we eat, and that seed food, containing so much potent, living quality should be an excellent means of maintaining its health.

Today there seems to be a noticeable deterioration in mental energies. With so much consumption of cola drinks, white hot dog rolls, ice-cream, candies, etc. by our teen-agers, is it any wonder that the colleges are complaining that there are not enough applicants for the more difficult courses of science, chemistry, etc.? Will there be enough technicians in the future to man the complicated Frankensteinian system of science that is being set up today? Researches must be set going to reevaluate all the factors of our nutrition insofar as it affects the operation of our minds as well as our bodies.

Is it possible that a body that is strengthened by consuming a certain portion of live seed food will be proof against cancer? Who knows? Nobody has researched it.

We once had an old parrot, about 90 per cent of whose diet was sunflower seed. And was he smart! He could sing a wonderful soprano, trilling in human fashion, without uttering a false note. When a knock came on the door he would always say, "Come in!" That is intelligence! There is many a cola-consuming teen-ager today who hears a knock on the door and who is too lazy to say, "Come in."

The value of seeds in connection with furnishing human mental energy should be investigated.

Seeds—Adding to Your Diet

Acorn

In *Seeds—Their Place in Life and Legend* by Vernon Quinn (Stokes & Co.) appears the following: "The same year, 1608, a colonist in Virginia was writing home to London of the strange uses the 'Salvages' made of seeds they gathered in their fall woods and fields. 'The Acornes, being boyled, at last affordes a sweet oyle, that they keepe in Gourdes to anoynt their heades and joynts.'

"Acorns, in those days, were a common food throughout all of America, wherever an oak tree grew. But the eating of acorns was by no means limited to the American Indians. Today in the mountains of Albania, and in other parts of the world, the poorer inhabitants live very largely on acorns. In Chaucer's day even the upper classes in England relished them. 'Thei weren wont lyghtly to slaken hir hunger at euene with acornes of okes'."

In a bulletin published by the Missouri Botanical Garden in 1924 the subject of acorns as food for modern man is discussed. Say the authors: "With modern kitchen equipment, acorn meal can easily be prepared at home. After husking the acorns they should be ground in a hand-grist mill or food-chopper. The meal is then mixed with hot water and poured into a jelly bag. The bitter tannin, being soluble, will be taken out by the water, but sometimes a second or even a third washing may be necessary. After washing, the wet meal is spread out to dry and is then parched in an oven. If it has caked badly, it should be run through the mill again before using.

"In cooking, acorn meal may be used in the same way as cornmeal. Its greatest fault is its color, muffins made from it being a dark chocolate brown; the taste suggests a mixture of cornmeal and peanut butter, and some people relish it at once, but others, it must be confessed, have to be educated to it. Because of the high oil and starch content of the acorn, it is very nutritious and is reported to be easily digested. Only acorns from white oaks should be gathered, as those from the black oaks are too bitter. Typical Missouri representatives of this group are the white oak, the swamp oak, the bur oak, and the chestnut oak.

"Muffins, ⅔ acorn and ⅓ oatmeal, are reported to be good."

We do not know in what part of the country the white oak family is most abundant. But if you are interested in trying some acorn bread, why not ask your county agricultural agent where you might find some white oaks in your neighborhood? Chances are whoever owns them would be glad to have you gather the acorns.

J. Russell Smith in his excellent book on nut-bearing trees, *Tree Crops,* (published by Devin-Adair, New York, N. Y.) tells us that possibly far more human beings have eaten acorns than have eaten wheat, down through the centuries. The acorn was certainly a staple food long before man ever became interested in planting and reaping. One reason for the highly nutritious quality of the acorn as food is its high fat content. As Dr. Smith points out, it is not just bread that you make from the acorns, but bread and butter.

In Europe, chiefly Spain, Portugal and Italy, acorns are as common in the diet as chestnuts are here. Some varieties can be roasted over the fire and eaten as a roast chestnut is. In Spain and Portugal oak trees are cultivated for their acorn crops which sell for high prices in the markets. Dr. Smith mentions that there are thirty-eight references to edible acorns in many parts of the world in the 1927 *Proceedings of the Northern Nut Growers' Association,* available from J. C. McDaniel, Secretary, Department of Agriculture, Nashville, Tenn.

We are told that ground acorns are used as coffee substitutes in some parts of the world. Their tannin content is supposed to make them powerful against chronic diarrhea. Of course to make them tasty the tannin must be removed.

Aniseeds

Aniseeds are used in pastry. Can be placed in apple sauce, stews, teas. The Romans ate aniseed cakes to aid the digestion. Then there is anisette, a liqueur that is supposed to "warm" the stomach. In Europe, especially in Germany, there are cakes with an aniseed flavoring. Anise is also used in soups.

Apple Seeds

A story in the Toronto *Globe and Mail* in the year 1941 (sorry, no further date available) tells of experiments on apple seed oil at the University of Oregon Medical School in which muscular diseases in laboratory animals were cured by the use of the oil. It was assumed that the vitamin E in the oil worked the miracle, for the cures went on even after all other Vitamin E had been removed from the diet.

At present, of course, we get vitamin E from wheat germ oil, a richer source. But it is well to keep in mind that all seeds contain vitamin E. And it is extremely difficult to get enough of the vitamin E in any other kind of food. Before you start to eat apple seeds in quantity, however, see the article on Editor Rodale's experience with them.

Bananas

The little dark spots on the inside of the banana are not seeds. The banana is seedless. This fruit has lost its seed through propagation for many generations by division. In its wild state it was almost filled from one end to the other with large seeds that were like stones, with just enough pulp in it to attract birds and wild animals.

Barley

Barley, a cereal popular in some parts of the world for bread-making, is used in this country chiefly for making beer. Fermenting barley results in malt which, in turn, is used in making beer.

We understand that barley used to have a medicinal purpose—being used to make hot poultices to apply to infections. It is perhaps the oldest cereal food. It was cultivated in China twenty centuries before Christ. It was also known in ancient Egypt, Greece and Rome and among the lake dwellers in ancient Switzerland.

Basil

Early herbalists believed that a decoction made from it would alleviate sadness. Basil leaves are flavorful with tomato dishes, salads, meats, sauces, and egg dishes.

Beans

Wherever possible, in the summertime, some beans should be eaten raw. Possibly in the winter, beans can be softened by soaking so that they can be eaten without cooking. Columbus ate cakes made of pounded beans and corn. Both are delicious in the raw state.

The iron in beans is in a much more available state than that in leafy vegetables. I quote from *Association of Southern Agricultural Workers Proceedings,* 37-38, 1937 pages 257-258:

"For many years it has been assumed that green leafy vegetables, especially spinach, were particularly valuable in the diet because of the assimilable iron which they contained. More recent investigations have revealed that while green vegetables are important sources of essential minerals and vitamins, a fairly large proportion of the iron which they contain may not be available for hemoglobin regeneration.

"A number of years ago this department began work on leafy vegetables to determine their actual value for hemoglobin regeneration. Turnip tops, mustard, collards, spinach and two varieties of lettuce have been tested for their anti-anemic potency. Composite samples of the dried ground vegetables were fed at a level of .25 mgs. of iron per rat per day six days a week, to groups usually of eight or more rats. At the end of 16 weeks the average hemoglobin for the different groups of rats was as follows: Those receiving New York lettuce 12.8 gms.; Grand Rapids lettuce 11 gms.; turnip tops 12.3 gms.; spinach 10.4 gms.; mustard 9.2 gms.; and collards 6.5 gms. A second lot of turnip tops from the California Vegetable Concentrate Company was fed to a group of rats whose hemoglobin averaged only 6.3 gms. at the end of 16 weeks.

"It was then decided to test cowpeas, a vegetable very commonly eaten in the South, both in the fresh and dried state. Two different composite lots were fed to two groups of anemic rats. By the end of the sixth week the average hemoglobin of both groups was 14.1 mgs. A third lot of cowpeas, also soybeans, butterbeans, and pinto beans have been tested for their anti-anemic potency. All hemoglobin reaching a level of between 13 and 14 grams by the sixth or seventh week, and remaining at about this level during the experimental period.

"The ash as well as the unashed vegetable was tested for its anti-anemia potency. The results indicated that a fairly large proportion of the iron in the unashed green vegetable was not available. By ashing the vegetable and feeding the ash in solution, all the iron was made available. Copper was also a limiting factor since the addition of copper increased the anti-anemic potency of both the ash and the unashed vegetable."

Berries

Strawberries are full of seed. They used to be prescribed for diabetics and arteriosclerotics because they are not too rich in sugar. The small seeds exert a mild stimulating action in the bowels. In raspberries the seeds are larger. Other berry seeds are currants, gooseberries and blackberries.

Buckwheat

Buckwheat is a cereal almost totally ignored in America. New York and Pennsylvania are the only two states which produce any significant amount of it. The blossom has a distinctive taste which in general people either like intensely or dislike just as intensely. Most of the buckwheat grown is used for flour to make hotcakes or pancakes. Unhappily it is generally quite thoroughly refined and plenty of other flours such as wheat are added to the buckwheat flour.

However, for those who like the flavor, there is probably nothing that can compare to a breakfast of buckwheat cakes, made from real, whole buckwheat flour, freshly ground. Raise the batter with yeast, to add B vitamins and flavor. Don't think of betraying a wonderful flour like this with baking powder! If you have a sweet tooth, pour some real genuine maple syrup over the cakes. This is an almost pure carbohydrate breakfast and we don't recommend it for frequent use. But for once in a while, it's a taste treat!

Many farmers plant buckwheat for its honey. The flower comes late after most other flowers are gone. And buckwheat honey has a completely distinctive flavor. After you have once acquired a taste for it, any other kind of honey may seem insipid. Buckwheat honey is dark in color, meaning that it is richer in vitamins and minerals than light-colored honey.

Buckwheat has recently come into prominence for quite another reason—as a source for rutin, the flavonoid which has been performing such marvels for patients with high blood pressure. Though buckwheat flour is a perfectly nourishing food we would not suggest using it as a source of rutin. The rutin is extracted from the buckwheat by a long chemical process and is highly concentrated. You can get your flavonoids from rose hip preparations and fresh fruits.

Cantaloupe

In this fruit there is a vast amount of seed that is thrown away. I could not find any data on it anywhere. It would be worth while experimenting with it. It enriches the garbage of many of our cities.

Caraway Seed

Caraway was well known to Egyptian priest-physicians before the book of Exodus was written. Culpeper says of it, "Caraway comfits once only dipt in sumgar syrup and a spoonful of them eaten in the morning fasting as many after a meal, is a most admirable remedy for those that are troubled by wind."

In Shakespeare's *Henry IV,* Squire Shallot invites Falstaff to a pippin and a dish of caraways. In Scotland to this day a saucerful of caraway is put down at tea to dip the buttered side of bread into and called "salt water jelly" . . .

Caraway seeds can be used in baked apples, apple sauce, soups, goulashes, and served to eat as is after meals. Try them with baked potatoes and in salad dressings.

Cardamom

The seeds of an oriental herb, cardamom, which have a pleasant, aromatic odor and an agreeable spicy taste. They are used in curries and as spices in cakes, liquors and so forth. In the east they are chewed, like betel nuts.

Carob Seed Pods

Strictly speaking, we do not eat the seeds of the carob. We eat the seed pods. The seeds themselves are too hard to eat. Carob pods are the fruit of the carob tree, related to the honey locust, also called St. John's bread and probably the food spoken of in the Bible as "locust."

Carob is a splendid food, rich in protein, carbohydrate, vitamins and minerals. It is an excellent substitute for sugar and for chocolate, since it is sweet and has a chocolaty taste.

Celery Seed

Celery seed peps up soups, stews and salads. This is one of the commonest of our seasonings. We can find nothing indicating the possible nutritive content of celery seeds, but we recommend them highly for their fine flavor, especially desirable for those who are on a salt-poor diet.

Coconut

All of the coconut inside the tough outer shell is a seed—the largest we have. Because they grow on beaches close to the sea, coconuts are bound to be rich in many minerals that may be lacking in land-grown seeds. Many of the most precious of these food elements are concentrated in the brown skin that clings so tightly to the white meat, so you should eat this skin when you eat coconuts.

In older times coconut meat was said to be very effective for ridding the body of intestinal worms. In tropical countries today it has the reputation of being good for disorders of the liver and stomach. But, then, in tropical countries where it grows, it forms the main staple item of diet and it contributes generously to the nutrition of all those folks wherever it is widely eaten.

Coriander Seeds

Coriander *(Coriandrum sativum)* seeds are crushed and used in cakes, bread, sausage, cheeses, baked apples, or with game or poultry. They are used in the food industry in making gin and curry powder.

The seeds were considered by the Chinese to confer immortality.

Corn

America's favorite and most famous grain. The history of corn goes back farther than we have any records. Apparently it was known to the very earliest inhabitants of the western hemisphere. We discuss corn in detail in other articles in this book. Don't forget one thing about it—how delicious it is raw—right from the stalk.

Cucumber Seeds

Cucumber seeds, we are told, had medicinal worth: "To such as are payned with the cough, if so many seedes be taken vp and vsed at a tyme, as may handsomely bee taken vp with three of the fingers, and these after the bruising with Commyne drunke in Wine, doeth in short tyme amend the same."

Cumin Seed

The fruits (or so-called seeds) of the *cuminum cyminum* are hot to the taste. They contain lots of tannin and are one ingredient of curry powder. In olden times they were eaten with bread, wine or water as a remedy for squeamishness! During the middle ages this was one of the commonest of the European spices. A stimulant and carminative (powerful against flatulence and colic) it is used today mostly by veterinarians.

Dill Seed

Dill *(Anethum graveolens)* is a delightfully tasty seed that adds so much to pickles, salads, soups, fish, meat, egg and vegetable dishes. Oil from dill has been used in the manufacture of gin. In the East it is ground and eaten as a condiment. Dill vinegar, made by soaking seeds in vinegar for a few days, is relished by many.

Dill is a very old herb, being well-known to our ancestors, who used to chew the seeds in church. In a medical botany of the 19th century dill seeds made into a tea were mentioned as a cure for obesity. Hiccoughs could also be cured, it was said, by boiling the dill seeds in wine, then tying them in a cloth and smelling them.

Elderberry Seed

The fruit of the elderberry bush, used widely today for wine and jelly, used to be prescribed for a reducing diet—"to consume the Fleshe of a corpulent Bodie" is the way the old herb books said it. We do not know how elderberries happened to achieve this fame. We do know that birds eat the elderberries ravenously so that one is lucky to find a bush that has not been completely denuded before he reaches it.

Fennel Seed

Fennel *(Foeniculum vulgare)* is sometimes made into fennel-water which is supposed to be a cure for upset stomachs. The seed is supposed to aid in the digestion of beans and cabbage. The volatile oil that comes from fennel is probably the same as that from aniseed.

In an old herb book we ran across the note that fennel tea (made from the seeds) will relieve colic in children. And is good for an eyewash. In cooking, fennel adds to the flavor of puddings, soups, cakes, sauerkraut and spiced beets.

Fig Seeds

Fig seeds, those tiny, crunchy specks in figs, are said to be curative of constipation. Often they pass through the digestive tract unchanged. One should make an effort to chew fig seeds carefully to get all the possible benefit from them.

Flax Seed

The flax plant *(linum usitatissimum)* was apparently found growing wild in this country by the early American colonists. Flaxseed oil (or linseed oil as it is generally called) is used widely in paints and varnishes, printer's ink and artist's colors. The oil is used in Eastern Europe as a cooking oil.

Old magic lore has it that flax seeds were the source of special magic, which changed as the moon changed. When they were gathered by the light of the full moon, they were used in brewing love potions. If you gathered them when the moon was dark, on the other hand, they could do harm to an enemy.

So far as diet is concerned, flaxseeds are a good source of the unsaturated fatty acids so essential to human welfare. We sometimes call them collectively vitamin F. They are also reputed to have a laxative effect. Some authorities believe them to be highly nutritious. The Indians of the Andes use them extensively as their favorite food—ground flaxseed with barley.

In ancient Greece and Rome flaxseeds were a great delicacy, munched between courses of a banquet much as we eat toasted nuts. The herb books tell us that tea made from flaxseed is good for respiratory disorders.

Grape Seeds

Some time ago a firm was established to make oil from grape seeds. We have no information on their food content but it seems likely that they contain valuable elements as do other seeds. It would seem best to eat them along with the grapes. Chew them carefully so that they can be digested. There is no evidence, incidentally, that appendicitis can be caused by eating the seeds of any fruit.

Hempseed

Hempseed is the seed of the hemp plant *(Cannabis sativa)* which is cultivated chiefly as a source of raw material for the manufacture of rope. The seeds are widely used in India and are considered more delicious than sesame seeds. Hashish, the drug, is made from hemp leaves and resins. Hemp seed is a fine bird food and the crushed seed is made into cattle food.

Hollyhock Seed

The Hollyhock seed was powerful against respiratory disorders, according to an ancient informant, "boyled either in milke or wine and orderly drunke doe remoue a hot cough, recover the Lunges blistered, and is a singular remedie against the consumption of the Lunges."

Lentils

The word *lens* which we use for a ground glass contrivance, was taken from the humble lentil, the sides of which are shaped about the same as a lens. The lentil is perhaps the oldest vegetable cultivated. Well known to all the ancient peoples, it figures in early mythology. And superstition.

One historical note concerns the early Christians who were worshipping in the catacombs during the time they were being persecuted by the Romans. They wished to have flowers growing before the altar, but no flowers would grow without light. They discovered that lentils and wheat would sprout and grow in the dark. So these two seeds were annually planted in earthen pots on Ash Wednesday. By Maundy Thursday they were high enough to be carried to the altar. Italians still observe this ancient rite.

The old herbalists were of two minds concerning the medicinal value of the lentil, some of them claiming it was beneficial as medicine, others condemning it as hurtful. However, we know today that lentils rank high among legumes and that they should form a more important part of the American diet. They can be used to advantage in any recipe that calls for dried beans. They mix well with tomatoes, onions, cabbage, vinegar, mustard, mushrooms.

Lettuce Seed

Lettuce seed was supposedly curative for a number of ills, but only if it was used without the patient's being aware of it! "The lettuce seedes brused and mixed with the white of an Egge applyed in plaister forme on the temples or forehead warme at the going to rest dooth marvelously procure sleepe." Lettuce leaves can be used, it seems, in case there are no seeds handy. But the leaves must be pulled up by the root by the left hand, before the sun rises and laid under the invalid's pillow so that the bigger end of the stalk and leaf lie toward the feet!

Lotus Seeds

We were enchanted to find lotus seeds listed in a book on the foods of the Eastern peoples. Imagine eating the seeds of that fabulous and exotic flower which appears so often in Egyptian and Hindu art! The lotus eaters, according to the Odyssey, were languid, dreamy and indolent because they ate lotus. Perhaps they ate the flower rather than the seed. We rather believe the seed would produce vigor and stoutheartedness, for it contains plenty of protein and minerals. Calcium, phosphorus and iron are all found in the lotus seed. Before you write in to ask, let us assure you that we know of no one in this country who has lotus seeds for sale!

Mustard Seed

Mustard seed is commonly used today in pickle recipes. The "hotness" of mustard seeds was recognized in the old herbals, for they were used for gargling a sore throat. They "amendeth the blistering of the mouth and asswageth the swelling of the throate. The person which every morning fasting shall swallow down two mustard seedes at a time shall be free that day from the falling sickness (epilepsy). The pouder of the seedes drawne vp by the nosthrills not onely procureth the creature to sneese, but marvellously purgeth and amendeth the braine."

Another herbal counsels using mustard seed against dimness of sight and spots and webs in the eyes. A mixture of mustard and vinegar would also quickly cure the bite of a venomous beast.

Or, for those with palsy: "The Mustard seedes retained under the tongue prevaile against the palsey of the tongue. The seedes do like profit against all kindes of palseys hapning in any parte of the body if a linnen bag filled with the seedes and boyled in wine be applyed on the grieved place."

Even today mustard is highly esteemed for making poultices. We have read recommendations in the most conservative of medical journals for using mustard baths for infants in a state of shock or convulsions. Of course the "hotness" of the mustard readily brings the blood to the skin when the mustard is applied.

Millet

Millet is a cereal, *panicum miliaceum,* botanically speaking, although when we speak of it we generally mean any of a number of related cereals. Its origin was probably Egypt. It is used in the form of groats and makes excellent bread especially when it is used in a mixture with wheat.

It is easily grown, even in very dry or cold climates. It is not used much for human food in our country, but is used extensively in the East. An interesting story about millet is told by Mark Graubard in his book *Man's Food* (Macmillan). Two African tribes, studied by a group of nutritionists, both had millet as their basic food. One tribe, superior in physique and health, was found to have an abundance of calcium in their diet. The other tribe, weak and sickly, was found to have a deficiency of calcium. So the millet was studied. That of one tribe contained 16 times as much calcium as that of the other. Was it the kind of millet, the kind of manure used, or the kind of land it was grown on? In our book on the food content of Far Eastern foods we find that one kind of millet is listed as having 20 milligrams of calcium, another as having 329 milligrams!

Nasturtium Seeds

Nasturtium *(tropaeolum majua)* is sometimes called Indian cress. Many people use both the seeds and leaves of nasturtium in salads or pickle the seeds, as one would a small cucumber.

Nutmeg

Nutmeg *(Myristica fragrans),* used widely today as a flavoring ingredient, had some therapeutic value, we are told in the old herbals. It was good against freckles in the face and it quickened the sight. We do not know whether the nutmeg was to be applied or eaten in order to do away with freckles.

Mace is a part of the nutmeg seed. These two spices have been known in Europe only since the twelfth century, making them fairly recent members of the spice family. They were used to fumigate the streets of Rome during the coronation of an emperor. The Dutch, coming into possession of the island of Banda, enjoyed a monopoly on the nutmeg trade by destroying all trees that happened to grow on any other island. Birds, however, swallowed the seeds of the Dutch trees excreted them elsewhere and thus spread the culture of nutmeg trees to other islands.

Nutmeg was used for its antiseptic properties in the early days. In fact, it made a fine embalming fluid.

Okra Seeds

Okra seeds, roasted and ground, have found use as a coffee substitute, supposedly a very tasty one. Oil is also extracted from the seeds.

One researcher has investigated okra thoroughly and bred it for its seeds. He found it not only rich in oil for industrial use, but he also bred a strain that would yield up to 2000 pounds of seed per acre with an oil content of up to 400 pounds. He states also that the okra seed is high in food value.

Parsley Seeds

Parsley *(Petrose linum sativum),* a plant rich and running over with vitamins A and C, was treasured in the old herbals for its power to "fasten loose teeth, brighten dim eyes and relieve a stitch on the side." We do not know the vitamin content of parsley seed. But the plant itself in large enough quantity in the diet could well provide enough of vitamins A and C to cure a case of scurvy (loose teeth) and night blindness (dim eyes). (See note on sprouting parsley seed in the article on *sprouting seeds* later in this book.)

Pepper

Pepper is the berrylike seed of the pepper plant which grows in hot humid climates. The method of curing the pepper determines whether you get white or black pepper. For centuries pepper was in such demand as an herb that it commanded a high price and was often specified as a tribute or fine. When the barbarian Alaric, king of the Goths, threatened Rome in 409, he demanded a price of 3000 pounds of pepper, among other tributes.

During the Middle Ages it became immensely precious in Europe. Medical men at that time believed that there were four "humors" which operated to produce health or sickness in the body—blood, yellow bile, phlegm and black bile. Blood was hot and moist and phlegm was cold and moist. If any one of the humors was out of order you could repair it by providing a medicine that would restore its original qualities. Hence pepper, being hot, could cure diseases in which the blood was thought to have become cold. It was used, too, for curing indigestion, mistiness of the eyes and other complaints.

How many spices you could afford in your food became a measure of snobbishness in Medieval Europe. We suppose that a large part of the reason for the craze for spices was that there was no refrigeration and little was known about preserving foods in other ways. Spices could be used as preservatives and also to conceal the taste of rancid or spoiled food. Then too, the perfumes of spices became valuable in an age when baths and personal hygiene were almost unknown.

At any rate, we are told that to this day poor children in some European countries taunt a richly dressed youngster as a "pepper-licker" —a phrase which undoubtedly goes back to the economics of the Middle Ages when only the rich could afford to have pepper every day.

Peony Seeds

Peony seeds were used as medicinal herbs in Greek and Roman times and later in Anglo-Saxon kitchen gardens. The flowers were used for flavoring and the seeds were carried as a charm against evil spirits.

According to an old herbal: "It is found by sure and evident experience that the fresh roots tied about the necke of children is an effectuall remedie against the falling sickness (epilepsy)." The seeds "to the number of fifteene taken in wine or mead is a speciall remedie for those that are troubled in the night with the disease called night Mare, which is as though a heavy burthen were laid vpon them and they opprest wherewith, as if they were overcome by their enemies or ouerprest with some great weight or burthen. And they are also good against melancholicke dreames."

Gardeners who specialize in plant personalities will tell you that peonies are extremely sensitive. They grow well only for those who appreciate them, say these experts. They do not like to be transplanted; one of our gardener friends tells us they will grow well only if you talk to them as you would to a child. This gardening lore seems to be tied in with their reputation against psychological ills.

Pine Cones

Dr. Smith in his book *Tree Crops,* quotes Dr. Robert T. Morris as saying that nuts in pine cones are near the head of the list of nut foods for human use. Dr. Morris states that there are about thirty species of nut-bearing pines between Quebec and Florida, that one species at least produces nuts the size of the average English walnut, others may be as small as a grain of buckwheat.

Many of the pine trees produce nuts that are edible either raw or cooked. Some of them are rich enough in starch to provide a staple starchy food for natives of South America, South Africa and Australia. Some of them are oily and may be pressed to yield a thick milky substance which can be kept for a long time and used essentially as a substitute for meat.

The reason why we know so little about these marvels of the conifer world is that, according to Dr. Smith, pitifully few of us are interested in tree crops—an error which Dr. Smith tries valiantly and emphatically to correct in his excellent book, *Tree Crops* which is published by Devin-Adair, New York.

We are told that pine cones were used freely by the old herb doctors, for almost any disorder. Fir cones were "wholsom and much nourishing whilst they are fresh, and although they be somewhat hard of digestion yet they do not offend; especially if they be steeped three or fower houres in warme water before the taking, to soake out their sharpnesse and oylinesse."

Pinon

The seed of the pinon pine. A pine nut, highly recommended as all pine nuts are, because they grow in the wild and so can't have been subjected to any chemical treatment.

Pomegranate

A fruit of ancient times. The flesh clings so tightly to the seeds that it must be sucked off. For this reason we do not generally do anything with pomegranate fruit except juice it.

The old Roman legend of Proserpine and Ceres involves the seeds of the pomegranate. You remember, Proserpine, abducted into the Underworld, refused to eat, mourning for her mother, Ceres, whom she thought she would never see again. Finally she ate six pomegranate seeds. When Ceres came to rescue her, it was decreed that Proserpine must stay one month in the Underworld for every pomegranate seed she had eaten. That is why, said the ancient storytellers, we have six months of summer (when Proserpine is on earth) and six months of winter (when she is in the Underworld).

Poppy Seed

Poppy seed is one of the better-known seeds in this country, since it is in wide use on breads and cookies. The seeds are so small that as many as 30,000 of them can be obtained in a single pod. Opium is not made from the seeds, but from the unopened pods of the poppy. But the tradition of sleepiness and death is continually associated with the poppy.

The poppy's name came from a custom of giving children the seeds mixed with their "pap," for "the Poppie seedes (after bringing to pouder) mixed with new milke as broth and given to children to drinke warme procureth them to sleepe." For adults, too, the poppy means sound sleep —"The Garden Poppie boyled vnto the thickness of honey profiteth vnto many griefs. The Seedes confected with sugar and eaten doe marvelously prevaile in procuring the weake patient to sleepe soundly."

Psyllium Seeds

Psyllium seeds, from the plant fleawort, are sold by the drug houses as a laxative. Their action is chiefly mechanical; the seeds swell to create bulk in the intestine (which of course occurs quite naturally in the digestive tract of anyone who eats foods in their natural state, rather than refined). The seeds lubricate, too, to a certain extent.

Rapeseed

The rapeseed comes from a plant of the mustard family and the seed has much the same characteristics as mustard seed. It is made into oil—not in wide use in this country.

Rye

Rye seeds have been found in tombs in association with weapons of the Bronze Age period, so we can assume that this is a very old cereal indeed. Bread made from rye flour is apparently less likely to cause allergies than that made from wheat.

One caution about eating rye products exclusively. Ergotism is a quite serious disorder caused by eating rye that has been infected with ergot, a disease. We read quite recently in a medical magazine of a theory that just the tiny amount of ergot that might be present in our carefully tended American rye might be enough to produce symptoms, if you are a heavy consumer of rye bread to the exclusion of other kinds.

Senna Seeds

Senna seeds were used in olden times for medicine. Infused in whey and then boiled they were a "physicke" against melancholy and many kinds of depression and sadness. Used as a laxative in modern times, they are generally combined with some aromatic herb to prevent griping.

Sesame Seeds

Sesame Seeds *(Sesamum)* used constantly over the centuries in the East, are almost unknown in this country. The Turkish candy, Halvah, available in some large cities, is made from them. Oil from sesame seeds, used in the East as a cooking and salad oil, contains a large percentage of the unsaturated fatty acids (vitamin F).

We think that sesame seeds almost equal sunflower seeds as a between-meal snack. And they can be ground finely and mixed with coconut or any other nut, poppy seed, honey, figs or any other healthful food to make a tasty candy. We have read of one case of allergy to sesame seeds, but we imagine this must be extremely rare, especially in this country.

Sorghum

Sorghum is a grain grown in much the same manner as corn. It is hardier than corn in that it will grow in regions that are consistently too hot and dry for corn. In other countries, in Africa and Asia, sorghum is used as food for both human beings and animals. In this country we feed it to the stock. It is said to have about 90 to 95 per cent the feeding value of corn. It should be supplemented with feeds that provide vitamins A and D, protein and calcium.

During the war when our sources of tapioca were lost to us, some enterprising food chemist discovered that a certain kind of sorghum could be used to replace tapioca. (Tapioca comes from the cassava plant. It is a root product, not a seed.) So a limited amount of the sorghum grown today is used for this purpose. Far more was used during the war to make alcoholic beverages.

Squash Seeds

The seeds from all kinds of squash and pumpkins have been known for centuries as good food. We have in our files a story written for us by a researcher who lived among the Maya Indians in Guatemala. The seed of the pepitoria squash has been one of their chief sources of protein and fats for centuries. Combined with corn, beans, fresh vegetables and fruits, the squash seeds round out an excellent diet and undoubtedly are responsible, at least in part, for the good health, fertility and excellent teeth of these people.

A learned Doctor from the Connecticut Agriculture Station made the headlines several years ago when he succeeded in breeding a squash whose seeds are "naked"—that is not covered with a tough hull. The gourd-like plant which he developed produced seeds which gave about twice as much oil per pound as the soybean and about one and one-half times as much as the cotton seed. Their protein value is high, too.

At the last report, which we read in 1948, the squash seeds were available in nut stores, toasted, buttered and salted. Readers should raise their own squashes and save the seeds or buy them unroasted and unsalted from a nut store.

Watermelon Seeds

We have several stories in our files on the potency of watermelon seeds in cases of kidney trouble. One is a story that appeared in the Allentown *Evening Chronicle* on January 1, 1946. A Mrs. Helen Kelly was near death in a hospital, according to this story, when her doctor decided to try watermelon seeds. He boiled three tablespoons of them in a quart of water resulting in a tea which stimulated the kidneys and brought this kidney patient back to complete health.

Apparently the same tea has been used in many other instances with success. We do not know why watermelon seeds should have any extraordinary effects on kidneys. But we are certain that they could do no harm and may indeed contain some substance that is a specific for kidney health.

We know that the protein of watermelon seed is worth while with a biological value of 73 and a digestibility of 92 per cent.

Seeds—Proteins of

We hear a lot these days about protein, foods containing it and the importance of protein-high foods in the diet. Vegetarians believe that they get enough protein in fruits, vegetables, nuts and cereals. Those who eat animal products declare that only in these foods can "complete proteins" be found, and so animal products must be included in healthful diets. What do we mean by "complete proteins?" Do any of the seed foods contain them? Can the seed foods be used as the only source of protein in a healthful diet?

Protein is the substance of which we are chiefly made. Blood, tissues, organs, skin, hair, nails, bones and body fluids are protein. Brain and nerves are protein. The proteins of which the body is made can be broken down into what we call "building blocks"—the amino acids. There are probably many more of these than have been discovered, but we know of some twenty or so. These amino acids, or building blocks of protein, are present in foods. When we eat these foods our digestive processes rearrange the amino acids, combining them in different ways, so that they can be built into body structure.

A grain of wheat or even a whole bushel of wheat grains do not look like a human brain. Yet after the wheat has been eaten, the amino acids it contained will go to form part of the protein of which the brain is made. Or the nerves. Or the blood.

Certain of the amino acids are absolutely necessary to health and life. We must have them to survive. So they are called the essential amino acids. There are ten of these whose names are: arginine, histidine, isoleucine, leucine, lysine, methionine, phenylalanine, threonine, tryptophan and valine. As researchers progress in their study of the proteins, it is quite possible they may discover that one or more of the other amino acids at present listed as "unessential" may also have important functions in the body so that it cannot be replaced. However, it seems that we may be able to manufacture within our bodies some of these unessential ones. We cannot manufacture the essential ones in our bodies, so they must be supplied in food. Animal proteins supply all of the essential amino acids. Of course the animal was made of protein, too, so it is only natural that the amino acids involved would be the same ones that we human beings find essential.

But in the case of foods of vegetable, seed or fruit origin, we find that most of them lack one or more of the essential amino acids or they contain it in such small quantity that it cannot be used by the body to put together another form of protein.

Corn contains less than half a gram of tryptophan for every hundred grams of corn. This is not enough to support life. In other words, one cannot live on a diet in which corn is the only protein, without suffering from certain diseases which indicate that there is an important protein missing. Peanut flour seems to rank high in most of the amino acids. But it is far below where it should be in methionine and tryptophan. Soybean flour which comes the nearest to supplying "complete" protein is still a little low in methionine and tryptophan.

So someone who depends on soybean foods for protein should go out of his way to eat some foods rich in methionine and tryptophan *at the same meal.* We stress the fact that the essential amino acids must all be eaten at the same meal. If you eat corn as your only protein at lunch and then use some food rich in tryptophan, such as eggs, at dinner time, the corn protein was wasted. For it does not tarry in your digestive tract waiting until some other food with just the right arrangement of proteins comes along.

The Arrangement of Amino Acids is Important for Good Diet

So eating a haphazard diet especially if you are a vegetarian, will not only bring ill-health, but will also result in wasting proteins which are the most precious elements in our food. The vegetarian who eats eggs or any other form of animal protein will not, of course, get into this difficulty. The vegetarian who takes brewer's yeast is even less likely to get into trouble, for the proteins of brewer's yeast are remarkably complete.

We sometimes hear of staunchly health-minded people who avoid all the refined foods, eat plenty of fresh raw fruits and vegetables, watch their diets closely and otherwise respect health rules. But they are not healthy. Perhaps, much oftener than we know, the reason is that they are not getting "complete" protein at their meals. That is, they are not getting enough of all the essential amino acids to keep rebuilding the worn-out protein cells of the body.

If you have several nutrition books at home you may find that the amino acid content of different foods varies in the different charts that are given by different authors. Of course no two pieces of food contain exactly the same amount of any food element, so naturally each researcher will get somewhat different results in his tests. But, in addition to that, we have word from eminent agricultural authorities that the protein content of our cereals is decreasing due to the fact that our soils are wearing out faster than we can rebuild them with our present methods of agriculture. So take this into account, too when you are figuring the amount of protein you expect to get from cereals and legumes.

To conclude what we have to say about the proteins of seeds—eat seed products along with a wide variety of other foods. They do not provide a healthful diet by themselves. Do not look to them to provide all the protein you need, unless you are a wizard at juggling amino acids and combining just the right ones at each and every meal. Laboratory researchers who have devoted their lives to this kind of juggling find it next to impossible to provide healthful diets using seed proteins as the only source of proteins.

On the other hand, most of us get far, far too little protein. The adult man should have 70 grams of protein every day. The average woman sixty. The requirement for children ranges from 40 (for one to three-year olds) to 100 grams a day for boys from sixteen to twenty. Even in prosperous times, even those of us who can afford to eat the best seldom get this amount of protein. Protein food is the most expensive there is. We crowd it out of the diet with refined carbohydrates, desserts, snacks, candy, sodas and all the other trash we put into our stomachs.

So, add additional protein to your diet using seed foods! Don't use them as a substitute for good meat and egg protein. But substitute them for the worthless foods you and your family may sometimes consume. Seed proteins are fairly inexpensive and while they are not "complete" proteins, still they add to the total protein you get in any one day and, when taken with foods that do contain whole proteins, they are well used by the body.

So substitute nuts or sunflower seeds for candy or soda when you're preparing snacks. Get in the habit of sprinkling ground sesame, sunflower seeds or nuts over salads, vegetable dishes, fruit cups. Have an attractive fruit bowl of nuts with a nutcracker ready on your living room table. Keep a jar of tasty seeds handy to munch on. If you're trying to decide between macaroni or beans for supper, choose the beans, for macaroni made from white flour contains little but starch. Get acquainted with soybeans which, more successfully than any other nonanimal food, can substitute for meat at a tiny fraction of the cost of meat. Try nibbling on fresh wheat grains instead of eating bread. Use seeds as they occur in nature and they will enrich your menus with additional protein.

Seeds—Poisonous

Many seeds are provided by nature with very effective protection against loss or destruction. Nature is, above all, interested in propagating everything that grows. So she takes good care of seeds, which carry the germ of the new plant. We are all familiar with the many devices that assure seeds of wide circulation—the dandelion's frothy silk that, swept by the wind, carries the seed and spreads it; the burr that sticks to passing animals and so broadcasts the tiny seed inside, the seeds that float on water, sail in air or scatter when they are brushed by passing animals.

Some seeds are protected by being poisonous. In this way nature saves them from animals which would eat them, for of course the animals soon learn which seeds can be eaten with impunity and which cannot. Some seed poisons are lethal to men and some to animals but not to birds or certain other animals. So far as we human beings are concerned, we need not concern ourselves especially about these seed poisons unless we are in the habit of breaking off and munching strange plants and berries as we walk through woods or meadows. Or unless we have young children or animals who may play near to where such seeds grow.

There have been many cases on record of children being poisoned by the seeds of the poison hemlock. This is not the hemlock tree, incidentally, but an herb which looks somewhat like Queen Anne's lace. The whole plant is poisonous to human beings—so poisonous that even a few seeds nearly always prove fatal. This is the hemlock that Socrates drank.

Water hemlock and spotted hemlock are other members of the same family, equally poisonous. Water hemlock, also called cowbane because of its poisonous effect on cows, looks not unlike celery and has seeds that look like anise seeds. Water dropwort, another poisonous plant, is in the same family.

Monkshood (aconite) is a lovely tall spike of blue flowers in the fall, more graceful and delicate than the delphinium. And deadly poison in all its parts. Now surely this is no reason not to plant monkshood for it will add charm to any garden. But don't plant it near the playpen and don't keep your flower seeds in the food cabinet. Foxglove or digitalis is another strong poison, especially the seeds. Of course the essence from them is used as a drug, for heart disease sufferers.

The "deadly nightshade" is the plant from which belladonna is made. All of the plant is poisonous to eat, but especially the seeds. Black nightshade is poisonous, too. And the berries of bittersweet—the lovely bright orange and red berry that vines over autumn walls. Lily of the Valley, wood anemone and laurel seeds are poisonous.

It's surprising how many seeds we list as poisonous that are being used in drugs today. The seed of the handsome castor oil plant is poisonous. Yes, of course, castor oil is made from the seed. And the same mother who warns her children from picking the seeds off the vine and eating them will probably resort to castor oil when "the children need a laxative" without giving it a second thought. The very fact that the seed of the castor bean is poisonous should make us hesitate a long time before ever taking castor oil as a laxative.

More Seeds to Beware Of!

Pokeweed has poisonous seeds. This bush has purple berries that country children used to make into "ink." The seeds of yew are another deadly morsel for human beings. Birds, however, eat them ravenously and harmlessly, as well as the pokeweed seeds. Henbane is a small, disagreeable weed whose seeds are deadly to hens as well as to human beings. The seeds were formerly made into oil and usd as a gargle to cure toothache! Apparently the juice contains some kind of narcotic.

Jimson weed, mandrake, Dog's Mercury, poison sumac, "snow-on-the-mountain," "burning brush" or "Spingle tree," poison ivy, mistletoe, holly, laburnum—all these have seeds that are poisonous to human beings. Wild cherries and peaches have a powerful poison *in the kernel inside the seed.*

One of the most unusual poisons is found in the fava bean which is grown widely in Europe for food. Just smelling the blossoms causes illness in some individuals and eating the beans can cause death. There have been about 1200 cases of *favism* in this country recently, mostly caused by eating the first young green beans. Some persons are so sensitive to the fava bean that they have attacks of favism each spring when the blossoms or the beans appear. The tendency seems to run in families.

Other individuals may eat the fava beans for years without ever having any trouble. We do not know how doctors interpret this peculiar poisoning that may emanate from the fava bean. It sounds like an allergy to us. And, unless you are in the habit of eating fava beans, don't give the matter a second thought. This is a definite family of bean, and is so listed in seed catalogs. So you needn't fear that you will ever get fava beans when you ordered snap beans.

A book entitled *British Poisonous Plants,* Bulletin No. 161 of the Ministry of Agriculture and Fisheries in England, a handsomely illustrated book, blithely lists hundreds of poisonous plants, including even wheat, rye, onions, barley, clover and scores of others. In fact, by the time we had finished reading, we had about concluded that almost anything, eaten in excess, can be poisonous. However the seeds we discussed in this article are, in general, the ones most likely to be encountered on a walk in the woods or fields. They should be avoided.

Seeds—Sprouting

Peoples of other lands and times, less surfeited with good food than we, have learned tricks for improving the nutritional content of their meals. Tricks which we would do well to study and emulate. Sprouting seeds is one of these. This practice has been known from earliest times, especially in the far eastern countries where sprouts are used as commonly as we use onions or celery.

Why should we sprout seeds? The sprouted seed contains more vitamins than the dry seed. It's just that simple. When the seed is given water and warmth, whatever it is in seeds that starts them to growing gets busy. The seed puts forth a tiny sprout, green and crisp. And as this sprout grows, vitamins are formed in it, right before your very eyes. A dried seed contains little or no vitamin C. But as sprouted seeds grow, their vitamin C increases. For instance, 100 grams of whole oats contain 11 milligrams of vitamin C. After they have germinated for 96 hours, they contain 20 milligrams. After they have germinated for 120 hours, they contain 42 milligrams. Dry peas increase from a vitamin C content of zero to 86 milligrams of vitamin C after 96 hours of germination.

The story of the other vitamins is even more astonishing. Seven parts of thiamin (a B vitamin) become nine parts in the sprouted wheat. And as for the rest of the B vitamins, listen to what happens to them: riboflavin increases itself by about four, niacin, pantothenic acid, pyridoxine and biotin just about double their content. And what about folic acid—that precious B vitamin which prevents pernicious anemia, that vitamin so scarce and rare in food that none of us ever get enough of it? Twenty-eight parts of folic acid in a wheat seed become 106 parts after sprouting! In addition, we are told by Dr. Francis Pottenger, Jr. of Monrovia, California, that the sprouts develop into complete protein capable of sustaining life. While you watch, then, protein is manufactured before your very eyes, along with vitamins.

Sprouting seeds is almost a brand new idea in this country, we suppose, because we have always had such a profusion of good, nutritious food available. So information about sprouting seeds is not easy to come by. However, during the last war when we were fearing further food shortages, Dr. Clive M. McCay of Cornell worked on the possibility of promoting sprouted soybeans as an all-around good nutritious food.

A report of his work occurs in *Science News Letter* for May 22, 1943. Soybean sprouts are rich in protein and fat, minerals, including calcium and usable iron and vitamins, he says. The Cornell workers developed easy methods of sprouting which involve nothing more complicated than a container from which drainage is possible. Place the beans in the pot and pour water over them. Be sure to let the water drain off and keep the beans moist and warm. Cornell students found that they had to develop a taste for the soy sprouts. But apparently plenty of seasoning would help so far as taste goes.

The best book we have found covering seed sprouts and how to sprout them is Catharyn Elwood's book, *Feel Like a Million,* which is an excellent all-round book on other aspects of nutrition as well. (This is published by Better Nutrition Institute, 2025 Park Rd., N.W., Washington 10, D. C.) Miss Elwood suggests several methods for sprouting and gives a number of recipes for using the sprouted seeds in tasty dishes.

Says she: "Sprouts from almost every bean (especially the mung and soya beans) peas, lentils, wheat, alfalfa, rye, corn and millet make delicious and nutritious additions to your vegetable bill-of-fare selection." She then goes on to describe several different methods of sprouting, all of them involving, of course, moisture and warmth. She tells us that "sprouts are ready for use as soon as the sprout is seen. The longer the sprout, the more nourishment. When the green appears, vitamin A and chlorophyll are developing. However, most sprouts are less delicious if too long. Here are my preferences:

"Wheat sprouts are most delicious when the sprout is the length of the seeds.

"Mung bean sprouts are best when 1½ to 3 inches long.

"Alfalfa sprouts are best when 1 to 2 inches long.

"Pea and soybean sprouts are good short or long.

"Lentil sprouts mold quickly so must be used when about one inch long.

"Sunflower seed sprouts are best when no longer than the seed. If longer they develop a strange objectionable sting in the throat after eating.

"When the sprouts have developed to the desired stage, put them in a closed jar in the refrigerator. They keep like any fresh vegetable for a few days if properly covered."

How to Sprout Seeds and Use the Sprouts

Some of Miss Elwood's recipes for sprout dishes involve: almond-mushroom chop suey, vegetable casserole, sprouts with eggs, chicken à la king with bean sprouts, and so forth. We strongly recommend your getting the book *Feel Like a Million* for its information on sprouts as well as the other splendid nutrition suggestions it contains.

Some years ago, Dr. Pottenger (to whom we referred earlier) wrote us about his own enthusiasm for sprouting seeds. He said, "Among those seeds which I have found most interesting are, of course, the common ones: wheat, rye, oats, barley, corn, alfalfa, clover and parsley. As you know, the list of seeds that can be used is long. The most tasty of the sprouts I have tried so far is parsley when used as a salad. As a breakfast food I prefer the alfalfa. Such common seeds as navy beans, red beans and so forth, when sprouted, require only ten to fifteen minutes to cook, instead of two to three hours. The mung bean also works up well either as a salad or as a cooked vegetable.

"I have experimented with many ways of sprouting, and have found that the methods commonly described in present-day periodicals have been entirely unsuccessful in my hands. With large quantities of seeds, however, the tray sprouter or Japanese method have worked very well, as has a modification of the Korean method, using a strawberry box. The Chinese way, involving the earthenware pot (or flower pot) was only fairly satisfactory, while milk bottles, mason jars and similar utilities only tend to enhance the growth of mold. I have had the greatest success by rolling the scattered seed inside a bath towel and dampening this roll from time to time.

"I have found that good seeds that get plenty of oxygen during the act of sprouting do not mold. Seeds of low sprouting capacity, an index of poor soil fertility, often succumb to this."

One final word about sprouting seeds comes from the *New York Times.* We do not have the date but we assume the article appeared during the war. In this article Roberta Ma recommends sprouting beans in a flower pot of two-quart size. Cover the hole in the bottom of the pot with a piece of crockery, she says. Wash thoroughly and soak a quarter of a pound of soy beans for about six hours, until they are plump and the skins burst. Then put the seeds into the flower pot. Sprinkle water on the seeds daily, perhaps twice a day or oftener, to keep them moist. In three or four days at room temperature the sprouts should be ready—just branching, without any show of green.

We hope that many readers will get into the habit of sprouting seeds regularly. It is economical, healthful and, really, not a lot of trouble. It's certainly less trouble than peeling vegetables or making cookies or frying foods in deep fat or any of those other kitchen tasks we used to engage in before we realized that they were not only unnecessary but positively harmful. Sprouting seeds takes no time at all, except for the few minutes of sprinkling them. All the rest they do by themselves with the help of nature. Why not start now to accustom your family to some new recipes, using sprouted seeds?

Seeds—Conclusion

By J. I. Rodale

Editor of *Prevention*

I believe we have opened up a new avenue of thought in the field of nutrition. We have been eating some seeds without being aware of what we were doing, or how to handle them to best conserve their life-giving elements. In this day of processed, refined, factoryized food, we have, in the form of seeds, a safety valve so to speak, because seeds are rich storehouses of vitamins and other rare as well as undiscovered substances.

When the eating of sunflower seeds will dissipate the blackness of my toenail, when they will enable me to be out in the snow without seeing pink, there must be a powerful element in them which must strengthen every part of the body. I have noticed that if I eat sunflower seeds every day, I can be at the beach without sunglasses.

To anyone bothered with constipation, the eating of seeds will be a boon. There must be dozens of other beneficial effects produced in the body by eating seeds of various kinds. And those of us who are worried about the effect of chemical fertilizers on our foods will now have an anchor, the secure feeling that seeds are a class of food which feel the effects of chemical fertilizers the least.

But we must not go overboard on the subject. Study it carefully. Eat more seed foods, but don't overlook your vegetables, meats, fish and eggs.

Eggs

I would like to dwell for a moment on eggs, the most wonderful food that God has created. An egg is just one big seed, and in it, as in the average plant seed, there is sufficient food to keep the emerging entity alive for several days. But there is a tremendous difference in the nutritional value of a fertile egg as compared with a non-fertile one. What is the difference? A hen can lay an egg without a rooster being present but such an egg will not hatch out anything. It is an infertile egg. It lacks the living germ. It is not a seed.

It is a commentary on the short-sighted policy of our Government that it encourages the production of such eggs. Because a fertile egg will spoil quickly in storage, due to the presence of the germ, the U. S. Department of Agriculture encourages poultrymen to keep roosters out of their flocks. This type of infertile egg has a higher economic value, but what about the nutritional needs of the consumer? The United States Department of Agriculture has nothing to do with that. "That is for doctors," they will no doubt say, if pressed. But I'll wager that the average doctor doesn't even know that a hen can lay an egg without a rooster's having a part in the transaction.

Yes sir. The average doctor does not know agriculture, and the average agriculturist does not know the simplest facts about human nutrition.

The egg is a seed, if it is a fertile one, and everyone should eat at least two of them a day. But try to discover a source where roosters are kept, if you wish to get the utmost nutrition out of your eggs. In future research I will go more deeply into the subject, for I have the medically researched evidence that a fertile egg is far more potent nutritionally in its effects on the health of the human body than an infertile one.

According to the latest researches, a heart case should not be told to avoid eating eggs because of their cholesterol content. It is not a matter of cholesterol as such, but the total fat consumption. The average American eats a diet which is 40 percent fat. That is why we have about the highest mortality rate in the world from heart disease. We must cut this fat consumption down to about 20 percent. My advice to a heart case is to eliminate milk and all dairy products such as cheese and butter. Eat eggs because they are seeds with certain living qualities that will help the heart case. This will cut down your consumption of fats. Also, cheeses and butter are heavily laden with salt, which is very dangerous to a heart case. To get the full value of the egg as a seed, consume it raw. Make an eggnog of the yolk only. The white of an egg contains avidin, a toxic substance if consumed raw. Cooking neutralizes its toxic properties.

Now, coming back to seeds generally, remember, I don't say to eat seeds exclusively. Be reasonable about it, as in everything else. And continue with your vitamin pills, bonemeal, etc.

If you are a city person, study seeds in the country in the summer when you go there for your vacation. Get acquainted with farmers who perhaps will ship you seeds during the winter and other seasons, seeds which you might persuade them to set aside for you without poison spraying.

Seeds is a subject regarding which very little has appeared in medical literature. This is the first time that it has been covered in such detail anywhere. It marks a new building block in the structure that we are rearing in a program to enable people to live the maximum number of years possible. It is not the last step. We are in the midst of a search. Gradually we will add more to our program. We may have to eliminate some too. But eventually we will come up with something that is very close to the Fountain of Youth. But of course man will never attain the utmost in perfection.

As Sir Robert McCarrison has said in his *Nutrition and National Health* (Faber and Faber, England):

"Given the will, we have the power to build in every nation a people more fit, more vigorous, more competent; a people with longer, more productive lives, and with more physical and mental stamina than the world has ever known."

Shoulder

Pain and stiffness in the shoulder have become so commonplace that quite a considerable number of articles in medical journals are devoted these days to the causes and possible cures of these disorders.

There are several reasons why our shoulders appear to be especially susceptible to strain and injury. First of all is our upright posture. Animals walk on four legs. But man walks on two, with the result that he has problems of posture which animals do not have. The whole construction of a shoulder seems to make it that part of us that can most easily be strained or hurt by our daily activity. Because man uses his hands almost constantly all day long, the shoulder has a lot of work to do. Then, too, much of today's kind of activity requires monotonous and often difficult use of the shoulder. We will discuss some of these circumstances later on.

Meanwhile there is the curious "syndrome" as doctors say, called variously painful shoulder, frozen shoulder, peri-arthritis (inflammation of the tissues around the joints) the shoulder-hand syndrome and so forth. Generally this kind of disorder appears first after the age of forty or so. It is common to both men and women. Sometimes it is serious enough to result in complete disuse of the shoulder which means a serious crippling of the individual's activity. *The Medical Journal of Australia* recently devoted several articles and a long discussion to this problem. Selwyn Nelson, M.D., of Sydney tells his physician readers that if pain is present only in the shoulder and in no other joints, no one should suspect rheumatoid arthritis, for it definitely is not that. He also describes a condition which, he says, is quite common among women at the time of menopause. It consists of a tingling sensation in the hand, occurring most often at night, which may be combined with pain in the upper arm and shoulder. There may be blanching and a feeling of coldness in the hands, too. He suggests relieving this condition by exercise that will improve posture. He also advises against the carrying of heavy shopping bags or anything heavy.

Richard Hodgkinson, M.D., also of Sydney tells us that all the many modern activities we engage in often demand an "extended and abducted" position of the arm to which the shoulder joint has not become accustomed. He tells us, too, that shoulder pain in later years is often caused simply by degeneration of the tendons. They are growing old. If an examination shows that there is no physical injury in the joint, he advises rest, pain pills and heat treatments as the best form of therapy. He concludes by saying "it is obvious, however, that there are many other causes of this condition which are not understood and much work is still required."

In the pages after these two articles, we have the report of the discussion that took place when these two papers were read before a medical society meeting. And we are inclined to agree with the comments of several of the physicians present who remarked that they were quite disappointed with the papers that had been read—actually, they asked, what more do we know about painful shoulders than we did before? They wanted to hear of new cures, new therapies.

Causes of Painful Shoulder

Mark B. Coventry, M.D., of Rochester, Minnesota, discusses painful shoulder in an article in the *Journal of the American Medical Association,* January 17, 1953. He says there are four possible causes: 1. muscular, which may mean overuse, fractures, dislocations, bad posture, tumors or calcification of joints; 2. nervous—caused by inflammation of nerves; 3. visceral—that is, the shoulder pain may actually originate in a gall bladder, heart or pancreas disorder; and 4. vascular—when there is a disorder of the blood vessels.

He discusses the possibility of occupational causes for shoulder pain. One patient of his worked in an overall factory and, when he had finished his particular operation on a pair of heavy overalls, he had to throw them over his shoulder onto a pile. Shoulder pain is also common among farmers after a session of especially heavy work such as silo-filling. But some occupational hazards are less obvious. One of Dr. Coventry's patients was a retired school teacher who had taken a job as a typist. The extended position of her arms as she typed all day was the cause of her painful shoulder. Another patient was a baker who decorated cakes. Apparently he stooped over a table, with his muscles tense, all day as he worked away at this very fine and intricate work.

Disuse can cause a painful or stiff shoulder, says Dr. Coventry. When a joint has been immobilized in a cast of course there is pain when you begin to use it again. On the other hand, when there is pain, you have a tendency not to use the shoulder, so that it becomes stiff. Then when you try to use it again, those creaking unused muscles give you such a twinge that you decide not to try to use them, thus leading to more stiffness.

Finally, says Dr. Coventry, there is the factor of the "peri-arthritis personality." A painful shoulder becomes stiff only if the patient does not use it and if the patient has a personality which makes him susceptible to this kind of disorder.

The "Peri-Arthritis Personality"

Three physicians of Madison, Wisconsin, discuss this kind of personality in greater detail in an article in *The American Practitioner* for May, 1953. They examined 300 patients who seemed to have psychosomatic illnesses and found that 60 of them suffered from pain and stiffness in the shoulder. Their ages ranged from 25 to 55 years; most of them were in their forties. The majority of them had other complaints along with their bad shoulders: headaches, some kind of chronic nose trouble, weakness and fatigue, dizzy spells, stomach trouble, heart trouble, or some muscular discomfort, such as muscular aches, cramps in the legs, and so forth. All of them, say our physicians, were tense and likely to over-react to physical stimulus—the kind of people who jump nervously at a hand laid on the shoulder or a leaf dropped on the hand. In most of these folks, an X-ray showed no physical injury or disorder in the shoulder.

Questioning elicited the discovery that in almost all cases the pain and stiffness had begun at a time of particular stress and heightened emotion. This does not mean necessarily some grave emergency. These people were the perfectionist kind who thought of themselves as self-sufficient, independent and energetic. They were all overly-conscientious. They lived well-planned lives, following rigid patterns of activity and any interruption of their well-laid plans brought frustration. But, gritting their teeth, they "carried on" bravely, all the time unconsciously resenting the fact that their responsibilities were too heavy.

In their daily work they did not use their hands or arms more than the average person, but they did everything with their muscles under tension which created a lot of resistance in the voluntary muscles which were working along at their usual speed and tension. "The protracted co-existence of these two opposing forces plus the vulnerability of the shoulder joint might explain why this structure is so frequently the site of this type of musculoskeletal disability," say the authors.

So these patients were given psychotherapy. We do not know of what this consisted. But we suppose that the psychiatrist or psychologist simply by talking to them managed to convince them that there was absolutely no need to be so tense, hurried and conscientious about the things they were doing. Actually no matter how hard we try none of us can be perfect. So if we plan to get something done by noon, let's try working at it in a relaxed fashion. If we succeed, fine, if not, then let's not get worried, tense and upset about it. Let's postpone it for the next day, without any regrets or self-blame. This is not a plea for laziness. But those folks who work (or play) at too intense a pitch are well aware of what they are doing. And if they wish to avoid ill-health they simply must learn to relax and not try so hard for perfection. In the case of the sixty patients, the psychotherapy worked wonders. They learned to take things much easier and, as their muscles relaxed, their shoulder pain disappeared.

All the articles in our file on painful shoulder mention the factor of personality. Whether you take it from the point of view of a psychosomatic personality—that is, someone who unconsciously interprets frustration or insecurity in terms of actual physical illness—or whether you decide that the muscular strain of such overly-conscientious people results in stiffness and pain in the shoulder, it boils down to the same thing—a defect in personality that somehow brings about a quite serious and common disorder.

Preventing Stiff Shoulder

Articles in our file discuss the use of various pain-killing drugs, deep X-ray, diathermy, injections of novocain and posture exercises. Of these, only the last gets an approving nod from us. Our field is not cure, but it seems to us that painful shoulder might be prevented by sensible rules of good health. We all know surely when we are overworking some particular part of us and we should know enough to stop before this overwork results in pain or stiffness. Yes, even if it means changing jobs, it would certainly be worth it.

Our research has shown us, too, that vitamin B is a preventive of muscle stiffness. Calcium helps prevent stiff muscles. And the diets of most of us are deficient in these two food elements. Brewer's yeast and bone meal are good sources.

Editor Rodale discovered something helpful in his own experience with shoulder pain. Several years ago he noticed that his right shoulder was painful. He thought it might come from doing so much writing with a pencil gripped hard in his hand. He switched to a typewriter and the pain disappeared. But he did not like to type, so he had to find some other solution. He began to use his left hand, rather than his right, whenever he could—in opening doors, putting on his hat, eating, brushing his hair, and so forth. As he gradually began to make his left hand do more of the inconsequential manual work, his right shoulder improved. Furthermore, he did a little research and found that the theory of using one side to rest the other side has long been known to primitive people. The American Indians practiced it in their long journeys by land. They marched part of the way using the right foot harder than the left, then shifted and made the left foot do more work. When you are eating dinner tonight, check and see if you are naturally chewing on just one side. You can bring on a fine case of malocclusion that way. So make a conscious effort to use both sides of your mouth in chewing—or chew first on one side, then on the other.

Interestingly enough, time and motion study experts, whose profession it is to get industrial jobs done with the least effort, the most production and the greatest saving of time, have found that one of their most important principles is to get both hands to share the work, so that neither of them becomes overly tired. Time and again, by proper planning, these experts have arranged a given piece of work so that both hands work at once or so that each hand works equally with the other, thus saving time, motion, money—and incidentally, making the job faster, easier and not so tiring for the worker.

One final caution. We noted throughout these medical articles how often the pain in painful shoulder occurred, or at any rate was worse, at night. It seems to us quite possible that an explanation of many of these cases might very well be incorrect sleeping positions assumed. As Editor Rodale has shown in his book *Sleep and Rheumatism,* no one knows exactly what is the best or healthiest position in which to sleep. But he has discovered a number of very significant things about ways *not* to sleep.

For instance, do you sleep with a pillow? Try sleeping without it. Give your blood a chance to circulate freely around your shoulders, neck and head, without the constriction of a pillow to interfere. Do you sleep with your arms crossed behind your head? What does the weight of your head do to the circulation in your arms and wrists? Do you often lie on one side with your whole arm flattened out beneath you? Don't you often wake to find that arm stiff and numb from lack of circulation? Do you ever sleep with one wrist crossed over the other and pressing down hard? All of these errors in sleeping positions and many more are reviewed, pictured and discussed in *Sleep and Rheumatism.* You can secure a copy from Rodale Press for 35 cents. The answer Editor Rodale has worked out is simply to re-educate yourself for sleep, by training yourself to sleep without constricting any part of your body and stopping the circulation. Perhaps this is one of the best preventives for "stiff shoulder."

Sinus

The sinus can be most easily defined as a hole in the head. Except for the fact that we have not just one hole in the head, but many. Sinuses, that is. Their purpose is surely not just to cause us trouble, yet sometimes it seems as though they had been created specifically for that.

Actually the sinuses in one's head are holes in the bones of the skull. They help to lighten the bony structure which would otherwise be quite a burden to carry around. In addition, they act as sound boxes for the voice. The vocal chords might be compared to the strings of a violin. The sinuses, then, are like the space enclosed in the violin proper in which the sound waves reverberate It is not by accident that many of our greatest singers have come from the sunny countries of the south, such as Italy, where vitamin D is plentiful and hence bony structure is good. The nasal passages, sinuses and throat of a Caruso have a great deal to do with the magnificence of his voice.

Here are the words of a famous sinus expert, describing the different sinuses and their location: Says Dr. Lucius Bush in his book *The Secret of Sinusitis and Headaches* (Liveright Publications) "Let us see how these sinuses are arranged. I mentioned previously the sphenoid sinuses, a pair of sinuses high up and toward the back of the nasal passages. The openings from these sinuses point almost directly forward. In front of them and slightly below are the posterior ethnoid sinuses which drain inwardly toward the nasal septum, the partition which separates one nasal passage from the other. There may be a half a dozen or more of these posterior ethnoid sinuses. In front of them lie the anterior ethnoid sinuses which drain mostly in an outward and downward direction. Both anterior and posterior ethnoid sinuses lie in the ethnoid bone about the middle turbinate (another bone). Near the anterior ethnoid openings are the openings of the frontal sinuses and antra. The frontal sinuses lie in the forehead above and between the eyebrows and their openings point downward, while the antra lie in the face under the eyes and drain upward into the nasal passages. In all, we find an average of fifteen or twenty nasal sinuses in the normal head. Some open outward, some inward, some up and some down."

There is no reason to remember all the names of the various sinuses, unless your doctor uses them in diagnosing your case and you want to have some idea of what he is talking about. What it boils down to is that all these various holes are grouped about your nose, and drain, one way or the other, into your nasal passages. Sinusitis and sinus trouble of any kind are involved chiefly with the drainage problem. As you can see from Dr. Bush's statement, the sinuses open up or down or out or in. We don't know why Nature (usually so efficient) should have bungled things so badly in relation to our sinuses. Unless, of course, we were meant to spend much more time on all fours, lying on our backs or standing on our heads, in which case fluid from all the sinuses would drain easily.

You see, the openings from most of these sinuses into the nasal passages are no bigger than the thickness of the lead in a pencil. The secretions that accumulate when one has a cold are thick and gummy. They can't get through! Dr. Bush explains the peculiar position in which the sinuses open by saying that we were meant to clear the sinuses of mucus by blowing our noses. Air can be blown forcibly through the nasal passage, says he, and it is blown over the fifteen or twenty individual sinus openings, if the nasal passage is normal. The passage of air creates suction which draws the liquid up so that it can be expelled by the air. So in the normal nose, it is easy to empty all of the sinuses simply by blowing the nose. Hence many people never have any trouble at all with their sinuses and don't know what it means to suffer the excruciating pain of sinusitis.

The sinusitis sufferer, on the other hand, has obstructed nasal passages for one reason or another and so fluid secretions collect in his head. The pressure of the fluid is what makes the pain. Someone whose nasal passages are narrow may be able to keep them well drained most of the time. But when a cold comes along and the mucus membrane inside his nasal passages swells, fluid may accumulate and sinusitis may be upon him.

Sinusitis

If you have a healthy and well-formed nose, you probably won't have sinus trouble. If you were born with nasal passages that are too narrow to perform their function, or if you have suffered from a blow on the nose, chances are that you have or may develop sinusitis.

The sinuses (cavities in the bones of the skull) open into the nasal passages. In some cases this small opening is at the bottom of the sinus; in some cases it is at the top or the side. Normally, blowing one's nose clears all secretions from the sinuses, for as the air passes over the sinus openings, the suction created draws the fluid out into the nose. However, if the passages of the nose are too small to accommodate the air, or if some injury to the nose has closed up those passages, the mechanism will not work and secretions begin to accumulate in the sinuses. Then, too, when you get a cold, the mucus membrane of the nose swells and may shut off the nasal passages. Most cases of severe sinusitis start from a bad cold.

Lucius M. Bush, M.D. in his book *The Secret of Sinusitis and Headache* (published by the Liveright Press, New York City, N. Y.) tells us that man has a long history of sinusitis. Ancient skulls show the effects of surgery which apparently was performed to ease the pain of sinusitis. In fact, Dr. Bush goes so far as to say that more than half of the human beings who ever lived have had acute or chronic inflammation of the nasal sinuses. He also believes that at least two thirds of the world's headaches are related to sinus disorder.

He tells us that the nasal membrane is extremely sensitive to all kinds of influences. A little loss of sleep, cold or wet feet or a draft at the neck may be all that is necessary to cause the membrane to swell and become congested. Many people even have some nasal congestion after a heavy meal. In head colds, the inflammation spreads along the mucus membrane into the sinus. It cannot get out since the membrane has swollen, so it causes more mucus, which produces pressure inside the sinus. The accumulated fluid becomes coagulated, thick and gummy. When there is enough of this fluid to overflow, it is forced out into the nasal passage, but the sinus is by no means drained. If the nasal passages are too narrow, or swollen with congestion from the cold, the rest of the mucilagenous matter remains in the sinus and causes more and more irritation.

Operations for sinus conditions are not notably successful. When surgeons make new openings into the sinus cavities the bones and cartilage tend to grow back together, so the project fails and the sinus fills up with fluid once more.

Dr. Bush has developed a unique method of treatment which resulted from a cold that he himself contracted. Using his finger, he pushed against the side wall of the nasal passage, which relieved the congestion in his nose. When it became stuffed again, he repeated the massage and found that gradually his nose cleared and he was able to breathe once again. Trying the treatment on his patients, he found that he could obtain a marked clearing of their noses and eventually complete relief from their symptoms of congestion.

One patient of his had breathed through one side of his nose for years. The nasal passage on the other side was almost completely blocked. After a number of treatments the passage opened and his breathing became normal once again. Polyps in the nose and sinuses also seemed to disappear when the proper ventilation was provided in these passageways. Dr. Bush also found that many patients suffering from asthma had narrowed nasal passage which he could manipulate to relieve the stuffiness in their heads.

Diet Can Prevent Sinus Difficulties

It is well to keep in mind how important diet is in the formation and maintenance of well-formed mouth and nasal passages. Prospective mothers can assure their children of good bone formation by eating diets in which refined foods are reduced to a minimum and vitamins A and D are plentifully supplied, as well as calcium and the other important minerals. Of course what the child eats while he is growing is important, too. Dr. Weston Price in his book *Nutrition and Physical Degeneration* available from The Lee Foundation for Nutritional Research, 2023 W. Wisconsin Ave., Milwaukee, Wisconsin presents priceless evidence that primitive peoples who have never known our "civilized" food, show, without exception, broad, well constructed mouth and nose formation. Just as soon as they begin to eat our diets, including white flour and white sugar products, the bone structure begins to change within one generation. Their teeth become crowded, the dental arch is small and narrow and their noses take on a narrow, pinched look.

The best book we know on the subject of sinus and diet is that by Egon V. Ullmann, M. D. entitled *Diet in Sinus Infections and Colds,* published by Macmillan Co., 60 Fifth Avenue, New York, N. Y. Dr. Ullmann believes firmly that modern diet is largely responsible for sinusitis. We have come to think of colds and sinusitis chiefly in terms of infections, says Dr. Ullmann, and our concept of infection has led us to believe that the infection—present through some mysterious means—is responsible for the cold and also for the feelings of ill-health that go with it.

Instead today, he says, "the trend is to look for constitutional changes which render our organism more susceptible to colds and their consequences. For want of a clearer definition we shall call the combination of constitutional weaknesses which so often leads to a series of colds, *lowered resistance* or a *rundown condition.*" The one symptom that is present in all patients with colds and sinus infections is acidosis, he continues. In other words, these patients have not been getting enough of the alkaline-forming foods in their diets.

Going further in his discussion of foods, Dr. Ullmann tells us that one of the early symptoms of vitamin A deficiency is lowered resistance to colds. Vitamin A is necessary to maintain the tissues in the skin of the body and the linings of body openings, such as the throat and nose. The mucus membrane in these linings is known to dry up considerably during the early stages of a cold. Exactly the same condition can be produced in laboratory animals by depriving them of vitamin A. Dr. Ullmann recommends natural vitamin A as it occurs in fish liver oil—not the synthetic vitamin. Vitamin A appears in most yellow and green foods, such as butter, carrots, salad greens and so forth, but there is a question as to how much of it is absorbed from these foods in a person who has any difficulty with his liver. So the wise thing to do is to take fish liver oil the year round, but especially during the fall and winter months when the cold danger is ever-present.

Proteins are important to a good diet, says Dr. Ullmann, and it is very difficult to get enough good, first-class protein without the animal foods—milk, meat, fish and cheese. However, it is well to remember that these foods are acid-forming in the body and must be balanced with foods that have an alkaline reaction. These are in general the fruits and vegetables.

However, there is one other group of foods that form acid in the body—the cereals. Dr. Ullmann gives in his book an excellent description of what happens to a grain of wheat in processing it to make bread. "If we consider the efforts other nations have to make in order to obtain the necessary amount of grain for their daily bread, it is a sorry sight indeed that the people of the United States who dispose of such wealth of grain do not make better use of it. But in the United States, a singular civilization, with all its habits and styles, is responsible for the restriction to bread made almost entirely of refined, white, wheat flour which is eaten either as toast or as any of the marketed products such as crackers, biscuits, rolls, buns, doughnuts, cakes, pies, puddings, waffles, wafers, etc. The consequences are lack of calcium and valuable minerals, a tendency toward acidosis, poor teeth, gas, constipation and sluggishness," says Dr. Ullmann.

He tells us that sufferers from colds and sinuses should keep to rye bread, graham bread and pumpernickel whenever possible. All of the cereals used should be unrefined. Sugar is another evil, says he, which should be omitted entirely from the diet if you would avoid colds and sinusitis.

Salt May Be Responsible for Sinusitis

Dr. Ullmann's chapter on table salt is the most interesting in the book. He tells us that almost all of us eat far too much salt. The amount of salt necessary to produce hydrochloric acid in the stomach is amply supplied in the food we eat, without any additional salt at all. Too much salt, therefore, can result in too much acid in the stomach which is believed to be a reason for stomach ulcer. Taking salt is merely a habit, says Dr. Ullmann. Experts tell us that more than eight grams of salt per day is injurious to the full utilization of the proteins we eat, yet many of us eat as much as 20 to 25 grams a day. Our kidneys cannot keep up with the job of eliminating this amount of salt, so it accumulates in our tissues.

However, from the point of view of sinus trouble, the reason for not eating salt springs from its relation to calcium in body metabolism. "If large amounts of sodium chloride are taken, a good deal of it will be stored in the skin, mucus membrane and other tissues and calcium will be liberated. Therefore each sodium molecule retained in the tissues will diminish the calcium effect. And this is important in preventing colds and other inflammation of the nasal passages." To prevent colds and sinus trouble, the diet should be what Dr. Ullmann calls "salt-poor"—not more than five grams of salt per day.

We are in one hundred per cent agreement with Dr. Ullmann's diet recommendations, particularly as they apply to salt, bread and sugar. In fact, we would go so far as to recommend no salt and no sugar at all for the individual who would avoid sinus infections. And as little bread as possible—only of the real whole grain variety. There are two excellent reasons for avoiding cereal products, especially in the case of children whose diet is likely to consist largely of cereals. First, they are acid forming. And secondly, they are so filling that they simply do not leave room for the fresh fruits and vegetables that are so necessary, both because they form alkaline residue in the body and because they are rich in vitamins.

Study the average cereal eater. You will find that he gets not nearly enough fruits and vegetables—that he has little interest in eating them at all.

How can one go about using the information we have given here to prevent or cure a sinus condition? First of all the diet we have outlined seems to us an excellent one whether or not you fear sinus trouble. By all means begin now to cut down on salt until gradually you are doing without it entirely in cooking and at the table. Of course this means no salty foods like potato chips, olives and so forth. Then, if you are eating much cereal food, cut down on that too. No more than one slice of bread per meal should be your rule, and less than that if possible. Of course the part of your meals that used to consist of bread should now consist of fresh raw fruits and vegetables.

If you are suffering from sinus trouble we think you should tell your doctor about Dr. Bush's discovery. He will want to get the book or write to Dr. Bush and find out more about it. In other words, we don't think you should try to give yourself this treatment, for the nose is a delicate piece of machinery and should be manipulated only by an expert. The name of Dr. Bush's book is *The Secret of Sinusitis and Headaches.* It is published by Liveright Publishing Co., 386 Fourth Ave., New York, N. Y.

Skin

Acne, psoriasis, eczema, seborrhea—even the very names of skin diseases are ugly. But not so ugly as the diseases themselves. There is probably no one thing that contributes so much to poor appearance as unhealthful skin. And there is surely no one thing that adds so much to the appearance of either a man or a woman as clear, smooth, alive skin, glowing with inner radiance that carries the beholder's eye over many minor defects in appearance. Truly, you can get away with a too large nose or mouth, a badly shaped face or a badly proportioned figure, if you have radiant skin.

Your skin displays the state of your health perhaps more than any other part of your body. We have shown the relation of vitamin A to skin health. Jon V. Straumfjord, M. D. writing in *Northwest Medicine* for August, 1943, showed that skin eruptions caused by vitamin A deficiency are very much like those of acne. They are nothing more or less than a hardening of the skin around the sebaceous duct—the small gland that produces oil for the skin. Dr. Straumfjord treated 100 of his acne patients with massive doses of vitamin A—he gave no medicine and prescribed no ointments or special skin care. Thirty-six of the patients became free from acne and 43 more were cured except for an occasional pimple. The oiliness of the skin also cleared up and a sheen and "good tone" took its place. Dr. Straumfjord believes that prevention of the disease may require much smaller doses of vitamin A than one needs to cure the disease, once it is started.

The fact that acne is commonest at puberty is a further indication that it may be the result of vitamin A deficiency. Most youngsters grow very rapidly at this time. All available amounts of vitamin A may be needed to supply this tissue growth and there may not be enough left to supply the needs of the skin which is also growing.

In another study reported in the *Journal of Investigative Dermatology* for April, 1950, Leonard E. Savitt, M. D. and Maxmilian E. Obermayer, M. D. tell us that they gave vitamin A for 18 months to a group of 65 college students, instructing them at the same time to continue with whatever self-treatment they had been using. Twenty of the students showed improvement ranging from slight to great; twelve showed no change and three showed an increase in the severity of the acne.

Dr. Merlin Maynard of San Jose, California, used vitamin D and calcium in treating 70 patients in one series and 60 in another. He reports on his experiment in *The Archives of Dermatology and Syphilology* for May, 1940. The results showed 75.6 per cent satisfactory results for the first series and 83.4 per cent for the second series. It is noteworthy that Dr. Maynard also placed his patients on a diet—lean meat, fresh fruits and green vegetables, with a minimum of carbohydrates. They were not permitted to eat sweets, chocolate, pastries, greasy or highly seasoned foods, or soda fountain items. It occurs to us that perhaps the diet had as much to do with the good results as the vitamin D had. If Dr. Maynard had included food supplements for the other vitamins and minerals, we believe he might well have had one hundred per cent success.

Multiple Vitamins for Skin Disorders

Another physician, Paul Kline of New York City, gave multivitamin preparations to his acne patients. In *The Archives of Dermatology and Syphilology* for November, 1950, he indicates that the relationship between the glands and the way vitamin A is assimilated is very important. The B vitamins, too, are involved in this process. When not enough of the B vitamins are present, the liver cannot perform its function in relation to the hormones, so vitamin A may be destroyed, rather than being used by the body. Adding vitamin E to the diet may prevent this from happening.

Dr. Kline treated 25 patients with multiple vitamin injections for eight months. Only one of them failed to show improvement. There was very little tendency for the acne to return once the injections were stopped. Of course, vitamin injections must be made from synthetic preparations. They are given in cases of disease so that as much of the vitamin as possible may be immediately put to use by the body. However, our point of view is, of course, that if one gets all the vitamins necessary in daily meals and food supplements, there will never be any necessity for vitamin injections.

Acne rosacea, which is a form of the disease more prevalent in middle age, has been cured with a diet rich in the natural B vitamins that occur in brewer's yeast and liver. Dr. Louis Tulipan of New York, reminding us that vitamin deficiencies may be present in persons who eat a perfectly balanced diet, because of failure of the digestive tract to absorb some kinds of food, tells us that he observed 96 patients for over eight years and came to the conclusion that acne rosacea is caused by lack of B vitamins in most or possibly all cases. In treating his patients Dr. Tulipan did not use synthetic preparations which contain only some of the B complex of vitamins. He used brewer's yeast, which is the natural source of all of them.

The B Vitamins and Vitamin C

We have other reasons, too, for believing that the B vitamins are extremely important for healthy skin. One of the symptoms of pellagra (a B vitamin deficiency disease) is dermatitis, or skin eruptions. An article in *The Journal of Investigative Dermatology* for January, 1953, gives us some indication as to why the B vitamins and vitamin C are concerned with skin health. This article by Teh H. Lee, Aaron Bunsen Lerner, M.D., Ph.D., and R. John Halberg, B.A., is concerned with the water soluble vitamins that are present in skin. They found that most of the B vitamins are present in considerable quantity and vitamin C is present, also.

Now perhaps we can see just why it is so necessary that vitamin preparations taken to prevent skin disorders should contain all of the known B vitamins. The fact that they all appear together in the skin certainly must mean that they work together there for the welfare of the skin as a whole. And it seems likely too that vitamin C along with the B vitamins would be concerned with all the various physiological functions that take place to keep the skin healthy.

A letter from a Turkish medical publication which appeared in the *Journal of the American Medical Association* for May 9, 1953 indicates that vitamins are important for skin disorders other than acne. The ten-year experimentation of Dr. Kemal Turgut covers lichen ruber planus and similar diseases which were promptly cured with 150,000 units of a vitamin A preparation. A boy with lichen spinulosus recovered with a daily dose of 100,000 units of vitamin A and a generous serving of carrots (rich in the vitamin) each day. A number of other patients with various kinds of skin disorders responded well to vitamin A therapy, including seven young women who had acne. In one case the patient had keratosis follicularis which disappeared when vitamin A therapy was begun, only to return as soon as he stopped taking the vitamin.

Vitamin F and Eczema

A. E. Hansen, writing in the *American Journal of Diseases of Children,* January, 1947, describes a series of 171 cases in which he found that the fatty acids were a valuable addition to his treatment of eczema. About 50 per cent of the cases which had responded to no treatment up to this time improved "markedly" when the essential fatty acids were given. Interestingly he found, too, that the diet of these children had been seriously deficient in this food element and that the eczema was often accompanied by respiratory infections as well.

Emotions Affect Your Skin, Too

Skin disorders may proceed from emotional causes, says Dr. D. Cappon, writing in the *Canadian Medical Association Journal* for June, 1951. Based on some 40 actual case histories from his own files and those of his fellow-doctors, the article presents evidence showing that skin symptoms—all the way from blushing to psoriasis—may be caused by the emotions. Dr. Cappon says that the holding-in of certain emotions may produce hives. He gives as examples a convict who developed hives daily just at the time he was locked in his cell after the day's exercise period, a manufacturer who developed an itching skin while he was watching his factory burn to the ground, a woman who would develop hives whenever she became angry with her husband under social circumstances where she could not relieve her feelings by scolding him.

Persons with asthma-eczema-itch complex are often, according to Dr. Cappon, apt to be "overanxious, needing to excel, above average in intelligence, over-dependent and over-protected." Sexual maladjustment, hatred of a cruel parent or a personality withdrawn into imaginary life often produce these conditions, he says. Fever blisters and cold sores can be produced by emotional upsets in patients who are usually submissive, obedient and sweet. Outbreaks of psoriasis also may be related to emotional disturbances, according to Dr. Cappon.

We are inclined to believe that vitamin deficiency probably comes first, then the emotional difficulty, then the skin disorder, for we know that lack of vitamins can bring about nervousness. In the case of the B vitamins alone, personality disturbances even to the point of insanity are one of the symptoms of pellagra, a disease of vitamin B deficiency. So perhaps the patients of the other doctors we have quoted developed as a result of their diet treatment much more adjustable and serene personalities along with their relief from skin eruptions.

Protein vs. Wrinkles

Protein foods may be the answer to the problem of wrinkles, according to a report by Dr. Charles S. Davidson of Harvard Medical School and Boston City Hospital at a symposium on various aspects of old age reported in *Science News Letter* for March 13, 1954. He believes that the glands may have the largest part in this so-called "withering" process. As one grows older, the glands gradually function at a decreased rate and so, perhaps, less and less protein is made available for the skin, muscles and so forth. But, on the other hand, perhaps the fact that older people tend to eat less protein is responsible for the slowing down of the glands and hence for the wrinkling of the skin. At any rate, it seems that the safest course, if you would avoid wrinkles, is to keep your diet high in protein, hence low in carbohydrates, to give your glands every opportunity to continue to function healthfully. After all, your glands, and your skin, too, for that matter, are both made of protein, so it seems only reasonable to expect that a high protein diet will keep them in good repair.

Editor Rodale recently had an interesting experience in regard to the use of salt and wrinkles in the skin. At a meeting of organic farmers he was discussing with one member the fact that we Americans use too much salt. The farmer stated that his wife had been put on a salt-poor diet by her physician, but that she absolutely refused to stay on it, declaring that she could not eat her food without added salt. Editor Rodale said, "Why not remind her that salt has a lot to do with the formation of wrinkles, because it tends to collect fluid around it in the body, which is, of course, very bad for the skin." The farmer went home and the next day reported back that for the first time in her life his wife ate a meal without dousing her food in salt. A possible improvement in appearance was powerful enough to interest her in giving up salt, even though the doctor's pronouncement about her health had not been.

Sunflower Seeds and Healthy Skin

We have long known that sunflower seeds have a most healthful effect on the skin. Just why we do not know. It may be because they are high in protein, or because they contain considerable amounts of B vitamins and vitamin A. Possibly one reason is that all their concentrated richness in food elements is easily available, since it is so simple to use them as a between-meal snack. Just like peanuts or popcorn, one handful of sunflower seeds leads to another, and if you are not careful you are likely to find you have eaten your way through a whole bagfull without noticing it. It's perfectly all right to eat as much as you want of this healthful food unless you are on a determined reducing diet in which case you had better restrict yourself to a couple of teaspoonfuls at a time, for the seeds are rich in calories. A reader tells us "After I had eaten sunflower seeds for about two months the eczema that I had on one side of my face disappeared. I had doctored for it for some time, but got no relief."

Food Supplements for Skin Health

Skin disorders are legion and volumes have been written on each one, so we cannot begin to cover them all in this article. But, in general, we would recommend a diet high in protein, low in carbohydrates and rich in vitamins A, B, C and D as well as calcium and unsaturated fatty acids, if you would have healthy skin. Fish liver oils are the finest supplement for vitamins A and D, rose hips for vitamin C and brewer's yeast or desiccated liver for all the B vitamins. Bone meal is your best natural source for calcium as well as other minerals. The unsaturated fatty acids are present in unrefined vegetable and cereal oils, as well as in some special food supplements.

Sleep and Rheumatism

By J. I. RODALE
Editor of *Prevention*

I would like to tell you the story of how I stumbled upon an interesting fact about neuritis.

Around 1940 I began to experience neuritic pains in the hands, arms and shoulders. There would be dull twinges and pains, and I found it extremely difficult to don my overcoat. If I raised my arms above a certain level the pain would increase. I couldn't turn my head without experiencing pain in the neck and shoulders. I would get up in the morning with a feeling in the shoulders and neck as if someone had sat on me all night, and my fingers had a numbness which made it difficult for me to tie my shoe-laces.

The doctor diagnosed it as neuritis, but its cause had him baffled, and in spite of months of medical treatments of all kinds, including osteopathy the painful condition persisted. As I look back now I can see that in this doctor's practice, he specialized in finding cures, but never spent any time in seeking causes. He asked me no questions about my daily life and habits in order to come upon some clue that might lead to the answer. I just kept coming and he kept treating it, mainly with diathermy, but nothing happened.

A friend of mine had about the same symptoms that I did and every time we would meet we would swap talk about our condition.

The Cause Discovered

One night I discovered the cause of my trouble. It was about 3:00 a. m. when I suddenly awoke from a disturbed sleep. My entire arm was numb from shoulder to finger tips. In fact it was practically paralyzed. I tired to think quickly, and noticed that I had been sleeping with my head on the paralyzed arm. I became convinced that this habit was at the bottom of all my trouble. My own hard head had been digging down on my arm for hours.

I stayed awake for a long time, thinking, and observing the actions of my arms and head. I would catch my arm attempting to move upward so that it could be a pillow to my head, but I fought against it. It took about a week to win complete control over them, and after that the habit was completely mastered. Never again did I sleep with my head on my arms, and miracle of miracles, the neuritis in my arms completely vanished.

I then went to see my friend who had the same condition I did, and when I related my experience to him, a light came into his eyes. He did not sleep with his head on his arms. In his case it was a way he had of folding back his left arm in a v-shape and sleeping with his body pressing on it. He now cured himself of this habit, sleeping with his arm spread out in a relaxed way, and within a week his neuritic pains completely disappeared.

When I saw how simple it was to cure these two cases I began to think of the hundreds of thousands of people who must be suffering from the same thing, and since in questioning people I found that a majority of them did sleep with their head pressing on *their* arms, I figured that I had a job to do. I had to share my knowledge with as many persons as possible. So I wrote a book on the subject in 1940, as well as several articles which appeared at that time in *Fact Digest* and *True Health Stories,* two magazines which I edited and owned. As a result hundreds of people have been cured of what I call pressure neuritis.

Medical Recognition of the Idea

I was surprised when in 1944, Dr. Robert Wartenberg sent me a reprint of an article he wrote in *The Journal of Nervous and Mental*

Disease (May, 1944) in which he mentioned my work in this field. I was surprised that a physician would mention the work of a layman.

A doctor friend of mine, a phlebitis specialist in New York, was incensed when he received a copy of my book, and said to me at our next meeting, "Why do you meddle in such things? You are not a doctor."

To give you another reaction from a doctor, may I quote from a letter received from Mrs. Susan Snyder, 135 Eastern Parkway, Brooklyn, N. Y. (Oct. 29, 1953):

"The doctor tells me that I have osteoarthritis. The pains I complained about—terrific headaches and pains from the back of the neck up and down to lower back as well as between shoulders completely disappeared after I arose and walked about for about a half hour. I asked my doctor (an M.D.) if it wasn't pressure pains. I suspected what your book confirmed. The doctor gave me some 'double talk' and said that the pain was due to adhesions, and he suggested 'radar' treatments. I went three times a week until your book opened my eyes. I was mad clean through. Why wasn't my doctor honest enough to tell me the pains were due to pressure exerted in sleep?

"I sent him your book and told him 'I know and so does Mr. Rodale that osteoarthritis is incurable (degenerated bones cannot be restored) but I am glad to have been corroborated in my suspicion that my pains were pressure pains and I didn't need a doctor for that'."

Mrs. Snyder turned over to me the answer from her physician. He said, "Proper sleeping habits are helpful in these conditions—but by no means curative—since they do not remove the, as yet, unknown cause or causes. Mr. Rodale over-simplifies the entire matter, principally through ignorance of the basic sciences relating to the human body. Improvement by any method of treatment may be only apparent, concurrent and coincident with a period of natural remission of symptoms—which usually recur in spite of the continuance of the temporarily 'miraculous cure'."

I make no comment except to say that my own cure has so far been in effect for over 16 years. Many others have had similar experiences. I have had hundreds of letters testifying to my method's efficaciousness in completely clearing up pressure neuritis.

Here is a typical case: One day I was in a broker's office and overheard the bookkeeper complaining to a customer's man that she had been having terrible pains in her arms and shoulders. "I have to go to my doctor this afternoon for vitamin B injections and dread going," she said, "and tomorrow I am supposed to go to my dentist to have my teeth x-rayed. The doctor thinks that it might be infected teeth, and I might have to have all of them extracted."

I walked over to her and related my own experience. When I explained that possibly head pressure could be the cause of her own trouble she was delighted to find an excuse for not going to the doctor or dentist. She at once admitted that she slept with her head on her arms. In about a week that girl was as free of pain as a new-born baby, without the benefit of any vitamin B injections. Of course not everyone who has pains in the arms and shoulder gets them from sleep pressures, but it is surprising how many cases do arise from this cause.

Some Letters

Here are a few letter received from readers who have benefited from my book on the subject. They are only a few chosen from hundreds:

Here is one from Bernard Singer, 16 Shanley Ave., Newark, N. J.:

"I had been experiencing sharp pains across the back occasionally. After reading your pamphlet I became aware of two faulty sleeping habits. I was resting my head on my right arm and my wife frequently threw one leg over my back as I slept. By avoiding these two faulty habits, I have found that my back-aches disappeared."

James M. Moore, Route 4 Greenville, Ohio writes:

"I had found my two big toes were becoming numb, with almost no feeling in them. By breaking myself of lying so that one leg was under the other, this situation has cleared up also. Now these toes have a normal feeling."

Mrs. C. C. Wacker, Wilton Junction, Iowa writes:

"I used to wake up more tired than when I went to bed, and so full of aches and pains that I was miserable—until I read your book *Sleep and Rheumatism*. Now I wake up refreshed. It's almost like a miracle. Others have been helped by your method through my telling them, including my husband who has been greatly benefited. So we decided to give four of these books as Christmas presents."

John H. Stevenson, 26 Southbridge St., Worcester, Massachusetts writes:

"Your book *Sleep and Rheumatism* has taught me how to get more rest in my sleeping hours. Now I get up in the morning without that swollen feeling in my hands, which our family doctor says is a sign of arthritis. We are hearing too much about that dreadful trouble, and I believe you have told me how to stop it."

Hugo Mayerhoefer, Salem, Oregon:

"My dear Mr. Rodale: Your book *Sleep and Rheumatism* told me exactly where 90 per cent of my rheumatism came from. However, none of the positions you illustrated fit my case and so it did me no good for about a year or so until I finally discovered that my collarbone, in sleeping on my side, pressed against some nerve and choked off the 'supply line' and a few weeks after noticed a change for the better. Twenty years suffering because my doctors didn't find the cause of my trouble. A million thanks to you."

Some Additional Facts

The sleep neuritis comes from pressure on nerves which damages them, and also from blood congestions caused by pressure on veins, but the amazing thing is how quickly the condition clears up when the sleep pressures are eliminated. You might ask, but how can I prevent myself from doing these things during sleep? The answer is that you begin by trying, and pretty soon your subconscious mind has learned a new set of sleeping habits. All you need do is to draw an imaginary line along your shoulders, and in sleep never let your arms go above that line, and keep your arms down at the sides, and as relaxed as possible.

In Germany, a survey made a few years ago showed that practically 100 per cent of the population aged between 40 and 50 were afflicted with some form of arthritis or neuritis, but this of course included very mild cases. Ask any person over 60 and you will find that they are suffering from vague bodily pains and twinges. Many of these cases are due to pressures exerted in sleep, although I have also found that some of it is due to sleeping on soft mattresses, which cause the spine to curve downward. Most of these people continue to suffer because cures are usually attempted with medication, whereas the cause is purely a mechanical one.

Dr. Emanuel Josephson of New York City who wrote a commentary on my book said that pressures on the arm and shoulder during sleep can lead to bursitis. The cause is injury to the lubricating system of the shoulder. There is a delicate sac in the shoulder joint which is moistened by an oily fluid. Pressure on the shoulder muscle during sleep can in some cases cause a breakdown of its lubricating system, giving rise to a case of subdeltoid bursitis and so many of these cases are usually operated on.

Many a drunkard has fallen asleep in a hall-way and because there are no pillows handy, used his arm for that purpose. But when one is drunk, the circulation and forces of the body are at even a lower ebb than in ordinary sleep, so that when the man is suddenly awakened, his arm is so paralyzed that he can hardly move it. Such cases sometimes have to be hospitalized, and in the big cities so many of them are brought into hospitals that this condition has been called Drunkard's Neuritis. It has also been called Saturday Night Neuritis, from the fact that so many workers are paid at the end of the week, indulging in wild bouts of drinking and sleeping it off under tables, etc.

Yet, though the doctors have handled so many of these drunkards, and knew that it came from sleeping on their arms, they did not think to associate it with other cases of arm neuritis. You can search high and low in the medical profession and nary a word will you find that the head pressing on the arm in sleep is the cause of these thousands of cases of pressure neuritis. Patients come to doctors with symptoms of waking up in sleep with arms paralyzed, and the doctors call it *Brachialgia Statica Paresthetica,* which means numbness in the arm during sleep, but always in their writing about it they state that it comes upon the person suddenly and that the cause is not known. I am wondering if what I have discovered is really *Brachialgia Statica Paresthetica.*

In the November 5, 1955, issue of the *Journal of the American Medical Association,* a physician asks a question of the editor. A patient of his, a 30 year old plumber, complains of his hands becoming numb every night during sleep. Upon awakening he has to shake his hands vigorously to do away with the numbness. There seems to be no evidence of disease that could be at the bottom of it. What could be the cause?

The editor replies. It is possible that this could be a scalenus anticus syndrome, the background for which could be a cervical rib and enlarged transverse process of the cervical spine, or even a hypertrophy of the scalenus anticus muscle. The editor advises an x-ray, and an injection of procaine solution into the affected muscles. The trouble could also be in the thyroid, says the editor, and advises quite a complicated and expensive procedure, including complete studies of the spine.

Then he says that sometimes such a condition has been vaguely diagnosed as *idiopathic nocturnal paresthesia.* This means a night-time numbness of spontaneous origin, which I will discuss in a little while.

Here are illustrations of the postures to avoid:

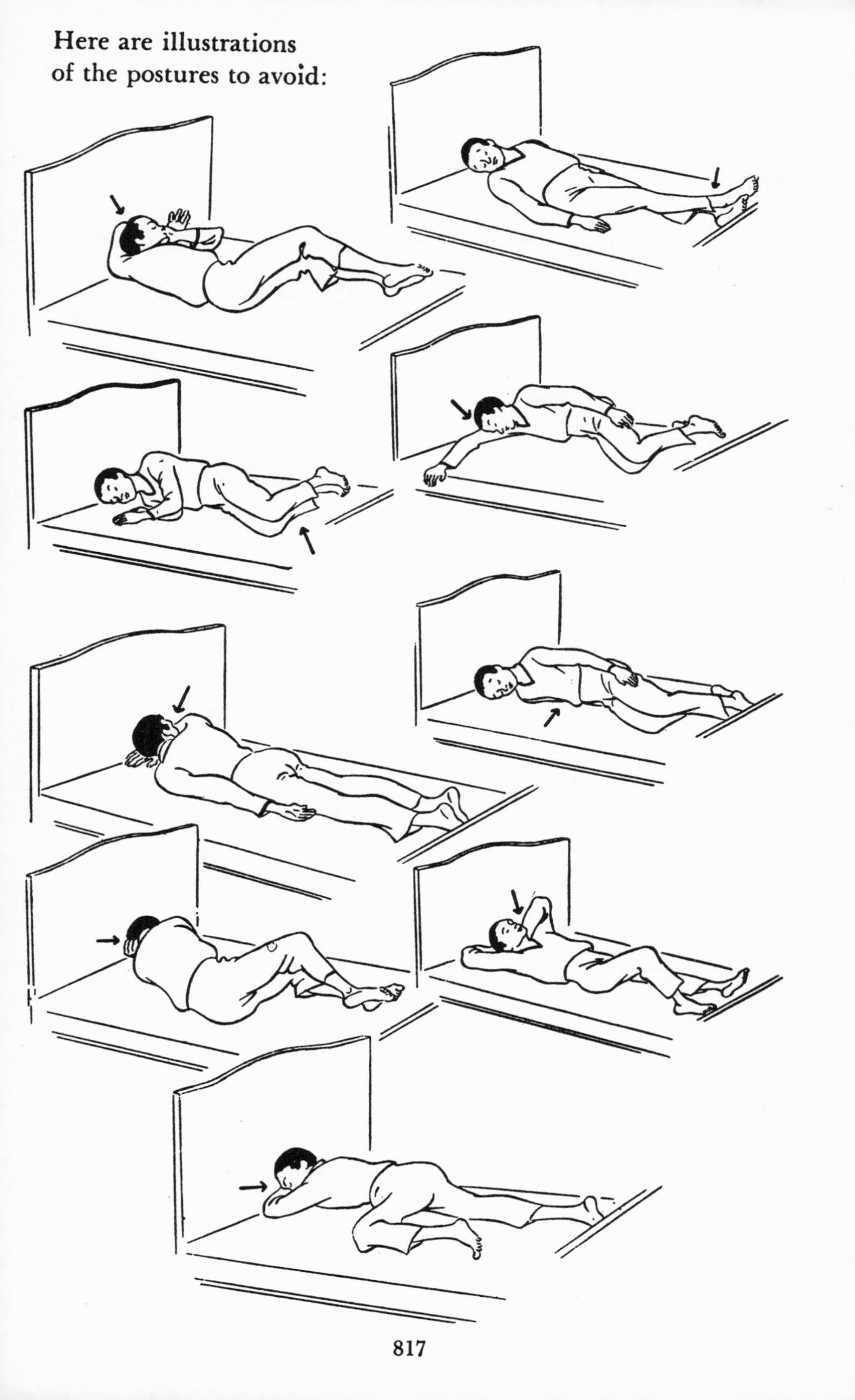

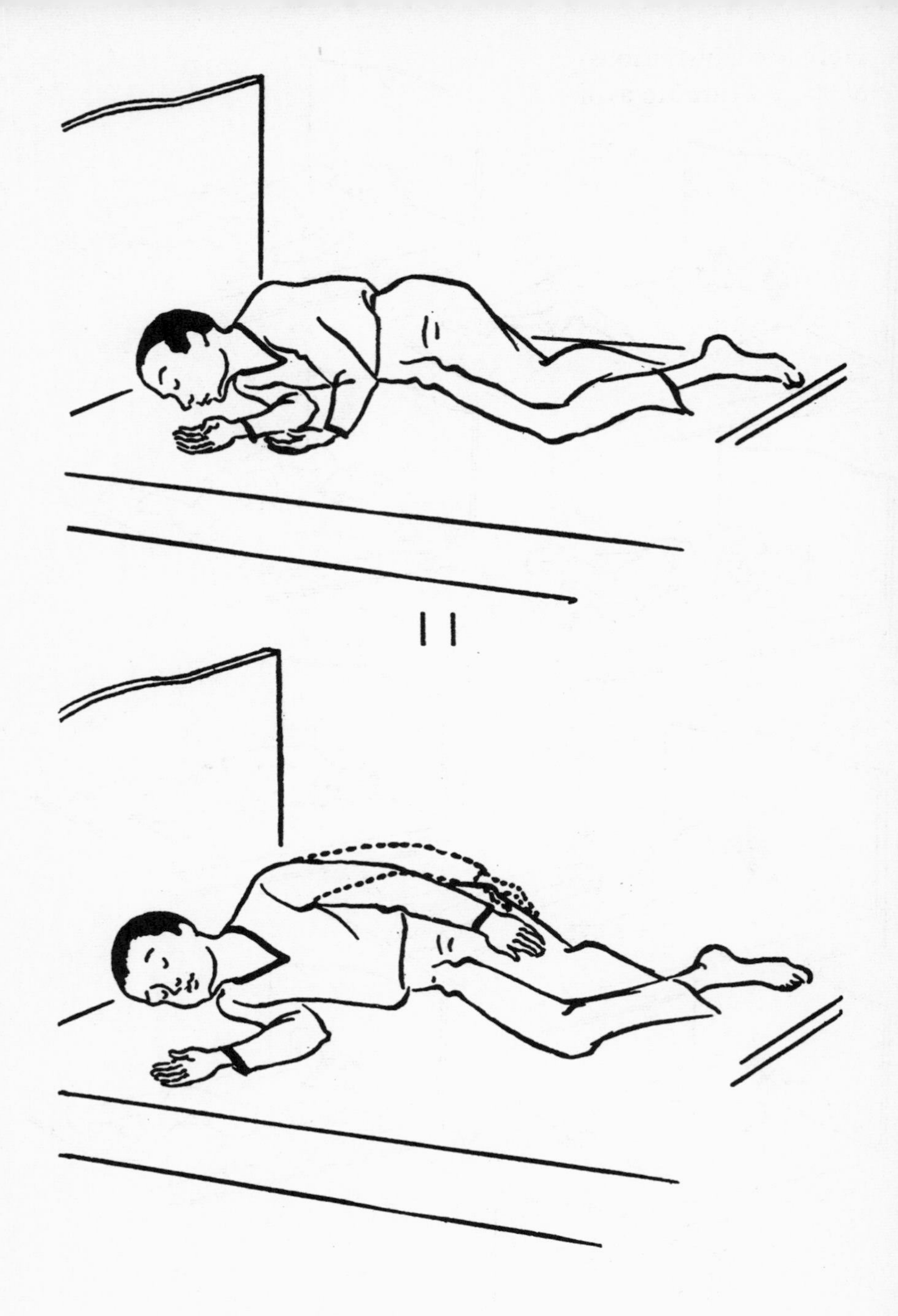

Here are illustrations of safe positions in sleep

Sometimes patients with this condition have what is called arteriospasm and for this, priscoline is given three or four times a day, as well as barbiturates. Also treatments with mecholyl every second day, ten times in all, have helped.

Now with all due respect to this editor's medical gobbledegook, which I have attempted to simplify, all that is probably the matter with this plumber is that he is sleeping with his head on his arms, causing pressures on nerves and the circulatory system. Sometimes people sleep with their arms curled up in positions which also cause stagnation in the circulation. All that is needed is about three nights of relaxed sleeping, with the arms down at the sides, and presto, no more *nocturnal paresthesia.* (Now he's got *me* talking that way.)

My little booklet *Sleep and Rheumatism* (35 cents) explains it all, and I have sent a free copy to the doctor who asked the question. We have dozens of letters from people who have read it and who have cured themselves in no time at all. In my work and in my travels in the last 25 years I have encountered at least 20 cases of people who had vague pains in their arms and shoulders, and in practically every case I later found that after they followed my simple instructions there was a complete cure—or as the doctors would say, a complete remission of symptoms.

Now what is this *idiopathic nocturnal paresthesia* that the editor mentioned? Years ago when I was doing a thorough research of the medical literature I made it my business to read as many articles on the subject as possible. It seems that *idiopathic nocturnal paresthesia* is a form of numbness in the arms which comes on during the night for no reason at all. It just as suddenly disappears and nobody seems to die from it. But the medical profession seems to be baffled as to its cause. The medical profession is so easily baffled, and then goes on to create elaborate, expensive cure procedures which pay them handsome premiums for their lack of desire, or energy, or what-have-you, in looking for causes. But from the experience that I had had in this field, my opinion is that there is no such thing as spontaneous paresthesia. The numbness must be caused by a pressure of one part of the body on the other. It can't be otherwise.

Just about that time I was invited to speak to a health group in Cincinnati, and part of my talk was to be devoted to pressure neuritis in the arms. In going over my papers the night before at the hotel, I found an article that had appeared in the May, 1944, *Journal of Nervous and Mental Diseases,* entitled *"Brachialgia Statica Parethetica." Brachialgia* means pain in the arms, *statica,* at rest, and *paresthetica,* an abnormal sensation, as burning, prickling, etc. This article was practically a complete review of what was known in this field. The author, Robert Wartenberg, M.D., even said in it, "Under the titles: 'Sleep and Rheumatism,' 'How I Cured Neuritis,' and 'Pain in the Finger,' etc., a layman, J. I. Rodale, wrote a book and magazine articles on this subject."

Again it was stressed that arm numbness could come about during the night spontaneously, without pressure being applied, and again I questioned it. Evidently my subconscious mind was reading the article along with me and differed with me, for during that night I had the most beautiful case of *idiopathic noctural paresthesia* you would ever want to see, and I am sure that it was my subconscious which did it, purely to teach me a lesson.

Now, I must tell you that a few years before, I had cured myself of a severe case of *pressure neuritis* in my arms by learning not to sleep with my head on them. I had learned this so thoroughly that it had become automatic. I suppose that that little imp which was my subconscious, stood watch for me while I was asleep to see that my arms did not go above my shoulder line. Thus my head would not be able to reach them.

But on this night of which I speak I know that I had a case of arm numbness brought about without any pressure. It was purely psychosomatic. It did not last very long, but there it was. The next morning I took my subconscious to task and spoke to it in no uncertain terms. "Subconscious," I said, "you and I are going to go through life together. We are going to read many medical journals and articles. We are going to have lots of fun, but don't take it personally or be too serious about it. Be objective! Remember what I tell you, now, because I don't want to have any more trouble with you. I don't want to insult you by telling you who is the master, but let us each know our place and function. I need you to remember things for me. Remember them well, but don't try any more experiments on my body."

That was about ten years ago and I have not had any similar trouble since. My subconscious and I have been the best of friends.

Sleeping on the Floor

By J. I. Rodale

Editor of *Prevention*

Many years ago I read somewhere that the late Bernarr McFadden, the well-known physical culturist, slept on the floor. He did it, of course, to prevent his spine from sagging downward in sleep. He knew that spinal abnormalities—curvatures and distortions—can produce disease, and that a strong, straight back is insurance that the nerves radiating outward from the spine will function efficiently, for the spine is the nerve switchboard that controls the health of man.

As a young man I dismissed this quirk of McFadden's as one of the things that only rabid physical culturists do, but as I went through life I heard more and more of people who were being advised by their physicians to sleep with a board under the mattress, to prevent it from sagging. This was because of their back troubles, and I could see that Bernarr was not far off the track. In fact, at the age of 40 I had to have my own board under the mattress because of rheumatic back pains.

It is amazing how many people are attacked with this affliction. In Germany a survey was made some years ago which showed that practically 100 per cent of the people over 50 had some form of rheumatism, although some were only mild cases. So many of the traveling public are suffering from back troubles that the Hotel Vier Jahrzeiten in Frankfort, Germany, will make your bed up on order—either soft, medium or hard.

The mattress makers were quick to cash in on the need for a harder sleeping surface and you will find dozens of orthopedic mattresses on the market. I have a typical advertisement in front of me. It says: "Throw that backache out of your life—designed to give you healthful sleep and ache-free days." This is true. These mattresses help. So does the board. But I found a better answer than either of these two devices.

I recalled old Bernarr MacFadden sleeping on the floor, and living to be way over 80, and parachuting off bridges. There must be something to this floor-sleeping business, I figured. So one evening I lay down on our living room rug and experienced a delightful half hour of soothing repose. I was surprised to find it so restful. I did it again on other nights and became convinced that sleeping on a hard surface was not as difficult as one would imagine. We know that half the world sleeps on the floor, or its equivalent. People in the vast regions of Asia, Africa, South America and other so-called uncivilized areas, have never even seen a bed. A G.I. friend of mine now stationed in Japan writes about a Japanese carpenter employed in the barracks, expressing great surprise when he saw his first bed there, which reminds me of the old Chinese lady who visited a family that slept on beds. She kept falling out of hers. Her subconscious mind had not learned the task of standing guard for her during sleep. The edge of the bed is a mental hazard which is unconsciously kept track of by the inner mind. Almost every child has fallen out of bed a few times until its subconscious mind became disciplined to the task of standing guard. In the same way one can learn to adopt non-pressuring postures during sleep, for the subconscious soon becomes habituated to the new "rule."

But there was something about sleeping on the floor that did not appeal to me. It was all right for Asia and Africa and for physical culturists, but I visualized one of my friends whispering to another, "Rodale sleeps on the floor"—not to mention what the good wife would say out loud.

The idea of sleeping on a real hard surface would not leave my mind. I kept thinking about orthopedic mattresses and under-boards, going over their advantages and disadvantages. There was still too much "give" to them. In either case the springs were somewhat compressed by the weight of the body and, since they had nowhere to go, especially in the case of the board, their increased tension kept pushing upward against the sleeper.

One day, an idea began to percolate. Why not put the board on top of the mattress instead of under it? I smiled. If I could do that, in effect, I would be taking the floor and putting it on top of the bed, thus sleeping on the "floor" but saving face—a sort of eating one's cake and having it too (although I never eat cake). This idea I liked, except that I did not relish sleeping on a plain board. I therefore figured that I would put a few blankets over it and sleep on the blankets.

I was weaving this idea in and out of my mind when one day I ran into Donald Goodman, of the Bethlehem Furniture Company, manufacturers of mattresses. By this time I had added something to my idea. "Donald," I said, "can you make a board, the size of my bed, with about ¾ of an inch of soft material over it, and cover both board and material with something to hold them together?" When I explained the purpose of the idea he entered into the spirit of adventure of the thing with enthusiasm and agreed to make it. In a few days I was called to see the contraption. But when I beheld it I was both amazed and delighted. The plant superintendent, Ted Collins, fortunately was a perfectionist and was not satisfied with a mere board. He had made it more functional, at the same time creating an article of commerce that had selling appeal. What he showed me looked in all respects like a real mattress. Had he just made a board, he said, it would have jiggled around on top of the bed during sleep. What he did was to mount the board on top of a wooden frame, placing the ¾ inch of soft material over the top of the thin board and encasing the whole device in an attractive, colorful mattress-covering material as shown in the illustration.

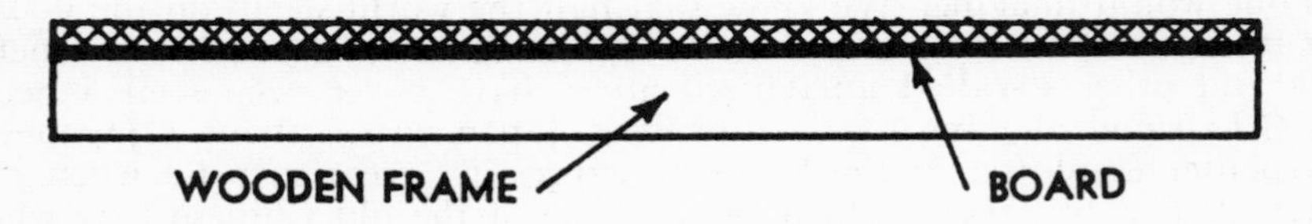

For all practical purposes it looked like a regular type of mattress, although it was an inch or two lower. But it did not have a single spring in it. The under-inside merely contained reinforcing struts of wood, to prevent the top board from bellying downward.

I tried it out right in the factory. In fact we all took turns lying on it, and unanimously agreed that it wasn't anywhere near as hard as we thought it would be. That night I slept upon it and must say that it gave me a fine night of rest. It seemed like the answer I had been seeking. It was as near perfection as I could ever hope to attain in a mattress. I tried it for a week, and when I was sure that I still was in love with it, I went to see Donald and told him that we had something we must share with the rest of the world.

Again Mr. Goodman entered into the proper spirit. He agreed to manufacture the new mattress, and asked me for my proposition. Personally, I told him, I did not wish to share monetarily in its manufacture. I gave the idea to him, lock, stock and barrel. I did not wish to be a sharer in a commercial project that had anything to do with health, vitamins, etc., as I did not want to become prejudiced in my writings. However, as a gentleman's agreement, there was a promise on his part to make occasional contributions out of his profits to the Soil and Health Foundation, of which I am president. This foundation, 99 per cent of whose income has been going as grants to universities, and whose charter prevents any officer from drawing a salary, is doing the spadework in research to show the dangers to human nutrition of using chemical fertilizers in growing our food crops. Its activities will soon be extended to take in general health research projects.

A patent is being taken out on the new mattress and an intensive sales campaign will be conducted on it all over the country. I am terrifically excited about this new development in sleeping. It could do a lot of good and I would like to see the idea widely adopted.

A few words more about the new mattress. I observed one marvelous hidden advantage in it. It is soft enough to prevent stagnation of the blood circulation, yet hard enough to offer a certain unlooked for benefit. The average person turns many times in sleep, sometimes fifty to a hundred times or more in a night. A softer mattress takes much more energy to make each turn in than a harder one, because the elbow digs down deeper, and it requires an effort to pull it out. It is like the difference between walking on a hard pavement or in very soft sand on an ocean beach. The hard surface of the new mattress provides a leverage which makes the turn easier. In this respect it causes a more restful sleep, because the turn can be made in a condition of semi-consciousness whereas on a very soft mattress and especially in the case of a susceptible individual, the turns can cause complete awakenings in every instance. A friend with whom I discussed this idea mentioned the fact that his wife had recently undergone surgery performed on her heart and had been advised by her doctor, until it healed properly, to sleep on the hardest mattress she could obtain, for the very reason that it would be easier to make the turns without straining her heart. Our new type of mattress would be perfect for such cases.

Another unexpected advantage, a wonderful feature, is the elimination of the little knots and indentations above each spring of the ordinary mattress. It has an absolutely straight, smooth top. There are no lumpy spots to bite into you, because there are no springs that require anchoring. You must sleep on such a surface to appreciate it. This top smoothness is the balancing feature that compensates for the loss of the springiness.

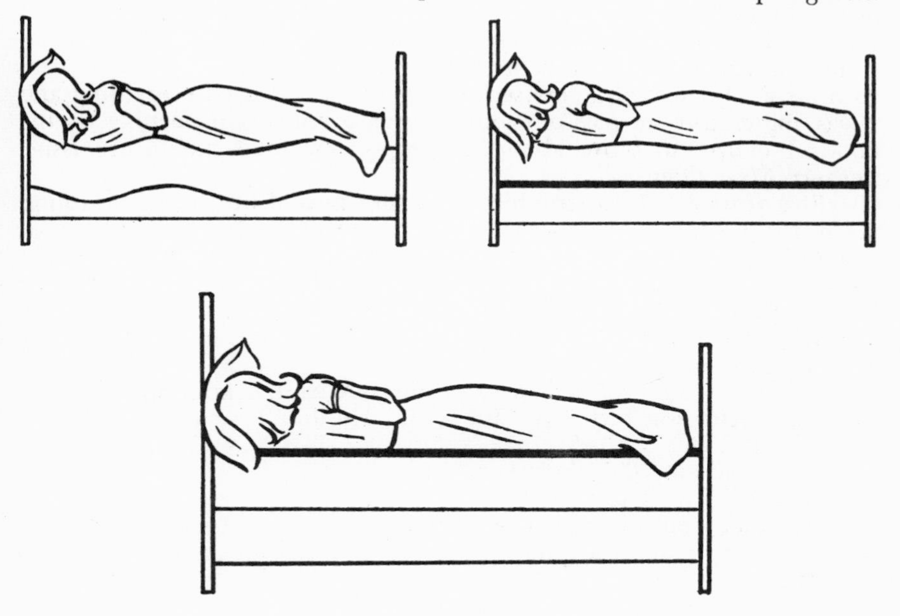

Life is a matter of habit. Sleeping on such a mattress takes a bit of doing, I will admit, but with a little perseverance you will master it, and gain a feeling that you are gradually rebuilding your back to what it was during your youth. The framework that God gave us should be carefully preserved. Wasn't it Thomas Edison who said, "The doctor of the future will give no medicine but will interest his patients in the care of the human frame?"

However, I wish to report one very serious drawback about this new mattress and it *is* serious. In a whole month of sleeping on it, it still holds good. You cannot *jump* into bed. I miss that. On the new mattress, I jumped into bed the first night, but never repeated the performance afterwards.

After the previous article was written, in rummaging through some old files, I discovered the following article which appeared in the April 1945 issue of *New Physical Culture.* Evidently my thinking regarding hard sleeping surfaces was influenced by it, because, even though I read it more than ten years ago, its basic idea must have remained tucked away in one of the inner recesses of my mind. Therefore, in reprinting this article herewith, with permission of *New Physical Culture Magazine,* now *Physical Culture Magazine,* Branford, Conn., may I express my admiration to the author, Carol L. Leeds for the fine scope of her writing on this all important subject—our daily bed.

I Sleep on the Floor

By Carol L. Leeds

Reprinted from *New Physical Culture*

Editorial Note: The recommendations in this article will seem rather revolutionary to the average reader, but soft beds are inclined to develop soft bodies, and emphasizing the great importance of this article, I have to admit that I firmly believe sleeping on the floor on one occasion practically saved my life. Through an accident I had to deal with a spinal defect of a very serious nature. I had tried everything and I was about ready to pass out, but I found a remedy in sleeping on the floor. I expect to write about this experience in some future issue. Bernarr Macfadden

Five years ago I was troubled by a shortness of breath, pain around my heart, and a weakened back that at times made it impossible to sit straight in a chair. I don't patronize doctors, as a rule, but after the pain became unbearable, I had to do something. And do it quickly for by now my back was so bad that I couldn't take a step without wincing in agony. It seemed, too, that my left leg was drawing up and gradually growing shorter.

And so I consulted a bone specialist. After ten minutes I decided that this doctor was certainly "different." He didn't prescribe pink pills or an operation.

"How old are you?" he asked.

"Forty-eight," I told him.

He quietly put his instruments away and sat down beside me, talking for almost an hour in a quiet unhurried way that at once inspired my confidence.

"You've got a muscular heart condition," he said. "Nothing serious, but enough to cause pain. Also, you have a slight curvature of the spine, and badly rounded shoulders from poor posture and poor sleeping position. Worst of all, you're developing sciatica and a misplacement of the sacroiliac from poor body posture.

"You see, the thin padding on the spinal column gets thinner as we grow older, thus exposing the sensitive nerve tissues that run up and down the spinal cord. So far, this condition is not serious, but may become so, if not given attention.

"A great percentage of older people develop sciatica in later life. They don't know it, but they could escape most of their misery if they would only throw away their feather-soft inner-spring mattresses that you see advertised everywhere in such glowing terms at such outrageous prices. I wouldn't give two cents for a soft bed, because I know I'd have to pay billions of dollars in pain and discomfort for all the years to come."

"What do you recommend?" I asked at last.

"That you sleep on the floor," he shot back, without a moment's hesitation. "Of course, if you're squeamish, you can sleep on fraction boards laid across your regular bed. But the floor is the best, and the most natural place for sleeping. The ventilation and air are better, too— as our Chinese and Indian friends wisely discovered years ago.

"When you sleep on the floor, the heart muscles retain their normal body position, and don't sag out of place and put extra pressure on the heart. Your backbone will get stronger and gradually adjust itself and become straight; also, your shoulder bones and muscles. Thousands of women have thrown vertebrae out of place by sleeping on soft mattresses. I tell you they're the biggest curse of modern civilization, and the chief cause of much of the sciatica backaches and sacroiliac troubles that plague older people today."

"What about medicine?" I asked.

He laughed. "A good hard, straight bed is the only medicine you need. But along with that, eat lots of plain wholesome foods, drink plenty of water and milk, and work up to a two-mile walk every day, even though, at first, the pain in your back seems unbearable."

As I rose to leave, I asked, "When shall I come again?"

He smiled. "Sleep on the floor for three months, with a heavy rug under you, and warmly covered. At the end of that time if you're not feeling entirely free from aches and pains, come back."

Frankly skeptical, I agreed. But inwardly I felt certain that mere sleeping on the floor couldn't overcome the backaches I'd had for years.

For my unique bed, I selected a corner, out of the draft, and I spread out a heavy rug. I used a small pillow, and blankets for warmth. The first night was torture. It seemed that every bone in my body was working through the flesh. The next night was somewhat more comfortable. The third night I really got some sleep, and I woke in the morning feeling much more rested than for weeks.

Long before the end of the month, my back showed great improvement. I had the comfortable feeling that every bone was squarely in the right groove, with no pressure on the nerves. Soon my backaches entirely disappeared. I discovered, too, that it was easier for me to hold my shoulders erect. The heaviness around my heart, caused by constricted and distorted muscles, became lighter, and at last, after three months, disappeared entirely.

With winter coming, I hesitated to continue sleeping on the floor, which is typically Californian and very thin, and I am subject to occasional colds. In response to my query, the doctor advised, "Get a low bed-frame and put fraction boards in the bottom."

Our handy man built the frame and stained it dark walnut. In the bottom, he put the discarded top of a billiard table that had cluttered up our garage for years. I spread my rug over it. It made an ideal bed—almost as good as the floor. Since it was raised four inches off the floor, I escaped the icy drafts. This is my winter bed. I still prefer the floor for summer use.

Nature gave man the good earth to sleep on. Indians, until they began using modern beds, were singularly free from backache and vertebrae misplacements. Yet civilized man still insists upon improving upon Nature's gift, and warps his bones and muscles all out of shape by sleeping on soft beds. When one considers that the average person spends one-third of all his time in bed, he can readily realize that a life-time of soft sleeping will finally distort his entire bone structure. If you don't believe it, rest your hand for a moment on a hard surface, and then on a soft pillow, and judge the results.

My suggestion is this: If you wish to avoid muscular heart trouble, sciatica, sacroiliac misplacements, curvature of the spine, and hunched shoulders, throw away your soft bed and sleep on the floor. I did just that. And at last I have learned the joy of having a good strong body, with every bone in its proper place, and with never an ache or a pain, month in and month out. . . . End

Hard Mattress

Most persons who have purchased the very hard Spine-a-Liner mattress have had unusually good results with it. Many glowing letters have been received by the manufacturer. But a few persons have had trouble with it. They don't seem to be able to get used to it, or they give up too soon. My advice to them is to place three blankets between the top of the mattress and the sheet. After a week or so, one of the blankets could be removed. A few weeks later the second one could go, and later the third one. In some cases, the last blanket could remain permanently. In fact, that is the way I like it. I still get the full effect of the hard mattress in keeping my spine from sagging during sleep.

It is the same with other desirable habits one wishes to cultivate. It sometimes takes time and scheming to learn to make them an integral part of one's daily routine. For example, many years ago I had trouble in learning to sleep without a pillow. So what I did was this: The first night I slept without a pillow only for as long as I could stand it, which was about ten minutes. I did the same each night. The time that I could stand it kept increasing gradually, until in about two weeks I was able to sleep all night long that way, and to love it.

Sleeping without a pillow prevents the jugular vein in the neck from getting crooked up and causing blood stagnation and retarded flow of it to the various places in the head where it is needed. This causes pains in the neck region to many susceptible persons. It is a wonderful experience to sleep without a pillow, once you have mastered the habit. But a strange thing has happened. Since I am sleeping on my hard Spine-a-Liner, I can sleep *with* a pillow. In fact, I find it gives me more comfortable sleep, and does not cause the pain in the neck which I had in the old days when I slept with a pillow. But when I sleep at a hotel on a soft mattress I find that I cannot get comfort during the night with a pillow, and sleep without it in such places. My body seems to sag down and being used to sleeping with my body projecting straight out, I get the feeling that I am in a hammock, and with a pillow, it throws my head up too much. Medical research should be done on this subject.

We received a recent release of the National Lumber Manufacturers Association (Washington, D. C.) which says: "Fort Lauderdale, Florida children are encouraged to sleep on the floors in the Broward County school system. Odd as it may seem, it's true—notably in the primary grades. The youngsters lie down on small blankets for a 20-minute rest period every afternoon."

The educational experts look at it from the point of view that the rest is good for the children, but overlook the fact that resting on the wooden surface is good for keeping backs straight. The lumbermen look at it from the point of view that a wooden floor is much better than a cement one, for sleeping on.

I sleep on my springless, hard-board mattress, made for me by the Bethlehem Furniture Company of Allentown, Pennsylvania, and I am getting to love it more and more. Sometimes I can hardly wait for sleep time in anticipation of the pleasure of being able to stretch myself out in such a straight line. A few weeks ago we had a family reunion at Atlantic City and do you want to know how I felt sleeping in the regulation hotel bed? It was as if I was sleeping in a hammock—absolutely and distinctly so!

. . . J. I. Rodale

Sleeping Pills

America is a nation of gadgets. According to an A. P. dispatch from Los Angeles the latest of these—most convenient little gimmick you can imagine—is an alarm-clock sleeping pill. The pill has three layers of different drugs. The first layer is nembutal which puts you to sleep. The second layer is butabarbital sodium which keeps you asleep and the third is dexedrine which "rings the bell in your brain" and wakens you after eight hours. The pills are on display at the California Academy of General Practice Convention. They must be obtained by prescription.

Now mind you, this is not a contraption dreamed up for a good gag on a comic radio program. This sleeping pill involves the infinitely complex and incredibly delicate tissues and cells of your nervous system and brain. So finely made are these tissues, so sensitive, that our most learned scientists have not even the slightest inkling of how they perform the perpetual wonders of thought, memory, emotion. Now we are turning loose among these vital threads of life a drug that will shock them into unconsciousness, another that will keep them unconscious and a third that will shock them into consciousness again. This will not happen just once in a lifetime, as a result of some dreadful unavoidable accident. It will happen every night inside the bodies of those individuals whose doctors prescribe this particular sleeping pill. If all the scientists who slaved for hours in laboratories to produce this monstrous medication had turned their talents to finding out why people can't sleep and preventing the sleeplessness, don't you think we'd be a little farther along the road to progress?

Smoking...and Respiratory Involvements

The *Reader's Digest* for January, 1950, published an astounding article on smoking in which the following aspects of the tobacco habit were reviewed: the effect of smoking on the throat membranes, on lungs, on stomach and digestion, on the skill of athletes, on the heart, on the blood pressure and the blood vessels, on Buerger's Disease patients, on cancer incidence, on mortality figures, on colds. Author Roger William Riis came to the inevitable conclusion that smoking does nothing but harm. His own personal testimony is as follows: "When I began research for this article, I was smoking 40 cigarettes a day. As I got into the subject, I found that number dropping. As I finish the article, I am smoking ten a day. I'd like to smoke more but my investigation of the subject has convinced me that smoking is dangerous, and worse—stupid."

Mr. Riis tells us that if you smoke a pack of cigarettes a day you take in 840 cubic centimeters of tobacco tar in a year. That means, he says, that you have exposed your throat and lung tissues to 27 fluid ounces or 15 full cocktail glasses of tobacco tar containing benzo-pyrene. The ugly, greasy tar that is left in your ash tray, on your fingers or in the filter of your cigarette holder is not nicotine. It is instead the "soot" that is left from the incomplete combustion of the tobacco—just as disagreeable and dangerous as the soot from your chimney. Many physicians agree that, as an irritant, it is more dangerous to heavy smokers than nicotine is.

He tells us that of 100 smokers examined in one test, Dr. Frederick B. Flinn found 73 with congestion of the throat, 66 with coughs, seven with irritation of the tongue. Dr. Emil Bogen reported on another 100 smokers, 30 of whom had mouth irritation and 30 of whom suffered from coughs. It appears that the way you smoke has something to do with how much injury you may encounter. The way you puff your cigarette, how long you hold the smoke when you inhale, how far down the butt you smoke your cigarette—all these have some bearing on how much irritation you are subjecting your throat tissues to. Rapid smoking, for instance, causes more irritation, because the smoke enters the mouth at a higher temperature.

Most of the nicotine escapes into the air when you smoke. About a third of it gets into your mouth where some of it is absorbed. Perhaps a fifth of what gets to the lungs is absorbed. Smoking one cigar gives the same effect as smoking about four or five cigarettes. The nicotine effect from a pipe is a little more than that from a cigar. The smoke coming into your mouth reaches temperatures up to 135 degrees Fahrenheit. The hotter your smoke, the more nicotine you absorb.

Says Mr. Riis, "In pure form nicotine is a violent poison. One drop on a rabbit's skin throws the rabbit into instant shock. The nicotine content of a trifle more than two cigarettes, if injected into the bloodstream, would kill a smoker swiftly. If you smoke a pack a day, you inhale 400 milligrams of nicotine a week, which in a single injection would kill you as quick as a bullet."

Quoting *Risk Appraisal* published by the National Underwriters Company, Mr. Riis tells us that "Habitual smokers have 62 per cent higher incidence of gas on the stomach, 65 per cent higher incidence of colds, 76 per cent higher incidence of nervousness, 100 per cent higher incidence of heartburn, 140 per cent higher incidence of labored breathing after exertion, 167 per cent higher incidence of nose and throat irritation and 300 per cent higher incidence of cough." Insurance companies make it their business to do careful research; their business depends on it.

Colds and Smokers' Asthma

So smokers have a 65 higher percentage of colds, 167 higher percentage of nose and throat irritation and 300 percent higher incidence of coughs! Surely this news should come as a surprise to no one. And we want to remind our readers, too, that "having a cold" is not the end of it. A cold, with its weakening effect on the body, may well predispose or lead directly to much more serious conditions.

An Associated Press News Release of April 17, 1953, quotes a Detroit physician, Dr. George L. Waldbott, as saying that there is a very definite disease known to medical science as "smoker's asthma." He told of a group of 58 cases of smoker's asthma, 28 of whom recovered immediately as soon as they stopped smoking, 24 others who recovered by discontinuing tobacco and taking other treatment as well, and the remainder of whom did not improve even after they gave up smoking.

He described smokers' asthma as "chronic inflammation of the Adam's apple area of the throat; wheezing, shortness of breath, a tendency to respiratory infections, constriction of the chest above the heart, and prolonged coughing in the morning, sometimes requiring several hours to clear the throat of mucus." He advised that other physicians should always make allowance for the possibility of "smokers' asthma" when they are diagnosing ailments.

Possible Effects of Your Tobacco Smoke on Others in the Family

Perhaps even more frightening is an article in the *Journal of the American Medical Association,* October 21, 1950, recounting the story of a one-year old infant brought to the hospital with a history of watery eyes, nasal discharge and sneezing. At the age of ten months she had had an asthmatic attack. When the baby's allergy tests showed that she was allergic to tobacco, her parents were questioned and it was found that her mother had been an incessant smoker for many years, smoking even while she fed, nursed and diapered the baby. All smoking was stopped in the house and within a few days the baby's symptoms disappeared completely.

A year and a half later the baby developed a dry hacking cough, and it was found that the mother had started to smoke again. When she stopped, the baby's symptoms once again disappeared. Asthma is a very serious ailment, especially in the case of a baby. The extreme difficulty an asthmatic patient suffers in trying to breathe can result in death. Yet, from the story above, it seems quite possible that many of our asthmatic children today are the product of a household constantly blue with tobacco smoke. Perhaps much of the watery eyes, nasal discharge and sneezing that cause more absenteeism from school than any other reason, may be traced to a family which smokes and encourages visitors to smoke. Surely even if parents will not make an effort to stop smoking for their own sakes, they should take into account the possible harm being done to children and other susceptible people who must breathe in the tobacco smoke they exhale.

Effect on Tubercular Patients and Post-Operative Patients

A question to the Editor of the *Journal of the American Medical Association,* September 30, 1950, asks whether or not smoking should be permitted in a tuberculosis hospital. The Editor answers that tobacco smoke causes "hyperemia of the mucous membranes"– that is, excessive blood congesting the membrane. He states that some specialists in bronchial diseases can tell from the condition of the membranes whether the patient is a one, two or three pack-a-day smoker. In addition, he says, smoking causes coughing which is of course much more harmful for a T.B. patient than for a healthy individual.

In *The Lancet,* 1: 368, 1944 (a conservative British medical publication), H. J. V. Morton writes on the incidence of pulmonary complications in patients who have undergone operations. Patients were grouped into three categories: smokers, light smokers and non-smokers. The first category included anyone who smoked 10 or more cigarettes a day. The conclusions were that smoking definitely increases complications of many kinds in patients who are undergoing operations. There were 257 patients in the study and results showed that the rate of complications for smokers was about six times greater than that of non-smokers. In addition Dr. Morton says that smokers are more likely to develop complications associated with serious constitutional disturbance.

Undoubtedly a thorough search of medical literature would reveal much more evidence of this same nature. Since the respiratory membranes—nose, throat, larynx and lungs—are more directly exposed and hence more irritated by tobacco smoke than other parts of the body, it seems only reasonable to assume that all the most pesky nose and throat disorders (including colds) would be more common in smokers than in non-smokers. Onces again, though, we must remember that families and friends are constantly exposed—though to a lesser extent—to the smoke of the tobacco user.

It's Not Just the Health Addicts That Are Concerned About the Tobacco Addicts

Smoking uses up vitamins that protect us against colds and other disorders—especially vitamin C and vitamin B. So the smoker, aside from irritating his nose and throat membranes, at the same time deprives them of food elements that might help to protect them against these poisons. Considering the fact that his respiratory membranes are pretty constantly in a state of irritation, is it any wonder that when the cold bugs attack, they find good pickings in these depleted, sick membranes? The weapons that might defeat them have already been used up and the smoker becomes easy prey for the sniffles, the tears, the fevers, the chills, the coughs, the hoarseness and perhaps finally the pneumonia.

When you show this article to some friend who may be a chain-smoker and who may have little regard for anything having to do with health, don't let him get away with sneering that we are cranks and crackpots. We didn't make up the figures on cold incidence among smokers just to frighten people. We don't have anything to sell in place of tobacco. The figures—65 per cent higher incidence of colds, 167 per cent higher incidence of nose and throat irritation and 300 per cent higher incidence of coughs—come from an insurance handbook put out by the National Underwriters Company.

We sent out some literature recently telling people about our series of articles on smoking. We were amazed to receive a reply—just one—doubting the quotes that we made, doubting that such an article as we quoted had ever appeared in a New York newspaper. So perhaps there really are people who are living wrapped up in a tight secure little cocoon of ignorance about what medical experimentation has shown in regard to the harmful effects of smoking. If you have a friend or relative like this, tell him to stop in at the local library and look through the *Reader's Guide To Periodical Literature*. All the magazine articles for the past fifty years or so are listed there. Ask him to look up smoking or tobacco or nicotine, and marvel, as we have, at the number of articles on the harmfulness of smoking that have appeared—and this in a country where many millions of dollars are paid out by tobacco companies for advertising in current periodicals! *Index Medicus* is a listing of all the articles in medical journals all over the world. Any one page of any one year of *Index Medicus* will yield enough information on the harmfulness of tobacco to cause the most hardened smoker to think a long, long time before he lights that next cigarette.

Smoking and Blood Sugar

"Plucky Strikes give you a lift" shrieks the billboard ad. "Scientific tests prove that Westerfields relieve fatigue" shouts the magazine ad. "Light up a Fall Mall and be the life of the party" croons the television announcer. And as the smoke curls up round his head, you can really almost see his eyes become brighter, his shoulders more erect, his smile more content.

We don't believe that Americans spend millions of dollars every year for cigarettes because they believe what the advertisements say about them. But actually what the advertisements say is true, in a distorted, back-handed kind of way. A cigarette *does* give you a lift. A cigarette *does* relieve fatigue in a pleasurable way. A cigarette *does* give you a spurt of energy you didn't have the moment before you put a match to that round, firm and fully-packed coffin-nail. Ever since the first European took his first draw on a pipeful of tobacco, scientists and medical men have searched for the secret of why tobacco should have a pleasant and relaxing effect. They have wondered, too, why the tobacco habit, once formed should be so tragically hard to break.

In our study of blood sugar we were delighted to run across several articles dealing with blood sugar and smoking. In 1934 Dr. Howard W. Haggard and Dr. Leon A. Greenberg of Yale University noticed that they were getting very unusual results among a number of patients involved in an experiment they were conducting. They were trying to determine ideal mealtime hours for children and adults—that is, how often during the day you should eat for maximum health. Their article in *Science*, volume 79, 1934, tells how they recorded the blood sugar level for several hundred subjects under many different conditions—fasting, frequent meals, infrequent meals and so forth. Some of the subjects showed wild fluctuations in blood sugar level—ups and downs on their charts that could not possibly be related to any of their meals. These folks were not suffering from any special emotional strain that might have caused the difference, and they were all adults. The two investigators thought of tobacco as a possible cause and found, sure enough, that all those subjects whose blood level fluctuated so noticeably had been smoking during the day.

Then they investigated the actual effect of smoking one cigarette. They found that, when blood sugar level is low, especially when it gets below the fasting level, a cigarette brings about an almost instantaneous rise in blood sugar which does not return to normal again for about 30 minutes. By further tests they determined that it is the nicotine in the tobacco that brings about this result. That explains why we smoke tobacco rather than anything else—such as corn silk or the leaves of some other plant. Why do we not smoke de-nicotinized products? Obviously because it is the nicotine in the cigarettes that gives us the "lift," the feeling of relaxation and well-being that comes from a rise in blood sugar. When the blood sugar is fairly high, for an hour or so after a meal, a cigarette does not produce this effect. However it always speeds up the burning of sugar in our bodies and so reduces hunger pangs temporarily.

Why should nicotine have this effect on blood sugar? It does not enter into the digestive tract; it is not assimilated by the body as food is. Animal experiments have shown that injections of nicotine stimulate the adrenal glands and these glands react by releasing blood sugar. So the entrance of the nicotine into the body sets off a chain reaction involving nerves, glands and blood sugar.

Tobacco—Induced Rise in Blood Sugar a Danger Sign

However, Dr. W. J. McCormick of Toronto explains that this release of blood sugar and the feeling of well-being that results do not mean at all that nicotine is good for you—quite the contrary. In his article "The Role of the Glycemic Response to Nicotine" in *The American Journal of Hygiene,* Volume 22, 1935, he tells us that there are other states that raise your blood sugar, too. A definite rise in blood sugar is noticed following administration of morphine, strychnine, cocaine, chloral hydrate, carbon monoxide, bichloride of mercury, ether and chloroform. The sugar level goes up in infectious diseases such as diphtheria, tuberculosis, syphilis, influenza and typhoid, and in cases of burns, asphyxia, hemorrhage and cancer. Your blood sugar also rises when you are angry, fearful or in pain. It can increase as much as 20 to 30 per cent within three to six minutes after one of these emotions hits you. The reason for this rise in blood sugar is that the fear, anger or pain stimulates your adrenals which prepare your body to take immediate action. This reaction is protective. If your fear arises from rounding a corner on a quiet street and coming face-to-face with an escaped tiger, the sugar swiftly pouring into your blood stream gives you the inhuman energy you need for that desperate 20-foot leap that carries you out of reach of the tiger's claws. So extra blood sugar in an emotional emergency supplies extra energy. And during the course of infections, the extra sugar in your blood provides fuel for the added oxidation your tissues need to fight the infection.

Perhaps many of you have noticed that your tolerance for tobacco is greatly reduced or perhaps lost altogether after a serious, infectious fever, such as influenza. In other words, the first "drag" on a cigarette after you're well may even knock you out. This is because the infection has made such demands on your body's supply of adrenalin that there is none left to carry through the job of raising blood sugar. So you become dizzy and nauseated. Isn't it possible, asks Dr. McCormick, that constant smoking also exhausts the adrenalin so that it is unable to provide protection against infection, when the germs come along?

Blood Sugar Protects the Body Against the Nicotine Poison

Dr. McCormick tells us that blood sugar is raised by nicotine so as to protect the body from the poison of the nicotine. But it is brought about by a different mechanism from that which raises blood sugar after eating. When blood sugar is used to fight poison, it is withdrawn from its storage place in the liver, thus depleting the body's supply. After meals, the added sugar in the bloodstream which produces the feeling of well-being, is on its way to this storage place.

It seems reasonable to us that the habitual smoker—the chain smoker, the individual who reaches for a cigarette the moment he is faced with a problem, the instant after he finishes a meal, the office worker who smokes constantly at his desk, and the housewife who carries her ashtray from room to room as she works—this individual gets along on an entirely artificial and dangerous kind of body chemistry. The vicious cycle set up goes something like this: the first cigarette in the morning stimulates the adrenals which release blood sugar from the liver. This means less blood sugar available for the body's use and within a half hour or so the effect of this first cigarette is gone. The smoker begins to feel a letdown. Nervously he reaches for another cigarette—another artificial rise in blood sugar with another "lag" later on. Unless something happens to intervene, such a pattern will probably go on all day with the result that this individual's body never gets a chance to catch up. All the nerves, glands and secretions involved in "operation blood sugar" are wearing themselves out all day long producing an artificial state of well-being, which nothing but another cigarette at definite intervals will prolong.

So the first puff on a cigarette (or pipe or cigar, of course) is, as Dr. McCormick says, "a burglar alarm" telling the sympathetic nervous system to release the blood sugar which will protect the body against this poison. If you could get enough nicotine in a given instant to paralyze this nervous system, so that the blood sugar would not be released, death would follow. Because of the small amount of nicotine entering our bodies when we smoke, the vicious cycle ensues—cigarette, blood-sugar-rise, "lag," another cigarette, another blood sugar rise and so forth.

As we have seen, a rise in blood sugar stills hunger pangs. So someone who is desperately trying to reduce is told to smoke, so that he will not be hungry. Dr. McCormick tells us that during famines in oriental countries, opium has been used for the same purpose, to decrease the craving for food when no food was available. But what a desperate gamble for any present-day American to take with his health! Says Dr. McCormick, "The 'lift' attributed to the cigarette is in reality a handicap which nature tries her best to counteract."

High Protein Diet May Help to Break the Nicotine Habit

We have long believed that addiction to smoking is similar to addiction to any other drug. Its helpless victim, once started on the cycle nicotine produces in his body, can no more free himself than an opium smoker or a cocaine addict can. While smoking does not reduce one to a morbid or drugged state, still its effects on health are of course extremely harmful and, as we have shown, so subtly habit-forming that it is well nigh impossible for the inveterate smoker to "pull himself together" and stop smoking just by using his "will power." We all know the old joke about the man who thought it was easy to give up smoking—he'd already done it 75 times!

We do not believe that people smoke just to be ornery, or just to be in style. Nor do we think people smoke because of an unsatisfied infantile urge to have something in their mouths, as psychologists have suggested. If this were true, why couldn't they chew a pencil and derive the same satisfaction? It has always seemed to us unfair and unkind to nag at the smoker and vilify him for his lack of will power when perhaps it is a flaw in body mechanics that causes him to smoke. Nor does the habitual smoker seem to us any more degenerate a member of society than the sweet-tooth-hound who wolfs down candy, cokes and cupcakes all day long. He too is trying to make up for some lack in his daily nutrition and is probably doing himself about as much harm with his sugary tidbits as he would do by smoking.

So it seems that the nicotine-produced rise in blood sugar is at least part of the reason why some people smoke and find they can't stop smoking. If you are a smoker and want to experiment with the theory, we'd suggest that you concentrate for a couple of weeks on keeping your blood sugar level high and see if this has an effect on your desire to smoke. This means eating meals high in protein and cutting down sharply on starches and sugars. In fact as you know, we advise eliminating all white sugar and white flour foods under any circumstances. You'll have to eat a breakfast high in protein. If you smoke at work you'll have to carry along a supply of snacks, preferably protein foods—a bag of nuts, sunflower seeds, a couple of hard-boiled eggs. When you feel the "lag" that means you need a "drag," reach for a walnut instead. If you're seriously trying to reduce, better skip the experiment until sometime later when the extra calories won't throw off your schedule.

Smoking and Cancer

The controversy over smoking and lung cancer that has raged so long in the newspapers might just as well be brought to a close, with a large and firm period to mark the end of the debate. So far as we are concerned, the final word has now been said on the subject and, no matter what further investigations may reveal, nothing can change the validity of this final word.

"The final word" is a book entitled *Smoking and Cancer,* published by Julian Messner, Inc. ($2.00). The author of the book is Alton Ochsner, M. D., former President of the American College of Surgeons, former president of the American Cancer Society and former president of the American Association for Thoracic Surgery. Dr. Ochsner begins his book with the ominous words "cigarettes cause cancer." He goes on to tell us that in 1954 some 23,000 Americans died from lung cancer. In 1955 about 25,000 Americans died from lung cancer. In 95 per cent of the cases death will be traceable to smoking. "The amount you have smoked daily and the number of years you have maintained the habit determine your chances of developing lung cancer," he says.

He describes a survey recently completed by Dr. E. Cuyler Hammond and Dr. Daniel Horn of the American Cancer Society. They studied the smoking habits of 187,766 men between the ages of fifty and seventy. They discovered that cigarette smoking is associated with an increase in the general death rate; heavy smoking nearly doubles the death rate from diseases of the coronary arteries and more than doubles the death rate from cancer. Even light cigarette smoking is associated with increasing death rates.

Dr. Ochsner goes on to discuss all the facets of smoking and disease that come up continually in every discussion of smoking. How come the death rate from lung cancer is lower among women? What about cigars and pipes—are they dangerous, too? What proof is there that smoking has anything to do with heart disease? Are filter-tips any advantage—do they lessen the risk? If cigarettes cause cancer, how come the tobacco companies can go right on advertising that their products are not harmful to health? If I stop smoking now, am I safe from cancer? How many cigarettes can I go on smoking daily without any risk? Dr. Ochsner answers all these questions and many more. He answers in confident, ringing tones. He leaves not a shadow or shred of doubt to comfort you, if you are a smoker.

If you give this book to someone who smokes, he's going to go on smoking at the risk of a terrible guilt complex and a session of horrendous nightmares, for the thought of lung cancer and other dreadful diseases will pursue him relentlessly. We handed the book to several of our smoking friends the day we got our copy. They glanced at it, asked a few questions about Dr. Ochsner's qualifications for writing it and then put out their cigarettes. When we met them the next day they told us they had stopped smoking. They haven't started again. We believe this book will probably do more to frighten people into giving up tobacco than any other single weapon in the battle.

The Nutritional Aspect of Smoking

It seems to us that Dr. Ochsner's chapter entitled *You Can Stop Smoking* is not up to the rest of the book. He himself has never smoked and he appears to attach little significance to the actual physiological reactions involved in addiction to a drug like nicotine. He takes no account of the fact that addiction to tobacco smoking may be the result of a semi-starvation diet, just as alcholism may be. We do not, of course, mean that people who smoke (or drink) don't get enough to eat. But many of them don't get the right things to eat. And the ever-present cigarette may be there to substitute for the B vitamins, the proteins, the minerals, the vitamin C, that the poor smoker is not getting in his three meals a day. Since smoking robs the body of vitamins, the smoker becomes more and more deficient every day and his craving for cigarettes grows.

We believe that it is far, far easier to give up smoking after you have made over your diet into a healthful one. Especially after you are getting plenty and more than plenty of the B vitamins and vitamin C. Your craving for cigarettes will lessen, your nerves will be calmer and you can face much more easily the difficulties of the first week or so of getting along without tobacco. So anyone who buys *Smoking and Cancer* should also buy *Twenty Ways to Stop Smoking* and *The Nutritional Way to Stop Smoking*. Both are by Editor Rodale and are published by the Rodale Press, Emmaus, Pa. They are attractive little books that sell for a dollar. If you have a friend or relative imprisoned in the fragrant toils of tobacco smoke, you couldn't do him a better favor than to get for him Dr. Ochsner's book *Smoking and Cancer, Twenty Ways to Stop Smoking* and *The Nutritional Way to Stop Smoking.*

Soap

A recent inquiry from an attorney came as a result of an article on detergents. This gentleman was representing a client who believed she had contracted a dermatitis from using a detergent. So little has been written in magazines in general circulation about the possibility of skin injury from detergents that the attorney could not find medical or scientific background for presenting his case.

We searched for material on the subject and found two very enlightening articles dealing with detergents, soaps and other cleansers in their relation to skin health.

Joseph V. Klauder, M.D., of Philadelphia, writing in the *Archives of Dermatology and Syphilology,* Volume 63, 1951, tells us that a total of 3,709 cases of skin diseases have been presented for claims for compensation under the Pennsylvania law since this law went into effect. Of these, 1,673 were occupational in origin; 2,036 were non-occupational. Of the occupational dermatoses 13.1 per cent were the result of "wet work"—that is, working in water, water and soap or water and detergents.

Dr. Klauder reviews standard tests of the ability of the skin to withstand such substances. The normal pH of the skin on the hands ranges from 4.5 to 6.5, so normal skin is acid. When the skin is bathed in sweat its acidity increases. Exposing the hands to alkali increases the alkalinity of their skin in proportion to the length of time they are exposed and the frequency, and the degree of alkalinity. The two persons in Dr. Klauder's article whose hands required the longest time to return to normal were two dishwashers whose hands of course were in soapy water most of their working time. It was discovered that not until 20 hours after their hands had been exposed to soap and water did the pH of their skin return to normal. This means that during their daily work their hands were constantly in an abnormal, alkaline condition, for the pH did not ever have time to return to normal on those days. On their days off they might expect a normal condition of the skin on their hands just as they were ready to go back to work!

Dr. Klauder studied the effects of many commercial detergents and reported on them: seven nonsoap detergents advised for dermatitic hands, 103 hand cleaners for industrial workers and 19 nonsoap detergents for kitchen and household purposes. Of the 103 hand cleaners, 94 were alkaline and 57 were gritty powders which contained one or more alkaline salt detergents.

The Normal Skin Is Acid

A. L. Hudson, M.D., of Toronto, Canada, writing in the *Canadian Medical Association Journal* for January, 1951, tells us more about the effect of soaps and detergents as well as different drugs, shampoos and ointments on the skin. We have somehow come to think of alkalinity as something to be highly desired. But when speaking of the skin, it is well to remember that alkalinity is not normal. Dr. Hudson tells us that normal skin has a pH from four to six, depending on the location of the skin and when it was last washed with an alkaline substance. In parts of the body where a great deal of perspiration is excreted the acidity is greater. And, naturally, in hot weather this pH goes even lower, for then there is more perspiration. This normally acid condition of the skin is spoken of as "the acid mantle." If one can maintain a constantly acid condition of the skin, one can prevent the development of contact dermatitis since the skin is much more susceptible to disease when alkaline.

Tests have shown that a skin area with a normal pH of four shows a pH of seven one minute after it is washed with soap and may require 70 minutes before the skin returns to its normal pH. When washing with some soaps it has been shown that this increased alkalinity may be present for as long as 3½ hours. We should keep in mind that when we talk of alkalinity in connection with soap, we mean all soap, because alkali is set free in water as soon as soap is put into it and the alkalinity of the solution may rise to as high as 10 or 11.

When there are certain kinds of disorder present in the skin, this change to alkalinity is more marked and more prolonged in the diseased area and the skin directly around it. In summer, when the skin is normally more acid it takes less time to return to the normal pH after using the soap. This may be the reason, says Dr. Hudson, why so many more people complain of dermatitis and eczema on their hands in winter. Variations in normal skin acidity occur according to: the character and quantity of perspiration, the prevention of evaporation of this perspiration, the amount of secretion of the oily glands of the skin which becomes alkaline as it is evaporating. So the acidity of the skin and, to a certain extent, the health of the skin, depend on the composition of sweat and how much of it is left unevaporated on the skin. Other conditions aside from washing with soap make the skin alkaline—dust, disintegrated sweat glands, seborrhea, psoriasis, tuberculosis, and several other skin diseases.

It seems obvious that medicines, ointments or soaps applied to any part of the body where the alkalinity is already high should, if possible, be acid, so that they may bring that part back to normal acidity rather than increasing the alkalinity. Especially in the case of fungus growths, such as cause athlete's foot, any medication used should make the skin more, rather than less, acid. Of course soap on athlete's foot is bound to increase the alkalinity still further and make the condition worse.

In testing soaps and shampoos, Dr. Hudson reports on Canadian products with which we are not familiar, but mentions several American products as well: Ivory soap has a pH of 7.5 which means that it is quite alkaline. French castile is somewhat better with a pH of six. Tide, the detergent, has a pH of 9.5—extremely alkaline. Drene shampoo has a pH of 6.5 and Halo a pH of four.

Dr. Hudson summarizes by telling us that the pH of the skin is the result of the physiological functions of the skin and is changed by certain environmental conditions and/or agents and by disease. Soaps increase the pH for relatively long periods and thus may make the skin much more susceptible to irritants or allergenic material. Once a dermatitis has been contracted, the use of soap will prolong it by keeping the skin alkaline rather than allowing it to return to its normal pH. So using soap or alkaline detergents is the most harmful thing you can do under these conditions.

If you have one of the skin conditions mentioned, you are probably being treated by a physician, so there is no further precaution you should take except to avoid soaps and detergents like the very plague. If your hands, feet and legs suffer in cold weather (and what housewife can honestly say she never has trouble with rough, painful hands in winter?) you would do well to take every precaution against exposure to soaps and detergents. It's awkward to use gloves for every kind of household task, but it's worth it in the end. So when you are doing laundry, washing dishes, cleaning and especially if you are using water outside in the winter, make certain that you do wear gloves, for you will be protecting your hands against painful roughness and possible skin disease.

Too many of us are likely to dismiss rough winter hands as "a bad case of chapping" and rub on some lotion which we hope will make them smooth again. Alkaline soaps and detergents, as we have seen, produce a definite unhealthy state of skin by the chemical action of changing the pH of the skin. And many kinds of disorders may result. You can buy lined rubber gloves these days which are much easier to work in, as well as to put on and remove. You can buy gloves with ridged fingers so that wet, slippery dishes will not slip out of your hands.

Some time ago we printed in *Prevention* the experience of an explorer in the tropical jungle who discovered that so long as he refrained from using soap, he, along with those natives who also did not use soap, was completely free from the many skin afflictions that tormented the other members of the party who used soap religiously. On the basis of this evidence, Editor Rodale began an experiment which he has continued up to the present—you guessed it, doing without soap. A daily shower or bath in clear water with the help of an efficient wash cloth has meant the elimination of any tendency to tender skin or skin disorders. Furthermore, he no longer uses soaps or shampoos on his hair, nor does he wash his hair, even with plain water. Every day he gives it a thorough, vigorous brushing. Dandruff has disappeared and his barber comments approvingly on the wonderfully healthy state of his scalp.

We would like to advise eliminating soap and detergent entirely, but in these days of coal soot and smog, we know that no housewife can get through her work using just water. But use as little soap or detergent as you possibly can. As for bathing, it seems to us quite unlikely that the average person, unless he does very grimy work, gets dirty enough to use any soap in his bath or shower. Try washing in plain water and see if you can't get rid of any wintertime eczema or other skin complaint.

Sodium

In the medical dictionary sodium is defined as "a metallic element of the alkaline group of metals. . . . Sodium occurs widely distributed in nature and forms an important constituent of animal tissues. . . . It is also a constituent of many medicinal preparations." It is well to keep in mind how widely distributed sodium is, for this is an important aspect of our consideration of this mineral.

We are most familiar with sodium as it exists in combination with chlorine as sodium chloride or common table salt. But it is well to remember that there are many other forms of sodium and that it appears in all foods. Sodium is the predominating element in body fluids that bathe different parts of the inside of the body. Potassium, which is closely related to sodium in physiology, exists mostly in muscle fibers and red blood cells. Sodium and potassium balance one another, you might say. That is, (just as in the case of calcium and phosphorus) sodium and potassium exist in the body in a certain proportion to one another. If something happens to disturb the sodium content, the potassium content is also disordered. Too much potassium in the diet results in loss of sodium. Too much sodium results in loss of potassium. And so forth.

Of course it has taken much research to discover what we now know about sodium and potassium and the part they play in physiology. Meanwhile for many centuries man has been eating salt and liking the taste of it, just as he likes the taste of sugar and spices.

Somewhere way back in history a man discovered a salt deposit, sprinkled some of it on a piece of food and discovered it gave the food a piquant taste. Since that time salt has become a commodity of great value—something rather difficult for us to conceive of today when a box of salt costs so little. But there are records of wars fought for possession of salt; there are nations of people among whom salt is so valuable that even wives and children have been traded for salt. It is noteworthy that these are nations whose diet is chiefly vegetarian. Among primitive peoples who are meat-eating, there is little or no desire for salt. In fact, primitive Eskimo tribes do not like the taste of it and will not eat food that has been salted. Among animals the herbivors (cattle, rodents and so forth) need salt because there is generally considerable potassium and little sodium in the vegetable foods on which they live. But carnivorous animals disregard salt and apparently have no need for it. This is because their food contains enough sodium, so they do not have any craving for it.

What Sodium Chloride Does in the Body

In *Clinical Nutrition* (published by Paul B. Hoeber, Inc.), Norman Jolliffe, M.D., E. F. Tisdall, M.D., and Paul R. Cannon, M.D., tell us that the main functions of sodium and chlorine in the body are: to control the volume of fluid and hence the presssure that exists between the walls of cells and the fluids that bathe them; to regulate the alkalinity or acidity of the body fluids. The way this mechanism works is by the action of the kidneys which excrete sodium or chlorine as the occasion demands. If the body is in a state tending toward acidity, the chlorine is excreted and the sodium retained. If the body is swinging too far toward alkalinity, the sodium is excreted and the chlorine is retained. In healthy people on a normal diet this mechanism functions almost perfectly. In disease, it may become disordered. Aside from these functions, sodium and chlorine appear to have no other role in nutrition, say the authors of *Clinical Nutrition.*

Considering that all these angles of health must be taken into account, it seems rather peculiar that up until recently we based our intake of salt purely on taste. And many people even today look at the plate of food set before them on the table (which has been heavily salted in the kitchen) and, without even tasting it, automatically pour on more salt from the salt shaker before they eat.

Our food comes to us already equipped with salt, remember that. Vegetables, cereals and fruits contain less salt than meat, eggs, milk and cheese. But all food contains *some* sodium. There seems to be no reason for believing that any salt at all should be added to food before we cook or eat it. Vegetables contain more potassium in proportion to their sodium content, so if you are a vegetarian and feel a real craving for the taste of salt, perhaps you are getting too much potassium in your vegetarian diet so that you need some added sodium to balance it. But if your diet contains animal foods as well—these are already high in sodium and low in potassium, and you certainly do not need to add more sodium at the table. Individuals who live practically entirely on animal products apparently have no difficulty in getting along without salt, as was demonstrated by the Arctic explorer Stefansson who gave up salt, after about two weeks of struggle with his acquired taste for it. Living on animal products in the far north, he found that, after he had overcome this initial craving, he felt no further need for salt and stated that he has known no person who enjoyed salt after being without it for half a year.

Possible Results of Eating Too Much Salt

Why should anyone trouble himself to give up salt? It's cheap, it tastes good, it makes meals more pleasant and it doesn't give you a stomachache or a headache. You don't get drunk on it; you don't break out in rashes; it doesn't take up much room in your stomach and you excrete any excess amount from the kidney or the pores of your skin. So why should anyone cut down on it?

Several years ago *Prevention* devoted an entire issue to the subject of salt (sorry, no copies are available) and turned up some amazing facts. We told of cases of cancer which were arrested on a salt-poor diet. We told of cases of deafness and sinusitis that were completely cured on a salt-poor diet. In cases of dropsy, heart disease, kidney disease, obesity, Meniére's Syndrome, headaches, insomnia and many more, salt-poor diets are now being prescribed by physicians, with remarkable results.

We know that part of the function of salt is to regulate the fluid content of the body. Anyone who has lived in a damp house in the summer knows what happens when salt and water get together. The salt attracts water. If you sprinkle only a few grains of salt on a table in a damp room, you will soon have a puddle of water around the salt grains. In the same way about one liter of water (1 quart) is present in the body for every six to seven grams of salt (about 1½ teaspoonfuls). We read somewhere the other day a statement that overweight is not the chief health problem of this country. Americans are not overweight, said this writer, they are waterlogged because of the enormous amount of salt they eat. It seems only reasonable that reducing would be much easier on a salt-poor diet, because there would be no excess water held in the body by excess salt.

The edema (swelling) that accompanies heart failure and kidney disease is now generally relieved by a salt-poor diet, rather than restricting water for the patient. In Bridges' *Dietetics for the Clinician* (Lea and Febiger, 1949) we find that excessive salt in food interferes with absorption and utilization, especially in the case of protein food. We also find a worthwhile suggestion for women who have difficulty during their menstrual periods. It has been found that before the menstrual period the body has a tendency to retain salt and, hence, water, resulting in a feeling of swelling and discomfort. This, we suppose, is due to one of the many changes that take place in body physiology at this time. Bridges recommends a pre-menstrual diet high in vitamins, relatively high in protein, with moderate carbohydrate and low fat and low salt content, with as little drinking water as possible. It is interesting to note that many physicians now place prospective mothers on salt-poor diets and find that labor seems to be much easier. We have published in past issues of *Prevention* the experiences of Dr. DeSnoo of Holland who believes that restricting salt is one important aspect of a successful and easy pregnancy.

Now perhaps our findings above may sound far-fetched. How could it be, you might ask, that after all these hundreds of years of salt-eating, we can possibly claim that disorders like deafness and cancer, headaches and obesity, difficult menstruation and complications of pregnancy, may be caused by too much salt in the diet? Remember, please, that salt has not always been as accessible as it is today. And there is no doubt about it, one does develop a taste for salt just as he develops a taste for anything else. So today most of us are using far more salt than we have any idea of. And who knows what the results might be in terms of body health?

We occasionally get letters from readers who are uneasy about taking bone meal because, they say, they are afraid they might get too much calcium. Now calcium happens to be a mineral that the body needs in relatively large quantities for many different functions. The American diet as a whole is remarkably deficient in calcium. Our national nervousness, our poor teeth, our many broken bones are indications of lack of calcium. Yet these same people who are afraid they might get too much calcium will eat food drenched in sodium chloride and will pour more sodium chloride on it at the table, without once questioning what too much sodium chloride may be doing to their bodies!

How Much Salt Do We Need and How Much Are We Getting?

What is the average human requirement for sodium? We do not know. Good health can be maintained on as little as one gram a day, according to *Clinical Nutrition*. Yet the average intake of sodium chloride today from all sources is about 8 to 15 grams per day. And some people eat as much as 20 grams (about 4 teaspoonfuls) per day! Jolliffe and his co-authors tell us that, since the kidneys control the excretion of salt, no serious sodium deficiency has ever been found in a normal human being as a result of low intake of salt. The kidneys are partially controlled by the adrenal glands, so a disorder of these glands, such as Addison's Disease, can cause the body to lose too much salt. In such a case, of course, the diet must contain more salt than would be normally required. But for those of us who are healthy, why should we permit ourselves to go on using such overdoses of a mineral that is not even a food in the sense that it is not actually used by the body in the process of building and replacing tissue, or supplying energy?

It is impossible to devise a completely salt-free diet, because sodium is present in all foods. The salt-poor diet (such as the famous rice and fruit diet for heart patients) is the closest we can come to it. We do not believe you should go out of your way to put together menus that will contain only foods low in sodium; if you are healthy and want to maintain your good health. But we do think you should learn as soon and as easily as you can, to get along without salt when you are preparing or eating food. It's really much simpler than you might think.

Remember, first of all, that all the food you eat contains some sodium. Then salt has already been added in the preparation of such foods as: salted meats and fish, potato chips, pickles, relishes, canned foods, commercially processed cereals and baked goods, salad dressings, olives, bouillon cubes, cheese (all cheeses contain salt except unsalted cottage cheese) and butter. We do not advise eating any of these foods. All have been processed. If you do eat them, you are getting lots of sodium in them. Your drinking water probably contains quite a bit of sodium. Your local board of health or waterworks can give you the exact figures. If your water is softened, either in your home or at the city waterworks, you are getting a considerable amount of sodium in your water, for sodium must be added to the water to remove the elements that make it "hard." We do not advise drinking water that has been "softened." In any case, there are so many chemicals added to city drinking water, that every city dweller would do well to buy bottled spring water for drinking and cooking.

Now look back to our opening paragraph in which we mentioned that sodium is contained in many medicines. (And incidentally, sodium rather than chlorine is the suspicious partner in the sodium chloride you eat.) Our medical dictionary lists three pages of names of medicines which include sodium, all the way from good old sodium bicarbonate (baking soda) to such things as sodium glycerinophosphate, which is used in cases of neurasthenia. Don't forget that baking powder contains sodium. And no toothpaste is free from it, so far as we can discover. Of course dentifrices aren't served as a course at dinner, but during a lifetime you may be sure you consume quite an amount of toothpaste.

Getting Along Happily With Less Salt

We are continually amazed at how many of our friends who are not health conscious have been placed on salt-poor diets by their physicians. If you or some member of your family has been told to omit as much sodium as possible, how are you going to do it? If you have been given a list of foods that are forbidden for you, abide by it. Your doctor knows what he is doing. If you simply want to cut down on salt as a matter of good health, just omit salt when you are cooking and remove the salt shaker from the table at meal time. You will really be surprised at how soon you will get over missing the salt at all. And you will be pleasantly surprised at the new taste sensation, for you will now be tasting the food itself rather than the salt you used to taste.

It seems especially difficult for older folks to learn to do without salt. We would not advise the use of a salt substitute, unless you can make absolutely certain that it is made of nothing but vegetables. Many salt substitutes contain sodium in one form or another, so you might as well use plain table salt as to use them. Herbs and other cookery tricks will help a lot. Most vegetables and meats are improved with a touch of onion, garlic, lemon juice, thyme, marjoram or parsley. Your local library has books on how to cook appetizingly with herbs. There are several excellent books on salt-poor diets. We would recommend *The Salt Free Diet Cook Book* by Emil G. Conason, M.D., and Ella Metz (published by Lear, New York). Your local bookstore can order it for you if it is not in your library.

Finally, here is a list of foods highest in sodium and foods lowest in sodium:

Highest: Biscuits, bread, butter, caviar, celery, cheese, clams, dandelion, crackers, egg-white, lima beans (dried), meat extract, olives, oysters, paprika, black pepper, raisins, spinach, turkey, all brined, pickled, smoked and salted foods.

Lowest: Cereals, cream, flour, fruit juices, fruit, honey, kidney beans, lettuce, macaroni, maple syrup, molasses, parsnips, potatoes, rice, squash, tomatoes, wheat gluten.

Soft Drinks

When summer weather is upon us, the all-this-for-a-nickel boys again step up their tunes. Radio and television fairly gurgle with soft drinks—and with a new enticement: Waistline watchers can now "refresh without filling"—with no risk of added poundage. Their ammunition aimed at the 30 million-odd obese adults in this country, the pop promoters are advertising the sugar-free drink which still contains all the beauties of its former self with the added glory of low-calorie content. But for those who respect their health, and are a bit wary about the explosives they pour into their stomachs, this means that even the slightest claim to any worth—nourishment—is gone. Take that away, dubious as it is, and what have you left?

Specifically, cola-type beverages contain the following ingredients—carbonated water, flavoring, sugar (or sugar substitutes), caffeine, and phosphoric acid.

Let's take these items one by one and see why the medical and nutrition journals, scientists, and conscientious parents are raising such a hullabaloo about these drinks—and later, why "big interests" are hushing the noise.

Carbonated Water—Harmless or Harmful?

This is the "fizz" that gives the appeal. From 89 to 93 per cent of a bottle of pop is water. The water is carbonated by putting in carbon dioxide under pressure, causing the bubbles. The carbon dioxide also increases the flavor, making possible a cheaper product. According to Harriet Morgan Fyler, Ph.D., writing in *Hygeia, the Health Magazine* for August, 1940, carbon dioxide in carbonated water is completely harmless and its "use goes back to remotest time." However, on the opposite side, Dr. Hunter H. Turner, in an article in the *Pennsylvania Medical Journal,* May, 1944, states that carbonic acid (in carbonated water) is decidedly harmful to the eye and that the increase in cases of myopia (nearsightedness) may well be caused by the "pernicious guzzling of carbonated beverages by young children today." Believe whom you will, but there is a doubt. There is also the question of the purity of the water used, which, if not properly inspected (though in the large concerns it must be), can cause untold harm through bacteria or chemicals.

Flavoring—Artificial or Real?

This may come from natural or synthetic sources or a compound of both. Chances are that the Florida-ripe orange luster gleaming from the bottle in your refrigerator comes from coal tar coloring, though perchance there's actually a portion of real orange juice used. But orange juice or no orange juice, you can probably rely on the presence of an added coloring agent, almost always made from coal tar. The government has certified these coal tars as safe for human consumption, in spite of the fact that other coal tar colorings are known to produce cancer.

We can remember a long bicycle trip we took over ten years ago in the height of summer. "Perishing" from the heat and exercise, and desperate for liquid, we stopped at the only "refreshment stand" within miles. Our only recourse was to a luscious-looking deep purple "grape" soda. Grape! There was never a more disappointing, literally sickening experience with food or drink. So if it's flavor you're after, here's a plug for the natural fruit itself—unfizzed.

Sugar—How Much Nutrition?

According to C. H. Manville, former Commissioner of the Food and Drug Department of Missouri, and an earnest defender of bottled carbonated beverages, tests showed that there was a percentage of 11.19 of sugar in 468 samples taken. This, he said, is enough to class these drinks as "food." However, in this line he went on to say that only sugar "refined to the highest degree of purity" is used. This means, of course, that every ounce of food value is refined out of the sugar, and that all the other food factors in the sugar cane are lost in the process. These other food factors are important for proper use of the sugar in the body. But aside from this, the argument for the nutritional value of soft drinks cuts its own throat. If the thousands of school children bloat themselves hourly in the winter as well as the summer months with this supposed "nutrition," how are their appetites for less exciting mealtime food? A carrot by comparison is bound to lose some of its glamor, especially if the stomach is full of "fizz." Would we have our children depend more and more exclusively on pop-bottle nourishment?

More technically, the concentrated sugar in soft drinks has a decidedly bad effect on blood sugar. When a bottle of pop gives you a momentary "lift," it is because the blood sugar level is raised. But almost immediately the level goes down, bringing on a need for another drink—and another. It is easy to see the dangers in this rise and fall, and it is clear that this constantly lowered blood sugar level opens up the road to countless disorders, of which two of the most serious are asthma and polio.

Sugar Substitutes—No Nutrition

The change to the use of sugar substitutes in soft drinks in the last few months will do more harm than good in the long run, as the manufacturers will be able to claim absolutely no food value in their drinks. The reason for their use, aside from their nonfat advantages, is that the substitutes, such as saccharin and sucaryl, are much cheaper to use than sugar (saccharin is 550 times sweeter than sugar). But all states have not sanctioned their inclusion in the beverages. Legislation by the sugar interests was secured at one time forbidding the use of saccharin, but now, with the onslaught of sucaryl which has won a place for itself, saccharin is again being permitted in some states, provided it is listed on the label of the bottle.

Caffeine, A Stimulant

According to the Council on Foods and Nutrition, cola drinks contain about two-thirds of a grain of caffeine per six ounces of beverage, or about one-third the amount in a cup of coffee. All doctors agree that caffeine is a stimulant, and even the cola advertisers stress the "lift" that comes from a coke. This "lift" which you always get from coffee, too, comes from the caffeine, as well as the sugar content. The cola manufacturers argue that since the caffeine content in their drink is only a fraction of that in coffee, it is harmless. But they do not add to their story the fact that children innocently drink bottle after bottle, day after day, thereby far exceeding the caffeine content in a cup or two of coffee.

The manufacturers also argue that parents permit their children to drink tea, which also contains caffeine. On this subject, a chemical bacteriologist from Holland, Dr. D. A. Mossel, tells us in *Nederlandsch Tijdschrift voor Geneeskunde,* for June 3, 1950, that tea is the least harmful of the drinks containing caffeine because the presence of another substance, called adenine, lessens the effect of the caffeine. Coffee does not contain this substance, but the milk used frequently in coffee acts as an "antagonist" to the caffeine. Dr. Mossel also states that experiments demonstrated that caffeine is much more harmful when taken in a cold drink than in a hot or warm one, and that the cola drinks, served ice cold (without milk), are the most dangerous of the three beverages.

Doctor George Blumer, of San Marino, California, states that excessive caffeine has been found to produce ulcers in animals and in some human beings, and that severe vertigo may also result. This is to say nothing of its common effects of heart and nerve stimulation.

Phosphoric Acid and Tooth Erosion

As its name suggests, this is a phosphorus compound, and inorganic phosphorus is known to be a toxic element. Its action on tooth enamel has been found to be especially destructive—its powers, one writer remarks, can be seen by the fact that this acid is used in industrial plants to dissolve rust.

In 1949, experiments were made at Cornell University by Dr. Clive McCay and Lois Will to determine the effect of cola drinks on teeth. Their findings aroused interest from doctors and nutritionists all over the country—and certainly, if known to the average person, should put a halt to all carefree soda drinking. They took four sets of rats, gave them a good diet and healthful surroundings, and gave each set a different beverage. The first group got tomato juice as their only beverage, the second orange juice, the third distilled water, and the fourth phosphoric acid and sucrose in the same percentage in which they are found in cola drinks.

The distilled water was the only drink that did not erode the rats' teeth. The phosphoric acid solution caused the most erosion, tomato juice the least. After six months, the teeth of those drinking the cola mixture had eroded right down to the gum line.

Answering those who might say, "Yes, but those were rats," experiments were made with human teeth suspended in a cola solution. In three hours, 1.4 milligrams of calcium per gram of tooth had been dissolved. In 336 hours, 14.6 milligrams of calcium had been dissolved.

Although we of course cannot see the enamel of teeth vanishing before our eyes in a matter of hours—as few of us soak our teeth in such a liquid so consistently—it is easy to understand what can happen to tooth enamel over a short period of time when it is frequently in contact with this acid. In their report in the *Journal of Nutrition,* November, 1949, McCay and Will state: "The erosion of the teeth by acids contained in such foodstuffs as lemon juice has long been recognized. . . . McClelland found he could decalcify teeth if they were left in a solution at a pH (acidity) of 4.5 for 12 hours. . . . In regard to more acid media he stated 'Certainly the presence of a reaction of 3.5 and below, even if existing for only a few minutes, is a potential source of damage to the teeth'."

The pH, or acidity, of the American cola drink is approximately 2.6. This is extremely acid as measured against a neutral liquid like water, which has a pH of 7. It is also more acid than the pH of 3.5 quoted above as being the danger mark for tooth erosion.

In answer to requests by readers for a comparison of the acidity of common types of carbonated soft drinks, *Consumer Reports* for July, 1950, published the following chart (the lower the number, the higher the acidity):

	Brands	*Aver. pH*
Colas	6	2.4
Lime, Lemon and Lemon and Lime	7	2.9
Ginger Ale	12	2.7
Grape	6	3.0
Raspberry	4	3.1
Cherry	7	3.1
Orange	11	3.2
Root Beer	4	3.4
Cream Soda	11	3.9
Sarsaparilla	5	4.0
Cocoa Cream	3	4.3
Club Soda	10	4.7

Going one step further in the experiments on teeth, Carey D. Miller, of the Foods and Nutrition Department of the University of Hawaii, tested the effects of many carbonated beverages on teeth, not limiting his experiments to the cola-type drinks. His results were reported in the *Journal of the American Dietetic Association,* for April, 1952. Flavored sodas, root beer, and other nationally advertised drinks were given to 129 rats with their food. Miller found that the amount of acidity in the beverage did not necessarily indicate the amount of erosion in the teeth—the degree of erosion even differed within the same drink among different brands. As a matter of fact, the erosion from two non-carbonated drinks—orange and strawberry—was greater than from the carbonated ones.

Miller believes that the presence of lithium in a drink seems to have some bearing on the amount of erosion. He found that one lemon soda without lithium produced 1.4 per cent erosion, while another lemon soda of the same brand with lithium produced only .9 per cent. However, in a past issue of *Prevention* we reported on the use of lithium in certain salt substitutes, the action of which was severe enough to cause several deaths. The Food and Drug Administration "recommends" that the use of lithium be discontinued in soft drinks, although its inclusion is evidently not forbidden to manufacturers. These facts, in spite of reports of less tooth erosion, should prevent an onrush to the pop bottles containing lithium. More than our teeth is at stake.

Harmful Chemicals in Processing

Aside from the contents of the soft drinks, there is a relatively new source of danger in the container. In 1953, Walter S. Mack, former president of Pepsi-Cola, and now president of Cantrell & Cochrane Corp., makers of Super Coola, Super Ginger Ale, Super Grape Soda, Super Club Soda, and Super Root Beer announced the revolutionary innovation of the use of the no-deposit, no-return can instead of bottles. Since that time the can business for soda pop has skyrocketed and many other beverage manufacturers have taken over the idea.

However, a carbonated beverage can present problems. *San Francisco Examiner,* for January 22, 1954, discussing the subject, states that "the pop would eat the liner and attack tinplate alloys of a conventional can. Pacific (Can Company, which started the boom) started with corrosion and acid-resistant steel. Then it developed a special organic coating, rolled on flat steel. Finally, a vinylite plastic lining is sprayed on after the can is fabricated."

All this shows a great deal of industry on the part of the can company, but even with its final product, who can determine the chemicals that have eaten away at the lining of the can and entered the beverage? The damage from this source alone can be considerable.

To date, we have no protection against chemicals in soft drinks. The Pure Food laws are not able to prohibit manufacturers from putting untested chemicals into food. Dr. McCay, of Cornell, testifying before Congressman James J. Delaney's Committee to Investigate the Use of Chemicals in Food Products in 1950, declared that the laws should be amended to require a list of ingredients and amounts on bottle labels (and now cans) of harmful products.

Difficulties in Combating Sales

With so much positive evidence against soft drinks, why is something not being done to prohibit their sale? First, the public is not fully educated to the facts. School boards continue to allow soda machines in the schools, and offer pop with school lunches; factory officials allow the machines in the factories for a handy "lift" for their workers; and parents innocently allow their children to drink as long as their nickels hold out.

The following astounding figures in the business end of the story give, perhaps, the best reason for the continued sale:

The retail value of the sale of soft drinks increased from $150,939,553 in 1935 to over $700,000,000 in 1949. In 1943, there were over 6,000 bottling companies in this country. In 1950 Pepsi-Cola had 66 plants in foreign lands, Canada Dry had 38, and Coca-Cola, the biggest of them all had 275 bottling plants—an increase from 65 in 1939. Over 100,000 people are employed in factories in this country. Sugar manufacturers supply over 250,000 tons of sugar to the industry each year. As well as the above, there are the flavoring concerns, the can companies, and the newspapers, periodicals, radio and television which are royally supported by their advertising. Even government officials who are looking into the matter are under strong political pressure to "go easy."

When you look at the picture of this mammoth enterprise, its relation to our economy, individual jobs, and its influence on so many unrelated concerns, it becomes frighteningly clear that the fight for our health must be hard and long.

Most children like milk shakes as well as soft drinks, or can be taught to like them as well. And milk shakes, especially those you concoct at home with your own blender, can be mighty nutritious. Aside from providing a lot of protein (which helps to regulate blood sugar) milk shakes properly made contain calcium, phosphorus and other minerals and most of the B vitamins in good quantity. Why not plan to keep the "makings" of some inviting milk shakes on hand from now on for the young folks of the family—fruit such as strawberries, peaches, bananas or dates, yogurt (which adds a lot to a milk shake) carob flour, wheat germ, brewer's yeast, honey, blackstrap molasses—all of these in the individual combinations your family likes best can provide frosty, delicious and healthful drinks, mixed either in your blender or with a hand egg-beater. Adults should use soybean milk, juice or water rather than milk. The section on milk explains our feeling that milk should be drunk sparingly by adults.

Soybeans

Have you discovered the soybean yet? In our search for a food high in protein, vitamins and minerals, practical, convenient, easy to prepare and economical, we could not ask for a better food than the soybean. The only food element in which it is notably short is vitamin C. And, as you might expect in dealing with such a versatile food, even vitamin C occurs plentifully in soybeans when you sprout them.

We Americans have only recently become acquainted with the soybean and its marvelous food value. The Chinese and other eastern people have known about soybeans for thousands of years. Without any knowledge of vitamins or minerals they have also discovered by experiment the most nutritious ways of preparing the soybean. We are told that, unless it is subjected to prolonged heat treatment, the soybean's excellent nutrition qualities are wasted. But the Chinese have used a series of processing methods on their soybeans, so they actually increase the food value and at the same time add greatly to the versatility of the food.

The soybean is germinated, producing sprouts—tender, succulent and crisp which may be eaten raw or lightly cooked. The soybean is fermented, producing soy sauce—the tasty condiment used so much in Chinese cookery. The soybean can be "infractionated" resulting in soy curd. Each of these is good food, rich in valuable nutritional elements.

In our country we process soybeans in other ways too. They can be made into flour which can be used much as grain flour is used. They can be made into a milk product which is in great demand for infants who are allergic to cow's milk. They can be made into oil which is one of our finest salad oils. Of course they can also be eaten fresh, as you eat other beans. And industries aside from food industries have found that soybeans can be used for making plastics and for other industrial purposes. The fact that by far the largest amount of soybeans is used for animal feed in this country indicates again, so clearly, our wastefulness in feeding our animals well while we let our people suffer from malnutrition.

High Protein Content of Soybean

Perhaps the most important single attribute of the humble soybean is its protein content. Soybean flour is 40 per cent protein and contains very little starch. A cup of cooked soybeans contains as much protein as ¼ pound of meat. So if you want an inexpensive food that can be substituted ounce by ounce for meat, the soybean is the answer to your search. Furthermore, the protein of the soybean is complete—that is, it is rich in all of the amino acids or forms of protein that are essential for good health. It is the only vegetable protein that can rightfully be called "complete."

As for minerals soy flour contains four times as much calcium as whole wheat flour. In a test done to determine the value of soy products, soy flour was used on one group of subjects, while wheat germ was used with another, in a diet where the soy and wheat germ were to enrich plain, unenriched white flour. The animals fed on the soy flour were as healthy in every respect as those fed on wheat germ. Other important minerals are present in ample quantities in soy beans, too.

Furthermore, soy beans have an alkaline response in the body. Many of us tend to be too acid because of the large amount of cereal products we eat, and because we will not eat enough of the alkaline-forming fruits and vegetables. Soybeans at mealtime will provide more alkalinity. The soybean is highly digestible. Apparently no one suffers from gas or other digestive disturbances after a meal of soybeans, as they may after eating other legumes. The soybean, like other legumes, enriches the soil in which it is grown, leaving valuable nitrogen which can be used by the crop that follows.

Another important element in soybeans is their oil. The oil is rich in lecithin and other fatty substances that are valuable, especially in combatting cholesterol deposits which lead so often to hardening of the arteries. Lecithin is also important for brain and nerve tissues. Soybeans are higher than almost any other food in pantothenic acid—one of the B vitamins which, it is believed, may play some part in keeping the hair color natural.

Our only problem with soybeans apparently is getting our families used to eating them, and devising ways to make them appetizing. Most westerners, not being accustomed to the taste, are inclined to decide that they don't like it. But almost any good general cook book will give you many suggestions for tasty soybean dishes. The taste is rather dull, so you have a chance here to let go with seasonings, herbs, onions, garlic, tomatoes, parsley, curry powder and whatever else you like in the way of flavorings. Adelle Davis in her excellent cook book *Let's Cook It Right* (published by Harcourt Brace and Co., New York) devotes a whole section to soybean cookery and gives a batch of mouth-watering recipes. Your state agricultural department may have free recipe pamphlets. Or try the Superintendent of Documents in Washington, D. C.

Here is an analysis of the vitamin and mineral content of about one-half cup of dried soybeans cooked:

Vitamin A	100 International Units
Vitamin B	
Thiamin	470-575 micrograms
Riboflavin	300 micrograms
Niacin	1 milligram
Pantothenic acid	1800 micrograms
Vitamin C	14 milligrams in the sprouts
Minerals	
Calcium	104 to 225 milligrams
Phosphorus	300 to 586 milligrams
Iron	8 to 10 milligrams
Protein	20 grams

Soybean Milk

A substitute milk used often when babies are allergic to cow's milk is soybean milk to which apparently few are sensitive. The reason for using a product of the soybean is, of course, the extremely high protein content of that legume. This is the only plant protein that is "complete" —that is, the protein of soybeans contains all of the essential amino acids or building blocks of protein, such as are contained in animal proteins like meat, eggs and milk. Soybean milk is high in calcium, phosphorus, iron and the B vitamins as well.

In the *Journal of Allergy,* for October 17, 1953, Douglas E. Johnstone and Jerome Glaser of Rochester, New York relate their experiences giving soybean milk to ninety-one children who were potentially allergic. That is, their family histories indicated that they were children who typically and probably would be allergic. Their histories were then compared with 65 of their brothers and sisters and 175 children unrelated to them who had apparently nonallergic backgrounds. Allergies developed in only 14 per cent of the children given the soybean milk, in 75 per cent of their brothers and sisters on cow's milk and in 52 per cent of the group that was unrelated to them.

In the *Indian Journal of Medical Research* for October, 1948, two different experiments are described, involving soybean milk, fortified with calcium phosphate. In one, the soybean milk was fed to a group of rats while cow's milk was fed to another group. The purpose was to test the use the animals made of the calcium in each kind of milk. It was found that the rats retained 82 per cent of the calcium and 87 per cent of the phosphorus of the soya milk. This compared very favorably with the retention of calcium of cow's milk. The growth of the rats on the cow's milk and the soya milk was practically the same.

Then both kinds of milk were given to children in an orphanage. By methods used in laboratories the calcium each child retained was measured. And, once again it was found that the soya milk was just as effective as cow's milk so far as the children's assimilation of it was concerned. In other words, it would appear that both milks are equally good food for children—or adults either, for that matter.

The taste of soybean milk is unusual and undoubtedly an adult or a child would have to learn to like it. An infant, of course, does not know what tastes he is supposed to like, so he would naturally take the soybean milk just as readily as the cow's milk.

A commercial brand of soybean milk purchased at the drug store showed the following mineral content, when it had been diluted to the strength one would normally use:

Calcium	.10%
Phosphorus	.05%
Potassium	.13%
Sodium	.05%
Magnesium	.02%
Iron	.0005%

A quart of the soybean milk in the diluted form in which it is drunk contained 2500 International Units of vitamin A and 400 Units of vitamin D. A quart of cow's milk contains about 2920 Units of vitamin A and its amount of vitamin D depends on whether it has been irradiated.

Spinach

Rich in iron, calcium, chlorophyll, vitamin A and vitamin C, spinach is one of those controversial foods that everybody likes to debate about. For a long time we believed that spinach was the answer to a lot of problems. It is rich in iron—so we fed it to the kids to keep their cheeks pink and their legs strong.

How did we feed it to the kids? We soaked it all afternoon in a large pan of water, then threw the water away and put the spinach through dozens of careful washings to remove sand. Then we boiled it in large quantities of water. After the spinach had boiled down to a soggy, slimy mass, we drained off all the water and then began to fuss with sauces and condiments to hide the taste and the appearance, for it was obvious that nobody in his right mind could ever be persuaded to eat a food that looked like this overcooked spinach.

During the soaking and boiling processes we lost most of the food value of the spinach, for the vitamins and minerals departed into the water. What was left was just soggy foliage. But we stuffed it into the kids. And Popeye with his can of spinach did his best to popularize it. But we all failed, for almost everybody agreed that if they had to eat spinach to stay healthy, they'd rather be sick.

Then the laboratory technicians made an interesting discovery about spinach. It contains relatively large amounts of oxalic acid, as do all the leafy vegetables of the same family—beet greens, swiss chard and so forth. The oxalic acid combines with the calcium in the spinach during the digestive process and forms oxalates which are not digested. So the calcium in spinach is generally not to be depended on, for it is probably in the form of an oxalate which will do you no good so far as your calcium supply is concerned. In fact, the oxalic acid in the spinach may well combine with other calcium in your digestive system and take it along, so that it, too, does you no good. So then the scientific magazines were buzzing with the tidings—don't eat spinach. It will rob you of calcium.

The real story on spinach seems to boil down to this: don't rely on spinach for calcium and don't eat spinach to the exclusion of other green vegetables. The fact that you lose a little calcium when you eat it doesn't detract from the fact that all the other minerals and vitamins are still there. If, however, you happen to have a spinach farm and you can't sell the spinach, don't decide you'll eat it all up yourself just to save it, for then you might come to grief.

Somewhere we met with the theory that oxalic acid in spinach is troublesome only if the spinach is cooked. If you eat it raw, this theory went, no calcium is lost and you get the full benefit of all the other minerals and vitamins. We don't know if the theory is scientifically sound or whether it's been tested in a laboratory. But it's an attractive theory, for why indeed should we spoil a fine vegetable like spinach by cooking it, when it's so tender, crisp and tasty eaten raw! Eat raw spinach in salads. If you must cook spinach don't soak it. Wash it hastily as possible as soon as you bring it in from the garden or the market. Keep it in the refrigerator tightly enclosed in your vegetable container. If you are going to cook it, use the least possible water, or no water at all. Adelle Davis in her excellent cook book, *Let's Cook It Right* (Harcourt Brace and Co.) advises cooking leafy vegetables only in their own juices, after you have carefully whirled them in a cloth bag to remove all water. They must be stirred constantly until the juices of the vegetables change to steam, then you can cover them and let them steam for a short time.

The vitamins and minerals in about four ounces of raw spinach or 1 cup of cooked spinach are listed below:

	Raw Spinach	*Cooked Spinach*
Calcium	81 milligrams	124 milligrams
Phosphorus	55 milligrams	33 milligrams
Iron	3 milligrams	2 milligrams
Potassium	780 milligrams	
Copper	.12 milligram	.26 milligram
Vitamin A	9420 International Units	11,780 International Units
Vitamin B		
Thiamin	.11 milligram	.08 milligram
Riboflavin	.20 milligram	.20 milligram
Niacin	.6 milligram	.6 milligram
Pyridoxine	83 micrograms	
Pantothenic acid	120-180 micrograms	
Biotin	6.9 micrograms	
Vitamin C	59 milligrams	30 milligrams

(In cases where the vitamin or mineral content of the cooked spinach is greater, this means only that the spinach is concentrated by cooking. A cup of cooked spinach represents a lot of raw spinach.)

Spleen

Editor Rodale calls the spleen "The junkyard." This is because one of its functions seems to be to store and destroy old wornout red blood corpuscles.

We have known about the spleen since times of antiquity and speculated about its possible function. Ancient literature is full of references to the spleen as the seat of the emotions—good humor and bad. Today the word means bad humor or irritability in our modern English. As one medical magazine puts it, the notion that the spleen is an organ of mysterious influence goes back to antiquity. And actually we don't understand much about it today.

The spleen is located against the under surface of the diaphragm and is so soft that it "gives" to make room for other organs that may crowd it. It looks like a large lymph gland and some of its functions are those of such a gland. It is important chiefly to the circulatory system of the body, and the blood. Blood is stored there—perhaps as much as one-fifth of the total blood in the body. This may be called into circulation from the spleen at any time.

We know that the various cells or corpuscles in the blood exist for a very limited time and are then worn out. It appears that the spleen's job is to dispose of them. It is also capable, we are told, of forming red blood cells in an emergency. Then, too, it forms the white blood cells that are found in lymph glands. Seemingly a very flexible and versatile organ, it aids in altering the relationship between the amount of plasma and cells in the blood, according to the various needs of the body. In other words, we suppose, if the body needs a bit more plasma, the spleen arranges things. And if it needs a few more blood cells, the spleen obligingly manufactures more.

Disorders of the spleen are always symptoms of disease somewhere else in the body. It becomes larger and softer in cases of acute infections, and in certain diseases such as malaria or leukemia it becomes permanently enlarged and firm. In malaria the spleen helps to deal with the parasites in the blood. Its function becomes so grossly deranged that it may become enormous. Other diseases in which the spleen is disordered are: *polycythemia vera* (a disease in which too many blood corpuscles are formed) anemia, liver disorders, heart disease, typhoid fever, polio, diphtheria, undulant fever (brucellosis), Rocky Mountain spotted fever, trench fever, tuberculosis and syphilis.

In cases of "hypersplenism" the spleen is enlarged and the blood immediately shows the effects in a diminution of one or more of the elements it contains—blood corpuscles, that is. In an article in *Industrial Medicine and Surgery* for August 1955, Steven O. Schwartz, M. D. of Chicago describes a number of cases of hypersplenism. In all these the blood was involved—anemia, Hodgkins Disease, leukemia and disorders of the bone marrow. It is interesting that several of the patients were suffering from arthritis and one of them had a history of five years of "black and blue spots." This sounds as if the patient were low in vitamin C, for bruises and discoloration can mean nothing else.

We also found a note in a physiology book indicating that a deficiency of vitamin A may bring about a defective development of the spleen resulting in later trouble.

Strawberries

Nature has a wise way of providing her creatures, both animal and human, with the food elements they need specifically at any given season. Thus rose hips ripen in the fall—extravagantly rich in vitamin C which, Mother Nature knows, her creatures will need in abundance throughout the winter. And one of the first foods of the early spring is the strawberry, also rich in vitamin C. Strawberries are apparently native to this country, for they were here when the first settlers came—wild strawberries, of course. But we defy anyone to produce a cultivated strawberry that matches in flavor the wild ones you pick after a day of hot sunlight.

Size has little to do with the taste of strawberries, small varieties being just as delicious as large ones. They should be bright red when you eat them, with no spots of white. After they are picked, they spoil much more rapidly than other fruits, so they should be eaten or frozen as soon as possible. If you leave the caps on, not so much vitamin C is lost in storage.

But once the caps are removed or the strawberries are sliced, vitamin C oozes away at a wasteful rate. If you cannot eat your berries immediately after they are picked or bought, put them unwashed and unhulled into the refrigerator and keep them there until just before eating time. Wash them as rapidly as possible, so that their temperature will not rise, cap them speedily and serve at once. If you are planning to freeze or can the berries, follow the same procedure of chilling them if you cannot go ahead with your plans at once.

It seems disgraceful even to speak of cooking such a delicacy as the strawberry, for there seems to be not the slightest excuse for it. Cooking of course destroys a large amount of the vitamin C of any fruit or vegetable. But jam companies still make strawberry jam and preserves, with, we might add, artificial coloring and probably artificial flavoring as well. If you have access to quantities of strawberries, for your own health's sake, freeze them, even if it means renting space in a locker or a neighbor's freezer. You can freeze them just as they are, or a little honey thinned with water can be added. They are one of the best food products for freezing and they retain all their vitamin C content through many months of frozen storage.

Wild strawberries are free for the picking in almost any meadow or pasture near where you live. And we can't imagine any pleasanter way of spending a fragrant sunny June afternoon than to have a wild-strawberry-picking party. True, they are small and it takes a lot of time to fill a basket. But we imagine (although we have not been able to find scientific evidence of this) that they must contain far more vitamin C than cultivated strawberries. And their flavor is so exotic and delicate that the French have made a business of providing wild strawberries (*frias de bois,* they call them) to gourmet restaurants and food stores in New York. They are flown from Paris every day during the season and sell for fabulous prices. Now how can you afford to ignore such delicacies which may be growing practically in your back yard? If you live in the city, ask your country friends if you may visit them during the season and pick their wild strawberries.

Here are the vitamins and minerals available from a half cupful of fresh or frozen strawberries:

Calcium	41 milligrams
Phosphorus	27 milligrams
Iron	.8 milligram (almost as much as raisins)
Copper	.02 milligram
Vitamin A	60 Inter. units
Vitamin B	
Thiamin	.03 milligram
Riboflavin	.07 milligram
Niacin	.2 milligram
Pyridoxine	44 micrograms
Pantothenic acid	260 micrograms
Biotin	4 micrograms
Vitamin C	50 to 90 milligrams (the average orange contains about 50)

Sugar—The Story of

The story of sugar seems to be one of the finest examples of man's inability to let well enough alone. Considering all the splendid and worth while improvements man has brought to his environment, it seems almost incredible that this same being, man, could also have invented and perpetrated one of the most serious and stupid mistakes in history—a mistake which, as one doctor of our acquaintance prophesies, may very well end our civilization within a few generations.

The story of sugar is a story of stupidity, greed and ignorance. It is the final devastating removal of man from his natural environment. We are talking now of white sugar—the sugar you buy at the grocery store—white, crystal, delicious, "pure." Throughout this book this is the sugar we mean when we say sugar. When we are speaking of *natural* sugars—from fruits, vegetables, honey and so forth, we will qualify them as natural sugars.

The chemistry of sugar is complex and we will not trouble you with it. There are many different kinds of sugars, chemically—fructose, glucose, sucrose, dextrose, lactose and so forth. They differ from one another in the chemical structure of their molecules. They are all carbohydrates. In other words, when you read or hear the word carbohydrate, as different from protein and fat, you will know that what is meant is sugars and starches.

The carbohydrates are the energy-giving foods, as separate from the proteins, which are the body building and repairing foods. We are told that 68 per cent of the food we eat is changed by the body into sugars to produce energy. The other 32 per cent is used for building and repairing the body. Not only sugars and starches but also fats and proteins can be changed by the body's marvelous mechanism into the kind of sugar that the body needs to produce energy. So it appears that we need sugar! Why therefore did we say that the story of sugar is the story of man's most colossal mistake? We do need sugar, yes, but the important thing is the *kind* of sugar we need.

Why Do We Like Sugar?

We have developed a taste for sweet things. Sweet things are delightful to eat. Melvin Page, D.D.S., in his splendid book, *Degeneration and Regeneration,* (published by the Biochemical Research Foundation, 2810 First Street, North, St. Petersburg, Florida) , tells us we were given a desire for sweet-tasting foods because, in natural foods, a number of very necessary food elements exist in combination with a sweet taste—vitamins and minerals, to be exact. Now a vitamin in the quantities in which it appears in food has no taste, so wise Mother Nature teams up a sweet taste with a number of vitamins. We need vitamin C if we are to live in good health for even one day. But we cannot pick vitamin C off a vine or tree and no amount of persuasion will get us to eat vitamin C if it has a disagreeable taste.

So vitamin C comes ready-packaged in cantaloupes, strawberries, guavas, oranges and so forth and we eat them actually because we have a need for the vitamins they contain. But we *think* we eat them because of the sweet taste. One-half cup of carrots is a compact little bundle of 4500 units of vitamin A, but nobody would eat them if they tasted bitter. So our taste for sweets is a reliable guide to foods that are good for us. But this guide is reliable only so long as the foods we have to choose from are natural foods that man, in his matchless inability to let well enough alone, has not tampered with.

What We Mean By "Refining"

Most of us are not familiar with sugar cane, so let's take as a sample grapes, which are rich in sugar. What could be more enjoyable than pitching in to a big dish of luscious Concords, purple and dewy and fresh from the vines! And healthy, too, for grapes come equipped with vitamins A, B and C, calcium, phosphorus, iron and many more food elements that are good for you, as well as all the substances your body needs to digest them.

Now suppose somebody—a chemist or scientist with a lot of degrees behind his name—came over to your dewy grape arbor and told you he was going to "improve" your grapes. He was going to put them through a process that would guarantee that they would keep practically forever, so that you could have them, in condensed form, on your table. You could flavor all your foods with their sweet taste, summer and winter. In addition he would "purify" your grapes. This purification process wouldn't mean much to you, except that you have come to believe that "purified" foods are somehow better, because they have no dirt in them, no germs, nothing extraneous. But, on second thought, what needs to be "purified" about your grapes as they come from the vine? Nevertheless your scientist proceeds with his terribly complicated and expensive process, which somehow, due to our technological genius, results in a product that is much less expensive than grapes, keeps indefinitely, tastes sweet and can be bought at any grocery store the year 'round.

Now we've solved all our problems. But have we? Let's look a little more closely at this very practical, sweet, inexpensive pretty-looking product you can use to your heart's content in cakes, candies, cookies, lemonade and coffee. Any vitamin B in it? Not an atom. Any vitamin A or C, any iron, phosphorus, calcium? Not a sliver. What then is left? Nothing at all is left but the sweet taste and the pure carbohydrate which will give you calories and nothing else. For your clever scientist has stripped the grapes of every vestige of food value and has left you only the sweet taste which, remember, was put there by nature to guide you to the healthful food elements that were in the original grapes. Would you say that the scientist was clever or would you say he had made a colossal mistake?

Nobody has yet discovered how to make a satisfactory, practical table sugar out of grapes. But the story above is precisely what happens in the manufacture of table sugar from sugar cane or beets. From the point of view of commerce, the refining of sugar is a stroke of genius, but from the point of view of human welfare it is one of the world's greatest tragedies.

History of Sugar

"Since we have no satisfactory knowledge of the beginnings of the culture of sugar cane, we can only infer that it was cultivated in northeastern India long before the Christian era. The earliest reference to sugar is contained in the comments made by several officers of Alexander the Great during his Indian campaign in 327 B. C." says Andrew Van Hook in his book *Sugar,* published by the Ronald Press, New York City. He goes on to say "It was still to be almost 1000 years before the consumption and cultivation of sugar began to spread beyond the borders of India. During this time, however, its sweet and honey-like nature became known and was mentioned by such writers as Theophrastus, Herodotus, Discorides and Pliny." So we see that human beings have arrived at eating sugar from sugar cane in recent times, in terms of man's life on earth. The Arabs and ancient Egyptians used sugar. The Chinese were using sugar when Marco Polo visited them in 1270-75. As history moved forward and the medieval crusades brought knowledge of eastern ways to western Europe, the use of sugar spread and eventually of course got to America. Among those Early Europeans only the very wealthy could have sugar on their tables, because it was expensive to import. In the western hemisphere sugar cane planting and slavery went hand in hand. In North and South America the tall sugar cane with its waving tassels was soon a familiar sight. "The sugar in those days was a highly impure and dark product which was shipped to the refining cities of the motherland countries for further processing," says Van Hook.

What exactly does he mean by that? He means that, to collect and ship the sugar, certain things had to be done to it, but in those days men didn't know how to remove all the dark colored substance (containing the vitamins and minerals). So their sugar was dark and sticky and difficult to handle—but much more nutritious than the white sugar we have today. It doesn't seem far-fetched to guess that none of us in the western world would be alive today if those old-timers had had the technical skill we have for "refining" foods.

As scientific knowledge developed, ways and means were discovered to refine the sugar still further. As refining processes grew more general, sugar became cheaper and more popular. In America the first refining plant was established in New York in 1689. By the middle of the nineteenth century sugar refining as we know it today had developed. Meanwhile someone had discovered that sugar might be made from beets which will grow in climates where sugar cane will not grow. And gradually the sugar beet refining industry began to grow. By 1940 the United States was producing well over two million tons of sugar per year *and consuming more than seven million tons!* A recent estimated value of the world production of sugar was two billion dollars, only a little less than the value of all the iron and steel produced in the United States. (Incidentally it is also interesting to note that the cigar and cigarette industry of this country was valued at one billion, two hundred million dollars in 1939.)

In 1939-1940 the people of the United States consumed 106.5 pounds of sugar per person—that means almost one pound every three days, *per person!* Taking into account all the babies and the sick people who dare not eat sugar, what kind of an average does that leave for the rest of us?

The Refining Process

There is no need to follow a piece of sugar cane through all the various complications of the refining process, but here are some of the substances used to produce those sparkling white crystals: lime, phosphoric acid, special clays known as diatomaceous earth, bone char, boneblack or animal charcoal. To powdered or confectioners sugar, corn starch or calcium phosphate is added to keep the sugars from caking. In producing lactose or milk sugar which is used mainly in infant foods, "the whey is first clarified with lime, decolorized with carbon and then concentrated and crystallized," says Mr. Van Hook. In refining beet sugar, lime, carbon dioxide and sulfur dioxide are involved in the "purification" process.

In harvesting sugar beets, the tops are carefully cut off while the beets are still in the field. The sugar beet industry has had some difficulty in disposing of its "wastes" which ferment easily. We put that word in quotations, for of course the "wastes" in sugar beet refining consist of everything that is worth while as food in the beet and beet top. But just as we finally learned that the germ and bran from refined wheat makes good food for cattle, so we discovered that cattle thrive on the "wastes" from beet sugar manufacture. Why shouldn't they thrive? In the wastes are concentrated all of the vitamins and minerals from the beets. Out of the whole procedure, the human beings involved—and this means you and me—get once again only the pure carbohydrate, stripped of all food value except calories.

The Food Value of Sugar

Following through on this whole senseless waste of good, healthful, wholesome food in a two billion dollar industry, do you get some idea what we mean when we use harsh and violent language in speaking of white, refined sugar? In the most sweeping evasion it has ever been our misfortune to meet in modern literature, Mr. Van Hook in his book *Sugar* has this to say about the food value of the product he is writing about: "In spite of its prominent place in the diet all over the world, the role of sugar as food has never been completely ascertained." Obviously, Mr. Van Hook, because it has no role as food. Applying even the most lax and generous interpretation to the words "food" and "nutrition" no one can show that white refined sugar has any place at all in the diet of any living thing. In speaking of the fashions in sugar all over the world, Mr. Van Hook says "In the United States a hard, white sugar of high purity is usually demanded, but in Europe considerable tolerance is allowed in respect to color. Native sugars (this means the sugars of those backward savages who are not as civilized as we) are soft, dark colored and impure, and the purity (that is, the per cent of sucrose in total dry product) is often as low as 60 or 70 per cent. *Whether or not American standards mean a superior product in nutritional value is questionable.*"

We italicized that last sentence to emphasize it, for it seems to us a masterpiece of understatement. Certainly any literate person with any nutrition chart before his eyes can readily see that American white refined sugar has absolutely no nutritional value whatsoever, so why do we need the half-hearted word "questionable?" So the uncivilized world which does not have our technical excellence has to be content with dark sugar which includes at least some (perhaps 30 to 40 per cent) of the original food elements of the beets and cane, while we civilized people deliberately choose to eat the pure, white worthless chemical left after refining.

Or do we "deliberately choose" to eat white sugar? Throughout all our research on sugar we found again and again the suggestion that the American public just won't have a dark sugar. No sir, they tell us, it must be "pure" and white as snow or Mrs. America will reject it scornfully. Mrs. America is a refined and cultured lady, they tell us, and her angel cakes must be white as moonlight, her boiled frosting pearly as Mt. Everest on a clear day, even the sugar she dumps into her morning coffee must glisten with silvery lights in her sugar bowl. Somehow we feel that this assumption is a libel on the good sense and practicability of Americans. We are absolutely certain that, if the gentlemen of the sugar industry would go to Mrs. America through the pages of her favorite magazines and in the commercials of her favorite radio and television programs, and would tell her the full story of sugar cane and beet sugar, would show her exactly what is subtracted from the cane and beet in the process of refining and would explain to her what is left in the pure white sugar she uses every day, Mrs. America would not only change her mind practically overnight about white sugar, but would march in a body to Washington and fight for legislation to make white sugar illegal!

And oh, what changes we'd have at the county fair and the mother's club bake sale! For the darkest angel cake would win the blue ribbon. And the cupcakes with the deep brown icing would sell best. To say nothing of the wonderful new opportunity for home economic experts to dream up new recipes requiring raw sugar, blackstrap molasses and honey!

Blackstrap Molasses As Food

What about blackstrap molasses anyway? Is it really the fountain of youth, guaranteed to banish any and all ailments and put hair on the chest of the scrawniest boy scout? No, we don't think so. But we know—because we read nutrition charts—that blackstrap molasses is a food, and a good food. Sugar is not. See for yourself. Here are the vitamins and minerals in one hundred grams of sugar and one hundred grams of blackstrap:

	Molasses	*Sugar*
Calories	220	400
	(All these are B vitamins)	
Thiamin	245 micrograms	0
Riboflavin	240 micrograms	0
Niacin	4 milligrams	0
Pyridoxine	270 micrograms	0
Pantothenic acid	260 micrograms	0
Biotin	16 micrograms	0

	Molasses (These are Minerals)	*Sugar*
Calcium	258 milligrams	1 milligram
Phosphorus	30 milligrams	trace
Iron	7.97 milligrams	.04 milligram
Copper	1.93 milligrams	.02 milligram
Magnesium	.04 milligram	0
Chlorine	317 milligrams	trace
Sodium	90 milligrams	.3 milligram
Potassium	1500 milligrams	.5 milligram

Where does molasses get all these vitamins and minerals? Obviously these are what is left when the sugar cane is refined. These are the vitamins and minerals Nature put in the original sugar cane to nourish you after you had discovered that the sweet taste is pleasant. But blackstrap molasses is "impure" scream the writers in the big popular magazines! That's right, folks, it is "impure." And the "impurities" are vitamin B, calcium, phosphorus, iron and other minerals which are completely essential to human nutrition. Blackstrap molasses doesn't taste as good as sugar until you get used to it. It doesn't look pretty in your sugar bowl. And blackstrap molasses that has been prepared for use in cattle food is not for human consumption of course. But blackstrap molasses for human beings (and most grocery stores carry it these days) is every bit as free from germs and dirt as any other food that must pass Federal inspection.

In the following pages we will show you what harm white sugar does to your body. It's not just something you can go right on eating, you know, so long as you eat good foods, too! Anything you put into your body that does not belong there is harmful, you may be sure. White sugar is a drug to which we Americans have become addicted. You will see in the following pages what devastating inroads on American health have been made by this particular drug. As you read, keep in mind that the average American (adult and child alike) consumes in toto about a pound of this drug every three days. Keep in mind, too, that white sugar and white flour (another completely worthless food) make up well over 50 per cent of the average American diet.

After you have read, dump the contents of your sugar bowl and sugar canister into the garbage can and start a new life!

Sugar, Disadvantages of

"You shouldn't eat so much candy, dear. It's not good for you. Well, just one more piece." And Mama hands Junior another piece of candy. Where did we pick up this idea that sugar is not good for us? Even those folks who stuff themselves on sweet things all day will mention meanwhile that they know it's bad for them. Have you ever talked to anyone who believes that eating sugar is good for him? "Oh I just can't get along without my dessert," he will tell you. But he won't add that the dessert is good for him.

So in your campaign to get your friends and relatives to stop eating sugar everyone you talk to will know in a sort of indefinite and reluctant way that sugar is not good for one's health. But, before you can get him to delete sugar from his daily meals, you will need a lot more definite and persuasive information than this. We hope that this article will provide you with the further information you need. We also suggest that the content of this article would make good material for a speech before the P.T.A. or mothers' club, or for a term paper in high school.

Isaac Schour, D.D.S., Ph.D., and Maury Massler, D.D.S., M.S., of Chicago have a lot to say about sugar and dental decay in an article in the *Journal of the American Dental Association* for July 1, 1947. These two investigators have contributed much to the literature on dental decay including a brilliant article in which they showed that fluoridated water is quite likely to be harmful to the teeth of badly nourished children, although it seems to postpone decay in children who are well nourished.

Refined Sugar and Dental Decay

In this particular article mentioned above, they discuss the situation in post-war Italy when 3,905 children were examined for dental decay and the figures were compared with dental decay in our country. In the Italian age group, 11-15 years, there was an average of 1.05 decayed, missing or filled tooth per child. In the same age group in the United States the average was 4.66 per child. On the other hand in four Italian cities examined, 53.4 per cent of the children between 11-15 years had no dental decay. In the United States only 9.5 per cent of the children in this age group had no dental decay. Figures on older age groups showed a similar story.

Discussing the reasons for this astonishing difference in tooth decay between Italy, a country which suffered greatly during the war, and the United States, where deprivation was certainly at a minimum, the authors point out that the amount of refined sugar available for Italian children was very limited. The Italian children were not especially well nourished, so apparently good nutrition is not the only essential for dental health. These Italian children lacked in their diets many of the healthful foods they should have had. But—and this is the crux of the matter—they also lacked refined white sugar, or at any rate did not have it in anything like the quantity in which it was available to American children. During the years 1930-34 the per capita consumption of sugar in Italy was 18 pounds, as compared to 103 pounds in America.

The investigators tell us that Clapp reported a remarkably low incidence of caries in young adult Italians who were born in Italy and who were living in Bridgeport, Connecticut. They had grown up on the Italian diet with a particularly low intake of sugar—about one-seventh that of American boys. On the other hand, Day and Sedwick examined the teeth of 500 children 13 years of age and of Italian descent (whose diet, presumably was now Americanized and high in sugar) and found no great difference between the prevalence of caries in this group and American children. This might lead to the supposition that dietary habits have a greater effect on the incidence of caries than does one's heredity, although the latter cannot be discounted.

The authors also remind us that the average Italian diet is high in carbohydrates. Spaghetti, bread and so forth make up a large part of it. Some experimenters have shown that carbohydrates produce the mouth acid that leads to tooth decay. But apparently in the case of the Italian children the carbohydrates made no difference. Even though they were badly nourished and their diet lacked many necessary foods, even though they ate a large proportion of carbohydrates in comparison to the amount of protein they had, still their teeth were infinitely better than those of American children who had been living on good diets—but had been eating large quantities of sugar.

One of the most complete discussions of refined sugar in relation to dental health comes to us in a symposium conducted by the California State Dental Association, April 24, 1950, and printed in the journal of that organization . . . *Sugar and Dental Caries.* In this 95 page booklet the speech most interesting to us was that of Dr. Robert C. Hockett of the Sugar Research Foundation, Inc., and the answer to his speech given by Michael H. Walsh, M.Sc., F.R.I.C., Instructor in Clinical Nutrition at the University of California.

A Noted Nutritionist Proves That Sugar Is Not Economical

Here are some excerpts from Dr. Walsh's brilliant rebuttal to the arguments that sugar is an economical food. . . . "If, as he (Dr. Hockett) asserts, sugar is the most efficiently produced food, why do not the commercial hog feeders, beef producers and poultry raisers feed their animals sugar in large quantities? . . . Surely if sugar were the most efficiently produced food, these scientists who are experts in animal nutrition would have advocated long ago the consumption of sugar in large quantities for the feeding of farm animals. . . . By efficiency (Dr. Hockett) means the ability to produce calories, and calories are identified as the only index of nutritive needs of man, without any regard for the need for nutrients such as essential amino acids, essential fatty acids, the many minerals and vitamins without which all the calories of sugar in the world are not only utterly useless as food but are physiologically harmful. What does it profit a man to have a million calories a year in the form of sugar if he does not have the essential nutrients to enable the sugars to be utilized?

. . . "When it comes to animal metabolism, every type of nutrient must be ingested—prefabricated, so to speak, and in that metabolism of animals—including humans—protein assumes primary importance because it is the essential raw material from which tissues are built. The most favorable development is obtained when proteins, fats, carbohydrates, minerals and vitamins are furnished to the animal organism simultaneously in amounts and proportions which we now know to be desirable; if there are to be limitations on the supply of these necessary foods, sugar cannot substitute for protein, fat cannot substitute for protein, but on the other hand, both fats and sugars can be and are derived from the metabolism of protein.

"Hence when it comes to human diets, there is no object in furnishing sugar unless appropriate amounts of proteins, fats, minerals, and vitamins are also furnished. Refined sugar, because of its highly concentrated form, and being completely devoid of essential proteins, vitamins and minerals, is now regarded nutritionally as a diluting agent of the modern diet. It is a displacer of other factors far more essential than sugar. Thus, the more sugar consumed, the less opportunity for getting essential nutrients into the diet. If sugar is furnished as a replacement of proteins, fats, minerals and vitamins, then serious physiological consequences follow. This is the essence and the crux of the physiological problem we have to deal with not only in dentistry but also in medicine.

"At this meeting the emphasis is on sugar and caries. To me there are far more serious disease problems to be dealt with than tooth decay. Far more teeth are lost today through periodontal (gum) disease than from tooth decay. There is growing and accumulating evidence that the patterns of food habits—including excessive sugar consumption—which are associated with dental decay in childhood, adolescence and early adult life are similar in structure to those of periodontal patients in later life. There is also coming to light, evidence of a dietary relationship between high sugar consumption and polio, rheumatic fever, arthritis and many degenerative diseases."

The Important Matter of Low Blood Sugar

What is some of this evidence Dr. Walsh refers to? First there is Dr. Sandler's fight against polio in North Carolina several years ago, when he brought to a standstill a polio epidemic that had frightened the residents so badly that many of them were willing to try out the diet he recommended. We have published this diet many times in *Prevention.* It is in the book, *Diet Prevents Polio* available from the Lee Foundation for Nutritional Research, 2023 West Wisconsin Avenue, Milwaukee, Wisconsin. The essence of the diet is a reduction of sugar.

Dr. Sandler forbids all forms of refined sugars (desserts, soft drinks, candies, and so forth) and even limits sharply the amount of fruit to be eaten. His theory (and we are entirely in agreement with it) is that low blood sugar makes individuals susceptible to polio. Low blood sugar is brought about by eating sugar, paradoxical as this may sound. Eating sugar brings up the blood sugar level for a short time, but then it plunges down far below normal. This makes you feel uncomfortable and you need something sweet again, so you have a soda, a piece of candy or a doughnut, and the blood sugar rockets up again, only to fall much too low a little later. As you can see, the net result is a vicious cycle of eating more and more sweets all the time, just to keep going.

Polio is not the only disease related to low blood sugar. Dr. E. M. Abrahamson in his excellent book *Body, Mind and Sugar* (published by Henry Holt and Company, New York), tells us that low blood sugar is far, far more prevalent in this country than its opposite—high blood sugar, which is diabetes. Recommending a diet very similar to that of Dr. Sandler, Dr. Abrahamson relates spectacular cures for asthma, alcoholism, neuroses, fatigue, rheumatic fever, ulcers, epilepsy, depression, and so forth—the list is encouraging.

What About Mosquito Bites?

Insect bites are probably not a very serious menace to health, except in countries where malaria is prevalent. But insect bites can spoil a vacation, cause loss of sleep, ruin one's appearance and otherwise be a pesky nuisance, especially when one is dedicated to avoiding insecticides. Over the years we have accumulated an amazing file of information on the relation of sugar-eating to susceptibility to insect bites. The only possible conclusion we can draw is that insects simply do not bite people who eat no sugar, we suppose because of the excellence of their blood chemistry. Here is a letter that came in the other day from a reader—a sample of many in our files: "A friend of mine was working in northern Canada where there was a settlement of Indians. It was during the black fly season and it was quite evident that the flies were concentrating on jabbing me, while the Indian chief who sat nearby was entirely free of them. My astonished friend asked why. The chief's reply was 'One month before the black fly season all Indians naturally know enough to leave all sugars from their diet'." We civilized Americans, with all our knowledge of chemistry, have not figured out a number of basic facts about nutrition that are well known to primitive people.

Editor Rodale confirms this story with an observation from his own experience. He visited Dr. Page in Florida and discussed his work on minerals and sugar. "When that was explained to me" he says, "I immediately realized that I wanted to have my blood as healthy as possible, and began to severely eliminate all these artificial sugars. It meant, however, that I could eat fruits and such things as honey and molasses in moderation.

"That summer I noticed that I was practically immune to mosquitoes. When all others were complaining about being bitten, I was not. And when I discussed this matter with an aunt of mine who has diabetes and who also has to forego artificial sugars, she said she has had the same experience. She does not get bitten by mosquitoes."

Here is a quick review of several other articles on other aspects of sugar consumption. J. W. S. Lindahl, M. Chir. F. R. C. S., writing in the December, 1951, issue of *The Practitioner,* says, "It has been suggested that one predisposing factor (in tonsilitis) is an unbalanced diet with too much sugar and starch in relation to protein and green vegetables and I believe there is much to be said for this theory."

Dr. Sidney A. Portis of the University of Chicago believes that a diet *low in sugar* will reduce fatigue, according to the *Journal of the American Medical Association,* Volume 142, 1950. Dr. Portis, a nervous and mental disease specialist, says that an excess of emotion stimulates the pancreas, resulting in low blood sugar.

Sugar and Vitamin B Deficiency

In the December, 1951, issue of *Prevention* Editor Rodale says, "I had a very interesting experience in meeting with a former aviation pilot who was active in World War II. He related to me an experience. He suffered from blackouts which lasted only a few seconds. But in a plane that would be very serious and dangerous. The doctors cured him by giving him vitamin B1. This would seem to indicate that airplane pilots should not eat the sweet foods such as ice cream, pies, pastries and others that contain artificial sugars, including cola drinks, because the chances are, if this pilot had been on a diet that did not take in these artificial sugars, he probably would not have suffered from these blackouts which were caused by vitamin B1 deficiency and cured by taking vitamin B1."

We stress over and over again the price we pay in vitamin B for eating white sugar. Natural sugars, as they occur in fruits and sugar cane, have with them the full assortment of B vitamins that are necessary for the assimilation of the sugars, and its use by the body. As we have seen, none of these B vitamins is present in white sugar. But, if the sugar is to be used by the body they must be present. So they are drafted—from nerves, muscles, liver, kidneys, stomach, heart, skin, eyes, blood. Needless to say, this leaves these organs of the body deficient in B vitamins. Unless a tremendous amount of vitamin B-rich food is taken, this deficiency will become worse and worse. As more sugar is eaten, more B vitamins are stolen.

Look around you. We are a nation of sufferers from "nerves," digestive disorders, tiredness, poor eyesight, anemia, heart trouble, muscular diseases and a hundred assorted skin diseases. How much of this suffering is due to lack of the B vitamins caused by the amount of sugar we eat every year? No one will ever be able to answer that question precisely, but we are willing to hazard a guess that nine-tenths of these troubles would disappear within a year of the time that white sugar was banned from our tables and from our food.

Do you suffer from any of the above complaints? Are you "nervous" and tired, do you have any kind of digestive disorder or skin disease? Are you willing to try an experiment to see just how much the eating of white sugar has to do with your complaints? For six months drop sugar from your menu. No halfway measures are permitted. You may eat *nothing* that contains refined sugar. This means no bakery products, no candy, soft drinks or chewing gum, no ice cream, canned fruit (unless it is packed without sugar), no sugar in your beverages or on your cereal. You may and should eat lots of fruit and vegetables, meat, eggs, cheese, nuts and fish. In addition you should certainly take brewers yeast or desiccated liver which contain all the B vitamins. For, if you have been in the habit of eating white refined sugar you are almost bound to have a serious vitamin B shortage.

For the first week or so you'll probably suffer gnawing hunger for sweets. Satisfy your hunger with something else. Eat an apple, a handful of nuts, a piece of cheese, a raw carrot. When you stop with friends at the soda fountain, order fruit juice or tea (with no sugar). Fresh fruit and Yogurt is a wonderful dessert and once you have become accustomed to ending a meal with fruit and Yogurt you'll wonder why you ever wanted all those gooey pastries and sticky pies and cakes. In another article we give you more hints on how to get along happily and healthfully without sugar.

Sugar—and the Calcium-Phosphorus Balance

An entirely different approach to the problem of sugar intake is presented by Melvin Page, D.D.S., of Florida, in his book *Degeneration—Regeneration,* published by the Biochemical Research Foundation, 2810 First Street, North, St. Petersburg, Florida. Says Dr. Page, "We have had up to now no device whereby which we could test the ability of our body-chemistry to withstand strains and exposure to disease. A measuring stick has now been found." He then discusses the importance of minerals in the diet and says "much research has led me to the discovery that the secret lay not in the amount of these minerals, but in their proportion to each other." The outstanding important element is the relationship of calcium to phosphorus in the bloodstream, which should be two and a half to one. "On the basis of 20,000 tests taken during the past 20 years, we can state that in clinical cases, in the adult, the critical point is reached when the calcium shows 8.75 milligrams per 100 cc of blood and when the phosphorus shows 3.5 milligrams per 100 cc of blood. Below these amounts for either calcium or phosphorus there is a withdrawal of minerals from the dentin and bone, and above these amounts a reserve is maintained.

. . . "There has been a great deal of talk about sugar being a cause of dental decay. Directly it is not, but indirectly it is." Dr. Page then relates the case histories of several patients whose blood chemistry he studied. In several of them he could find no reason for sudden changes in an excellent blood chemistry, until they confessed that just recently they had gotten into the habit of eating candy and sweets. He then tested the blood of other patients and immediately gave them candy to eat. Within two and a half hours there was a difference of nine points in the usable calcium and phosphorus in their bloodstreams.

Arthritis, Cancer and Sugar

Pyorrhea, an inflamed condition of the gums is actually a form of arthritis, says Dr. Page, although it is not called that because of its location in the body. "In a series of several hundred arthritics," he says, "nearly all consumed large quantities of sugar. Sugar disturbs the calcium-phosphorus balance more than any other single factor. It disturbs it in the direction of higher calcium and lower phosphorus. When the effect of the sugar has worn off, there is a rebound in the opposite direction, for action equals reaction.

"Someone might ask, why not use sugar to maintain better equilibrium of calcium and phosphorus levels. . . . First of all, it cannot be done effectively without taking just the right amounts at frequent intervals and secondly the method increases the deficiency already existing—adding fuel to the fire so to speak. Sugar is a drug and at times can be used for the purpose of raising the calcium level and lowering the phosphorus level. But its use would be for temporary effect only." In summing up his thoughts on nutrition, Dr. Page lays down two rules: 1. Our diet must not contain any harmful things; 2. It must contain all things necessary to the human body. If these two rules are obeyed, health can be attained and maintained, for adequate nutrition means calcium-phosphorus balance and good health. Refined sugar is not necessary. Refined sugar is harmful, so a sugar-eater has violated both rules for health.

"What is the result of a total discontinuance of sugar?" asks Dr. Page. Do we fail from loss of energy? Do we become tired and worn? Does our food become tasteless? Sometimes we have all these symptoms but only for a few days. A readjustment must take place in the body. We have to learn all over again to use our built-in resources.

"It is remarkable how soon we do this. How soon we feel better than we ever did. How soon our tastes recover their sensitivity so that we find flavors in food that we never realized were there. . . . You know you cannot hear ordinary conversation in a boiler factory. Neither can you taste ordinary flavors when the strong chemical sugar is making such a din. . . . Recently Dr. Otto Meyerhof of the University of Pennsylvania Medical School and the 1923 Nobel Prize winner in medicine stated that possibly growth of cancerous tissue might be stopped if biochemists could find a safe way to curb the appetite of tumors for sugar." This article, incidentally, appears in the magazine *Drug and Allied Industries,* Page 28, Volume 35, number V, May, 1949.

"We believe that the sugar level of the blood is even more important than Dr. Meyerhof states. We do not remember seeing a single cancer case who had a correct sugar level, yet in most non-cancer cases this is easily obtained by means of a sugar-free diet alone." He then describes a case of skin cancer of the face which cleared up entirely within a few months when the patient gave up drinking daily twelve bottles of a widely distributed soft drink.

Here are some more quotes from Dr. Page's book:

Sugar and Civilized Man

"The two greatest changes in nutrition have been from the whole grain flours to white flour, from few sweets and those natural, to refined sugar and that in large quantities. These two things, white flour and sugar, are the most common and the most harmful elements in our diet. They have been in use only one hundred to one hundred and fifty years, which is a long time if you think in terms of your life and mine but not when you think in terms of civilization as a whole. In plant life alterations can be developed or new species brought into being but it is a process of selection and repeated reproduction involving generations of plant life. Changes in man come just as slowly if not more so because though we use scientific methods to produce plants, we are hit-and-miss about the propagation of man. To make radical dietary changes in one hundred to one hundred and fifty years is to court disaster. The human mechanism is not adapted to such rapid changes. Our bodies are capable of adaptation but it must be a slow process covering generations.

"Sugar, the ultra-refined sweet, has had every element but sweetness removed and is lacking in both minerals and vitamins. It is a popular item of diet, especially in America. As previously noted in the discussion on dental decay, it has a deleterious effect on the calcium-phosphorus levels, the health indices, of our bodies. A brief explanation of the relationship of sugar to our bodily processes may make clear the reason for this harmful effect. Sixty-eight per cent of the food we eat is broken down through bodily chemical processes into sugar. Sugar, water, the amino and fatty acids, and mineral salts in solution are capable of permeating the intestinal wall and directly entering the blood stream. If we take refined sugar, a general requirement of the American table, into our systems, it does not need to be changed greatly in order to permeate the intestinal wall. It is nearly ready to enter the blood stream and it does so in a flood. And as in any flood, some one must come to the rescue to prevent disaster. . . . If there is more than one teaspoon of sugar in the entire blood stream or less than one-half teaspoon, we court disaster. . . . But we are most remarkably built and the liver and the pancreas form a rescue team and turn this sugar into glycogen and store it for future use. Now that may be very well in an emergency, but think of the abuse which most of us inflict on our systems daily. It is astonishing that any of us are well. And when you consider that the intake of sugar increases the calcium assimilation and that resistance to degeneration and bacteria are dependent upon the maintenance of a proper ratio between calcium and phosphorus, you can not but be impressed by the necessity to use this drug with care. As mentioned earlier, nine chocolates can throw the calcium-phosphorus levels out of balance within two and one-half hours and keep them below the margin of safety for immunity to dental decay at least thirty-two hours. Seventy-five per cent efficiency of the human machine will maintain good teeth but that is too low a degree to prevent the occurrence of other degenerative diseases. It would be laughable if we were to represent machines in the open market as only seventy-five per cent as good as they could be made.

There Are Exceptions

"You can all point to So-and-So who is healthy and takes sugar by the carload in his coffee or So-and-So who just lives on soda pop—one bottle of pop generally contains four teaspoons of sugar—and still keeps well. This is true, firstly, because there are exceptions to all rules and secondly, because many do not begin to pay for their extravagances until late in life. But look at their children and grandchildren. Do they hand down bodies as strong as those which they inherited? Natural sweets such as honey, molasses and maple syrup can be used within reason. They do affect the calcium-phosphorus levels but since they are not pure sweet and do contain essentials of diet, their presence among our foods is not as injurious as refined sugar. In generations past sugar was never found alone. It was always accompanied by other materials that the body needed. Sweet is just the label on the package.

"A scientific experiment with the sea-anemone, a water organism, provides an amusing illustration of the folly of being misled by labels. Sea-anemones live on meat but it is the creatine in the meat which attracts them. That is their one sense of taste. However, if the meat from which the creatine has been extracted is placed in the water, the sea-anemones ignore it, but if blotting paper soaked in creatine is placed within reach, they eat it with relish. They eat the label and leave the substance. Silly isn't it? But how about us?

"When we use free sugar we do so at the expense of the other essentials to the body. Our total caloric intake of food may not be changed, but the proportions of the heat producing and cell-replacing ingredients are considerably altered. In this respect the use of sugar creates a deficiency in these other materials. In every instance where a patient has habitually used refined sugar, deficiencies have existed in the other factors of an adequate nutrition, particularly as regards the vitamin B complex."

Sugar, Doing Without

Some time ago we asked *Prevention* readers to share with us their experiences in getting along without sugar. The response was so overwhelming that we published as many of the letters as we could. And long after the article had gone to the printer, letters continued to pour in! Here are some of them—joyous testimonials from folks freed of a lifelong addiction:

T. A. Lamb of Beaverdam, Virginia, writes us: "We have neither bought nor used any refined sugar since the days of rationing and now we have a family of six boys. We use no candy, commercial ice cream or other foods to which we know that refined sugar has been added. When friends send candy to the boys at holiday time we give them a quarter each to buy other toys and give the candy to the dog. Incidentally, the dog has more health sense than most people, for he just licks it a little and leaves it.

"As a result, the boys have had no sign of tooth decay or pain, but pass from baby teeth to second teeth as the trees exchange their old leaves for the new. Also we are almost free from colds the year 'round. Of course we think there are other factors, too, such as raw whole milk, fruit and fruit juices, plenty of vegetables and especially potatoes baked in the jackets. Also, we use no white flour, flesh or flesh products except a weekly meal of fish or seafood, no salt except vegetable salt and of course no tea or coffee.

"Now to offset this loss (?) of sugar we use plenty of natural raw honey on our cereals with whole milk, avoiding those cereals to which sugar has been added. We also keep a box of raisins of the unsulphured variety open before the boys to which they can help themselves at all times. This or other raw fruit is all they ever eat between meals. Occasionally, we make ice cream or other sweets, always with honey as the medium of sweetness."

Mrs. John Lienhard of Glenview, Illinois, writes: "I buy a sixty pound can of honey from an organic farm near us. I make my own bread from freshly ground whole wheat flour. I never make cake or pies or sweet desserts. We use fresh fruits and vegetables or frozen fruits in winter. . . . Eliminating all sugars and most starches from our diet we have no trouble whatsoever about overweight. . . . We get most of our proteins from organically-raised grains, cereals, eggs and so forth. I serve liver once a week and a serving of beef if I can afford it. . . . Our doctor is much interested in our diet for we all are in the best of health—high blood counts, good clean, clear, firm skin, radiant health. Amazing, says the doctor. Yet we are on a salt-free diet, sugarless diet, starch-free as we can make it—a minimum of meat. We try to eat living food, not dead food and we buy direct from organic growers."

Home Made Ice Cream Without Sugar

Here is comforting information from Mrs. Alice M. Green of Cloverdale, California: "Having a terrible sweet tooth, it was hard for me to give up candy and desserts. We used raw sugar in place of white for some time, also honey, but gradually used less and less. *(Editor's note:* as we say elsewhere in this book, the craving for sweets soon disappears on a good diet.) At present we use no sugar and little honey in any food, and seldom give it a thought. We eat dried fruit such as dates, raisins, figs, etc., to satisfy our desire for desserts.

"In hot weather we often crave ice cream and we worked out two recipes that we enjoy ever so much. One is for pineapple ice cream. We open a can of unsweetened pineapple juice and add about the same amount of rich goat's milk (cow's milk will do) pour into a glass baking dish and put into the freezing compartment. Several times during the day we stir it thoroughly. It makes a most refreshing and wholesome dessert. It is so simply and quickly made that even as busy as we are we can take a few minutes to prepare it. The other recipe is date ice cream. I pit from 12 to 20 dates, depending on the size and how sweet you want your ice cream. These I liquefy in the blender with top goat's milk. When it is completely liquefied, I pour it into the glass dish and it is ready for the freezing compartment. This is sweeter than the pineapple and is indeed delicious."

The following wonderful letter came in with no name or address, but we are certain the writer will not mind our sharing it with you: "We thought we were using much less candy and sweets than most people, but we have always had our share of allergies, colds and sickness. Our doctor is very much for preventive medicine if he can get his patients to try it. When I asked him how to keep from having colds he said 'leave sweets alone.' For over a year I left out all sweets, only occasionally using honey in cookies, pie or dessert. I had better health than I had had for years. Still had an occasional cold, but less severe. . . . When I make bread, I save out a loaf and roll out about one-fourth inch thick. I spread is generously with applesauce, raisins and nuts. Then it is rolled up and cut as in cinnamon rolls. These are sprinkled generously with finely ground coconut and baked after they rise. We sprinkle coconut on our bread pudding or use rice and raisins for a festive appearance and brown in a warm oven. We have a rule in our family that we do not eat between meals, thus eliminating many of the snacks that most children eat."

Sugar-Craving Like Alcoholism

Tom Straub of Port Hueneme, California, says "Prior to my breakdown I was a heavy sugar consumer. Lots of sugar in my coffee, sugar in cereals, rich cakes. As my health improved I suddenly noticed that I did not want sugar. I did notice, however, for many months, under conditions of fatigue, I would find myself reaching for the sugar bowl, not as a conditioned reflex, but from a desire for the sugar. I am inclined to think the same applies to the so-called alcoholics, because I have noticed among my friends that they are more inclined to drink under conditions of what might be called nervous or emotional fatigue.

"I do not use any sugar substitutes, but rely on my system metabolizing blood sugar from my day-to-day food. I have toyed with blackstrap molasses and honey but did not notice any perceptible improvement. I feel that sugar consumption and alcoholic consumption are closely related to fatigue of the endocrine glands, and the proper way to kill the desire for sugar is to eat strong wholesome foods and keep on eating them until the body improves to where the glands can metabolize the blood sugars from the various carbohydrates and fat reserves."

From Mrs. L. E. O'Keefe of Springdale, Arkansas, comes this refreshing note: "It is all of 25 years since we became convinced that our family would do better without most of the white-sugar, white-flour products. Our first move was to eliminate store candy and bakeshop products; also commercially-made ice cream. We found the use of honey the most satisfactory. I learned to can all our fruit unsweetened and then when we open it we add liquid honey and sometimes cream. We even deepfreeze some of our fully ripe fruits without added sweetening and for a change in the way of serving we often run a package of frozen fruit through the food chopper, then add honey, just drizzle it over the fruit ice. This makes a good evening dessert for hot days. In our immediate family we do not use any white sugar at all, but keep it for the pleasure (?) of our guests, though quite often we find our guests like to eat as we do."

An End To Sinus Trouble

H. C. Edinborough of Banning, California, writes: "We never took sugar into account until my dentist lent me Dr. Weston Prices' book *Nutrition and Physical Degeneration,* available from The American Academy of Applied Nutrition, 6238 Wilshire Blvd., Los Angeles 48, California.

It really opened our eyes to the relationship of foods and health. But what really changed our eating habits was your stories about sugar in *Organic Gardening* and *Prevention.*

"My wife and boy—especially my wife—have suffered from sinus trouble for years. Her sinuses had grown shut and it took a number of operations to open them up. But in spite of all kinds of treatments there was still some infection, congestion and pain. She noticed that milk and cheese made the trouble worse, so dairy products were dropped. Little did we realize that the combination of sugar and milk was causing the trouble. When sugar was completely removed from the diet, there was no trouble at all with dairy products.

"All was well up to this point, but now, how to wean our sweet tooth! (It is remarkable how the two words "sweet" and "tooth" got put together.) . . . I had little trouble cutting out sweets but not so with my wife. She craved white sugar. As long as she ate at home she planned her meals and avoided granulated sugar and sweetened with natural sugar. She got along quite well until she would eat a cup cake, pie or something at a party, then she would come home and walk the floor, or just give in and go on a sugar binge. *(Editor's note:* We repeat, sugar is a drug.) She realized for the first time that she had been drunk on sugar for years and was reminded of the alcoholics who can't stay away from the stuff once they get a taste of it. So from then on it was total abstinence for her. She can tell by the reaction in her system and her cravings when she has used anything but natural sugars in her diet.

"I must add that her health is greatly improved. Besides dropping white sugar and bleached flour from our diets, we eat our own organically-grown vegetables and use bone meal, wheat germ and brewer's yeast. *(Editor's note:* Another reason why the Edinboroughs can get along without sugar easily now—their bodies are getting enough minerals and vitamins.) We have learned many of these good things from the pages of *Organic Gardening* and *Prevention.* Your magazines have helped point the way to continued good health. We always pass their message on to others."

Fedor Mausolff of Chicago is a 17-year-old dancer. How often have you heard that sugar is an absolute necessity for any kind of strenuous exercise? But listen: "How do I get along without sugar? I still (after four years) find sugar tempting and good tasting. I am a tumbler and do ballet as a hobby. After a workout I have found it bad to take anything sweet. It makes my muscles become sore and lowers my endurance, I think. If I take any before a workout then I feel weak and discouraged. Also I do not sweat as easily as I do when no sugar is taken."

Mrs. A. C. Brookey of San Antonio, Texas, uses honey and brown sugar. She tells us: "I use honey in hot tea and really like it better. When the problem of iced tea came up (which we use a lot during hot weather), I sweeten it while it is hot. This is delicious and makes it more convenient when serving. *(Editor's note:* A sprig of fresh mint cheers up a glass of iced tea wonderfully, too!)

Mrs. S. N. Smith of Montpelier, Indiana, cans fruits in their own juices without water, or sugar. She bakes apples stuffed with a date, fig or some raisins. "I thought I could never eat pumpkin without sugar," she says, "but found if you mix some raisins or figs or dates with the pumpkin it is very good. Cooked breakfast foods need no sugar if a few of these dried fruits are added. Use a little honey mixed with water, diluted peanut butter, and lemon juice for a good mayonnaise. Sweet potatoes need no sugar—try them as they are. *(Editor's note:* This comment shows how different food habits grow up with you. We had never heard of using sugar with sweet potatoes until we read Mrs. Smith's letter. We always eat them baked, whole, in the skins.) When I am where sweets are served I sometimes eat a small amount if I feel it is necessary. I put treat candy in my purse when no one notices!"

A Cure For Stomach Ailments

A lady from Ontario, Canada, who asks to remain anonymous, says: "I want you to know that by eliminating from my diet white flour, white sugar and all foods containing either of these, I have been cured of a stomach ailment which had made my life miserable for many long years. More than one good doctor treated me and for a short time I would be better, but the trouble always returned. It was from reading your *Prevention* articles I learned of the evils of these foods and my permanent recovery followed. I cannot tell you how thankful I am to you."

Here are some brief comments from letters we do not have space to print in full:

From Mrs. Rosa N. Morrill (aged 88) of Venice, California: "I do not think any substitute for sugar is required, if one includes in one's diet figs, dates, prunes, raisins, and so forth. I sometimes eat a little honey or a bit of maple sugar."

From Dr. M. D. Stevens, Coral Gables, Florida: "We discontinued using sugar some 20 years ago without trouble at all. We don't drink cocoa, tea or coffee. However, we use honey whenever we have postum."

From Mrs. D. W. Hopwood of Santa Barbara, California: "I use a lot of herb teas—strawberry, red clover, shave grass and camomile. In these I put honey—not just any honey but a good grade of natural honey from the health food store. . . . Another product that is not well known but a wonderful food, as well as a sweet, is carob meal or St. John's bread in flour form." (Thank you, Mrs. Hopwood, for sending us on a quest for carob flour on which we had an article some months ago.)

Mrs. J. P. Atkins of Muscatine, Iowa, tells us that a serious illness started her hunting for a healthful diet. At present "I need no sugar substitute, but I have black figs, dates, raisins and prunes. I cook with pure sorghum and honey. . . . When I go to birthday dinners where I am confronted by three big cakes, I nibble on the lemon sponge." Mrs. C. M. Condron of Homer City, Pa., has been "off white sugar for two years, *positively*. I use raisins and blackstrap molasses wherever I can in baking and I use honey and maple syrup in some cases."

Mrs. Herbert P. Rogers of Burbank, California, has not eaten sugar for three years—"Has this paid off? It certainly has! The past two years neither my husband nor I have had a cold of any kind, even though colds have reached epidemic proportions around us."

If you're a sugar-eater and can't face the thought of doing without it, don't these letters give you courage and hope? It's not so hard, really, to throw the poisonous stuff out of your life entirely, and it needn't ruin your social life or get you labeled as a "crank" if you do as Mrs. Smith does and "put the treat candy in your purse," or do as Mrs. Atkins does, and "nibble at the lemon sponge!"

Sugar—Blood

By MELVIN E. PAGE, D.D.S.

Author of *Degeneration–Regeneration,* published by Biochemical Research Foundation, St. Petersburg 4, Florida

Dr. Abrahamson has written a book called *Body, Mind and Sugar* (published by Henry Holt and Company, New York). In it he brings attention to a very prevalent condition, Hypoglycemia. He states that according to his observations there are about four times as many such cases as there are cases of too high blood sugar (Hyperglycemia).

Hypoglycemia—Too Low Blood Sugar

When there is a disturbance of the mechanism which controls the blood sugar level this level will be either less than it should be or more than it should be. The correct level under normal working conditions should be very nearly 100 milligrams of sugar to 100cc of blood.

There are several undesirable results from a chronic low level of sugar. Lack of energy is the most common symptom. Many people are accused of laziness when their real trouble is hypoglycemia. More serious results are epileptic seizures. Not all epileptic seizures are due to this factor however. Brain injuries are a common cause. Some cases of schizophrenia, a form of insanity, are due to or at least concomitant with low blood sugar.

There are other results which are not uncommon at all but whose true cause is not so commonly recognized. The true story of one individual will perhaps show you that many people have hypoglycemia with serious results to themselves. Perhaps you will recognize a friend or even yourself as falling within this category like "Joe" in this story.

When Joe was a youngster he was an average student in school. Not the best nor the worst. He was athletically inclined and did well in all the physical activities of school and YMCA. In high school he began to have a harder time to get through some of his courses, especially the classes that occurred just before noon and the first part of the afternoon.

The trouble was that from eleven o'clock to twelve it was hard for him to pay attention to the teacher. He felt lightheaded and dizzy. He attributed this to hunger so it became a habit with him to eat some malted milk tablets at eleven. This helped some.

At the first afternoon class he was so sleepy that it was hard for him to pay close attention to the teacher. Even biting his lips didn't help much. However, he got through high school and went to college.

At college the same thing happened only to a greater degree. As a result Joe failed those classes which occurred at eleven and at one. He was hauled on the carpet by the dean. Neither he nor Joe could explain the situation. It was decided that Joe should take an enforced vacation from school until he would or could study harder.

Joe went West to teach in a country school. Since the school was many miles from town it was necessary for Joe to live in the schoolhouse and cook his own food. Hunting, his recreation, was also the source of supply for the major portion of his food.

That this life apparently was good for him was proven when he returned to college two years later. His scholastic standing was completely different at this time. He made good grades and did even better than before in athletics.

It wasn't until years later that the real story was unfolded. As a boy at home Joe had the diet of the average American. That is, he had milk, meat, vegetables, bread, fruit and, of course, pie, cake, ice cream and candy. At college he had even more pies, cakes, etc. But in the West he had no desserts for two years. Sweets were the secret of his trouble and their omission the cause of his recovery.

The chief cause of hypoglycemia is the use of sugar. Sugar, such as candy, cake, pies, etc., calls for extra effort on the part of the blood sugar regulating mechanism. In time, this results in wide swings in the amount of insulin produced by the pancreas. The eating of sugar causes the pancreas to put out extra insulin to take the excess sugar out of the blood. At first this production overruns the need and a low blood sugar results usually just before the next meal.

A low blood sugar creates appetite and then one eats too much with the attendant sleepiness. The extra food eaten has to be stored and the individual gets fat. In short, the appetite is for the purpose of raising the blood sugar. Opposed to this type of individual are those who have high blood sugars with a small appetite. They either burn their food up too rapidly or have such a small appetite in the presence of the elevated blood sugar that they do not gain weight, so generally speaking these people are thin.

Dr. Abrahamson finds that the cure of hypoglycemia is to eat no sugar or sweets of any kind. Our experience with many such cases over a number of years leads us to the same conclusion. Sometimes there are other factors involved but the major one is civilized man's use of sugar.

Hyperglycemia—Blood Sugar That Is Too High

An opposite condition to hypoglycemia is hyperglycemia. We consider any blood sugar level above 100 mg. per 100cc, when the patient is on a basic diet, to be too high. The basic diet is one which is mainly protein, with some fat and only those vegetables having a five per cent carbohydrate content. Coffee is also omitted before the testing of the blood, as caffeine raises the blood sugar. Any deviation from this diet two days prior to a blood test could easily prevent the real sugar level from being discovered.

When a higher or lower sugar level than normal is discovered under these conditions it means that the chemical regulators of the body are out of order.

Sometimes it is no more possible to correct such a condition by diet than it is to make an automobile run well by only changing the gasoline, water, and oil to a better grade. The timing system or the carburetor may be out of order. They may have been out of order from the very beginning, and until adjustments are made, the engine will not burn the fuel efficiently no matter how good the fuel.

When the blood sugar level is above a point of approximately 180 mg. one finds sugar in the urine. This is called diabetes mellitus. This may be due to much sugar in the diet, or to lowered function of the pancreas. There are cases, however, when other glands are at fault and a correction of these glands may eliminate the diabetes.

Another type of diabetes is called diabetes insipidus which is due to a deficiency of the posterior pituitary gland. This is subject to correction by the use of posterior pituitary substance by mouth. This gland may be weak because of inheritance, but again sugar in the diet makes the gland weaker and the diabetes worse. The chief symptom is excessive thirst and frequent and copious urination.

Sometimes diabetes of whatever nature can be cured by diet and endocrine supplementation, but when the disease is severe it can usually only be held in check by medical treatment. Early discovery and treatment is of the greatest importance. The earlier the discovery the greater the chance of recovery.

As with other diseases, the most important objective is prevention. An efficient body chemistry is nature's way of protecting us from disease. How do we get an inefficient body chemistry, and how do we make an inefficient body chemistry efficient?

First, some of us inherit a better body chemistry than others. We can keep it that way if we know how and make the effort. And it is an effort, for the civilization of which we are so proud has its detrimental side, too. We have so changed our foods by our technological advances that we have surrounded ourselves with a man-made environment detrimental to our well being. We must increase our knowledge and intelligence so that some of us at least may be able to separate the good from the bad, otherwise the future of this civilization will be rather limited.

I believe the use of sugar to be about the greatest evil of our civilization. Its use increases in direct ratio to the general prosperity of the people. In the time of George Washington the annual consumption per capita was eight pounds—now it is well over 100 pounds.

Our bodily mechanisms are unable to cope with sugar as we use it. It throws such a load upon the endocrines which are the regulators of our chemistry that they get out of order. The time it takes to do this is from one to three generations at the rate of our present consumption. We can live awhile upon the normal chemistry we inherited, but commonly we pass on to our children less than we have received from our parents.

An old saying based upon thousands of years experience is that "civilization signs its own death warrant." It would be more accurate to say that civilization based upon technological advance without corresponding mental advances throws our environment out of balance. It isn't that we have too much civilization, but rather that we do not have enough.

Sugar and Insect Bites

By J. I. Rodale

Editor of *Prevention*

Very few physicians are aware of what sugar actually does to the blood chemistry, and very little appears in modern medical literature regarding it. But, in searching for a yardstick to measure the ability of our bodies to withstand the strains of exposure to disease, Dr. Melvin Page made a startling discovery. Regarding it, he says, "Much research has led me to the discovery that the secret (of health) lay, not in the amount of minerals in the blood, but in their proportions to each other. The outstanding important element is the relationship of calcium to phosphorus in the bloodstream, which should be two and a half to one.

". . . There has been a great deal of talk about sugar being a cause of dental decay. Directly it is not, but indirectly it is." Dr. Page then relates the case histories of several patients whose blood chemistry he studied. In several of them he could find no reason for sudden changes in an excellent blood chemistry, until they confessed that just recently they had gotten into the habit of eating candy and sweets. He then tested the blood of other patients and immediately gave them candy to eat. Within two and a half hours there was a difference of nine points in the usable calcium and phosphorus in their bloodstream.

Pyorrhea, an inflamed condition of the gums is actually a form of arthritis, says Dr. Page, although it is not called that because of its location in the body. "In a series of several hundred arthritics," he says, "nearly all consumed large quantities of sugar. Sugar disturbs the calcium-phosphorus balance more than any other single factor. It disturbs it in the direction of higher calcium and lower phosphorus. When the effect of the sugar has worn off, there is a rebound in the opposite direction, for action equals reaction."

He says further: "A brief explanation of the relationship of sugar to our bodily processes may make clear the reason for its harmful effect. Sixty-eight per cent of the food we eat is broken down through bodily chemical processes into sugar. Sugar, water, the amino and fatty acids, and mineral salts in solution are capable of permeating the intestinal wall and directly entering the blood stream. If we take refined sugar, a general requirement of the American table, into our systems, it does not need to be changed greatly in order to permeate the intestinal wall. It is nearly ready to enter the blood stream and it does so in a flood. And as in any flood, someone must come to the rescue to prevent disaster . . . If there is more than one teaspoon of sugar in the entire blood stream or less than one-half teaspoon, we court disaster . . . But we are most remarkably built and the liver and the pancreas form a rescue team and turn this sugar into glycogen and store it for future use. Now that may be very well in an emergency, but think of the abuse which most of us inflict on our systems daily. It is astonishing that any of us are well. And when you consider that the intake of sugar increases the calcium assimilation and that resistance to degeneration and bacteria are dependent upon the maintenance of a proper ratio between calcium and phosphorus, you cannot but be impressed by the necessity to use this drug with care. As mentioned earlier, nine chocolates can throw the calcium-phosphorus levels out of balance without difficulty within two and one-half hours and keep them below the margin of safety for immunity to dental decay at least thirty-two hours. Seventy-five per cent efficiency of the human machine will maintain good teeth but that is too low a degree to prevent the occurrence of other degenerative diseases. It would be laughable if we were to represent machines in the open market as only seventy-five per cent as good as they could be made."

The fact that there must be a balance between the calcium and phosphorus in the blood was known to Louis Berman, M.D. who as far back as 1932 said, "A lack of balance in the calcium-phosphorus intake means not only the badly grown bones and physique of rickets, but also the badly grown brain of spasmophilia (a tendency to spasm, tetany and convulsions)." This comes from Dr. Berman's book *Food and Character* (Houghton-Mifflin, 1932) which is a remarkable piece of writing and which could have been a blueprint for an effective program of disease prevention, but it has been entirely ignored.

The work of Dr. Peter Bernfeld of Tufts College Medical School is further proof of the delicate effects that food has on our blood stream. In studying the electrophoretic blood patterns of hundreds of persons he has found no two exactly alike. They are what might be termed "electric blood prints" and could almost be used by the police for identification purposes, except, he says, for the fact that some aspects of the pattern change with the health and the diet of the person. Thus a person who was a sugar eater and suddenly dropped it from his diet, would experience a significant change in his electrophoretic blood pattern, probably due to the correction in the calcium-phosphorus ratio.

I know a physician in Philadelphia, who is helping people by testing their blood specifically for vitamin deficiencies and prescribing the lacking vitamins. I have seen three cases in which this physician helped immensely. A few weeks ago I personally took a friend to see this doctor, to see how it was done. This patient was suffering from hay fever, and the doctor took some of his blood and tested it right before my eyes on a spectroscope. The blood of this patient showed all kinds of deficiencies. Then the doctor looked at me with a peculiar gleam in his eyes and said "Look here, Rodale, you are supposed to be eating food raised organically and you therefore should have a good blood chemistry. Now I've got you here, let me take some of your blood and test it."

I said, "Sure, go ahead."

When he tested some of my blood, he looked at me and said: "Rodale, this is about the best blood I have seen in the year and a half I have been doing this kind of work, and bear in mind that I have been testing blood of healthy people, as well as sick ones, for many persons come here for routine checkups."

But the one thing he particularly showed me was my calcium-phosphorus relationship. He said he rarely comes across a case where it is as close to two and one-half to one as mine was. My calcium was 10.00 and my phosphorus was 4.575 milligrams. The patient that I brought along had calcium 8.895 and phosphorus 4.620. Considering that I am on a strict nonsugar diet this brought home forcefully the fact that sugar *does* distort the calcium-phosphorus relationship in the blood.

I cut sugar from my diet about seven or eight years ago and after a few months began to notice a startling thing. I became immune to mosquitoes. They just wouldn't touch me, when all others were complaining about being bitten. When I discussed this matter with an aunt who has diabetes, and who has had to forego artificial sugars, she said the same thing, she does not get bitten by mosquitoes. This may sound incredible. How can a mosquito detect a difference in blood chemistry in such a short interval of time? Well the time isn't as short as you might think. I did some research on the subject and found that a mosquito does not bite you on the wing. He lands first, then he takes a certain stance, probably one which will enable him to do the job efficiently. No doubt through some well developed sense, during this preparatory period, he gets a taste or smell of the blood. If it isn't to his liking, he sheathes his needle and goes his way without a jabbing. A mosquito seems to be a censor, determining whether there is too much or too little of certain chemical elements in the blood. Incidentally it is only the female mosquito that bites, the male's mouth parts are not adapted to biting.

I would like to quote from an article called "Down the Pike," by E. S. Bayard which appeared in the *Pennsylvania Farmer* of May 28, 1949. It throws additional light on the subject of diet and mosquitoes:

"Many years ago in Western Canada the late Herbert Quick and I went to a church event where ice cream and other good things were served. The air was full of mosquitoes and there was a smudge fire in each corner of the yard where the good things were supplied. Mr. Quick and I ate with two Indian women who admired his books. Not a mosquito was on the arms or face of either lady. I was told that this was because they ate no sugar—but that may not be the real reason. In the black fly season in Canada I knew a man and his sister who ate at the same table in the inn in which I was. The black flies filled up on the brother's neck until blood ran down over his white collar whenever the full fly dropped off. And no fly would touch his rosy sister!"

Captain Albert W. Stevens, of the U. S. Army Air Service, writing in the April, 1926, *National Geographic,* under the title "Exploring the Valley of the Amazon" said:

"These Indians . . . were not bothered in the least by mosquitoes or gnats. Their fine brown skin, smooth and satiny, showed no evidence of insect attack although they wore nothing for protection. We developed a theory that their failure to use either salt or sugar so changed their blood and perspiration that they were not attractive to insects.

"The Indians later on met our main party, but Hinton and I never saw them again. We mentioned to members of the expedition the peculiarity which had so impressed us and we were informed that our savage friends, when last seen, were slapping mosquitoes with great energy. This seemed to us to bear out our supposition that when they began to eat white man's salt and sugar, their insect troubles began."

Here is a letter that came in the other day from a reader: "A friend of mine was working in northern Canada where there was a settlement of Indians. It was during the black fly season and it was quite evident that the flies were concentrating on jabbing me, while the Indian chief who sat nearby was entirely free of them. My astonished friend asked why. The chief's reply was 'One month before the black fly season all Indians naturally know enough to leave all sugars from their diet'."

We civilized Americans, with all our knowledge of chemistry, have not figured out a number of basic facts about nutrition that are well known to primitive people. When you figure that mosquitoes are the carriers of such dread diseases as malaria and yellow fever the question arises could many lives have been saved if this mosquito-repulsing idea were generally known. And even today there are still places in the world where there is some malaria and yellow fever, where some good can be done if this fact about sugar could be disseminated abroad. U. N. Health Department—please take notice!

I was amazed the other day to read in *Time* magazine (January 17, 1955) an item quoting Dr. Fred L. Soper, director of the Pan American Sanitary Bureau. He said, "Yellow fever is not a dead duck. It has not been conquered, and it has not been eliminated as a permanent threat to the U. S." A mosquito, *Aëdes aegypti,* which carries the yellow fever virus, is known in a broad belt reaching from El Salvador through Mexico into our South, going from Arizona to New Mexico and across to Virginia and North Carolina. The disease could flare up at any moment.

The American Academy of Pediatrics had their 20th annual meeting which was reported in the *New York Times* of October 24, 1951. Among other subjects discussed, was the question of flea bites. Doctors were advised to consider them as a possible cause of certain skin troubles. But they overlooked certain researches which indicate that where the body is well nourished, fleas will not find conditions palatable to their appetites. It seems that a flea thrives on a diseased or deficient skin.

In experiments with dogs, where doses of vitamin B were given, the fleas left for other parts. No flea will inhabit the skin of a dog unless he has a vitamin B_1 deficiency. Dr. Leonard Haseman, an entomologist of the University of Missouri, in the September 6, 1950 issue of the *Journal of Economic Entomology* said, "Scrawny, underfed animals seem to be more attractive to and more heavily infested with lice."

In a further discussion of insect bites at the Pediatrics meeting previously mentioned, but not referring to fleas, Dr. Earl D. Osborne, of Buffalo, referred to a research which indicated that if vitamin B_1 were given to individuals in quantity, by mouth, it acted as an insect repellent. Now here is an astonishing aspect of this mosquito-sugar relationship. Giving vitamin B_1 is proof that sugar does something to attract insects, for it is a known fact that white sugar uses up vitamin B_1 in the body. Thus people who use sugar are not only distorting the calcium-phosphorus relationship of their blood, but are also destroying vitamin B_1.

A World War II aviation pilot used to suffer blackouts, which would last only a few seconds, and the doctors would help him with shots of vitamin B_1. This would seem to indicate that airplane pilots should stay away from ice cream, pies, soft drinks, candies, and should not put sugar in their coffee. They should conserve their body stores of vitamin B.

I have heard that in Maryland cows have been wearing pants. The farmers were driven to that recourse by a plague of blood sucking flies. I feel certain that these flies are attracted to the cows because of imbalances in their blood chemistry brought about by artificial practices in their feeding. A study no doubt will reveal that by bringing the diet of the cow back to its original primitiveness, the cow's blood would return to normal and would be distasteful to insects generally.

The medical profession seems to be blissfully unaware that a distortion of the chemistry in the blood, brought about by variations in the diet, could affect the biting propensities of mosquitoes. Some time ago an Associated Press dispatch told of the case of a Mrs. Berger of Lindsey, Ohio, who is so sensitive to mosquito bites that she had to be injected with a serum prepared from dried mosquitoes. So she had all the boys in town chasing mosquitoes at a penny apiece. But had her doctor told her to eliminate sugar from her diet it no doubt would have been just as effective or more so. But there would be no recurring fees as in the case of serum injections.

The medics have done some work on mosquito bites. In the *Journal of the American Medical Association,* May 17, 1952, is an article entitled "Local Effect of Compound F on Reactions to Mosquito Bites." I don't know what compound F is, but if it runs true to form it must be pretty potent stuff. (I have since found that compound F is 17-Hydroxy-Corticosterone.) The article showed that if compound F was injected into the skin of a person sensitive to the bite of a mosquito, the bite did not act up over the area where the injection was made. So to get results, a person would have to be injected all over his body, I presume.

There is a proprietary product on the market called Bite-Ban which is supposed to prevent mosquito bite. The instructions on the box say, "Adults: Two pellets, four hours apart, day before exposure, two pellets morning and night, during exposure. For best effects, Bite-Ban should be chewed or dissolved without water, or only a sip." Splendid for children, says the box. It also advised that Bite-Ban is harmless. I love it when chemical manufacturers call their product "harmless," without giving long-term, thoroughly researched proofs.

The box says that Bite-Ban contains *stavesacre,* and not knowing what *stavesacre* was I consulted my medical dictionary. *Stavesacre* it said, was *staphisagria.* Then I looked up *staphisagria* and found that it was the poisonous seed of the *delphinium staphisagria,* or louse-wort. It said that the plant and its seed are poisonous and narcotic, and sometimes used for killing lice. I have since found out, however, that Bite-Ban is a homeopathic preparation, which would indicate that the *staphisagria* is present in an extremely diluted quantity. However, regardless of the dilution, who wants to take a louse-killer to prevent mosquito bites, when a sugarless diet will be more thorough, for Bite-Ban has been effective in only about 60 per cent of the test cases.

The story of an interesting mosquito study done in Jamaica and reported in the *British Medical Journal* of May 19, 1951, begins: "While it has been known for a long time in a general sort of way that some individuals are more attractive to mosquitoes than others, little attempt has been made to follow up the wider implications of this and see whether any particular age group is more attractive than the others."

In my opinion the "wider implications" should first have taken in the question of differences in the chemistry of the blood of people as a basis for the mosquitoes' preference, rather than mere age. In the

Jamaican research it was found that babies are bitten by a certain species of mosquito *(A. albimanus)* much less frequently than older children or adults. For each bite made on a baby, there would be from 20 to 30 on its mother. Now if these investigators had been more thorough they would have asked themselves, why do mosquitoes show less of a predilection for babies than for grown-ups. If they had been nutrition-minded they might have speculated on the fact that a baby is usually born with a natural blood-chemistry, and that as it grows older and eats the common type of over-refined diet, its blood-chemistry becomes more and more distorted until finally it is distorted enough to attract a mosquito. By the time mother begins to heap sugar onto its cereal, and gives it chocolate drinks and ice cream, its blood becomes "interesting" enough to attract mosquitoes. But this *British Medical Journal* article, in not one sentence, considers or theorizes on the body make-up of a baby as compared to older people. It sticks to age statistics and mathematics. This is fragmentation with a vengeance.

A few months after this article appeared in the *British Medical Journal* a physician (B. W. Hughes) who read the original article wrote a letter to the editor (September 15, 1951 issue) in which he said, "I am in medical charge of a solely European military families hospital. During the last rainy season 28 per cent of all Army children got malaria—only 6 per cent of all Army wives were infected." Since malaria comes from the bite of a mosquito this will give us another opportunity to show that mosquitoes prefer individuals who like sugary food. On the average children consume more of this type of food, including lollipops, ice cream, candy, etc. Many of the Army wives no doubt are on reducing diets, shunning sugar foods on account of their fattening quality.

So we see pretty much evidence that the mosquito prefers an unhealthy blood. There is much other proof that insects generally have been evolved over millions of years to aid nature to keep things in order, to destroy unwanted vegetation, to act as a censor, to destroy diseased and weakened life of all sorts.

Sulfur

Sulfur is a non-metallic element which occurs widely in nature, being present in every cell of animals and plants. One-fourth of one per cent of the body consists of sulfur. About half the total body sulfur is concentrated in the muscles, the skin and bones contains about one-eighth of the total, and half of one per cent of the brain solids are sulfur. Four to six per cent of the body sulfur is in the hair. The blood contains 1.2 milligrams of inorganic sulfate per 100 milliliters.

Our chief concern with sulfur in human dietetics is the fact that proteins contain sulfur. Carbohydrates and fats do not. This means that proteins contain two substances—nitrogen and sulfur—whose waste products must be excreted by the kidneys rather than the lungs, as is the carbon dioxide produced when carbohydrates and fats are burned in the body furnace. Nitrogen and sulfur are closely rated in foods, occurring in approximately the ratio of 16 parts of nitrogen to one part of sulfur.

Nitrogen and sulfur are acid-forming. That is, the waste products resulting after the body has used these two elements give an acid rather than an alkaline reaction in the urine. In contrast to this, calcium, sodium, potassium and magnesium have an alkaline reaction in the body. One of the most important angles of metabolism (the whole process of burning and using food) is keeping a proper balance between acidity and alkalinity. Some authorities believe that the healthy body itself is equipped at all times to maintain this balance, so that, no matter what you eat, the ratio between acid and alkaline will always be correct. Other nutritionists say that one must exercise a wise choice of food to help the body preserve this balance. We are inclined to agree with the latter point of view. In other words, although protein, rich in sulfur and nitrogen, is essential to life since all body cells are made of it, still one must eat the right amount of foods containing alkaline elements for good health. Meat, milk, cheese, grains, eggs and nuts—the protein foods—should be balanced with plenty of fresh vegetables and fruits which are alkaline in their reaction.

The sulfur we take in our food is contained—practically all of it—in several amino acids or building blocks of protein. These are cystine and cysteine, ergothionine and methionine. Of these, methionine is absolutely essential for health. It must be supplied in food, for the body is unable to synthesize it. Since our bodies need sulfur for proper functioning, we are inclined to rate as "high-grade" protein those foods which contain large quantities of methionine and the other essential amino acids. These are largely foods of animal origin—milk, meat, eggs and so forth. The protein contained in plants such as grains and legumes does not have such a high content of these important amino acids.

How Does the Body Use Sulfur?

No one is exactly sure of all the functions performed by sulfur in the body, but we do know that it is contained in certain hormones—that is, substances given off by body glands—such as insulin, the hormone of the pancreas, and the anti-pituitary hormone. We know too that sulfur exists in two vitamins—thiamin and biotin which are essential for health. Apparently the sulfur in the body is used as an important part of certain enzyme systems that have to do with oxidizing, or burning foods. During this process, according to Dr. Henry C. Sherman of Columbia University in his book *Essentials of Nutrition* (Macmillan, 1948), the sulfur is converted to sulfuric acid. Even a diet that is fairly moderate in protein results in the formation of two grams of sulfuric acid which is then changed to sulfates in order to be excreted. It is believed that the liver uses these sulfates, which are waste products of digestion, to detoxify poisons produced by the putrefaction of food in the intestine.

It is difficult to conceive of a diet lacking in sulfur, since it is so widespread in nature and since all of us are bound to eat some protein, regardless of how little we regulate our meals. However, a diet lacking in methionine—the amino acid that contains sulfur—can have serious consequences such as anemia, a hemorrhaging disease of the liver, the inhibition of hair growth, and what is called a negative nitrogen balance, which means that the kidneys are not secreting urine as they should. The matter of growth of hair is extremely important in some agricultural pursuits such as raising sheep. It has been found, for instance, that wool contains about 3.55 per cent sulfur and the amount of wool on sheep is increased when the amino acids containing sulfur are added to their diet, regardless of how good the diet was before.

The Harmfulness of Some Kinds of Sulfur

Sulfur which does not appear in animal or plant food has no place in human metabolism and is, from all we can learn of it, extremely harmful. As you know, this is true of other elements as well. Fluorine and iodine occurring naturally in foods are used by the body to good advantage. But fluorine or iodine not occurring in foods can be poisonous. It seems that nature always presents us with a package in the matter of food—sulfur does not appear by itself, but in small dispersed quantities well mixed with plenty of other things. Man has a tendency to ignore these careful precautions of nature and to believe that he can safely use all chemical elements isolated from the substances that accompany them in nature.

Our concern with sulfur as a poison is chiefly brought about by the age in which we live—the age of coal and petroleum from which so many products are made that we are constantly exposed to the unhealthful effects of sulfur which occurs in these two products. Coal smoke contains sulfur and the least that can be said about breathing coal smoke is that it is not healthful. As we have pointed out many times in these pages, coal smoke—in the concentrations which we breathe during the winter months—is strongly suspected as a cause of cancer. Sulfuric acid which occurs in smog, due to coal furnaces as well as countless industrial processes which give off this corrosive acid into the air, may well be one of the main reasons for the ever-increasing rate of lung cancer. We know that cancer is an occupational disease of chimney sweeps who are constantly exposed to coal soot from chimneys.

In addition to the hazards of smoke, sulfur is ever-present in other substances to which we are exposed daily. In drying fruits such as apricots, prunes and so forth, sulfur is used to retain the color and some of the nutritive quality of the fruit. We strongly advise buying dried fruits that have not been sulfured. If the package does not indicate whether the fruit has been treated with sulfur, don't buy it until you have contacted the processors to find out. There is no law against sulfuring fruit, so they will not hesitate to tell you whether or not it was used in the preparation of the fruit.

Many coal tar products (and we are always warning against coal tar products in these pages) are processed with sulfuric acid during their manufacture. Saccharin, aspirin, alum (and hence some kinds of baking powder) are made with sulfuric acid. Alum is used in commercially-processed pickles and maraschino cherries. In many cities the water is treated with alum, as well as chlorine. Copper sulfate (a sulfur compound) is also often used in purifying water supplies. It is an insecticide, too, so we may be sure we are getting copper sulfate in fruits and vegetables we buy. The sulfa drugs which used to be so popular as a remedy for infections are made of sulfur. Of course more recently information about the damage the sulfa drugs can do has just about ended their popularity. We could go on and on enumerating products made from inorganic sulfur which we meet every day of our lives. But you get the idea, we're sure.

What steps should you take, then, to make sure you are getting enough organic sulfur in the food you eat and are not getting too much inorganic sulfur either in food, air, medicine or water? The table at the end of this article indicates those foods that are richest in sulfur. In all probability you are eating them every day.

As for avoiding sulfur compounds, we would suggest that you study the labels of all food you buy, looking for sulfur or coal tar substance that may have been used in its preparation. When you see a preservative listed on a label, shun that food. You will know it by the long, chemical-sounding name. To avoid sulfur insecticides, eat organically-grown food if you can. If not, scrub and pare all fruits and vegetables. Use bottled spring water for drinking and cooking. Throw out of your medicine cabinet (and don't replace) all the coal tar medicines, salves, ointments and pills that may contain sulfur as an ingredient or may have been manufactured with the use of sulfuric acid.

Foods Rich in Sulfur

Bacon	Cereals	Fish	Onions
Beans, dried	Cheese	Fowl	Oysters
Bran	Clams	Horse-radish	Peas, dried
Brussels sprouts	Cocoa	Meats	Swiss Chard
Cabbage	Crackers	Mustard, dry	Watercress
Cauliflower	Eggs	Nuts	

Tea

"In order to rightly estimate the advantages of tea, we must not look at its value abstractly, but on the influence it exercises on the country at large. We look at its use as one of the greatest counteracters of intemperance, for the man who enjoys his tea with his family is not a person who seeks the stimulus of the tavern, and in the lower classes the public house and the gin-shop. These are pitfalls purposely placed to entrap the footsteps of the unwary. Few are so heedless as to fall into a pit if exposed to their view; but the warmth of the fire, the brightness of the lights, the temporary excitement of the draught are as flowers strewn over the chasm beneath. We do not go as far as to say that good and cheap tea would in any decided manner remedy this evil. But we do say this, and every man who has bestowed a thought upon the subject will agree with us, that the man who enjoys a good cup of tea and can get it, with its necessary concomitants, fire and comfort, at home, will not be in much danger of turning out after the labors of the day to seek the poisonous excitement of the drinking house."

So said an anonymous writer in London in a little booklet called *The Tea Trade,* published in 1850. It seems that, not only in England but in other countries as well, tea has been introduced and promoted for the express purpose of luring wayward fathers of families away from stronger drinks. A Chinese legend tells us that tea was first used in China in 2737 B.C. However, it is first mentioned in Chinese literature in 350 A.D. Its use spread rapidly through China and Japan under the guidance of the Buddhist priests who were trying to combat intemperance. The United States at present consumes only about seven-tenths of a pound of tea per person annually, where the British use about ten pounds.

The tree which produces tea looks a little like myrtle and blossoms like a wild rose. When the leaves are being picked, the end ones—that is, the newest and tenderest ones—are picked for high-grade tea. The next leaves down on the branch for the next grade of tea and so forth. In all about 3,200 leaves or "shoots" are necessary for one pound of tea. There are over 2,000 possible blends.

In processing black tea the leaves are "withered" with heat, then rolled and allowed to ferment. For the green tea, the leaves are withered in hot pans, then rolled and dried. Oolong tea is partially withered at ordinary temperatures before it is dried. The fermentation of black tea removes some of the tannin, so that a cup of black tea properly made contains less tannin than a cup of green tea.

It appears that the criterion for excellence in tea is the amount of caffeine contained in it in relation to the amount of tannin. The aim seems to be to achieve a tea high in caffeine and low in tannin. It is suggested that the best way to do this is to infuse the tea only five or six minutes and then immediately pour it off the grounds. Milk in tea nullifies the effect of some of the tannin, so tea with milk is better for you than plain tea. For making tea, the water should be freshly boiled, the water and tea put into a hot teapot, then the brew poured off into another hot teapot. And, of course, teapots should always be of crockery, glass or china, never metal.

Tea contains caffeine, tannin or tannic acid and essential oils. The caffeine is the stimulating element, the tannin gives tea its color and body and the oils give it flavor and aroma. Tea contains 2.5 to 5 per cent of caffeine and 7 to 14 per cent of tannin. The tannin in concentration has an unpleasant effect on the mucus membranes of the mouth and digestive tract, but in the concentration in which it appears in a cup of tea it is not believed to be harmful. It is of course, the same substance used widely in medicine as an astringent and for skin diseases and burns.

Whether Or Not You Should Drink Tea

In general everything we had to say about caffeine in relation to health applies to tea as well as to coffee, except that the caffeine content of tea is not so high. Then too, it appears that there are fewer people in this country in danger of becoming tea addicts. There are, of course, people who drink tea in quantity, people who simply cannot get along without their tea. These folks are caffeine addicts just as the coffee drinkers are.

There is one aspect of tea which should be mentioned, because of the recent controversy over water fluoridation. Tea, as we drink it, is extremely rich in fluorine. A government booklet tells us that cheap grades of tea may contain as much as 398.8 parts per million of fluorine. Many of our foods contain fluorine in its natural form, in combination with other food minerals. So far as we have been able to determine, this naturally occurring fluorine is not harmful, any more than naturally occurring iodine in foods is harmful, in spite of the fact that a concentration of purified iodine, not combined in a food product, is of course poisonous.

If fluorine is indeed powerful against tooth decay as the "experts" would have us believe, how does it happen that the English people, drinking such quantities of fluorine in their daily tea, do not have wonderful teeth? As a nation, the British people have notoriously bad teeth. So far as we know, the "experts" who are promoting fluoridation, have never explained these curious facts.

We would say, however, if the water in your locality is fluoridated, you would do well to stay away from tea because tea-drinking is bound to add considerably to your fluorine intake. And the fluorine in tea does not appear with other minerals as it does, for instance, in the case of bone meal. We quote W. J. McCormick of Toronto, Canada, as saying "An optimal intake of foods rich in calcium is desirable (for protection against the toxic effects of fluorine) such as milk products and green salad vegetables. A surplus of these in the diet provides the calcium necessary for neutralizing the fluoride as previously explained. Bone meal, as a dietary supplement, should have similar effect."

So, if your local water supply is fluoridated and you still feel that you cannot get along without your tea, perhaps bone meal as a food supplement would be your best safety bet.

Teeth

Prevention of dental caries in children—what an encouraging ring the words have! We were interested in this article by N. J. Ainsworth, M.C., MRCS, LRCP, FDS, RCS, in the *British Medical Press* for April 23, 1952, mostly because of the word "prevention" used in the title. We found the article was a review of all the varous theories that have been advanced on the cause and prevention of tooth decay.

Our modern thinking on tooth decay seems to start with W. D. Miller who in 1882 carried out many experiments and wrote many articles on his theory that decay is caused by mouth acids produced by bacteria living on carbohydrates. First, he believed, the enamel is destroyed by decalcification, then the dentine and the underlying parts of the tooth are attacked by the acids. For many years proponents of this theory worked hard, isolating bacteria from saliva and trying to find ways of neutralizing the acid formed in the mouth.

In 1918 May Mallenby, working with laboratory animals, published the results of her experiments which showed that adequate calcium, phosphorus, vitamin A and especially vitamin D in the diet were all necessary for creating good structure of teeth. She also showed that a diet lacking in vitamin D caused a defective structure which later on would yield readily to decay. So Mellanby concluded that structure is the main deterrent to decay and that, if teeth are well formed, they will have few caries. She also discovered—and this, we think, is immensely important—that "a diet of high calcifying properties, given *after* the eruption of teeth whatever their structure, could prevent or retard the onset of caries, or if the disease had already developed, bring about the deposition of well-calcified secondary dentine and ultimately the arrest of the carious process." In other words, Mellanby's research shows us without any doubt that good diet will stop tooth decay—no matter how late in life this diet is resorted to. Mellanby also showed in her experiments the ravages caused by a diet high in cereal products and low in vitamin D and calcium. Cereal foods contain a substance which is antagonistic to calcium, so a diet very high in cereals will not be a healthy one, unless plenty of calcium and vitamin D are included as well.

Early in the century a researcher named Leon Williams invented the slogan "clean teeth do not decay," thereby ushering in the era of the toothbrush and toothpaste, along with all the extravagant and wholly irresponsible claims that go with them. Dr. Ainsworth tells us this slogan was shouted from the rooftops of all the dental hospitals in England and America for a generation and "echoed rather half-heartedly (by the children) for children are realists and the retort that no amout of brushing seemed to reduce the number of holes found each holiday was difficult to answer." While it is possible, of course, to remove particles of food from around and between teeth, using a toothbrush or dental floss, we cannot possibly make our teeth bacteriologically clean, so long as they are in our mouths, washed by saliva.

Later experiments showed that saliva that has been mixed with sugar for six hours, reaches an acidity capable of dissolving tooth enamel. Eating a cube of sugar will increase the acidity of the saliva within a matter of minutes. Eating soft sweets will raise the acidity within 20 minutes.

So the recommendation then became to eliminate carbohydrates in general and sugar in particular or to remove them rapidly from the mouth after they are chewed, or to eradicate the acid-forming bacteria of the mouth.

Mouth Washes and Tooth Pastes

Working on this latter proposition, one researcher tested all the various substances that might be used in mouth washes and found of course that nothing will guard the mouth against bacteria for longer than a few hours. Hydrogen peroxide, formaldehyde and such substances are the ones found most effective for bacteria-slaughter, understandably enough, since these are also quite dangerous substances for human beings.

Most recently two investigators found that there appeared to be less decay in mouths where the ammonium concentration was high. As a result of later experiments several researchers suggested the addition of ammonium phosphate to dentrifices, warning that one should not depend on this substance alone to prevent decay but that dietary measures also might be necessary.

Although tests have shown reduced decay in some persons using ammoniated toothpastes, the investigators themselves often suggest that this may be the result of the increased attention to toothbrushing encouraged by the experiment. Dr. Ainsworth also points out that, in spite of anything accomplished by an ammonium toothpaste, the acidity of the mouth is still raised to a decay-producing level within two minutes after rinsing the mouth with glucose (a sugar solution). So even if you use an ammoniated toothpaste, immediately after a meal, this might be too late to prevent decay, if you have eaten foods containing glucose or sugar at the meal.

"To sum up the conflicting evidence, the case for ammoniated dentifrices seems 'not proven'," says Dr. Ainsworth. Penicillin in toothpaste has been shown to produce some reduction in decay in an experiment by H. A. Zander in 1950. However, since the use of penicillin results in the production of strains of bacteria resistant to penicillin, there seems to be little point to its use in toothpastes, for any protection would surely be very temporary.

Dr. Ainsworth then discusses the prevention of decay by the use of fluorides, painting them on the teeth, or putting them in drinking water. More and more evidence is piling up to indicate that, while fluoridation of water may reduce or delay dental decay in very young children, its effects on the health of older people, infants and ill people have not been studied sufficiently to warrant taking a chance on artificial fluoridation of water. Dr. Ainsworth believes that applying fluorides directly to the teeth, while it is a tedious process for the child, may bring reduction in decay.

Finally he takes up the subject of soil and tooth decay. The organic farming theory, he says, "has a few enthusiastic advocates but no general support because it is difficult to devise proofs and impossible under present conditions to apply the principle generally." As readers of our magazine know, we believe there is ample proof right now of the wonderful results in good health obtained by eating organically grown food and Dr. Ainsworth himself quotes Sir Albert Howard and several other experts as to the effects of organically grown food on animals and people. Farming organically means returning to the soil all those elements taken from the soil, but returning them in the natural, slowly soluble forms in which they occur in nature. That is, using ground phosphate rock rather than a phosphate fertilizer, using compost (decayed leaves, grasses and manures) rather than a commercially prepared fertilizer that acts too quickly on the soil and may not offer the soil nutriments in the proper proportion.

It is our opinion, supported by numerous observations, as well as experiments reported in books, that an individual living entirely on organically raised foods will have little or no difficulty with dental decay.

Dr. Ainsworth concludes his article with a quote from Weston Price, that famous dentist who made a trip around the world 20 years ago and reported in his book, *Nutrition and Physical Degeneration* (available from The American Academy of Applied Nutrition, 6238 Wilshire Blvd., Los Angeles 48, Calif.), on the many nations of the world living on natural foods, to whom tooth decay is all but unknown. Dr. Price says: "We have accordingly today supporters of a variety of viewpoints. There are those who say that caries are of bacterial origin; others consider them to be all or partly nutritional, and there are others who would say that food has little or nothing to do with it. Some would expect to accomplish control of caries by prophylaxis procedures; others believe that prophylaxis cannot prevent dental caries or at least that it is not adequate alone. Some would persuade the public that particular brands of washes and dentrifices can accomplish the desired results. Others would put primary emphasis upon the mechanical phases, such as the method of using the brush, the coarseness or hardness of foods eaten, etc. As in all health problems we get our standards from Nature. When we study Nature, we find that animals throughout the passing periods have been largely immune to dental caries, that many races of humans have been immune, and that limited groups are today immune. These immune peoples, whether of the past or present, have had very little knowledge of the tooth brush, mouth washes or dentrifices.

"From the above it is suggested that progress when it is made, must be through a better understanding of the natural laws as involved in nutrition and external environment of the teeth, as these vary with susceptibility and immunity to dental caries."

Teeth and Diet

In a report entitled *Control of Tooth Decay,* the National Research Council discusses our present knowledge of tooth decay and suggests rather hesitantly that diet may have something to do with it. Fluoridation, of course, is safe, cheap, simple and sure, giving the impression that fluoridation is probably the best answer, according to them. But they do mention diet and they do suggest a proper diet for reducing tooth decay. As usual, they give only about half of the picture.

In their suggested diet you are to be sure to get protein, green leafy and yellow vegetables, citrus fruits or tomatoes and berries, and whole or enriched cereals. Now, with such a limited recommendation as this, any school child would eat almost precisely what he is eating now—the same diet that is ravishing his teeth and making him a dental cripple by the time he is grown. He could live on white bread sandwiches, cokes, cake, candy, ice cream and all the other refined carbohydrates with a piece of carrot or fruit from time to time. We wonder why such a diet continues to be recommended. Mothers read it, check on their family's diet, and then go happily on, convinced that diet has nothing to do with decay, for this diet is just what their children are eating!

As a matter of fact, there is a great deal of literature available showing exactly what kind of diet *does* decrease tooth decay. We wonder why this kind of diet is not recommended by organizations and institutions who want to be helpful. In the *Medical Journal of Australia* for June 20, 1953, there is the story of a group of children who live on such a diet. They range in age from four to nine years. The majority of them have been living in the institution, Hopewood House, since the earliest months of life. In general, their surroundings are "healthful"—that is, they have regular meals, good clothing, supervised exercise. They live as much as possible as though they were in their own homes, rather than an institution. The home is located on a 750-acre estate in the southern highlands of New South Wales.

The diet the children eat consists of: wholemeal bread, wholemeal biscuits, wholemeal porridge, wheat germ, fruits, fresh and dried vegetables, (cooked and raw), a small amount of meat, butter, eggs, cheese, milk and fruit juices. Every child takes vitamins and is allowed a little honey or molasses, and occasionally nuts.

We quote from the *Journal,* "As far as possible, food was taken uncooked and/or with a minimum of preparation, the idea being to present the food in its natural state. Notable for their absence from the diet were such items as sugar (white and brown), white flour products (including cakes and sweet biscuits) and any combination of these items. No tea was used. The water was drawn from the town supply. *This water has been examined for the presence of fluoride but none was detected.*" (Italics are ours)

Tests and examinations were made of all the children for a period of about five years. It was found that, of 81 children, 63 had no tooth decay. This proportion of children without decay is far in excess of those in other groups throughout Australia, Canada and New Zealand. The teeth of the group as a whole were remarkable for the very small number of decay spots. No child had more than six teeth needing care. The rates of decay beginning and proceeding in the mouths of these children were very far below those of the population in general. Say the authors, B. Lilienthal and his associates, "The outstanding difference in the environment as between this group of children and groups living in the population at large is the nature of the diet. Foods containing refined carbohydrates (for example, sugar, white flour) are either excluded from the diet or eaten in very small amounts." We suppose that the refined foods "eaten in very small amounts" are simply those the children may get at school or from visitors. Their noonday lunch is provided by the home, however, so three meals a day are good, unrefined foods.

How To Get Such a Diet for Us All

In a later issue of the *Journal* (July 24, 1954) we were interested in reading a discussion of this article by H. R. Sullivan and N. E. Goldsworthy of the Institute of Dental Research of the United Dental Hospital, Sydney. They say "This desirable state of freedom from caries presumably can be attained by any person who is prepared to adjust his dietetic habits or those of persons in his charge so that the carbohydrate intake satisfies nutritional requirements but does not greatly exceed them and is obtained from the products of wholemeal flour and other cereals and carbohydrates, *in their natural state.* (That is not refined or processed.) Under the conditions of western civilization the use of refined carbohydrates, including white flour products has become an accepted, almost basic, part of the dietary pattern. Therefore, in order to satisfy nutritional requirements and to prevent caries, a sustained effort is needed if we are to establish a new dietary pattern."

The rest of the article is an attempt to outline how we might go about attempting to revise present-day diets to bring them nearer to the kind of diet the children ate at the Hopewood House. By the end of the article the authors have just about convinced themselves that it cannot be done. And here are some of the reasons:

1. The disease of dental decay is neither fatal nor crippling so people don't get very upset about it.

2. People in different social strata have fixed ideas about food which are difficult to change.

3. Cultural patterns in different national groups are hard to change (those who *had* to eat black bread in the old country are determined to eat white bread in America, etc.). Then, too, there are such insurmountable difficulties in supply at local and world level, that foods simply must be refined so that they can be cheaply distributed to the consumer.

We do not believe these reasons are sound. It is our firm conviction that if our food processors could be persuaded to give us unrefined food (regardless of how many changes had to be made in production, marketing and transportation facilities), if all our mighty magazines, newspaper, radio and television networks took up the message and promoted unrefined food, within a year practically everybody in the country would have changed over. It wouldn't be any harder than that. But so long as the merits of refined, degerminated, worthless, lifeless foods are preached day and night in every piece of reading material we pick up and every commercial we hear on the air, then just so long will it be impossible to revise our diets into healthful ones.

Why Not Tax Sugar?

We found what we believe is an excellent suggestion in the *Journal of the American Medical Association* for October 16, 1954. In a report from Sweden, we learn that the Ministry of Health in that country has outlined many voluntary measures that could be taken to reduce tooth decay there. The medical and dental professions were invited to co-operate in promoting health education on the radio and in the press.

The Ministry went on to recommend discouraging the use of candy, and other sweets and producing sugarless bread which could be easily recognized by the consumer. It was also suggested that taxation might prove effective in reducing the consumption of sugar. It might even be a good idea, says the report, to select for very high taxes those products that contain most sugar—such as candy.

Could this possibly be the solution we have been looking for? Tobacco and alcohol are taxed and this does not seem to reduce their consumption. In fact, it has been suggested that the vast income from taxation on tobacco and alcohol is one reason why government agencies appear to be loath to make statements on the possible harm these two categories of poisons can do. No, people who want to drink and smoke will continue to do so, were the taxes even higher than they are.

But taxing sugar seems to us a little different. Especially if we make it clear why the tax is there. We are sure that thousands of mothers do not know the harm that sugar is doing their children. It is cheap and accessible, so why shouldn't they have as much of it as they wish? If sugar is taxed and the price of everything made from sugar goes up as a result, won't it bring home to people as nothing else could the danger that lies in our present high consumption of this white drug? We believe that Sweden may have something there and we hope the project of taxing sugar goes through so that other countries can study the results. This will be one step on the road to doing away with all refined foods!

Teeth—Gums

Human teeth are set in a membrane called the periodontal membrane, which is composed of many tough fibers which hold the tooth firmly in the alveolar bone which supports the tooth and anchors it to the jaw. The gums are the tissues that cover the alveolar bone. They are made of the same kind of tissue as the lining of the mouth, cheeks and lips.

Healthy gums are pink, tough and hard—not as hard as teeth, to be sure, but not soft and cushiony. They are smooth and fit tightly around the base of the tooth. They can be brushed without bleeding. In fact, really healthy gums should never bleed unless of course they are subjected to some unusual injury. Unhealthy gums may be red, swollen, tender and bleed easily. One of the first signs of unhealthy gums is gum recession—that is, the gums begin to pull away from the teeth. They do not lie so closely around the base of the tooth, but seem to be pushed back leaving a little pocket where bacteria can take over and trouble start.

The toothpaste ads which used to claim that four out of five have pyorrhea were not so far off as you might believe for it is estimated that far more teeth are lost from pyorrhea than from tooth decay and we know that tooth decay is almost universal in this country. Pyorrhea is a form of chronic gum disease in which the gums are involved first, then the alveolar bone that holds the teeth in the jaw bone, and finally the teeth themselves which become loose and must be extracted. The gums are swollen and tender and bleed easily. Whereas tooth decay is a disease widely prevalent among young people, pyorrhea is much more common among middle-aged and older folks.

Trench mouth, or Vincent's Disease, is another disease of the gums which may also involve the tissues of the inside of the mouth and throat. This frequently occurs among people who have pellagra, a disease caused by deficiency in vitamin B. Although it is apparently brought on by a germ that is highly contagious, it seems to affect only people whose resistance is low—because they have been ill, or have undergone some other great emotional or physical strain.

Tartar on teeth is apparently one of the causes of gum disease. Lack of vitamin C may be a cause of tartar, the thick deposit that forms on teeth. There is also ample evidence that pyorrhea can be prevented by plenty of vitamin C in the diet. In fact, pyorrhea may be an evidence of getting not quite enough vitamin C, just as scurvy is evidence of getting not nearly enough!

Other researchers have shown that vitamin A is essential for gum health, as it is, indeed, for the health of all body tissues. In addition it appears that plenty of calcium in the diet is important for healthy gums. Infants and children usually get enough calcium from the milk they drink and vitamin C from their fruit juices. But as they grow older and choose their own foods, they neglect those which are rich in vitamins and minerals. Most adults today are suffering in general from what doctors call "multiple deficiencies"—that is, lack of all the vitamins and minerals. Repairing that lack will prevent gum disease, we believe.

So the most important food elements for gum health appear to be vitamins A, B and C and bone meal. Brushing your teeth correctly will help keep your gums healthy and eating foods that require pretty vigorous chewing is beneficial, too. Fresh raw fruits and vegetables are in this category. Sunflower seeds must be chewed quite vigorously and in addition they appear to contain many elements that aid in keeping gums healthy, As a matter of fact, we can't recommend them too highly.

Not only do sunflower seeds contain vitamins and minerals aplenty, as we show in our booklet *Sunflower Seeds, the Miracle Food,* but eating them is splendid exercise for the gums and the teeth. Especially if you buy them with the hulls on and crack the hulls with your teeth to get at the kernels. In many parts of the world sunflower seeds are eaten as a snack, the way we eat popcorn and peanuts. The hungry nibbler leaves a trail of hulls behind him.

Teeth—Daily Habits and Tooth Brushing

Why do we get what dentists call "periodontal disease"—or disease of the gums? How does it happen that more teeth are lost from gum disease than from all other reasons combined? In recent years the science of periodontistry has achieved ever greater importance. For many Americans, especially those who are past middle age, are faced with the prospect of losing all their teeth, not because of diseases of the teeth but because of unhealthful gums!

Dr. Sidney Sorrin, D.D.S., Associate Professor of Periodontia at the New York University College of Dentistry, has done excellent work in discovering and presenting to the dental profession many highly significant facts about the how and why of gum disease.

In an article in *The Journal of Dental Medicine* for January, 1955, Dr. Sorrin and his associate Dr. Marvin Simring list the possible causes of gum disorders. They may come under the heading of (1) functional—that is, how one's teeth perform their functions of biting and chewing. Teeth that are too big or too small for their supporting gum structure, teeth that do not meet properly in a "bite" so that much of the force of the bite is lost, teeth that are clenched or ground because of nervous habits are likely to be responsible for lots of gum trouble.

In addition, (2) irritants on the inside of the mouth may help to bring on gum disorders. Impaction of food, tartar on the teeth, mechanical irritants such as dentures that don't fit and hence rub against the gums, chemical irritants, atmospheric irritants (mouth breathing) improper tooth brushing—all these may help to bring on trouble with gums. Then, too, there are the possible systemic reasons—having to do solely with bodily health—faulty nutrition which may mean that the body is too acid or too alkaline, that there is vitamin or mineral deficiency or both; chronic diseases; gland disorders; anemias; allergies or sensitivity to drugs; pregnancy; psychological causes.

Vitamin C is the single most important food factor for gum health, vitamin A and vitamin B being almost as important, as well as calcium and the other minerals that are so necessary for bone health. (Much of our trouble with gums arises from the fact that jawbones disintegrate and wear away so that the whole mouth and tooth structure are thrown out of alignment. American diets are notoriously short on calcium, so necessary for healthy bone structure.)

Here is one of Dr. Sorrin's case histories—a woman patient, aged 39, who came to him with an extremely bad case of gum disease. Her gums had receded and eroded, they bled at the slightest touch, and they were filled with pus. He tells us that this patient had always used an upward, downward and circular method of tooth-brushing. She had the following abnormal habits: pencil-biting, bobby-pin biting, bone chewing, hang-nail biting, biting on nuts. Her diet was unbalanced, with large quantities of cake, pies, pastries and candies being eaten. She also told Dr. Sorrin that she had pains in her elbows and knees, slight heart trouble and used laxatives constantly. Furthermore, she had high blood sugar, low blood pressure and anemia. So it seems that her gum disorder sprang from completely inadequate diet, poor mouth hygiene, especially so far as tooth-brushing was concerned and bad habits of which she was probably unaware but which apparently had a lot to do with the poor condition of her gums.

In another article in this book we discuss tooth-brushing, giving Dr. Sorrin's ideas as to exactly how the teeth should be brushed, if you want to avoid gum trouble. For cases of malocclusion—that is, where the "bite" is not right, your periodontist should be consulted. And incidentally, this is a job for a specialist, not your regular dentist. He can adjust dentures or plates or he can grind certain teeth down so that your two jaws will be able to work efficiently together again.

As for the habits that can be so harmful to teeth, here is a list of the commonest ones. Check over it carefully. And better check with your family, too! Perhaps you actually do some of these things without being aware of it.

Habits That May Do Serious Damage

First of all, Dr. Sorrin cautions against the use of dental floss, saying that you may do far more harm than good by using it. You may defeat your own purpose by injuring the gums further. Dental floss should be used only by dentists, says Dr. Sorrin. Now check your score on these:

1. *Neurotic habits:* lip-biting, cheek-biting, toothpick-biting, tongue pressure against teeth (that is, pressing or thrusting your tongue against your teeth) fingernail-biting, pencil- or pen-biting, biting on ear parts of eyeglasses, playing with bridges or dentures (slipping them nervously in and out of place) clenching teeth for control of emotions, biting on straws, matches, etc.

2. *Occupational habits:* Thread-biting, keeping pins or needles in the mouth, holding nails between teeth, cigar-biting (cigar workers may do this) using a reed in playing a musical instrument, any occupation in which the patient grinds his teeth in rhythm with the work at hand, package-wrappers who constantly keep cord between their teeth while packing parcels, stone-cutters, bricklayers, plasterers (dusts erode their teeth), bending wire with teeth while making artificial flowers, etc., etc., etc. Probably every manual occupation carries some risk, if at any time you hold anything in your teeth while you are working.

3. *Miscellaneous habits* (and these are the ones most of us are guilty of): pipe-smoking, biting on various objects such as safety pins and hair pins, biting or chewing a cigarette holder, opening tops of bottles with the teeth (yes, apparently there are some people who do!) cracking nuts or bones with teeth, chewing of cigars and/or tobacco, abnormal sleeping or reading habits (with the fingers pressed against the teeth), mouth breathing which dries out the mucus membrane in the front part of the mouth, pressure on the teeth from the hand when the head rests on the hand (how often do all of us do this, when we are sitting at a table!) thumb-sucking, chewing on one side of the mouth only (a very common habit), wedging of toothpicks between teeth, opening bobby pins with the teeth, biting the end of a tobacco pouch string (where the individual closes the pouch by holding one end of the string in his mouth while he is rolling or filling his pipe).

It seems surprising, doesn't it, that a learned dental researcher should have to take the time to point out in the pages of a learned dental magazine that such habits are harmful and very destructive to teeth and gums alike! Yet how often are any of us conscious of doing any of these things? How many of us had any idea of the harm they might do?

Dr. Sorrin says, to the dentists to whom he is addressing his remarks: "The eradication of an established habit is easier if the patient becomes conscious of the involuntary habit, realizes its harm and cooperates in its elimination by the exercise of will-power or by the adoption of a harmless substitute. After the habit is discovered, the means of correction must then be determined. In some instances, for example, the teeth can be ground so that it will be impossible for the patient to resume the abnormal position of the teeth."

A word to the wise is sufficient. We are sure that readers will make every effort to correct habits such as these and will watch their children and other members of the family to make sure that such habits do not develop.

Tooth Brushing

Fashions in tooth-brushing come and go. We used to be told that we should brush our teeth straight across horizontally. We don't know who invented this method, but it seems apparent that it couldn't work, using the average toothbrush, because the brush would not be able to penetrate between the teeth where most of the food debris lodges.

Then came the advice to brush teeth up and down, vertically, so that the brush would get to all the cracks and crevices between the teeth. Then someone suggested brushing with a circular movement.

Dr. Sorrin, whom we quote on gum disorders in another article, has utmost confidence in a completely different method of toothbrushing, which at the same time massages the gums. Here is a complete review of

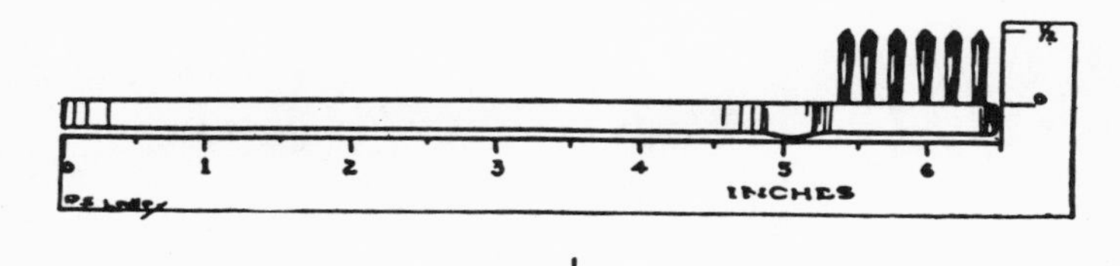

1

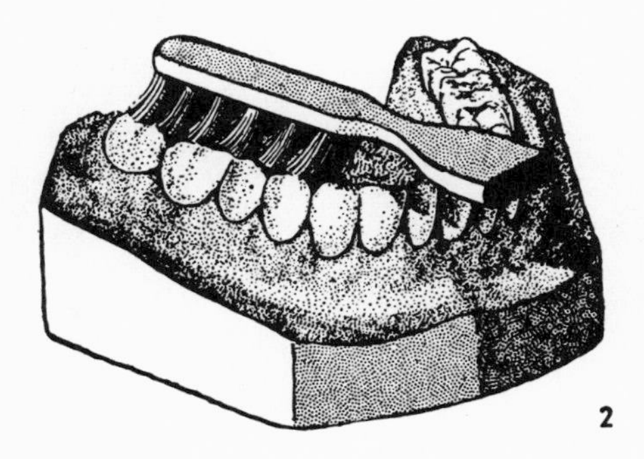

2

the method which Dr. Sorrin advocates, along with pictures illustrating exactly how it is done:

First, the toothbrush should have a short working head, long stiff bristles and a long handle. See figure 1.

How to brush the chewing surfaces. Before massaging the gums, clean the chewing surfaces of the teeth by scrubbing or pressing the points of the bristles into the grooves. This also serves to prepare the brush for gum massage. See figure 2. If you are using a plastic-bristle brush, the chewing surfaces should be cleaned after the gums are massaged.

Placing the brush. Place the bristles of the brush flat against the teeth, the bristles being parallel to the teeth and pointing toward the gums. See figure 3. The bristles should cover the teeth and 1/8 inch of the gums. Point the bristles upward on the upper teeth and downward on the lowers. If the bristles are placed flat against the teeth with the flat of the brush handle and the base of the bristles against the chewing surfaces and the bristles pointed toward the gums, the brush will be in the correct position.

Pressing the brush. Turn the brush to an angle of 45 degrees by twisting the handle until the outer row of bristles touches the gums, producing just enough pressure to bend the bristles. See figure 4. Your gums should blanch slightly (that is, turn a little pale) at the pressure, for the blood is driven out of them.

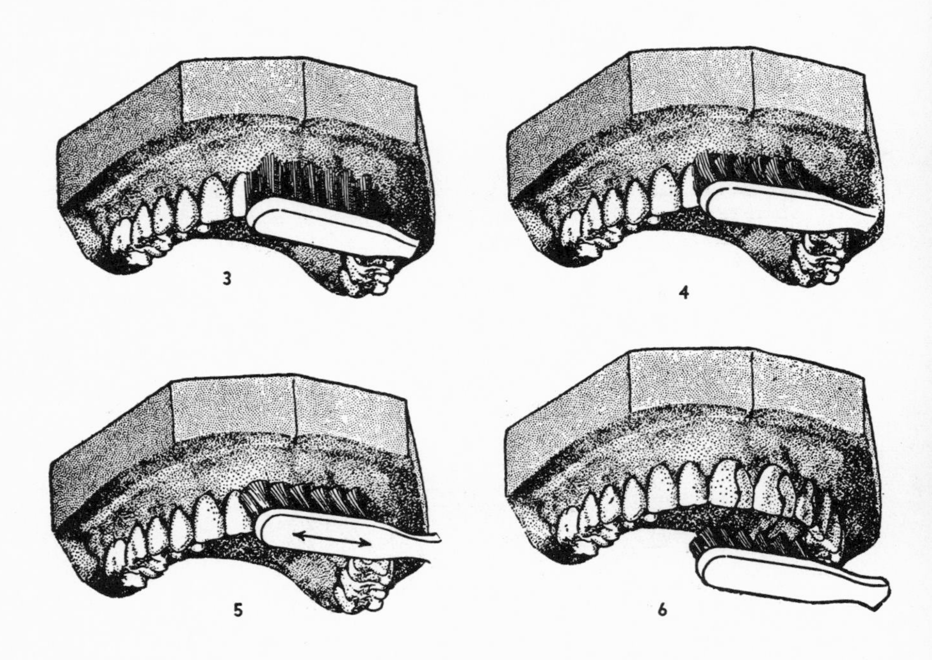

Pumping the brush. The handle of the brush is moved from side to side causing the bristles to bend, *but not to move from their original position.* The movement is taken up by the sway in the bristles only. See figure 5.

Pulling the brush. Continuing this movement, gradually draw the brush toward the chewing surfaces of the teeth. Repeat four times in the same area. Then move to a new area until all the teeth have been brushed. Overlap some teeth in each area. See figure 6.

In figures 7, 8, 9 and 10 you will see how these movements of the brush are carried out in brushing the inner side of the upper teeth.

In figures 11, 12, 13 and 14 you will see how to brush the outer surfaces of the lower teeth and in figures 15, 16, 17 and 18 the inner surfaces of the lower teeth.

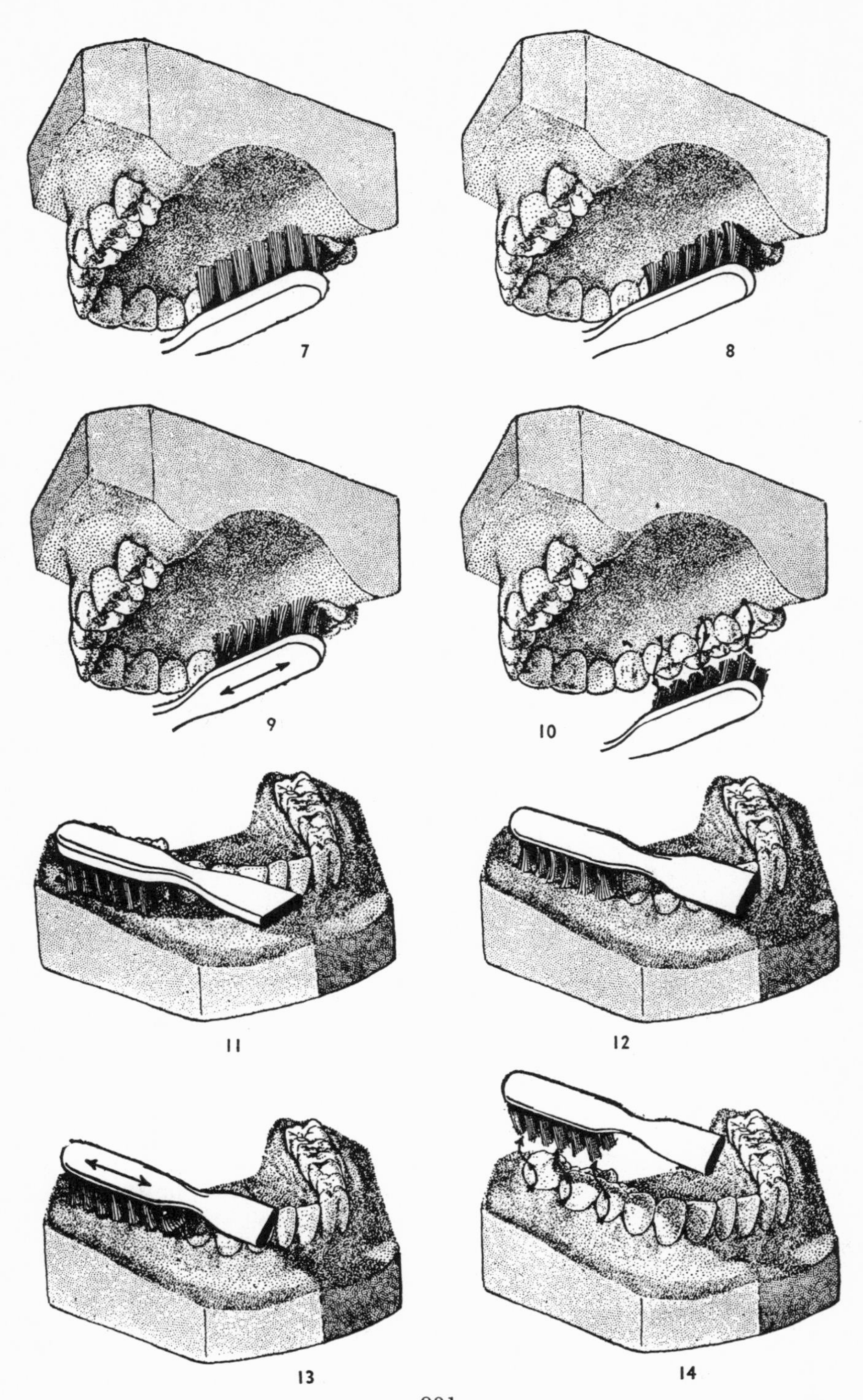
7
8
9
10
11
12
13
14

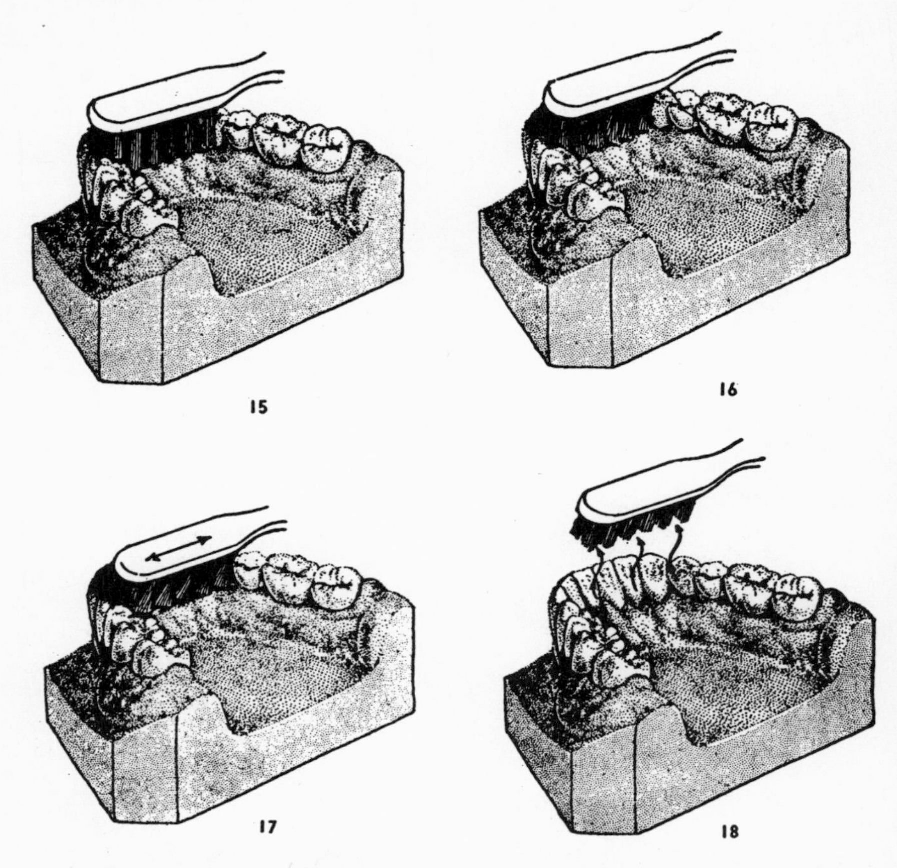

Here are some further directions which you should be certain to observe:

1. Always start with a thoroughly dry brush. Have three brushes in use at all times. Allow each to dry 24 hours before using it again. Hang the toothbrush where it can dry. Do not keep it in a closed container.

2. Discard the brush when the bristles become too soft (usually 2 to 3 months). Rinse brushes carefully. The bristles will harbor germs unless they are thoroughly clean and dry.

3. When you are brushing your teeth, do not start with the brush too high on the gums.

4. Do not scrub the gums. The ends of the bristles must not move from their original position when the brush is pumped.

5. When you brush the front of the lower front teeth, hold your lip away to prevent injury to it.

6. Should any sore spots develop, you are brushing incorrectly. Go over the instructions again. If your gums have been bleeding, they may continue to do so for a few days after you first begin your brushing program.

Teeth—Toothpaste

Toothpastes May Cause Decay

According to Dr. Albert Schatz, co-discoverer of streptomycin and Dr. Joseph J. Martin, both of the National Agricultural College, Doylestown, Pennsylvania, there is a very real possibility that dentrifices in current use may actually increase tooth decay rather than preventing it. According to these two researchers, acids, long believed to cause tooth decay, may actually help to prevent it. "For almost a century," said Dr. Schatz, according to a clipping which he sent us, "most people have tried to blame tooth decay on lactobacilli and other bacteria . . . but the acid theory has never been conclusively proven, and efforts to prevent decay by neutralizing or eliminating fermentation acids from the mouth have not been very successful."

They go on to explain that since teeth contain both mineral and organic matter, they concentrated on the organic part of the teeth in their research. They believed that bacterial destruction of tooth organic matter must be important in tooth decay, but where were the bacteria? Finally they isolated microbes from the mouth which fit the picture of tooth decay by bacterial action. And it appears that the destructive action of these bacteria may be held in check by the lactobacilli and other acid-producing bacteria in the mouth.

Present-day dentrifices are designed mostly to counteract or prevent acid in the mouth. Since the decay-causing bacteria discovered by Drs. Schatz and Martin thrive best under alkaline conditions, then the toothpastes are only making matters worse. Actually we have the assurance of the American Dental Association that no toothpaste has the slightest beneficial effect on teeth. They have tested them all, they say, and while they give a pleasant taste to the mouth they do nothing to promote tooth health. So, in view of the new discovery related above, don't you think it would be wise and economical to eliminate toothpaste entirely and brush your teeth with plain water?

Thirst

Since the earliest days of human history man has known that water is vital to him every day. Civilizations have risen and fallen depending on their water supply. Was thirst first developed as a sensation when the ancestors of present-day animals left their homes in the sea and came to live on land? We do not know, yet we know that fishes drink water.

Yet in spite of the fact that man has always known what the sensation of thirst means, we have never found out how it is brought about in the body. The experts tell us that thirst may be the result of dry mouth tissues and of course we are all familiar with the sensation of thirst that arises when the mouth is dry. Yet we know, too, that we can be thirsty without a feeling of dryness in the mouth. The occasional person born without salivary glands does not suffer from abnormal thirst. Does thirst then result from dehydration inside the body cells? Does it spring from a sudden or a gradual change in the osmotic pressure of the fluids inside the body? Is it related to a change in the volume of blood or other body fluid? Apparently not. Or, perhaps we should say that it may be related to any or all of these, or it may not.

Thirst may result from diarrhea, vomiting, excessive sweating, hemorrhage or polyuria (the excretion of excessive amounts of urine). It is common in certain disorders such as diabetes, hyperthyroidism or some disturbance of the salivary function. We all know, too, that thirst—or at any rate a dry mouth—may result from extreme fright or anxiety. We may become thirsty after taking a drug such as atropine.

A person or an animal who is dehydrated will drink only enough water to replace 70 to 80 per cent of the total water deficit. If the stomach is extended in an experiment (with a blown-up balloon, for instance), the sensation of thirst is prevented. It is possible that we may be desperately in need of fluid without feeling thirsty. Such circumstances happen sometimes in cases of food poisoning. It is also true that persons who drink water to excess for some psychological reason may bring on symptoms like those of a diabetic. Yet in spite of all the knowledge about thirst we have gathered over the centuries, we still do not know exactly what the mechanism is that causes a report to go up to the brain "I'm thirsty."

How much fluid should we drink in a day to keep in good balance, if we have no way of guiding our intake by thirst? Animals, so far as we can discover, drink only when they are thirsty. They generally drink after they eat, suggesting that the moisture is needed to help out in digestion. It has been estimated that we need about two or three quarts of fluid daily. However, this does not mean we must drink this much water or other fluid. Fruits are anywhere from 75 to 90 per cent water. Vegetables contain from 75 to 95 per cent water. Drinking excessive amounts of water will probably dissolve and carry away part of the water soluble vitamins in the digestive tract which is, of course, not healthful.

In cool air the average human being loses about 500 to 600 cubic centimeters of water daily in perspiration (17 to 20 fluid ounces). He may lose 400 to 500 cc in his breath and 600 to 700 cc in urine. Losing ten per cent of the body's fluid will result in serious symptoms. Losing twenty per cent may prove fatal.

Considering how much of the food we eat consists of water, it seems sensible to make any other liquid intake count from a nutritional point of view. In other words, does it not seem unwise to drink much plain water or beverages such as coffee and tea that do not contribute something to health? Vegetable juices or the water in which vegetables have cooked are, we believe, the best answer. Or fruit juices well enough diluted with water so that their acid content does not endanger the tooth enamel.

Thumbsucking

Thumb-sucking in infancy and early childhood is apparently only one-half of a habit. If the other half is caught and removed, the thumb-sucking will automatically stop, writes a contributor to the *British Medical Journal* for April 7, 1951.

Placing of the thumb in the mouth is, of course, the more serious half of the habit. Its dangers to the shape of the growing mouth and to the formation and structure of the infant's teeth when they are cut, are well known. What, then, is the second and more innocent half of this habit?

Mr. J. H. Badcock, of Suffolk, England, found it to be in "the fumbling by the child's other hand of something soft and warm, a soft toy, the blanket, a 'woolly' kept for the purpose (or sometimes its own hair), without which the child will not go to sleep. When trying to effect a cure this should always be looked for and when possible removed, possibly at the expense of one or two disturbed nights. I have known the taking away of a 'woolly' to stop the habit without other means."

Sounds simple enough, doesn't it? Watch, therefore, the other hand of your child, if he or she is addicted to the pleasure of tasting his thumb. If that other hand is caressing a toy or some other equally removable object, try placing it just out of reach. Put up with the complaints that are sure to follow for a few nights at least, and tell us what happened.

Thyroid Gland

Some people are thin, nervous, highstrung and do everything rapidly. Some people are chubby, slow-moving and inclined to be lazy. One reason for these differences in personality may well be the difference in makeup and health of the thyroid gland. Like all other glands in the body, the thyroid has a definite function to perform and accomplishes this by releasing into the blood stream a hormone—thyroxine—which affects other parts of the body. Thyroxine determines growth, regulates the burning of food in the body, influences emotions and personality and is related in some important ways to reproductive functions. Storing most of the iodine in the body, the thyroid uses it, along with a protein substance, tyrosine, to form the hormone, thyroxine.

Other glands in the body are related to the thyroid in function—the pituitary and the sex glands, for instance. The parathyroids are small glands embedded in the thyroid. Their function is not clearly understood as yet, but we do know that their complete removal means death to many forms of animal life. Their partial removal causes a serious decrease in the body's store of calcium. The assimilation of phosphorus is also upset. Acidosis may result and difficulty in assimilating carbohydrate foods is certain to result. It is believed that the parathyroids probably secrete some hormone that preserves the balance between calcium and other minerals in the body.

From radioactive studies we know that when iodine is given by mouth, it is brought to the thyroid in the blood stream where, within several hours, it is manufactured into other complex chemical compounds and sent once more into the blood stream. You can see from this how important it is to the thyroid that you have enough iodine in your diet. If you do not, the thyroid may enlarge, in an effort to continue to manufacture enough thyroxine. Or, if the iodine content of the diet remains constant, but some condition arises which causes the body to require more thyroxine, the thyroid may enlarge. Puberty, pregnancy, childbirth and menopause are conditions that for some reason require more thyroxine, so the thyroid gland is very often slightly enlarged at these times. After the emergency is over, it may decrease in size once more, or it may continue to grow (especially if not enough iodine is present) into a colloid goiter. A simple goiter may become more serious and develop into toxic goiter. Or a goiter may become cancerous. In cases of simple goiter the thyroid gland may still manage to manufacture enough thyroxine to prevent visible signs of goiter—that is, swollen throat, bulging eyes and so forth. But there may be difficulty in swallowing, hoarseness, cough and harsh breathing.

In persons whose thyroid glands produce too little thyroxine, the regulatory machinery is thrown out of gear, the person puts on weight, and his heart beats more slowly, resulting in poor circulation which causes his skin, hair and nails to become unhealthy. His memory may become faulty and he may be anemic. He generally feels cold when everyone else is comfortably warm. Someone whose thyroid gland produces too much thyroxine has opposite reactions. His heart beats faster, he becomes nervous and fidgety and has a tendency to feel too warm most of the time.

"Taking thyroid" means taking, by doctor's prescription, a thyroid preparation made from the thyroid gland of an animal. This produces somewhat the same effect in one's body as would occur if one's own thyroid were stimulated to produce more thyroxine. For this reason, thyroid should be administered only under a doctor's supervision, for just a little too much will increase heart action greatly and speed up metabolism dangerously. You have probably seen "reducing pills" advertised which contain thyroid—extremely dangerous preparations to take, for if someone takes them who does not need extra thyroxine, or if just a little too much is taken, results can be fatal. It is unwise to take thyroid preparations, even under a doctor's supervision, for a very long time, because this may result in so much thyroxine that one's own thyroid does not need to manufacture any more, so it may atrophy and become completely useless. Since "taking thyroid" means taking into one's body a synthetic or foreign substance, it is best not to take it except, of course, in dire emergency.

Aside from iodine, vitamins A, B and C are important for proper functioning of the thyroid gland. A deficiency of vitamin A or C may induce goiter when there is not enough iodine in the diet. In animals it has been found that a deficiency of the B vitamins may decrease the output of thyroxine as much as 80 per cent, resulting in a serious shock to the thyroid as well as all the mechanism the thyroid regulates.

Tomatoes

A rosy, ripe, fragrant tomato fresh from the vine on a hot summer day—what could be more refreshing, or, for that matter, what could be more packed with healthful vitamins and minerals? We can buy tomatoes the year 'round these days, but there is a big difference between the pale, tasteless soggy variety we buy in winter and spring, and the luscious crisp beauty we picked from the vine in the sentence above! And, as you might suspect, winter tomatoes and ones grown in hothouses just don't contain the same food value as summer tomatoes.

Tomatoes picked when they are green, then shipped and ripened on the way are quite inferior in vitamin content to those that are picked ripe from the vine. To attain the maximum vitamin content, the tomatoes should be ripened in bright sunlight and not picked until they are completely ripe. Ethylene gas is often used to ripen commercially-grown tomatoes, picked green. This gas speeds up the production of the bright red tomato color.

The amount of vitamin A in a tomato differs with the variety and also with the growing method, weather, kind of soil and so forth. Tomatoes may be stored for 10 to 14 days at a temperature of 60-90 degrees Fahrenheit without spoiling, if they are picked when they are mature in size but green in color. However the vitamin C content is much greater when they are ripened on the vine in full sunlight. Apparently the sun itself increases this vitamin C content. So it is best to harvest tomatoes just after several days of bright sunshine, if possible. Also it is best to stake tomatoes, so that the vines are kept off the ground. Staked tomatoes contain more vitamin C than those which have been allowed to tumble on the ground.

In commercial canning of tomatoes, when vacuum methods are used, very little vitamin C is lost, for the cans or bottles are sealed before they are heated, so no vitamin C can escape. When you can tomatoes or tomato juice at home, you are bound to lose much vitamin content in the steam from your canning kettles. So, actually commercially canned tomatoes generally contain more vitamins than home-canned ones. However there are other things than vitamins to consider, too. Tomatoes you buy in a can may have been fertilized and insecticized with all kinds of chemicals. Your own home-grown ones have been grown organically. In addition, some chemicals are added by commercial firms in the canning process. Calcium chloride may be added to firm the tomatoes, sodium chloride will surely be added and probably quite a few other chemicals have been used in the contents of any can of tomatoes you buy.

If you have a freezer and want to preserve garden tomatoes for winter eating with the very least possible loss of vitamins, we'd suggest freezing them or juicing them and freezing the juice.

One of the finest qualities of the tomato is its versatility. Cooked or raw, juiced or whole, used alone or in any of a myriad of recipes, the tomato pays its way in health, for it is richly endowed with the food elements you need.

Here are the vitamins and minerals in one small tomato:

Vitamin A	1000 International Units
Vitamin B	
Thiamin	75 micrograms
Riboflavin	60 micrograms
Niacin	.6 milligram
Pyridoxine	60 micrograms
Pantothenic acid	110 micrograms
Biotin	4 micrograms
Inositol	46 milligrams
Folic acid	12-14 micrograms
Vitamin C	13-30 milligrams
Calcium	11 milligrams
Phosphorus	27 milligrams
Iron	.6 milligram
Copper	.06 milligram
Sodium	3 milligrams
Cobalt	10 micrograms
Fluorine	3-5 micrograms

Tongue

"Now let me see your tongue," says the doctor almost any time you visit him with an undiagnosed ailment. No one is quite sure why the tongue is such an excellent indicator of the condition of the health, but apparently there are many diseases whose clearest symptoms may appear on the tongue.

Of course the tongue serves other purposes, too. You cannot talk without using your tongue, although there are cases on record of persons who learned to make themselves understood vocally after their tongues had been removed. Your tongue is also an important organ in the process of eating. It shifts the food around in your mouth so that it mixes properly with the saliva. When you swallow, your tongue presses against your teeth and the roof of your mouth so that the food will be carried back rather than forward.

Some people—and not necessarily orators—have very mobile tongues that they can turn completely upside down in their mouths. Others are "right-tongued" or "left-tongued" according to the way they naturally use their tongues in eating or talking.

Taste is perhaps one of the most important functions of the tongue. The many little taste buds on the surface of the tongue register four different taste sensations—sweet, sour, bitter and salt. The buds for tasting sweet and salt are towards the front of the tongue, the sour-registering buds are along the sides and those that register "bitter" are at the back.

Anesthetizing the tongue wipes out taste sensation in the following order: bitter is the first to disappear, then sweet, then salt and sour. Taste blindness is common and hereditary. In these cases, the sensation of "sourness" is the one most commonly lost. The taste of "sweetness" is the one least commonly lost.

The whole subject of taste is a fascinating one and not too well understood. We know that smell apparently has a great deal to do with taste, for some foods appear to have no taste if we eat them with our noses held shut. Sour tastes are much more sour after we have eaten something sweet. Some people have more sensitive taste apparatus than others. In tests it has been found that benzoate of soda (a preservative) can be tasted in food by about 25 per cent of the people tested. A very small quantity of chlorine or phenol in water cannot be tasted by the average person. But putting the same amount of both together in the water brings a very disagreeable taste sensation.

Modern researchers believe that taste is not just a luxury, meant to give us pleasure with our food, but instead was given us as a guide to those foods that are good for us nutritionally. Another excellent reason for eating foods in their natural state, so that we can be guided by the pleasant tastes that nature has put there to lead us to foods that we should be eating. Another good reason for not eating refined foods such as white sugar, where all the nutritional part of the food has been removed and only the sweet taste left!

No one knows exactly what causes a "coated" or "furred" tougue. Some researchers believe it indicates a lack of hydrochloric acid in the stomach or some other disorder in the digestive system. Others believe that the coating on the tongue may simply be a natural accumulation that occurs mostly at night when the tongue is not being used for talking or chewing. Others believe that a coated tongue represents a stagnation of food particles among the little papillae or nodules that occur on the surface.

The reason the doctor looks at your tongue is because it gives a handy and almost infallible indication of certain unhealthful conditions. In kidney disease, for instance, the tongue may be red and cracked. If you have liver or gall bladder trouble, it may look yellow. In feverish conditions, it may be coated and dry. Normally it should be pink and clean. And not too shiny.

The tongue is perhaps most efficient in revealing symptoms of vitamin deficiency. Swelling, burning or needle-pricking sensations in the tongue may indicate deficiency of the B vitamins. In a patient suffering from a deficiency of niacin (a B vitamin) the tongue is bright scarlet, dry and painful. It may also look "bald" or shiny. In a deficiency of riboflavin (another B vitamin) the tongue may look very clean and shiny, but be bright magenta in color. And the little nodules on the surface may be atrophied and useless. In dogs, a disease where the tongue turns black indicates deficiency of B vitamins.

A deficiency in amino acids (the various protein substances in food) can result in an abnormally red tongue. Iron deficiency, too much smoking, irritating "hot" food or drink can cause troublesome disorders of the tongue. Irritating dentures or broken teeth can produce sores on the tongue. Oral treatment with certain of the antibiotic drugs can result in harm to the tongue. Cancer of the tongue occurs so much more frequently in men than in women that we cannot help but lay at least some of the blame on pipe-smoking.

If you have chronic or frequently recurring sores on your tongue, it would be best to see a doctor, as serious conditions such as cancer may spring from just such a small beginning. If you are interested just in maintaining the good health of your tongue, we would suggest ample B vitamins and vitamin C in your diet, as these are the two food elements most concerned, apparently, with the health of this organ.

Tonsils

Of recent years there has been a change of heart within the medical profession in regard to the tonsil. It seems we have passed that stage when a tonsil was only something to be removed as speedily as possible. Nowadays there is a trend away from tonsillectomies. Medical magazines publish more and more articles urging a return to moderation in regard to tonsil operations.

Part of our original trouble in dealing with diseased tonsils consisted in the fact that we did not know why they were there to begin with, so it seemed best to get rid of them once they began to be troublesome. An infection of a finger or a nose calls for the most careful kind of treatment because we know the value of these appendages and would not dream of lopping them off until we had exhausted all possible means of treatment. But tonsils have been removed since the days of Hippocrates and, we understand, some five hundred years earlier by the Asiatic Indians who were highly skilled in medicine.

Today we know that tonsils and adenoids have a very specific function. According to *Today's Health* for May, 1951, tonsils are normally protective organs and should not be removed. There are two main tonsils which are located at the opening of the throat and the pharyngeal tonsils (adenoids) which are up near the top of the nose cavity, behind the nose. There is a very definite reason why the tonsils are located as they are, present-day researchers believe. For nowadays we realize that they are a part of the system of lymphatics, with the important job of catching, destroying and disposing of infection before it can go any deeper into the system. Most of the germs we take in come through the throat and nose. So swollen and inflamed tonsils are not necessarily "infected." They may instead only be indicating that they are doing their job of trapping infections and helping to build immunity for the future.

In 1943 an examination of 1,000 eleven-year-old New Yorkers revealed that 610 of them had had their tonsils removed. The remaining 390 children were referred to school medical officers who advised that all but 65 should have a tonsillectomy. In England today one Regional Hospital Board alone has a waiting list of 15,000 children—all candidates for tonsillectomies. Yet in spite of these figures, and in spite of the very lucrative aspect of tonsil operations, the swing today is away from "having them out."

An article in the *Journal of the American Medical Association* for March 28, 1953, declared that there are only four conditions under which tonsillectomy should be considered as absolutely necessary: 1. frequent attacks of tonsillitis with fever, illness and sore throat, 2. recurrent attacks of peritonsillar abscess—that is, abscess in or about the tonsils, 3. recurrent or persistent cervical adenopathy—that is, disease of the neck glands, and 4. such enlargement of the tonsils and/or adenoids that breathing, speaking and so forth become difficult.

Apparently no one has ever been able to show statistically that colds, sore throat and other disorders of the breathing apparatus are less frequent after the tonsils are removed. In fact, the evidence appears to show that individuals who never had their tonsils "out" have fewer such infections. This seems reasonable, since the tonsils are there to protect against infection. Furthermore, it seems important to remember that the body makes every effort to replace the tonsil tissue after it has been removed, for in many, many cases it grows back again most persistently and stubbornly. The tonsils are present at birth and grow larger until about the age of three to five, after which the size of the tonsils themselves is gradually reduced and adenoids disappear almost completely. So it must not be assumed, because the tonsils of a child this age seem large, that they are therefore harmful—they are naturally large at this age.

It may surprise you to know that the mortality figure for this so-called "simple" operation is considerable. In the *Journal of the American Medical Association* for February 13, 1954, figures are given from the year 1922 showing a mortality rate of 16.9 per cent which was gradually reduced to 12.7 per cent in 1931. The risk involves reaction to anesthesia, hemorrhage, shock and the possibility of inhaling part of the diseased tissues. Naturally today improved operating techniques and the use of antibiotics decreases the risk. But it is still there.

Says Dr. Jan Stewer in *The Lancet* for January 23, 1954, "Do we really know what ill health can be caused by the tonsils? When they are inflamed how does one know whether the infection is endogenous (from within the body) or exogenous (from without)? Repeated attacks are taken as evidence of endogenous infection, but is this true? There's no difficulty in finding children whose recurrent infections are just as common after operation as before; the only difference is they have tonsillitis when they have tonsils, and pharyngitis, bronchitis or pneumonia when they haven't. It's just possible that the tonsils are there to prevent their having bronchitis or pneumonia!"

One important aspect of tonsil removal is the grave danger of polio, especially if the tonsils are removed during polio season. Many, many medical articles have warned of this danger, for the polio contracted after tonsillectomies is generally the most serious kind—bulbar polio.

Many writers in medical journals today plead for prevention of tonsillitis rather than operation. In general they suggest the use of antibiotics to treat infected tonsils. We recommend instead a program of good nutrition. We know well that vitamin A protects against infections. Bicknell and Prescott in their monumental book *The Vitamins in Medicine* (Grune and Stratton, 1953) tell us that the duration of an attack of tonsillitis is less in adolescents treated with vitamin C than in children who did not receive the vitamin. Surely if colds and other infections respond to vitamin C, tonsillitis should be no exception.

One further note: Dr. J. W. S. Lundahl, writing in the December, 1951, issue of *The Practitioner,* declares that "acute tonsillitis results from a combination of infection and lowered resistance, local and general. Measures should therefore be taken to improve the general health. It has been suggested that one predisposing factor is an unbalanced diet with too much sugar and starch in relation to protein and green vegetables, and I believe that there is much to be said for this theory."

Tuberculosis

We are accustomed to thinking of tuberculosis as a disease that has been largely conquered through the modern therapy of rest, good food and drugs. It is surprising therefore to learn that tuberculosis is still the leading cause of death among Americans between the ages of 15 and 38. It has been estimated that about 500,000 residents of this country have active pulmonary tuberculosis at this time. True, mortality rates from the disease have decreased. They declined 90 per cent betewen 1900 and 1950. And the mortality in 1950 was only half that of 1945.

However, although not so many people die of tuberculosis as in past years, still the case rate for tuberculosis increased substantially in this country, as well as in the British Isles and Canada, from 1940 to 1950. Perhaps the decrease in mortality, then, only reflects the better care, the hospitalization and the other means of therapy that are available today. Frank Carey, Science Reporter for the Associated Press, stated in a release, October 7, 1953, that there is still grave danger of tuberculosis among our infant population. Quoting Dr. Edwin L. Kendig, Jr., of the Medical College of Virginia, he tells us that "in recent years the decline in tuberculosis morbidity and mortality rates has led to some faulty thinking and some actual neglect on the part of many practicing physicians." Of 1,480 answers to a questionnaire sent out, only 55.5 per cent of the physicians queried stated that they employ a tuberculin test on infants. So T. B. may be far more prevalent than we know among infants. He also stated that, of one group of about 600 children seen at a clinic during a four-year period, 11 per cent had already contracted tuberculosis. That's a mighty high percentage in these times.

Esmond R. Long, M.D., writing in the *Annals of Internal Medicine* for November, 1952, states that the known prevalence of the disease has declined little in the last 20 years. We can count on an average of about 120,000 new cases each year. There are 102,000 hospital beds for tuberculosis patients in this country and the annual cost of the disease is calculated at 350 million dollars. The average cost for one case of tuberculosis is about $15,000.

Today's search for a tuberculosis drug is largely confined to the antibiotics. Hardly a month goes by without an announcement in the papers of a startling new wonder drug for T. B. The headlines are bold and, since the stories are so seldom followed up later on, we do not know of the dismal conclusions eventually written to these stories. With each new drug, it seems to be only a matter of time until the germs become resistant to the antibiotic. The next procedure is to combine this medicine with one or several others. If the aftereffects are not too serious for the patient, this kind of treatment may go on for some time. But eventually, the smart bugs (which are bent on survival, remember) develop strains resistant to all the combinations of antibiotics and a somber report is made in medical journals that such and such a drug has also failed. Some of these new drugs that you have read about are: streptomycin, diamino-diphenyl-sulfone and related compounds, para-aminosalicylic acid, thiosemicarbazones, neomycin, viomycin, the hydrazides, etc. Usually they are reported in the newspapers under a set of initials, because of the complexity of their names. Thus para-aminosalicylic acid is called PAS, etc.

What About Tuberculosis Prevention?

We do not for a moment discredit the splendid work that is being done in developing drugs which may conquer tuberculosis. Much of the work is being done in the laboratories of the big drug companies. But as usual our interest is in what is being done to prevent tuberculosis. We find numerous clippings in our file headed "Prevention of Tuberculosis" and read through them eagerly, only to find that at present prevention is apparently thought of only in terms of vaccine, so far as most of the medical profession is concerned. BCG (Bacillus Calmette-Guerine) named after its discoverers, has been used widely in foreign countries and to a lesser extent in this country. The idea is the same as that behind smallpox vaccination. Inject the germs of T. B. into individuals who have not been exposed to it and they will develop a certain amount of immunity to the germs when they do meet up with them. This seems not too distressing an alternative, especially for nurses and attendants at sanatoria who are constantly exposed to contagion.

But is that really the only method available to us in preventing T. B. on a world wide scale, among infants, children and grown-ups alike? There is overwhelming evidence that T. B. is a disease of malnutrition. In fact more than any other disease (except for scurvy or beriberi or other direct deficiency diseases) there is common agreement among researchers that T. B. is prevalent where nutrition is bad. Much work has been done to show which elements are lacking in a diet that predisposes to T. B. Yet in spite of this, how much publicity is given in this country to the idea of preventing T. B. by a proper diet? Granted that much tuberculosis occurs in slum regions where it is probably difficult to educate overworked mothers in methods of planning healthful diets. But all these people *do* eat. In good times like the present they spend enormous amounts of money for food. Why should not some effort be made to see that they buy the right food—the kind of food that will prevent T. B.?

Vitamins A and C in Tuberculosis Prevention

Take vitamin A, for instance. We have known for a long time that this vitamin is seriously deficient in T. B. patients. We have infallible proof from the two world wars. In the first, Denmark suffered an extremely high rate of T. B. deaths while she was selling her foods (especially fats, rich in vitamin A) to Germany. As soon as these foods were consumed by Danes rather than being exported, the rate dropped. During the second war, nutrition in England was good. And, although housing, hygiene and other conditions commonly blamed for tuberculosis were very bad, the rate of deaths from T. B. did not increase. But in Germany, after the war, when nutrition levels were extremely low, tuberculosis death rates soared—and the Germans are people commonly thought to be highly resistant to T. B. Must we have more proof than this?

We know that the need for vitamin A increases greatly in fevers, which is believed to be the reason why T. B. patients suffer from lack of vitamin A, which is evidenced by night blindness and other symptoms. We are told that an enormous amount of vitamin A (100,000 units) daily is necessary to keep the level of the vitamin in T. B. patients up to that of normal people. In addition countless surveys have shown that vitamin A is deficient in American diets—not deficient enough to put people to bed from vitamin A deficiency, but enough to bring on a state called "sub-clinical" deficiency, just enough to lower their resistance to diseases, for example.

We have also known for many years that vitamin C is deficient in T. B. patients. *Nutrition Reviews* for April, 1947, tells us that as much as 1000 milligrams of vitamin C must be given to T. B. patients every day to keep their body supply of the vitamin at a normal level. Investigations of laboratory animals have shown that in cases of re-infection with T. B. germs, the cells and tubes of the lungs are filled with an accumulation of vitamin C, which explains why the vitamin is so lacking in the blood of victims. Now they tell us that we cannot assume from this that quantities of vitamin C will cure or prevent T. B. But why can't we? Isn't it obvious that the body, trying to protect itself against the germs, concentrates its strongest fighting force in the lungs, where the disease is concentrated? If this force is vitamin C, why is it not possible to prevent and cure T. B. with massive doses of vitamin C? We know from animal experiments that a vitamin C deficiency predisposes to the disease. Massive doses of the vitamin increase the weight of tuberculous animals and decrease the severity of their T. B. symptoms. Why then do we not publicize *these* facts about preventing T. B. rather than the always discouraging news about new wonder drugs!

Jolliffe, Tisdall and Cannon in their classical book *Clinical Nutrition,* published by Paul B. Hueber, Inc., tell us that it has long been assumed that malnutrition predisposes to T. B. Tuberculous animals are afflicted with scurvy unless they are given large amounts of vitamin C. Protein and vitamins A and C are the food elements missing, whose lack in a diet predisposes to tuberculosis, say these experts on the subject of nutrition. In the *American Journal of the Diseases of Children,* April, 1951, we find an account of premature children born to tuberculous mothers. The authors tell us that premature births are common among these patients—*not because of the tuberculosis, but because of the impoverished nutritional status of the mothers.*

Protein vs. Tuberculosis

Speaking of the necessity of protein in preventing T. B., we have an article from *Diseases of the Chest* for April, 1950, by Benjamin P. Sandler, M.D., in which he discusses treating 38 patients with a high-protein, low-carbohydrate diet. Results were significant; improvement in cough, strength, weight, appetite and so forth. Dr. Sandler attributes this success to the fact that the diet adjusted the patients' carbohydrate metabolism so that their blood sugar level was more nearly normal. We stress all the time the importance of high-grade protein in the diet and the fact that most Americans eat far, far too many carbohydrates, especially in the way of white sugar and white flour products. Says Dr. Sandler, "A normal carbohydrate metabolism with concomitant normal liver glycogen stores is an essential and fundamental mechanism on which other defense mechanisms rest." How often, in T. B. prevention literature, do you see any mention of a high protein diet as an essential?

Now we come to what we think is the most significant study on tuberculosis and nutrition that has been done up to now. And, interestingly enough, we find this experiment mentioned in every book on nutrition, so we know that it is very widely known and highly thought of. It involves 1100 men whose health histories were followed for a period of seven years. The survey was done in a low-income section of Philadelphia where there was a large Negro population. T. B. is about three times as prevalent among Negroes as among whites, so it was decided to concentrate on Negro subjects for this study. Over the years, as these men presented themselves at the clinic, a whole series of tests was made on blood corpuscles, bone density, chest X-rays, and the blood content of vitamins A and C as well as calcium and phosphorus.

The study is reported in the *American Review of Tuberculosis* for October, 1951. Horace R. Getz, Esmond R. Long and Howard J. Henderson, who did the survey, tell us that they also studied as closely as possible the exposure to T. B. experienced by each of these subjects. They were all between the ages of 20 and 45. Twenty-eight people in the group developed T. B. during the years of the investigation. Putting together all the information available from the tests made, the researchers discovered that these 28 individuals were average in all the tests made except for their status in regard to vitamin A and vitamin C. They were at the bottom of the list in this regard. "All cases of clearly active disease occurred in persons with markedly substandard values for vitamins A and C prior to the development of tuberculosis." And apparently exposure to T. B. germs had little to do with contracting the disease.

Has this information appeared in widely distributed press notices? Is it included in bulletins sent out by the Tuberculosis Association? Do doctors, magazines, radio programs urge the use of more protein, vitamins A and C to prevent tuberculosis? We do hear considerably more about diet than we used to. But it is all in vague, general terms. "Eat plenty of eggs and green leafy vegetables; drink milk." This is about the extent of the diet advice that percolates through to most people today. But no one tells them of the widespread deficiency in this country of vitamins A and C. No one tells them of all the enemies of these two vitamins—sleeping pills, mineral oil, cigarettes and all the other menaces to which many of us are exposed which actually destroy these two vitamins in the body. Nobody tells them that the carotene contained in yellow vegetables cannot be transformed into vitamin A by many people, due to disorders in their metabolism. And most of all, nobody tells them that stuffing on soft drinks, candy bars and other worthless carbohydrates all day long is bound to result in deficiencies of all the vitamins, for these foods simply dilute the diet and do not leave enough room for the worth while foods. And finally, no one, except the health magazines, tells them to take food supplements to make up for the vitamins lost in the transportation, storage, refining, and processing of our modern food. Anyone who does advise food supplements is labeled a faddist. If the amount of money spent in this country on soft drinks and candy alone were spent instead for a high protein diet and natural food supplements for vitamins A and C, it seems to us that tuberculosis would soon be a disease as obsolete as the black plague.

For your own protection and that of your family, especially if you are subject to respiratory disorders, won't you make certain you will be safe from tuberculosis by eating a diet high in protein (meats, eggs, and poultry, fish and nuts) rich in raw vegetables and fruits. And won't you make doubly certain by taking natural food supplements for those elusive vitamins A and C which are so important for our resistance against diseases, tuberculosis among them? Fish liver oils are the richest sources of vitamins A and D. It doesn't matter whether you take them in liquid or perle form. Just make sure they are made entirely from fish liver oils, with nothing synthetic added. Vitamin C can be bought very cheaply in synthetic form. It's called ascorbic acid, generally. And it's made synthetically with none of the added elements that naturally go along with vitamin C in foods. We do not advise you to buy it. Natural vitamin C supplements are made from rose hips, green peppers and other foods rich in this substance. They are more expensive, because they are difficult to prepare so that all the vitamin C will be there in concentrated form. But they are well worth the money you spend.

Ulcers

"Life is so hectic these days that even the small fry get ulcers," says an International News Dispatch from Kansas City. "Dr. W. E. Hendrickson of Poplar Bluff, Missouri, estimated today that 50,000 children from one to six years of age are suffering from gastric ulcers. The physician said even peptic ulcers no longer are rare among children. Hendrickson placed the blame on increased family tensions."

So now the kids are worrying themselves into ulcers! We read some place the other day that stomach ulcers are just about as common among pigs as they are among human beings. This is probably the first you ever knew that pigs, too, were the "worrying kind." One of these days some statistician will publish the figures on heart disease among children, along with a learned conjecture that "it's the pace" of present-day kindergarten and grade school that leaves our children cardiac cripples.

Fifty years ago most kids grew up on the farm. They got out of bed long before dawn to do the chores. They walked miles to school where, as like as not, their teacher licked them soundly just for the exercise. They walked home again, did the chores again and fell into bed too tired even to get into mischief. Who is to say what "family tensions" existed then? But in those days did anyone ever hear of a child below the age of six with a stomach ulcer?

Editor Rodale has covered the question thoroughly in his book *This Pace is Not Killing Us* (Rodale Press, Inc. $1.00), showing that our lives are easier today than ever before and that actually the emotional and nervous strains of times past were just as great as ours today. The only difference is that in those days folks were able to cope with their stresses and strains without developing ulcers, or heart trouble or nervous breakdowns. How? We believe the food they ate was largely responsible.

Here, for instance, is a quote from the Los Angeles *Examiner* for April 4, 1952: "Britain's health officers believe that the treatment of the nation's food with chemicals is having a serious effect on the people's health. After a national inquiry, they blame the increase in stomach ulcers and similar illnesses on greater use of chemicals to sweeten or preserve foods, color them, and extend the fat content." Many people, in this country as well as in England, never have the opportunity of eating anything at all that is free from chemicals. Every mouthful of food they take has been refined, processed, degerminated, pasteurized and chemicalized until it resembles food only in the name and perhaps in the number of calories it contains.

Recently there was a great commotion over a new method of healing ulcers—the cabbage juice treatment. In the September, 1950, issue of the *Journal of the American Dietetic Association* appeared the article that started the hullabaloo. Garnett Cheney, M.D. of the Department of Medicine of Stanford University wrote of treating 65 patients with raw cabbage juice. No medicine was given. The average amount of cabbage juice given per day was one quart. Many of the patients took one quart of fresh cabbage juice for as long as 6 to 12 weeks without any discomfort. Several of the patients had a little difficulty with gas and bloating. But the large majority downed their quart of cabbage juice every day with no trouble at all. The juice was made in a juicer. But Dr. Cheney says it can be prepared (with a little more trouble) in an osterizer or even in a plain hand meat grinder. The pulp that results must then be squeezed through a cloth to obtain juice. The juice was taken in conjunction with meals, and also in midmorning, midafternoon and before retiring.

Is It the Rawness and Freshness of the Cabbage Juice That Does the Trick?

Dr. Cheney stresses over and over again that the juice must be freshly made, and must not be heated. His theory is that the "factor" which cures the ulcer (called "vitamin U" during this experimental period) is very sensitive to heat. Whatever juice is not taken at one time should be refrigerated immediately until it is used. Other vegetable juices or fruit juices may be added to it to increase its palatability. But the main ingredient should of course be the cabbage juice. Fresh celery, tomato, pineapple or citrus juice added in small quantities will improve the taste. Incidentally, all but three of the fifty-five patients who used the cabbage juice treatment were free from symptoms in from 2 to 5 days.

Dr. Cheney believes that "there is an anti-peptic ulcer dietary factor which is readily destroyed by heat. Cabbage in the form of the head, leaf or juice is only one source of this factor." He also reminds us that the whole subject is in the experimental stage and should be carried out only under a physician's direction. We wonder what has happened in the years since this article was published in 1950. Have any more experiments been done? We have seen no reports on any.

Possibly there is something to the theory that some magical anti-ulcer substance exists in cabbage juice. Certainly we doubt whether all the health-minded folks who regularly juice some cabbage or other raw vegetable and drink it ever get stomach ulcers. But we are inclined to believe that it is not the cabbage itself that creates the magic—but the fact that it is, *that it must be*—raw. Probably for many people who suffer from ulcer, this quart of raw cabbage juice may be the first morsel of uncooked food they have had to eat for years and years. Consider for a moment the children below the age of six about whom we spoke at the beginning of this article. How many of them live on a diet like this: breakfast—cereal, white toast, pasteurized milk (everything here has been cooked); lunch—sandwich, soup and pudding, or stewed fruit (everything here has been cooked); dinner—meat, potatoes, cooked vegetables and pastry or cake (everything here has been cooked). Between meals they have soft drinks and cookies or crackers and jelly.

It is interesting to note that, after Dr. Cheney has relieved the symptoms of his patients, he puts them on a convalescent diet which includes raw fruit or vegetables at every meal and considerable raw fresh vegetable juice. We are sorry to see that he also allows bread products made from white flour and desserts made with white sugar. We are sure his patients would have a much more successful and rapid convalescence if just these two items were omitted.

A Diet to Prevent the Recurrence of Ulcer

D. T. Quigley, M.D. of Omaha, Nebraska, gives his ideas of a diet that will prevent the recurrence of ulcers in *The Nebraska State Medical Journal* for April, 1945. Dr. Quigley says "peptic ulcer is a deficiency disease reflecting a relatively high intake of refined carbohydrates and an inadequate amount of all vitamins and food minerals. A high vitamin and mineral diet should be prescribed along with cod liver oil concentrates and all water soluble vitamins, the concentrates to be used in large doses for a limited time, the high-vitamin-high-mineral diet to be kept up for life."

The patient treated by Dr. Quigley is not sent back home to continue eating whatever he was eating before—which is obviously what gave him his ulcer to begin with. He is put on a diet that may seem strange and unbearable at first to the former ulcer patients. Perhaps the foods you may *not* eat on this diet are more important than those you may eat. Dr. Quigley forbids "all canned and packaged foods. They are stale and worthless." "The so-called enriched flour is still lacking in many vital elements and so it is a menace to these patients since it engenders a false sense of security. It should be forbidden the ulcer patient for life. Sugar furnishes calories without vitamins or minerals. It is slow poison for the ulcer patient. . . . All foods containing sugar or white flour are permanently forbidden."

The foods permitted are "milk, meat, raw fruits and vegetables, eggs, cheese, whole wheat and sea food. . . . Any fruit or vegetable that can be served cooked or raw should always be eaten raw. . . . Most persons eat too much salt and there is a constant lack of proper balance between sodium and other alkalis in the blood of the average person." He also stresses the fact that vitamin and mineral supplements should be taken at all times.

Doesn't it all seem related—the incredibly high incidence of stomach ulcers in children who have been brought up on cooked, refined, processed foods, the discovery that there is a magical "something" in raw vegetable juices, especially cabbage juice, that will cure ulcers, and the revelation by a Nebraska physician that a recurrence of the ulcer can be prevented by a diet which includes no processed or packaged foods, and nothing that has been refined, degerminated or meddled with in any way.

Let's put our expectant mothers on this kind of diet. Let's put our infants and children on this kind of diet and wipe out stomach ulcers in future generations! Let's all start eating this kind of diet today to prevent stomach ulcers as well as other degenerative diseases!

Underweight

Being too fat is distressing both from the point of view of health and happiness. But being too thin is almost as great a problem, as those of us know who grew up to the derisive catcall of "Hey, skinny!"

Excessive thinness is not attractive. And it may produce unusual fatigue, nervousness and a predisposition to many ills. It is considered quite healthy to be slightly underweight. Deaths from most of the degenerative diseases—heart and blood vessel disorders, diabetes, cancer, and so forth—are much fewer in that group of people who consistently maintain their weight at a little below "normal." But some diseases such as tuberculosis claim most of their victims from among those who are very thin.

We put the word "normal" in quotes above for we have the idea that many of us tend to measure our degree of over—or underweight by the tables that are put out by the insurance companies according to age and height. But what is underweight for one person may be normal for another, so it is not wise to go entirely by the standard tables when you are figuring out just where you stand. These tables are compiled not from any ideal weight but from averages over the country as a whole. So if you happen to be 35 years old and five feet six inches tall, the table does not mean that 142 is the ideal weight for you. It means simply that this is the average or "normal" weight for others of your age and height all over the country.

So don't spend too much time worrying if you show up quite a bit underweight according to the tables. It seems that it is perfectly natural and healthy for many people to be thin. Doctors call these people "sthenic." They have good muscles and the average amount of endurance and stamina. They have good resistance to disease, they are poised and emotionally stable. They have a well balanced nervous system, but their bodies somehow just don't deposit fat. If you are this kind of person, don't worry about your underweight. You will probably live to a healthy old age untroubled by the high blood pressure, and diabetes that make your stout neighbors' lives unendurable.

The other kind of thin person is called "asthenic." Such a person lacks endurance, is easy prey to fatigue and diseases, is nervous and physically weak. He is not able to meet the demands made on him by society either from a physical or personality standpoint. Usually such an individual has a narrow, shallow chest, poor posture, flabby muscles, and a weak digestion. Subconsciously he fights the idea of taking more food, for he is convinced that food does not agree with him. So he continues to grow thinner. If you are an "asthenic" type of thin person, you would do well to increase your weight if you can, for obviously your body is badly nourished and the outcome may not be a happy one.

Medical literature and the books on library shelves are full of suggestions on losing weight. Almost every month a new book on reducing is published, a new reducing diet appears at regular intervals in monthly magazines, radio programs advertise countless diets and reducing medicines that line the shelves of drug stores. In fact it seems that the plight of the overweight person gets much more attention than that of the thin one. One good reason for this is the large number of Americans who are overweight. Underweight is not nearly so general a problem. But there is another reason, too. It is pretty generally agreed that the overweight person can reduce by simply eating less. But it does not follow, apparently, that the thin person can gain weight by eating more. Throughout all the research we did in medical journals we found very, very little material on the subject of gaining weight. And what articles we found specified that there is no one formula for success. Serious underweight is a hard problem to lick.

How Is Your Appetite?

There is general agreement on the fact that there are two kinds of underweight—exogenous and endogenous. That is, some people are thin simply because they don't eat enough of foods which will put on weight. This is exogenous underweight—coming from circumstances *outside* the body. But others are thin apparently from some reason that has nothing to do with how much food they eat, for they may have good appetites and (without gaining a single pound) may eat as much as others in their family who are overweight. This is the endogenous underweight—arising from something *inside* the body.

In the case of the first group the answer is simply to eat more food. Yet perhaps we had better not say "simply" for sometimes there are complex reasons why people do not eat enough, just as there are complex reasons why others eat too much. Faulty habits of eating are perhaps as responsible as anything else for inadequate intake of food. An example is the child who gets up too late to eat breakfast, wolfs down a few bites for lunch because he is eager to get back to playing, and hastens through dinner with one eye cocked toward the television set. In the case of children, of course, the parents must play the biggest part in correcting bad eating habits, for the child cannot possibly foresee what difficulties may result later from these habits. But how can he be taught good food habits by a father who habitually gulps a cup of coffee for breakfast, skips lunch or eats a sandwich while he stands up at a drug store counter and then finds himself too exhausted to do justice to dinner? Or a mother who also skips breakfast and can't be bothered to make lunch because no one else is home at lunchtime?

Children and adults alike should be taught the importance of food and of mealtimes. Three times a day at least, all other activities should be dropped completely for meals. Meals should be eaten in a quiet, unhurried and unworried atmosphere, regardless of what television programs are at hand or what other activities are pending. Mealtime should above all things be a pleasant time—no scolding, no worrying, no arguing, no recitals of bad news should ever be permitted within ten feet of a dinner table. Meals should be served at regular hours. If dinner is delayed an hour beyond the regular time children and adults alike will be so hungry that they are bound to be grumpy and cranky. If they have taken the edge off their appetites with crackers or candy, the worthwhile food served at the meal may go uneaten.

Persistent worry, psychological upsets and a feeling of being unwanted or unloved can result in lack of appetite. In fact, the whole phenomenon of psychological disorders getting in the way of appetite has become so common that it has been given a medical name—*anorexia nervosa*—nervous lack of appetite. As the appetite dwindles, and the individual eats less, his stomach shrinks accordingly, he has a desire for less and less food. As his body loses nourishment he may develop an extremely serious condition that can result in death—death from starvation actually, although there is plenty of food around him.

In the case of children, one nutritionist, Jean Bogert, has put the matter quite directly in her book, *Nutrition and Physical Fitness* (Saunders, 1949) —we do not let our children decide on what clothes to buy, whether or not they wish to go to school or what time they go to bed, so why in the world should we leave it up to the children to decide what they will or will not eat? Obviously this is a matter needing mature judgment. And the child who is allowed to have as much candy, soft drinks, chewing gum and ice cream as he wants between meals will not have any appetite for the meats, vegetables and fruits which he should be eating at his meals.

Bringing back appetite to adults is a little harder to accomplish. And sometimes it necessitates a firm hand and as much will power as the overweight person needs to refuse food. One element that should be kept constantly in mind is that a lack of vitamins—B vitamins particularly—results in loss of appetite. We have yet to see or hear of the thin person without appetite who can hold out against a whopping big dose of brewer's yeast or desiccated liver daily. He has no choice. Regardless of "nerves," stubborness or a deep psychological hatred of food, three or four weeks of brewer's yeast or desiccated liver therapy *will* give him an appetite—it's bound to—unless there are conditions of ill health present that prevent him from absorbing the B vitamins.

Of course we should not have to remind you that food should be attractively served to tempt the appetite of a thin person. A rest (yes, we mean lying down!) from five minutes to a half hour before and after meals will bring enough relaxation that food may appear attractive again. If appetite has been poor for some time, it will take a while to establish normal eating habits again. The stomach must be stretched so that no feeling of disagreeable fullness results. Snacks in mid-morning and mid-afternoon as well as something to eat before going to bed may be the answer, for it is hard to eat enough at only three meals, if you have been accustomed to nibbling on meals.

Now throughout all this discussion of how to get thin persons to eat more, we have not touched on *what* they should eat. Not so many years ago the theory was that since sweet and starchy food make a fat person fatter, therefore a thin person should eat lots of them to gain weight. In fact one medical article that we found, written only about 15 years ago, advised all kinds of starchy foods—spaghetti, macaroni, bread and butter—for gaining weight. But more recently the thinking has been that, just as high protein diets regulate metabolism so that the fat person loses weight, so high protein diets are valuable for gaining weight. True, the thin person need not watch calories on foods like potatoes, beans, butter and so forth. But he should certainly not try to put on weight by eating lots of refined cereals, foods like noodles, spaghetti, cake, pie, or foods that are high in refined sugars such as candy, ice cream and so forth. A diet high in protein and starchy vegetables (prepared to retain all their vitamin and mineral content) with a minimum of sweets and plenty of butter and vegetable oils should certainly result in weight-gaining.

Some Deterrents To Food Absorption

The second kind of thin person who wants to gain weight presents a much harder problem to solve. This is the individual who has a good appetite and eats as much as the average person but who still remains scrawny and bony, in spite of everything he can do. In the book *Diseases of Metabolism* edited by Garfield G. Duncan, M.D. (W. B. Saunders Company, 1952), there is a full page list of factors which can produce undernutrition. Skipping those which have to do with lack of appetite, and purely mechanical causes such as bad teeth, diseases of the mouth and diseases such as peptic ulcers and so forth, we find quite an extended list of conditions that prevent absorption of food, which might be what is wrong with our thin person who cannot gain weight no matter how much he eats.

Here are some of them: 1. Those which increase destruction of food before the body has assimilated it—lack of hydrochloric acid in the stomach, or the taking of alkaline medicines such as bicarbonate of soda.

2. Those which interfere with absorption of food—absence of normal digestive secretions, dysentery, colitis and other diarrheal diseases, sprue, vitamin deficiencies, drugs which prevent absorption, such as mineral oil, cathartics and so forth.

3. Those which interfere with utilization or storage—impaired liver function, alcoholism, hypothyroidism, therapy with one or another of the sulfa drugs, or X-ray therapy.

Now how does such information apply to those of us who are underweight? Well, have you had an illness during the past ten years or so for which your doctor prescribed sulfa drugs? If so, it is quite possible that these drugs affected a very important part of your digestive tract—the intestinal flora—those friendly bacteria that dwell inside you and help in the digestion of food and the synthesis of some vitamins. This might be an excellent reason why you are short on B vitamins and why you are not assimilating your food as you should. Do you take mineral oil? If so, you're bound to be suffering from a shortage of all the fat-soluble vitamins—A, D, E and K, for these are dissolved and carried away in the presence of mineral oil. Do you suffer chronically from any condition involving diarrhea? If so, perhaps a great deal of your food is excreted without being assimilated, so that no matter how much you eat your food is doing you little good.

Or perhaps you have not been eating correctly and so you have a real deficiency of many vitamins. This will prevent you from making proper use of your food. People who are underweight should try as much as possible to eat concentrated foods.

Food supplements are a highly concentrated food. For instance, let's say you are underweight and have been taking mineral oil and so are short on vitamin A. Don't try to get all that vitamin A from carrots. Although carrots are good food for many reasons, you must eat more than one cup of diced carrots to get the amount of vitamin A that is contained in a few perles of a commercial vitamin A product. Carrots are quite low in calories, so they will not help much in your weight building program.

Most advice on gaining weight will tell you to avoid bulky foods that are low in calories, such as salad greens. Under no circumstances would we advise cutting out raw green leafy vegetables—you must have them. But you can cut down to, say one salad a day provided you get plenty of vitamins C, A and B in food supplements. That would mean taking rose hips, fish liver oil and brewer's yeast or desiccated liver—highly concentrated sources of these three vitamins.

Do You Know How To Save Energy?

Finally authorities are agreed that the most common reason for underweight among people whose appetites are good is a waste of nervous and muscular energy. If they are children they are striving to be the best student in the class or the captain of the team. If they are adults, they are perfectionists in everything they do—driving themselves all day long, never relaxing, and too busy to waste much time sleeping. If this is your difficulty, the only way to solve it is to begin to take it easy. Don't rush. Do everything with the least possible expenditure of energy. Don't walk if you can ride. Don't stand if you can sit. Don't sit if you can lie down. The more energy you use up in everyday activities the more fat you are burning. And you need your fat. You need it to pad your bones. You need it to provide support for your abdominal organs so that they will not become displaced. And you need it against some possible future day when an illness may use up even more fat and energy than you expend when you are healthy.

In general then, this would be our advice for those of you who are worried about being underweight.

1. Watch your diet. Don't try to gain weight by stuffing yourself on desserts and candy. A diet high in protein—meat, fish, nuts and eggs—is best for you, along with plenty of vegetables and fruits, fresh and dried.

2. Relax and stop burning up so many calories in your daily activity. Take naps. Rest before and after meals if possible. Be sure that you eat three good, big meals a day and have wholesome snacks between meals and at bedtime (if this does not spoil your appetite).

3. Eat concentrated natural foods high in calories. Remember, though, that refined foods—white breads, bakery goods and refined cereals—will do you no good and may do you considerable harm. Make certain you are getting enough vitamins and minerals by taking food supplements—the most highly concentrated foods there are. Take fish liver oil for vitamin A, brewer's yeast or desiccated liver for vitamin B and rose hips for vitamin C.

The Metropolitan Life Insurance Company publishes a handy little book called *Overweight and Underweight* which contains calorie lists of foods. You can send for it at their New York office. Or you can send to the Superintendent of Documents in Washington, D. C., for a copy of the Department of Agriculture Handbook No. 8, *Composition of Foods* which gives the protein, vitamin and mineral content of all foods, as well as the calories.

Undulant Fever

The disease we know today as undulant fever or brucellosis may have been known as long ago as 400 B. C. We are told that Hippocrates described an intermittent fever which may have been this. Undulant fever existed along the shores of the Mediterranean for five or six hundred years. In the eighteenth century it was studied by the medical profession. It was then called "Malta Fever."

Brucellosis is caused, supposedly, by a germ called the *Micrococcus melitensis*. It is found in the liver, kidneys, spleen, lymphatic glands and salivary glands, in the blood, bile, urine and in milk. The disease is very widespread around the world, apparently. It seems certain that the disease is transmitted from food animals to human beings. Apparently milk from infected cows, if it has not been treated to kill the bacteria, may cause the disease in susceptible persons.

Its symptoms are rather varied. Edwin C. Mick, M.D. of East Orange, N. J. writing in *Archives of Pediatrics* for April, 1955, tells us symptoms of a number of his patients who were suffering from brucellosis. Extreme fatigue, abdominal pains, and pains in other parts of the body, especially joints, loss of sleep, night sweats, loss of appetite and weight, digestive disturbances were the symptoms. In every case, recurrent fever was a symptom. Some of the patients had had brucellosis since childhood. In others it was of more recent origin.

Dr. Mick describes twelve cases of his own. Then he tells us that from reading articles by Dr. W. J. McCormick he decided to use vitamin C as therapy for these patients. Dr. McCormick of Canada has successfully used large doses of vitamin C on many kinds of infectious diseases. Dr. Mick gave his patients as much as 3000 to 6000 milligrams of vitamin C a day, after all other medication had failed to show any results.

These are his reports on patients after they had taken the vitamin C:

1. Fatigue all gone. Abdominal pain gone. Occasional pains in joints. All other symptoms have disappeared.

2. Except for a slight skin eruption he is symptom-free.

3. No further symptoms.

4. Free from all symptoms. Tremors gone. Numbness, pain, mental depression gone. Normal appetite. Working full time.

5. This patient had brucellosis since childhood. Dr. Mick is certain that, because of her acute intestinal disturbances, she did not absorb the vitamin C, for she showed no response.

6. This patient, too, had the fever from childhood and apparently did not absorb the vitamin.

7. Pain in legs eliminated. Headaches absent. No pain in eyes. Fatigue much diminished. New outlook on life.

8. Definitely improved. Almost free from pain. Appetite improved.

9. Sleeping normally. Nausea gone. Fatigue reduced. Temperature normal.

10. All pains gone. Fatigue almost gone. Temperature normal. Nausea gone.

11. Fatigue rapidly disappearing. No further swelling of ankles or dizziness.

12. Less fatigue. Pains gone. Symptom-free.

Dr. Mick quotes Dr. McCormick as saying that he had found ascorbic acid (vitamin C) better than any or all of the antibiotics for infectious diseases, bacterial or viral.

In New Jersey, alone, says Dr. Mick, there are estimated to be 30,000 new cases of brucellosis yearly. Some authorities believe that as much as 10 per cent of the entire rural population of this country is infected. In a booklet entitled *Crippler in Disguise,* published by The National Society for Crippled Children, Dr. Alice C. Evans states that the number of sufferers from brucellosis in this country must be around eight million. Since milk is pasteurized in this country, says Dr. Mick, the number of cases in countries where raw milk is drunk must be staggering.

Another Way to Get Brucellosis

Another very interesting aspect of the cause of the widespread incidence of brucellosis comes to us in an article from Brazil, *Rev. Assoc. Med.* for July, 1955. This article says that brucellosis is one of the diseases that may be transmitted by a blood transfusion. Trying to determine the frequency of brucellosis in donors that come to the blood bank at the Hospital of the University of Sao Paulo, the writers of this article performed tests on the blood of a number of healthy persons. They found nine positive reactions among 839 donors. That does not seem very high, but the number of donors who might have contributed brucellosis infection to the blood bank does not indicate of course what might happen to those who have blood transfusions from that particular blood bank. How much infection is needed to cause brucellosis in persons who are already ill who receive blood transfusions?

The Brazilian magazine goes on to say that although the transmission of brucellosis by the transfusion of blood has been demonstrated in rare cases, the problem is of little practical interest because the disease is not common there. (In Brazil, that is.) Even so, those who slaughter hogs, workers in refrigerators, butchers and veterinarians, and all those with suspected brucellosis should be rejected as donors, or should be tested before being allowed to donate blood.

Could our present mania for blood transfusions at the slightest excuse have anything to do with the fact that brucellosis is apparently widespread? At any rate, we have proof once again of the marvelous effectiveness of vitamin C against bacteria, even in cases of long-standing infection.

Uterus

The uterus, or womb, is the main organ involved in the reproductive system of the female. It is a small pear-shaped organ, suspended in the abdomen by ligaments. It is located between the bladder and the rectum and hangs with its narrow neck downward, joining the vagina. The cervix is that part of the uterus that opens into the vagina. At the top of the uterus are two openings connected to the Fallopian tubes which are joined to the ovaries.

It was not until quite recently that we understood much about the female reproductive mechanism, especially the phenomenon of menstruation. Until recently it was generally believed that ovulation took place during menstruation. Now we know that ovulation takes place between the periods of menstruation. Ovulation is the process by which an egg from the ovary descends the Fallopian tubes into the uterus. It remains there only for about 24 hours, if it is not fertilized by a sperm cell, from the male.

Meanwhile, as soon as the egg appears in the uterus, two hormones or body secretions, (progesterone and estrogen) immediately begin to prepare the uterus for the possible advent of an embryo. They set up a temporary gland arrangement which brings about certain chemical changes in the lining of the uterus so that the newly fertilized egg can be nourished. If fertilization does not occur, there is no need for this arrangement, so the temporary gland stops functioning, the tissues which have been laid down on the lining of the uterus slough off, the blood which has collected disperses. This process is what we know of as menstruation and it occurs approximately every 28 days in women past the age of puberty and before the age of menopause.

If fertilization does occur, the sperm cell enters into the egg and forms an entirely new cell, with a new nucleus—the beginning of a new human being. By the end of the tenth day after fertilization, this new cell burrows into the wall of the uterus and begins to grow. It is surrounded by the placenta, a protective covering of tissue which leaves the mother after the child is born and is called, then, the afterbirth. The placenta protects the growing embryo from any poisons that may be in the mother's system. Accumulations of fluorine have been found in the placentas of mothers who live where water has been artificially fluoridated. Since fluorine is a poisonous substance it seems reasonable that the placenta accumulates it in order to protect the unborn child.

The embryo, which is called a fetus after it is about ten weeks old, lives in a bath of amniotic fluid which fills the inside of the uterus and protects the embryo from shock, equalizes pressure and provides a comfortable, cushiony bed. As the time for childbirth approaches, the sac containing this fluid ruptures, thus providing the mother with one indication that the baby's birth is not far off. Contractions of the uterus result in "labor pains." Pressure on the fluid-containing sac causes the cervix, or mouth of the uterus, to open, and birth begins.

After childbirth, the uterus contracts again and gradually is reduced to about the size of a lemon. Stimulation of the breast, when the baby nurses, aids in this process, so that mothers who nurse their children regain their figures more rapidly than those who do not.

The menstrual cycle brings about great changes in the body's chemistry. Often it is the occasion of considerable discomfort. The Fallopian tubes, the vagina and the vulva become congested with blood and the vaginal secretions increase. Sometimes the nose and vocal cords become congested, too. The breasts may become slightly painful and there may be a heavy feeling of discomfort in the back, loins and abdomen. Despondency, irritation, lack of appetite, headaches, all these are rather common symptoms of menstruation. It goes without saying that the healthier one is, in general, the less discomfort she will notice during menstruation.

Emotional Life and Menstruation

Apparently emotions are closely related to menstruation. Any great change in climate or living conditions, a new job or new home or an emotional upset may cause a stopping of the menstrual cycle. This is apparently quite common and nothing to worry about. When menstruation begins (anywhere from the age of ten to about sixteen in our part of the world), there may be considerable irregularity before the cycle is established. We are told that Eskimo women do not begin to menstruate until they are twenty years old and that menses cease during the long Arctic nights. Perhaps this is a provision of nature for conserving strength among women subjected to considerable hardship during their daily life. In tropical countries where the living is easy the age of the "menarche" as it is called comes much earlier.

Considering the part it plays in the average woman's life, it is not surprising that the uterus should be subject to disorders. Among modern women in our country cancer of the uterus is a veritable plague. The operation of removing the uterus is called hysterectomy. In some cases the ovaries are removed as well, if there appears to be any indication that they may also be susceptible to cancer. Several medical reports in our files give evidence of grave damage done by the use of various medications in douches. Potassium permanganate is the chief offender. But it goes without saying that great caution should be used in exposing the delicate membranes of the female reproductive tract to any form of drug or medicine, unless it is specifically ordered by the doctor.

Animal experiments have shown that vitamin E is extremely important for the health of the reproductive system as a whole. Animals on diets lacking vitamin E cannot have normal pregnancies. Degenerative changes occur in the uterus and miscarriages are common. In some species, the unborn fetuses are re-absorbed into the mother and never born. Although there is some disagreement among nutritionists today about the necessity of vitamin E for human reproductive function, it seems to us quite logical to assume that it is as important for us as for animals. And many researchers have prevented abortions in women by the use of vitamin E. It seems that vitamin C is also important for the health of the uterus, for it improves the tone. Vitamin A, so necessary for the good health of all tissues, must not be lacking in the diet. Deficiency brings about a degeneration of the tissues of the uterus. So we safely say that a good diet, with special attention to vitamins E, C and A, will be your best guarantee of good health for this most important body organ.

Varicose Veins

Nobody dies of varicose veins. Most people who have them don't even consult a doctor or get put to bed. Yet we are told by one authority that they occur in practically everybody after middle age. There is no doubt that they cause untold suffering both because they are painful and because they are disfiguring. Yet most of us go along, unconcernedly accepting varicose veins as the natural and troublesome companion of middle and old age; we get bandaged or "stripped" and somehow hobble along until the next time we notice how extremely bad our varicose veins have become. And, peculiarly enough, varicose veins—a degenerative disorder if there ever was one—are becoming quite common among young folks.

What are they and how do they come about? We are told by Dr. R. Rowden Foote in his book *Varicose Veins* (published by Henry Regnery Company, 20 West Jackson Blvd., Chicago 4, Illinois) that no four-footed animal has ever had varicose veins. So we must assume that at least part of the reason why human beings have them is that we walk upright. This means that the trip from our hearts to our toes is a long one for the blood to make, when five or six feet of "us" is standing bolt upright and all the force of gravity is pulling downward on the bloodstream. Animals' legs are thin, bony and spry. Human legs are plump and clumsy in comparison. Legs which are subject to varicose veins are apt to be especially plump, for obesity often accompanies the disorder.

Imagine for a moment the job our hearts must do to pump fresh, red, oxygenated blood through the millions of arteries and capillaries all the way down to our feet. Then imagine the job of pumping that blood (heavy and thick with impurities gathered on the way) back up to the heart again through the veins, with gravity pulling the other way.

There are two different kinds of veins that run through our legs. And while varicose veins may occur anywhere they are most common in legs, for obvious reasons. Deep in the center of the leg, surrounded and supported by muscle and tissue, lies one large vein. And on the outside of the leg, not far beneath the skin, lies another series of veins. These outside veins have little support from muscles or bones. And these are the ones that most frequently become varicose. The word *varicose* comes from the Latin word meaning *twisted.*

And twisted it is, elongated, too, and knotty, bulbous, inelastic and diseased. Inside the leg veins there are valves—little flaps of tissue which swing shut after the blood has moved along up the vein, and so prevent the blood from falling back. In the varicosed vein, these valves fail to function. There may be local patches of clotted blood and sometimes chalky deposits on the vein wall. The inside lining of the vein has become diseased, so the elasticity is gone and many are the complications that may ensue.

Some of the reasons for varicose veins (aside from the original one of being an upright-walking human being) are found in faulty daily habits. Here is one disorder of which we can say with full confidence that you yourself can prevent varicose veins as much by your daily habits as by any other single thing.

Daily Habits That Predispose You to Varicose Veins

Let's say you wait for a bus on a certain corner every day. You're usually prompt and the bus is usually late. You stand. Perhaps while you read your paper or talk to a friend, you stand in the same position for a half hour or more—which is the worst thing you could do if you would prevent varicose veins. When you are standing, there is nothing to help the blood flow and your heart labors, the valves in the veins struggle and a little more stress is added to what these veins must endure every day while you wait on this corner.

Now on the other hand, let's say you walk briskly to the next corner, or even the next, or even all the way to work, what happens inside those veins that were taking on a predisposition to varicosity? The exercise helps to send the blood moving along at a fine rate, the valves close properly, the blood gets back to the heart easily and meanwhile the good oxygen that you have been breathing is right there in your lungs to help purify the blood once again.

There are many places where we must stand, it seems—if the bus is crowded, for example, or while we wait in line at a theater or a market. Then, too, there are many places where we must sit for long periods of time—on a bus or plane trip, for instance. It is well to remember that moving around as much as you can under circumstances like these will help immeasurably, not just to prevent varicose veins, but to make you feel rested and alert.

Those in occupations where standing is essential should, if possible, find some way to sit or move around at least part of the time, or find another job. Dentists, barbers and beauty operators could find suitable stools so that they could sit during most of their working day. Many states have laws requiring that salespeople have a place to sit when they are not attending to a customer; some cities even allow their policemen to sit while they are directing traffic! But what of the housewife who stands all day over an ironing board, a sink or a stove? There is no excuse for her to punish her body this way and she is inviting varicose veins as well as a host of other ailments. Sit down, lady, when you work! Today's household equipment provides almost anything you want in the way of comfort while you are working. There is no necessity to stand, no matter what household chore you are doing!

Another way we bring varicose veins on ourselves is with tight clothing. Tight garters of course hinder blood flow, even if they are not tight enough to be uncomfortable. Tight girdles or belts the same. Crossing your legs for long periods of time brings the same result. How many times in the movies have you found when it was time to leave that one or both of your legs was "asleep" with pins and needles prickling when you tried to move it?

Editor Rodale has shown in his booklet *Sleep and Rheumatism* (Rodale Press, price 35 cents) that crossing one part of the body over another during sleep is apt to cause rheumatism or neuritis, because the circulation is stopped or slowed down in that part of the body. How much more would this be true of the feet and legs when they are at right angles to the floor, and the blood, trying to force its way against gravity back up the veins, encounters a solidly crossed knee shutting off the only passageway!

Complications and Medical Treatment for Varicose Veins

Varicose veins may very possibly develop into something more serious if they are neglected. Usually because the flow of blood is scanty due to the bad condition of the veins, a slight cut or bruise will bring an ulcer. Varicose ulcers are a common occurrence. Phlebitis is an inflammation of the inside wall of a vein. This occurs perhaps most frequently in pregnancy partly, we are told, because of the alterations in blood flow that come when the baby begins to develop in the mother's womb, or perhaps because of the disturbance of gland function. Later in pregnancy it is believed that the pressure of the extra burden the mother carries tends to shut off the flow of blood from the legs and hence causes phlebitis.

The medical treatment of varicose veins is the ultimate in horror, we believe, although all the surgery is considered minor and complications are few. The main object seems to be to close off, by one method or another, the varicose veins. Before this is done, of course, the physician must be sure that the big vein running up the middle of the leg is open and functioning well. Otherwise gangrene would result, for the blood would then have nowhere to go. Bandaging the leg, or wearing an elastic stocking either closes off the offending vein entirely or gives the weak, twisted walls of the vein sufficient support that discomfort is avoided.

Varicose vein surgery may involve either injecting the vein with something extremely deadly and irritating so that it collapses. Or removing it. Now of course we have come to think casually of having teeth removed. Many people have only one kidney. Internal organs are removed right and left these days by knife-happy surgeons. But we are sure no reader likes to contemplate having a portion of his anatomy cut out, no matter how troublesome it has become. And this happens to be a vein through which blood is returned from the feet to the heart!

Of course if nature had planned that only one vein was necessary for this purpose, she would have given us only one. Removing anything in the body means additional stress and strain on the organs that must carry on the work. So having a varicose vein removed means added work for the remaining ones. While the operation is simple and done usually under local anesthesia it is certainly not to be recommended to any health-minded person, unless everything else has failed.

What do we mean by "everything else?" First of all, has every effort possible been made to overcome whatever circumstance might have contributed to the varicose vein—long hours of standing, lack of exercise, tight clothes? Then, look to nutrition. For the veins, like every other part of the body, are made up only of what we put into our mouths—nourishing or otherwise.

Vitamin C is absolutely necessary in quantity to hold together the cells in tissues. It is largely responsible for forming the cement that performs this job. Can slight deficiency of vitamin C be one of the major causes of varicose veins? We know that one of the surest symptoms of scurvy—the disease of vitamin C deficiency—is bleeding from different parts of the body. The cell-cement in the smallest blood vessels gives way and the blood pours out. Perhaps deficiency of vitamin C not quite extreme enough to cause bleeding can weaken the walls of the veins so that they give and sag and twist unhealthfully into the shape of a varicose vein. In the book mentioned above by Dr. Foote there is very little information about diet in these conditions. Dr. Foote does say, however, that "so many patients suffering from varicose ulceration are in a low state of health and the healing of their disability may be hastened by getting them as fit as possible. It is not at all uncommon to find anemia to be present and it is, therefore, advisable to examine the blood in all cases where the ulcer has been present for any length of time. We also find that many of these patients are deficient in vitamins and healing may be accelerated by attention to this point, especially if large doses of vitamin C are added to their diet. . . ."

Vitamin P, a fairly recent discovery, accompanies vitamin C in foods. (It also goes by other names—flavonoids, rutin, hesperidin, etc.). It is used in serious blood vessel disorders to prevent degeneration of the small blood vessels which may result in clotted blood, strokes or apoplexy. "Varicosed conditions have responded dramatically when adequate vitamin P (rutin) has been supplied," says Catharyn Elwood in her excellent book on nutrition *Feel Like a Million* (published by Crusade For Better Nutrition, Dept. P-4, 279 E. 4th St., Logan, Utah). Vitamin P is present in the white sections of citrus fruit. Juicing the fruit and straining the juice before you drink it strains out all the vitamin P. Could today's abundance of varicose veins among young people be due partly to the drinking of strained citrus juice?

We know that an abundance of vitamin E is an absolute essential for the health of the blood vessels. And we know that this vitamin is very carefully removed from our food when it is processed. So it seems likely that lack of it could be responsible for much of our difficulty with varicose veins.

In their book *Alpha Tocopherol (Vitamin E) in Cardiovascular Disease,* (Ryerson Press, Toronto, Canada) Drs. Wilfrid and Evan Shute describe a number of cases of what they call "indolent ulcers" or varicose ulcers of the lower leg which responded well to the administration of vitamin E. It was a long hard pull in most cases, for the ulcers were well established.

The Shutes have this to say "It will be seen that we, too, have had a great deal of difficulty in handling these indolent ulcers. Alpha tocopherol (vitamin E) is not the general, final and complete answer in many instances. The same thing, of course, can be said about every other type of treatment that has ever been advanced. What can be said for alpha tocopherol is that it often wins where every other measure has failed, and that it offers some hope of prophylaxis against (that is, prevention of) future recurrences."

We think this is an important enough statement to warrant adding vitamin E to your diet (at mealtime and in food supplements). This vitamin is richest in vegetable and cereal oils like salad oils, wheat germ oil being especially rich in it, as well as wheat germ itself, beans, eggs, sweet potatoes, greens. We believe in addition that it is wise to take fifty or so milligrams of vitamin E as a food supplement, if you are perfectly healthy and want to stay that way.

Here is a letter from a reader, telling us of using vitamin E for varicose veins. Walter Weck, Jr. of Long Branch, N. J. says, "One of my wife's friends developed very bad varicose veins early in her second pregnancy and after delivery one leg swelled up with phlebitis. Eventually she submitted to having her veins injected by her doctor and had the usual immediate relief. However, almost immediately after becoming pregnant the third time, the swollen veins reappeared, worse than before! Leg cramps would develop every day late in the afternoon and she had to be off her feet completely in the evening. We suggested vitamin E. Her doctor neither approved nor disapproved, so she tried it. Within three days the aching had eased and by the end of the first week of vitamin E, the swollen veins had all but disappeared."

One final suggestion for those of you who would avoid varicose veins. Your feet and legs take a terrible beating all day long, no matter what kind of work you do. They always suffer from being so far away from the center of things, biologically speaking. It helps immeasurably to rest every day with your feet as high or higher than your head. It's not difficult really. Just provide your house with plenty of stools or hassocks and always raise your feet to one of these when you sit down. Lie on your couch or bed with pillows beneath your knees and feet, or park your trotters up on the wall while you lie comfortably at an angle on your favorite couch.

If you like gadgets there's a lot of fun and healthfulness to be had from a "slant board." This is a scientifically designed appliance which you can regulate to get your feet as high or as low as you want them while you lie at a delightful angle on the board. You can get a clumsy approximation of the slant board by placing a thick, wide board on the floor with one end raised on a stool or a box, but the slant board is adjustable and good-looking.

It doesn't matter how long you rest with your feet higher than your head. As long as it's comfortable is about right. And you'll notice, after you get up, that your feet and legs feel rested and your head, from which gravity pulls the blood all day long, feels alert and fresh. Of course, it's the gradual rush of blood carrying food and oxygen and carting away all the day's waste material.

Vitamins—When to Take Vitamins

By J. I. Rodale, Editor of *Prevention*

What I offer here is not scientific, because it deals with the experience of only one individual, but it has some value because you can repeat my experiment and see if the same results are obtainable in your case. The idea goes back several years when I was keeping records of my pulse before and after meals. I noticed that after one particular meal my pulse shot up much more than it should have, and for no accountable reason. After a bit of reflection, however, I recalled that I had overlooked taking my vitamins at that meal. In other words, I figured, in some way, vitamins added to food cause it to be more thoroughly digested.

What is the reasoning behind this statement? Digestion requires the aid of the pump—the heart. If there is some difficulty at a particular meal, the heart has to pump more, which is reflected in more beats of the pump per minute. Could it be possible that vitamins act as catalysts with food, causing it to be more thoroughly digested and absorbed by the bloodstream, thus putting less of a load on the heart? If this is so, think what a help the taking of vitamins at meals could be to the average heart case! The important point at issue is, that if the results I have obtained are generally applicable, then it is extremely important that we divide our daily vitamin ration into three portions taking some at breakfast, some at lunch, and some at dinner.

But let us get to our experiment, which was done with respect to my lunch, and its effect on my pulse. Every day for ten successive days, before I ate, I took my pulse. I took my pulse again one-half an hour after the end of the meal and again one hour after the end of the meal. I tried to have meals that were as uniform as possible, using meat-balls as the base of six lunches, and broiled chicken for the other four. There were, of course, such things as peas, carrots, lettuce, fruit, parsley, etc.

In connection with the meat-balls I experienced some trouble. Years ago I had discovered that when I ate anything with onions my pulse would jump up unusually, and I found that the meat-balls, being made with this tear-causing vegetable, accounted for the big rise in the pulse in some of the meals with meat-balls. But since the onions were present in the meals *with* as well as *without* vitamins, the conditions were averaged out and did not distort the end results.

Now, if you will look at page 936 you will see a table in which are recorded the pulse readings of the ten meals. On the average where vitamins were taken with the meals, one-half hour afterward my pulse had risen an average of only 3⅗ beats per minute, whereas where vitamins were not taken it jumped by 7⅖ beats or 105 per cent higher. At one hour after the meals, where vitamins were taken, the pulse rose by but 5⅖ beats, but where they were not taken, the average jump at this time was 12⅕ beats, or 126 per cent higher. These are extremely significant increases and in my own case distinctly show two things: one—it pays to take the vitamins I am taking, and two—it proves that I should take my vitamins with my meals.

I am sure that anyone will admit that the proper digestion of food is of terrific importance to the human body, because it is the first step in the chemical process which is at the bottom of all body processes. The raw materials for these processes must be in the proper condition, just as the building blocks must be, if a good building is to be erected. But I would like to draw attention to a certain condition in which it is extremely important that attention be given to perfect digestion of food, and that is obesity. In my opinion overweight, with few exceptions, can be usually attributed to two basic errors, overeating and defective digestion. The food is not thoroughly digested. Some people have referred in an amateur way to the fact that the food "does not get burned up," but they are on the right track; of course, the glands enter into the picture too.

But all I know is that as soon as I began to take fairly good doses of natural vitamins and reduced my intake of food somewhat, such a startling change occurred in my appearance, due to the reduced weight, that I must attribute the greater part of it to the vitamins and to the better digestion of my food, due to the fact that I took my vitamins at mealtime. And I must say that it was pleasant music to hear the ah's and the oh's of my friends, some of whom accused me of taking pills. They didn't know how right they were!

What I wish to imply here is that it may be generally possible, if people will reduce and take a whole array of "our kind" of vitamins at meals, that due to the better digestion, or due to some hidden factor produced by the vitamins, there may be an improvement in the biological set-up which will prevent that haggard, face-drawn appearance so common in reducers. At least that is what happened to me, and I offer it for all it is worth, with a prayer in my heart that it will work for others too. Prayers are not scientific, but let us see anyhow. I might say also that I can now eat more than I used to without it all immediately turning into fat. You mustn't forget, of course, that I usually walk an hour a day. Perhaps that is part of the biologic process.

I have never been in favor of the all-in-one vitamin for several reasons. One of them is that you cannot tailor the quantity of each vitamin. The other is that vitamins should be taken at each meal, and in proper quantities of each type, in order to keep the pulse down. Remember that the late Dr. Raymond Pearl, the famous medical statistician of Johns Hopkins, found that on the average those people who died young had a higher than average pulse.

There may be some who will say that the whole experiment was distorted by the fact that I knew what I was doing, that my mind, therefore, affected the pulse by the power of mind over matter. I do not know what to answer them. I must say, however, that as the years roll on and I see the increasing benefits in better and better health from my vitamins, I get a general undercurrent of a feeling that seeps into my subconscious mind and adds another strong force impelling me to feel better. Is it a crime, then, for my mind as well as my vitamins to improve my health? So long as I am not telling myself a lie, so long as I am improving myself physically from year to year, and so long as I know that some of it comes from my vitamins, let my mind add another quota of physical improvement to my body.

Another aspect: Could these results have been obtained with synthetic vitamins? I wonder, but am not sure. I would not like to try this experiment for I have already done my share on this particular one. Perhaps some physician might be interested in doing it with his family or some other group, putting one-half of the people on natural vitamins, and one-half on synthetic. In the meantime, perhaps some readers of this book might wish to try it, using the regular natural vitamins. Let me know what happens.

Coming back to the subject of the proper digestion of food in order to reduce weight, there seems to be some evidence that thorough mastication of food is of great help in reducing. This seems to fit in with what I have found about vitamins and reducing—namely, good digestion. We can see, therefore that the taking of vitamins at meals and the thorough mastication of food will make Jack a thin boy much easier than otherwise.

Incidentally, you don't have to chew meat, fish or eggs, as much as starchy foods. The animal foods are more or less digested in the stomach.

	Meals With No Vitamins			*Meals With Vitamins*		
Date	Pulse at Start	½ Hour After Meal	1 Hour After Meal	Pulse at Start	½ Hour After Meal	1 Hour After Meal
Feb. 14	72	82	90	..	..	..
15	..	..	..	76	84	84
16	76	90	84	..	..	..
17	..	..	..	73	76	85
18	72	72	77	..	..	..
19	..	..	..	68	72	70
20	70	75	90	..	..	..
21	..	..	..	73	74	74
22	68	76	78	..	..	..
23	..	..	..	72	74	76
Total	358	395	419	362	380	389
Average	71⅗	79	83⅘	72⅖	76	77⅘

With Vitamins
½ Hr. (72⅖ from 76 = 3⅗)
Without Vitamins
½ Hr. (71⅗ from 79 = 7⅖)
Net Increase 3⅘
105%

With Vitamins
1 Hr. (72⅖ from 77⅘ = 5⅖)
Without Vitamins
1 Hr. (71⅗ from 83⅘ = 12⅕)
Net Increase 6⅘
126%

Vitamins and Minerals—Habits

By J. I. Rodale, Editor of *Prevention*

There is no question that the habit of taking vitamins and minerals is going to be with us for a long time, because of the poor quality of the food we get in the markets and because of what we do to that food when it comes into our homes. The vitamin manufacturers are probably safe for a hundred years but if they are good businessmen they will set up a reserve to take care of the day when agriculture will learn how to grow food crops that contain all the vitamins and minerals, and, for the time when the nutritionists in our universities will tell us how we can get enough of the proper parts of the plants and the animals that will give us the full range of vitamins and minerals. In that day no one will waste money for vitamins and minerals.

In the meantime we must get some of our vitamins and minerals out of bottles, and we must learn how to adjust ourselves mentally to this condition. We must understand that we takers of vitamins by no stretch of the imagination can be considered hypochondriacs, that the vitamins and minerals that we take are foods, not drugs, and that they are merely restorations of valuable substances which are lost in today's methods of growing and processing our food crops. This is not an attempt at debt rationalizing. An impartial examination into the facts will reveal the unhappy truth of what I have said.

The first problem we have to deal with is how to answer the friend who sees six bottles of vitamins and minerals on your table and lets off something skeptical about it, sometimes doing it only with his eyes. Here is the way I have answered this type of person on occasion. There are certain peoples in Europe who are known to live to extremely old ages, like the Bulgarian peasant, and who subsist on only two or three types of food. If they were to come into a modern American kitchen and see the dozens of different boxes, cans and bottles that the average housewife uses, it would be *their* turn to be doubting Thomases. They would really smile at the silly array of Condiments, the baking powders, the manufactured whipping creams, the synthetically produced sauces, and many other bottled and canned things that masquerade under the word food.

In the Bulgarian home everything is thrown into one pot and his diet is 90 per cent made up of this wholesome dish which includes a few bones. None of this *bottle* and *can* nonsense for the Bulgarians, so many of whom live to be over 100—far more in terms of percentage than is true among us Americans.

Then here is another angle to the six bottles that our maid automatically brings to our dining room table at each meal. In our case they are merely substitutions for six other bottles that the average household has on its table. We have no salt or pepper shakers, no white sugar bowl, no bottles of ketchup, Worcestershire sauce or mustard. Ketchup usually contains benzoate of soda and mustard, in carefully controlled experiments, have been seen to inflame the lining of the digestive system. No sir! I want none of the condiments or saturatives which disguise and pervert the God-given taste of foods. You can decide for yourself which six bottles are the better. This is a wonderful answer to give to a skeptic and it usually knocks the props right out from under him.

Here is another problem. Some people think it too much trouble to open six bottles at each meal. There are two ways to overcome this chore. There are tiny bottles that you can purchase from your druggist that are only large enough to contain the vitamins to be taken at one meal. You can sit down and fill 15 or 20 of these at one time which means that you open a bottle once instead of 15 or 20 times—You can also take one of these little bottles to the office or wherever your job is, or on trips. The second method would be to take from only two bottles at each meal, but the entire day's portions, varying the vitamins taken at each meal. I don't care for this idea too much, however, because I believe the digestion benefits more and the assimilation is more effective if the entire range of vitamins is taken at each meal. I have proved this in my own case in connection with a study of my pulse.

With regard to these tiny bottles one can buy small flat leather carrying cases in drug supply houses which contain a dozen or more of these bottles, usually used by physicians for pills. One of my daughters gave me one as a birthday gift. These are excellent for use when traveling.

A word of caution about preserving the nutritional value of vitamins and minerals. They should be kept in the refrigerator, if possible. I recently visited a friend and noticed that all of his vitamin bottles were on a kitchen table at a point where the sun shone directly upon them. Of course, since the glass of these bottles was brown, the light rays of the sun could not penetrate. But what was the heat doing to them? I touched the bottles and found them to be extremely warm. Such vitamins, in my opinion, have lost most of their value. Have a special stocky square tray, in which the bottles can be piled one upon the other and reserve a permanent spot for it in the refrigerator.

Another problem is the changing methods and policies of the vitamin manufacturers. For example, a friend of mine who has been taking a vitamin D and A product made from fish liver oils for years, a famous brand made by one of the largest drug firms, suddenly found after he had taken half the perles in his last bottle, that its label carried a new story. It stated that it was made by chemical formula and nothing was said about fish liver oils. He had purchased it without taking the time to carefully read the label. He immediately threw what remained of them into the waste paper basket.

It would be a good thing if our readers shared their knowledge in regard to anything of interest they have learned about the use and abuse of vitamins. If you have something of importance that you have observel will you kindly write us?

Vitamins, Conservation

We get letters frequently from readers who tell us that they do not see the sense in taking food supplements. Vitamins and minerals are supplied naturally in foods, they tell us. If you eat a good diet with as few refined foods as possible and lots of fresh fruits and vegetables, nature has assured you of plenty of vitamins and minerals. Almost every day we get letters of a different kind, from readers who are eager to take food supplements, but are completely confused as to how much they should take. "The label on the bottle suggests six tablets a day," say these readers, "but how do I know whether I actually need that much or whether that is enough for maximum health?"

The subject of this article is to try to answer both these kinds of readers. We will try to show you in this article just one angle of the problem of whether or not you need food supplements and if so, how much. We are going to tackle the subject from the negative point of view. Rather than telling you what additional food supplements will do for your good health, we are going to tell you what happens to many of the vitamins you eat (and take in food supplements) to deflect them entirely from their job of supplying you with certain essentials.

When mankind was young, living in the forests and fields, his enemies were climate, wild beasts, certain poisonous plants and famine. So long as he could find or grow enough food of the right kind he could be certain of complete nourishment, for neither the wild beasts nor the climate could rob him of this nourishment. Today we have a different set of enemies. Climate is a small consideration in our health. Wild beasts have all but disappeared, we avoid poisons that occur in nature, and food is plentiful. But in the process of becoming civilized and industrialized, we have stirred up a host of new enemies which are waiting at the most unsuspected corners to pounce on us, and rob us of good health.

It works like this. All of us today, no matter how excellent our diets, are coming into daily contact with man-made substances which, science is now discovering, have a detrimental effect on various food elements. If you are a person who can say honestly that you never have any contact whatsoever with any of these substances, you are indeed fortunate. But we must still doubt your word, unless you are living quite alone in a wilderness.

We started out to do research on the subject of vitamin enemies in several excellent books: *The Vitamins in Medicine* by Franklin Bicknell and Frederick Prescott (published by Grune and Stratton, 1953), *Biological Antagonism* by Gustav J. Martin, (published by the Blakiston Company, 1951) and *Vitaminology* by Walter H. Eddy, (published by Williams and Wilkins Company, 1949). Then, too, we came upon a splendid summary of the subject in a booklet published by J. B. Roerig and Company, 1953. This is called *Vitamin Antagonists* by John J. Miller of the Research Department of this company. Before we had completed even one of these books we found we had too much material for one article. It seems that the lists of vitamin enemies are practically endless. And every day's scientific and chemical research probably turns up more.

Keep in mind, please, that we are referring only to substances or circumstances that are known to destroy vitamins or the efficiency of vitamins in human food or the human digestive tract. We will leave for a later article all the information available concerning the effects of white sugar, refined white bread and other refined and processed foods on our vitamin store. These are all old familiar enemies. We want to tell you now of enemies of which you may be unaware.

Do you know, for instance, some of the natural enemies of vitamins? Light tends to destroy all of the vitamins. Some of them are more sensitive to light than others. A bottle of milk left on a doorstep in the sunlight may lose 50 per cent of its riboflavin, (one of the B vitamins) within several hours. Oxidation of foods (the browning of a cut apple or peach) destroys vitamins speedily. Cooking, even at low temperatures, destroys some vitamins. Pasteurization of milk destroys vitamins. Soaking foods or throwing away the water in which foods have been cooked results in serious loss of vitamins. Leaving vegetables at room temperature before cooking them destroys vitamins. Storing foods, especially in warm temperatures and in light, destroys vitamins.

Drugs Versus Vitamins

Now we come to the general subject of drugs and their action on vitamins—and we relate this story with a full realization of the fact that readers, we know, stay away from drugs as much as possible. John Miller in *Vitamin Antagonists* says "Supposedly harmless drugs operate very largely through interrupting enzyme reactions; hence they are strong antagonists. . . . Such toxic metals as lead, arsenic, mercury and bismuth—all of which are used as drugs—not only inhibit enzymes by displacing the mineral-catalyzing portion of the enzyme, but also greatly increase the urinary excretion of vitamins." In other words, there is an important relation among vitamins, minerals and enzymes. All three of them must be present and work together if your body is to have any good effects from the vitamins it takes in. Drugs throw this relationship completely out of gear and cause the vitamins to be wastefully excreted without doing any good.

Here are some samples of drugs that harm you. The sulfa drugs are notorious as enemies of all good and true vitamins. One after another the vitamins are wiped out in the presence of the sulfa drugs. Certain anti-malaria drugs (paludrine and daraprim) destroy one of the B vitamins. Thiamin (an important B vitamin) can be washed from the body by an excessive intake of fluids (as when you are drinking lots of liquids for treating a cold). In addition, drugs which produce diuresis (excessive urination) destroy thiamin. In cases of edema or urinary diseases, mercury compounds are given to increase urination. And down goes the thiamin store of the victim!

Drugs which have a toxic action on the liver destroy niacin, another B vitamin. Any medicine of an alkaline nature, such as bicarbonate of soda or any of the various advertised anti-acids destroys B vitamins, for they can exist and function only in a neutral or acid medium. All of the water soluble vitamins (the B vitamins and vitamin C) are absorbed by such substances as aluminum hydroxide, fuller's earth and magnesium trisilicate. Charcoal used in medicines absorbs the water soluble vitamins, so that they are not available for use by the body. Anesthesia (local or general) and analgesics, or pain killers, are enemies of vitamin C. Procaine, gold and lead used in medicines, phenytoin (a drug given to epilepsy patients) and any medicine containing mercury destroy vitamin C. Vitamin C is also made ineffective by insulin, ammonium chloride, the anti-histamines (which many people take for colds), thioracil, thyroid extract, atropin, adrenalin, amidopyrine, chloroform, chloretone, paraldehyde, medicines containing arsenic, and the sulfa drugs. If you are healthy it is easy to dismiss this list of drugs with the comment that you take hardly any medicines so why should you be worried. But stop and look again at the labels of any medicines you do take or give to your children. If the label does not indicate the contents, ask your doctor. If you are taking any of the above drugs in any form, you are losing vitamins daily, no matter what quantities of vitamins you are getting in your daily food.

Sedatives, Laxatives, Antibiotics, Bleaching Agents

Sedatives and narcotics are virulent enemies of the vitamins. Are you or members of your family addicted to any of the following: nicotine, alcohol, morphine, barbiturates (the drug used in sleeping pills), aspirin, or any similar pain-killing drug that contains salicylic acid, or phenobarbitol? Nicotine uses up vitamin C and causes the wasteful excretion of niacin. This does not necessarily mean that you yourself must smoke, in order to be harmed by tobacco. When those around you are smoking, you are bound to inhale some of the tobacco smoke.

Laxatives of any kind destroy vitamins. The water soluble ones dissolve and carry away vitamins B and C. The oily kind (like mineral oil) destroy the fat soluble vitamins—A, D, E and K. Miller has this to say about antibiotics (by this we mean penicillin, aureomycin, chloromycetin and so forth): "Antibiotics in great variety owe their effectiveness to gastrointestinal bacterial destruction which means either loss of favorable bacteria which synthesize vitamins or development of unwanted bacteria which prevent the growth of favorable bacteria and even produce intestinal toxins (poisons) that in themselves destroy vitamin activity." Many of our most important vitamins are manufactured by the friendly bacteria in the intestines. So even if you lack some vitamins in your diet, you still may get along, for your own body may be manufacturing them for you. But a whopping big dose of antibiotics (for a cold, maybe) destroys these vitamins as fast as they are manufactured and may so disturb the intestinal bacteria which manufactures them that it may take a long, long time for you to get back to normal.

In this respect, we had better keep in mind, too, that antibiotics are being used today in ever greater quantities in animal food. They make the cows, pigs, sheep and chickens grow faster, so it is profitable for the farmer to feed them. Needless to say we take in quantities of antibiotics in meat, milk, cheese, butter and other foods of animal origin. Cheese makers in some parts of the world are having trouble making cheese out of milk from cows that have been fed antibiotics. The antibiotics destroy the bacteria that are responsible for making the cheese. So, of course, they will also in time and in enough quantity destroy the friendly bacteria that live in our intestines, synthesizing vitamins and helping in the digestion of food.

Bleaching agents used in food destroy vitamins. Agene, which was used in this country to bleach flour, destroys vitamin E. The chlorines, persulfates or peroxides that are being used continually in foods destroy fat soluble as well as water soluble vitamins. We can't tell you all the foods that are bleached, but we do know that an increasing number are now subjected to this process, apparently because food processors believe we will not buy their foods unless they are light in color.

Insecticides Versus Vitamins

If you will stop a moment and think about insecticides you will realize that an insecticide does its deadly work of destroying insects by causing some kind of change in the body physiology of the insect. There is every reason to believe that this same process takes place in human beings when we eat even such small quantities of the insecticides as are found on our fruits and vegetables. We know definitely that one insecticide, lindane, works by destroying the insect's ability to use inositol, a B vitamin. Now human beings also must have inositol. The more lindane residue we get in our food the less inositol our body will have to work with. Lindane is the insecticide used so commonly in food markets and restaurants in a contraption that sprays it gently out into the air so that it settles on everything around and kills flies. At the same time it settles on the food you buy, and, make no mistake about it, you cannot wash all of it off.

There is one other angle to the insecticide problem that had not occurred to us before. Miller tells us "Britten and Fairing have reported that a considerable proportion of residual insecticides in sprayed fruits reacts chemically with the fruit on cooking. The nature of the residual chemical products, and whether they are more or less toxic than the unchanged insecticides are not yet known."

In other words, if you stew your peaches because you are afraid of the insecticide residues, you may be making an even more poisonous brew, when the heated insecticide combines with the fruit. It may take a dozen more years of scientific research to find out all the details about this particular angle of the problem.

Do you drink chlorinated water? Chlorine is a powerful oxidizing agent as well as a bleaching agent. When your local dose of chlorine is strong enough that you can smell it when you turn on the faucet there is every reason to believe that the amount of chlorine you ingest may be destroying all those vitamins that are particularly susceptible to oxidation.

Finally, in the line of man-made hazards, we must remind you of the various industrial products that surround us and bring us grief due partly to their action in destroying vitamins. Benzene (a solvent used in so many products that we cannot list them all) destroys vitamins. Trichloethylene is a vitamin enemy. The lead used in paint, fumes from many cleaning fluids, vapors from chemical or processing factories in the neighborhood and smog—all these carry substances harmful to your store of vitamins.

Your Own Condition Determines Your Absorption of Vitamins

One last reminder of many conditions that may make it impossible for your body to use whatever vitamins you give it. An abundance of hydrochloric acid in the stomach is necessary for utilizing many vitamins. Bile is necessary for using the fat soluble vitamins. If you suffer chronically from any diarrheal condition or other gastrointestinal disorder you are throwing away quantities of vitamins, which simply disappear in your intestine without doing you a bit of good. All the water soluble vitamins are lost in excessive sweat, so if you work at heavy labor in a high temperature, you are losing vitamins constantly. Exposure to cold, hemorrhages, burns and severe exercise cause immediate and excessive loss of vitamin C. Rancid fats in the diet destroy vitamin E. Pickling, curing or salting foods destroys all vitamin C in them, so you cannot rely on such food for the vitamin you obtain abundantly in fresh vegetables and fruits. Raw white of egg contains avidin, a substance that is a fatal enemy to biotin, a B vitamin. Raw fish (yes, we mean raw clams or pickled herring) contains a substance that destroys thiamin, another B vitamin.

It's a pretty frightening array of facts, isn't it? Most of us must eat fruits and vegetables that have been picked days, weeks or months before we buy them, so that their vitamin content is low, meats that have been stored for goodness knows how long, milk and cheese that has been processed until most of its vitamin content is gone, cereals that are milled, processed and refined until practically all food value is destroyed, fats that have been hydrogenized and doctored up with synthetic preservatives. And in addition to all this, we are exposed constantly, day after day, to conditions and substances that rob us of still more vitamins. What do you think? Do you not agree with us that it is absolutely essential to take natural food supplements to replenish to some extent those vitamins that have been stolen from us?

Now as to what quantities of these you should take—this becomes a very complex question indeed, in the light of what we have said above. To what extent are you exposed to nicotine, barbiturates, antihistamines, antibiotics, aspirin and so forth? Is your digestive tract in such perfect health that there is no danger of your not assimilating vitamins? How often in the past have you taken sulfa drugs and other medicines that destroy vitamins? Is the food you eat completely free from vitamin-killing insecticides?

Questions like these can be answered only by you. And your answers determine to a large extent the quantity of food supplements you should take. It's a long job and a hard one to sit down and figure out just how you live and what you eat and hence what vitamins you especially need in larger-than-recommended quantities. *The daily minimum requirement* (DMR on the labels of food supplements) *is determined by laboratory experiments in which an effort is made to discover the least possible amount of any one vitamin necessary to keep one from being ill. That is all it means.* Naturally, these experiments are carried out without exposing the animals to any of the vitamin enemies we meet every day. Nutritionists in general agree that maximum good health results from getting many times that minimum amount in food or in food supplements. Our recommendations for everyone, young or old, well or ill, are: take fish liver oil for vitamins A and D, brewer's yeast or desiccated liver for the B vitamins, rose hips or other natural preparations for vitamin C, wheat germ oil and/or a natural vitamin E preparation and bone meal for minerals.

Vitamins, Choosing

When the mailman dumps his sack of mail every morning at our office, we find we have a certain percentage of letters from earnest and puzzled readers who write us that they are not well. Then they describe the nature of their symptoms or tell us the name of the disorder they have and ask "What vitamin shall I take to get well again?"

We are very happy to hear from readers. We are glad to give them all the help we can in planning their diet so that they can eat as healthfully as possible. But we are not permitted to prescribe for their illnesses, even if we could. It is illegal for anyone but a licensed doctor to treat the sick. But quite apart from the legal considerations, is the fact that there just isn't any answer to the question—"What vitamin shall I take?" It doesn't matter whether you are sick or well there is no "vitamin" as such that will mean the difference between robust health and illness.

Health is a lot of other things aside from vitamin pills. Let's explain a little further. Take a look at this letter from Mr. Sickly. His mother taught him very early in life that fruits and vegetables are excellent foods. So he eats lots of salads and raw fruits; he gets plenty of sleep and exercise, he doesn't smoke or drink. How does it happen then, he asks us, that he gets headaches, always feels tired and is susceptible to colds. "What vitamin shall I take," he queries.

There is no vitamin that will stop your headaches, fatigue and colds, Mr. Sickly, because, although you neglected to tell us, your diet is really just about as bad as it could be. You eat in restaurants most of the time, which means that the fresh vegetables you get have been prepared and losing vitamins for hours before you sit down to dinner. You eat lots and lots of bread with every meal. You eat stewed fruits for dessert, fondly thinking that is healthful, but the fruits have been prepared with sugar syrup. You eat little meat because you have trouble chewing it, and no poultry. Eggs disagree with you. Actually what you need is *all* the vitamins and minerals with a whopping lot of good complete protein thrown in!

Eating too much bread may be solely responsible for the colds. Eating too little protein may well be responsible for the headaches and fatigue. You may be getting far too little vitamin C because of the way your fruits and vegetables are prepared, Mr. Sickly, and you are bound to be lacking in vitamin B because you eat lots of refined cereal products and sugar.

On the other hand, maybe your headaches and fatigue result from boredom. Perhaps all you need is to develop some new interests and hobbies; make some new friends; go out more in the evenings. Do you see how wasteful and foolish and downright misleading it would be to tell Mr. Sickly "Take such-and-such a pill every day and you'll soon feel fine." He won't unless he makes a lot of quite drastic changes in his way of life.

What About the Way You Work?

Mrs. Conscientious writes us that she has been told she must have an operation for varicose veins in her legs. She thinks she eats a good diet, but she has her own beauty parlor business, which means she is on her feet about 12 hours a day. After work she comes home and does all the housework, so she really doesn't get much sleep. Weekends she helps her husband in his garage. This means she is on her feet most of the weekend too. Now, no matter how good a diet Mrs. Conscientious might work out for herself, no matter if she took every vitamin pill being made, she could not possibly remain a healthy person with this kind of daily schedule. And the surprising thing is not that she has varicose veins, but that she did not develop them much sooner. You cannot punish your body year after year, Mrs. Conscientious, and expect it to snap back to perfect good health with the addition of a few vitamin pills. Diet is important, but other habits may be equally important.

Let's take a look at a letter from Mr. Pampered. He's retired. Overweight, too. Has had difficulty with his heart, so he's pampering himself. Has a wonderful old-time German cook whose cooking is so delicious that he knows there could be nothing wrong with his diet. Takes great care not to exert himself. What vitamin shall he take that will put an end to his heart trouble? No vitamin will do that, Mr. Pampered.

First of all, Mr. Pampered, your fine cook is probably serving you pies, cakes, waffles, hot cakes, ice cream, noodles. She probably never heard of salads, scorns raw fruits, overcooks all vegetables, and roasts all the goodness out of meats. And besides that, Mr. Pampered, what are you doing sitting in that deck chair watching your gardener? You probably don't get five minutes of good honest exercise a day, let alone the hour or two you should have, if you want your heart and blood vessels to function properly.

No vitamin pill is going to solve any problem for Mr. Sickly, Mrs. Conscientious or Mr. Pampered. Taking vitamins will help. But taking vitamins and ignoring a proper diet, taking vitamins and getting no exercise, taking vitamins and continuing to work under circumstances that you know are harmful—these examples demonstrate the wastefulness of taking vitamins at all.

Taking Single Vitamins Alone is a Mistake

Now, so far as the vitamins themselves are concerned, there is no such thing as "taking a vitamin" in nature. Nature's foods come equipped with many different vitamins to each different food. And for a very good reason. The vitamins, the minerals, the enzymes and the hormones all work together with equal responsibility in this big assembly line that is the body. And you know how assembly lines work. The first fellow on the line has to perform his job or the second job can't be done. No matter if you have three or four fellows trying to get the second job done, it can't go forward without the first fellow's cooperation. Taking mineral pills is wasteful unless you have, somewhere in your diet, the vitamins that work with these minerals in body processes.

For instance, calcium and phosphorus must be accompanied by vitamin D or they will not be absorbed. So, if you believe your trouble comes from too little calcium, it may have nothing to do with the amount of calcium you get, but may be entirely tied up with the fact that you get little or no vitamin D. Vitamin A and vitamin E react on one another. Vitamin A may not be used at all by your body, unless you are getting enough vitamin E at the same time. There is a B vitamin you need, too, if you want to be able to store vitamin A. That is choline. And you should not take any of the B vitamins alone—you should always get them in a food product where they are accompanied by the other B vitamins.

Do you see how immensely complicated the whole thing is—every element in nutrition interlocks with other elements, so that you are simply kidding yourself to think that taking one vitamin alone will solve any problem.

Check on Your Own Health Program

What then is the answer? We believe that the answer is prevention—preventing disorders, diseases and vitamin deficiencies before they get started. First of all, check the healthfulness of your environment on things other than food. Do you get enough sleep? By this we mean do you wake up in the morning, well rested, before it's time to get up? If not, you're getting too little sleep. Do you exercise enough? If you are a housewife, laborer, or farmer, you can skip over this one. But if you are an office worker, chances are you get little exercise in the open air. We don't insist that you take up tennis or swimming. But walk every chance you get. If it's practical, walk to and from work. If not, take time in the evening or before breakfast to stretch your legs in the open air.

Are you working too hard under conditions that are unhealthful? There's no answer for this one, except to change jobs. Are you drinking city water full of chlorine, fluorine and a score of other chemicals? Perhaps some friend in the country will supply you with spring water, for drinking and cooking. If not, buy bottled spring water.

Are you watching your posture? Do you stand, sit and walk with your head and chest high, your abdomen pulled in, your buttocks tucked beneath you? Do you wear comfortable clothing, low heels, no piece of clothing that scratches, draws or pinches? Do you walk barefoot whenever you can? Are you careful to steer clear of all the many poisonous compounds that surround us these days—the cleaning fluids, insecticides, drugs? Do you avoid medicines—especially medicine chest remedies, like boric acid and bicarbonate of soda—like the very plague?

A Healthful Diet Program

Now finally, how do you eat? We believe that you *can* work out a healthful diet, even in this chemical age. First of all, eat all organically grown food if you can. If you can't, make as much of your food as possible organically grown. Get plenty of protein. Eat protein at every meal, and make certain you have a high-protein breakfast. Protein foods are, in general, meat, fish, eggs, poultry and nuts.

Eat nothing that contains white flour or white sugar. These two worthless foods have probably done more to undermine the health of present-day Americans than any other foods. If you want more information on the damage they can do send for our bread booklet (*Better Bread for Better Health,* price 50c) and our sugar booklet (*Sugar, the Curse of Civilization,* price 50c).

Eat as much fresh raw fruits and vegetables as you can get away with. Eat all fruits and vegetables, don't get into the habit of "liking" only a few. Eat little bread and cereal. If you must buy ordinary baker's bread, we'd advise that you eliminate bread altogether from your diet. Even if you make your own from real whole grain flour, or get bread that is healthfully made from real whole grain, don't eat more than three slices a day. Avoid all processed cereals. Ignore canned and processed foods as if they simply didn't exist. If you can't get fresh meats, fruits and vegetables, get frozen ones. Far more of the vitamins and enzymes are saved when foods are frozen.

Now these suggestions just about cover our recommendations for a healthful diet. Even if you are eating just such a diet, we believe you will not be getting all of the vitamins and minerals you need. For this reason we recommend taking food supplements, that is, foods high in certain vitamins and minerals which have been concentrated so that you get more vitamins per ounce of food in these supplements than in the food you eat at the table.

All of the other things that accompany the vitamin in the food are present in the food supplement. For instance, we advise eating rose hip supplements for their vitamin C content. But they also contain the rutin, hesperidin and other elements that should be eaten along with vitamin C. Then, too, they contain vitamin A, some of the B vitamins, vitamin K and vitamin P.

We believe everyone—old or young, sick or well—should be taking all these food supplements every day: fish liver oils for vitamins A and D, brewer's yeast or desiccated liver for the B vitamins, rose hip or green pepper supplements for vitamin C, wheat germ oil, natural vitamin E, and bone meal for minerals.

This is the answer we should give to this impossible question "What vitamin shall I take?" but we would urge that you listen to this answer even if you are in a wonderful state of health. Don't wait—*Don't Wait* until something goes wrong before you begin to be concerned about your health.

Vitamins, Getting Too Much

"I want to give my child rose hips with every meal. Will that be too much vitamin C for him?"

"Someone told me fish liver oil can poison you if you get too much of it. How can I know how much to take?"

"Four tablespoons of brewers yeast! Why, wouldn't that give me too much vitamin B and mightn't that be harmful?"

Questions like these are asked often in letters to us. And it is understandable that folks would have such questions. We have stressed the fact that vitamins are powerful agents, that they are necessary in very small quantity only, unlike proteins, fats and carbohydrates. We have talked about the miracles that the merest fragment of one or another of the vitamins has brought about. So, understandably, anyone who is eating a good diet and taking a lot of food supplements might begin to worry about whether or not he is getting too much of these powerful substances.

There *are* cases on record of people getting too much of some of the vitamins. So we feel that a full discussion of this matter would be valuable.

First we must remember that there are two different basic kinds of vitamins—water soluble and fat soluble. The ones that dissolve in water are excreted by the kidneys if there is any excess of them. So there seems little reason to fear that getting enormous quantities of these could be dangerous. And indeed, there are no records of harm befalling anyone taking massive doses of vitamin C, one of the water soluble vitamins.

The case of the B vitamins is a little different because there are a lot of them. And while no one has ever come to grief taking large amounts of all of them in a natural food source such as brewer's yeast, it is perfectly possible to do yourself harm by taking large quantities of one or several of the synthetic B vitamins *without the rest of them.* So that is what you must watch out for.

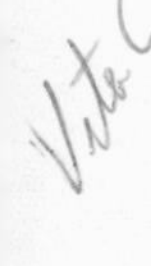

What do we mean by "massive doses" of vitamin C? Was the reader who asked about the possible harm of a rose hip tablet at every meal speaking reasonably? So far as we know, the most vitamin C that can be crammed into a natural food supplement tablet is 100 milligrams. Synthetic vitamin C comes in tablets containing as much as 250 milligrams. Although the minimum daily requirement for vitamin C is officially about 70 milligrams, doctors have given as high as 6000 milligrams "to saturate the tissues" with vitamin C and no harmful effects have been seen.

In experiments, extremely high doses of vitamin C have been given over a period of several months to old people and to sick people. With no unpleasant results whatsoever. So you can easily see that taking three tablets a day, each containing 100 milligrams of vitamin C, just as it appears in food, could not possibly do any harm.

In this connection, we sometimes get letters from readers who say "I find that I am allergic to ascorbic acid. I just can't take it, no matter how I try. How can I manage to get along without it?" The answer is, of course, that you can't get along without it. Nobody can. Every cell of your body must have vitamin C every moment of the day and night. So there is just no such thing as "not being able" to take vitamin C. If anybody really were unable to take vitamin C he would have died long before he got a chance to write a letter about it.

We think that the readers who have written us about vitamin C must mean that they are allergic to citrus fruit since that is the food most commonly associated in our minds with vitamin C. Of course you may be allergic to citrus fruit, but it is not the ascorbic acid in the citrus fruit that you are allergic to! You must, then, find another source of ascorbic acid—green peppers, parsley, watercress, rose hips—and, of course, in addition, some natural food supplements made from one or several of these sources.

So far as the B vitamins are concerned, we know definitely that one or several of these does no good unless you have the others that should go along with it. Furthermore, taking one by itself or several without the rest may do you serious harm. This is the reason why we protest so sharply against the use of synthetic B vitamins. Scientists have not as yet identified all the B vitamins. So, since we do not know what they are, we obviously cannot include them in synthetic vitamin B tablets. But we do know that they all come together in foods like liver, brewer's yeast, wheat germ and so forth.

Eddy and Dahldorf in their book *The Avitaminoses* (published by Williams and Wilkins) tell us that the interrelationships among B vitamins are complicated and numerous. Riboflavin is poorly absorbed unless thiamin is present. Giving large amounts of niacin by itself produces sudden and unexpected symptoms in laboratory animals. This shows us that the so-called "enrichment" of cereals is bound to have a devastating effect eventually. For *all* of the B vitamins are removed when flour is refined and only two or three are replaced synthetically.

Scientists who specialize in this field know that those of us who regularly eat "enriched" cereals are building up an imbalance of these B vitamins which may be responsible for harmful results later on. Those of us who take synthetic B vitamins are courting trouble. So, the rule is a simple one—if you get your B vitamins from a natural source you can't possibly get too much. Taking them from a synthetic source you are almost certain to get the wrong amounts.

Fat Soluble Vitamins Can Be Stored in the Body

Now about the fat soluble vitamins. We are more likely to find complications here for the fat soluble vitamins are stored in the body. They are not excreted every day as the water soluble ones are. So of course they are more likely to cause trouble.

Vitamin D is the worst offender in this respect. For a long time there has been considerable controversy as to whether the harmful effects of enormous doses of vitamin D came from the vitamin itself or from impurities in the solution in which it was given. Some of the vitamin D preparations seem to be more toxic than others.

However, Dr. Eddy in *The Avitaminoses* states "It is apparent that the danger of over-dosage is remote when the usual preparations of vitamin D are used." The early symptoms of vitamin D "poisoning," as it is called, are: nausea, loss of appetite, vomiting, cramps, diarrhea, tingling in the fingers and toes, dizziness and so forth. Of course these are symptoms of many other disorders, too. When you get too much vitamin D your body does not use calcium properly any longer and this is what causes the complaints. In some way not understood by physiologists vitamin D controls calcium and phosphorus in your body. If there is not enough vitamin D this machinery will go awry. If there is too much, it will go wrong in a different way.

How much is too much vitamin D? Practically all of the cases of overdoses related in medical journals are concerned with children who have been taking several times the prescribed dose of cod liver oil, or adults whose doctors were giving them vitamin D in massive doses to see what the effect on their state of ill-health would be. For laboratory animals, 100 times the "protective" dose is harmful. Four thousand times the protective dose is definitely injurious and 40,000 times the protective dose is strongly toxic. Applying this to human beings, damage might follow 1000 times a curative dose of 3000 units—which would involve taking 30,000 grams or about a thousand ounces of cod liver oil—a near impossibility.

Doctors have given as high as 5,000,000 units a day over a period of two weeks. They have gotten unpleasant symptoms on doses as low as 200,000 units a day.

The recommended daily minimum of vitamin D for children is 400 units. Officially, adults are not supposed to need vitamin D at all unless their habits of life shut them off entirely from sunlight. For the sun manufactures vitamin D on our skin, you know! And 400 units a day is a far cry from 200,000 units a day! So we think there is very little chance of any of us getting too much vitamin D if we are taking natural products—fish liver oil, in this case, and paying attention to how much we take.

Vitamin A comes in fish liver oil, too, and there have been records of people getting too much vitamin A. Polar bear liver is richer in vitamin A than any other substance. Foolhardy explorers in arctic regions who have ignored warnings and eaten polar bear liver have suffered from vitamin A poisoning. Bicknell and Prescott in their book *Vitamins in Medicine* tell us that ¾ pound of this liver may contain as much as 7-8 million units of vitamin A. Symptoms of poisoning are nausea, vomiting, diarrhea, drowsiness, sluggishness, desire to sleep.

Other case histories of vitamin A poisoning have usually involved children whose mothers have given them spoonfuls rather than drops of concentrated vitamin A, thinking that it is the same as fish liver oil. Of course fish liver oil contains other things than vitamin A and vitamin D, so a teaspoonful of fish liver oil would contain far less vitamin A than a concentrated preparation containing nothing but vitamin A.

Then there are cases of patients whose doctors prescribed massive doses of vitamin A for some condition of ill health. The patient who goes on taking such medication for months or years is likely to run into serious trouble. Twelve cases of chronic vitamin A poisoning were reported in this country in 1950—surely not a very large number considering the number of people who regularly take vitamin supplements. So it is pretty obvious that taking the usual vitamin supplement, especially when it is a natural food like fish liver oil, can become hazardous only if one pays no attention at all to the amount of the supplement he is taking.

One further note about vitamin A. As you know, the vitamin itself occurs only in food of animal origin—fish livers, butter, eggs, liver and so forth. Carotene, which appears in green and yellow fruits and vegetables, is made into vitamin A inside the body. In counting up the amount of vitamin A you get each day, however, it is wise to keep in mind that vegetable juices (being highly concentrated) yield a very high amount of vitamin A.

We talk a lot about using vitamin E to prevent heart and circulatory disorders. Doctors who prescribe vitamin E for heart patients sometimes use massive doses of this vitamin. The two specialists who have done most work on this treatment, Dr. Wilfrid and Evan Shute of the Shute Clinic, London, Ontario, Canada, warn against using large amounts of vitamin E if you suffer from high blood pressure. The vitamin has a tendency to raise blood pressure when it is given in large doses to someone not used to it. This seems to be the only situation in which vitamin E could prove to do harm—and this would be brief, but disquieting.

If your blood pressure is high, therefore, take vitamin E with great caution, starting with a small amount and increasing it very gradually to make certain that all goes well.

There is no record of other vitamins causing any harmful effects in large quantities. So we could summarize by saying that only vitamin D and vitamin A (and this in enormous quantities) are known to be possibly harmful. And the B vitamins, taken separately and not in a natural combination, are known to be harmful.

Here, just for review, we give you a table of the various vitamins whose daily *minimum* requirement has been officially set, along with the suggested optimum intake for good health, and the limit of dosage at which each may become dangerous.

	Recommended Optimum Intake	*Possible Toxic Dosage*
Vitamin A	Adults, 5000 I. U.	50,000 to 100,000 (normal persons not suffering from deficiency)
Vitamin B		None
Thiamin	Adults, 1.2 milligrams	(unless taken separately from other vitamins)
Riboflavin	1.8 to 3.3 milligrams (depending on daily activity)	None (if given without other B vitamins)
Niacin	Adults, 10-18 milligrams (depending on physical activity)	None (unless taken separately from other B vitamins)
Vitamin C	70-75 milligrams	None known
Vitamin D	Adult need, except under extraordinary conditions seems to be minimum. Curative dose if one seems to be deficient ......3000 units	One thousand times that amount

Vitamin A

The fountain of youth! Since time immemorial man has been seeking it. And today the birthday of anyone over 80 rates a newspaper notice with the inevitable question "To what do you owe your long life?" How varied are the answers! For every ten people who declare "I lived this long because I never touched liquor or tobacco" there are bound to be ten more who attribute their longevity to "a daily glass of beer and pipeful of tobacco." For every 90-year old farmer who states he lived so long by keeping busy, there seems to be a 95-year old watchman who knows that the only way to live to a ripe old age is to "take it easy."

And no doubt all of the answers are partly right. For surely each of us has his own peculiar make-up and, up to a certain point, what is one man's meat may be another man's poison.

But it seems to us that by now we should know more than we do about growing old healthfully and happily, especially since our population is showing a steady increase in individuals over the age of 65.

It should not be too difficult, it seems to us, to determine by experiments with rats which elements in food lead to longevity and which do not seem to be related to long life. We are fairly certain of one thing—longevity appears to have some relation to heredity. In a volume entitled *Vitamins and Hormones,* published by Academic Press appears an article by Dr. Clive M. McCay of the Laboratory of Animal Nutrition at Cornell University.

Dr. McCay tells us he believes that heredity influences longevity. He tells us of one experiment at Cornell in which the careful records kept of each litter of rats indicated that a small number of the mother rats were responsible for a large per cent of the long-lived rats, and a small group of mother rats was responsible for the short-lived ones. In human experience it appears, too, that children and grandchildren may expect to live long if their ancestors did. Since there is absolutely nothing we can do about heredity, it would seem best for those of us who descend from short-lived parents to take special care with diet and other aspects of living so that we may bequeath to our children a longer expectation of life.

Dr. Henry Sherman of Columbia University has done a most intensive study on diet and longevity. His experiments were originally reported in *The Proceedings of the National Academy of Science,* volume 31, page 107 and volume 35, page 90 and *The Journal of Nutrition,* volume 37, page 467. Of course the experiments have also been discussed as the classical experiments in this field by almost every writer on nutrition since that time. As you know, the life span of a laboratory rat is only a few years, so that many generations of them can be studied in one man's lifetime. The rats used for these experiments were a community of the Osborne-Mendel strain. Their history showed that they were very normal, happy rats. There was nothing unusual at all about them. They had been living and thriving on diet A (whole wheat and milk) for 67 generations. So there can't be any question in anybody's mind about whether or not this diet was adequate. Hadn't it kept hundreds of rats healthful and fertile over 67 generations? (Remember, please, that rats make their own vitamin C, so they do not need the assortment of fresh fruits and vegetables we human beings need.)

Adding Twice and Four Times the Usual Vitamin A

Now suppose, said Dr. Sherman and his associates in this experiment, we should increase this adequate diet with considerably more of one of the vitamins, then we might get some idea of how longevity might be increased. So they took one group of the rat family and doubled their allowance of vitamin A. The gentleman rats survived for a five per cent longer time and their wives lived 10 per cent longer than any of their relatives on the "adequate" diet they had been eating over the years.

Then for one group of rats the amount of vitamin A in the diet was once again doubled without making any other change in the diet. Rats getting this quadruple quantity of vitamin A every day lived (for the males) 10 per cent longer and (for the females) 12 per cent longer than the other rats.

But, you may ask, of what use would these extra years be if you lived them in a state of senility, being a burden to those around you and not able to enjoy yourself? *The added years were not senile years.* It's difficult with rats to decide on a criterion of "useful life." With these rats it was observed that the reproductive life of the females was increased in even larger proportion than the length of life.

In terms of human beings this means that double or quadruple amounts of Vitamin A might bring about a 15 to 20 per cent increase in years of life, and an even greater increase than that in active and useful life. Roughly estimated it seems that we might expect to live to the age of 110 or 120 without any difficulty, and to be "in the prime of life" up to the age of 70 or even older. Incidentally when Dr. Sherman and his associates doubled the vitamin A ration once again they found there was no further improvement. So it seems that you cannot go on and on adding vitamin A to the diet and increasing the benefit. There is, it appears, a level beyond which your body cannot use extra amounts of vitamin A. But it seems certain that this level is far, far higher than we have been led to believe up to now.

Many readers write in to ask us how much they should take of the various food supplements. Of course we always tell them to go according to the instructions on the label. These suggested doses are based on recommendations of the Committee on Foods and Nutrition of the National Research Council. They indicate the amount that apparently will keep an individual in good health, or at any rate will prevent symptoms of vitamin deficiency. In other words, the amount listed in the official daily minimum recommendations is the amount the rats were getting over the first 67 generations of their lives. We have seen that quadrupling this amount of vitamin A resulted in a very significant increase in length of useful life.

Many researchers feel that the daily minimum requirements have been set far too low. But here we have definite proof of how much too low they are—at any rate in the case of laboratory rats. And there is no reason to believe that the same would not be true of human beings. The recommended minimum of vitamin A is 5,000 International Units daily for an adult man or woman. Is it possible that 20,000 units daily would result in much better health and much greater length of useful lives? Until experiments with human beings have demonstrated this, we cannot say for sure. And this means we will never be able to know, for certainly human beings cannot be as rigidly controlled in their diet as rats and we doubt if there is any human being who would consent to be the subject of a nutritional experiment all his life. However there seems to be no reason for not taking 20,000 units of vitamin A per day if you want to, and perhaps your own lengthened life will give you the answer.

Why Vitamin A Food Supplements Are So Essential

We must point out several other angles involved in the vitamin A story. If you are depending on your meals alone for vitamin A, keep in mind that vitamin A itself does not occur in foods. Carotene, which does occur in foods, (yellow and green foods chiefly) is made into vitamin A by the body. If, through any disorder, you are not able to convert carotene into vitamin A and you are not taking any food supplement that contains vitamin A itself, then you will surely suffer from a deficiency.

It was recently discovered and reported by two New York physicians that diabetics are unable to transform carotene into vitamin A. This experiment, too, was performed with laboratory rats. All the rats were fed carotene rather than vitamin A. Then studies were done which showed that the diabetic rats had only one-fourth as much true vitamin A in their bodies as the non-diabetic ones. But when true vitamin A, as in fish liver oil, was fed, both the diabetic rats and their healthy controls showed an equal amount of vitamin A. Dr. Albert E. Sobel and Abraham Rosenberg of the Polytechnic Institute of Brooklyn, who made the announcement of these experiments, said, "these studies carry the clear indication that the diabetic rat must receive some source of preformed vitamin A, such as fish liver oils, rather than the usual carotene source, such as vegetables. The discovery that the conversion of carotene to vitamin A is impaired in experimental diabetes can be regarded as the first step toward the discovery of an agent to control the premature aging of the arteries found in individuals suffering from diabetes mellitus."

Once again we have a link between vitamin A deficiency and aging! Now surely anyone who suffers from diabetes should be taking a fish liver oil supplement to prevent night-blindness, skin disorders and the other symptoms of vitamin A deficiency, and those of us who suspect there is anything wrong with the function of our livers should also be taking fish liver oils, for liver disorders, too, interfere with conversion of carotene (in food) into vitamin A in the body.

Note please that the rats in Dr. Sherman's experiment were not kept on the just adequate vitamin A diet until they began to approach middle age, and were then given the double and quadruple doses. No. They were fed from birth on the bigger doses. And the lesson here is plain for us to see. Most of us are not even conscious of our health, or of how we are taking care of it, until middle age or perhaps a little earlier when we contract some annoying disease, or begin to notice lines in our faces, or gray hairs, or bad teeth, and all of a sudden we scramble desperately around trying to make up for all the years we have ignored our health. Dr. Sherman's experiment does not show what will happen to rats whose diet is enriched with vitamin A late in life. But it does show that those which grow up with it reap worth while benefits. So our suggestion would be, if you have children, give those youngsters the best possible start towards a long and happy life by increasing their vitamin A, either in meals or supplements or both. And for those of us who are middle-aged or older, who knows? Perhaps increased vitamin A will postpone those wrinkles, gray hairs, and other signs of aging for another ten, fifteen or even twenty years! At least there's no reason not to give it a try!

Vitamin B—Biotin

This vitamin has become especially noteworthy because of its relationship to another substance—avidin, which occurs in the whites of eggs. Avidin has the power of "binding" biotin so that it is not available for our bodies to use. A great deal of research has been done to discover more about this peculiar combination, so that we may understand more about the way in which other substances may act to cancel out the good effects of other vitamins.

Biotin exists in small amounts in all higher animals and in plants. It exists in a "free" state in fruits and green vegetables. In grains, nuts and other vegetables, it is chemically "bound" with other substances. Biotin is insoluble in both fat and water and can be released for food only in the process of digestion. It has been known for some time that biotin is necessary for health in both animals and man, but its exact chemical function is not as yet understood, so no one has suggested as yet any minimum daily amount that human beings should have for perfect health.

A deficiency of biotin produces symptoms somewhat like those produced by too little of other vitamin B's—lassitude, sleepiness, muscular pain, loss of appetite, pallor, dryness of skin, a feeling of distress in the region of the heart and disturbances of the nervous system. A severe deficiency brings about mental depression which may become serious enough to develop into mild panic. In animals a peculiar loss of hair, called "spectacled eye" results from biotin deficiency—the animals lose the hair around their eyes, so that the bald rings of skin left resemble spectacles. Baldness and spasticity also result in animals who do not obtain enough biotin in their diets. Death results from severe prolonged deficiency in laboratory animals.

Since biotin is present in so many foods which are common in man's diet, biotin deficiency among human beings apparently is unknown or at least has never been observed as such, unless it has been induced in volunteers for experimental purposes. Studies seem to indicate that some of the biotin we need is manufactured within our intestines. How then is it possible for any of us to have a deficiency of this vitamin? The consumption of too much avidin may use up all our supply of biotin so that we may suffer from a deficiency. In addition, the taking of sulfa drugs may prevent the manufacture of biotin within our bodies.

Sulfa Drugs May Produce Biotin Deficiency

In the book *Vitaminology* by Walter H. Eddy, Ph.D., published by the Williams and Wilkins Company in 1949, we find that "ordinary doses of sulfonamides do not seriously impair the intestinal synthesis of biotin, but the effect varies with the type of sulfa drug and the size and duration of the dosage. Large doses of sulfsuxadine, for example, can almost completely inhibit the synthesis of biotin in the colon. Whether this constitutes an actual menace to man is not certain but severe biotin deficiency in animals by use of sulfa drugs has been produced in less than six weeks."

Biotin is very necessary for growing tissues, so pregnant women and nursing mothers should have ample biotin in their diets. Biotin is present in human breast milk. Scientists believe that biotin may be involved in regulating the assimilation of fat and/or carbohydrate in our bodies. In the cells, it helps to regulate the way in which carbon dioxide is handled. Manganese, a mineral, is used in this process, too. And potassium is closely involved with biotin in the blood stream, although it is not clearly understood just how or why.

So, as with the other B vitamins, we find that biotin is necessary for daily human activities and that it works in conjunction with other food elements. Especially since we know so little about the action of biotin in the body, we should guard against ever taking it by itself as a food supplement. We should rather take it in combination with the other B vitamins, as it appears in food substances, such as liver, milk, brewer's yeast, eggs, molasses and so forth.

Other B vitamins are: niacin, thiamin, riboflavin, pyridoxine, choline, folic acid, inositol, pantothenic acid. In general, they are necessary for the welfare of our digestive tracts and nervous systems. They occur together in the same foods and they work with one another in close relationship, so that an over-abundance of one may result in a deficiency of another. The B vitamins are all destroyed or removed by our present methods of milling grain and refining food, so it is almost impossible to obtain enough of them from daily meals, unless you are eating right out of your own garden and farm. This is why we advise taking all the B vitamins in natural food supplements such as desiccated liver and brewer's yeast.

Foods Rich in Biotin

Food	*Micrograms of Biotin*
Bananas	4 in 1 medium banana
Beans, dried lima	10 in ½ cup, steamed
Beef	4 in 2 slices roast beef
Carrots	2 in 1 cup carrots
Cauliflower	17 in ¼ small head of cauliflower
Cheese	2 in 5 one-inch cubes
Chicken	5-10 in 3 slices of chicken
Corn	6 in ½ cup steamed corn
Eggs, whole fresh	25 in 2 eggs
Grapefruit	3 in ¼ medium grapefruit
Halibut	8 in 1 piece halibut
Liver, beef	100 in 1 piece of liver
Milk	5 in ½ cup
Molasses	9 in 4 tablespoons
Mushrooms	16 in 7 mushrooms
Onions	4 in 2 medium onions
Peas, fresh	2 in 1 cup of steamed peas
Peanuts, roasted	39 in about 100 peanuts
Salmon	5 in ½ cup salmon
Spinach	2 in ½ cup steamed spinach
Strawberries	4 in ½ cup strawberries
Tomatoes	2 in 1 small tomato
Wheat, whole	5 in 10 tablespoons
Yeast, brewer's	75 in 3 tablespoons

Vitamins—Biotin and Raw Eggs

What Is the Evidence for and Against Eating Raw Eggs?

Many benefits can be derived from eating foods raw, so that all their nutritive value is preserved. All food suffers some loss of vitamins, enzymes and minerals when it is cooked, even at a low temperature. When the temperature is high, as in roasting or frying, much greater loss is suffered.

An advertiser, described on the back cover of *Prevention* magazine laboratory experiments involving raw egg white and its effect on health. Raw egg white is injurious to laboratory animals, he said, but egg white heated to 170 degrees is one of our finest proteins. Our mail bag for the next few weeks bulged with indignant letters from readers—about half of them folks who regularly eat raw eggs and were upset because our advertiser claimed they were harmful; the other half were persons who were trying to include more raw food in their meals as a result of our article. These folks were upset because we had advised them to eat raw foods and now, it seemed to them, we were contradicting ourselves.

Here are some samples of protests: "Your advertisement has caused considerable consternation in my home. My wife and son have been taking two raw eggs, well beaten, with a glass of orange juice as a substantial part of their breakfast. . . . My wife says she never felt better. Also how about the habit many laborers have of swallowing whole raw unbeaten eggs?" Another reader sent us a clipping about a prospective channel-swimmer who eats six raw eggs a day to "build up his wind." A third letter went like this: "The article on raw egg white is doubtful in truth. For years I have eaten two raw whole eggs every morning. I am eighty-four years old. I doubt if raw egg whites are poisonous."

Although it means a lot more work for us, we are always delighted to find ourselves in the middle of a controversy, so we got to work in our library and did some extensive reading on the subject of eggs. It seems that during the research that went on around the discovery of the vitamin biotin there was renewed interest in the fact that laboratory animals do not do well on diets that include a lot of raw egg white. Now egg white is a protein and proteins are essential for life and health. Other proteins seem to be far more valuable as food when they are eaten raw. So what could be the cause of this peculiar reaction to egg white? Was it some poison in the egg white that disappeared when it was cooked? Or was it something else in the diet that did not get along with the egg white?

Actually in the laboratory experiments, animals on very good, nutritious diets invariably showed symptoms of great distress if the diet contained a high amount of raw egg white. The animals lost their hair, became sluggish and nervous and contracted a dermatitis chiefly around their eyes, noses and paws.

Foods rich in the B vitamins prevented these symptoms. But which of the B vitamins was involved? By feeding carefully controlled diets in which trials were made with each of the known B vitamins, it was finally revealed that the newly discovered vitamin biotin was the victim. Further research showed that there is a substance in egg white, called avidin (the hungry protein) which binds the biotin in our digestive tract so that it cannot be utilized by our bodies. The laboratory animals were consuming an amount of egg white which used up every vestige of biotin, so that they suffered from a severe biotin deficiency.

Experiments Show Harm Done By Raw Egg White

As word got around in the scientific journals, researchers looked further into this strange phenomenon. A group of workers at the University of Wisconsin tried nutritious diets plus egg-white on five different kinds of animals—chicks, rats, rabbits, monkeys and guinea pigs. Their results are reported by J. G. Lease, H. T. Parsons and E. Kelly in *The Journal of Biochemistry* for March, 1937. They found that the first four animals showed similar symptoms of baldness, skin eruptions, swelling, scaliness and redness about the eyes, ears, paws and mouth. In the rat only there were nervous symptoms as well. The guinea pig showed the least reaction to the egg-white. The diets fed were healthful, nutritious diets, containing plenty of all the necessary vitamins. However, about 40 to 50 per cent of the daily ration was dried, uncooked egg white.

In 1939 E. Uroma published an account of the reaction of children to raw egg white. In *Acta Societatis Medicorum Fennicae Duodecim*, Volume 21, 1939, he described feeding one raw egg daily for from one to three weeks to 48 children between the ages of one week and seven months. It was found that the blood of three of the children developed antibodies against the egg white—seeming to indicate that some poisonous substance was present and the antibodies were mobilized to fight it. Two of these children also developed a slight eczema on the face and neck. This breaking out disappeared when the eggs were omitted from the diet. It began to appear that raw egg white had indeed a very serious effect on the health of human beings.

Then came the famous experiment that provided final proof of the harmfulness of raw egg white. V. P. Sydenstricker, S. A. Singal, A. P. Briggs and N. M. DeVaughn of the University of Georgia School of Medicine set out to produce the so-called "egg-white injury" in human beings and, if possible, cure it by administering biotin. Their experiment is reported in *Science* for February 13, 1942. Seven human volunteers agreed to the test. This is the diet they were placed on: polished rice, white flour, farina, cane sugar, lard, butter and lean beef. This diet contains practically no biotin. Then the volunteers were given vitamin and mineral supplements to make up for the vitamins and minerals that were missing from their food, so that whatever symptoms they showed could not possibly be the result of some other vitamin deficiency. Then they were given each day enough raw egg white to make up 30 per cent of the total caloric intake.

Only four of the volunteers followed through to a satisfactory termination of the experiment. This is what happened: during the third and fourth week all four developed scaliness of the skin, without any accompanying itching. In the seventh week one man developed a dermatitis over his neck, hands, arms and legs. During the seventh and eighth week all the volunteers developed a gray pallor of their skin and mucus membrane and later extreme dryness of the skin, with additional scaliness.

After the fifth week they all developed other kinds of symptoms as well—depression which progressed to extreme lassitude, sleepiness and, in one instance, a mild case of panic. All experienced muscle pains, excessive sensitivity to touch and localized sensations such as numbness, tingling, "pins-and-needles" and so forth. After the tenth week they began to lose their appetites and feel nauseated. Two of the volunteers complained of distress around their hearts and an electrocardiogram revealed that their hearts were not normal. The blood of all showed a decrease in hemoglobin (the red pigment that carries oxygen to the cells) and in red blood corpuscles, even though their diet was planned to prevent anemia. The cholesterol content of their blood was also very high. When biotin was given to them, the symptoms disappeared within several days.

Now the conditions of this experiment are exaggerated, of course, as this kind of test necessitates. In real life, it is hardly possible that anyone eating such a diet as these volunteers were eating would at the same time be taking raw eggs and vitamin supplements. Since the symptoms of the human subjects were so similar to those of animals deprived of biotin, it seems we are safe in assuming that a biotin deficiency can indeed be induced in human beings who eat a great deal of raw egg white.

Possible Relationship Between Biotin and Cancer

Somewhat later, interest was aroused in the possibility of biotin having something to do with cancer formation. It was found that certain kinds of cancer contained more biotin than normal tissue. Biologists reasoned that if an excess of biotin caused the cancer, they might prevent it by feeding raw egg white whose avidin content would neutralize the biotin. Three researchers at the University of Wisconsin experimented with rats, feeding them a diet that included butter-yellow, a cancer-causing substance. Then they fed one group of the rats raw egg white, another group raw egg white plus biotin, and a third group cooked egg white, in which the avidin had been destroyed by the heat. Of the rats which ate the cancer-producing diet to which nothing had been added, 77 per cent developed liver tumors. The rats on any or all of the other diets developed from 10 to 18 per cent of liver tumors, which indicated that something in the white of egg protected them against tumor growth. The authors comment on the fact that the egg white exerted this protective effect equally well whether it was fed raw, or with biotin, or cooked to overcome the effect of the avidin. It would seem from this experiment that the peculiar relationship of biotin and avidin has nothing to do with cancer formation, even though signs of severe biotin deficiency appeared in those rats who received raw egg white in their diets, without any extra biotin.

Our study turned up numerous other experiments on biotin-avidin, but nothing that gave us any more of a clue as to just where we should stand on the raw egg white controversy. Our favorite book on animal nutrition, *Nutrition of the Dog* by C. M. McCay of Cornell University (published by Comstock) tells us that as early as 1898 it was discovered that the feeding of raw eggs was often followed by vomiting and diarrhea in dogs. It was also found that from 30 to 50 per cent of the raw egg white could be recovered from the dog's feces, indicating that he had digested only 50 to 70 per cent of it. On the other hand, tests showed that the same dog digested 90 per cent of cooked egg white. One researcher thought that this might be due to the rapid rate at which raw egg white leaves the stomach—the digestive juices simply do not have time to digest it. Raw egg starts to leave the stomach almost as soon as it reaches it. An hour and a half after it is eaten the egg white is well on its way through the small intestine. Boiled egg white, on the other hand, remains in the stomach two or three hours, until well digested. Knowledge of this fact about boiled egg white is valuable for someone on a reducing diet. If you eat your eggs hard-boiled, they will stay in your stomach longer and ward off those uncomfortable hunger pangs.

Helen T. Parsons and a group of fellow workers showed in an article in *Proceedings of the Society of Biological Chemistry,* volume 31, page 77, that in rats the effects of raw egg white could be prevented by including certain amounts of brewer's yeast or dried liver in the diet.

Dr. McCay is one of the country's outstanding animal nutritionists. In his recommendations for feeding dogs, he advises *that you should not feed raw eggs,* but feed whole, hard-boiled eggs, shell and all. He admits that no one knows why the raw egg white is not digested properly by dogs. He also mentions that it is better digested if it is thoroughly beaten or thoroughly mixed with milk before it is eaten.

Why Should Raw Egg White Be Harmful?

We have only one possible solution for the egg-white question—and this was suggested to us by a *Prevention* reader. Wild animals do not of course cook their food. Many wild animals eat bird's eggs. Nature provides ingenious and extremely successful ways of protecting new young life in various species. Could it be that avidin has been placed in egg white so that animals which prey on eggs will discover that the egg white eventually makes them ill and will be forced to find other kinds of food? Can avidin in egg white be just one of mother nature's ways of maintaining the proper balance among all the different kinds of life? Perhaps, who knows, if there were no such substance as avidin, birds would long ago have become extinct and the valuable functions they perform—scattering seed, pollinating flowers and destroying insects—would have suffered.

However, if it is possible for any animal to perceive the potential harm in raw egg white, you would think that dogs would refuse to eat it; whereas there is nothing they enjoy more than a fresh raw egg, even if they must steal it from the chicken house and break the shell themselves. So far as we know, however, no one has ever done any research on how many whole raw eggs any one dog will eat during a given time, if he is left to his own devices. Maybe he is able to sense just when to stop in order not to do himself harm. But, if this is so, why did the laboratory animals in the experiments above not refuse to eat the raw egg white after it had begun to produce unpleasant symptoms in them?

There is one other possible explanation, too, for why our 85-year old friend mentioned in the early part of this article might go on eating raw eggs for many more years in perfectly good health. You will notice that in all of the experiments in which raw egg white produced unhealthy symptoms, *only the egg white was fed.* No one tried to induce "egg-white injury" by feeding whole eggs. So perhaps we were intended to eat raw eggs, and "egg-white injury" is another example of what happens when we eat part of a food and throw away or change another part. We were meant to eat foods whole, undivided, unrefined and untampered with—of this we are certain. We know that egg yolk contains large amounts of biotin—perhaps enough to protect our 85-year old friend over all these years from any deficiency he might suffer if he ate just the whites alone. Perhaps egg yolk contains other substances, too, aside from biotin which protects against the hungry protein, avidin.

What do we advise, then, to our anxious reader whose wife and son eat two raw eggs for breakfast every day? We would not advise them to stop it entirely at once. We would be inclined, however, to advise changing the menu frequently—eating raw eggs perhaps once or twice a week and boiling or poaching them on other days. We do not like to give way an inch on our recommendation of eating as much food raw as possible, for we know that this is sound and sensible from every health point of view. We know that it takes a lot of raw food, every day, every meal, to make up to our bodies for the roasting, frying, boiling, toasting and broiling procedure we put most of our food through before our digestive juices get a chance to work on it. But perhaps we have not as yet developed such a state of nutrition that we can withstand the possible injurious effect of raw egg white.

But maybe those of us who are in excellent health and those of us who are getting ample supplies of B vitamins in our food supplements might be able to eat quantities of raw eggs without any ill effects whatsoever. But, if you have a suspicion that your supply of B vitamins may be deficient, better poach or boil those eggs, and take only an occasional eggnog.

We are deeply grateful to the following *Prevention* readers for translations from European medical journals:

Erna Borm of Tacoma Park, Maryland.

Dr. C. S. Green of Rexburg, Idaho.

Vitamins—Riboflavin and Psoriasis

Riboflavin and Psoriasis

The B vitamin riboflavin taken by mouth and by injection seems to help some people with psoriasis, stubborn skin disease, reports Dr. Merlin Maynard in the *Journal of Investigative Dermatology*. One quarter of the patients treated reported that their skin condition was completely healed. The rest found some improvement. As long as two years later, the disease had not returned in those who reported cures. Riboflavin is a mighty important member of the B complex, especially necessary for a healthy skin. Of course the only truly beneficial way of taking any B vitamin is in some natural food product which contains the rest of the B vitamins as well—liver, wheat germ, green vegetables. If you can't stand liver, won't eat salads and like the taste of white bread too much to give it up, then your only answer is the food supplement, desiccated liver, a recommended daily dose of which contains .35 milligram of riboflavin, along with all the other B vitamins, just as Nature planned and proportioned them.

Vitamin C

It seems pretty certain that for many thousands of years before human beings learned how to cook their food, they lived largely on raw fruits, berries, nuts, roots and whatever game they could find—eaten raw. Such a diet was rich in vitamin C. Since human life must have begun in a warm climate, there was little variation between summer and winter—fresh foods were available the year 'round. If mankind had continued to live this way, we would probably never have known there was any such a substance as vitamin C—for it would be so plentiful in our food we would never have a chance to study a vitamin C deficiency.

Since, for so many years human diet contained plenty of vitamin C, there seems to be little doubt of its importance to our well being. A substance which, for millions of years, has been used by every tissue and cell of every human body, cannot be neglected without serious harm resulting. However, as civilization progressed, vitamin C gradually decreased in our food. Men moved to northern lands where fresh foods were not available in the winter. They developed elaborate ways of preparing foods, most of which destroyed vitamin C. They began to take long sea voyages and go on long marches for which they had to carry provisions—dried, preserved foods in which there was, for practical purposes, no vitamin C at all.

As we became more and more adept in preserving foods, we lost more and more vitamin C. Today even with the enormous markets in our cities, with our elaborate system of transportation, with all our knowledge of food requirements and our scientific means of weighing and measuring things like this, we are undoubtedly getting far less vitamin C today—all of us—than our early ancestors got when they ate the fruits right off the trees, the berries off the bushes and the roots and grasses right out of the ground thousands of years ago.

If it were possible to change human physiology within a matter of several thousand years, this modern lack of vitamin C would not be so serious. But the process of adaptation is a long, long process and the cell that has, for millions of years, used a certain substance for performing a certain physiological task cannot be fooled into using something else. So there is no substitute for vitamin C. It is just as important for human welfare today as it was millions of years ago. Perhaps it is even more important today. For today we are surrounded by a myriad of poisons (unknown years ago) which vitamin C helps to neutralize. And in the process the vitamin is used up. So perhaps we actually need far more vitamin C than our ancestors did.

The Functions of Vitamin C

Let us see what are some of the uses the body has for vitamin C. When you glance over them quickly you become convinced that this is certainly the most important food element there is, for it appears to be involved in almost everything that goes on inside us. First of all, it is a carrier of hydrogen to all the cells of the body. Just as the red blood corpuscles carry oxygen, so vitamin C carries hydrogen. So for every chemical change involving hydrogen that goes on in our bodies, we must have vitamin C. Then, perhaps even more important, vitamin C is necessary for the formation of "collagen" which is the cement that glues together the various cells into tissues. It is important in the formation and upkeep of skin, tendons, bones, teeth, cartilage, connective tissue —in fact, every part of us contains some of this protein material which can be formed only if vitamin C is present.

The amount of oxygen our tissues need depends partly on vitamin C. The function of our blood vessels and heart goes smoothly only if there is ample vitamin C present. Wounds heal quickly in individuals whose vitamin C intake is high. Infections are less common. Under conditions of stress, such as extreme cold or heat, fatigue or anxiety, vitamin C is used up rapidly and must be replaced through diet. This appears to indicate that vitamin C is extremely important to the health of our adrenal glands, which are always involved under conditions of stress. And sure enough, the adrenal glands are storehouses for vitamin C. It is also believed that vitamin C assists in manufacturing the adrenal hormone, so important for so many different body emergencies.

Many investigations indicate that vitamin C seems to have a lot to do with the body's use of cholesterol. This is the fatty substance that collects on the inside of blood vessels and apparently causes hardening of the arteries. Could today's heavy toll of heart and vascular diseases be at least partly caused by deficiency in vitamin C? The strength of the capillary walls depends on vitamin C. If they are fragile there is far greater chance of hemorrhage which may result in a "stroke," or death from a brain or heart hemorrhage. Vitamin C is sometimes necessary in large quantities for recovery from anemia, suggesting that it takes an important part in the formation of red blood corpuscles in the bone marrow. Then too, vitamin C is used in many combinations with other food elements—vitamins and minerals. Certain of the B vitamins are closely tied up with vitamin C in their working. Iron, copper and other minerals have certain definite effects on vitamin C in the body's workings. Deficiencies in vitamin C may show up in the form of tooth decay, pyorrhea, gum infections, lack of appetite, anemia, undernutrition or susceptibility to infection.

How Was Vitamin C Discovered?

We talk so glibly about "discovering" vitamins that you might think the scientist comes upon the vitamin already labelled. Taking apart an orange or a green pepper, he suddenly finds a substance spread over the surface which he puts under a microscope and peers at. At any rate, this is the way they do it in the big scientific scenes in the movies and television, excitedly the scientist (always handsome and garbed in a spotless and very becoming white lab coat) calls in his assistants. "I've discovered vitamin C," he tells them modestly.

How very, very different are the actual facts! As the story of the conquest of scurvy shows, doctors have believed for hundreds of years that there was some substance in fresh fruits and vegetables that could cure or prevent scurvy. Of course they had no idea of what it was and no chemical means for identifying it. Actually it was not until about 20 years ago that vitamin C was tracked down, isolated and taken apart, so that we know of what it consists.

The story is told entertainingly by Charles Glen King, one of the discoverers of vitamin C, in *Nutrition Reviews* for January 1954. Dr. King was working at the University of Pittsburgh under very difficult conditions. Finally he and his assistants managed to produce a substance that, by all the tests, seemed to be vitamin C. It also seemed to be exactly the same substance produced by two other scientists a little earlier. As Dr. King and his colleagues prepared a manuscript on their discovery, they read a press release from Norway indicating that another scientist had identified vitamin C as an alkaloid substance having little or nothing to do with the stuff Dr. King had produced. So it seemed necessary to wait until they could get more information about this Norwegian product.

Two papers were prepared for scientific journals. Dr. McCollum, the famous nutrition expert, heard Dr. King read one of these papers at a scientific meeting and congratulated him for having "given us a pure compound as a vitamin." After the scientific papers had been printed, word came from Hungary that two researchers, Svirbely and Szent-Gyorgyi, had prepared a substance from adrenal glands which they called "hexuronic acid." This, too, protected animals from scurvy. Was this the food element they were all looking for?

Testing this substance, King found that it seemed to have the same properties as his vitamin. A German scientist succeeded in isolating from citrus fruit something that cured scurvy, too. Two English workers confirmed the fact that the Hungarian product cured scurvy. Then Szent-Gyorgyi and his colleague made and distributed widely a substance they got from green peppers. By this time it was clear that all of them had been working on the same substance. No matter what name you might call it, this arrangement of molecules containing such and such an amount of carbon, hydrogen and oxygen in such and such a combination was the elusive food element that doctors knew hundreds of years before could cure scurvy.

Synthetic Versus Natural Vitamin C

Then, having broken down the chemical composition of vitamin C it became necessary to devise ways of putting all these molecules together again to synthesize pure ascorbic acid, or vitamin C. Here the question arises—what is the difference between synthetic vitamin C and natural vitamin C? After they have broken down vitamin C into all its parts, scientists can then assemble all these parts, chemically. Why isn't this synthetic vitamin as good as the natural vitamin which occurs in food? Some scientists and nutritionists will say that it is. But others know full well that it is not.

Researchers found that the "pure" synthetic vitamin could not perform the near-miracles they might achieve using foods high in vitamin C. The answer was that another compound comes along with vitamin C in most foods—something called originally vitamin P. This was not, of course, in the synthetic vitamin C, for it had not as yet been discovered; its presence was completely unknown. But after this substance (also called hesperidin, flavonoids, rutin, vitamin P, etc.) had been discovered, we found that it helps vitamin C in its work and that anything vitamin C can do, the two of them together can do much better.

Now do you see the reason for not depending on synthetic vitamins? The drug companies will declare to you that their synthetic vitamin C is exactly the same thing as the vitamin C in rose hips or green peppers. And so it is, chemically. But it is not accompanied by all the other things in the rose hips and the green peppers that make the vitamin C work so much better. It may be hundreds of years before we find out what are all the various things in rose hips that make their vitamin C such a wonderfully good source for human beings. Until then, how can you possibly get these things in a synthetic vitamin? We don't even know how many of them there may be, let alone what any of them are!

This is your answer to the vitamin salesman who tries to sell you a synthetic vitamin, telling you it is "just as good" as a natural one.

Vitamin C and Acne

The author of a paper in the *Archives of Dermatology and Syphilology,* volume 70, page 363, 1954, gave massive doses of vitamin C to 53 acne patients, 43 of whom improved. Fifteen of these had been treated for months or years by all the usual methods, without success. Ten patients failed to improve and seven did not return for a check-up.

The vitamin C consisted of an eight-ounce glass of citrus juice twice daily as well as three grams (3000 milligrams) of ascorbic acid per day. We assume that this was synthetic ascorbic acid, since nothing in the article indicates that it could have been from natural sources.

In addition, the patients were put on a diet free of chocolate, nuts and peanut butter, were told to clean their skin three times a day and were given *lotio alba* to apply at night. As we know, vitamin C has a lot to do with skin health. It has also been found that persons deprived of vitamin C entirely are likely to suffer from a worsening of their acne, if they are subject to it. It seems as if plenty of vitamin C in the diet might play a big part in preventing acne. And it is well-known that the diet of teen-agers (most susceptible to acne) is likely to be short on this vitamin.

Vitamin C—Pyorrhea and Kidney Stones

Kidney stones and pyorrhea! What do these two things have in common? One is a disease of the gums and mouth tissues—a chronic inflammation. As it becomes more serious, the teeth are loosened and eventually fall out. In the other condition, stones, sometimes called gravel, form in the kidneys. If they are not removed by surgery, they may cause inflammation of the kidneys. Or they may stop off the channels leading from the kidneys so that the patient dies of uremia.

What have these two conditions in common? Well, first of all, pyorrhea is generally associated with the formation of tartar—that thick, unpleasant substance which forms on the teeth. The collected tartar irritates the gums, especially in those places in the mouth where it's hard to reach with a toothbrush. The irritated gums become sore and as more tartar collects the soreness spreads. Kidney stones are of course a kind of deposit too—calcium, apparently, which is not used properly by the body and hence collects in places where it should not.

So apparently both pyorrhea and kidney stones begin with an unhealthful condition in which deposits are formed. Dr. Sigurd Ramfjord of Oslo, Norway is quoted in a United Press dispatch as saying that gum disease afflicts from 80 to 90 per cent of all adults and is responsible for the loss of more teeth than cavities. He said that the slow deterioration of gums usually goes unnoticed because it is painless, but it is the principal cause of loss of teeth in persons more than 30 years old. Kidney stones, too, are widely prevalent and, strangely enough, seem to occur in certain geographical areas, as if there were something about the soil or the air or the climate that made the people there more susceptible to kidney stones.

We are told that pyorrhea is practically universal in Newfoundland and is accompanied by heavy deposits of tartar on the teeth. In the British West Indies on the contrary (where fresh fruits are available the year round) pyorrhea is practically unknown. Kidney stones are common among the people of Tibet, West China, India, Labrador and Newfoundland. There are other localities of the world where they are unknown.

Dr. W. J. McCormick in an article in the *Journal of the Canadian Dental Association* for August, 1946, tells us that the eastern peoples in the localities mentioned above live chiefly on rice, barley flour, butter and tea, with few or no vegetables or fruits. In Labrador and Newfoundland white flour, fish, game, lard, oatmeal, tea and sugar make up the bulk of the diet. Fresh fruits and vegetables are all but unknown, especially during the winter months, and the winters are long in Canada.

Dr. McCormick tells us further that the teeth of people living on these diets are covered with tartar. Even very young children have heavy tartar deposits on the teeth. This might happen, he says, because lack of vitamin C leads to a breakdown of the body tissues, including those of the mouth. The mucus lining scales off and, mixing with remnants of food, creates the unsightly and unhealthful deposit that clings so tenaciously to the teeth, resulting in pyorrhea and inflammation of the mouth tissues which have already been seriously weakened by lack of vitamin C.

How Lack of Vitamin C May Affect Mouth and Kidney Tissues

Is it not possible, he asks, that the urinary tract goes through the same process when there is not enough vitamin C in the diet—the mucus lining scales off and forms the nucleus of the stones? And if this is true of kidney stones, might it not also hold true for gall bladder stones, and stones in the appendix, pancreas, prostate gland, mammary gland, uterus, ovaries and even the calcium deposit that brings about hardening of the arteries and arthritis? We have shown in other articles in this book that vitamin C deficiency indeed appears to be related to hardening of the arteries and deposits of cholesterol—the substance generally involved in gall stones.

Observing his own patients, Dr. McCormick found that cloudy urine containing phosphates and pieces of sloughed off mucus from the walls of the urinary canal went hand-in-hand with vitamin C deficiency. Giving large doses of vitamin C (much larger than one would get even in a daily diet relatively high in vitamin C) he could clear the urine within a matter of hours. During this treatment his patients reported to him *that the tartar deposits were clearing from their teeth and dentures.* Nurses in hospitals reported that patients whose urine had formerly caused calcium deposits on the urinary vessels found that the utensils remained free from calcium deposits. He interjects at this point a reminder that these particular patients were also getting a diet and dietary supplements high in the complex of B vitamins. So undoubtedly the vitamin B should have some of the credit, but Dr. McCormick feels certain that it was the vitamin C which was responsible for the change in the appearance of the urine. And the disappearance of the tartar.

As is the case with infectious diseases, the incidence of kidney stone has, in recent years, shifted from children to adults. Can this be because mothers, conscientiously stuffing their infants with vitamin C, almost universally ignore the small amounts of vitamin C their older children and adult members of the family may be getting?

Dr. McCormick quotes J. W. Joly in his book *Stones and Calculus Disease of the Urinary Organs* (C. V. Mosby Co. 1929): "I believe the hypothesis that stone is a deficiency disease is the most plausible and probable that has yet been advanced. It explains not only all the principal features of the condition today, but also the changes in incidence during the past years. I believe that vitamin starvation acts primarily on the renal epithelium (lining of the kidneys) and through it on the colloidal mechanism of the urine; also that once this mechanism is deranged, stone formation must follow as a direct result of the laws of physical chemistry."

Pyorrhea and Vitamin C

J. A. Sinclair, D.D.S. in an article in the *Journal of the American Dental Association* for October, 1939, tells us that vitamin C deficiency destroys the body's ability to rebuild tissues and fibers such as the tissues of the gums. He tells us that he completely cured two patients of pyorrhea by giving them 150 milligrams of vitamin C daily for 30 days. Paul E. Boyle, D.M.D. and his associates, in the same journal for November 1937 tell us that among 66 patients examined at the Harvard Dental School more than half had far less vitamin C than normal in their blood. And all of these patients had marked disease of the gums. "Ten of these patients in the low level range were given pure vitamin C by mouth and showed clinical improvement in the (gums), coincidental with increase in the blood ascorbic acid."

Anna P. Boudin, D.D.S. writing in the *Medical Woman's Journal* for April, 1943, tells us that a diet completely lacking in vitamin C produces extensive inflammation of the gums, however, in many cases, giving vitamin C alone will not bring about a cure. Generally when the vitamin C intake is low, multiple deficiency is present, she says. So an all 'round good diet should be prescribed, which will result in plenty of vitamin C, along with the rest of the vitamins.

A case of gingivitis is discussed in a letter to the editor of *Oral Hygiene* for January, 1955. J. R. Russell, D.D.S. of San Diego, California states that he is treating gingivitis with 100 milligrams of vitamin C and 100 milligrams of niacin (a B vitamin) at each meal. When the vitamins are discontinued for any length of time, the swelling of the gums returns. We think these patients would undoubtedly get along better on natural vitamin C and all the members of the B complex of vitamins, as they are found in brewer's yeast or desiccated liver.

Join Our Experiment!

A number of readers have written us about the problems of tartar on the teeth, which, as we know, can easily lead to pyorrhea and loss of all the teeth. If you are bothered by deposits of tartar on the teeth, follow carefully the chart given on page 973, which indicates which foods are rich in vitamin C and about how much each of them may contain. Keep track of the approximate amount of vitamin C you get each day.

Whether in food or food supplement, see that you get at least 150 milligrams of vitamin C every day, without fail. If you get 75 with your meals, take a natural vitamin C supplement to make up the other 75 milligrams. Don't eat it all at once, at one meal, for it takes your body about four hours to make use of as much vitamin C as it can handle at one time. So spread it out over the day. Then watch what happens to the tartar deposits. If you visit your dentist during this time, ask him to check on the tartar and see if there is an improvement. If you smoke, there is probably no use in your conducting the experiment, for this amount of vitamin C would be rapidly used up by the tobacco.

Vitamin C—The Universal Remedy?

Here are some notes from our files on various disease conditions (other than those we discuss elsewhere in this book), in which vitamin C has been tried and found useful in curing the particular ailment for which it was used. Remember, please, that we are not suggesting that you use vitamin C to cure yourself in case you are suffering from one or several of these ailments. But you can certainly take this information to your doctor and ask him to prescribe vitamin C for you. And of course you can take plenty of vitamin C in your meals and food supplements now to make certain that you will not ever succumb to the disorders we mention below.

Vitamin C and the Eyes

There is abundant evidence that vitamin C is plentiful in the healthy lens of the eye. It is absent or nearly absent in the diseased lens. In the answer to a letter to the editor of the *Journal of the American Medical Association* for December 16, 1950, we find this information: Vitamin C plays an important part in the nutrition of the eye tissues. The healthy lens is particularly rich in this vitamin, while eyes that have cataracts contain little or none.

In the *British Medical Journal* for November 18, 1950, there is a review of 51 cases of small corneal ulcers—that is, ulcers of the cornea of the eye. About half of the patients received 1500 milligrams of vitamin C every day, while the other half received a tablet containing nothing of medicinal value. In those who received the vitamin C there was no significant difference in the healing of the superficial ulcers, but the deep ulcers healed much more rapidly.

In *The Eye, Ear, Nose and Throat Monthly,* volume 31, page 79, a doctor gives his formula for preventing cataract and checking its progress once it is formed. He gives his patients a special diet which includes the tops of vegetables—in other words, garden greens, one pint of milk and two eggs daily. In addition each of his patients got vitamin supplements—chlorophyll tablets and vitamins C and A.

Cataracts are a disease of later years. And we suspect that one very good reason why they form may be that older people get out of the habit of eating eggs, leafy green vegetables and other foods that are rich in vitamins and minerals. It's so much easier and cheaper to live on white bread, soft, starchy desserts and coffee or tea. Surveys show that older folks especially are deficient in vitamin C. They also appear to need more of this vitamin than the younger people.

The Thyroid and Vitamin C

According to *Iodine Facts,* volume 1, 1940-1946, Sir Robert McCarrison, the famous British nutritionist, found in his researches in

India that individuals who were deficient in vitamin C had a fourfold increase of iodine in the thyroid gland. Iodine is one of the ingredients of thyroxin—the hormone manufactured by the thyroid. When there is too little or too much iodine in this gland, we know there is something seriously wrong with the body metabolism. This observation of McCarrison's appears to show that vitamin C is most important for the good health of the thyroid gland.

Stomach Ulcers

Eddy and Dahldorf in their book *The Avitaminoses* (published by William and Wilkins) tell us of a group of ulcer patients put on the usual bland ulcer diet. One third of these had capillary fragility within 16 days. In 70 per cent of these, vitamin C produced a cure. Another researcher found that of 18 ulcer patients 15 had vitamin C blood levels far below normal. In another group of 20 patients, 18 were found to lack vitamin C in their blood. Is it because the diets they are eating are grossly deficient in vitamin C, or is it that they cannot utilize vitamin C properly? We think it is probably a combination of all three, but certainly the most important fact is that the usual ulcer diet is practically void of vitamin C. On the other hand, if a lack of vitamin C in the diet has had something to do with the formation of the ulcer in the first place—and we believe that it does—then how foolish it seems to prescribe a diet of milk, crackers, and soft bland foods in which there is little or no vitamin C!

The Healing of Wounds Large and Small

Vitamin C is absolutely essential for proper wound healing. The rations of the Armed Forces in World War II contained 75 milligrams daily of the vitamin because it is known that the vitamin is mobilized into the tissue around a wound to help in the healing process. In animals on a vitamin C deficient diet it was noted that the healed wound was much more likely to open once again. Human volunteers, too, have found that wounds heal slowly when vitamin C is deficient in the diet and are inclined to open once again under stress.

The Adrenal Glands and Vitamin C

The adrenal glands, located just in front of the kidneys, are the source of adrenalin which is released into your body whenever you are under stress of any kind—fright, anger, pain, heat, cold, fatigue, things like that. The graying of hair appears to be related to the adrenal glands. So perhaps stress and strain, through their action on the adrenal glands, may actually produce gray hair.

There is an abundance of vitamin C in healthy adrenal glands—a great deal more than you will find concentrated in any part of the body. Why? Is it just stored there? This seems unlikely. Is it necessary for the proper functioning of the adrenal glands? It seems so. As long ago as 1940 several researchers reported that the hormone released by a certain part of the adrenals cannot be formed there unless vitamin C is present. This seems to us to be ample reason for getting enough vitamin C every day, even if the body had no other use for it at all.

Fertility and Vitamin C

Phillips and his colleagues, writing in *The Journal of Biological Chemistry,* volume 130, page 145, 1939, have produced evidence that vitamin C encourages the motility of spermatozoa. In experiments with bulls they were able to induce sperm motility by injecting vitamin C. When the vitamin C in the blood fell below a certain point, the result was impotence.

Motility of sperm is of course extremely important for fertility. If the sperm are alive and moving rapidly, they are healthy and the chances for conception are good. If the sperm are slow and sluggish, conception may very well not take place. How many of our tragic childless marriages of today are the result of too little vitamin C in the diet?

Hay Fever, Allergies and Asthma

In 1942 researcher H. W. Holmes made a report in *Science,* volume 96, page 497, that gave promise of relief to hay fever victims. He gave daily doses of 200-500 milligrams of vitamin C for a period of a week. Then the treatment was stopped. If the symptoms appeared again, the vitamin was given again, in large quantities. Holmes declared that these massive doses of vitamin C protect not only against hay fever but also against food allergies and asthma.

Perhaps this is one reason why the Abrahamson diet for correcting low blood sugar does so much for hay fever and asthma patients. The individual on this diet must do without sweet and starchy food. This adjusts the level of his blood sugar. At the same time it forces him to eat far more of vegetables and fruits than he otherwise would. So perhaps the additional vitamin C in the diet is another reason for its success.

The Health of the Liver

Lack of vitamin C damages the liver. Researchers do not know exactly how vitamin C works to keep the liver in a healthy condition, but they believe that the normal mechanism in which the liver engages, turning carbohydrate and protein into a form that can be used by the body is slowed down when there is not enough vitamin C present.

Prickly Heat

Frederick Reiss, M.D., writing in the *Journal of the American Medical Association* for March 10, 1951, describes a condition always associated with prickly heat which he says is connected with a vitamin C deficiency. He gave his patients 900 to 1000 milligrams of vitamin C which cured the condition. He says that small doses ranging from 200 to 300 milligrams were effective only when the hot weather subsided and perspiration decreased. This physician believes that hot weather depletes the body's store of vitamin C, through perspiration. Vitamin C is water soluble, so it seems reasonable that the body would lose it in perspiration. Perhaps lack of vitamin C lost this way may be the main contributing factor to prickly heat.

Vitamin C for Some Kinds of Anemia

The Lancet for October 31, 1953, concluding an article on vitamin C in relation to anemia, has this to say: "Thus good evidence has been provided that if the diet is deficient in ascorbic acid (vitamin C) for long enough, anemia will result. Slight deficiency of ascorbic acid is common enough and cases of true scurvy still turn up—especially in old people living alone . . . Clearly if this deficiency is unrecognized and untreated, the anemia may resist the usual hemantics (medicine given to increase the hemoglobin in the blood). It is good to know, too, that the habit of prescribing iron and vitamin C together has some scientific support." The article refers to the fact that iron, whether in food or medicine, is better absorbed by the body if it is given along with vitamin C.

Vitamin C and Menstruation

It is interesing to note, in connection with capillary fragility, that several things are involved. According to Bell, Lazarus and Munro, writing in *The Lancet,* for August 10, 1940, "Apart from abnormal influences—fever and administration of heavy metals—two factors influence capillary fragility in health—menstruation and ascorbic acid. In women near the menstrual period, the petechial count will be raised." The petechial count involves the number of small blood vessels that break beneath the skin when it is subjected to pressure.

It seems from this comment that menstruation may cause a drain on vitamin C and perhaps vitamin P as well. Since capillary fragility is greater at this time it would seem to be wise for women to increase the amount of vitamin C they are getting as the time for their regular monthly period draws near.

Burns Treated with Vitamin C

A number of physicians have used vitamin C in the treatment of burns with startling results. Writing in the *New York Journal of Medicine* for October 15, 1951, D. H. Klasson tells us that vitamin C alleviates pain and in minor burns hastens the healing period. It reduces the time interval necessary for skin grafting. This in turn reduces the chances of infection and long convalescence. Sixty-two cases of burns formed the basis for Dr. Klasson's conclusions.

Insect Bites

A friend of ours got bitten by a yellow jacket the other day. She is especially sensitive to insect bites and usually swells up like a balloon and stays that way for days if a wasp or a bee stings her. The yellow jacket involved was from a particularly vicious swarm that had raised welts on several of the neighbors who swatted at them.

The varmint got our friend on the end of her finger. As soon as she felt the searing pain on its way up to her elbow she went into the house and got several tablets of natural vitamin C, plunked them in a cup with a dab of water inside and put her finger to rest on the tablets. As they dissolved in the water, the pain subsided, and within twenty minutes or so, the finger was normal again. No pain. No swelling. Vitamin C has been used by physicians to treat black widow and snake bites. Of course massive doses are used in these cases.

Vitamin C for Cancer

E. Schneider, writing in *Deutsche Medizinishe Wochenschrift* volume 79, page 15, 1954, relates how he gave vitamin C (1000 to 2000 milligrams daily), along with vitamin A, to about a hundred early and advanced cancer patients. There was general improvement—a reduction in the size of the tumors, increase in body weight, lowered blood sedimentation rate, a better nutritional state, reduction in hemorrhage and ulceration. He did not cure the cancers with vitamin C. But he got as good results in improving the condition of the patient as others have gotten with potent measures that have had drastic after-effects.

Foods That Contain Vitamin C

Here is the vitamin C content of those foods richest in the vitamin.

Food	*Mgs. of Vitamin C*
Asparagus, fresh green	20 in 8 stalks
Beans, green lima	42 in ½ cup
Beet greens, cooked	50 in ½ cup
Broccoli, flower	65 in ¾ cup
Broccoli, leaf	90 in ¾ cup
Brussels sprouts	130 in ¾ cup
Cabbage, raw	50 in 1 cup
Cantaloupe	50 in ½ small
Chard, Swiss, cooked	37 in ½ cup
Collards, cooked	70 in ½ cup
Currants, red	40 in 1 cup
Dandelion greens, cooked	100 in 1 cup
Grapefruit, fresh	45 in ½ grapefruit
Grapefruit juice, fresh	108 in 1 cup
Grapefruit juice, canned	72 in 1 cup
Guavas	125 in 1 guava
Honeydew Melon	90 in ¼ medium
Kale, cooked	96 in ¾ cup
Kohlrabi	50 in ½ cup
Lemon juice	25 in 1 tablespoon
Lime juice	18 in ¼ cup
Liver, beef	30 in 1 slice
Liver, calves	25 in 1 slice
Liver, chicken	25 in ½ cup
Liver, lamb	20 in 1 slice
Loganberries	35 in 1 cup
Mustard greens, cooked	125 in ½ cup
Orange	50 in 1 medium
Orange juice, fresh	120 in 1 cup
Orange juice, canned	80 in 1 cup
Parsley	70 in ½ cup
Parsnips	40 in ½ cup
Peas, fresh cooked	20 in 1 cup
Peppers, green	125 in 1 medium
Peppers, pimento	200 in 2 medium
Pineapple, fresh	38 in 2/3 cup
Pineapple juice, canned	25 in 1 cup
Potatoes, sweet	25 in 1 medium
Potatoes, white, baked	20 in 1 medium
Potatoes, white, raw	33 in 1 medium
Radishes	25 in 15 large
Raspberries, black	66 in 1 cup
Raspberries, red	23 in 1 cup
Rose hips	500-6000 in 100 mg.
Rutabagas	26 in ¾ cup
Spinach, cooked	30 in ½ cup
Strawberries, fresh	50 in ½ cup
Tomatoes, canned	20 in ½ cup
Tomatoes, fresh	25 in 1 medium
Tomato juice, canned	48 in 1 cup
Turnips, cooked	22 in ½ cup
Turnips, raw	30 in 1 medium
Turnip tops, cooked	130 in ½ cup
Watercress	54 in 1 bunch

Vitamin D for Growth

Vitamin D is of utmost importance to children, for they are growing and their bones and teeth must be made from minerals which they can secure only from their diet and which their bodies will be able to use only if they have sufficient vitamin D. Country children who are outdoors all summer and take cod liver oil in the winter seldom have rickets. But city slum children who see little of the sun, and whose mothers know nothing of nutrition, may grow up deformed, small in stature, with little chance for beauty, for their faces are narrow, their legs bowed, their jaws under—or over-developed, their teeth crowded into dental arches too small to contain them, their foreheads bulging. So vitamin D is the beauty vitamin. For how can a child attain the wide chest and hip structure, the normal mouth structure, straight legs, strong back and good posture that go with beauty, unless the proper minerals are present, along with vitamin D to create this handsome bone structure? In one sense, vitamin D is the most important of all vitamins, for with all the others, the conditions caused by a deficiency can be corrected. But once a bone has stopped growing, nothing will make it grow again, once a leg bone has been bowed, no diet will straighten it out, and once a jaw structure has grown small and misshapen, no vitamin can transform it.

So modern mothers give their children fish liver oil which is richer in vitamin D than any other substance. It goes without saying these days that any doctor delivering a baby advises fish liver oil right from the beginning of the baby's life. And most babies in our country these days reach the age of four or five without contracting rickets. But all too often the dose of fish liver oil is discontinued too soon. Remember that children keep on growing until they are fully mature. And for good growth, sound teeth, long straight limbs and strong backs, fish liver oil should be part of their diet until full growth has been achieved. Aside from the matter of beauty, vitamin D is important for health in later life. For if the body structure of a chest is narrow, diseases of the chest are likely to be more easily contracted. A woman with a narrow pelvic structure (caused by lack of vitamin D in childhood) is almost certain to have a difficult time in childbirth.

Vitamin D In Pregnancy

Facial asymmetry in newborn babies may be the result of osteoporosis (softness) of facial bones and also the position of the child in the mother's uterus, according to Elena Boder writing in *The Journal of Pediatrics* for May, 1952. In her opinion, the surest preventive is ample vitamin D for the mother during pregnancy.

The reasoning behind this would seem to be that with enough vitamin D and minerals in her diet, the mother can provide her child with the equipment for making strong bones, so that not even the pressure of an unnatural position in the uterus can force these bones into asymmetry.

Vitamin E

We think of vitamin C preventing scurvy. Vitamin B_1 prevents beriberi. Rickets can be caused by lack of vitamin D. And each of these vitamins is also involved in the good health of other parts of the body. We need vitamin C for preventing colds and other infections. Vitamin B_1 is necessary for nerve health. All of the vitamins are versatile; not one of them is needed for just one single purpose. Nature is more economical than that.

The more we read about vitamin E the more convinced we become that this is surely the most versatile of all vitamins. And yet, up to now, official bodies have said that there is no positive indication that vitamin E is essential in human nutrition. Another way of putting it is to say that we get plenty of vitamin E in our food, so there is never a need for taking vitamin E as a supplement.

We have published a lot of information about the use of vitamin E in heart and blood vessel conditions. This work with vitamin E is being carried on in North America chiefly by Evan and Wilfrid Shute, two brothers, M.D.'s who were instrumental in founding the Shute Institute at London, Ontario, Canada. The latest issue of their magazine *The Summary* (published by the Institute) is another testimonial to the versatility of vitamin E. This hundred and ten page magazine of closely printed text describes cases in which vitamin E has been used, sometimes successfully, sometimes without much success. But the incredible thing about the story is the number of different and supposedly wholly unrelated conditions in which vitamin E may bring relief.

The first article talks about gangrene treated with vitamin E. The gangrene of Buerger's disease, that of arteriosclerosis and that of diabetes are all discussed. In many of the case histories given, the final report goes something like this: "Healed in 1½ years," "healed in three months," "ulcer healed" and so forth. Of course there are cases where vitamin E did not cure the gangrene. No drug and no vitamin works in every and any circumstance. But the fact remains that in many of these cases—dire cases where no other treatment had benefited, vitamin E brought about swift change for the better. The diabetic patients did the best of the three groups. Surprisingly enough, fifty per cent of the diabetic cases reduced their insulin intake while they were taking vitamin E. Most of the patients in all three groups came to the Shute Institute with fully developed gangrene and long histories of trouble of this kind. Many of them had had amputations. In many cases the patients lived far from London and had to be treated by mail over long distances.

Vitamin E for "Female Troubles"

The next chapter is on vitamin E in obstetrics and gynecology. Vitamin E appears to be most successful in treating male sterility and many of the different complications of female reproductive organs, especially at the time of the change of life. As Dr. Evan Shute says, "Whatever is said as to the great number of menopausal women who have no or only slight menopausal complaints, of the large number who need only sedatives and/or reassurance, and on the fact that estrogens are indicated for only a minority, the fact remains that almost every practitioner in the world automatically administers estrogens with or without a barbiturate to women who complain of hot flushes at this epoch. No therapeutic practice has become more universal in the last 25 years." Estrogens are the female sex hormones which, everyone agrees, frequently cause most annoying after-effects by bringing on the patient's menstruation periods again, only postponing the time for the final menopause. Then too, it is generally agreed that female sex hormones, used indiscriminately, can cause cancer in those who are susceptible to it.

Dr. Shute tells us that vitamin E "does not often give as complete relief from hot flushes as do the estrogens. But it does give good help in many cases, is especially valuable for the headaches and migraine of the climacteric, is unique in the relief it provides for vulvar senility and does not produce untoward vaginal bleeding." Vitamin E is also very valuable in preventing thromboses or blood clots after operations. "Once used," says Dr. Shute "it will never be replaced by any of the currently popular but dangerous anticoagulants. The writer has not used anything but vitamin E for this purpose for the last eight years." Restoring normal circulation after five years of phlebitis is almost inconceivable, he says, but occasionally vitamin E has achieved a reduction in the amount of crippling.

In discussing vitamin E in heart disease, Dr. Shute points out some of the excellent reasons for using vitamin E that are not apparent at first glance. Being treated with vitamin E, the heart patient who is desperately ill can still remain at home and have his own doctor, rather than some strange and busy specialist. The Shute Institute has rarely had four patients in London hospitals at any one time, and generally has one or none, in spite of the fact that it refuses no heart or blood vessel patient, no matter how desperate his case may be.

Finally, says Dr. Shute, "It is the kindliest treatment any cardiovascular patient can achieve, and also the cheapest for him and his community. It is the most helpful medicine to appear in our day on the horizon of the largest group of ailing persons. It even does a great deal to restore the general practitioner to his proper and unique place in the care of the sick. It is pre-eminently his drug."

Other Conditions That Are Helped

In a series of brief notes on reports in other medical magazines, we find mention of many other conditions treated with vitamin E. There are several reports on diabetes with the comment by Dr. Shute "Vitamin E plugs the leak in the insulin dyke." There is an interesting article on hemorrhage in the newborn which was prevented by giving the mother vitamin E while she was in labor. There are discussions of the use of vitamin E and choline (a B vitamin) in muscular dystrophy. There is the story of a German physician who has been treating gastric ulcers with vitamin E for eleven years with great success. Another German report concerns burns from x-ray which responded well to vitamin E. This same doctor used it for acne rosacea with excellent results in some patients. Another German physician used vitamin E in treating gum disorders. He injected it into the gums. There was great improvement in all 76 patients treated.

If your doctor is hesitating about prescribing vitamin E, suggest to him that he send for a copy of the current issue of *The Summary* published by The Shute Foundation, London, Ontario, Canada.

In the April 23, 1955, issue of *The Lancet,* a conservative medical journal of England, there is an article about the use of vitamin E for pain during menstruation. E. Blanche Butler and Edith McKnight, who wrote the article, believed that pain just before and during menstruation might come from the constriction of blood vessels in the uterus during this period. They believed that vitamin E might relieve the pain by preventing the spasm of the blood vessels.

Their investigations were made at the University of Wales where they worked with 100 women students between the ages of 18 and 21. All were in the same good health, all ate the same diet and had the same living habits generally. Their menstrual periods were regular and normal except for the fact that they had considerable pain before and during the period. Fifty of the girls were given 50 milligram tablets of vitamin E three times daily. The other fifty took pills that looked exactly the same but contained nothing.

Over a period of three months the girls reported their symptoms. In most cases those who were taking the vitamin E showed improvement —in some individuals within the first month. In addition it seemed that the vitamin E had a cumulative effect. Twenty of the girls became entirely free from pain in the premenstrual and menstrual period. This result was obtained in eight of them during the first month of treatment and for the remaining 12 girls the rate of improvement was slower. In some cases there were relapses during the second month. At a routine physical examination a year later some of the girls who had taken part in the experiment and had received the vitamin E tablet said their pain had returned after the experiment was over. They asked for a supply of vitamin E that they might continue to take it on their own. Altogether 70 per cent of the young women taking the vitamin E showed improvement, as against only 29 per cent in the controls.

Why should vitamin E have such remarkable powers—even greater, it seems, than the other vitamins? We do not know. But one explanation occurs to us. For many thousands of years human beings have been eating grains. Whole grains are our richest source of vitamin E, aside from vegetable oils. So down through all the centuries many of today's most troublesome diseases were unknown—muscular dystrophy, heart and blood vessel diseases, and so forth. We do not say that these are caused only by a deficiency in vitamin E. Undoubtedly there are more reasons. Undoubtedly other food elements that are lacking today are important for preventing these diseases

But from *The Annual Review of Bio-Chemistry,* volume 23, 1954, quoted in *The Summary:* "After treatment of flour with chlorine dioxide under commercial conditions (bleaching, that is) the tocopherol (vitamin E) content was reduced about 70 per cent, compared with untreated flour. Since flour is a staple article of diet and since chlorine dioxide has replaced agene as the more commonly used flour improver in the United States, the available vitamin E in the diet may be significantly decreased through its use." Doesn't it sound to you as though the Shute brothers may be replacing in daily diet something that has been lacking for a long time—and this is the secret of the versatility of vitamin E!

Vitamin P

Actually very little is known about vitamin P. It was discovered by Szent-Gyorgyi in 1936—or rather, he announced at that time that apparently some substance was present in certain foods which had an effect on the fragility of blood capillaries. A great deal of work has since been done with no very conclusive results. Paprika and lemon peel were the two foods which Szent-Gyorgyi found to contain some substance, other than vitamin C, which prevented hemorrhaging.

He discovered this by giving vitamin C to animals which suffered from scurvy. Some of them did not improve. But when paprika or lemon peel were given, the hemorrhaging of these animals stopped, indicating that some substance present had strengthened the capillaries. Citrin is the name given to this particular vitamin P.

Rutin, another vitamin P, was originally obtained from California poppies. Recently buckwheat has been found to be the most economical source. A great many theories have been postulated to determine how vitamin P works in the body, but no definite conclusions have been arrived at. It is known that adrenalin, a hormone produced in the body, regulates the tone or health of the capillaries. Perhaps vitamin P works with adrenalin, or perhaps it takes part in the body's assimilation of tyrosine, an amino acid which is necessary for the formation of adrenalin. These are only two of the many theories as to the place of vitamin P in the body functioning.

Vitamin P has been used in treating the following diseases: non-thrombopenic purpura (a disease in which small hemorrhages take place in the skin), hemophilia (in which blood will not clot), nephritis, ascitic cirrhosis (a swelling and inflammation of an organ), eczema, glaucoma, and rheumatic gout. Results have been good in some cases and indifferent in others—in other words, not conclusive. One researcher used vitamin P in the treatment of psoriasis in 45 patients with these results: 30 patients improved, 12 did not change and 3 grew worse. Used in treatment of hypertension, vitamin P may be of value in controlling the fragility of the capillaries, and hence preventing hemorrhaging, but it does not cure or improve the hypertension.

Uses For Vitamin P

However vitamin P is effective in controlling the hemorrhaging of laboratory animals which have been exposed to X-ray. If it is given before the X-ray exposure, it protects animals from these bad aftereffects on capillaries.

In addition, we know that patients who suffer from multiple vitamin deficiencies also have great capillary fragility. In other words, when you are deficient in one vitamin you are generally deficient in several others, because many vitamins occur in one kind of food. If you are not eating that food—or any of the foods in which that vitamin occurs, you will suffer from deficiency of more than one vitamin. In addition, the vitamins work together in a very complex manner inside your body. So a deficiency in one generally means a deficiency in several others as well. In such a condition, there is bound to be capillary fragility—that is, the capillaries, or tiny blood vessels rupture easily, causing bruises and hemorrhages.

From this we can see that the food we eat certainly has a definite effect on the health of the small blood vessels. Perhaps a deficiency in other vitamins helps bring about the deficiency of vitamin P which may cause the blood vessel walls to become fragile.

Some good sources of this not-so-well known substance, vitamin P, are: oranges, lemons, grapes, plums, black currants. Other sources in which it is a little less plentiful are: grapefruit, apricots, cherries and blackberries.

The Federation of the American Societies for Experimental Biology have voted to discontinue the use of the term vitamin P on grounds that the existence of such a vitamin has not been substantiated. This does not mean, of course, that such a substance does not exist. It means rather that research up to the present time has not indicated that this substance is necessary for health or that a deficiency of it will result in any disease. In order to qualify as a vitamin, any substance must fulfill these two requirements.

Other Possible Vitamins

There are a number of other so-called "factors" that have been called vitamins tentatively until more is known about them. L1 and L2 are lactation factors—substances that seem to be necessary for proper nursing of young. These substances were extracted from liver and yeast. Vitamin M is a substance needed by monkeys for building blood. Later investigation showed that folic acid (one of the B vitamins) contains vitamin M. Vitamin U is a substance found in alfalfa, kale, fresh milk and greens, raw egg-yolk, wheat bran, liver fat, soybean and olive oils. This is an anti-ulcer factor. It prevents ulcers in laboratory animals. It has also been discovered in cabbage juice and is thought to be the substance responsible for the remarkable cures of human stomach ulcers with raw cabbage juice. Vitamin J is a substance found in fruits that cures pneumonia in laboratory animals.

Then there are substances called "the animal protein factor," the "summer butter factor," the "grass juice factor" and vitamin B14 on which research is going forward. But we do not know enough about them at present to decide whether or not they should be called vitamins, or whether they are simply food elements that have been undiscovered until recently.

Although all these factors are apparently important to good nutrition, it seems safe to conclude, until we have more information about them, that the best plan is to strive for a wholesome all-around diet that will include all of the known vitamins in ample quantity. Probably in this way we will be getting enough of the now unknown factors as well. Raw fruits and vegetables should be a large part of your daily diet—organically grown if possible. Vegetables should include both the green, leafy kind and yellow vegetables such as carrots and sweet potatoes. You should eat plenty of protective protein foods—meat, especially organ meats like liver and heart—poultry, fish and eggs. You should eliminate from your diet all foods made from white flour or white sugar, for these rob your body of B vitamins. We do not recommend extensive use of cereals—most of us eat far too much of this kind of food. Experiments have shown that cereals tend to deplete the body's store of calcium, unless plenty of vitamin D is taken along with the cereals. If you do eat cereals, make certain that they are completely whole grain, as freshly ground as possible—with no added "enrichment" or "fortification."

Finally, to make certain you are getting plenty of all the necessary vitamins, the following natural food supplements should be on your daily menu: fish liver oil for vitamins A and D, brewer's yeast for vitamin B, rose hips for vitamin C and wheat germ oil for vitamin E.

Vitamin P, New Discoveries About

The story of vitamin P is the best example we know of illustrating the superior value of natural vitamins over synthetic ones. Vitamin P is a substance that occurs along with vitamin C in foods. So when you take synthetic vitamin C made in a laboratory you don't get any vitamin P of course. But when you eat foods rich in vitamin C or take vitamin supplements made from natural foods such as rose hips or green peppers, the vitamin P comes right along with the vitamin C. And we have discovered that in countless situations where vitamin C alone is not effective, the combination of the two will work wonders.

In February of 1955 a meeting was held in New York to honor Nobel Prize winner Albert Szent-Gyorgyi who has done such outstanding work on vitamin C and vitamin P. At the meeting researchers spoke on their experiences with vitamin P, or, as they called it, "the bioflavonoids." Actually we should not speak of the bioflavonoids as a vitamin until their status has been clarified. Our official scientific body which determines terminology like that has decided that the bioflavonoids are not a vitamin. Until we discover that they occur in the human body, then we should not speak of them in terms of being a vitamin.

What are the bioflavonoids? They are brightly colored substances that appear in fruits, along with vitamin C. They have also been called citrin, hesperidin, rutin, vitamin C-2, vitamin P, flavones, flavonols, flavonones and so forth. These names are important to biochemists but do not have to concern us. It's up to the researchers to separate and sort, study and test these various substances. We need only to be grateful for the work they are doing, and make the most we can of their discoveries.

At the meeting in February Charles E. Brambel of Mercy Hospital, Baltimore, spoke on the use of the bioflavonoids in anti-coagulant therapy. Because of the tendency of blood to coagulate too easily in certain heart and vascular diseases, doctors give medicines that they call "anti-coagulants" designed to prevent blood clots or thromboses. Coumarin is one of these. Coumarin keeps the patient's blood in such a state that it cannot clot and stop up a blood vessel. But you can see that such a medicine might cause some difficulty. What if it keeps the blood in such a free-flowing condition that the patient has hemorrhages instead? Dr. Brambel has studied 2000 patients using anti-coagulant medicines. Five per cent of them developed bleeding complications. One hundred milligrams each of hesperidin (bioflavonoids) and vitamin C were given four times daily. The areas where the hemorrhages had been cleared rapidly. Dr. Brambel tells us that hesperidin and vitamin C together accomplish this, whereas neither of them alone will do the job.

Treating Rheumatic Fever and Miscarriages

Dr. James F. Rhinehart of the University of California spoke at the meeting on the subject of rheumatic fever. It is his belief that vitamin C and the bioflavonoids have considerable value in the treatment of rheumatic fever. Dr. Carl T. Javert of Cornell University spoke of using vitamin C and bioflavonoids to prevent miscarriages. In a study of 1334 patients, he found that 45 per cent of three groups tested were deficient in vitamin C. This is in contrast, he says, with normal nonpregnant women, *only one-third of whom are deficient in vitamin C.* (Note that last statement. Our nutrition "experts" keep on telling us that we get enough of all the vitamins in a well-balanced diet and yet figures like this, for "normal" women keep cropping up.) Giving large doses of vitamin C and the bioflavonoids to 100 pregnant women with histories of habitual abortion, he achieved a successful pregnancy in 91 per cent. These patients took a diet rich in vitamin C (350 milligrams) plus a supplement containing vitamin C and the bioflavonoids—making a total of 500 milligrams of vitamin C per day. The vitamin C or the bioflavonoids alone did not do the job. But the combination of the two worked the miracle.

Dr. Robert Greenblatt of the Medical College of Georgia also reported on using vitamin C and the bioflavonoids for habitual abortion. A group of women who had never been able to carry their children and bring them into the world alive were examined to determine the state of their capillaries—that is, the tiny blood vessels that spread through every inch of our bodies. It was found that they suffered from capillary fragility—that is, the walls of these tiny vessels burst easily, causing bruised areas. Vitamin C and the bioflavonoids were given to them with excellent results. Eleven of thirteen patients with two previous abortions delivered live infants.

Dr. George J. Boines of Wilmington, Delaware, spoke on using these two food substances for curing polio. He said that tests indicated that all 400 patients with acute polio were found to have abnormal capillary fragility, indicating that they needed vitamin C and the bioflavonoids. They were given 600 milligrams of vitamin C and 600 milligrams of hesperidin daily until the state of their capillaries improved. Eight per cent responded in the first five weeks. Appetites improved within the first week and by the second week there was increased warmth to touch in the involved arm or leg.

The Relation of Bioflavonoids to the Capillaries

What are the capillaries and why are they so important? We have some rather startling information on this. The capillaries—those tiny, fragile blood vessels—exist in such profusion in the human body that if the capillaries of one man were stretched out in a single line they would reach two and a half times around the globe! According to one expert "This vast ocean of capillaries provides the working barrier separating the blood from the cellular elements and tissues. Across the walls of the capillary must pass all life-giving ingredients found in the blood" whether they are in the form of gas or solids.

The most important part of the capillaries is the layer in their walls which contains the intercellular cement. Any change in the composition of this cement is bound to have a tremendous effect on how substances pass through the capillary wall into and out of the blood. The composition of the cement is influenced largely by vitamin C and the flavonoids. So you see why the vitamins are so important and why the capillaries are so important.

According to researchers who have experimented with these two food substances, there is no diseased state in which the capillaries are not harmed. And, too, there is no diseased state that will not be improved by improving the state of the capillaries. Habitual abortion, rheumatic fever, rheumatoid arthritis, diabetes and diabetic retinopathy, hypertension—in all of these there is one common symptom—the capillaries are failing. So in all of these vitamin C and the bioflavonoids should be used.

While none of our reseachers declare that other methods of therapy for these various diseases should be abandoned, they do claim that *"the combination of vitamin C and the bioflavonoids benefits every condition in which it has been tried and should be considered by physicians as 'supplemental therapy' of value in virtually all diseased states and specific in action with respect to some."*

Those are strong words—"of value in virtually all diseased states," but actually why should they not be used? We are talking of two substances which, when used together, keep the walls of the blood vessels healthy. Every cell in your body depends, every second of the time, on the materials that are brought to it through the blood vessels. So what could be more important?

Bioflavonoids and Infections

Vitamin C and the bioflavonoids have been used successfully in the treatment of colds. A group of nurses at Creighton University School of Medicine was given tablets containing the two substances and then checked for a year against another group which got nothing. The treated nurses had fewer colds by about 55 per cent and their colds lasted only an average of 3.9 days compared with 6.7 days in the untreated group. In the *American Journal of Digestive Diseases* for July, 1954, Morton S. Biskind and W. C. Martin reported on 22 patients who had respiratory infections varying from a simple cold to influenza. Twenty of them recovered in an 8 to 48 hour period after treatment with the bioflavonoids and Vitamin C. The patients got 600 milligrams of each of the two substances every day. Vitamin C alone or the flavonoids alone did not produce results. But together they did.

A bibliography of the medical articles on the subject of bioflavonoids and vitamin C, compiled by the Sunkist Growers, lists 511 separate pieces of information on this subject—an imposing list, which shows the immense interest that has been aroused in the subject within the past fifteen years or so.

How Can You Get Bioflavonoids in Your Diet?

Where are you going to look in food for the bioflavonoids? The substance used by many researchers comes from citrus fruits—it is contained in the white skin and segment part of the fruit—not in the juice. We are told that the edible part of the orange contains a tenfold concentration of bioflavonoids, compared to the quantity in strained juice. In the fresh peeled orange there are 1000 milligrams of bioflavonoids and about 60 milligrams of vitamin C. In the strained orange juice there are only about 100 milligrams of bioflavonoids. Here we have one excellent reason for not juicing citrus fruit; eat it instead. And when you eat it, don't do as the cookbooks tell you to do and remove all the white layers under the skin and around each segment of fruit. That's where the bioflavonoids are. Lemons, grapes, plums and black currants, grapefruit, apricots, cherries and blackberries also contain flavonoids. You will get probably enough to maintain health if you eat lots and lots of fresh raw fruit, especially if you can eat it fresh from the tree or vine.

But how are you going to get bioflavonoids in your food supplements? Natural vitamin C food supplements made from rose hips or green peppers contain the bioflavonoids for of course they occur along with the vitamin C right in the foods from which these supplements were made. Or you may find natural food supplements with added bioflavonoids. The flavonoids may be called rutin, hesperidin, vitamin P.

Here's the story of something that happened to a friend of ours. She had developed arthritis and the doctors were talking to her about cortisone. They told her there was nothing else that could help. She got interested in some synthetic vitamin C plus hesperidin tablets that a friend was taking. She took them for quite a while with only slight benefit. We asked her why she didn't try the natural vitamin C (rose hips) in which of course the hesperidin was contained. She began to take them and was free from her arthritis within a few weeks. Each time she has tried to go back to the synthetic vitamins, the sore joints threaten to return. But her natural vitamin C tablets keep her completely healthy. She is taking at present about 750 milligrams a day.

Water—Body Fluids

When you drink a glass of water the water goes to your stomach and part of it is absorbed directly into the blood stream through the stomach walls. The rest goes to the intestines where it helps to keep the food in a liquid state while it is being absorbed. This, too, is then absorbed into the blood.

Is your blood dangerously thinned, then, when you drink water? For a few moments, but after that the liquids are rapidly distributed to other parts of the body. Does a large drink of water have any tendency to raise blood pressure? You would think, since part of the water goes directly to the blood, that the added liquid in the blood vessels would cause them to distend and pressure might then rise. But so marvelously is your body geared to keep the water balance constant that taking up to six quarts of liquid a day does not change your blood pressure in the least. The average daily intake of fluids is about 1½ to 2 quarts.

Where does the water go that is not in the blood? Every one of the many billions of cells in your body contains fluid and is surrounded by fluid. In addition, much of the water we drink is used to make up saliva, blood serum, spinal fluid, gastric juice, bile, pancreatic juice, tears, sweat and so forth. Losing large amounts of one or more of these juices is likely to dehydrate you. In vomiting, for instance, you lose large amounts of digestive juice and saliva. Patients with diarrhea lose dangerous amounts of water in their very liquid bowel movements.

"Water is continually shifting about the body, so as to provide a vehicle for digestive juices and other secretions, to transport nutriments and carry off waste products," say the editors of *Bridges' Dietetics for the Clinician.* The body must be continually adjusting the "water balance" as physiologists call it. By this they mean that we are constantly losing water and so we must always be replacing it. But we dare not take in too much and we dare not let water accumulate in any spot where it is not supposed to be.

The chief danger in heart failure is the danger of literally drowning in one's own body fluids. When the heart becomes too weak to pump blood to the kidneys, they in turn cannot dispose of waste water, so it accumulates. Ankles, feet and legs swell.

Then as much as a gallon or more of fluid may accumulate in the chest cavity and abdomen, so that life for the victim of heart failure becomes a losing battle against bloating. One reason why salt-free diets are prescribed for heart patients is that one ounce of salt holds in solution as much as three quarts of water. That is, so long as there is an excess of salt in the body, there will be large amounts of water, too, held there by the salt.

The fluid inside the cells and outside the cells of the body is continually being moved and shifted. It conveys every substance that moves from place to place. It is necessary for absorption, diffusion and secretion. And it enters into many chemical reactions in the body. The lymph is that fluid which circulates through the lymph glands as the blood circulates through blood vessels. Lymph apparently moves quite rapidly from one part of the body to another, for dyes injected into the leg appear in lymph ducts in the chest in about a minute's time.

The way your body adjusts its water balance in a normal day's time goes something like this: You may take in 1500 cc. in fluids, 800 cc. in so-called solid food, and the combustion process in your body may release another 300 cc. of water. This totals 2600 cc. You may lose in urine 1500 cc., in vapor from the skin and lungs 1000 cc. and in the feces 100 cc. This also totals 2600, so your water balance is perfect on that day. During periods of excessive sweating you may lose as much as 5000 to 15,000 cc. An attack of diarrhea may account for the loss of 5000 cc. A bad case of vomiting might cause you to lose 5000 cc.

One final word about sweating. It is generally accepted among scientists that one rapidly acclimatizes himself to a hot temperature, so that he will lose less and less body fluid in perspiration. Then, too, as one becomes accustomed to heat, less salt is lost in perspiration. For instance, some heat-resistant animals who have lived continually in the tropics have arrived at the point where they secrete almost pure water, rather than a salty fluid.

In general individuals who eat little salt find that they are not thirsty in the hot weather. We wonder what is the effect on all the body fluids of drinking water which contains chlorine, fluorine, alum and all the other hundred or so chemicals which may be in city water. When you consider the complexity and delicacy of the set-up which regulates the body fluids, doesn't it seem that all the chemicals we are continually imbibing might eventually do serious damage?

As you know, we recommend using as little salt as possible—none at all in cooking or at the table. If you suffer from a heart condition this is most important. If you have been dehydrated (that is, through vomiting or diarrhea) many valuable minerals have been lost as well as fluid. Calcium, potassium, phosphorus, all these should be replaced as soon as possible with a natural mineral supplement, such as bone meal.

The more research we do in medical journals, the more we discover about the complete uselessness of table salt in our diets and the great possibility for harm that it holds in store. Do begin to "taper off" on salt right away. After a few weeks, you'll find you don't miss it at all!

Weather—Hot

When summer rolls around once again, life assumes an entirely different aspect for most of us. Out come the garden tools, the tennis rackets and golf clubs, the shorts, the suntan oil. We take to the out-of-doors. Those of us who have long vacations can plan on plenty of time at the beach or in the mountains to get old man winter's kinks out of our systems. Those of us who must stay on the job can look forward to long, cool summer evenings and much more relaxation than we obtain during other seasons of the year.

Yet a glance at any summer newspaper of past years will readily show that health hazards are, if anything, increased during summer months. In spite of the fact that there is no snow on the roads, automobile accidents are not less frequent. Sunstroke and heat prostration account for about as many disabilities as coasting accidents or falls on the ice in the winter. We are more healthy in summer—there can be no doubt of that. The ultraviolet rays of the sun increase the health-value of summer food, and we all benefit from being out of doors. We tend to shake off tension and worry.

Yet in spite of all this, there are hazards peculiar to summertime that must be guarded against. It has been found, for instance, that hot weather, especially humid hot weather, is especially trying for heart patients. As stated by G. S. Berenson, M.D., and G. E. Burch, M.D., in an article in *Modern Medicine* for June 15, 1952, "Patients with congestive heart failure cannot tolerate excessively warm atmospheres." They go on to tell us that human beings exposed to hot humid environment find that the elimination of their bodily heat is impaired, so that blood vessels dilate, causing more work for the heart and perhaps bringing serious consequences for the heart patient. "As the exposure is continued, the subject becomes irritable, weak, faint and complains of being extremely hot. Later the central nervous system is affected, producing headache, visual disturbances, restlessness, as well as muscular tremors." Patients with chronic pulmonary diseases also suffer more than average from hot weather, say these researchers.

Aside from heart patients, however, it behooves all of us to take it easy—or take it easier—during the hot weather. With so many attractive sports beckoning, with so much to be done in the yard and garden, we have a tendency to overdo things and then blame our feeling of fatigue and listlessness on the heat. Eagerly we ply ourselves and our families with iced drinks. It is generally agreed that we need considerably more liquid intake during hot weather, to make up for the fluid our bodies lose in perspiration. But the kind of drink we take is important, too. Sweet drinks—and this includes lemonade and iced tea as well as soft drinks—do not make us cool. Rather they increase our feeling of discomfort, for they supply added calories, and a calory, anyway you look at it, means heat. Alcohol contains more calories than many foods, so an alcoholic drink, no matter how plentiful the ice it contains, is bound to make you feel much hotter.

Don't Take to Soft Drinks

Every summer when we see the vast quantities of soft drink cartons that are bought every day at our local market, we feel that we cannot stress too strongly the very serious harm done to the human body by this modern concoction of man. A soft drink—any soft drink—contains nothing of benefit to good health. It is a mixture of refined sugar, acid, artificial flavoring and coloring. The phosphoric acid in the cola drinks has been found to deplete the calcium of the teeth. The sugar has an extremely bad effect on the blood sugar level of the body, by raising it suddenly (hence the "lift" you feel from a soft drink) then plunging it down far lower than it should be. This lowered blood sugar has been mentioned by many researchers as a possible cause of polio, asthma and epilepsy, to mention but a few diseases in which low blood sugar levels prevail.

Children who play to the point of exhaustion in the hot summer sunlight and then gulp soft drinks are inviting polio. In addition the sweetness of the drinks lessens their appetites so that they do not and will not eat the protective foods that are just as necessary in summer as in winter.

Make no mistake about it, you need protein, vitamins and minerals regardless of the weather. Salads, and fresh raw fruits and vegetables are absolute daily necessities in summer time. But, since they are so easily available from the garden or so inexpensive at the store you will probably not slight them. However you may have a tendency to avoid the so-called "heavy" foods such as fish, meat, poultry and eggs. Remember that you cannot substitute cookies or sandwiches or even fruit drinks or vegetable snacks for good quality protein. So continue to serve your usual amounts of the protein foods during the summer months. If you seem to feel cooler eating cold meat rather than hot meat, then do. But there is no physiological basis for this feeling. If soup with a meat and marrow-bone base does not appeal in summer time, then substitute cold jellied consommé so that you will still get the benefit of the proteins and minerals of the soup.

Keeping Cool

Just keeping cool is mostly a matter of evaporation—that is, helping the air to evaporate the heat and moisture from your body. Light, porous clothing helps. Avoid tight belts, collars or jewelry. Actually shorts are the most sensible garb for summertime, any time you can be this informal, for they permit the most circulation of air about your legs and hence help in the job of evaporation. A lukewarm shower or bath will cool you off more successfully than either a cold or hot one.

Quite apart from the general state of your health, it is best to avoid strenuous exercise in hot weather. Nine chances out of ten you are not accustomed to it and an hour on the tennis court or behind the power mower can be a serious shock to the system of an individual accustomed to sitting behind a desk the rest of the year. Don't undertake long hikes, lengthy sessions of swimming, rowing or other sports unless you are accustomed to strenuous sports the year 'round.

What About Suntan?

A press release from the *U. S. News and World Report* for May 22, 1953, quotes Dr. John M. Lynch of the National Institute of Health as saying, "it's pretty generally agreed now that sunning confers no special health benefits. Overdone, it can be harmful. You will do well to avoid getting severe sunburn. No great danger immediately but it appears that cumulative effects of too much sunning, over many years, can encourage skin cancer." There are other reasons, too, for avoiding heavy tan. As you know, the body manufactures vitamin D from some substance in the sun's ultraviolet rays. This is the reason why children in northern climates should take cod liver oil in the winter—to supply the vitamin D they are not receiving from the wintry rays of the sun which cannot penetrate their heavy winter clothing. So of course, it is good for you to be exposed to the summer sun to some extent, for you can store some vitamin D for the dark days of next winter.

Animals wisely do some sunning every day. But no animal will voluntarily stretch himself in full summer sunlight for hour after hour, as we human beings do. He takes his summer siesta in the shade. In order to protect the body from too much of the ultraviolet radiation, the skin tans or, in the case of blondes and redheads, reddens so that no more radiation can penetrate. Once you have achieved a dark tan no more radiation gets through and you may suffer from a serious depletion of vitamin D during next winter. So it seems best, then, to avoid tanning. If you get out of the house just the average amount of time in the summer, you will be exposed to enough of the sun's rays, even if you stay in the shade, to provide you with ample vitamin D. And of course, the hazards of blistering, peeling and possibly infected patches of sunburn are to be avoided at all costs.

A clipping from *Time* for March 5, 1956, tells us that suntan oils may cause inflammation at the very time they are protecting the skin against sunburn according to dermatologist Wiley M. Sams of Miami. Some ingredients of the oils can filter out part of the ultraviolet rays, but at the same time sensitize the skin to other rays. Knowing our firm stand against cosmetics, readers will readily understand that we do not recommend suntan oils.

We must insist, too, on the advisability of continuing your food supplements in summer time. The water soluble vitamins—B and C are lost in perspiration. So if you are doing very heavy work it might be wise to increase your B and C food supplement. Minerals are also lost in perspiration. It is quite true, too, that prolonged heat constitutes a condition known among physiologists as "stress" and, generally speaking, requirements for all the vitamins and minerals are raised by "stress." So, while you can count on getting more vitamins and minerals in your summer, sun ripened foods, don't make the mistake of letting your good nutrition go into a slump during the summer months.

Weight—Obesity In Children

A problem in obesity that is not generally treated in family magazines is the problem of the obese child. Before we get into discussion of a diet that is effective and not too great a burden on the child's self-control, let's take a moment to consider some of the elements in his environment that may produce obesity in a child.

It is quite generally accepted today that heredity has nothing whatever to do with one's weight. It is true that obesity seems to "run" in families and chances are that if both parents are overweight the children will be overweight, too. But this does not indicate that the obesity is inherited. An article by Max Millman, M.D., in *Today's Health* for August, 1950, shows us that fat people with obese parents can reduce successfully if they want to, just as children of thin parents can. Obesity running in families incriminates rather the food and eating habits that are established in a household.

If mother bakes the best chocolate cakes and the most frequent French fried potatoes on the block, because she enjoys them, and if Pop brings home from the office almost daily boxes of chocolates because he likes to eat them, the odds are that parents and children in that family will be overweight. If soft drinks, doughnuts, ice cream and cookies are available and encouraged at all times for between-meal snacks, Junior follows his parents' example and his weight goes up as theirs does. Then too, if salads are by-passed by the adults, Junior and his sister come to think of them as unattractive. If candy and cake are offered as rewards for good behavior, then these weight-building delicacies become highly desirable to the children.

Dr. Millman discusses the very frequent emotional basis for overeating. Food is the most easily obtained solace for emotional upset. "Worry, fear, anxiety and fatigue will cause one person to lose his appetite completely; the next may react by overeating. 'When you are emotionally upset, do you eat more or less?' A large majority of several hundred fat people answered 'more.' They admitted that whenever they became nervous or upset, they just couldn't stop nibbling or chewing. This explains the truism that many people worry themselves into obesity" says Dr. Millman. He cites the case of a 16-year old boy who was afraid of the rough games his classmates engaged in. He was ashamed to confess his fears, of course, and took to overeating as a defense mechanism. Once he was fat he was not expected to engage in the games, so he kept on overeating, to escape the dangers that he feared but could not admit.

Lack of security may also result in obesity. The boy or girl who crams sweets all day long may be making up for some real or imagined lack of love or attention. An older brother or sister of whom his parents are obviously very proud may cause a younger child to overeat for compensation. Then, too, there is the matter of habit, and many children as well as adults find it actually unbearably difficult to get along without candy, sugar or chocolate. "In this respect food differs very little from tobacco or alcohol. Excessive drinking is to be condemned, of course, but it is safe to state that too much food has shortened the lives of many more people than has too much alcohol," says Dr. Millman.

Chubbiness and even fatness used to be regarded as a sign of health in children. Today we know differently. But we may not know when weight reduction should start. How can you tell whether your own child has arrived at a point where you should take steps to reduce his weight? William A. Reilly, M.D., of San Francisco, writing in the *Southern Medical Journal* tells us that a child is obese if his weight is 20 or more per cent above the normal weight for his size and age, if the child is over six years of age and if the obesity has been present for at least some months.

The Child Must Cooperate For Program To Be Successful

The first step to take if you decide that a reducing program is in order is to talk to the youngster about it and get his agreement to your program. No child enjoys being called "fatty" and a careful and sympathetic discussion is the first necessity for his wholehearted cooperation. If you cannot arrive at a satisfactory agreement with him possibly some other member of the family for whom he has great respect (an athletic uncle or, in the case of a girl, a slim and pretty aunt) can do the trick. Or perhaps your family doctor can find arguments that will convince the child.

There are two methods of planning a reducing diet, says Dr. Reilly, the quantitative one and the qualitative one. If you use the first you must count calories. This means getting yourself a reliable calory guide to foods and preparing and serving to the child all food according to the list. A good book to start with is the *Agriculture Handbook Number 8*—Composition of Foods, Raw Processed, Prepared. You can obtain this free from the Superintendent of Documents or the Department of Agriculture in Washington, D. C. In this, foods are listed according to calory content as well as protein, fat, starch, and vitamin and mineral content. "Calory reduction should be gradual," says Dr. Reilly. "The caloric intake can be reduced by 250 calories every three to five days until the normal figure is reached."

This seems to us like the hard way of doing things, for the mathematics you get into figuring calories includes not only the food your child eats at home, but also whatever he eats away from home and you may find it extremely difficult to keep an accurate record. Besides there is a chance that high calory foods containing little food value may take up too large a part of the diet, at the expense of the child's health. And, too, if the calory count is kept low enough in any given day to allow Junior a rich dessert for dinner, you are not improving his food habits. And going without the dessert will be harder the next day.

A quantitative diet seems to us much easier to manage and at the same time much less likely to result in deficiencies which might inhibit growth, bring on tooth decay and other serious difficulties. The diet suggested by Dr. Reilly seems excellent to us, with just a few changes. The child is allowed to eat all he wants of certain foods and *none at all of certain other foods.*

HERE ARE THE FOODS ALLOWED:

Meats: Steak, chops (except pork), lamb, veal, mutton, beef roast, brains, chicken, turkey, squab, wild duck, sweetbreads, kidneys, liver.

Fish and Shellfish: Any fish except salmon, shad, sardines and caviar. Dr. Reilly allows shellfish, too, although we believe shellfish are not to be recommended.

Fresh Vegetables: Lettuce, tomatoes, celery, carrots, cauliflower, cabbage, mushrooms, string beans, cucumbers, squash, turnips, radishes, beets, pumpkin, spinach, asparagus, artichokes, onions, sprouts, eggplant, okra.

Fresh Fruits (without cream or sugar): Oranges, lemons, strawberries, watermelon, blackberries, loganberries, peaches, pears, cantaloupe, Persian melon, honeydew, raspberries, pineapple, grapefruit.

Pickles and Condiments: (We would warn against too much salt which is especially harmful in obesity.)

Clear Soups

Desserts (Any kind, one moderate helping, says Dr. Reilly.) As you know we do not advise for anyone, no matter what his weight, any dessert made with white flour or white sugar.

Beverages: Tea, coffee and carbonated beverages. Here is where Dr. Reilly makes his most serious mistake, we believe, in not even limiting carbonated beverages. Considering the amount of sugar they contain as well as their untold capacity for doing harm, these would be the first "foods" we would prohibit on any diet for child or adult.

Dairy Products: Eggs, skimmed milk, cottage cheese, buttermilk. Don't be shocked at this recommendation for skimmed milk. All the food value of whole pasteurized milk is contained in skimmed milk, except for the fat. Less than one-half cup of powdered milk contains all the nutriments of a quart of fresh skimmed milk. The youngsters will probably enjoy mixing up a milkshake of powdered milk, water and molasses and real vanilla flavoring.

FOODS FORBIDDEN ENTIRELY ON THE REILLY DIET ARE:

Meats and Fish: Bacon, ham, pork, sausage, caviar, goose, tame duck, salmon, shad, sardines.

Dairy Products: Butter, whole milk, cheese, condensed milk, cream (and we add ice cream).

Sweets: Sugar, honey, jellies, chocolate, syrups, jams, candy, cocoa. (and we add pastries, cakes, cookies, doughnuts, etc.).

Starches: Bread, crackers, rolls, biscuits, muffins of any kind whatever (this means white, brown, graham, rye, gluten, bran, zwiebach), potatoes, noodles, corn, baked beans, fresh peas, macaroni, vermicelli, lima beans, parsnips, spaghetti, rice.

Fruits: Bananas, prunes, ripe olives, grapes, apples, plums, nuts, figs, apricots, dates, cherries, canned fruits.

Cereals: Mush, hot cakes, porridge, breakfast foods, waffles.

Cream Soups

Fried Foods

Several advantages of the above diet are that the obese youngster need suffer no hardship at the dining table by having to watch the other folks eat a different and more appealing meal, for a whole family will benefit from eating such a diet day in and day out. If other members of the family must have cream, butter, beans, cheese, etc., for some special dietary reason, they can have these served inconspicuously or eat them between meals.

Dr. Reilly goes on to suggest diet supplements and, we are sorry to say, drugs, to aid in the reducing program. He admits that some of the drugs may cause nervousness and sleeplessness. We of course do not advocate any drug for reducing purposes and we have our own ideas about diet supplements which will guarantee that Junior will not become deficient in any of the necessary food elements. Bone meal will give him calcium, phosphorus and other minerals. Brewer's yeast or desiccated liver will supply all the B vitamins (and incidentally he doesn't need so many B vitamins since his intake of sugar and starch has been cut down so drastically). Rose hips tablets will give him vitamin C, and fish liver oil perles will contribute vitamin A and D in natural form.

" 'Policing' is very necessary," says Dr. Reilly, "especially in the early months; all obese patients need much interest, convincing and sympathy to gain their cooperation in this trying routine." We suggest that the routine won't be nearly so trying if everybody in the family cooperate by giving up the same foods and eating the same high-protein, nourishing diet we have just prescribed for Junior. In addition to serving just about the most nutritious fare that can be imagined, you will also be initiating excellent food habits which, when once established, may govern your child's diet for the rest of his life.

Wheat Germ Oil and Stress

By

Professor Dr. William Halden

We are all well aware that people living under "stress" need more oxygen and more of the other elements essential to the proper functioning of our bodies. Runners, football players, channel-swimmers—men like these need more oxygen. Not only do they need more oxygen, but their internal mechanisms must be exactly regulated for the proper use of the oxygen they take in. One of the chief aids for proper oxygenation of the body is an ample supply of vitamin E. This vitamin assists in all the reactions connected with the coming of oxygen into our cells, tissues and organs.

There is an interrelation between vitamin E and vitamin A which also helps in reactions having to do with oxygen. Vitamin A is protected from being oxidized and destroyed by vitamin E. Mutually, large amounts of vitamin A have what biologists call "a sparing action" on vitamin E. That is, if you have plenty of vitamin E in your diet you can get along with less vitamin A and vice versa.

Probably not many of us are full-time athletes, so why should we worry about the proper oxygenation of our tissues? There are other forms of "stress" than athletics. Growing old is a form of stress. Older people need more of all the food elements because the functions of their bodies have slowed down. Professor H. C. Sherman of Columbia University is famous for his insistence that elderly people should have much more vitamin A than younger people. Increasing the vitamin E in the diet (for instance using whole grain bread rather than white bread, or taking vitamin E) would thus result in increasing the aging individual's store of vitamin A, as well as vitamin E.

We are told that there is plenty of vitamin E in the usual diet. Don't worry about vitamin E; it's all around you; you won't have any shortage of it if you eat a moderately well-balanced diet, we are told. But is this actually the case? The Dutch nutritionist, C. Engel, in an article entitled "Vitamin E in Human Nutrition" in the *Annals of the New York Academy of Sciences,* volume 52, page 292, 1949, discussed the average amount of vitamin E in the Dutch diet in 1949. Here is the chart of his findings:

Foodstuff	*Grams per Day*	*Calorie Values*	*Vitamin E (milligrams)*
Milk	350	190	0.10
Meat	50	125	0.30
Fish	15	22	0.15
Eggs	10	16	0.30
Cheese	15	51	0.09
Butter	15	118	0.33
Fat	9	84	0.01
Dark Bread	400	924	5.60
Cereals	30	105	1.02
Potatoes	450	414	0.45
Vegetables	182	93	4.60
Fruits	70	27	0.01
Oils (Margarine)	20	153	2.00
Sugar	55	214	...
		2,614	14.96

You can readily see that by far the largest amount of vitamin E came from vegetables and whole grain bread. Cooking oils and cereals in general contributed the next largest amount. The vitamin E contained in vegetables is assimilated only to a comparatively low degree (about 15 per cent) if it is not administered with fatty substances, whereas the vitamin E from cereal grains, wheat germ or dark bread is completely absorbed by the intestinal tract and made available to the body.

Comparing some various natural sources of vitamin E, we can see that there is no other foodstuff containing as much of this vitamin as wheat germ and its oil. Here is a chart showing the amount of vitamin E in the various foods:

Food	*Milligrams of Vitamin E per hundred grams*
Wheat germ oil	320
Wheat germ	30
Wheat grains	2
Whole grain bread	1.3
White bread (patent flour)	0.1
Rye germ oil	250
Barley germ oil	240
Linseed oil	113
Soybean oil	110
Cotton seed oil	81
Corn germ oil	91
Rape seed oil	56
Peanut oil	20
Coconut oil	8
Meat	1 to 3
Liver	1.6
Cabbage	6
Lettuce	6

Wheat germ contains about 10 per cent oil and this is characterized by its high content of other fatty substances that should accompany the vitamins in order to make a complete functioning unit of the whole. For instance, unsaturated fatty acids "(vitamin F)" occur in wheat germ oil. These are balanced by tocopherols or vitamin E. Then there is lecithin, so important for the prevention of fatty livers and cholesterol-clogged blood vessels.

In wheat germ as a whole the protein is of special importance, too. Wheat germ protein contains much more methionine than white-flour protein. Methionine is that amino acid, or part of protein, which contributes most to human welfare. There is also much more lysine, another extremely important amino acid. These are two more sound reasons for always using whole grain products rather than white, refined products.

To summarize some of the highlights of vitamin E, whose richest source is wheat germ, we may point out the following facts. "Vitamin E is the most important non-specific conditioning agent of the body" according to K. C. P. Hickman, one of the pioneers in vitamin E research. Vitamin E acts as a carrier of electrons—the tiniest particles of electricity —and also as a moderator of the process of oxidation in the body, preventing the super-oxidized fatty acids from depositing on the walls of arteries.

People who eat lots of fat in their diets require even more vitamin E than those who eat less fat, for the body must have sufficient vitamin E in order to use the fats properly. This should be especially important for Americans, for their diet is, generally speaking, richer in fat than that of any other nation. Hence they should have more vitamin E to use the fat properly.

There is also an interrelation between the vitamin E requirement and "stress." Strenuous muscular activity raises the requirement for vitamin E. Other stresses, such as old age or illness, also cause the body to need more vitamin E. Whenever there is an increase in the amount of oxygen the body uses there is a greater requirement for those substances that help to regulate the way the body uses oxygen. These are riboflavin (vitamin B2), vitamin C and vitamin E. All of them are electron-carriers of the highest value.

The function of the liver as a central organ for regulating how we use our food is greatly aided by an ample supply of vitamin E, as well as the welfare of the glands such as the adrenals, the action of the heart and the purity of the blood vessels—all these profit from vitamin E and from the administration of one of its most abundant sources—wheat germ.

Editor's note: Readers making their own bread from whole-grain, freshly ground flour get wheat germ in their bread. Even when this source of supply is available, we recommend taking wheat germ oil as a food supplement. As it is our belief that all of us—and especially those of us who fear heart or blood vessel disorders—should also be taking vitamin E in concentrated natural form.

Wheat Germ Oil and Endurance

This article is reprinted from the Urbana (Illinois) *News Gazette*, March 14, 1954, by permission of the editors and the author, Ed Gorman, News Editor

A teaspoonful of wheat germ oil, taken daily in conjunction with exercise, has been shown to increase men's physical capacity and endurance by as much as 51.5 per cent.

That and many other findings which point to wheat germ oil as a "valuable nutrient supplement" are being reported scientifically for the first time by Dr. T. K. Cureton, head of the University of Illinois Physical Fitness Laboratory.

The reports are based on experiments carried on at the University for more than four years on more than 200 men, including varsity wrestlers, swimmers, youths selected at random from a fraternity house, and middleaged men who were in poor physical "shape" when they began a training program.

The studies were conducted under grants from the VioBin Corp. in Monticello. Heretofore, they have been kept under wraps because, Dr. Cureton said: "We wanted to make sure."

Now, he disclosed, 10 scientific consultants have recommended publication of the results in scientific journals.

Cureton reported the findings Saturday with this assertion:

Valuable in Diet

"Wheat germ oil is a valuable dietary supplement to men doing hard exercise, and it has possible application to competitive sports. We have tried it sufficiently to believe that this is true. It provides something that enables men to bear hard stress and continue to do hard labor without deteriorating. It particularly affects physical endurance and heart response."

Wheat germ oil, he explained, was tested in a continuing search for something that will give men extra drive and energy. Alcohol, benzedrine, caffeine, cocaine, digitalis, gelatine, fruit juices and hormones have been tried in the past and discarded as ineffective, Cureton said.

Until the wheat germ oil tests were run, Vitamin B complex offered the most encouraging results but, Cureton declared, the evidence in behalf of it was "contradictory at best."

Wheat germ oil, however, has proved "consistently effective" in all the experiments run in the UI laboratory, where men run on a treadmill until they drop and undergo other tests of physical capacity while doctors measure heart action, oxygen consumption, blood pressure and other body functions.

Other Tests Used

The treadmill is only one of many tests in which men's performance was measured in the experiments. It, however, well illustrates the credit given by Cureton to wheat germ oil.

Eight middle-aged professors who combined wheat germ oil with physical training gained 51.5 per cent in the time they could run on the treadmill before they were exhausted. They had no opportunity to practice on the treadmill in between tests. They were tested for a first time, given 12 weeks of other types of exercise along with wheat germ oil, and then tested again. They did not go near the treadmill during the interim.

At the same time, a matched group of men—matched in age and in run-time after the initial test—gained only 19.4 per cent after receiving the same physical training without the wheat germ oil.

These, Cureton emphasized, were sedentary professors, unaccustomed to great physical exertion before they began training in the laboratory.

Works on Athletes

Equally convincing evidence, according to Cureton, was obtained in tests with athletes already at the peak of training—such as the varsity wrestlers and swimmers.

Cureton said it has been well established that men cannot be kept at a peak of physical condition indefinitely—that most of them reach a "plateau" after about 12 weeks of hard training and begin to slump.

However, when the athletes were given wheat germ oil after they began their slump, the scientific measurements of their performance jumped up to new peaks. At the same time, a "control group" which did not receive the wheat germ oil continued their slump.

Results were particularly noticeable in the increased strength of "T waves" measured in electrocardiogram tests of their hearts, Cureton said. He explained that the "T waves" measure the electrical energy of the heart's contraction.

"Never before in any experiment," said Cureton, "have I seen a subject train hard for 12 weeks, reach the plateau, and then go on to a higher peak."

Exercise Needed

Dr. Cureton emphasized, however, that few if any of these results can be obtained unless the wheat germ oil is coupled with physical training. On the other hand, wheat germ oil and exercise together produce results not obtained by physical training alone.

His explanation is that exercise opens up the tiny blood vessels (capillaries) of muscles and heart tissues, increases the blood flow of arteries, and allows the nutrient to reach the muscle and tissue where it is needed.

"The exact nature of this mechanism in wheat germ oil has not been determined, but we have established that it is significantly effective as a dietary supplement," Cureton said.

Editor's Note:

In all previous experiments with vitamins, researchers have been forced to use as subjects persons who either were ill or who were kept on a controlled diet to induce vitamin deficiencies. This is necessary because a natural diet includes at least some of all known vitamins. Processors of wheat germ oil have known for many years that it is a good source of natural vitamin E. They have also known that wheat germ oil is one of the richest natural sources of essential fatty acids. Yet these values are relatively insignificant in the light of our new knowledge of wheat germ oil. Wheat germ oil is an unrefined vegetable oil, derived from wheat. The average diet contains very little, if any, unrefined vegetable oil. The values in wheat germ, which also may be present in other vegetable oils, are denied to the average American.

For a number of years it was thought by scientists that vitamin E was the distinguishing and important feature of wheat germ oil. However, when vitamin E was crystallized in pure form (that is, made synthetically) it was found that vitamin E and wheat germ oil do not produce the same clinical results. An earlier University of Illinois study, published in 1951 showed that wheat germ oil contains also a "survival factor" which aids young animals to survive.

Other Studies

The Montreal Neurological Institute has published the results of ten years of study on the use of wheat germ oil in the treatment of certain forms of muscular dystrophy. Positive results were obtained. Dr. Wayne Silbernagel of Columbus, Ohio, reported that a concentrate of wheat germ oil reduced miscarriages in pregnancy from 14 per cent to three per cent. A report published in the scientific journal *Endocrinology* credited wheat germ oil with hormonal effects—that is, having the same effects as the hormones produced by the body's glands.

Some experimenters are now making an effort to show that wheat germ oil contains a factor that influences glycogen metabolism. The theory is that all these effects may be explained by a new discovery that the sugar chemistry of the body is involved. Glycogen is a form of sugar in blood which provides energy of muscles. Such a discovery would indeed revolutionize many of our ideas of blood chemistry and its proper maintenance!

INDEX

B

C

D

E

F

G

H

I

J

K

L

M

N

O

P

Q

R

S

T

U

V

W

X

Y

Z